Dermatopathology A-Z

Vladimir Vincek

Dermatopathology A-Z

A Comprehensive Guide

Springer

Vladimir Vincek
Department of Dermatology
College of Medicine
University of Florida
Gainesville, FL
USA

ISBN 978-3-030-13264-4 ISBN 978-3-319-89486-7 (eBook)
https://doi.org/10.1007/978-3-319-89486-7

Softcover re-print of the Hardcover 1st edition 2018

This Springer imprint is published by the registered company Springer Nature Switzerland AG
The registered company address is: Gewerbestrasse 11, 6330 Cham, Switzerland

This book is dedicated to my parents, who provided me with an enriching childhood, to my wife for all of her patience, understanding, and support, and to my children for some unforgettable moments that always brighten my days.

Preface

The field of dermatopathology can be overwhelming unlike any other part of pathology because of the sheer number of different skin diseases. There are hundreds of different skin entities, many of which have multiple variants.

The goal of this book was to help dermatologists and pathologists master the field of dermatopathology through a visual approach. The majority of dermatologists and pathologists, including myself, have a visual learning style and value a good image over a thousand words. Being able to notice visual details and tuning in to similarities and differences makes an expert.

The book is alphabetically organized, so that one can rapidly locate a disease and gather a visual image and succinct pathological description. I tried to make the book comprehensive with all skin entities known to myself, although I am sure that some very rare entities were probably missed. As the emphasis is on visual learning, the great majority of diseases (with the exception of some extremely rare diseases) are illustrated by images from two different cases. The reason for this is that no two cases of the same disease have identical histomorphology. It is important for the audience to visualize variations in disease presentation. Also, for every case, low, medium, and high power images are shown as this is how dermatopathologists develop diagnosis under the microscope and build their visual image of the disease histomorphology.

On the other hand, although the book is comprehensive, the text was kept succinct for the purpose of focusing only on the diagnostic criteria needed for diagnosis. The goal was to describe all diseases in no more than five lines that are easily memorized and then accompany the text with high-quality images. That way, a novice to the field can quickly learn diagnostic criteria and memorize the images. On the other hand, an experienced dermatopathologist or surgical pathologist can quickly refresh his/her visual memory by reviewing images of two cases of the particular disease.

It is difficult to define the success of the book. However, for me it will be if any of the book's images help a resident solve an unknown slide or a diagnostician renders the correct diagnosis.

Gainesville, FL, USA — Vladimir Vincek

Acknowledgment

I am immensely thankful to Dr. Mehrdad Nadji who taught me how to think as a pathologist and Dr. George Elgart who taught me how to become a better dermatopathologist.

I also thank all of my colleagues and residents who have helped me build my personal collection of dermatopathology slides and images used to create this book.

Special thanks to my colleagues Drs. François Aubin, Andrea Azaola, Jisun Cha, Ko-Ron Chen, Monica da Silva-Nunes, Christopher Demarco, Fernando Toledo de Oliveira, Mohamed Desouki, Jerad Gardner, Murat Gokden, Lena Gowring, John Griffin, Lawrence Hall, Koremasa Hayama, Shivani Kandukuri, Viktorya Kazlouskaya, Christine Ko, Ivanka Kovalushyn, Larissa Larsen, Jason Lee, Konstantinos Linos, Mar Llamas-Velasco, Bogdan Lytvynenko, Kelly Magliocca, Kiran Mothaparthi, Annie Morrison, Melissa Piliang, Tania Gonzalez Santiago, Mary Stone, Claudia Vidal, and Julie Wu who were kind enough to provide me with images or slides of some unique disease entities that I did not have in my collection.

I also want to express my gratitude to Dr. Christopher Demarco, my fellow at the time, who read the first draft of the book and gave me very helpful suggestions, as well as to Dr. Claire Haycox and my daughter Sara, who helped me tremendously with editing. And I would like to thank Connie Walsh, Rebekah Collins, and Asja Rehse of Springer for their efficient and professional help with editing.

Vladimir Vincek

Contents

Dermatopathology A 1

V. Vincek, *Dermatopathology A–Z*, https://doi.org/10.1007/978-3-319-89486-7_1

Abscess

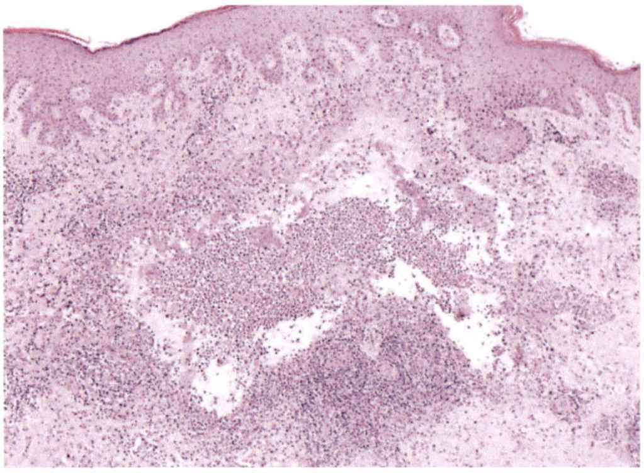

Fig. 1.1 Dermal aggregate of inflammatory cells

Histopathology (Figs. 1.1, 1.2, and 1.3)
- Dermal or subcutaneous nodule composed predominantly of neutrophils
- Central necrosis and surrounding scarring and chronic inflammation usually seen
- Look for remnants of ruptured follicle/cyst, foreign body, necrotic tumor, or organisms as underlying causes for abscess formation
- The presence of eosinophils suggests an insect bite as the possible cause

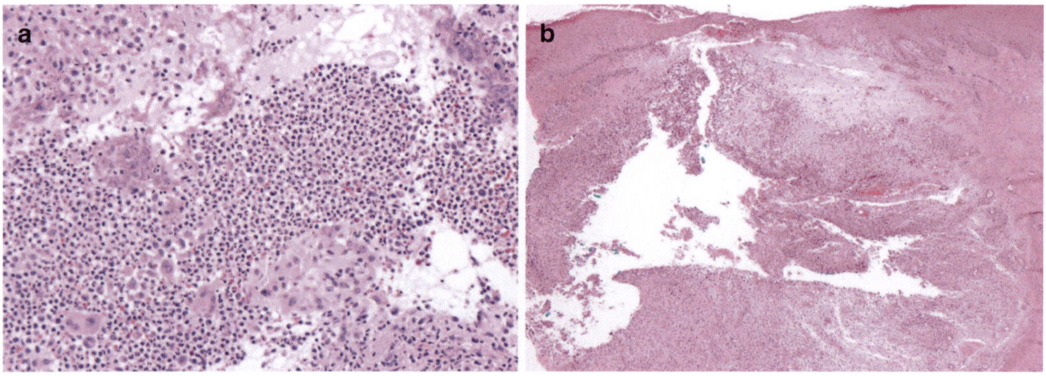

Fig. 1.2 (**a**, **b**) Central aggregate of neutrophils surrounded by scarring and mixed acute and chronic inflammation

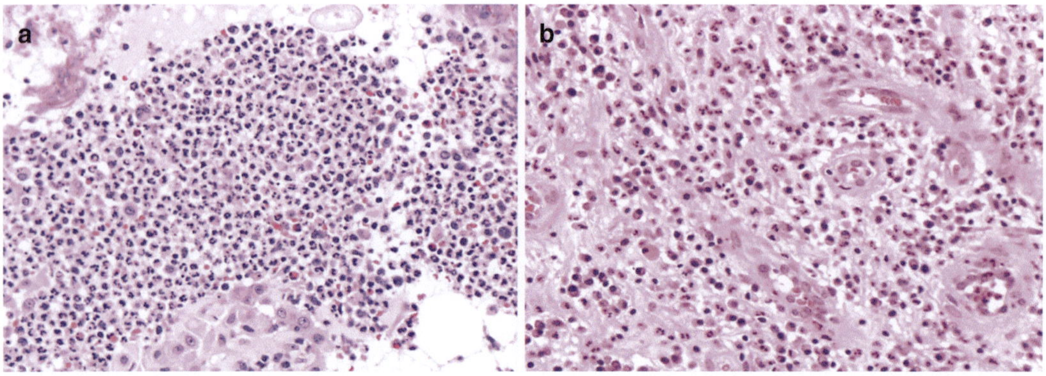

Fig. 1.3 (**a**, **b**) Most of the cells are neutrophils with some admixed lymphocytes, histiocytes, and reactive endothelial cells

Acanthamoebiasis

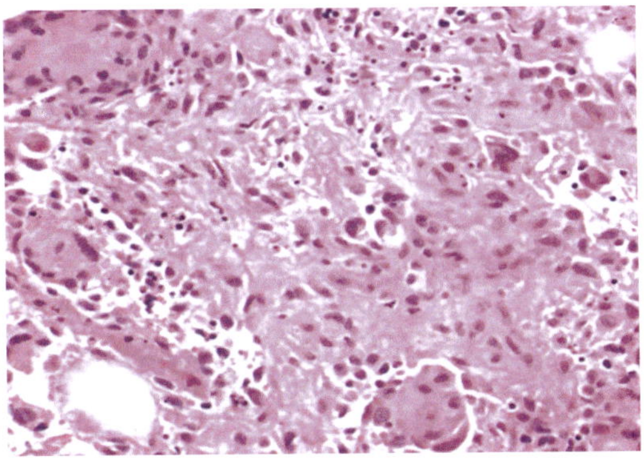

Fig. 1.4 Granulomatous inflammation with focal necrosis

Histopathology (Figs. 1.4, 1.5, 1.6, and 1.7)

- Ulcerated skin with central extensive necrosis and pseudoepitheliomatous hyperplasia at the margins
- Abscess/granulomatous inflammation in the ulcerated area
- Trophozoites with "bull's-eye" appearance and cysts with wrinkled membrane are present within the giant cells

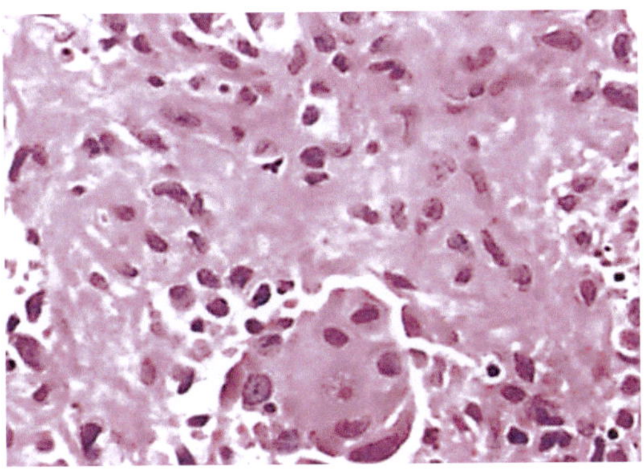

Fig. 1.5 Trophozoite within multinucleated giant cell with surrounding necrosis and histiocytes

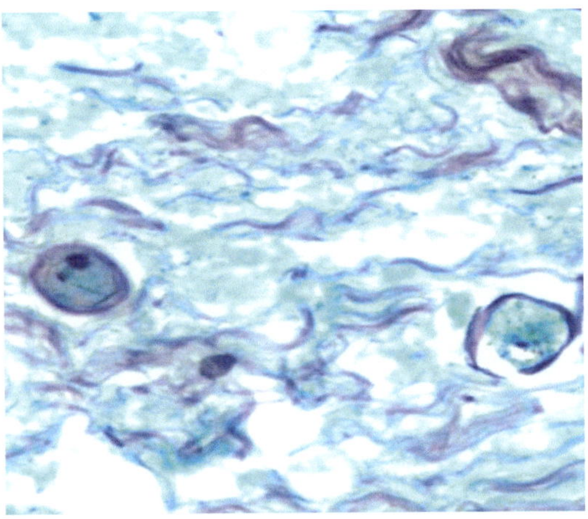

Fig. 1.6 Trophozoite with "bull's-eye" appearance (left) and cyst with wrinkled membrane (right) (GMS stain)

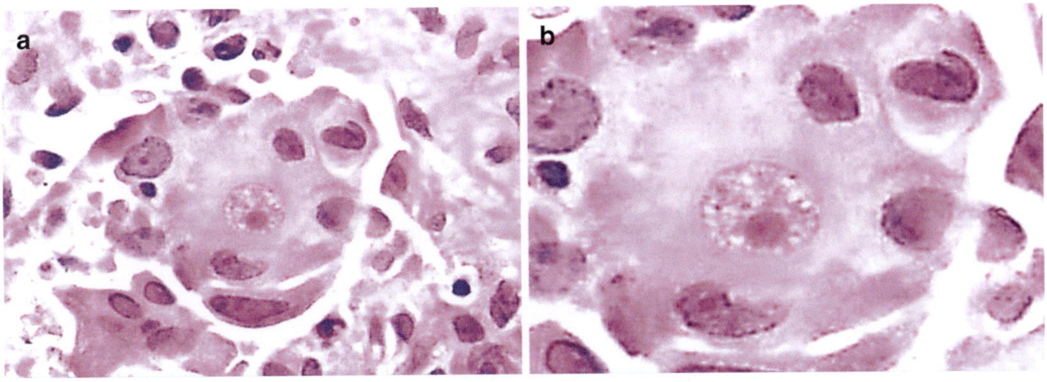

Fig. 1.7 (a, b) Trophozoite with "bull's-eye" appearance present within multinucleated giant cell

Acantholytic Acanthoma

Histopathology (Figs. 1.8, 1.9, and 1.10)
- Well circumscribed indented lesion
- Epidermal hyperkeratosis, papillomatosis, and acanthosis
- Acantholysis with dyskeratosis in the upper two thirds of the epidermis
- Preservation of lower one third of the epidermis

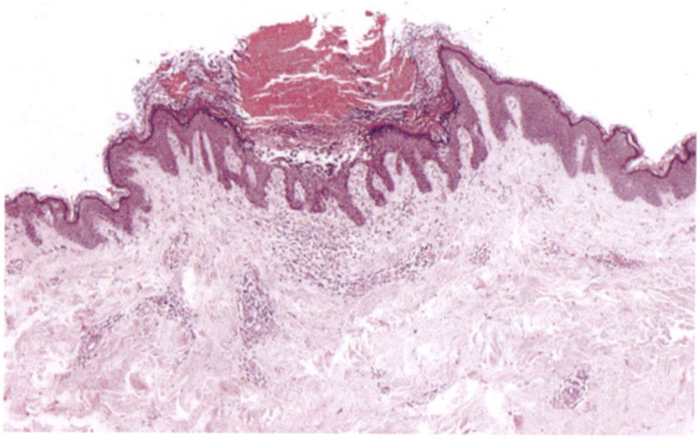

Fig. 1.8 Symmetrical epidermal lesion with well-defined lateral edges

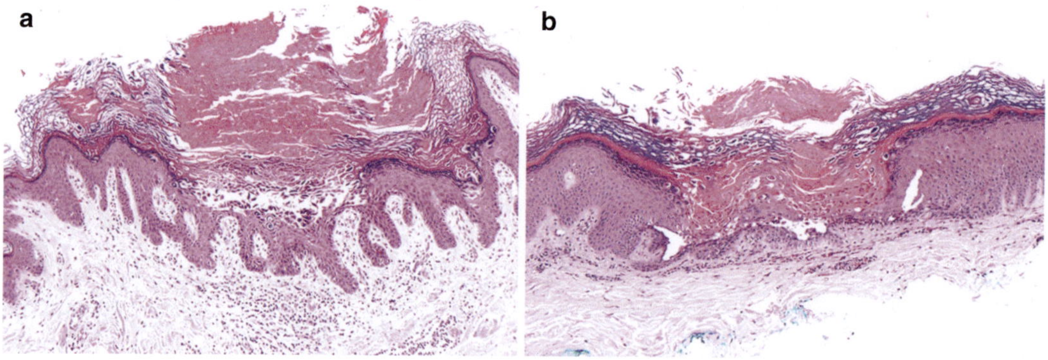

Fig. 1.9 (**a**, **b**) Hyperkeratotic, acanthotic epidermis with epidermal papillomatosis

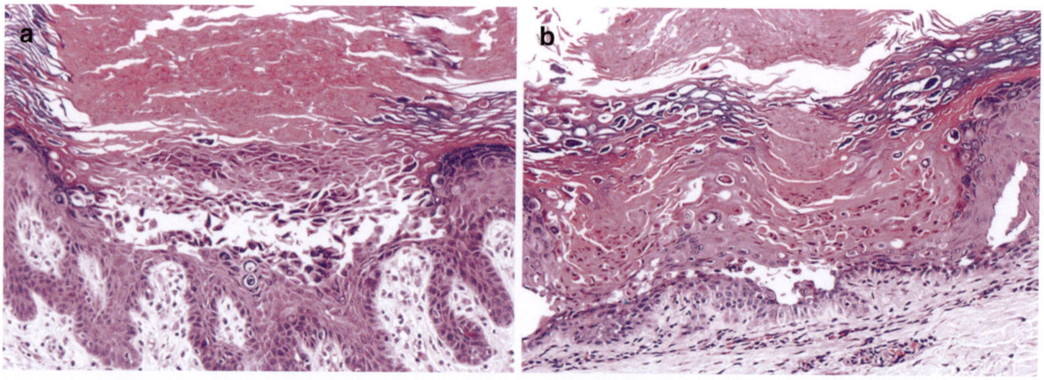

Fig. 1.10 (**a**, **b**) Acantholysis with dyskeratosis in upper 2/3rd of the epidermis with preservation of the basal epidermis

Acanthosis Nigricans

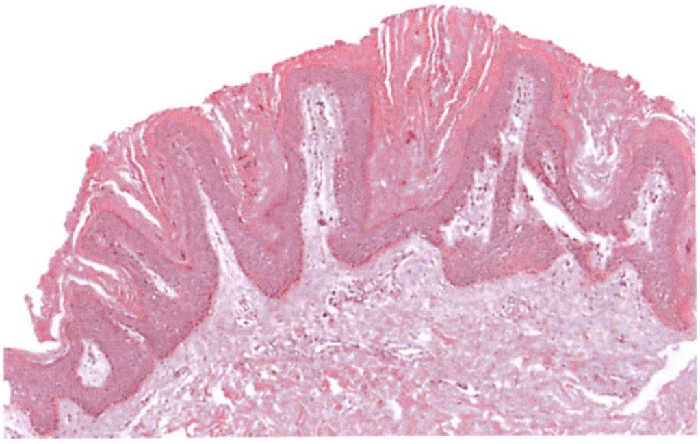

Fig. 1.11 Epidermis with papillomatosis and hyperkeratosis

Histopathology (Figs. 1.11, 1.12, and 1.13)

- Hyperkeratosis with a mildly acanthotic to atrophic epidermis
- Slight increase in epidermal hyperpigmentation
- Epidermal papillomatosis with a squared off appearance

P.S. name is a misnomer as epidermis is usually not significantly acanthotic or hyperpigmented. *Tripe palms* are variant that has 90% association with internal malignancy

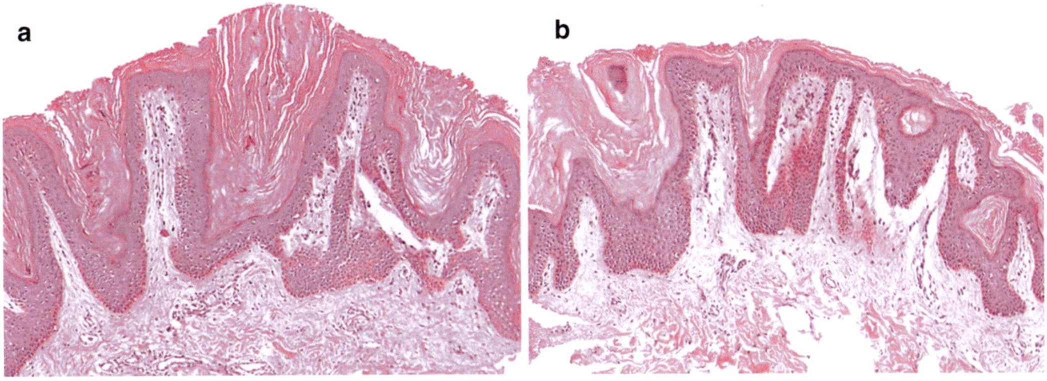

Fig. 1.12 (**a**, **b**) Squared off, slightly irregular papillomatosis with mild atrophy of epidermis

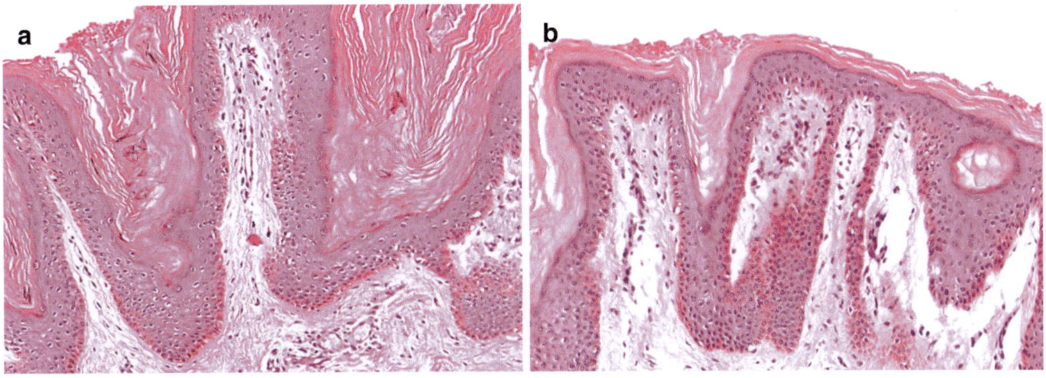

Fig. 1.13 (**a**, **b**) Mildly increased basilar hyperpigmentation

Accessory Tragus

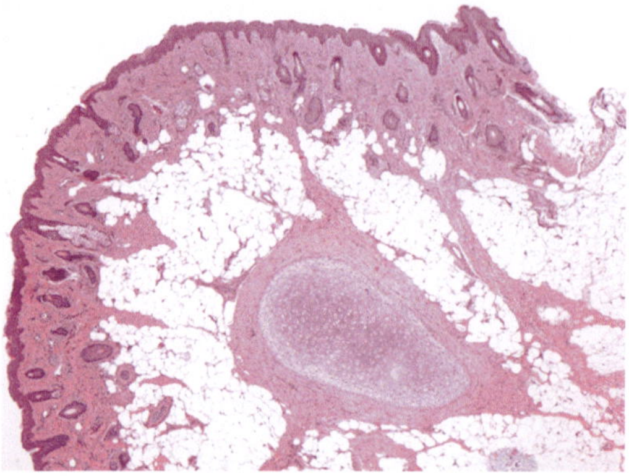

Fig. 1.14 "Skin tag-like" polypoid lesion with central cartilage and adipose tissue

Histopathology (Figs. 1.14, 1.15, 1.16, and 1.17)

- Polypoid "skin tag-like" appearance
- Numerous vellus hair follicles
- Core of adipose tissue and mature cartilage
- Cartilage may not always be present and therefore villous hairs in the polypoid lesion may aid diagnosis

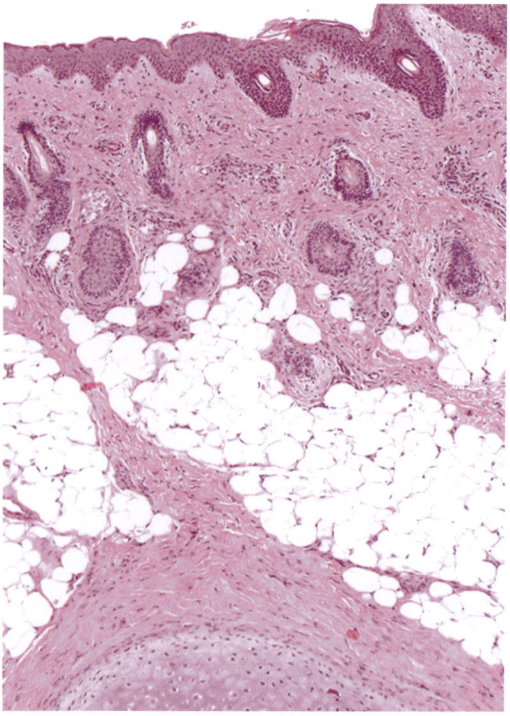

Fig. 1.15 Numerous vellus hairs and central mature cartilage

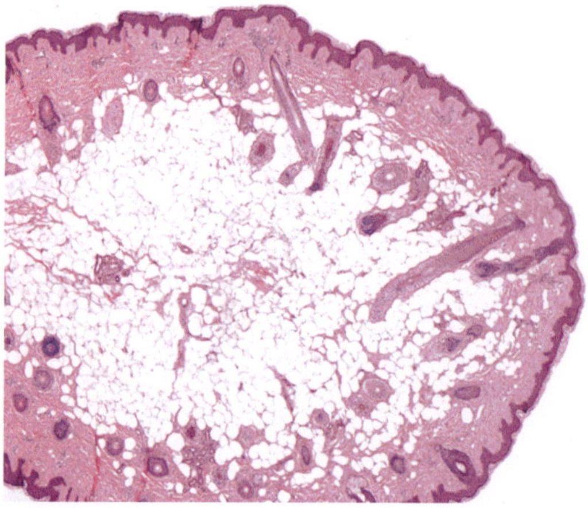

Fig. 1.16 Polypoid lesion with absent cartilage

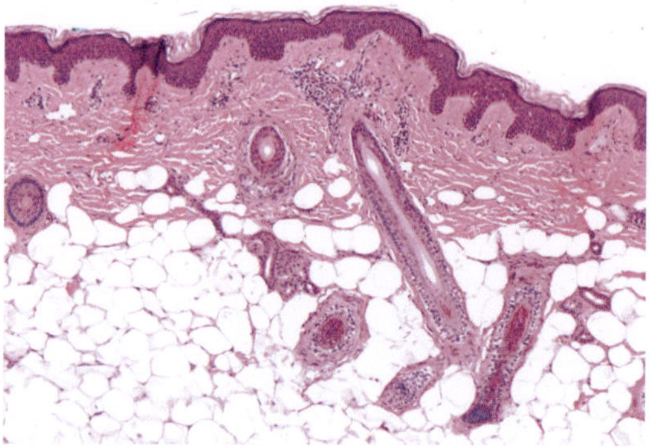

Fig. 1.17 Vellus hairs and adipose tissue

Acne Agminata

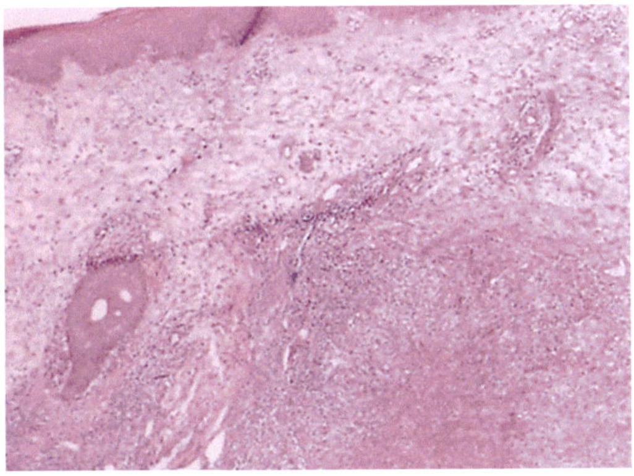

Fig. 1.18 Large epithelioid granuloma adjacent to hair follicle

Synonym: Lupus Miliaris Disseminatus Faciei

Histopathology (Figs. 1.18, 1.19, 1.20, 1.21, and 1.22)

- Epithelioid granulomas with central caseating necrosis
- Granulomas present in upper dermis and perifollicular
- Variably sized granulomas and variably sized central necrosis
- Occasional disruption of hair follicles

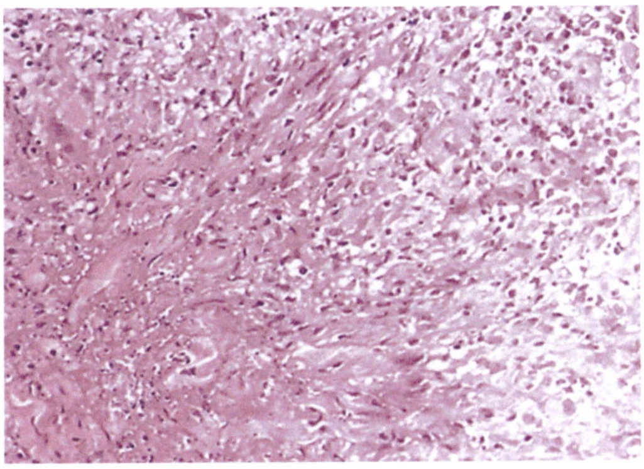

Fig. 1.19 Irregular caseating necrosis

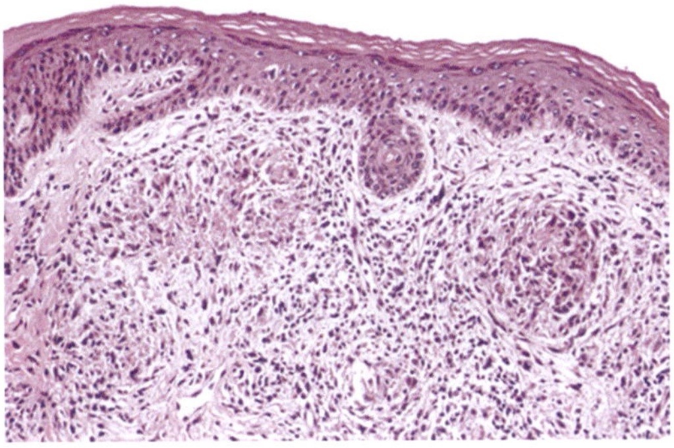

Fig. 1.20 Small granulomas present in the papillary dermis

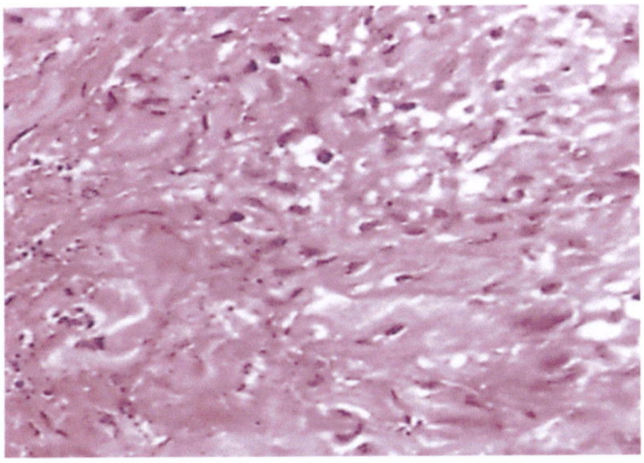

Fig. 1.21 Necrotic area surrounded by histiocytes and lymphocytes

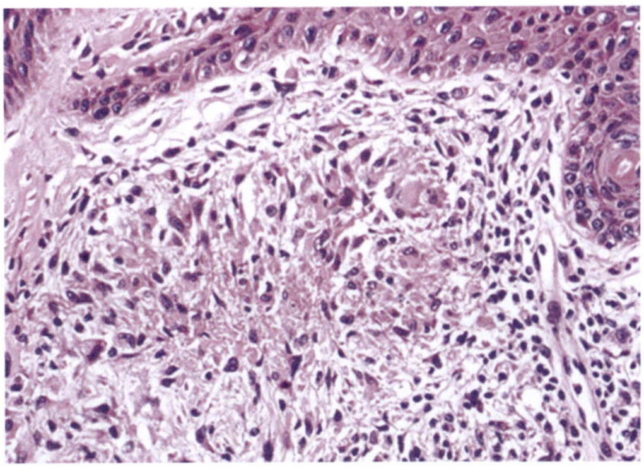

Fig. 1.22 Epithelioid granuloma with central necrosis

Acne Conglobata

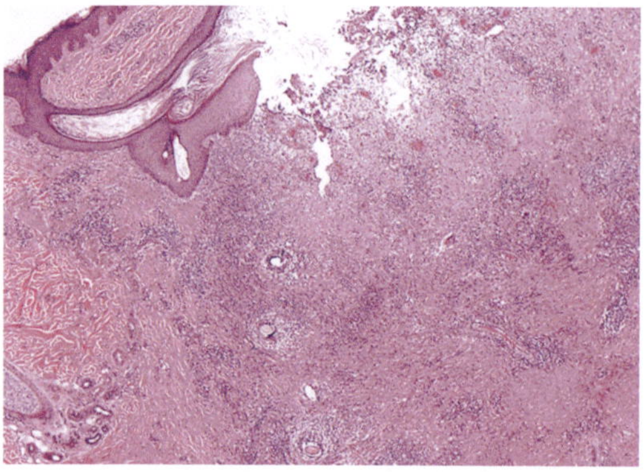

Fig. 1.23 Sinus tract formation lined by squamous epithelium and surrounding abscess formation

Histopathology (Figs. 1.23, 1.24, 1.25, 1.26, and 1.27)

- Ruptured hair follicles with naked hair shafts in dermis
- Superficial and deep dermal abscesses
- Keratin in dermis with surrounding foreign body reaction
- Sinuses tract formation

P.S. similar histology to *Hidradenitis Suppurativa*

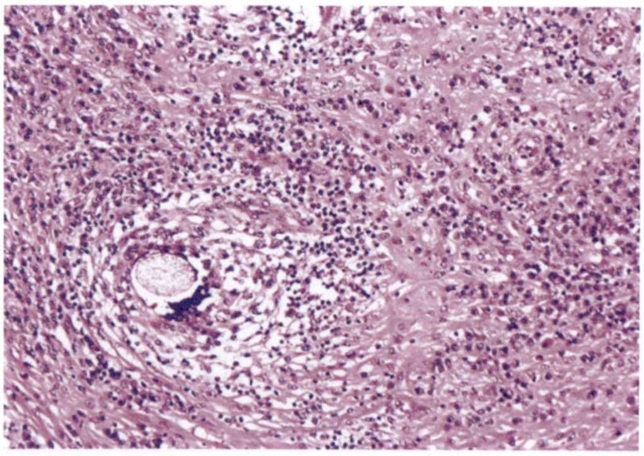

Fig. 1.24 Ruptured hair follicle with surrounding exuberant acute inflammation

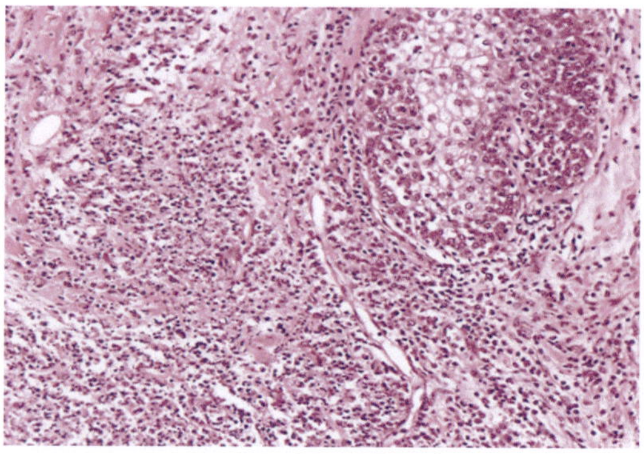

Fig. 1.25 Neutrophilic aggregate forming an abscess

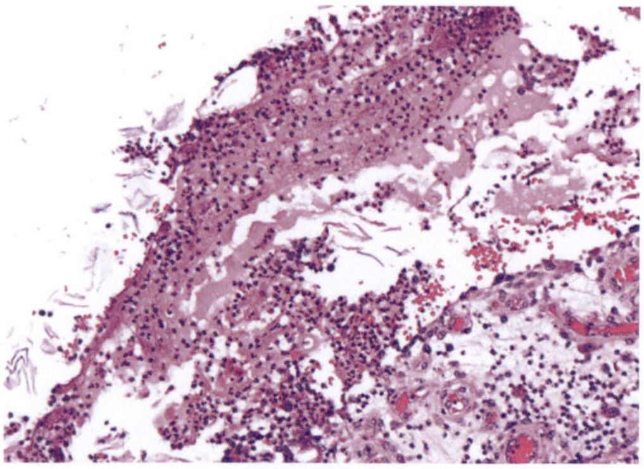

Fig. 1.26 Keratin foreign body reaction

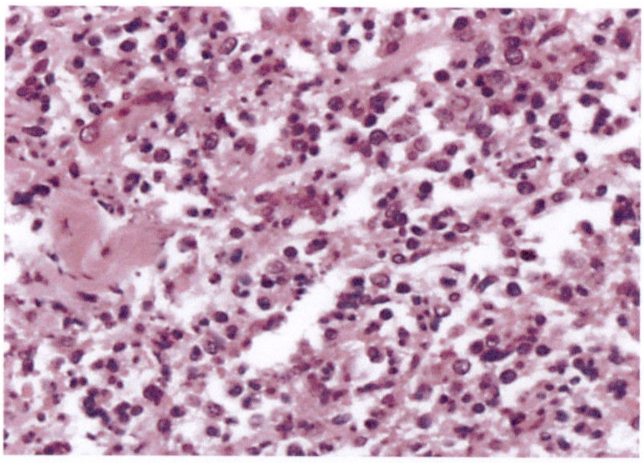

Fig. 1.27 Abscess with focal necrosis

Acne Fulminans

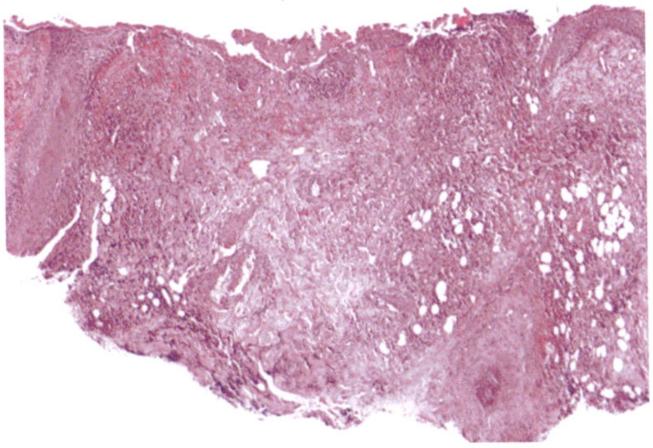

Fig. 1.28 Epidermal necrosis with ulceration

Histopathology (Figs. 1.28, 1.29, 1.30, and 1.31)

- Epidermal ulceration and necrosis
- Extensive acute inflammation in the dermis
- Destruction of follicles and sebaceous glands with abscess formation
- Dermal fibrosis and scarring

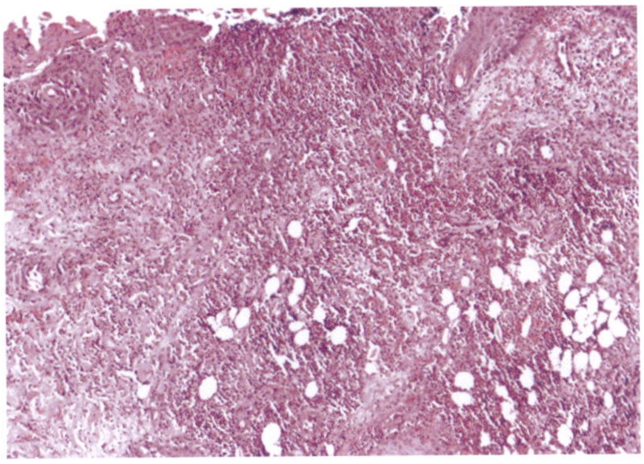

Fig. 1.29 Exuberant dermal acute inflammation with destruction of hair follicles and sebaceous glands

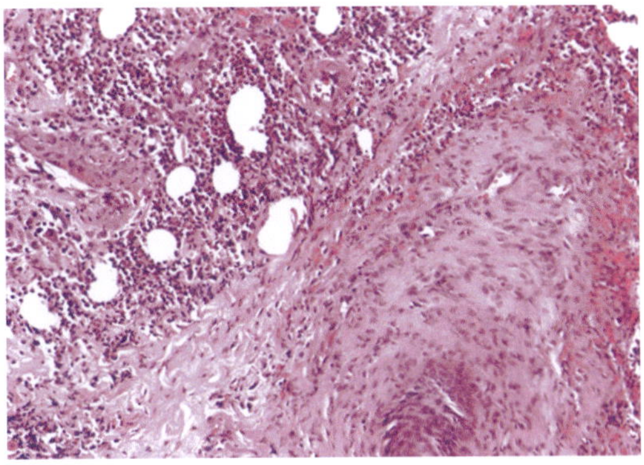

Fig. 1.30 Dermal scarring

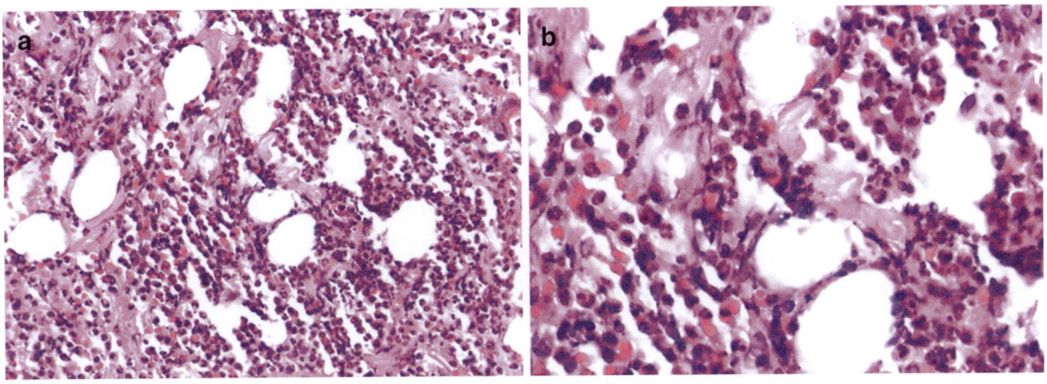

Fig. 1.31 (**a**, **b**) Abscess formation with predominant neutrophils and focal necrosis

Acne Keloidalis Nuchae

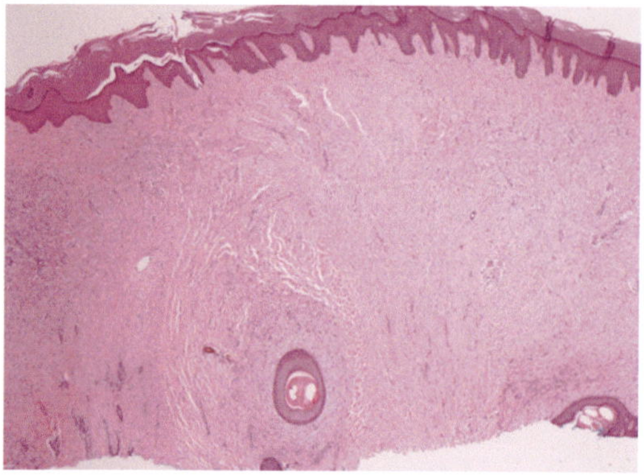

Fig. 1.32 Scalp skin with notable decrease in hair follicles

Histopathology (Figs. 1.32, 1.33, 1.34, 1.35, and 1.36)

- Early findings of hair follicles dilatation and acute, neutrophilic inflammation
- Established lesion with destruction of hair follicles with free hair shafts in dermis
- Dense scar and fibrosis with lymphocytic and plasmocytic inflammation
- Collagen bundles are "keloid-like" with dark pink color but without increased thickness of keloid collagen

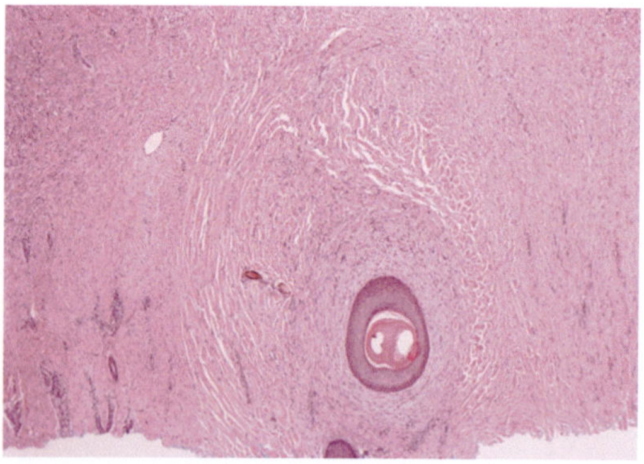

Fig. 1.33 Scarring of hair follicle with perifollicular fibrosis and multiple inner root sheaths

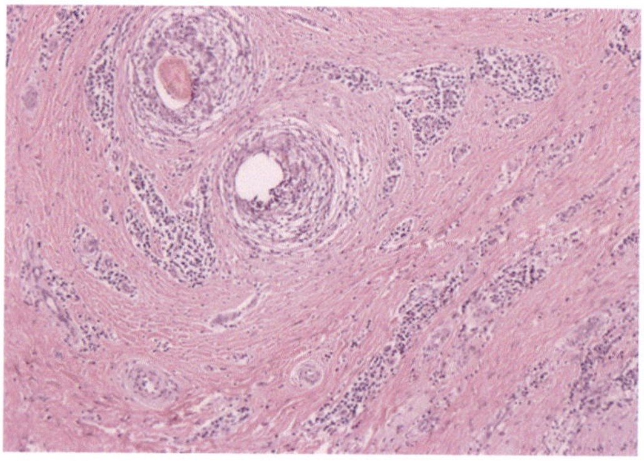

Fig. 1.34 Free hair shafts in dermis

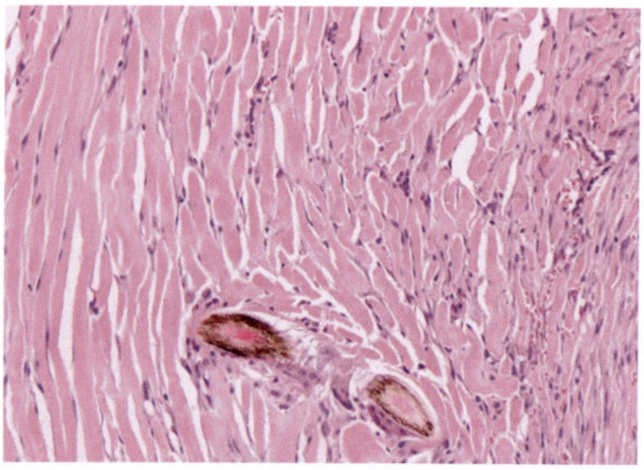

Fig. 1.35 Darkly pink "keloid-like" collagen but not as thick as keloid collagen

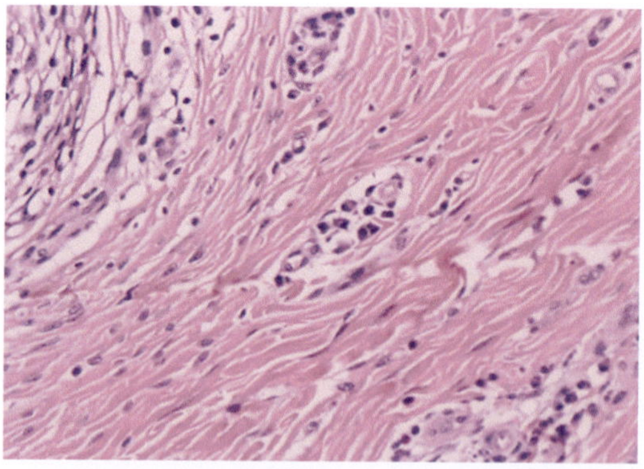

Fig. 1.36 Fibrosis with lymphocytes and plasma cells

Acne Vulgaris

Clinically and histologically acne vulgaris can be divided into two groups:

Noninflammatory (comedones) (Figs. 1.37, 1.38, and 1.39)
- Dilated hair follicle
- Follicle is filled with keratin
- Bacteria may be present in follicle (*P. Acnes*)
- Sebaceous glands are usually prominent
- Lack of significant perifollicular inflammation

Inflammatory (Figs. 1.40, 1.41, 1.42, 1.43, and 1.44)
- Ruptured dilated hair follicle
- Acute follicular and perifollicular inflammation
- Keratin in the dermis with foreign body reaction may be present

P.S. histologically lesions of *Acne Aestivalis* (acneiform variant of *Polymorphous Light Eruption*) present similarly to inflammatory acne vulgaris

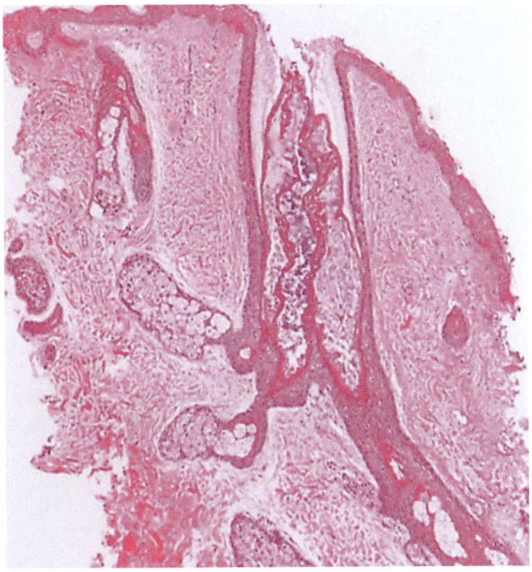

Fig. 1.37 Dilated hair follicle with prominent sebaceous glands and lack of inflammation (**comedone**)

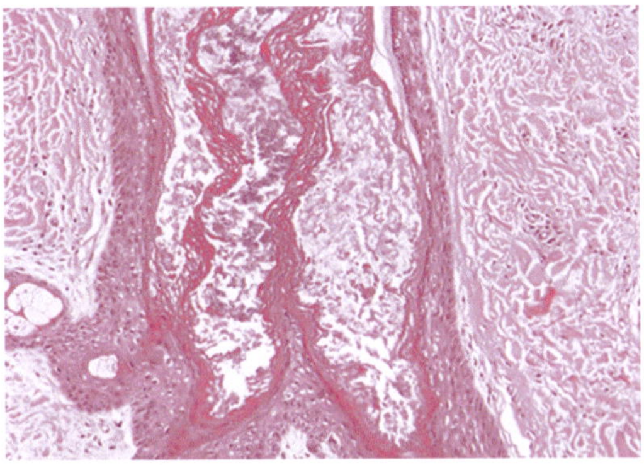

Fig. 1.38 Dilated follicle is filled with keratin

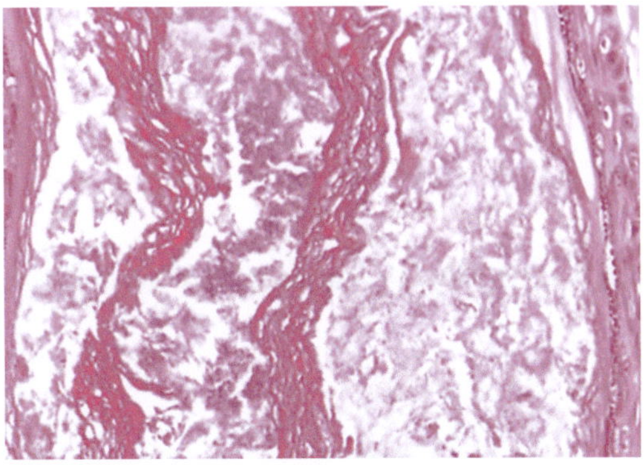

Fig. 1.39 Bacteria are present within the hair follicle

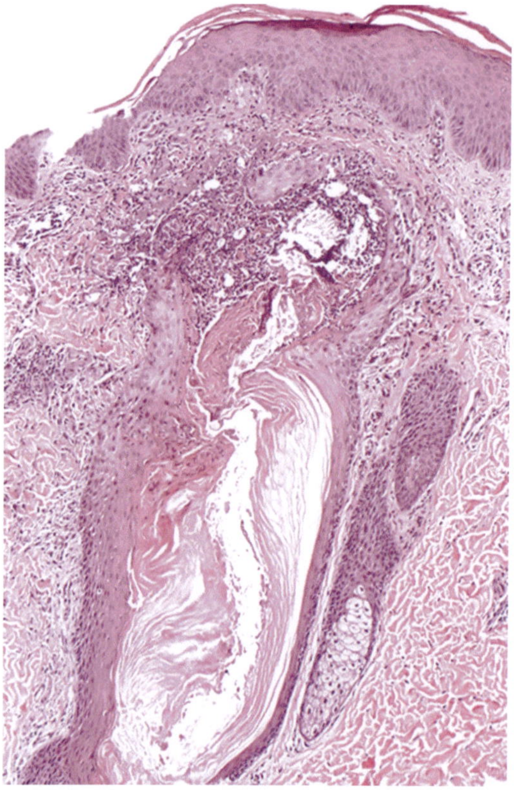

Fig. 1.40 **Inflammatory acne vulgaris** with dilated, partially ruptured hair follicle

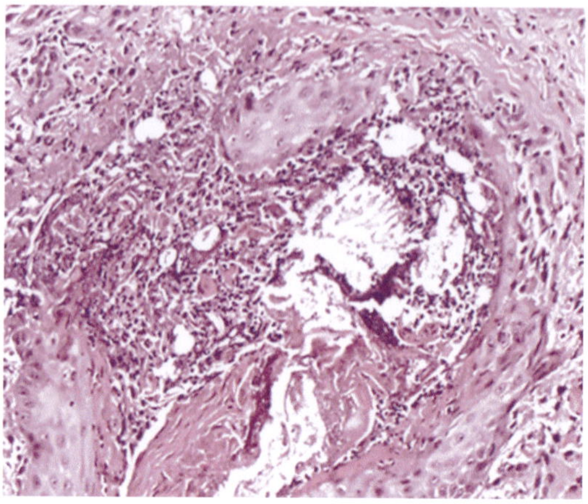

Fig. 1.41 Keratin granuloma and neutrophilic inflammation

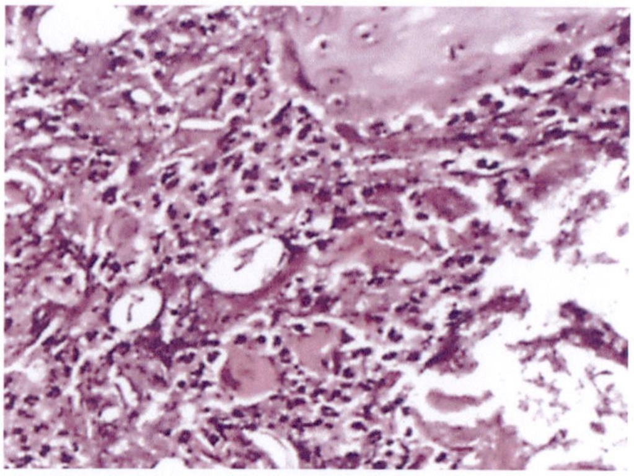

Fig. 1.42 Foreign body reaction due to flakes of keratin

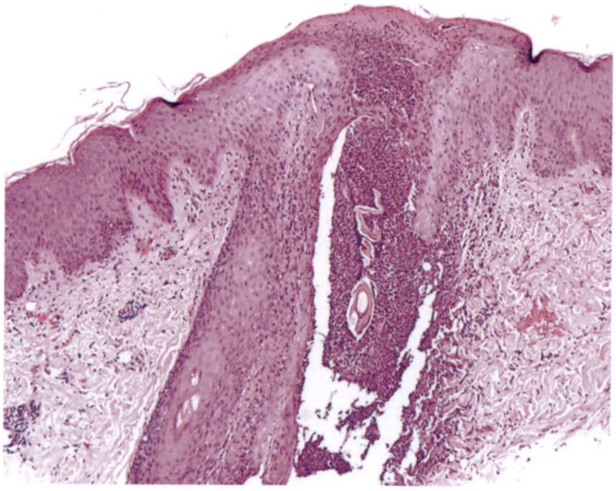

Fig. 1.43 Dilated hair follicle with follicular and perifollicular inflammation

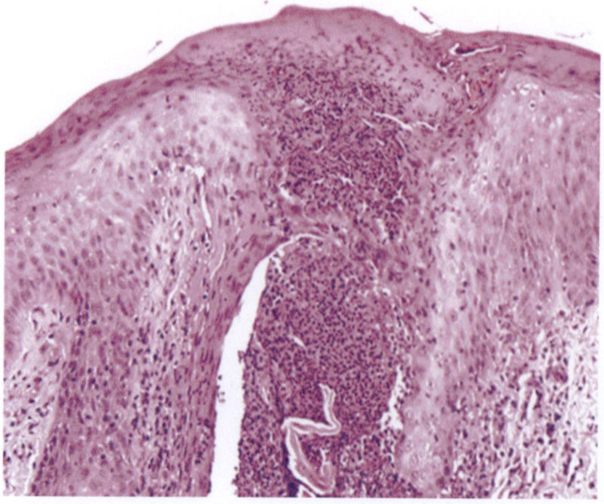

Fig. 1.44 Dilated follicular infundibulum with neutrophilic pustule formation

Acral Fibrokeratoma

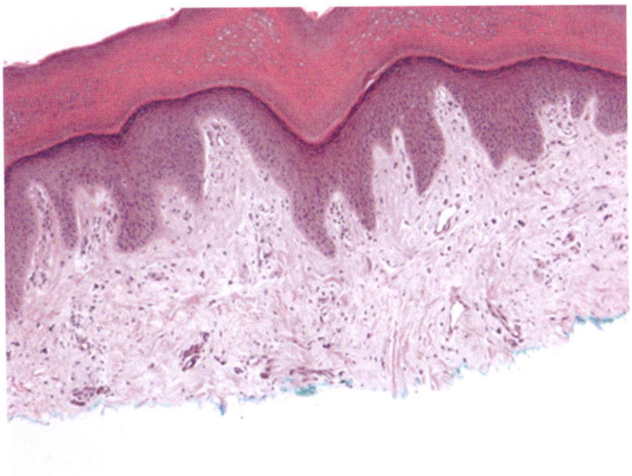

Fig. 1.45 Acral skin with dermal fibrotic lesion

Entities with similar histology are *Acquired Digital Fibrokeratoma* and *Periungual Fibroma.*

Histopathology (Figs. 1.45, 1.46, 1.47, 1.48, and 1.49)

- Hyperkeratotic and acanthotic epidermis
- Thickened collagen bundles
- Increased fibroblasts which may be angulated or multinucleated
- Variable increase in dilated capillaries

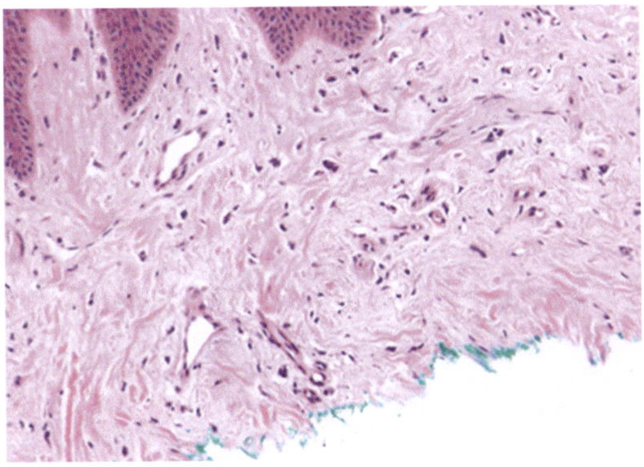

Fig. 1.46 Increased number of dilated capillaries within a fibrotic dermis

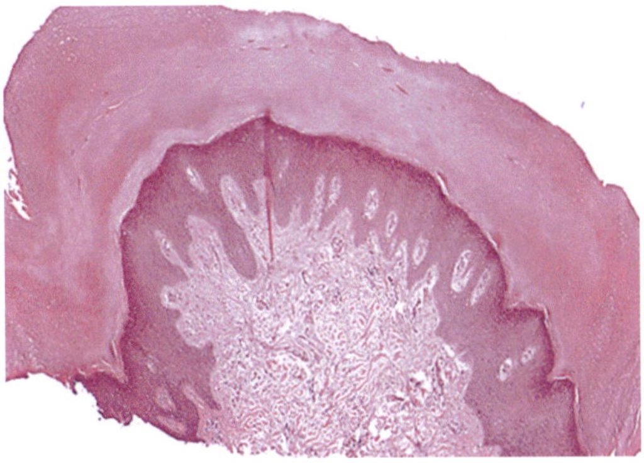

Fig. 1.47 Polypoid acral skin with fibrotic dermis

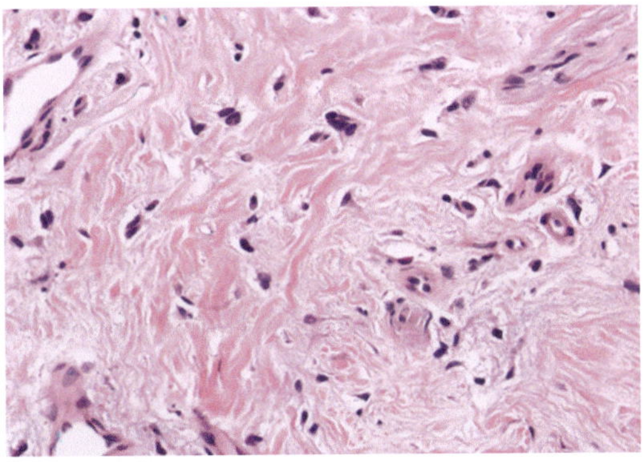

Fig. 1.48 Angulated fibroblasts, some with multinucleation

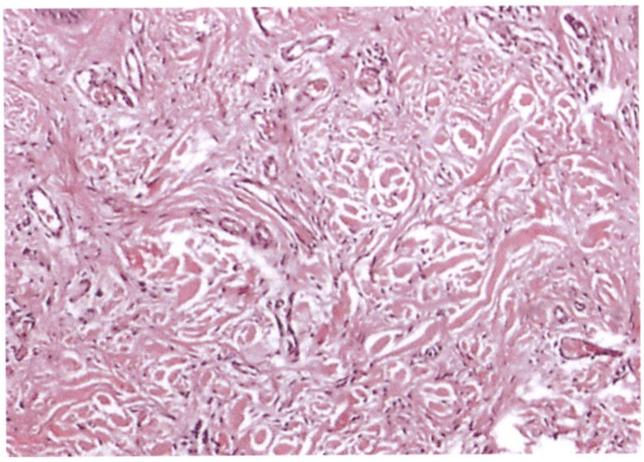

Fig. 1.49 Thick collagen bundles and dilated capillaries

Acral Fibromyxoma

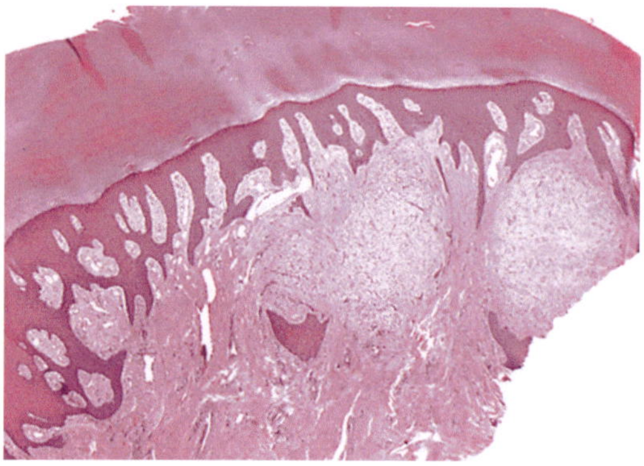

Fig. 1.50 Acral skin with dermal, non-encapsulated myxoid nodules

Histopathology (Figs. 1.50, 1.51, and 1.52)
- Majority are subungual or periungual
- Well-defined, non-encapsulated dermal and subcutaneous nodules with Grenz zone sparring papillary dermis
- Moderate number of spindle cells in nodules surrounded by loose myxoid stroma
- Mast cells are frequent and number of vessels is variable
- Spindle cells positive for CD34 in 70% of cases, CD10+ in most of the cases

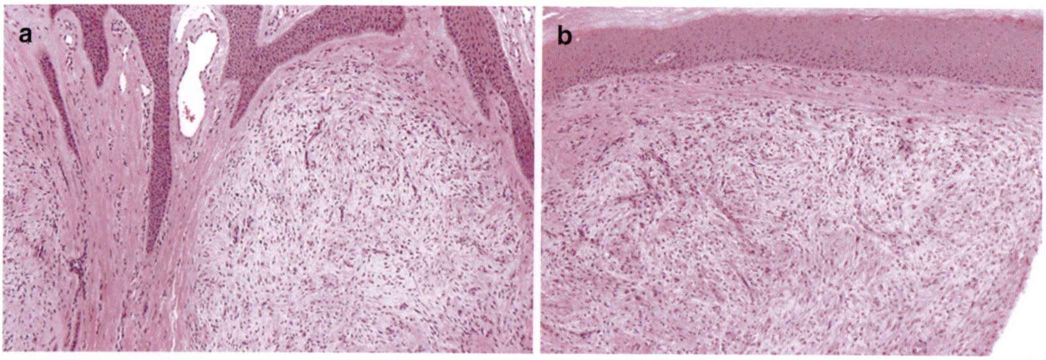

Fig. 1.51 (**a**, **b**) Grenz zone of normal collagen separates tumor nodules from the epidermis

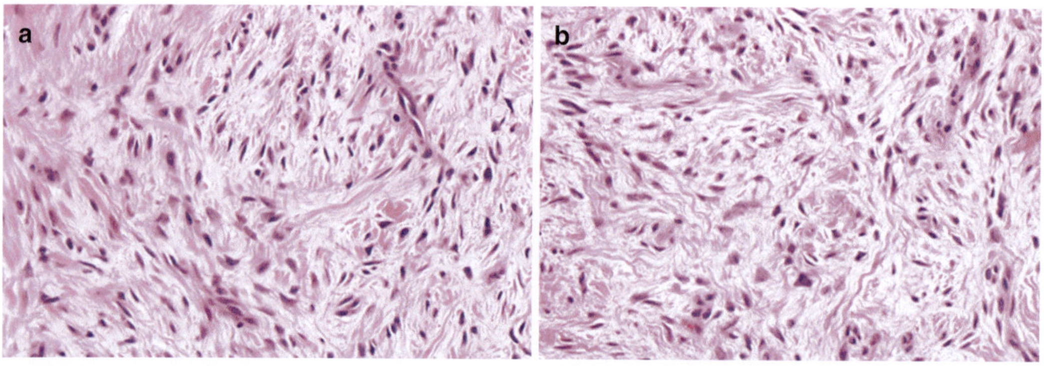

Fig. 1.52 (**a**, **b**) Spindle cells present within myxoid area; occasional mast cells are present

Acral Persistent Papular Mucinosis

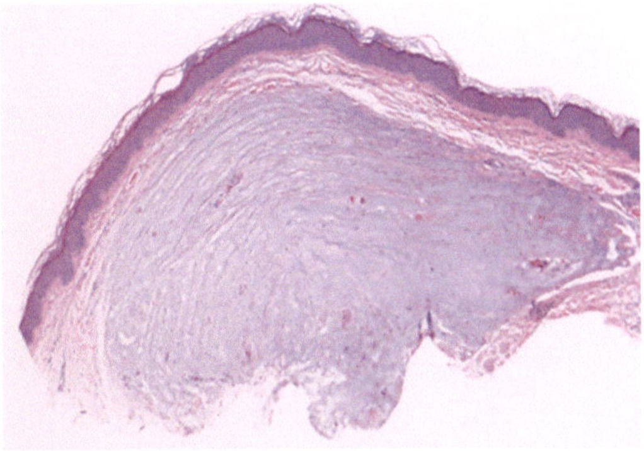

Fig. 1.53 Well-circumscribed nodule of mucin

Histopathology (Figs. 1.53, 1.54, and 1.55)

- Well-circumscribed non-encapsulated nodular deposit of mucin
- Nodule predominantly in upper and mid dermis
- Grenz zone sparing papillary dermis
- Increased fibroblasts in nodule

P.S. it is rare subtype of *lichen myxedematosus*

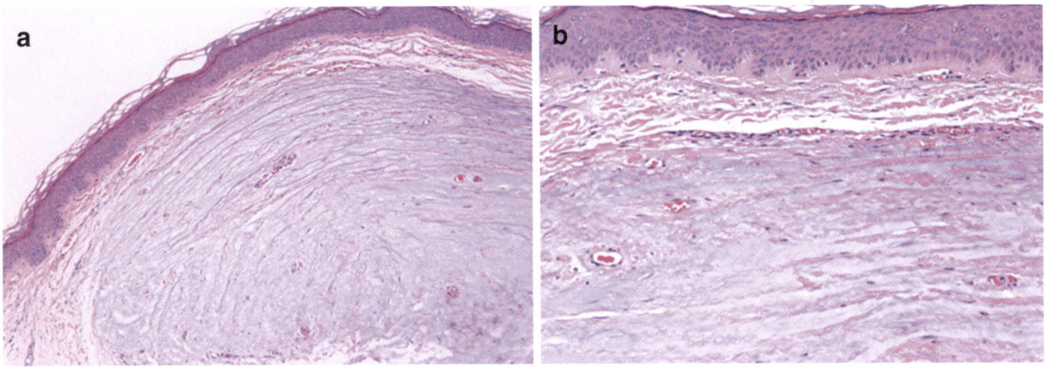

Fig. 1.54 (**a**, **b**) Nodule of mucin in upper/mid dermis with Grenz zone sparing papillary dermis

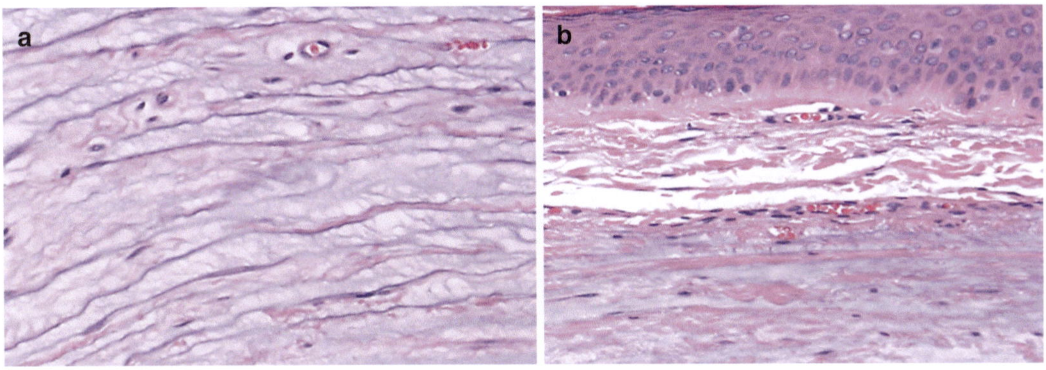

Fig. 1.55 (**a**, **b**) Large deposits of mucin with spindled fibroblasts

Acroangiodermatitis

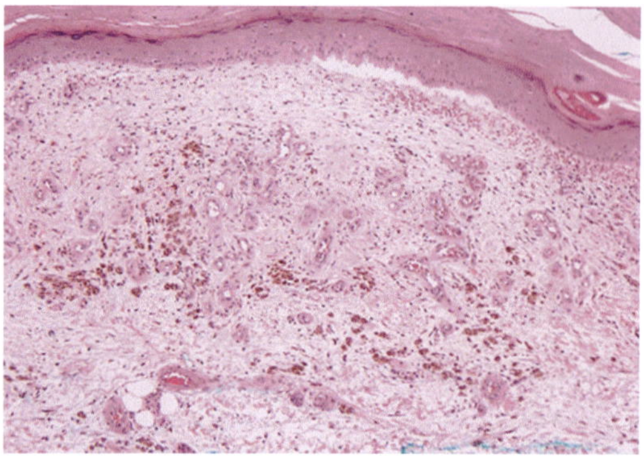

Fig. 1.56 Hyperkeratotic epidermis with dermal vascular proliferation

Synonym: Stasis Dermatitis

Histopathology (Figs. 1.56, 1.57, 1.58, 1.59, and 1.60)

- Epidermal acanthosis and hyperkeratosis
- Lobular proliferation of small dermal vessels
- Plump endothelial cells surrounding round vessel lumens
- Red blood cell extravasation
- Dermal hemosiderin in older lesion

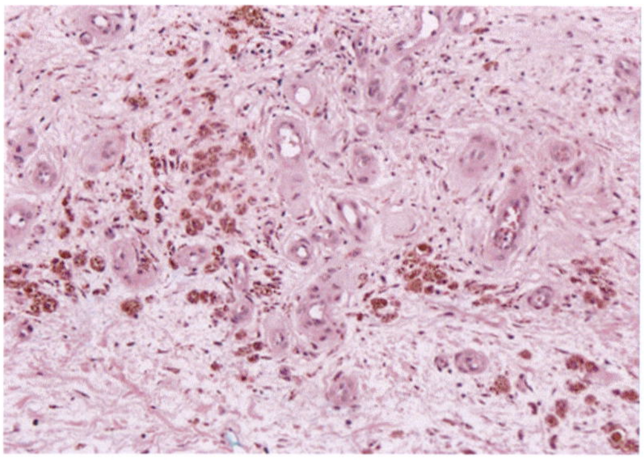

Fig. 1.57 Lobular proliferation of capillaries

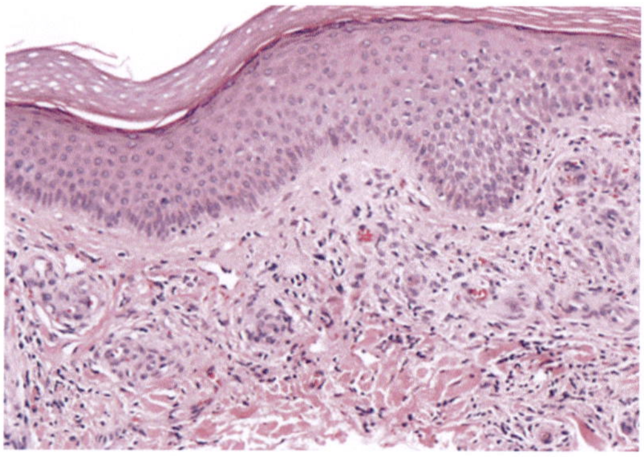

Fig. 1.58 Dermal vascular proliferation

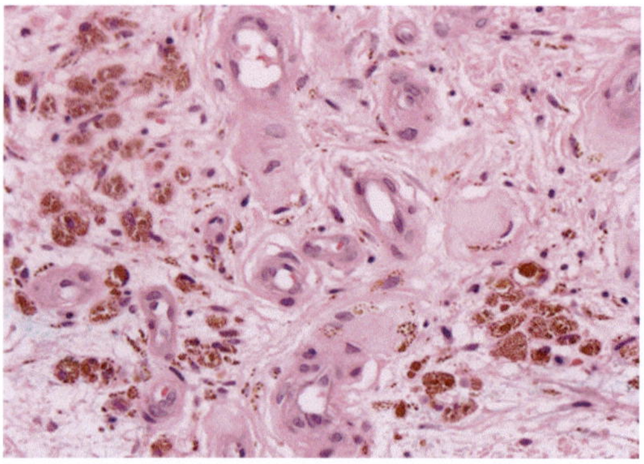

Fig. 1.59 Plump endothelial cells and dermal hemosiderin

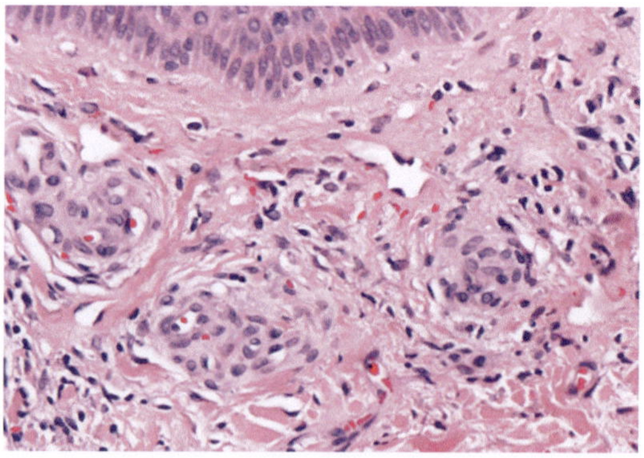

Fig. 1.60 Red blood cell extravasation

Acrochordon

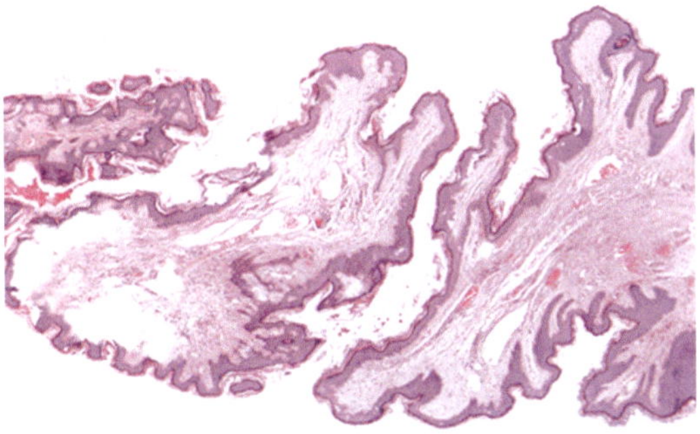

Fig. 1.61 Multiple polypoid lesions with lack of adnexal structures

Synonym: Skin Tag

Histopathology (Figs. 1.61, 1.62, 1.63, 1.64, and 1.65)

- Polypoid appearance
- Epidermis is hyperkeratotic and variably acanthotic
- Stroma can vary from dense sclerotic to loose collagenous
- Larger lesions may have a core of adipose tissue
- Lack of adnexal structures

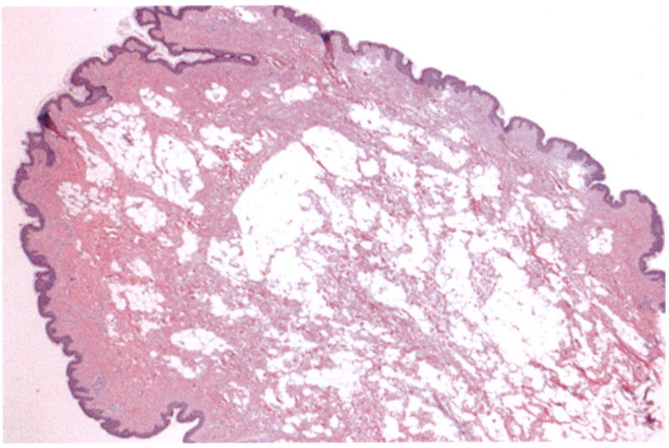

Fig. 1.62 Polypoid lesion with central core of collagen and adipose tissue

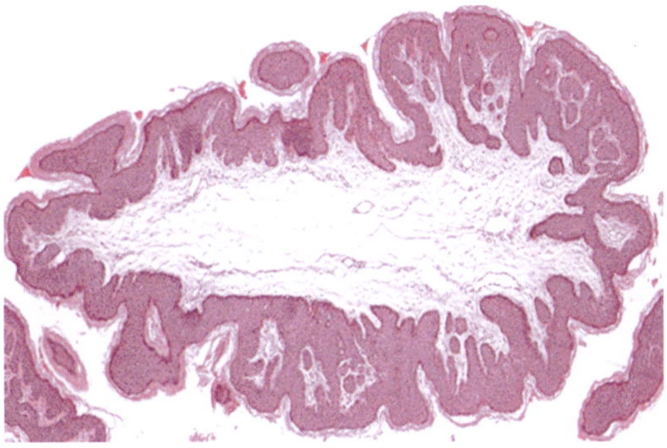

Fig. 1.63 Hyperkeratotic acanthotic epidermis with loose fibrotic core

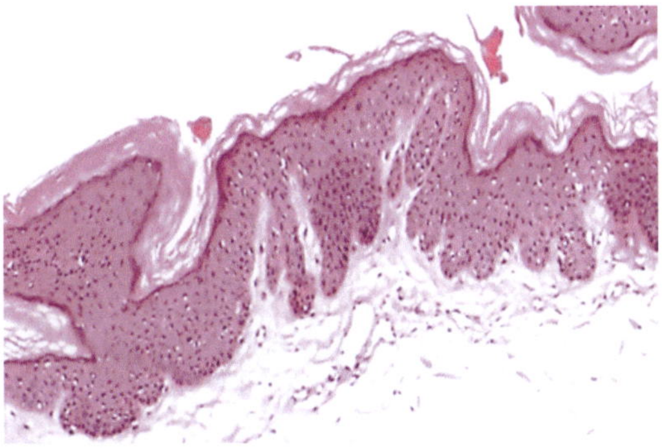

Fig. 1.64 Hyperkeratotic and acanthotic epidermis

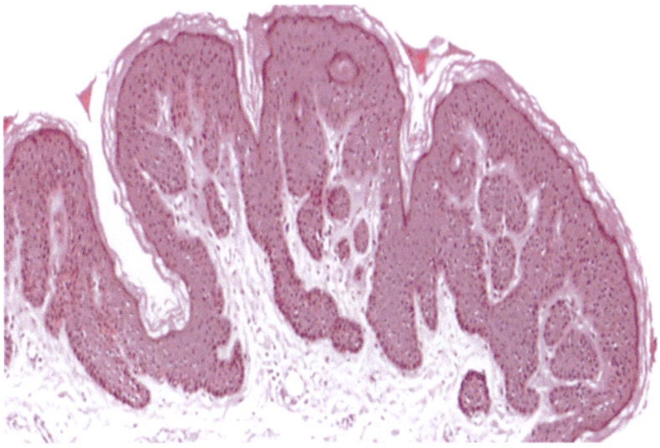

Fig. 1.65 Acanthotic "seborrheic keratosis-like" epidermis

Acrodermatitis Chronica Atrophicans

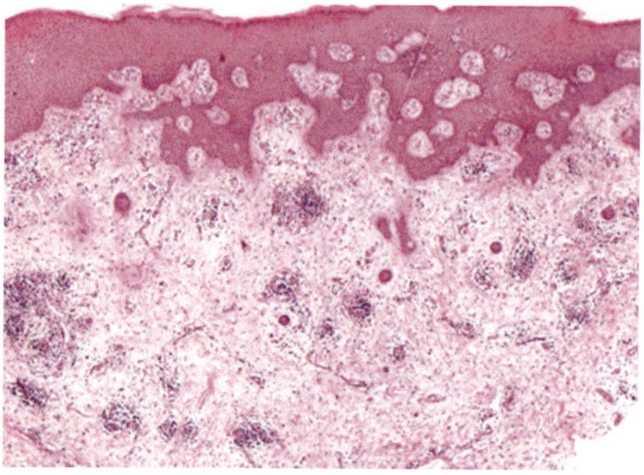

Fig. 1.66 **Initial lesion** with perivascular inflammation and myxoid stroma

Histopathology

Early lesions (Figs. 1.66, 1.67, and 1.68)
- Initial inflammatory stage with perivascular lymphocytic and plasmocytic inflammation
- Background myxoid to edematous stroma

Established lesions (Figs. 1.69 and 1.70)
- Epidermal atrophy with effacement of rete ridges
- Dermal atrophy and fibrosis
- Adnexal structures are reduced or absent

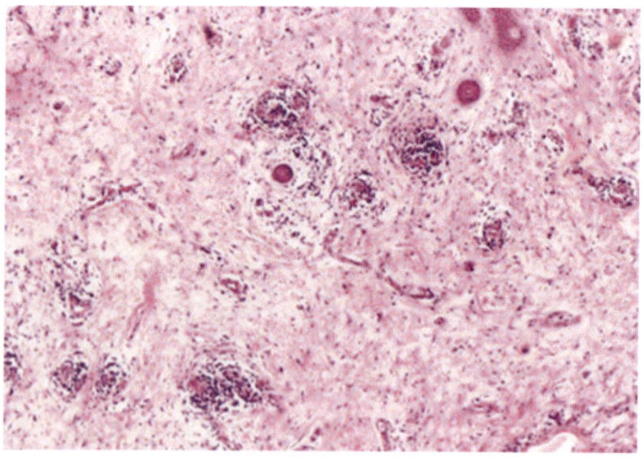

Fig. 1.67 Tightly cuffed perivascular lymphoplasmocytic inflammation

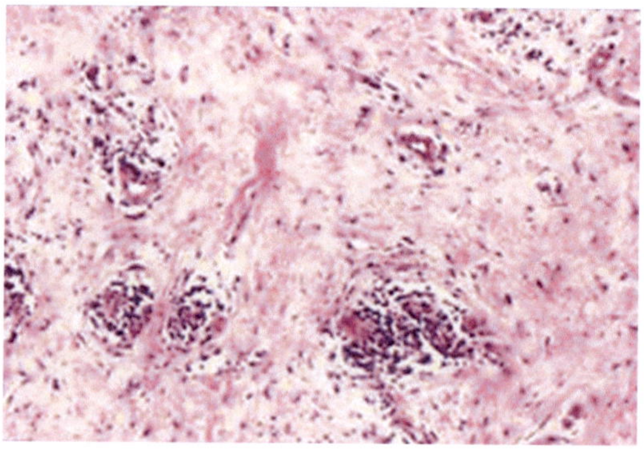

Fig. 1.68 Edematous to myxoid background

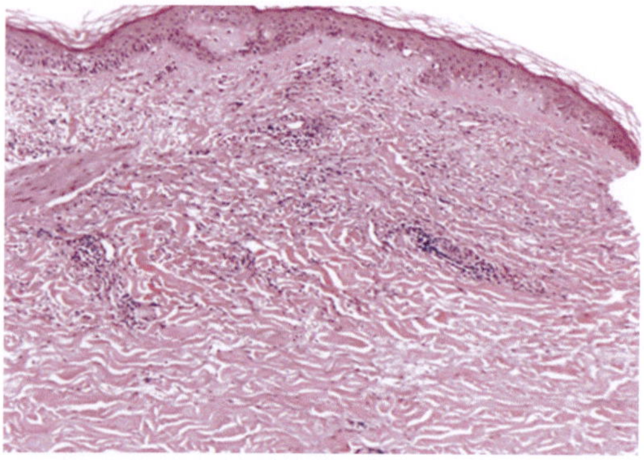

Fig. 1.69 **Established lesion** with epidermal atrophy, absent adnexal structures, and focal inflammation

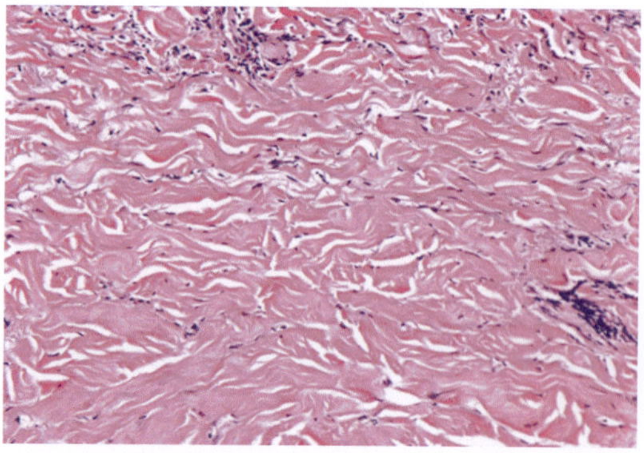

Fig. 1.70 Dermal fibrosis

Acrokeratosis Verruciformis of Hopf

Histopathology (Figs. 1.71, 1.72, and 1.73)

- Epidermal hyperkeratosis, acanthosis, and "church spire-like" papillomatosis
- Lack of dermal inflammation

P.S. associate with Darier's disease

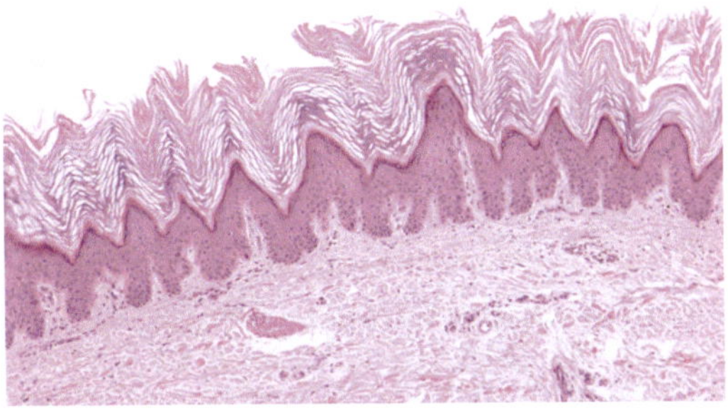

Fig. 1.71 Uniformly wavy acanthotic epidermis

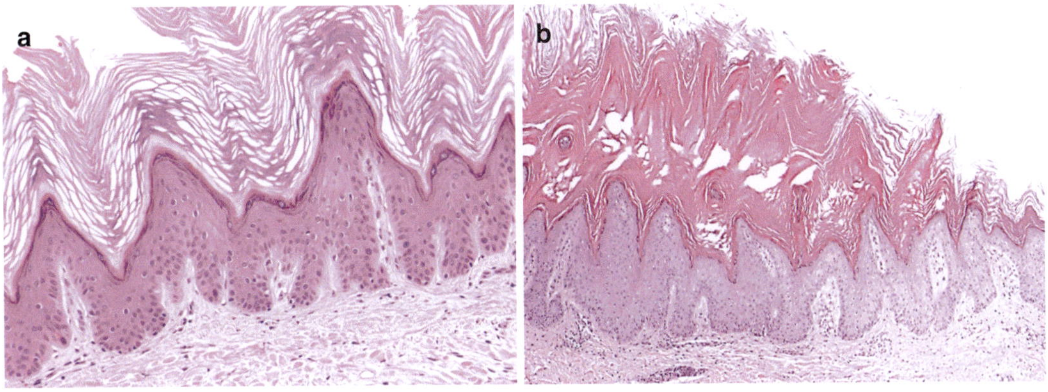

Fig. 1.72 (**a**, **b**) Significant hyperkeratosis with "church spire-like" papillomatosis and normal appearing epidermis

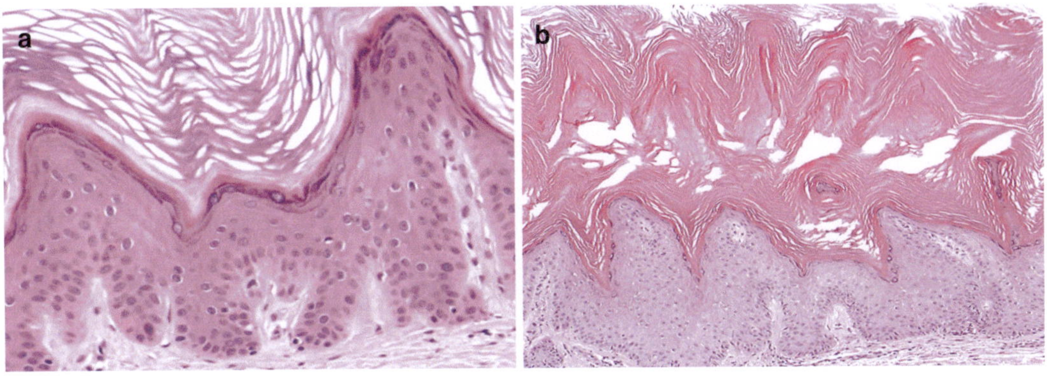

Fig. 1.73 (**a**, **b**) Normal appearing granular layer and lack of parakeratosis

Acrospiroma

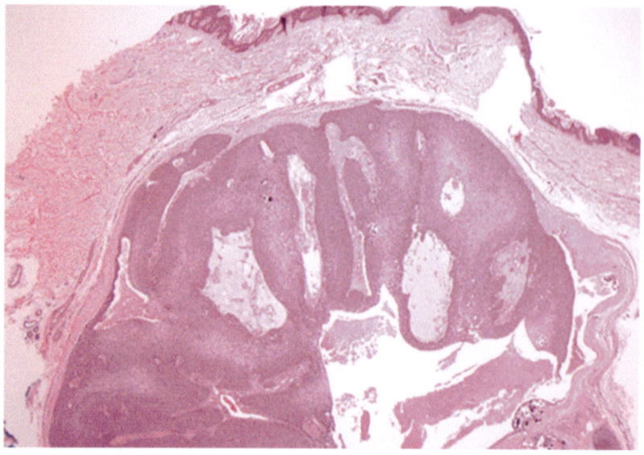

Fig. 1.74 Dermal, well-demarcated, non-encapsulated nodule with broad pushing borders

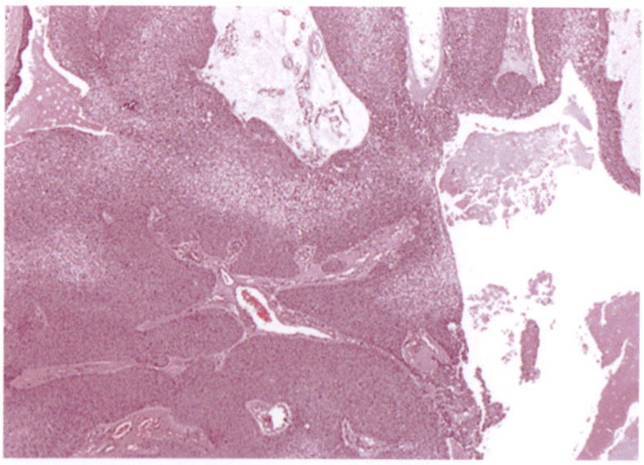

Fig. 1.75 Solid cellular areas with large cystic areas

Synonyms: Eccrine Acrospiroma, Hidradenoma, Solid-cystic Hidradenoma

Histopathology (Figs. 1.74, 1.75, 1.76, 1.77, 1.78, and 1.79)

- Dermal well circumscribed non-encapsulated tumor with broad borders pushing into subcutaneous fat
- Epidermal connection can be present
- Solid cellular tumor areas with cystic spaces and ductal structures
- Two cell population of larger cells with clear and smaller cells with darker cytoplasm
- Sometimes a single cell population will predominate
- Stroma is often vascular and hyalinized
- Tumor can frequently show squamatization and/or mucinous changes
- Ductal structures frequently seen (highlighted by EMA and CEA)
- Focal spindle cell epithelial cells can be seen

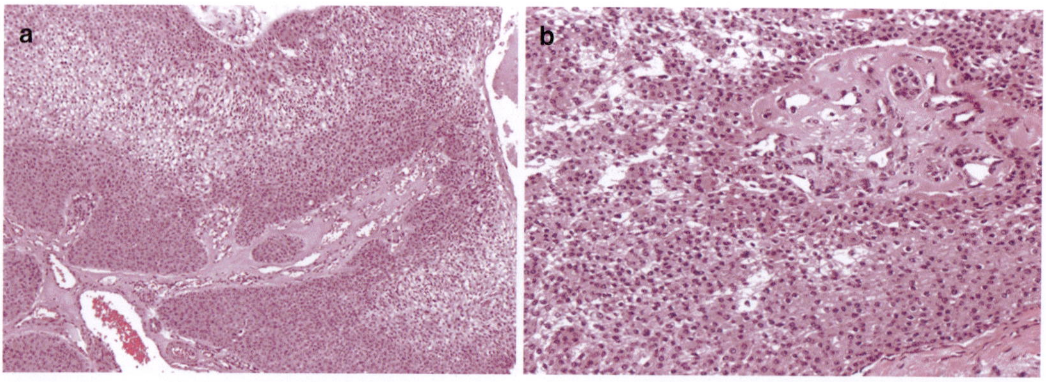

Fig. 1.76 (**a**, **b**) Admixed, pale and dark uniform cells with hyalinized pink collagen within and around tumor nodules

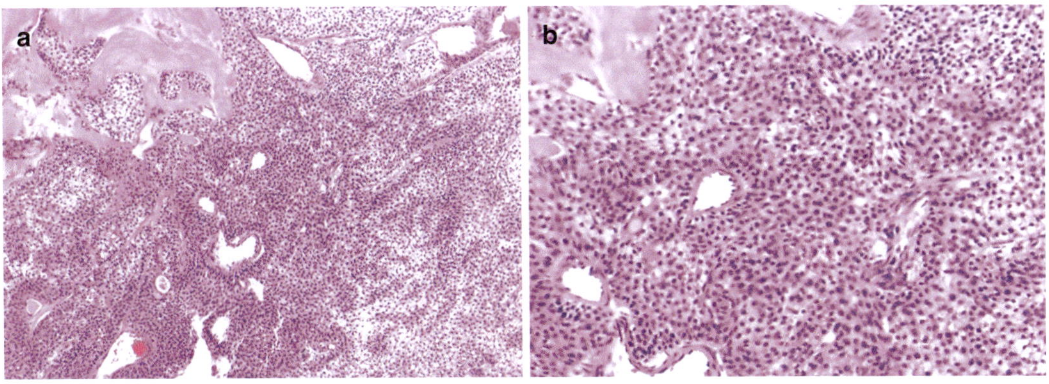

Fig. 1.77 (**a**, **b**) Uniform, admixed pale and dark cells with surrounding pink hyalinized stroma

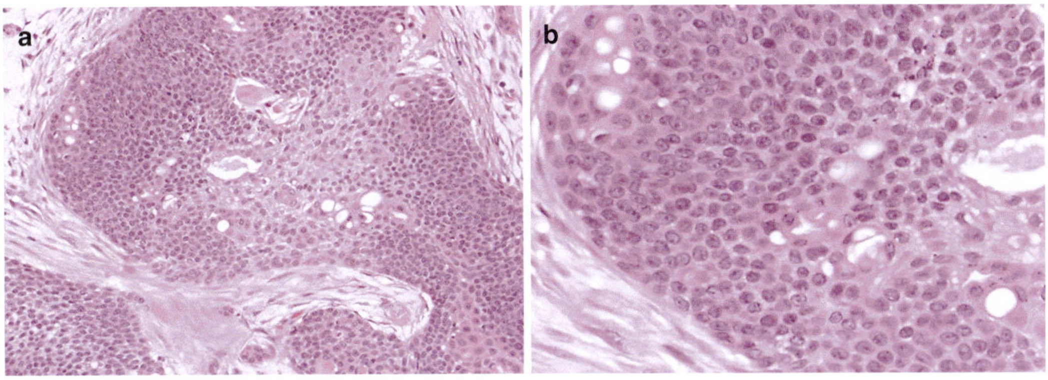

Fig. 1.78 (**a**, **b**) Scattered, variably sized ductal structures present within tumor nodules

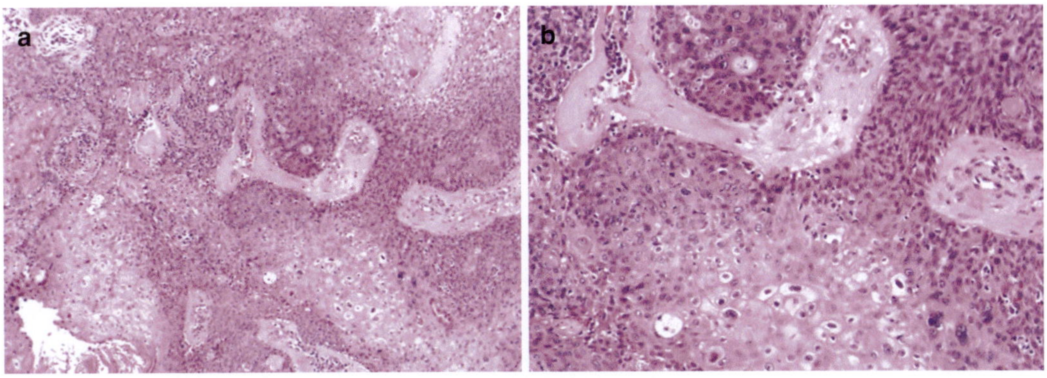

Fig. 1.79 (**a**, **b**) Foci of squamous metaplasia with pleomorphism are present

Actinic Cheilitis

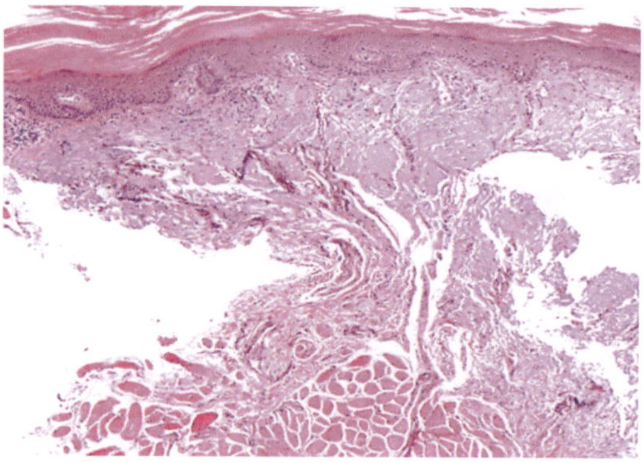

Fig. 1.80 Mucosal epithelium with hyperkeratosis and severe solar elastosis

Histopathology (Figs. 1.80, 1.81, and 1.82)
- Mucosal epithelium with frequent squamous metaplasia
- Acanthosis, hyperkeratosis, parakeratosis, and hypogranulosis
- Atypia of keratinocytes but lacking full thickness atypia or dermal invasion
- Marked solar elastosis
- Chronic inflammation commonly present

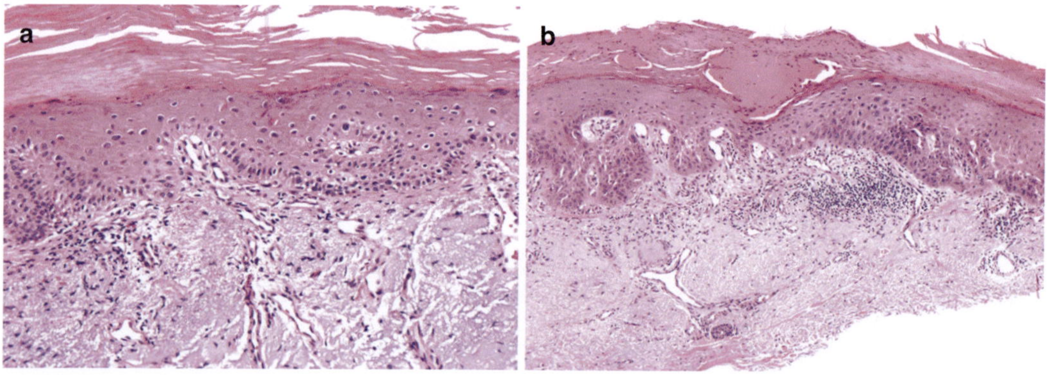

Fig. 1.81 (**a**, **b**) Keratinocyte atypia in lower epidermis with underlying solar damage, inflammation, and telangiectasias

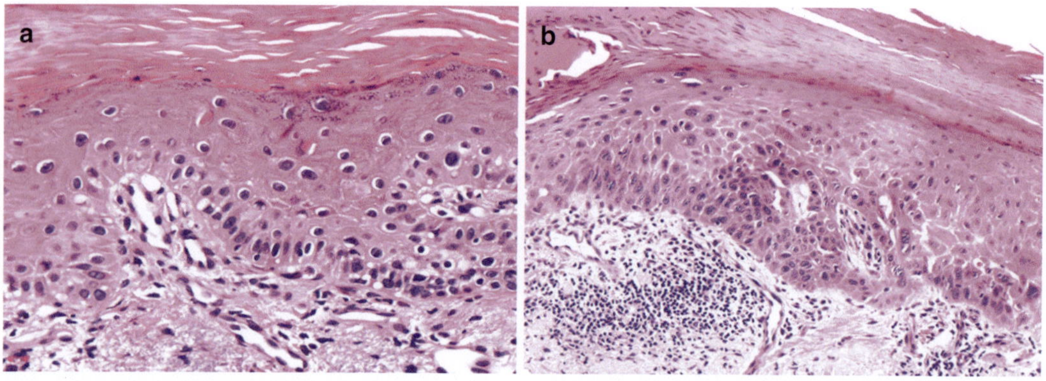

Fig. 1.82 (**a**, **b**) Scattered parakeratosis, hypogranulosis, and keratinocyte atypia without full-thickness atypia

Actinic Granuloma

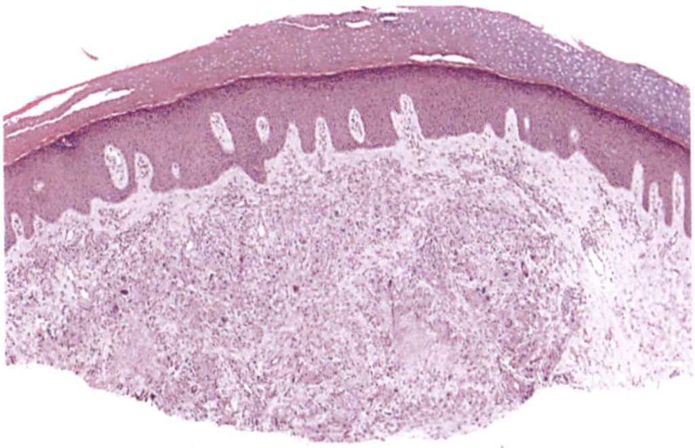

Fig. 1.83 Dense, diffuse dermal infiltrate with foci of palisading

Synonym: O'Brien Granuloma

Histopathology (Figs. 1.83, 1.84, and 1.85)

- Dermal infiltrate of histiocytes and multinucleated giant cells
- Inflammation may be distributed diffusely between collagen bundles or form palisaded granulomas
- Damaged elastic fibers within multinucleated giant cells or within center of palisaded granulomas
- Lack of increased dermal mucin

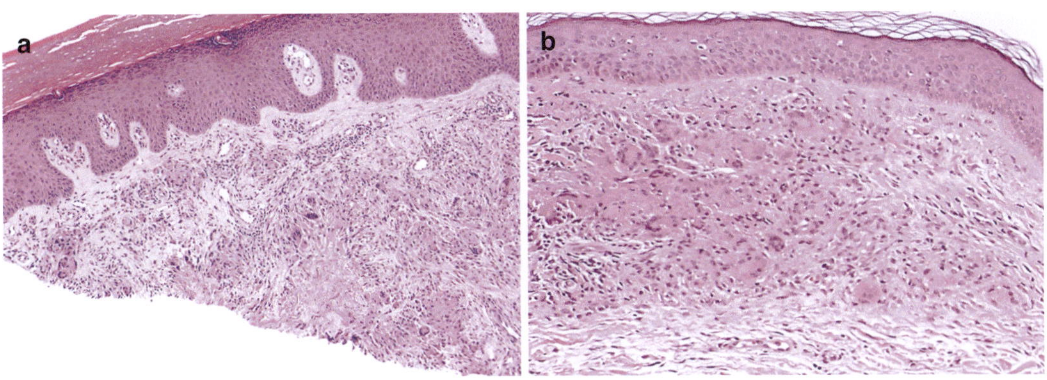

Fig. 1.84 (**a**, **b**) Infiltrate of predominantly histiocytes and multinucleated giant cells with surrounding solar elastosis

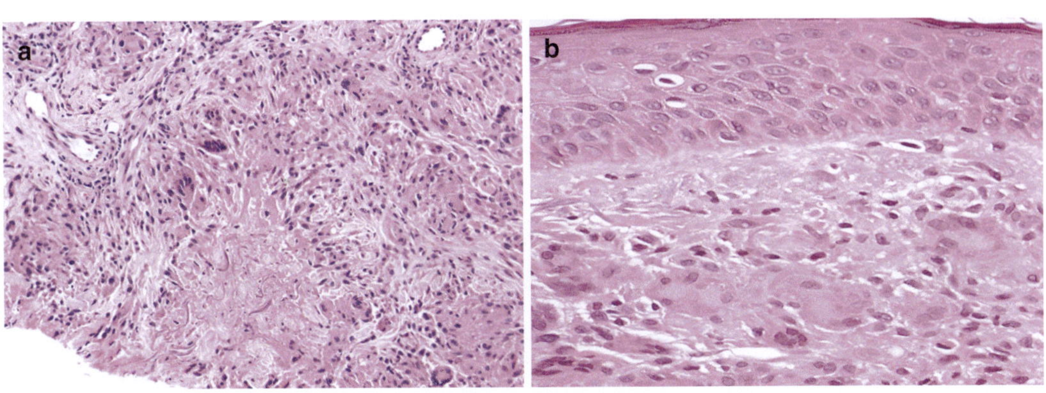

Fig. 1.85 Elastic fibers surrounded by palisaded granuloma (**a**) and engulfed by multinucleated giant cells (**b**)

Actinic Keratosis

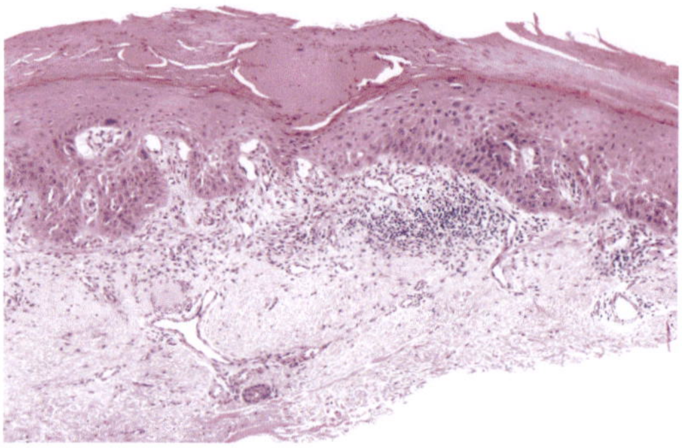

Fig. 1.86 Hypertrophic actinic keratosis with epidermal acanthosis, dermal solar elastosis and telangiectasias

Histopathology (Figs. 1.86, 1.87, 1.88, 1.89, 1.90, 1.91, 1.92, and 1.93)

- Acanthosis, hyperkeratosis, focal parakeratosis, and/or hypogranulosis
- Keratinocyte atypia in lower two thirds of epidermis
- Solar elastosis, telangiectasias, chronic dermal inflammation

P.S. variants include hypertrophic (Figs. 1.86 and 1.87), lichenoid (Fig. 1.88), acantholytic (Fig. 1.91), atrophic (Fig. 1.89), and pigmented (Fig. 1.90)

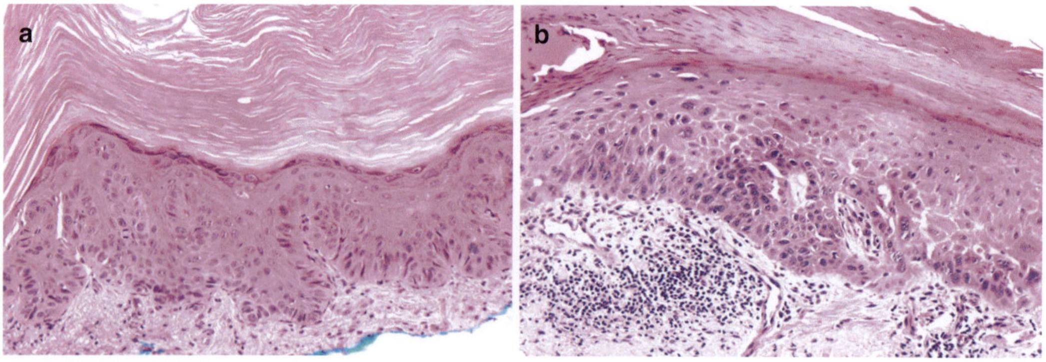

Fig. 1.87 (**a**, **b**) Atypical keratinocytes in the lower portion of the epidermis with dermal chronic lymphocytic inflammation

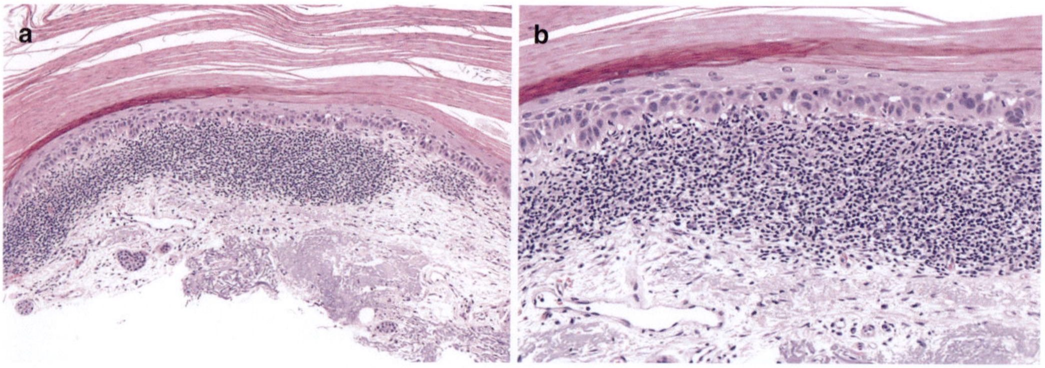

Fig. 1.88 (**a**, **b**) **Lichenoid actinic keratosis** with atypia of basal layer keratinocytes and band-like lymphocytic inflammation

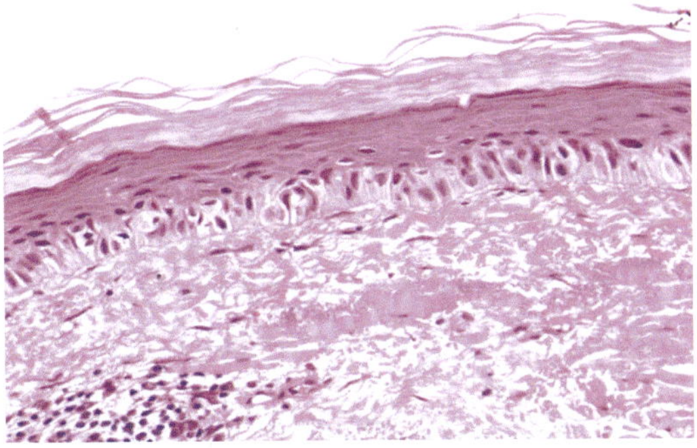

Fig. 1.89 **Atrophic actinic keratosis** with atrophic epidermis and atypia of basal layer

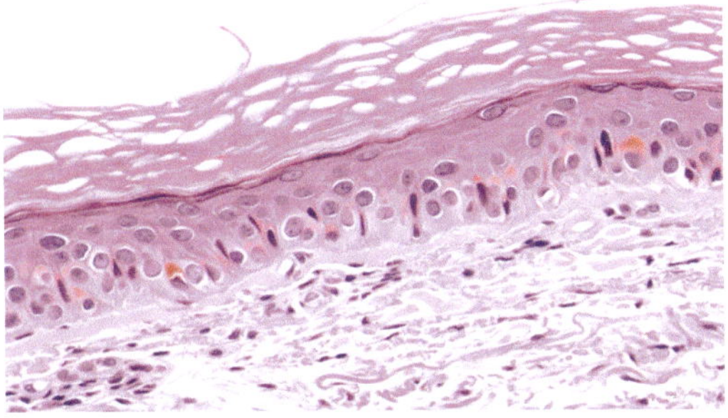

Fig. 1.90 **Pigmented actinic keratosis** with basal layer pigmentation

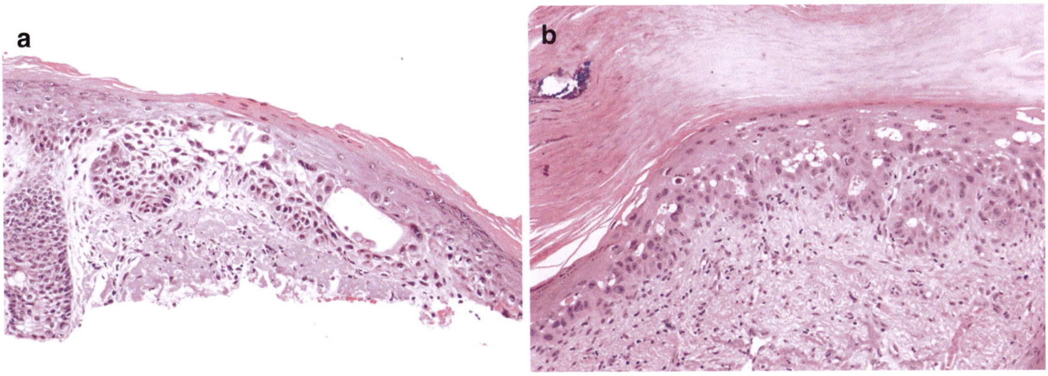

Fig. 1.91 (**a**, **b**) **Acantholytic actinic keratosis** with atypia and separation of keratinocytes in the lower half of the epidermis

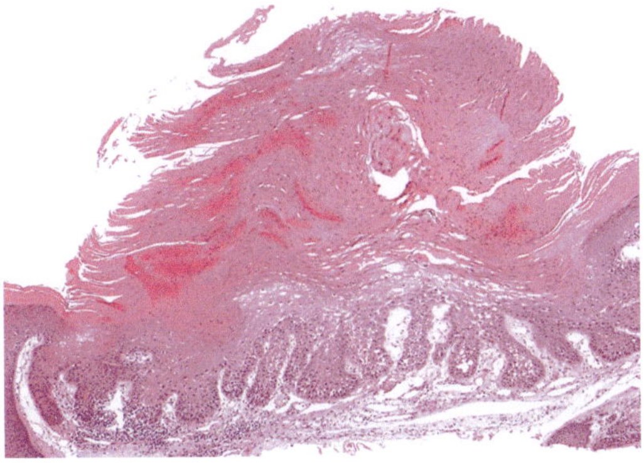

Fig. 1.92 Actinic keratosis with **cutaneous horn**

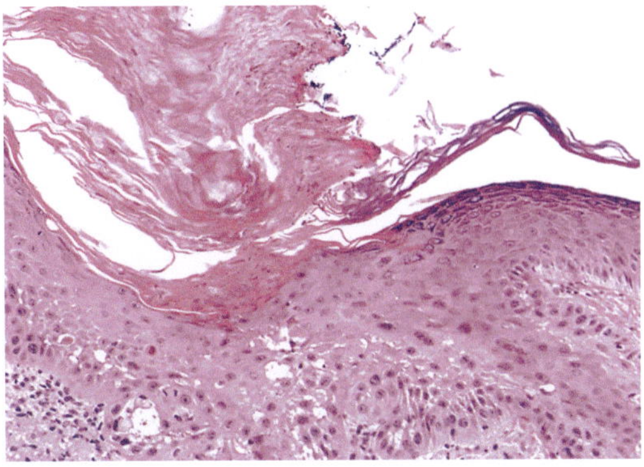

Fig. 1.93 Actinic keratosis with **pseudo-cornoid lamella**

Actinic Prurigo

Histopathology (Figs. 1.94, 1.95, 1.96, 1.97, and 1.98)
Acute: epidermal spongiosis, papillary -dermal edema, and perivascular lymphocytes (*PMLE-like*) (Figs. 1.94, 1.95, and 1.97).
Chronic: hyperkeratosis, acanthosis, papillary dermal fibrosis (*prurigo nodularis-like*) (Figs. 1.96, and 1.98).

– Large lymphoid germinal centers can be seen in lip and conjunctival lesions

P.S. idiopathic familial photodermatosis seen most commonly in American Indians. The histology is nonspecific

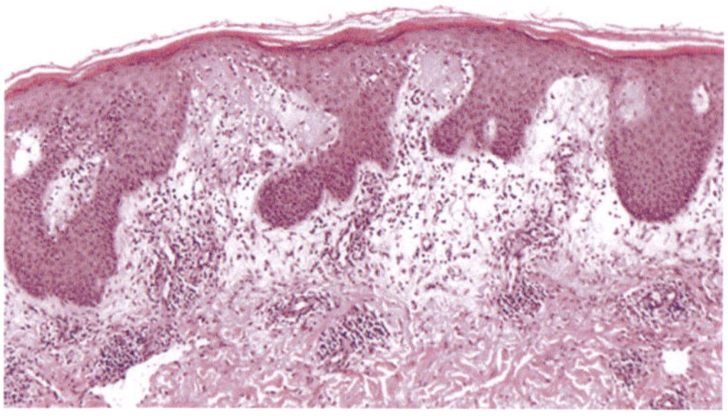

Fig. 1.94 **Acute** actinic prurigo

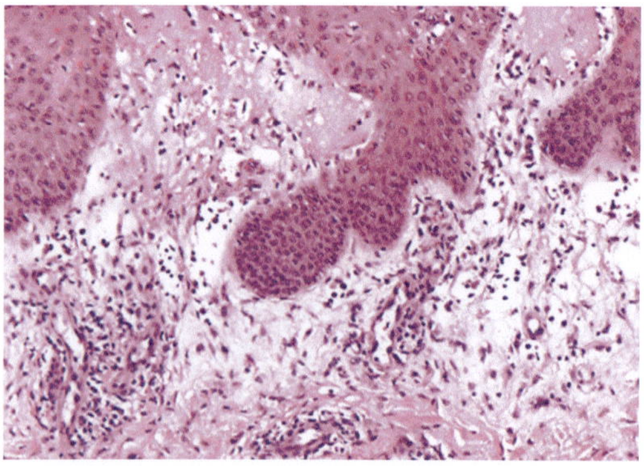

Fig. 1.95 Mild epidermal spongiosis and papillary dermal edema

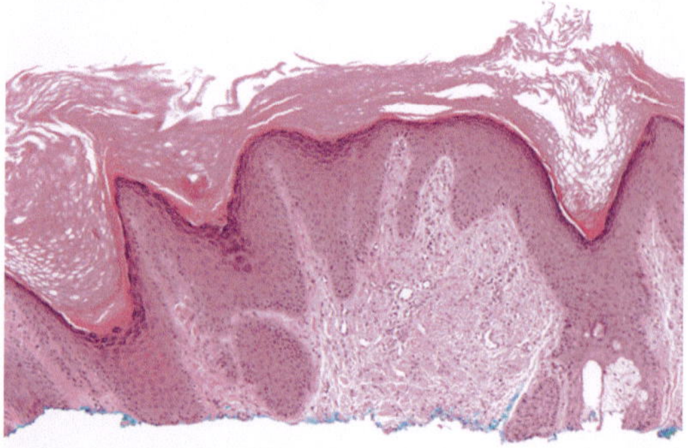

Fig. 1.96 **Chronic** actinic prurigo

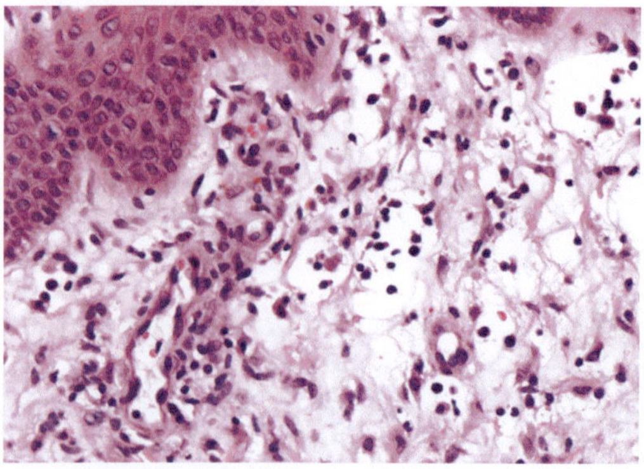

Fig. 1.97 Dermal edema with perivascular lymphocytic infiltrate

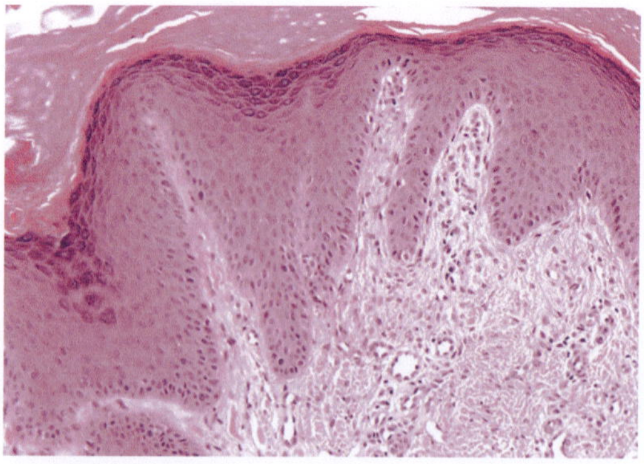

Fig. 1.98 Hyperkeratosis, acanthosis, and dermal fibrosis

Actinic Reticuloid

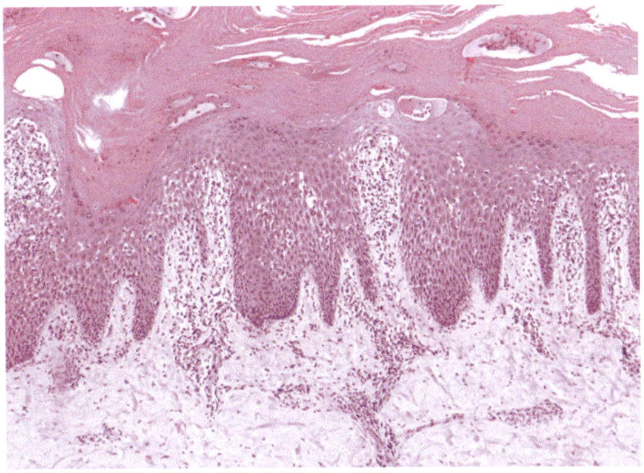

Fig. 1.99 Acanthotic psoriasiform epidermis

Synonym: Chronic Actinic Dermatitis

Histopathology (Figs. 1.99, 1.100, 1.101, 1.102, and 1.103)
- Epidermal psoriasiform acanthosis
- Epidermal exocytosis of lymphocytes
- Chronic dermal lymphocytic infiltrate with mild atypia of lymphocytes
- Papillary dermal fibrosis

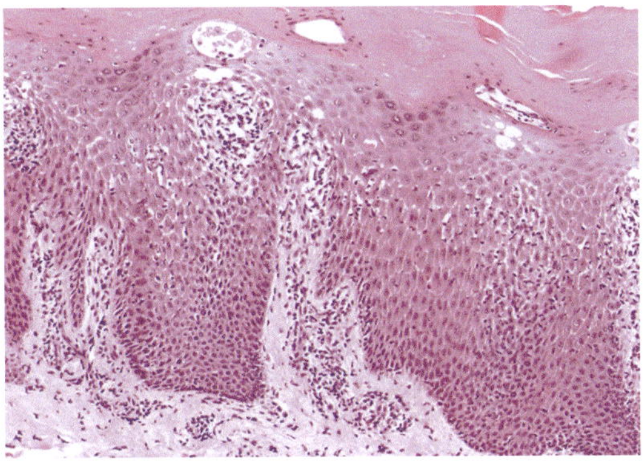

Fig. 1.100 Epidermal lymphocytes are forming aggregates

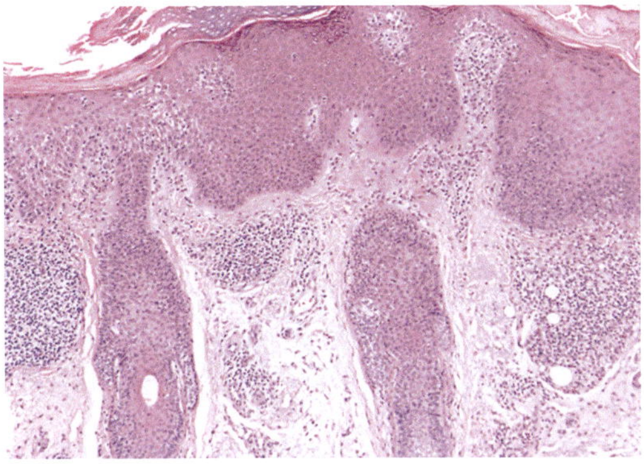

Fig. 1.101 Psoriasiform acanthosis with dermal fibrosis and lymphocytes

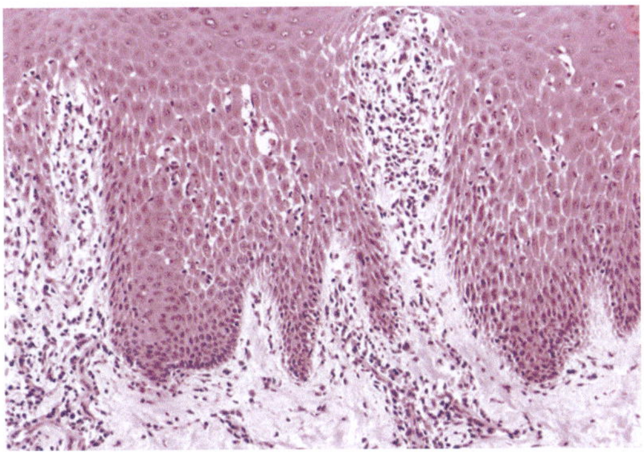

Fig. 1.102 Lymphocytes are present in the epidermis while dermis is fibrotic with atypical lymphocytes

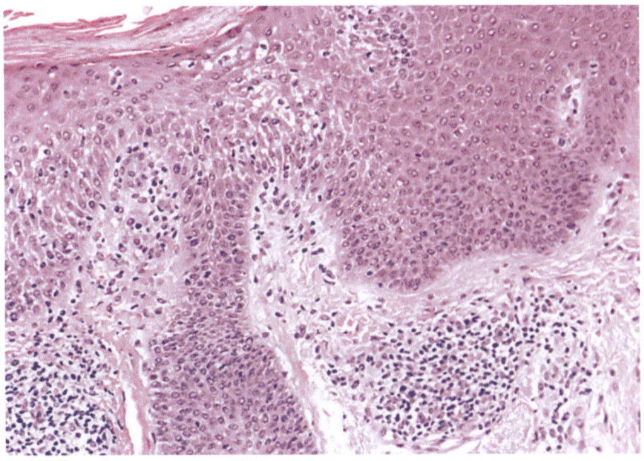

Fig. 1.103 Epidermal lymphocytic exocytosis

Actinomycosis

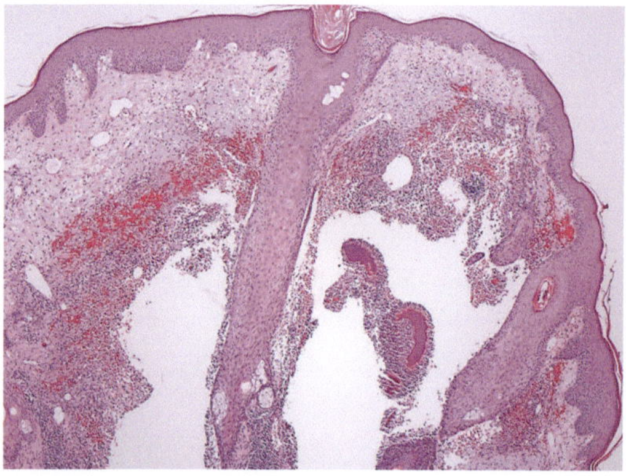

Fig. 1.104 Dermal abscess

Histopathology (Figs. 1.104, 1.105, 1.106, and 1.107)
- Dermal/subcutaneous abscess
- "Sulfur granules" composed of filamentous bacteria
- *Actinomyces israelii* is the most common bacterial species
- Splendore-Hoeppli phenomenon may occur around edge of grains

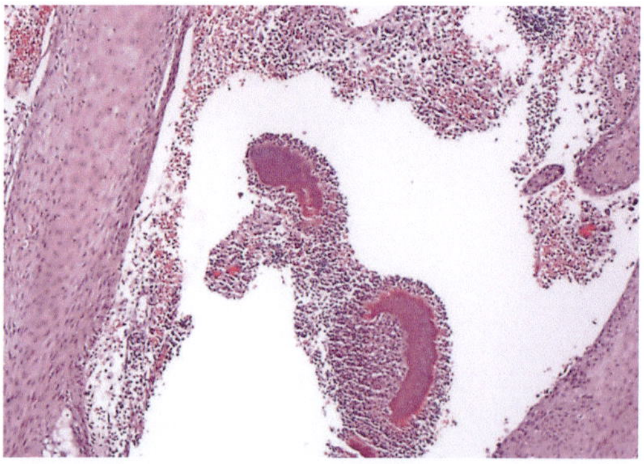

Fig. 1.105 "Sulfur granules" within dermal abscess

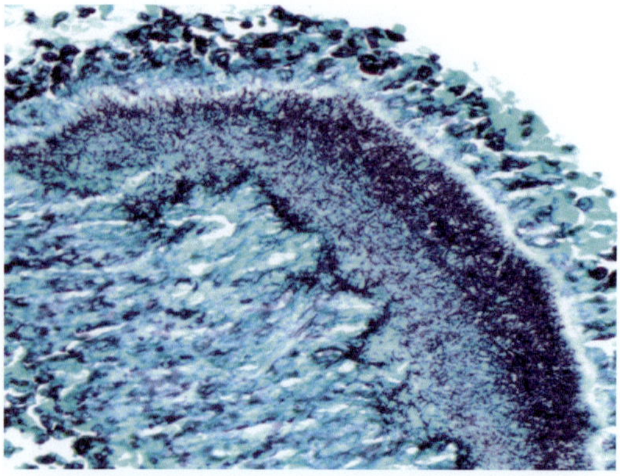

Fig. 1.106 GMS stain outlines filamentous branching organisms

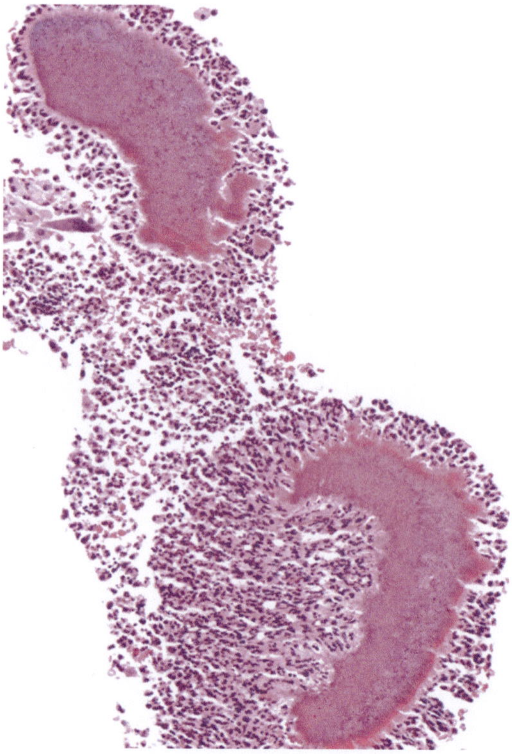

Fig. 1.107 Bacterial colonies in the center of the abscess

Acute Generalized Exanthematous Pustulosis

Synonym: AGEP

Histopathology (Figs. 1.108, 1.109, 1.110, 1.111, and 1.112)

- Epidermal spongiosis with intra- or subcorneal neutrophilic pustule
- Dermal mixed inflammation with neutrophils and occasional eosinophils

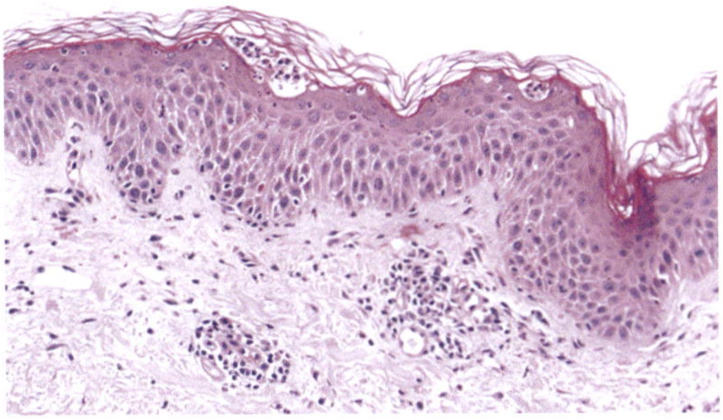

Fig. 1.108 Spongiotic epidermis with pustules

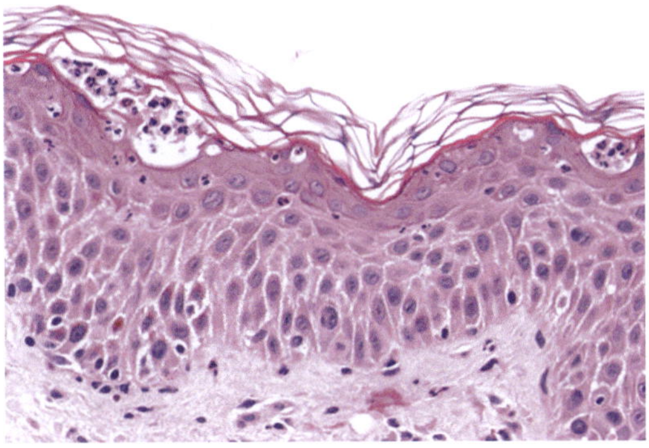

Fig. 1.109 Intracorneal neutrophilic pustules

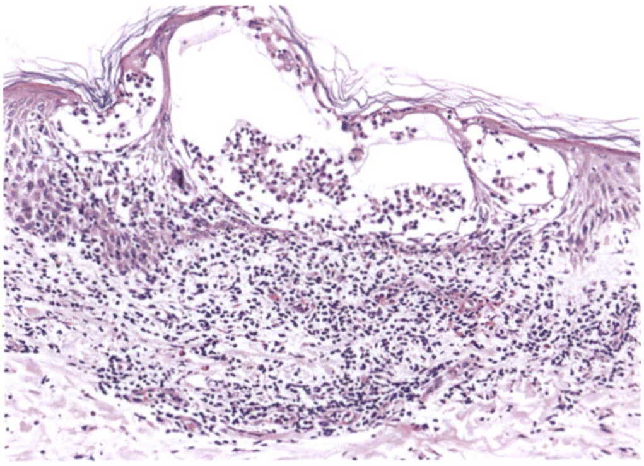

Fig. 1.110 Subcorneal neutrophilic pustule

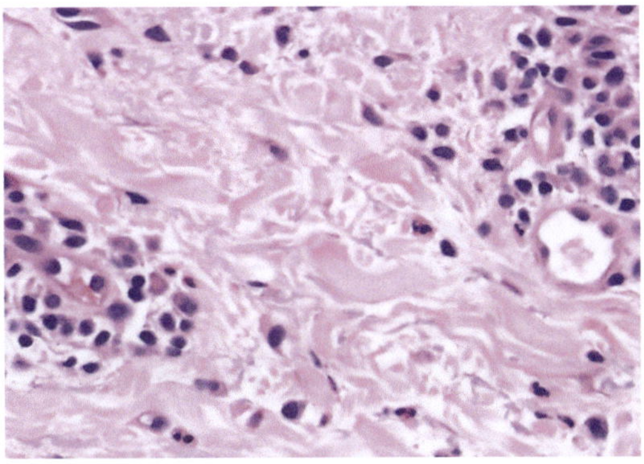

Fig. 1.111 Perivascular lymphocytic infiltrate with scattered neutrophils

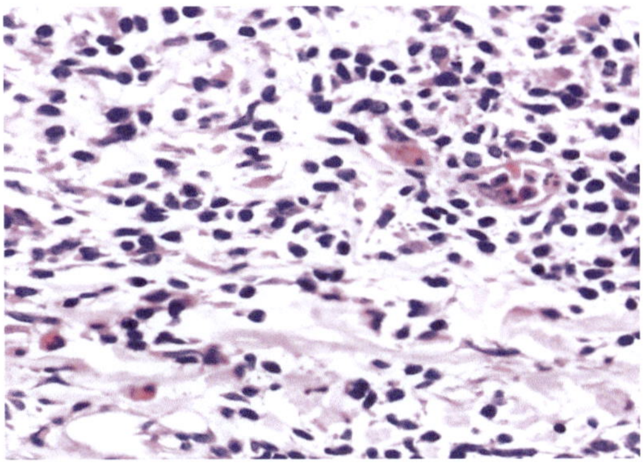

Fig. 1.112 Dermal infiltrate with scattered eosinophils and neutrophils

Acute Lupus Erythematosus

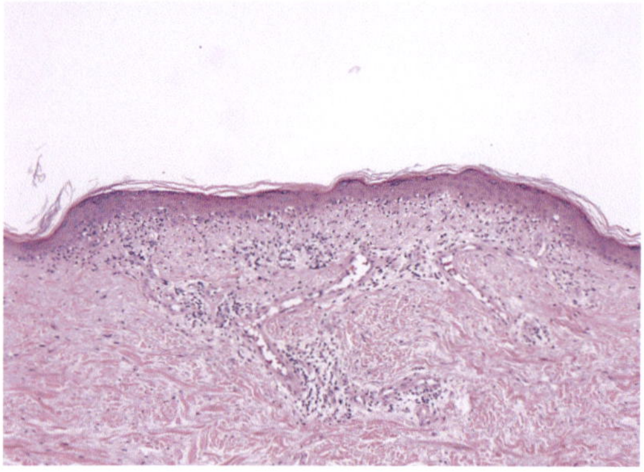

Fig. 1.113 Atrophic epidermis with mild inflammation

Histopathology (Figs. 1.113, 1.114, and 1.115)
- Mildly atrophic epidermis
- Vacuolar interface changes
- Basement membrane thickening
- Mild increase in dermal mucin
- Mild perivascular and interstitial lymphocytic infiltrate

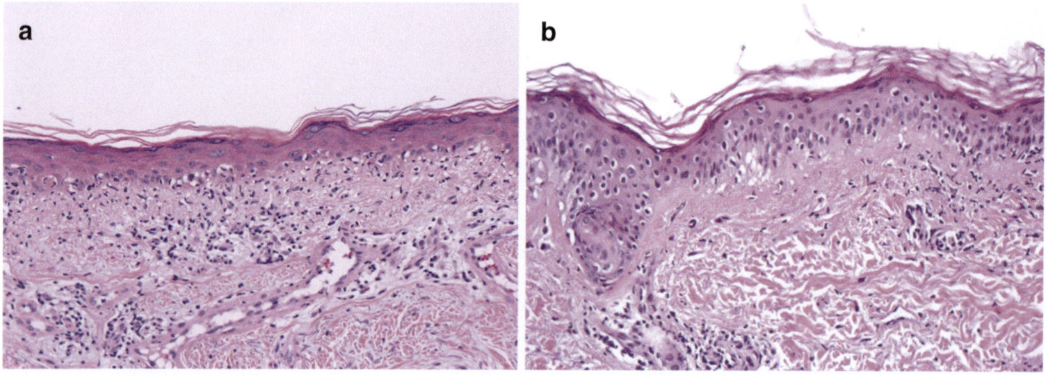

Fig. 1.114 (**a**, **b**) Mild vacuolar interface changes with perivascular and interstitial lymphocytic dermal inflammation

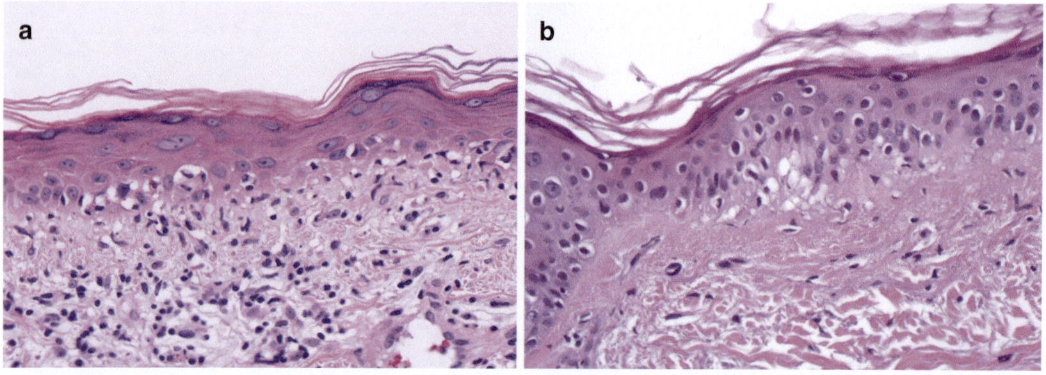

Fig. 1.115 (**a**, **b**) Epidermal atrophy with vacuolar interface dermatitis and mild increase in dermal mucin

Adenoid Cystic Carcinoma

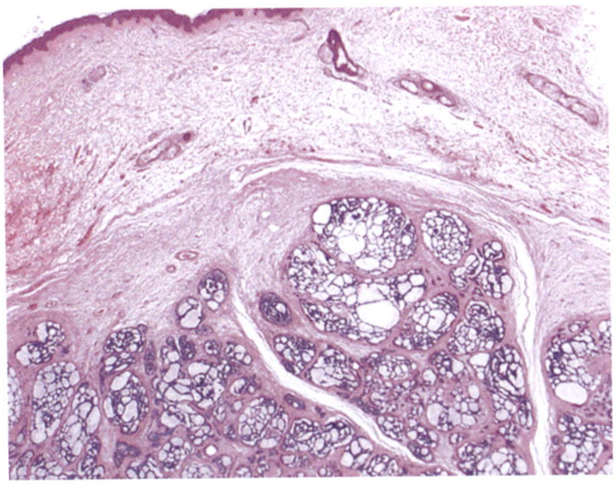

Fig. 1.116 Nodules in the deep dermis and subcutis

Histopathology (Figs. 1.116, 1.117, and 1.118)

- Nodules in the deep dermis and subcutis
- Lack epidermal connection
- Multiple ducts present giving a cribriform appearance
- Small, monotonous appearing blue cells
- Perineural invasion is common
- EMA and CEA confirm ductal lineage and Alcian Blue confirms mucin in lumens

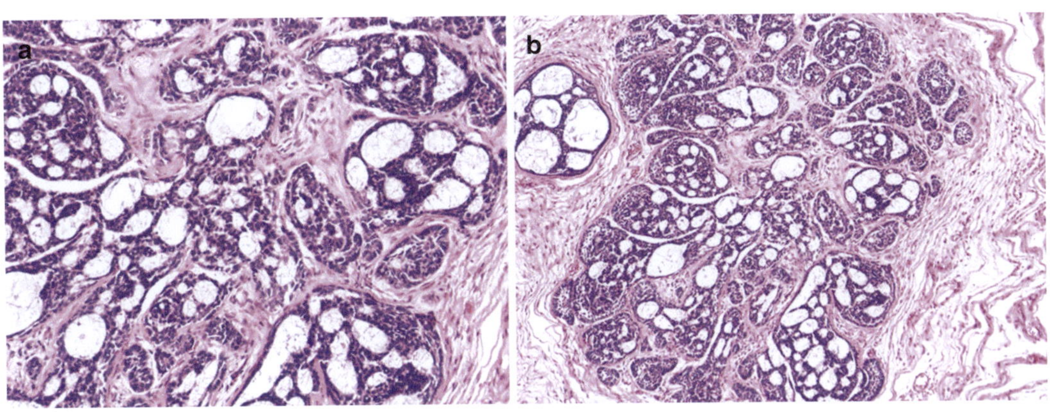

Fig. 1.117 (**a**, **b**) Basaloid nodules with cribriform ductal differentiation

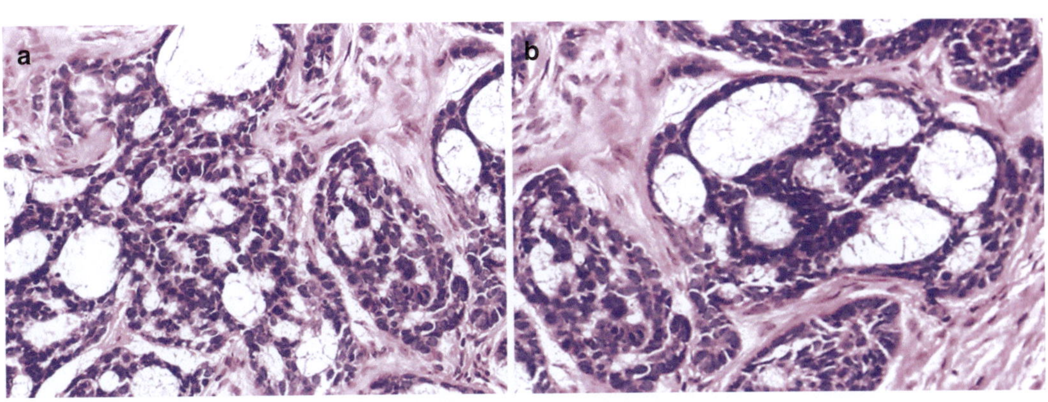

Fig. 1.118 (**a**, **b**) Smudgy, dark, atypical cells lining ductal spaces are filled with mucin

Adult T-Cell Lymphoma/Leukemia

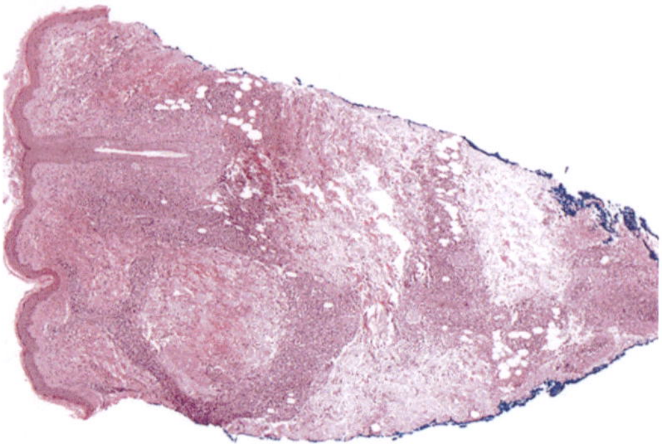

Fig. 1.119 Dermal and subcutaneous lymphocytic infiltrate

Histopathology (Figs. 1.119, 1.120, and 1.121)

- Variable histological patterns including perivascular (most common), nodular, or diffuse with atypical lymphocytes that can range from small, medium, to large
- Epidermotropism with Pautrier microabscesses sometimes present making distinction from mycosis fungoides difficult
- Atypical lymphocytes are typically CD3+, CD4+, CD25+, with positive staining for HTLV-1

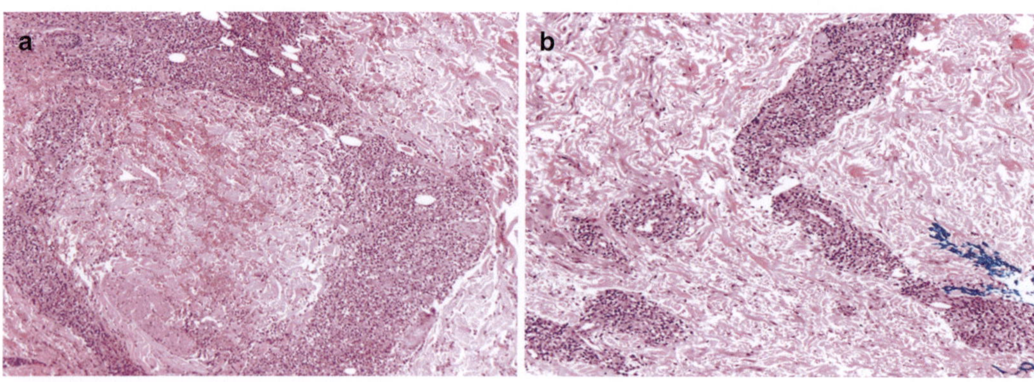

Fig. 1.120 (**a**, **b**) Atypical perivascular infiltrate of lymphocytes

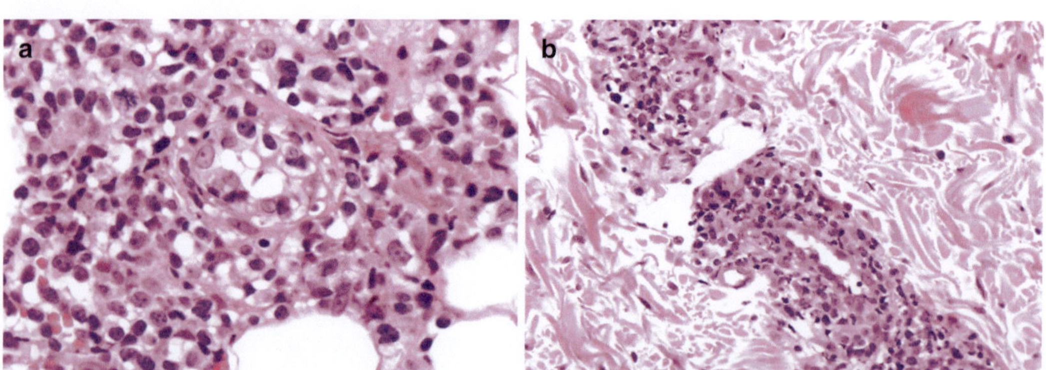

Fig. 1.121 (**a**, **b**) Dense, small to medium sized, perivascular atypical lymphocytes with scattered mitoses

African Tick Bite

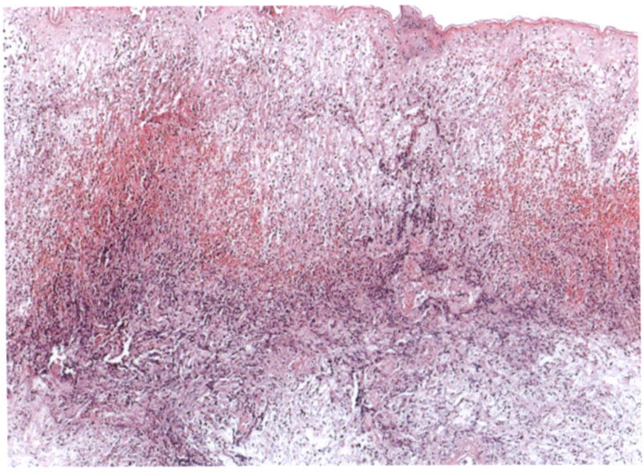

Fig. 1.122 Necrotic hemorrhagic skin

Histopathology (Figs. 1.122, 1.123, 1.124, and 1.125)

- Epidermal and dermal necrosis with extensive acute inflammation
- Necrotizing vasculitis with neutrophils, histiocytes, and lymphocytes
- Fibrin thrombi are commonly seen

P.S caused by *Rickettsia africae* and transmitted by *African tick bite*

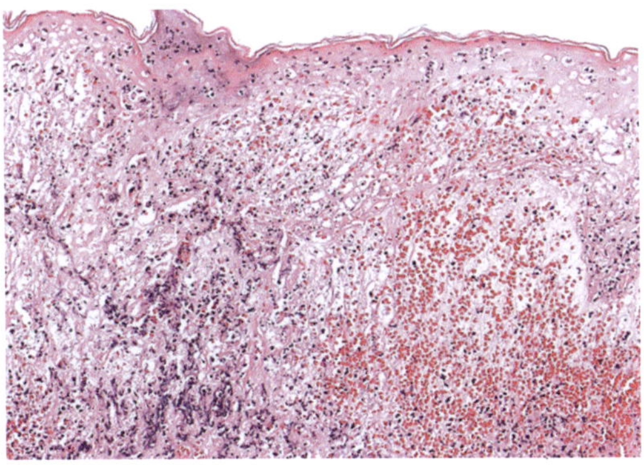

Fig. 1.123 Epidermal and dermal necrosis

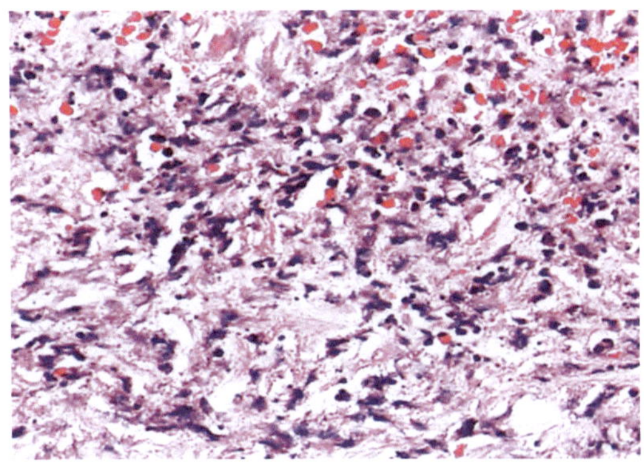

Fig. 1.124 Extensive neutrophilic inflammation

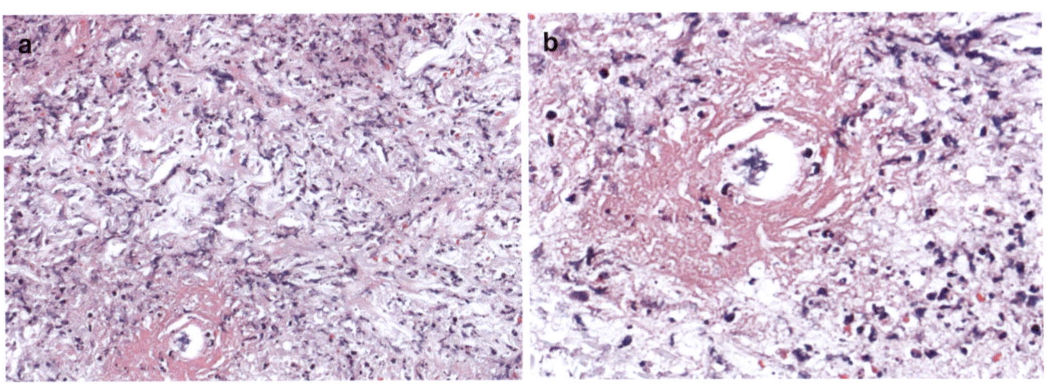

Fig. 1.125 (a, b) Necrotizing vasculitis with fibrinoid degeneration of the vessel wall

Aggressive Digital Papillary Adenocarcinoma

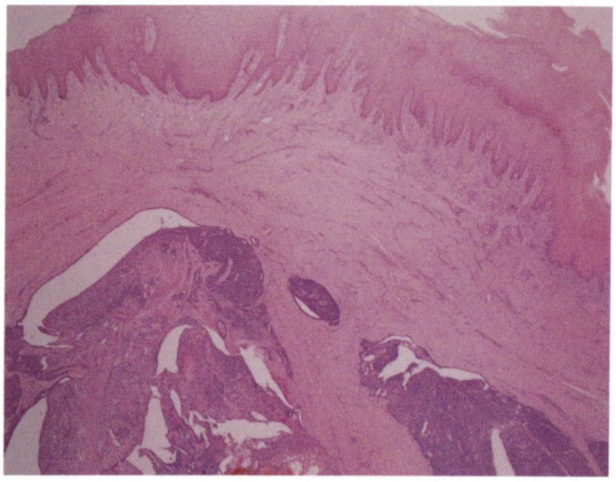

Fig. 1.126 Acral skin with nodulocystic infiltrating tumor

Synonym: Papillary Digital Eccrine Adenocarcinoma

Histopathology (Figs. 1.126, 1.127, 1.128, 1.129, and 1.130)

- Variable histological presentation with dermal nodules with glandular, papillary, tubular, and solid areas
- One to two layers of cuboidal cells with dark vesicular nuclei and eosinophilic cytoplasm are lining papillae/ducts
- Papillae have fibrovascular stroma, vary in size, and show infiltrative growth with common mitoses and necrosis
- Tumor is EMA+ with surrounding p63+ myoepithelial cells

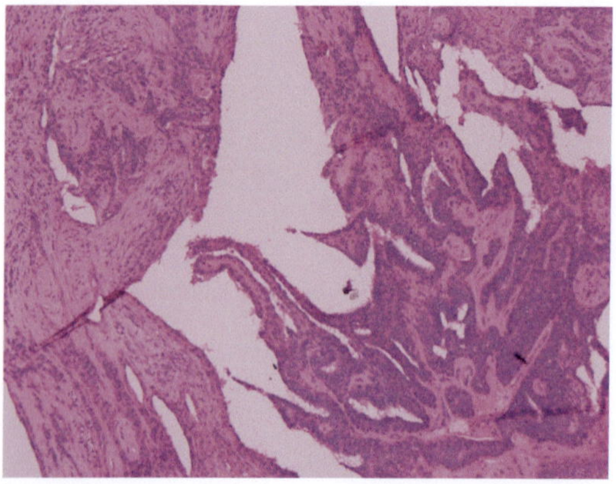

Fig. 1.127 Admixture of tumor papillary and glandular structures

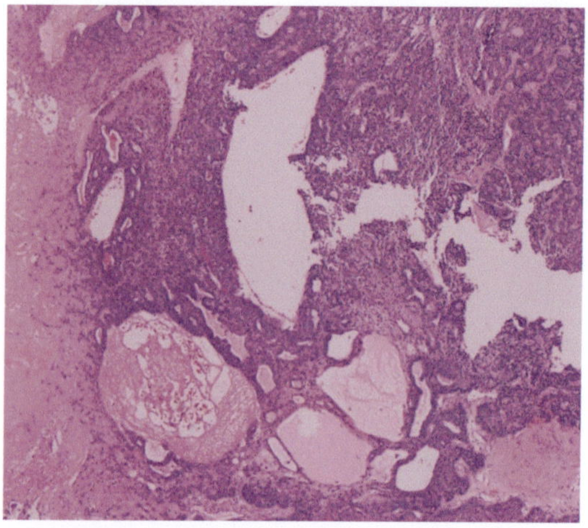

Fig. 1.128 Large areas of necrosis are present

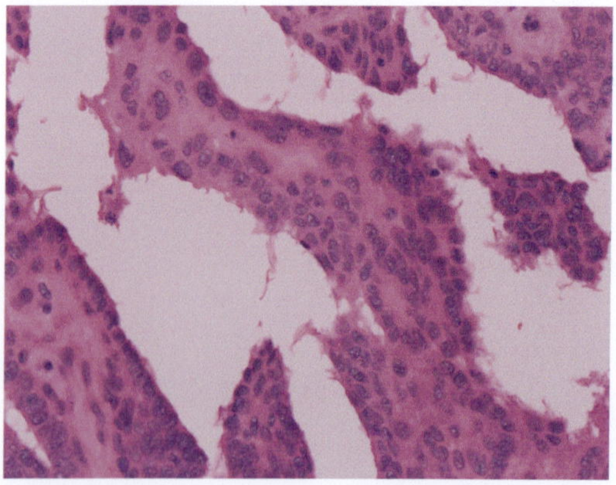

Fig. 1.129 Atypical papillae contain fibrovascular stroma

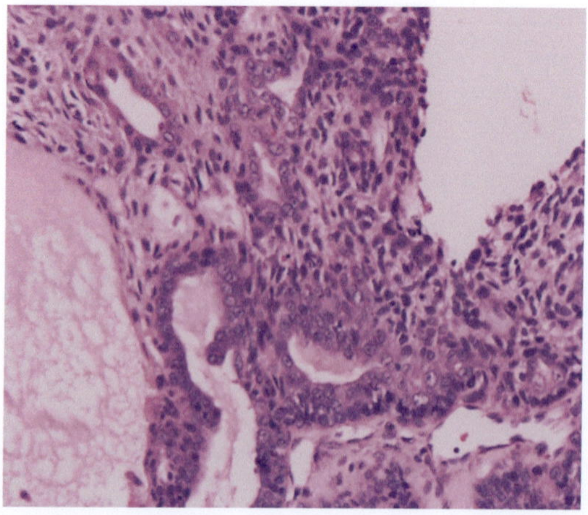

Fig. 1.130 Papillary and ductal structures lined with cytologically atypical cells

Albinism

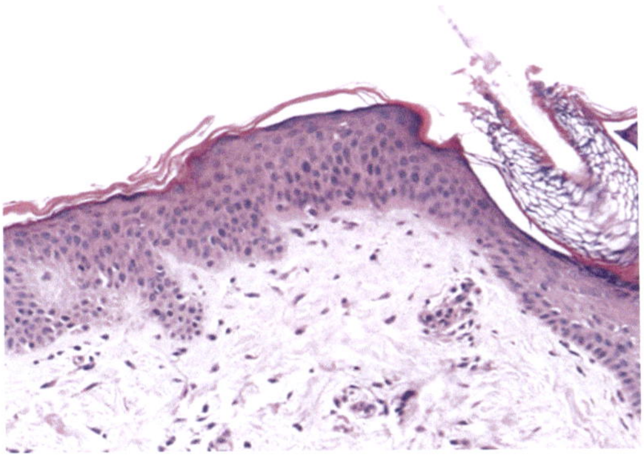

Fig. 1.131 Skin appears normal on H&E slide

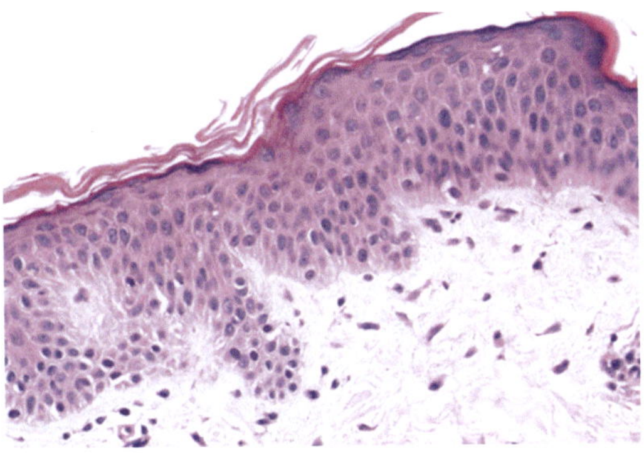

Fig. 1.132 Epidermal melanin is decreased considering that a patient is African American

Histopathology (Figs. 1.131, 1.132, 1.133, and 1.134)

- Normal skin appearance on H&E slides
- Basal layer melanocytes are present in normal number
- Melanin content is decreased or absent

P.S.

- **Progressive Macular Hypomelanosis** has almost identical findings as albinism
- **Chédiak-Higashi syndrome** has same histology as albinism and has additional presence of giant melanosomes
- **Tuberous Sclerosis (Ash-leaf Macules)** has similar findings as albinism but melanin amount is reduced and not completely absent
- **Idiopathic Guttate Hypomelanosis and Hypomelanosis of Ito** has similar findings as albinism but has reduction and not complete absence of both melanocytes and melanin

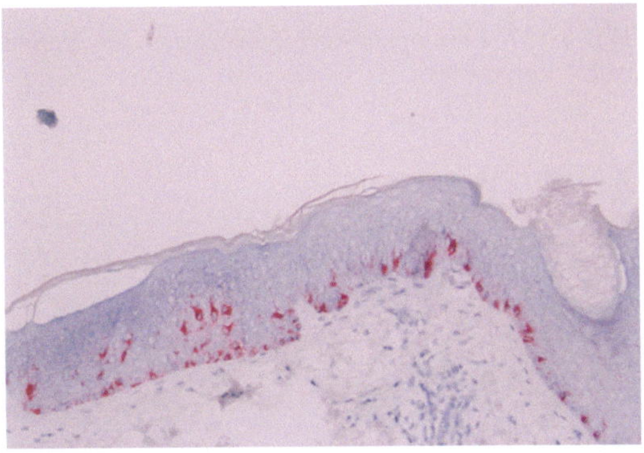

Fig. 1.133 Melan-A stain detects normal number of epidermal melanocytes

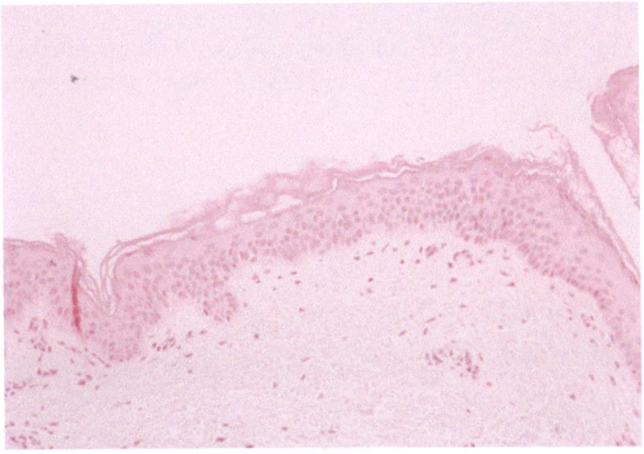

Fig. 1.134 Fontana Masson melanin stain demonstrates an absence of epidermal melanin

Allergic Contact Dermatitis

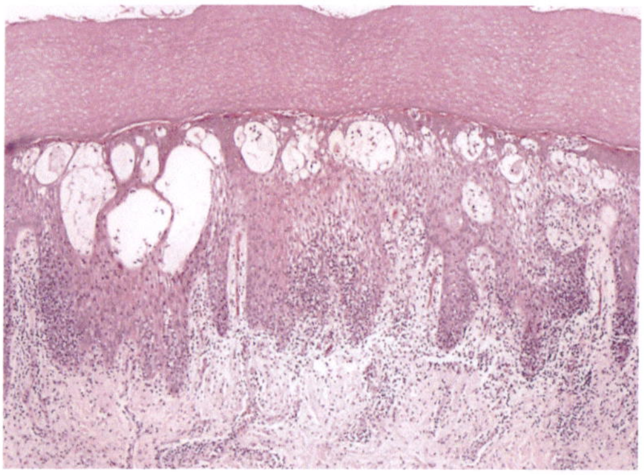

Fig. 1.135 **Acute/subacute** allergic contact dermatitis

Histopathology

Acute—epidermal spongiosis with vesiculation and dermal, perivascular inflammation composed of lymphocytes and eosinophils (Figs. 1.135, 1.136, and 1.137)

Subacute—psoriasiform acanthosis with spongiosis and perivascular lymphocytic inflammation with scattered epidermal eosinophils (Figs. 1.135, 1.136, and 1.137)

Chronic—epidermal acanthosis, hyperkeratosis, and focal parakeratosis. Dermal fibrosis with perivascular lymphocytic infiltrate and occasional eosinophils (Figs. 1.138 and 1.139).

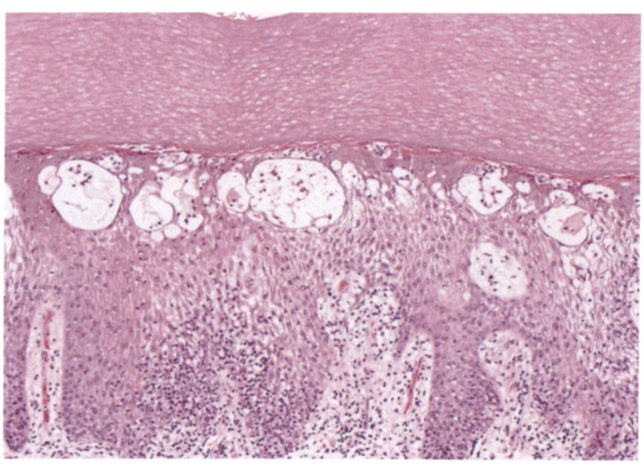

Fig. 1.136 Epidermal spongiosis with intraepidermal vesicles and dermal lymphocytic inflammation with eosinophils

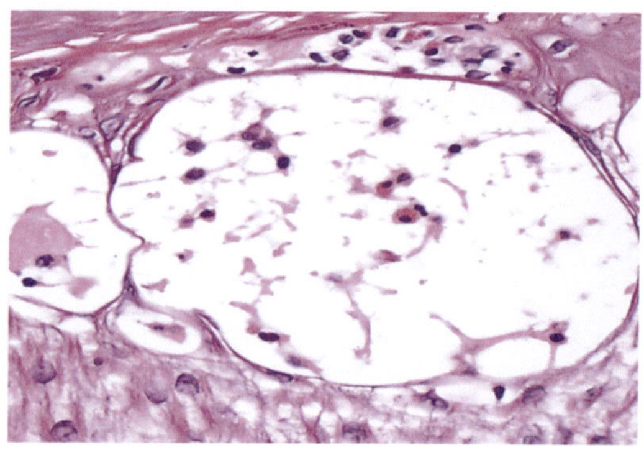

Fig. 1.137 Eosinophils and lymphocytes are present within the vesicles

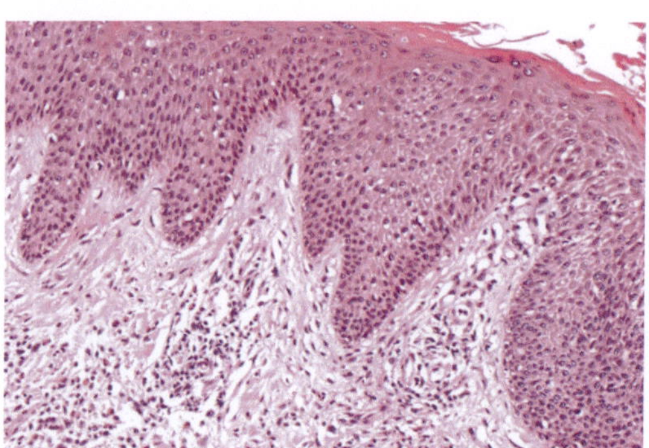

Fig. 1.138 **Chronic** allergic contact dermatitis with acanthosis and hyperkeratosis

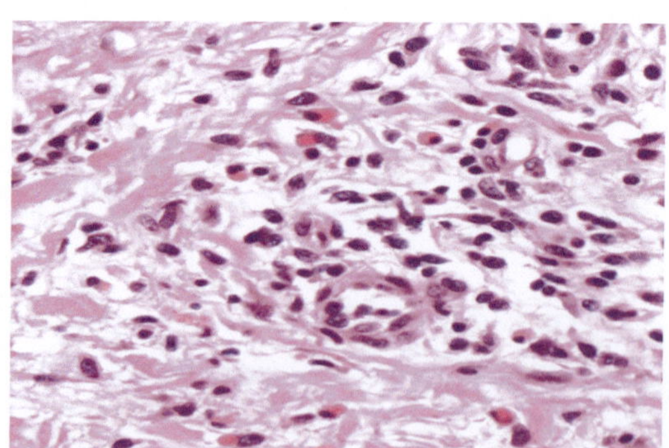

Fig. 1.139 Dermal fibrosis with lymphocytic infiltrate and eosinophils

Alopecia Areata

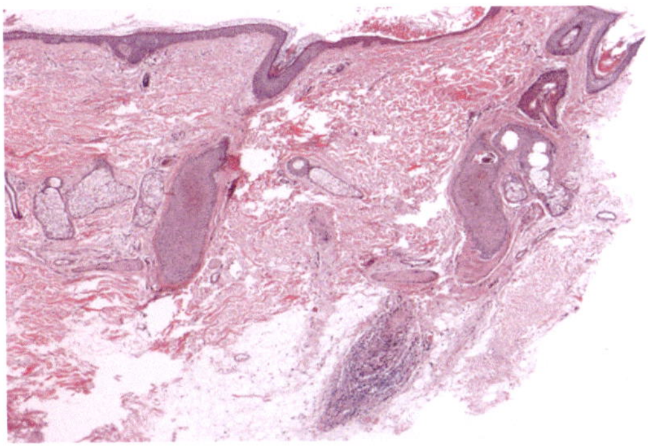

Fig. 1.140 Decreased number of anagen hair

Histopathology (Figs. 1.140, 1.141, 1.142, and 1.143)

- Decreased anagen to catagen/telogen ratio
- Lymphocytic, perifollicular infiltrate around hair bulb
- Fibrous tracts formation and pigment incontinence sometimes but scarring is absent

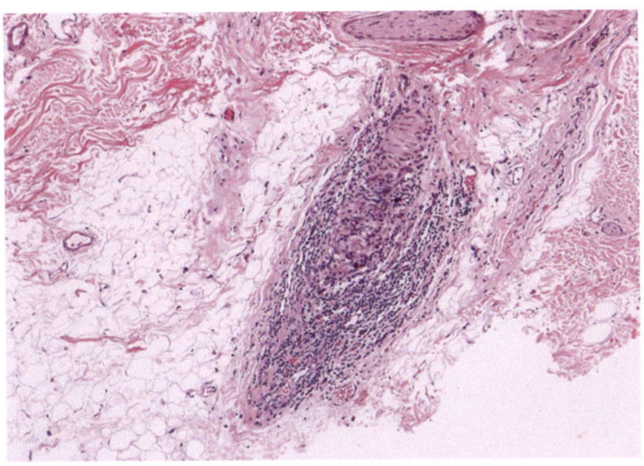

Fig. 1.141 Peribulbar lymphocytic inflammation

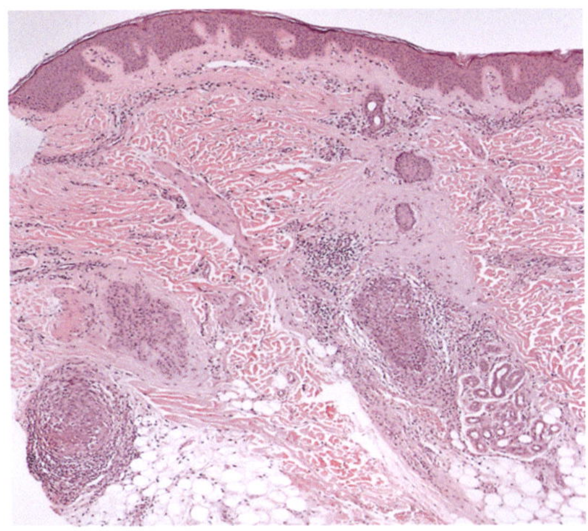

Fig. 1.142 Fibrous stellae are seen

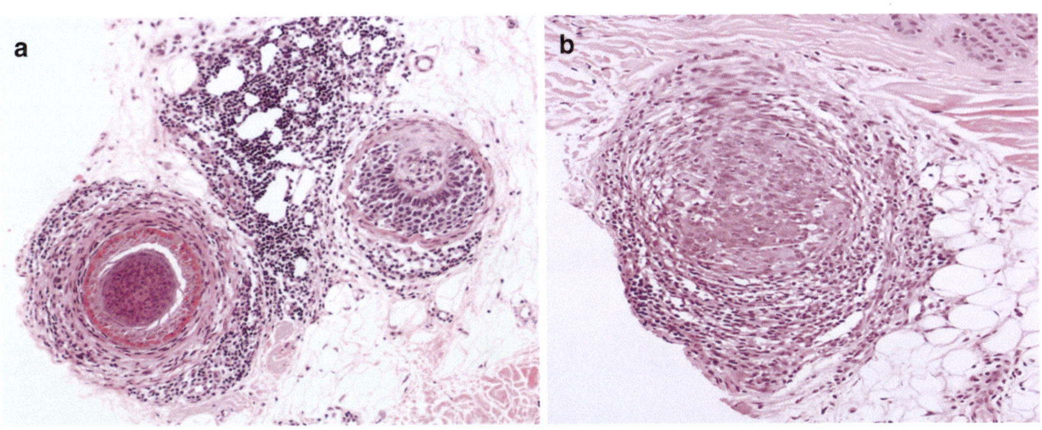

Fig. 1.143 Horizontal (**a**) and vertical (**b**) sections with lymphocytic, perifollicular inflammation of lower segment and hair bulb

Alpha-1 Antitrypsin Panniculitis

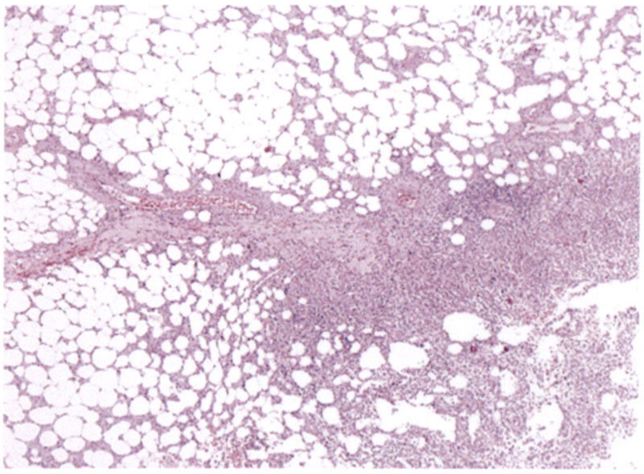

Fig. 1.144 Predominantly septal panniculitis with spill into lobules

Synonym: Alpha-1 Antitrypsin Deficiency Associated Panniculitis

Histopathology (Figs. 1.144, 1.145, 1.146, 1.147, and 1.148)

- Focal acute septal or mixed septal/lobular panniculitis that is primary neutrophilic
- Necrosis and septal hemorrhage common
- Infiltrate starts in septae and spill into lobules

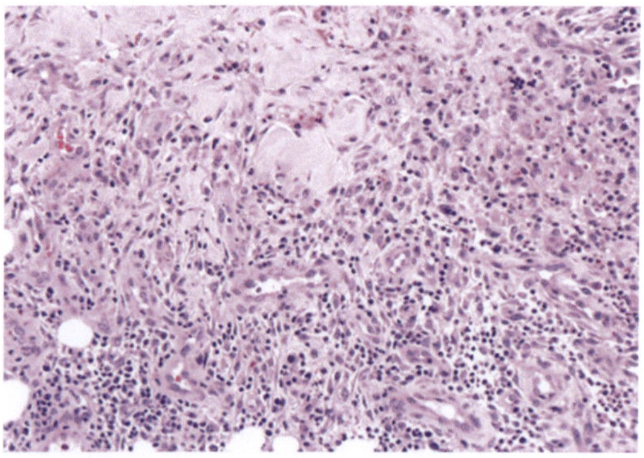

Fig. 1.145 Septal neutrophilic panniculitis

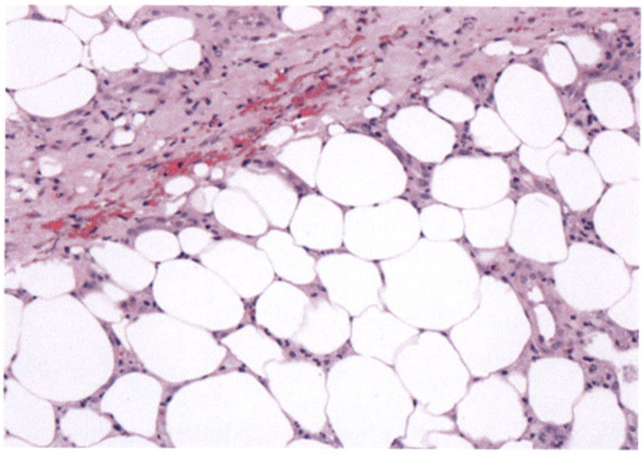

Fig. 1.146 Septal hemorrhage

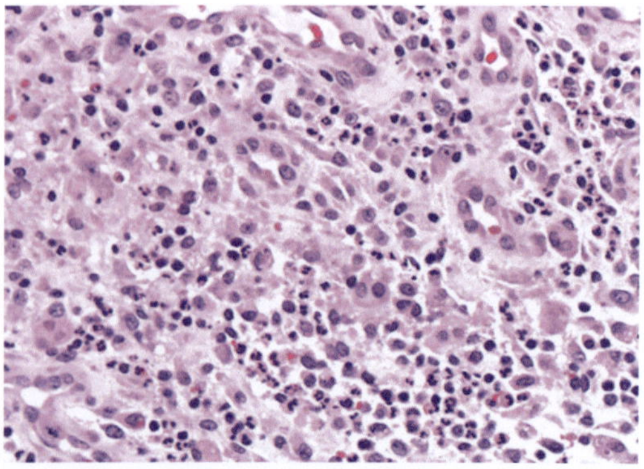

Fig. 1.147 Dense neutrophilic infiltrate with focal necrosis

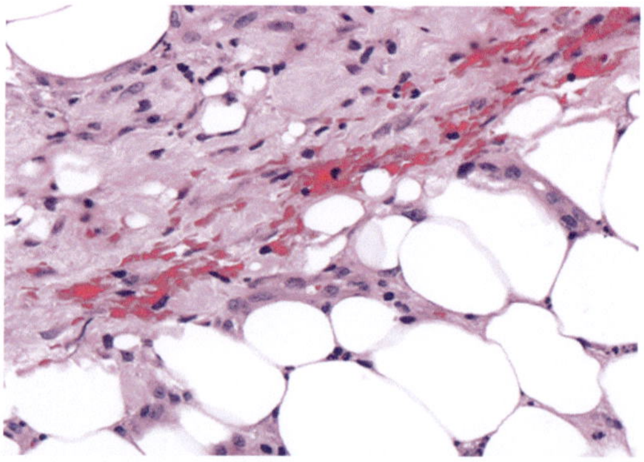

Fig. 1.148 Septal inflammation extending into lobule

Alternariosis

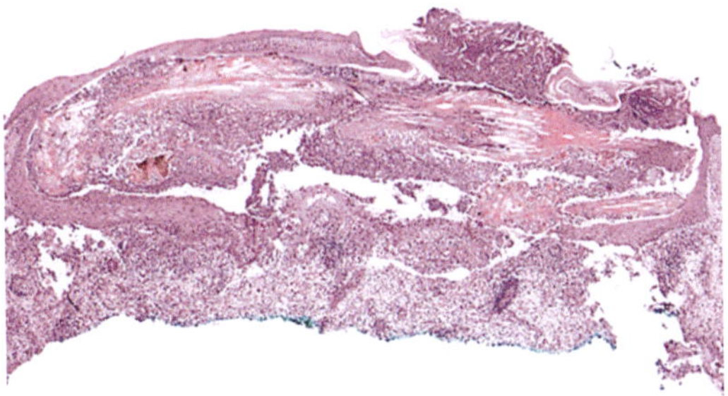

Fig. 1.149 Skin with foreign body and inflammation

Alternaria is a saprophytic fungus that is primary plant pathogens and therefore are usually associated with plant foreign body (splinter).

Histopathology (Figs. 1.149, 1.150, 1.151, 1.152, and 1.153)

- Acute inflammation and foreign body giant cell reaction to plant splinter
- Pigmented spores and branching, septate hyphae
- Spores with a double contour and often in clusters

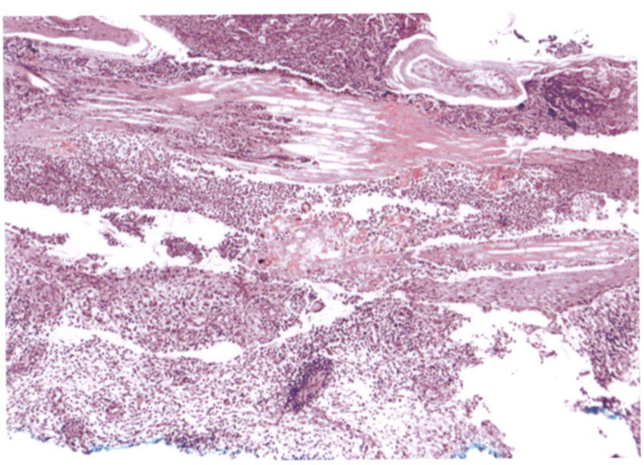

Fig. 1.150 Plant material with exuberant acute inflammation

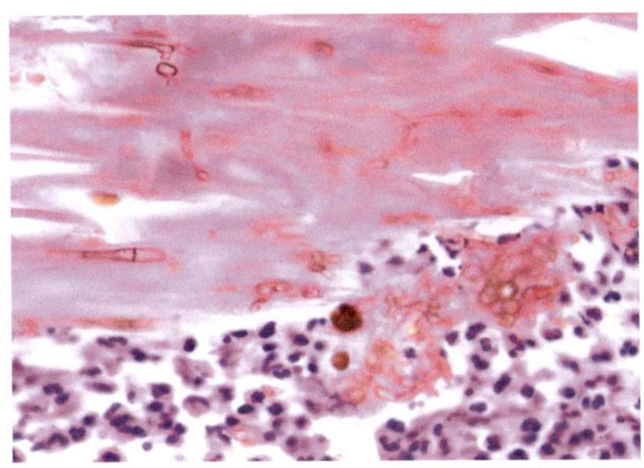

Fig. 1.151 Pigmented, branching, septate hyphae with spores

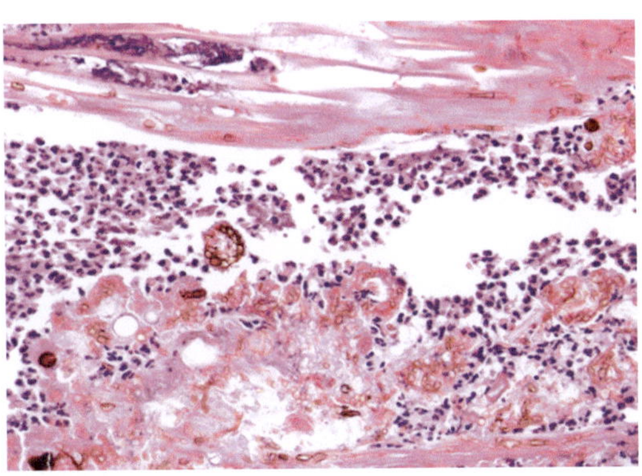

Fig. 1.152 Splinter with acute inflammation and pigmented fungi

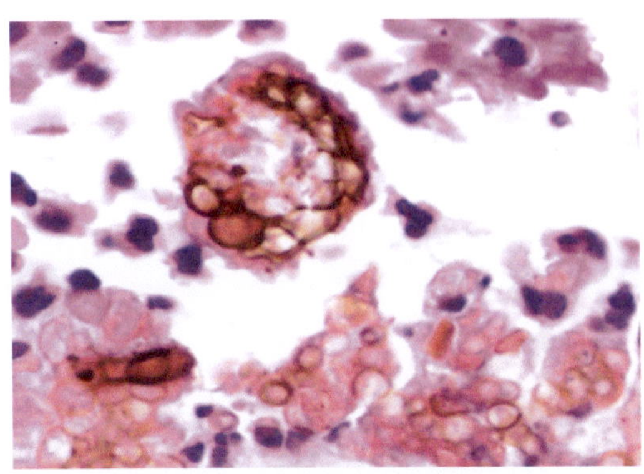

Fig. 1.153 Clustered, pigmented, double walled spores

Amalgam Tattoo

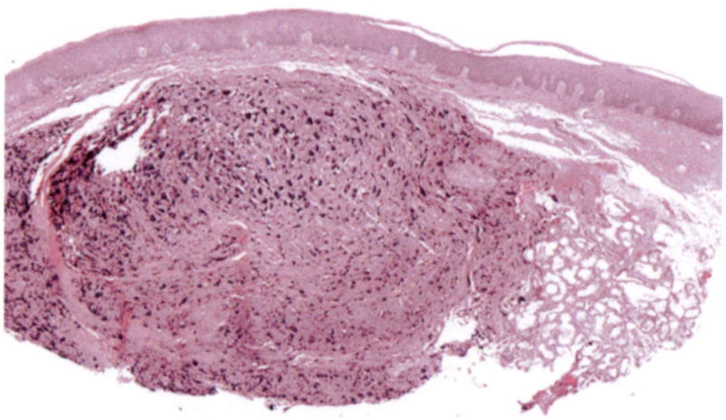

Fig. 1.154 Oral mucosa with submucosal pigmented nodule

Histopathology (Figs. 1.154, 1.155, 1.156, 1.157, and 1.158)

- Oral mucosa with submucosal dark pigment
- Amalgam usually surrounded by dense fibrous tissue
- Minimal to mild lymphocytic inflammation
- Occasional foreign body giant cell reaction
- Adjacent salivary glands usually present

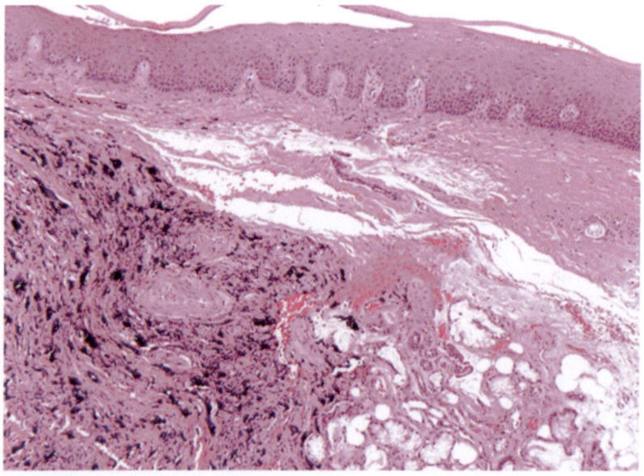

Fig. 1.155 Dense fibrous tissue with dark pigment

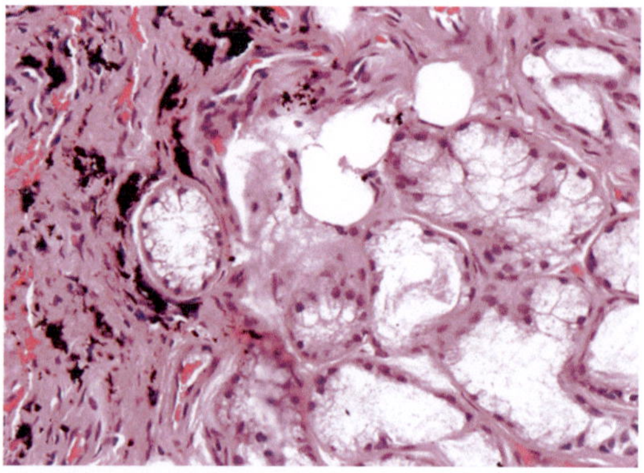

Fig. 1.156 Dark pigment adjacent to salivary gland

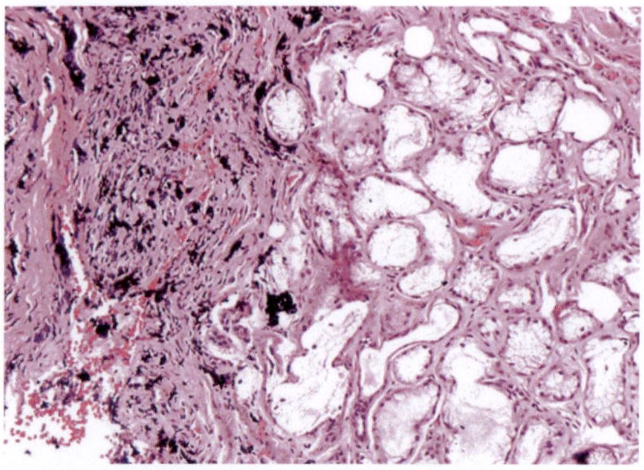

Fig. 1.157 Fibrous tissue surrounds amalgam

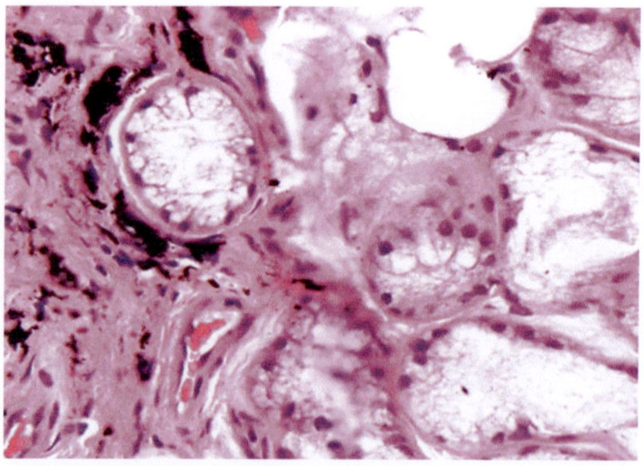

Fig. 1.158 Minimal inflammation

Ameloblastoma

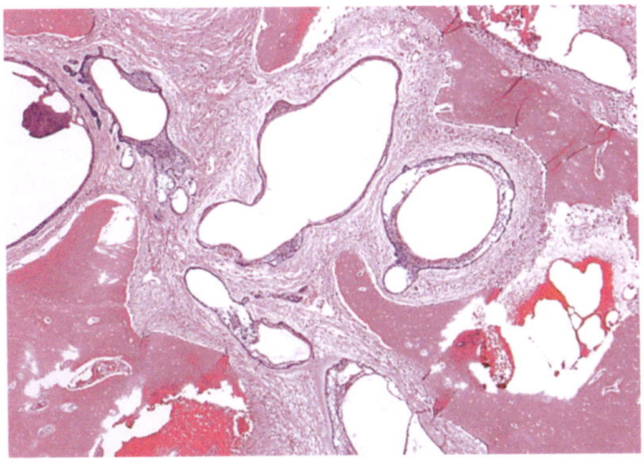

Fig. 1.159 Cystic, basaloid tumor invading bone

Histopathology (Figs. 1.159, 1.160, 1.161, 1.162, and 1.163)

- Nodules of odontogenic tumor composed of central, pale cells and peripheral, palisaded, basaloid cells with minimal to severe atypia
- Cystic and "jigsaw puzzle" appearance with bone invasion is common
- Resembles basal cell carcinoma but lacks myxoid stroma and retraction
- BRAF, RAS, SMO and FGFR2 mutations in 88% of cases

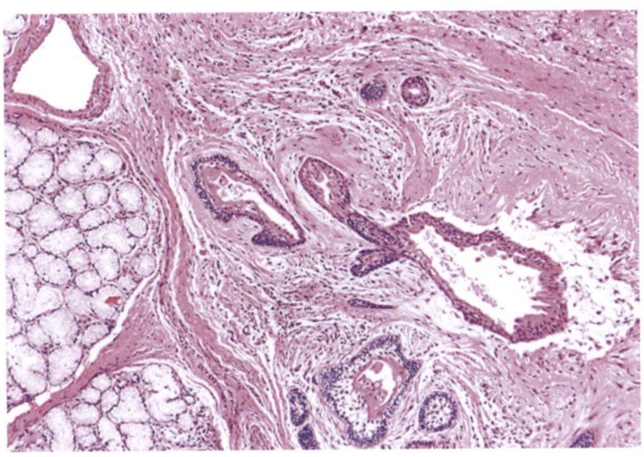

Fig. 1.160 Basaloid tumor with peripheral dark and central pale cells

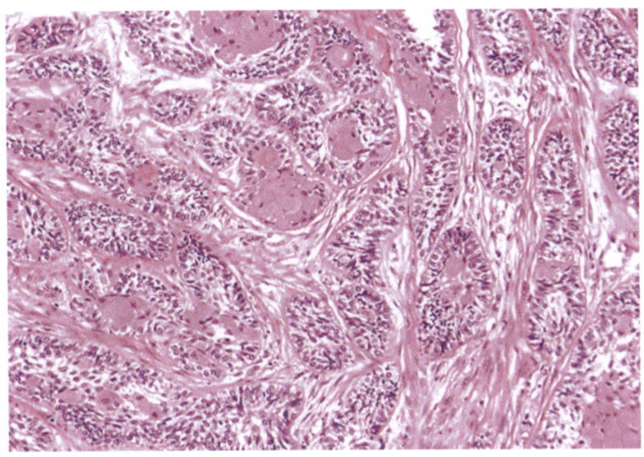

Fig. 1.161 Tumor islands organized in "jigsaw puzzle" pattern

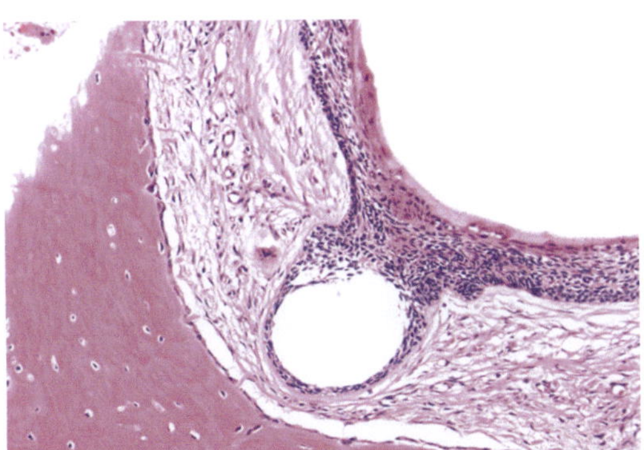

Fig. 1.162 Bone (left) and tumor cells (right) with peripheral palisading, fibrotic stroma and no retraction

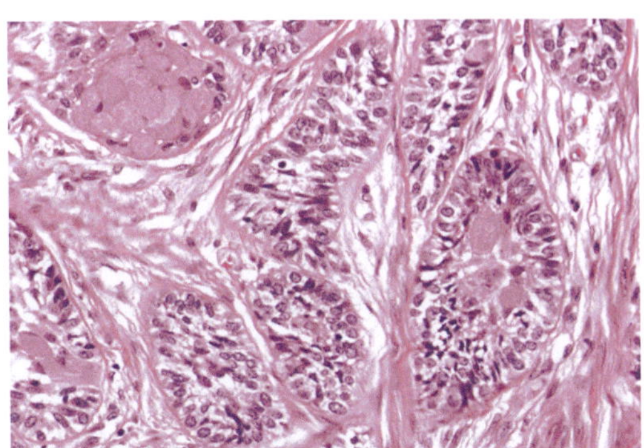

Fig. 1.163 Peripheral palisading but no stromal retraction. Central cells demonstrate squamous metaplasia

Amyloidosis

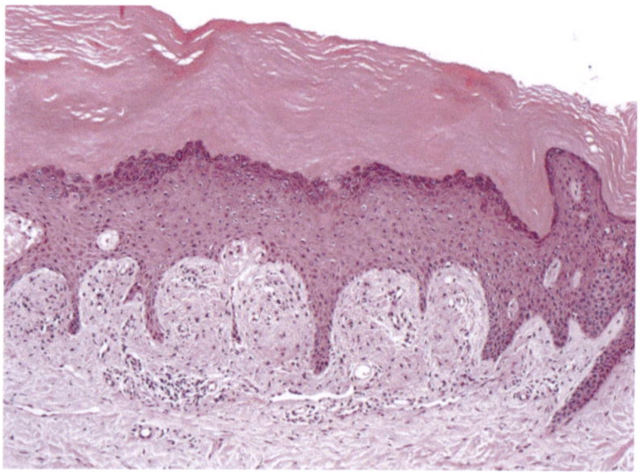

Fig. 1.164 **Lichen amyloidosis** with hypertrophic acanthotic epidermis and dermal amyloid

Histopathology of amyloidosis (Congo red, crystal violet, thioflavine T, scarlet red, pagoda red +):

Lichen amyloidosis (Figs. 1.164, 1.165, and 1.166)

- Usually pretibial lesion with hypertrophic epidermis with eosinophilic, faceted amyloid deposits in the papillary dermis. Pigment incontinence is commonly present.

Macular amyloidosis

- Usually back lesion with normal epidermis and scant globular deposits of amyloid in the papillary dermis with common pigment incontinence

Nodular/plaque amyloidosis (Figs. 1.167 and 1.168)

- Large mass of amyloid in the dermis and subcutis

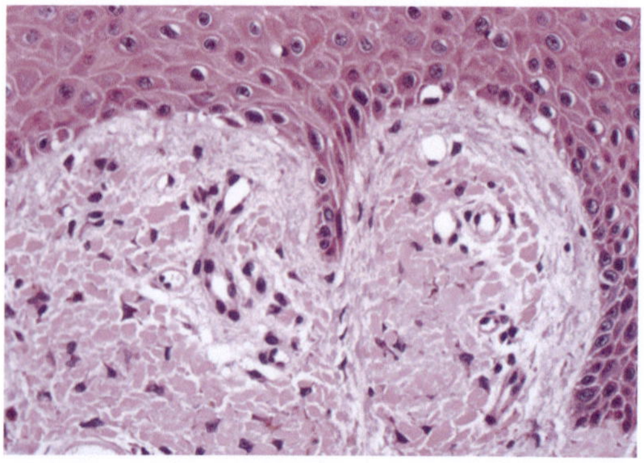

Fig. 1.165 Amyloid deposition in the papillary dermis

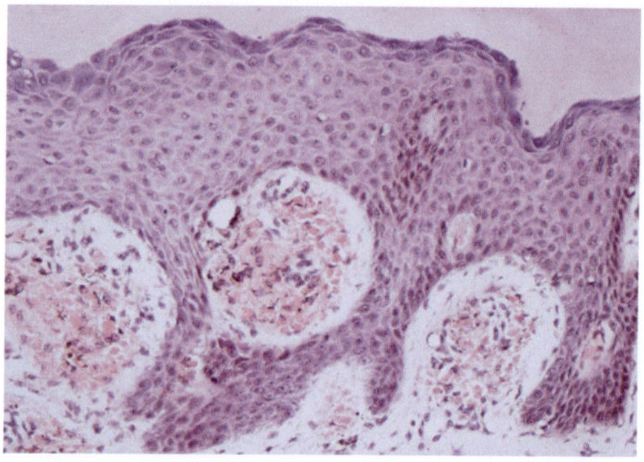

Fig. 1.166 Congo Red staining of lichen amyloidosis

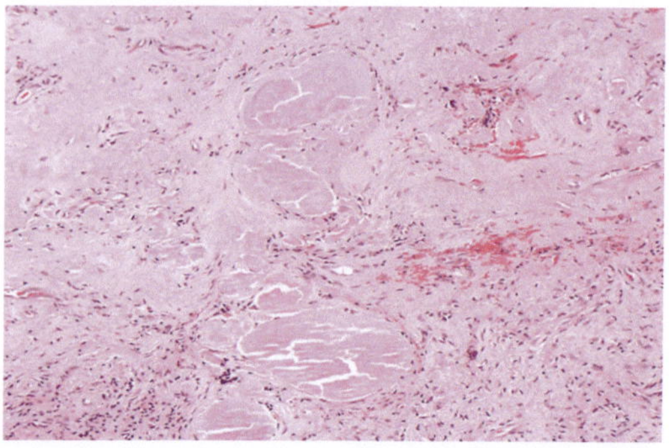

Fig. 1.167 **Nodular amyloidosis** with large amyloid deposits

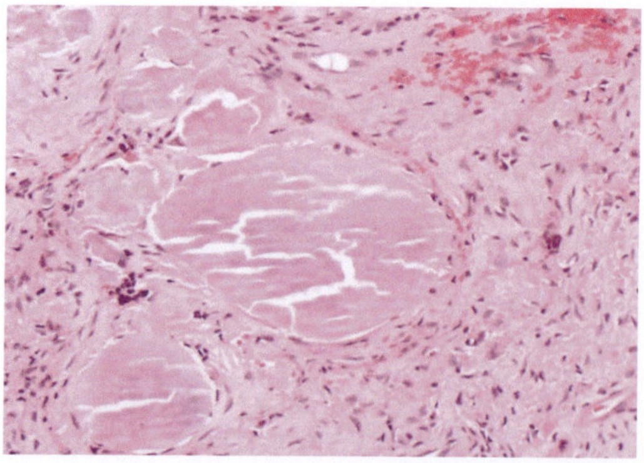

Fig. 1.168 Amyloid deposits surrounded by fibrous stroma

Androgenic Alopecia

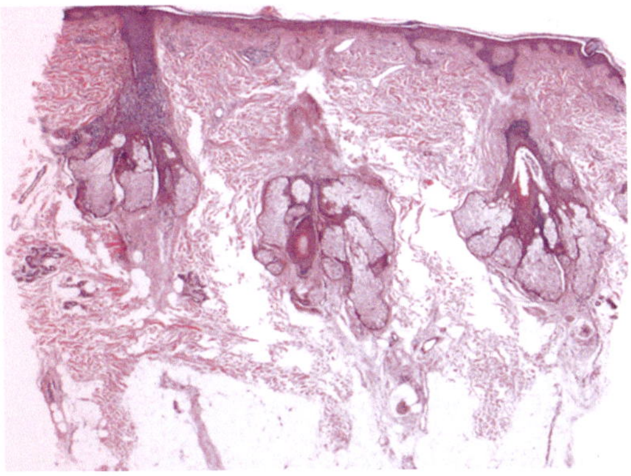

Fig. 1.169 Multiple vellus hairs with no terminal hairs

Histopathology (Figs. 1.169, 1.170, 1.171, and 1.172)

- Decreased ratio of terminal to vellus hair
- Miniaturized hair follicles
- Retention of normal sebaceous glands giving appearance of hyperplasia
- Increased number of follicular fibrous tracts

P.S. these biopsies were taken from author's own bald spot by a brave dermatology resident

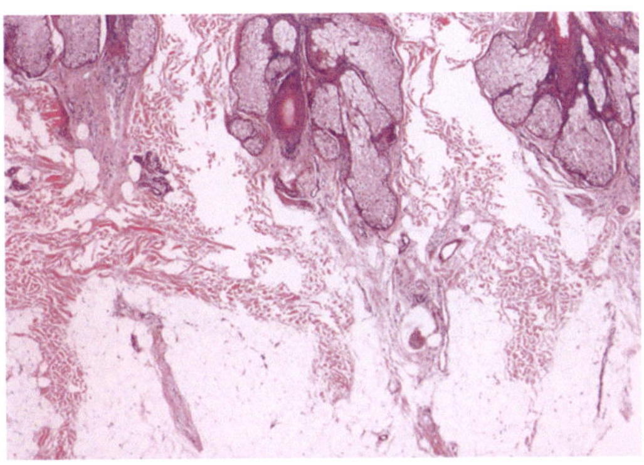

Fig. 1.170 Prominent sebaceous glands without terminal hairs

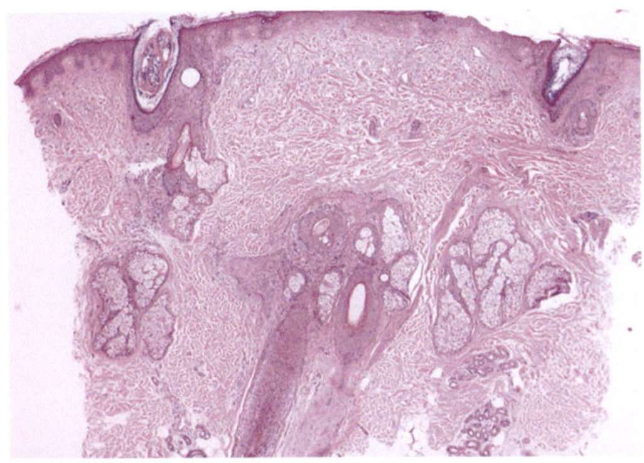

Fig. 1.171 Few terminal hairs with reduced ratio when compared to vellus hair

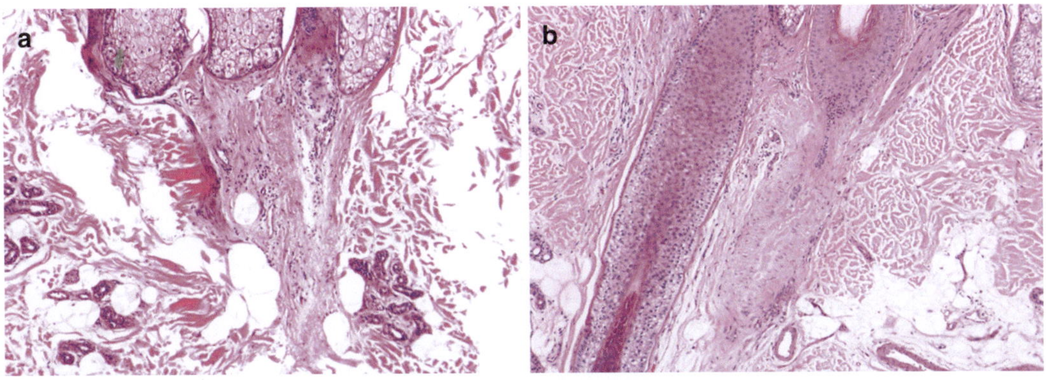

Fig. 1.172 (**a**, **b**) Fibrous stelae (streamers) extends below miniaturized hair follicles

Anetoderma

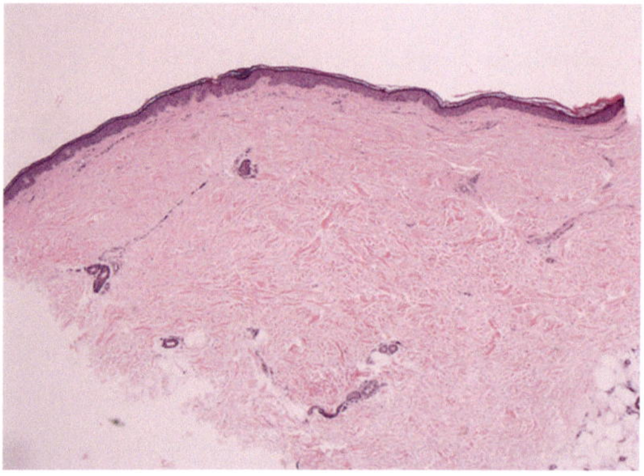

Fig. 1.173 "Normal" appearing skin

Synonym: Macular Atrophy

Histopathology is very subtle and clinical correlation is necessary:

Early lesion:

- Mild nonspecific lymphoplasmocytic, perivascular infiltrate

Established lesion:

- Normal appearing skin with minimal inflammation on H&E, but decreased or absent elastic fibers with elastic stain (Figs. 1.173, 1.174, 1.175, and 1.176)

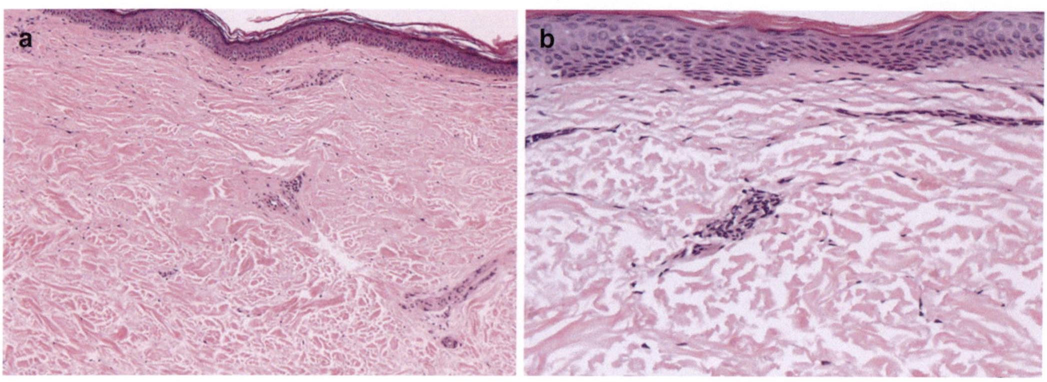

Fig. 1.174 (**a**, **b**) Focal, mild, perivascular infiltrate

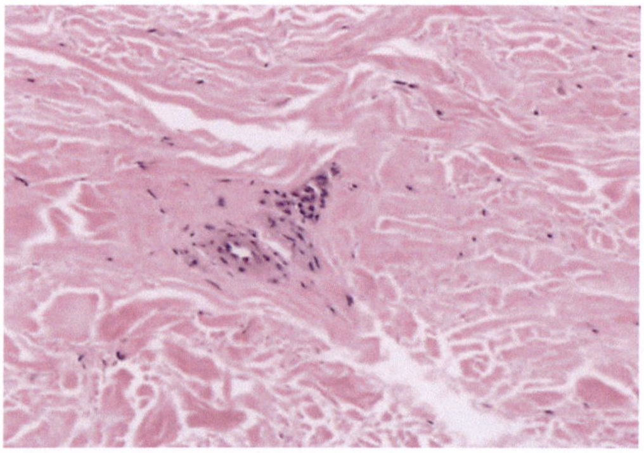

Fig. 1.175 Lymphoplasmocytic perivascular inflammation

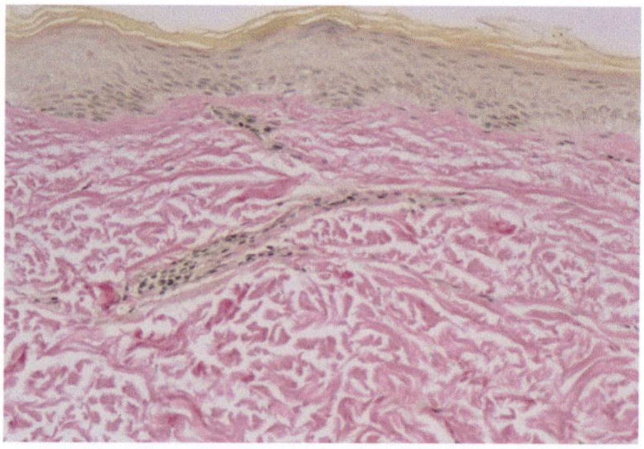

Fig. 1.176 Absence of elastic fibers (VVG stain)

Angiofibroma

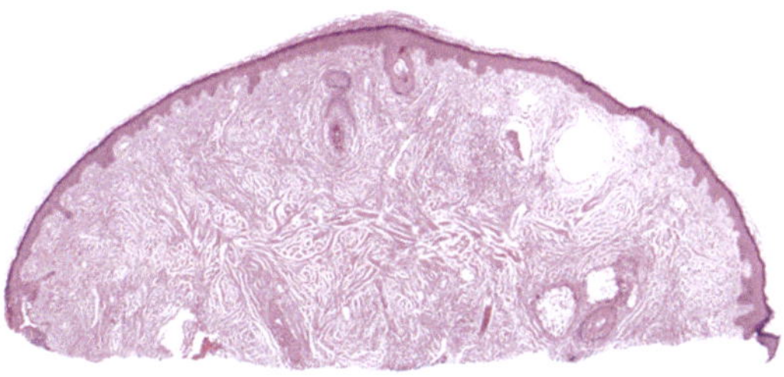

Fig. 1.177 Dome-shaped lesion

Synonyms: Adenoma Sebaceum, Fibrous Papule of the Nose (Face), Pearly Penile Papule

Histopathology (Figs. 1.177, 1.178, 1.179, and 1.180)

- Elevated dome-shaped lesion with dilated thin vessels in the upper portion of the dermis
- Thickened stroma with collagen bundles often perpendicular to the epidermis and around follicles
- Spindled and stellate fibroblasts that sometimes can be multinucleated (factor XIII+, CD68+)
- Multiple lesions associated with NF2, MEN1, Tuberous Sclerosis, Birt-Hogg-Dubé syndrome

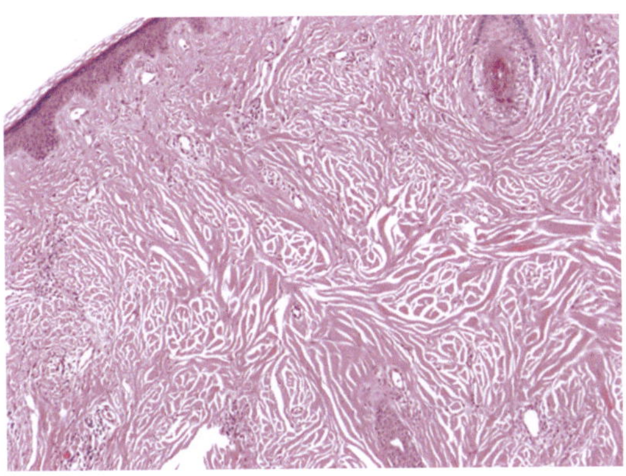

Fig. 1.178 Prominent stroma with thick collagen bundle

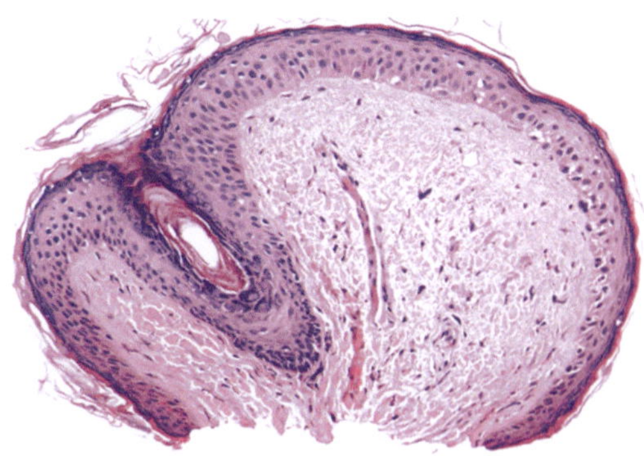

Fig. 1.179 Small sclerotic papule

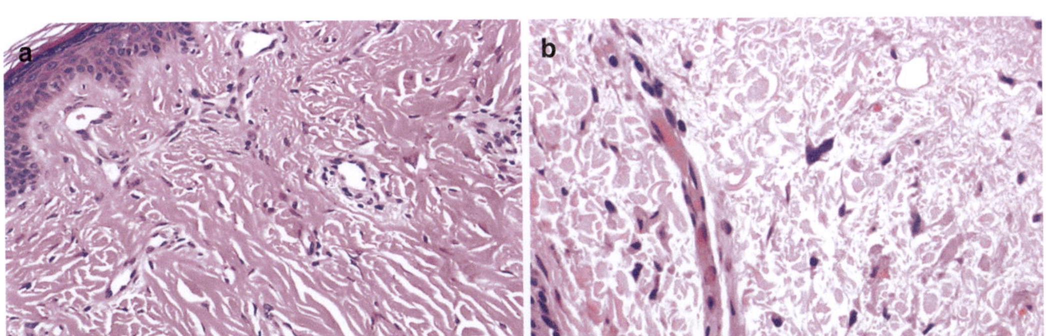

Fig. 1.180 (**a**, **b**) Stroma with multiple dilated small vessels and reactive fibroblasts some with irregular shape

Angiokeratoma

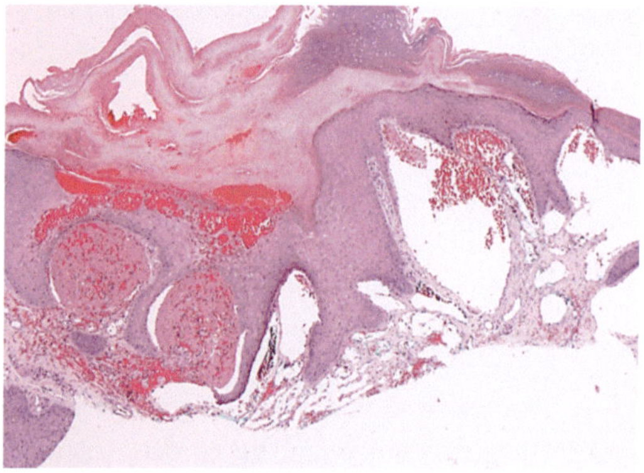

Fig. 1.181 Hyperkeratotic acanthotic epidermis with irregular papillomatosis

Histopathology (Figs. 1.181, 1.182, 1.183, and 1.184)

- Epidermal acanthosis, papillomatosis, and hyperkeratosis
- Dilated vascular channels in the papillary dermis
- There is an impression that vascular channels are pushing into the epidermis
- Vascular channels are usually congested
- Thrombi can form within vessels

P.S. *angiokeratoma corporis diffusum* is associated with Anderson-Fabry disease

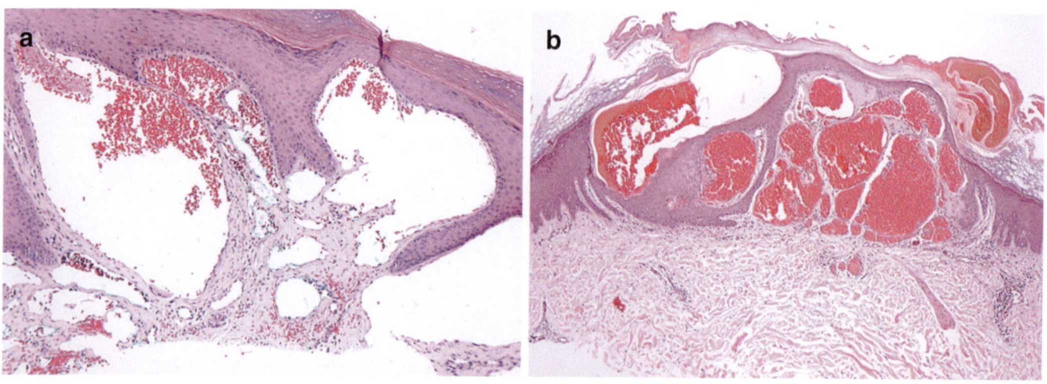

Fig. 1.182 (**a**, **b**) Dilated vascular channels that are pushing into the epidermis

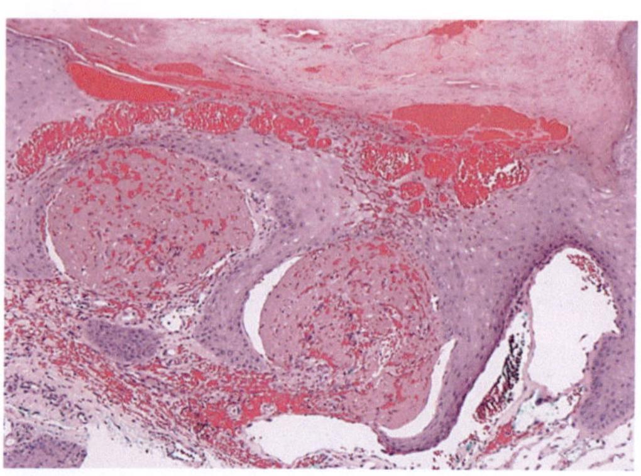

Fig. 1.183 Thrombi are present within two vascular channels

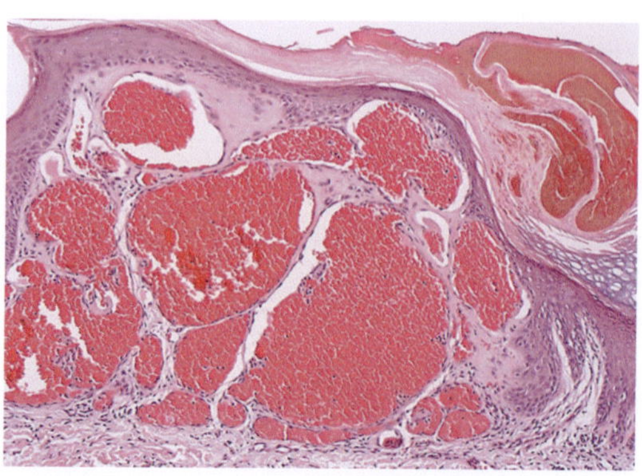

Fig. 1.184 Vascular channels are congested

Angioleiomyoma

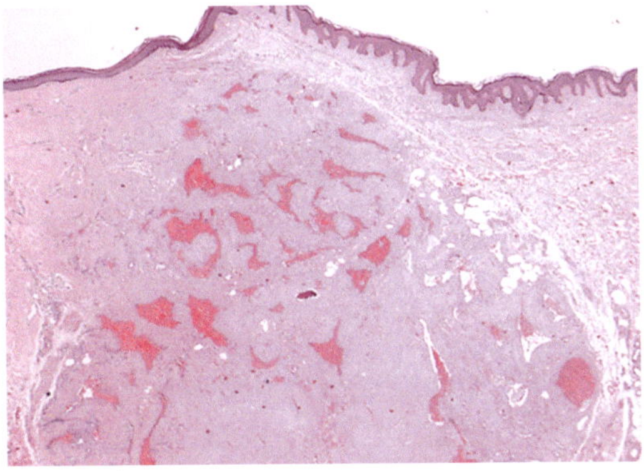

Fig. 1.185 Well circumscribed nodule

Histopathology (Figs. 1.185, 1.186, and 1.187)

- Well circumscribed nodule with fibrous pseudocapsule
- Consists of interlacing bundle of smooth muscle
- Numerous vascular channels
- Stroma can show myxoid changes
- SMA+, desmin+, caldesmon+

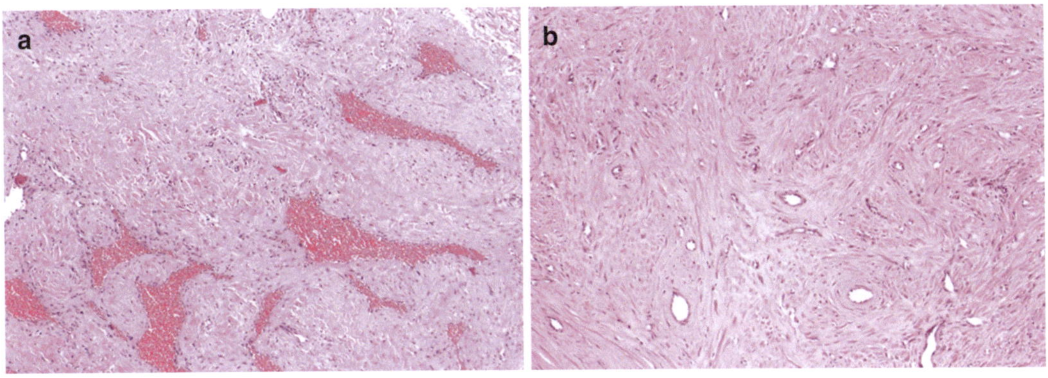

Fig. 1.186 (**a**, **b**) Interlacing bundles of eosinophilic smooth muscle

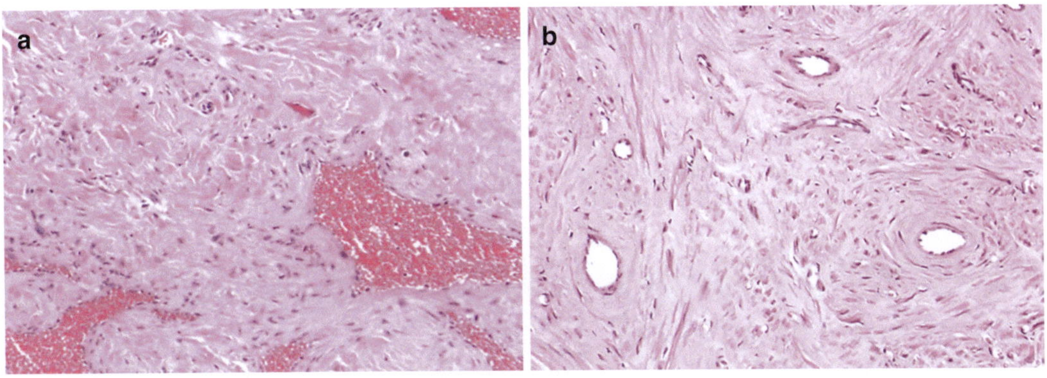

Fig. 1.187 Numerous congested (**a**) and not congested (**b**) small dilated vessels in between smooth muscle cells with elongated nuclei and no atypia

Angiolipoma

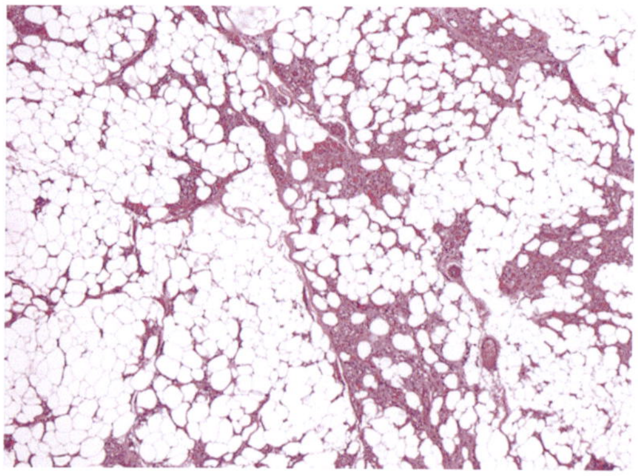

Fig. 1.188 Adipose tissue with prominent vessels

Histopathology (Figs. 1.188, 1.189, 1.190, and 1.191)

- Subcutaneous nodule
- Mixture of adipose and vascular tissue
- Adipose tissue is mature with no atypia
- Vascular tissue must comprise more than 5% of overall tumor and consists of capillaries
- Capillaries are concentrated more around the periphery of the tumor and small thrombi can be present

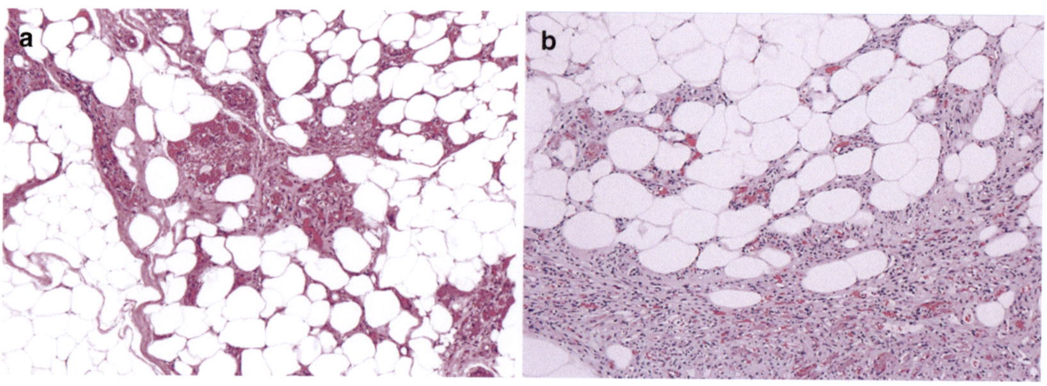

Fig. 1.189 (**a**, **b**) Admixture of mature adipocytes and small capillaries

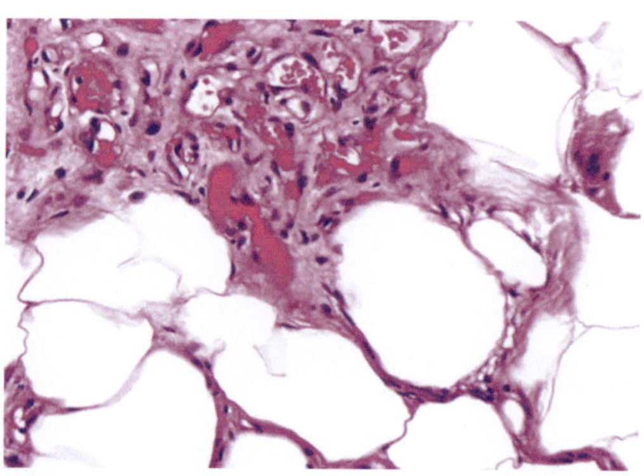

Fig. 1.190 Capillaries are congested and few are filled with thrombi

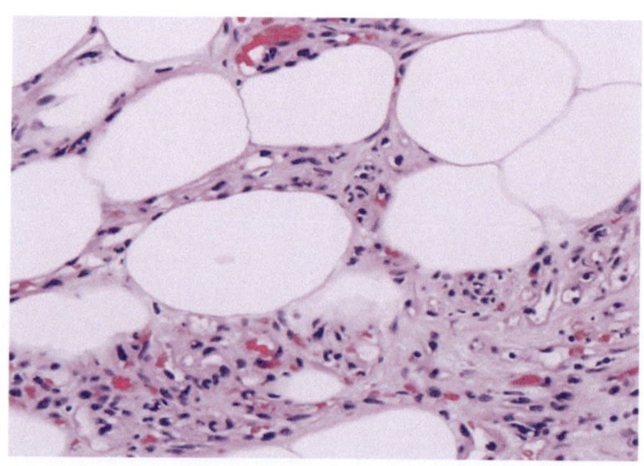

Fig. 1.191 Endothelial cells and adipocytes with no atypia

Angiolymphoid Hyperplasia with Eosinophilia

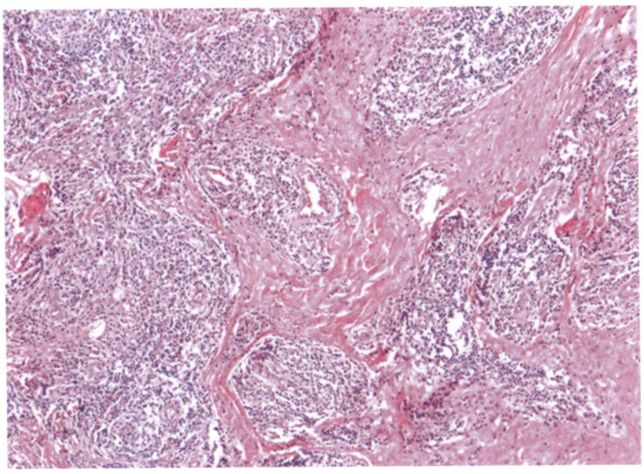

Fig. 1.192 Vascular tumor in fibrotic stroma

Synonym: Epithelioid Hemangioma

Histopathology (Figs. 1.192, 1.193, 1.194, 1.195, and 1.196)

- Variably sized vessels with plump, enlarged endothelial cells, some with hobnail nuclei and cytoplasmic vacuoles
- Variable number of lymphocytes, plasma cells, and eosinophils
- Variable perivascular fibrosis ("onion skin")

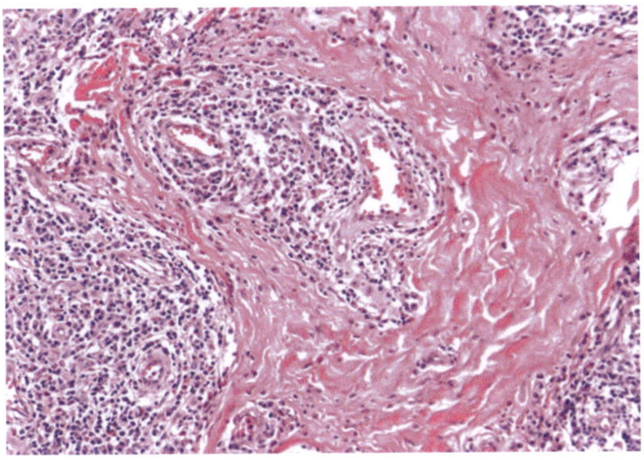

Fig. 1.193 Vascular channels and inflammatory cells in fibrous stroma

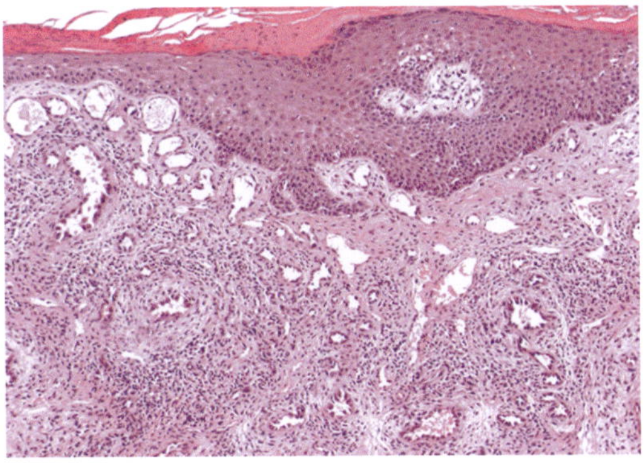

Fig. 1.194 Enlarged endothelial cells with "hob nailing"

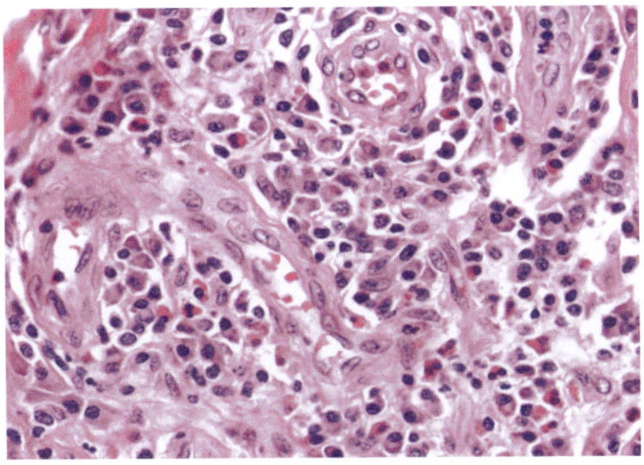

Fig. 1.195 Lymphocytes, plasma cells, and eosinophils surround plump vessels

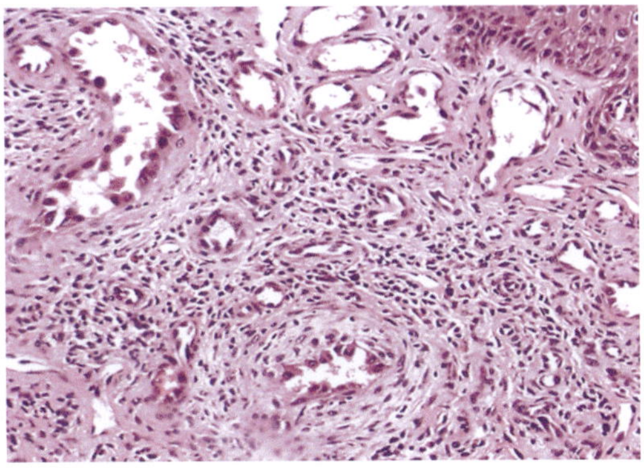

Fig. 1.196 Perivascular "onion skin" fibrosis

Angiomatosis

Proliferation of blood vessels involving large areas of the body with limbs being a favorite site.

Histopathology (Figs. 1.197, 1.198, and 1.199)

- Diffuse subcutaneous proliferation of vascular channels (mostly veins and capillaries)
- Vascular elements are admixed with fibroadipose tissue

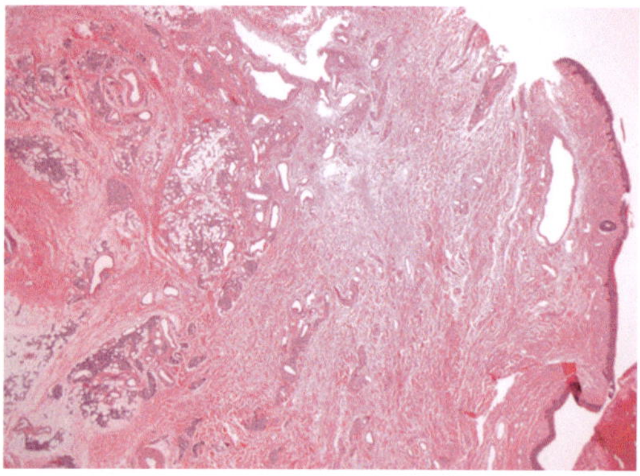

Fig. 1.197 Irregular diffuse subcutaneous vascular proliferation

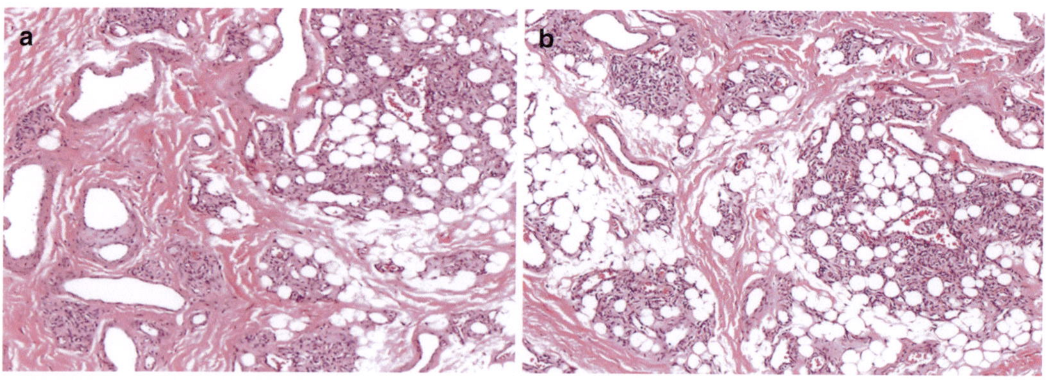

Fig. 1.198 (**a**, **b**) Vascular channels are admixed with mature adipose tissue and thickened fibrous stroma

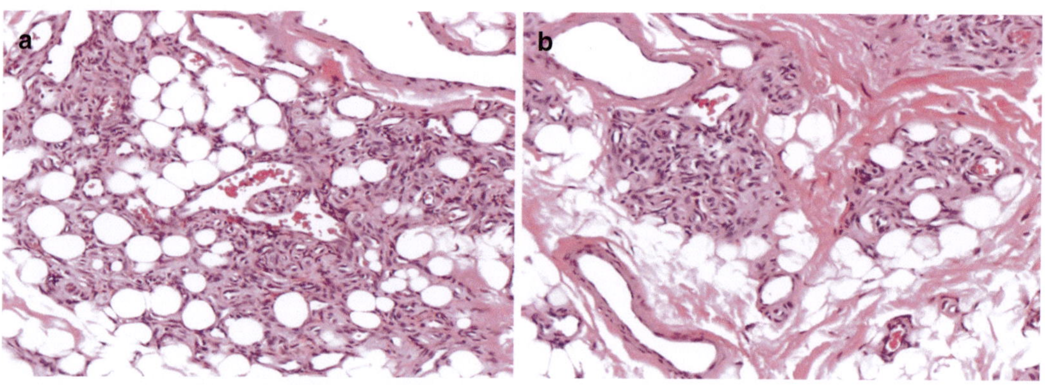

Fig. 1.199 (**a**, **b**) Mixture of capillaries, veins, and cavernous vascular spaces

Angiomyofibroblastoma

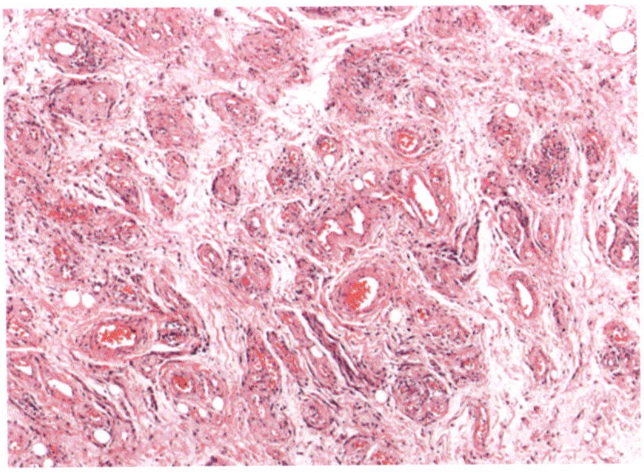

Fig. 1.200 Benign appearing vascular proliferation

Histopathology (Figs. 1.200, 1.201, and 1.202)

- Subcutaneous nodule of vulva or scrotum
- Prominent thin walled vessels in edematous stroma
- Spindle shaped or rounded myofibroblasts with eosinophilic cytoplasm present in the stroma
- Myofibroblasts (desmin+, SMA+, ER+, PR+) are concentrated around vessels
- Mast cells can be seen
- No cytological atypia or mitoses

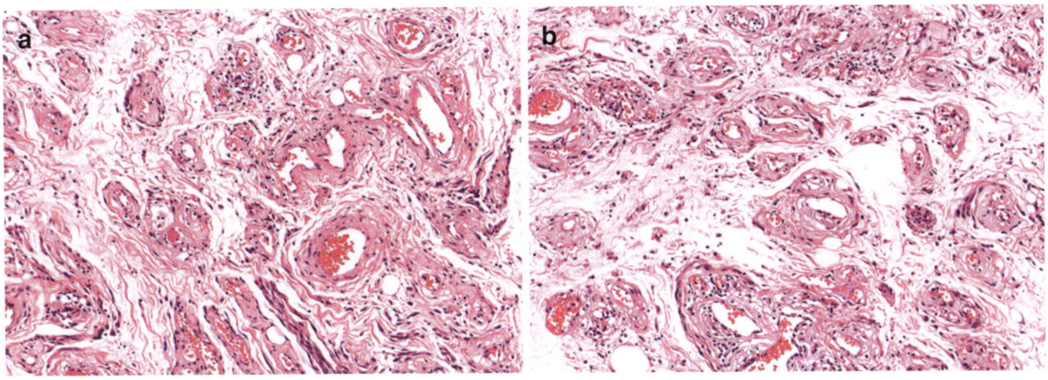

Fig. 1.201 (**a**, **b**) Small and medium size vessels in edematous stroma

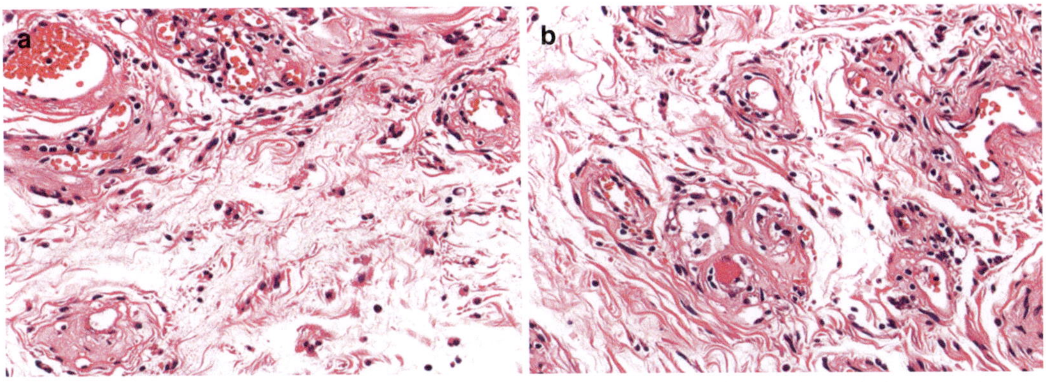

Fig. 1.202 (**a**, **b**) Rounded and spindle shaped myofibroblast with no atypia are present in stroma

Angiomyolipoma

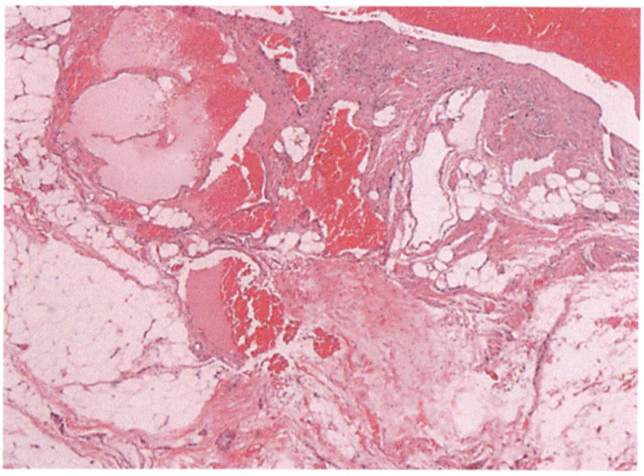

Fig. 1.203 Poorly defined subcutaneous tumor

Histopathology (Figs. 1.203, 1.204, and 1.205)
- Subcutaneous poorly defined tumor
- Consists of bundles of smooth muscle, vascular channels of various sizes, and mature adipose tissue
- HMB45 is negative in cutaneous tumors but is positive in renal lesions

P.S. cutaneous lesions are not usually associated with *Tuberous Sclerosis*

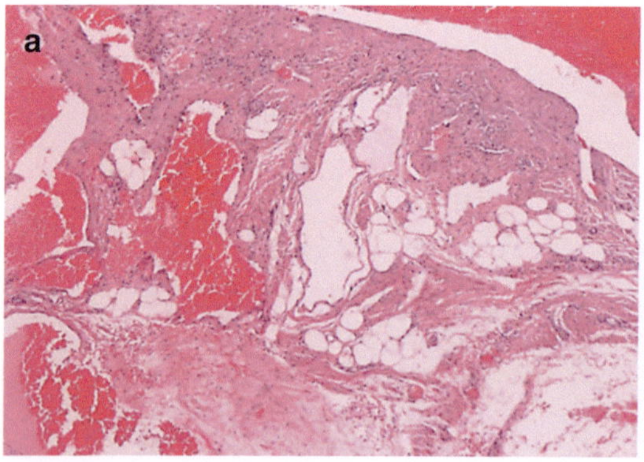

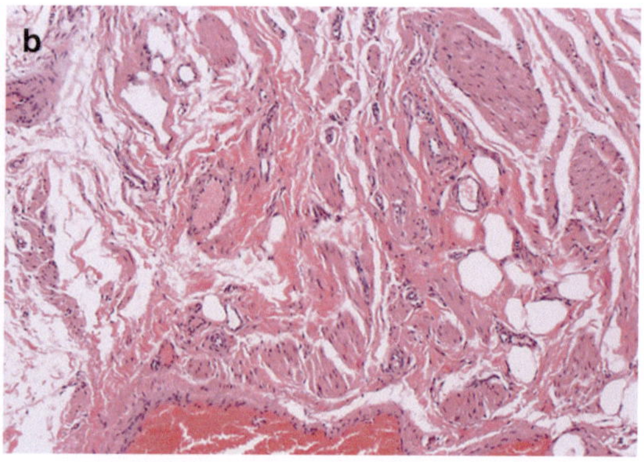

Fig. 1.204 (**a**, **b**) Vascular channels of various sizes admixed with smooth muscle bundles and surrounded by mature adipose tissue

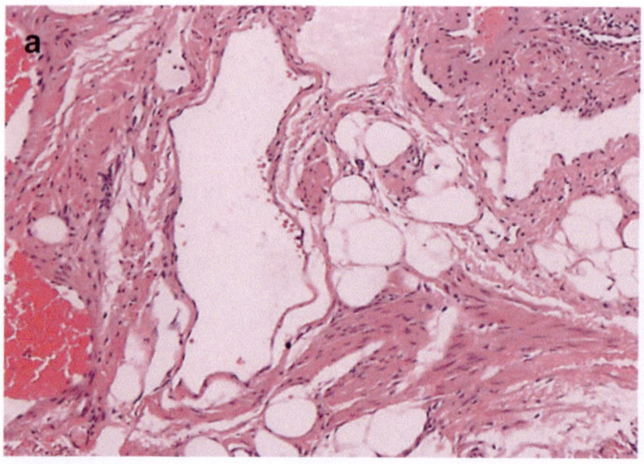

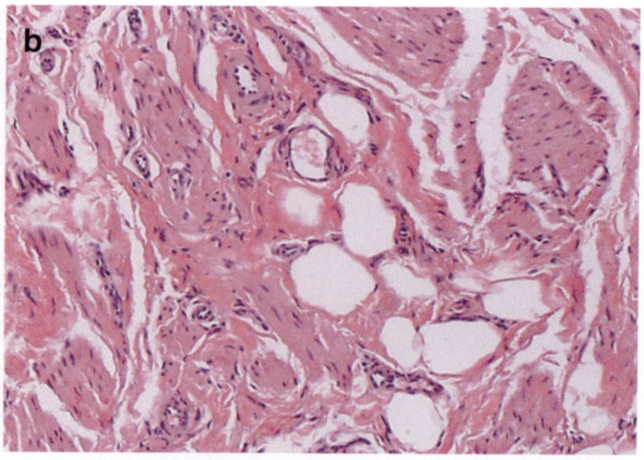

Fig. 1.205 (**a**, **b**) Muscle bundles are haphazardly oriented and adipocytes appear entrapped

Angiomyxoma

Synonym: Superficial Angiomyxoma

Histopathology (Figs. 1.206, 1.207, 1.208, 1.209, and 1.210)

- Poorly circumscribed lesion
- Myxoid stroma with variable number of spindle or stellate fibroblasts
- Prominent capillaries

P.S. multiple lesions may be associated with *Carney Complex*

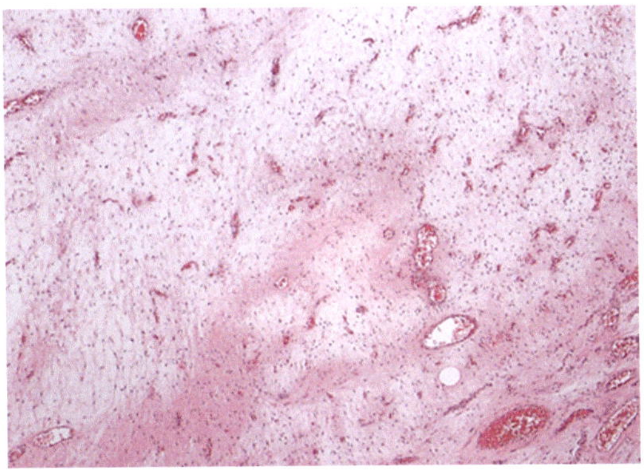

Fig. 1.206 Poorly defined myxoid tumor

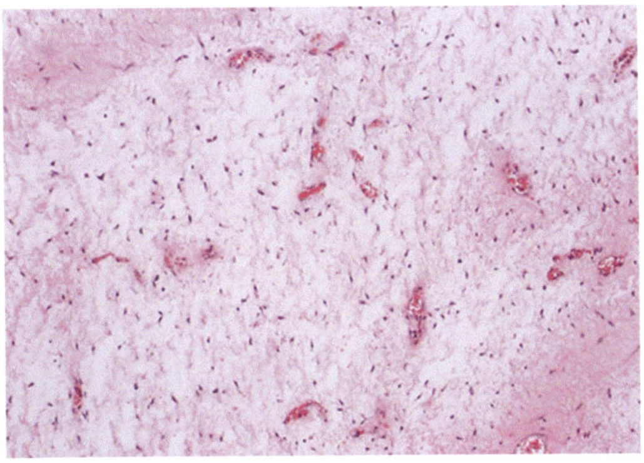

Fig. 1.207 Myxoid stroma with increased number of capillaries

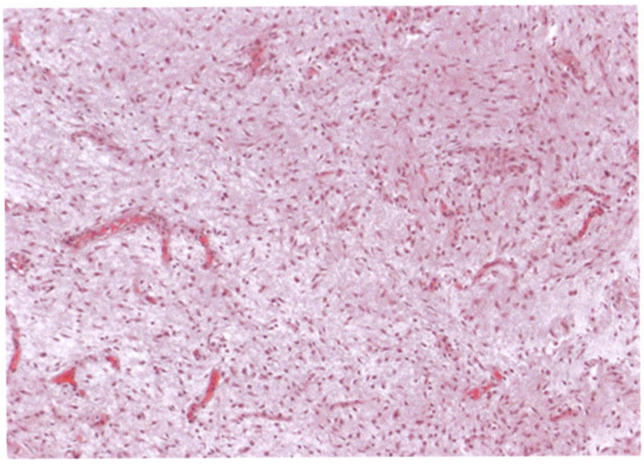

Fig. 1.208 Less myxoid tumor with more prominent fibroblasts

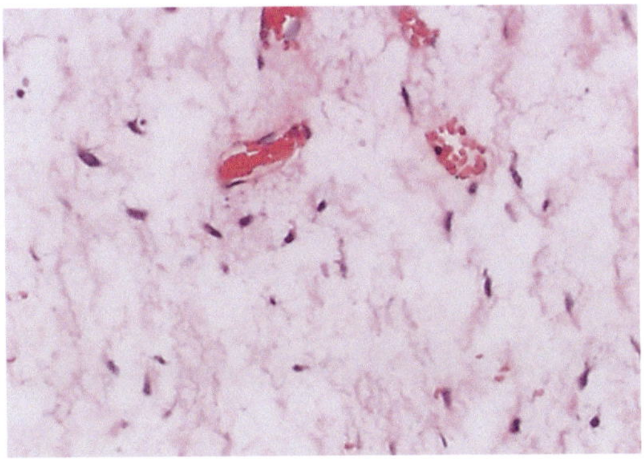

Fig. 1.209 Scattered fibroblasts in myxoid stroma

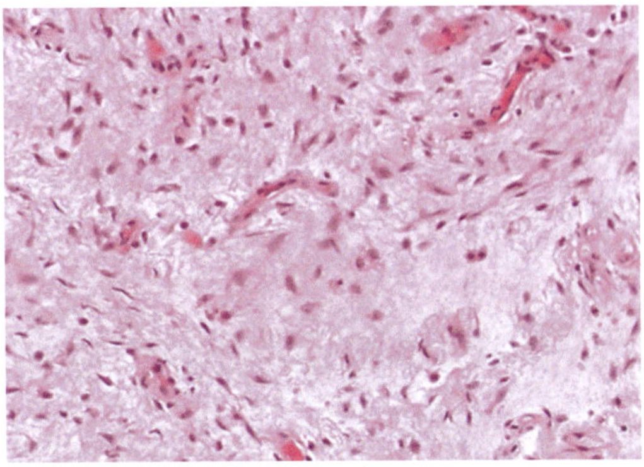

Fig. 1.210 Spindle and stellate fibroblasts

Angiosarcoma

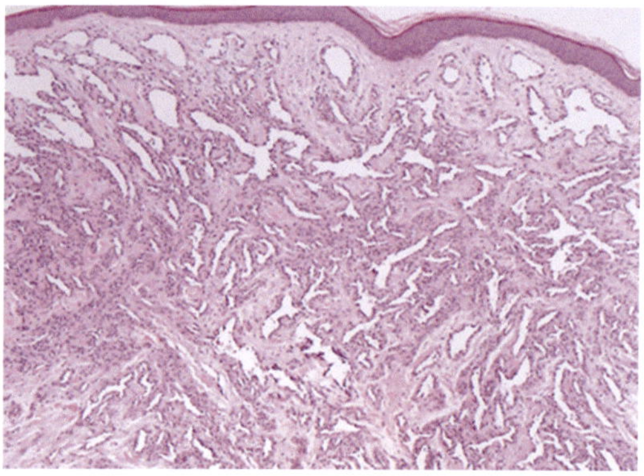

Fig. 1.211 Infiltrating vascular tumor

Histopathology (Figs. 1.211, 1.212, 1.213, 1.214, and 1.215)

- Poorly circumscribed, infiltrative tumor
- Irregular vessels dissecting collagen, some with "staghorn" pattern
- Epithelioid endothelial cells with "hobnailing" of nuclei
- Vessels can be more "slit like", resembling Kaposi's sarcoma, but without spindle cells in between vessels
- Tumor cells are CD31+, CD34+, factor VIII+

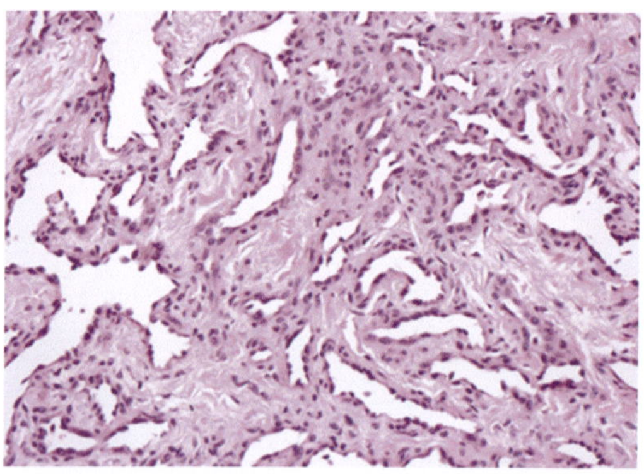

Fig. 1.212 "Staghorn" shaped blood vessels dissecting collagen

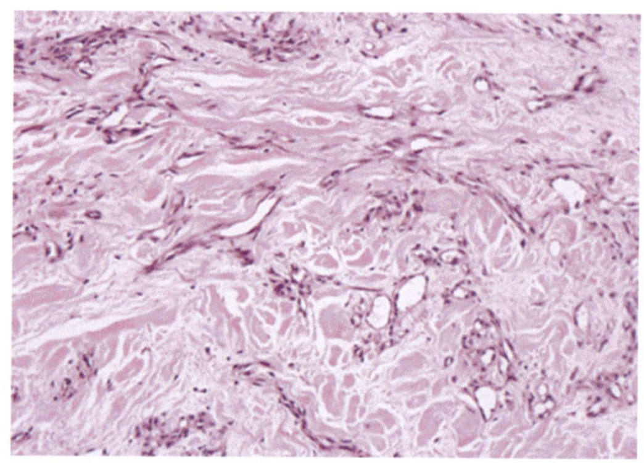

Fig. 1.213 Vessels with "slit-like" appearance

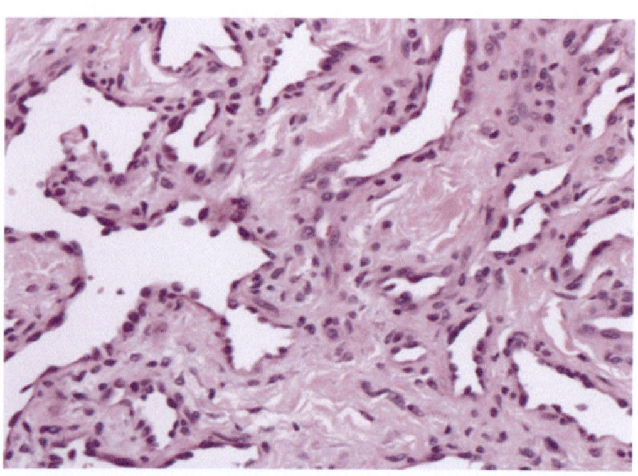

Fig. 1.214 Prominent endothelial cells with "hobnail" appearance

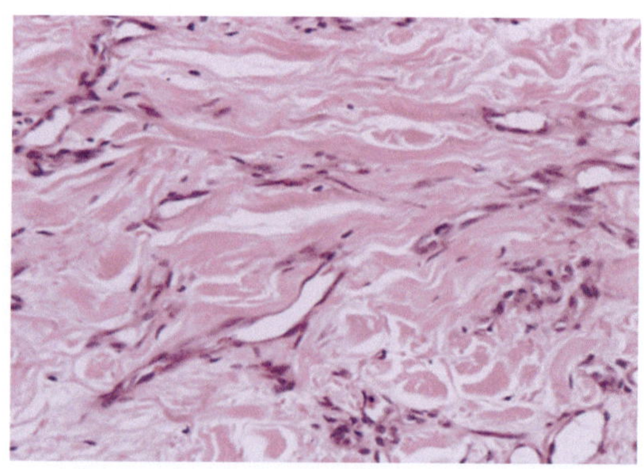

Fig. 1.215 No spindle cells in between vessels

Aplasia Cutis

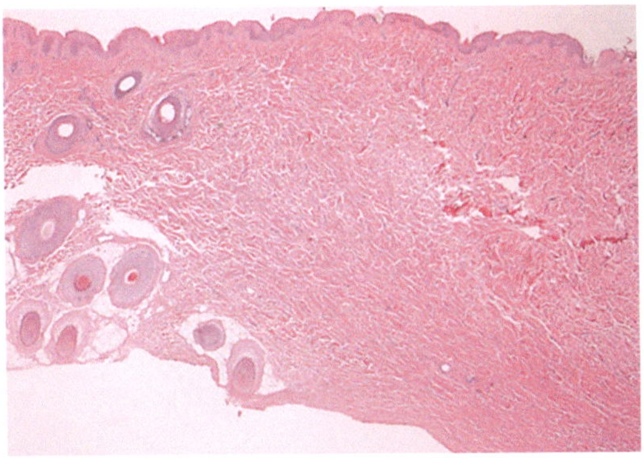

Fig. 1.216 Dermal scar

Histopathology is that of the scar and therefore clinical correlation is necessary:

Early lesion:

- Ulcer with loss of epidermis and dermis

Established lesion:

- Healed area with atrophic epidermis and scar with absence of adnexal structures (Figs. 1.216, 1.217, and 1.218)

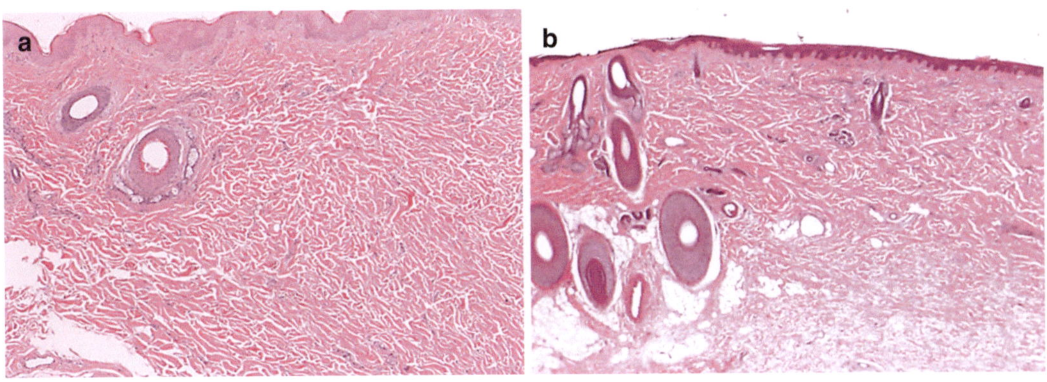

Fig. 1.217 (**a**, **b**) A biopsy from the edge between an area of developed skin to the left and congenitally absent skin to the right

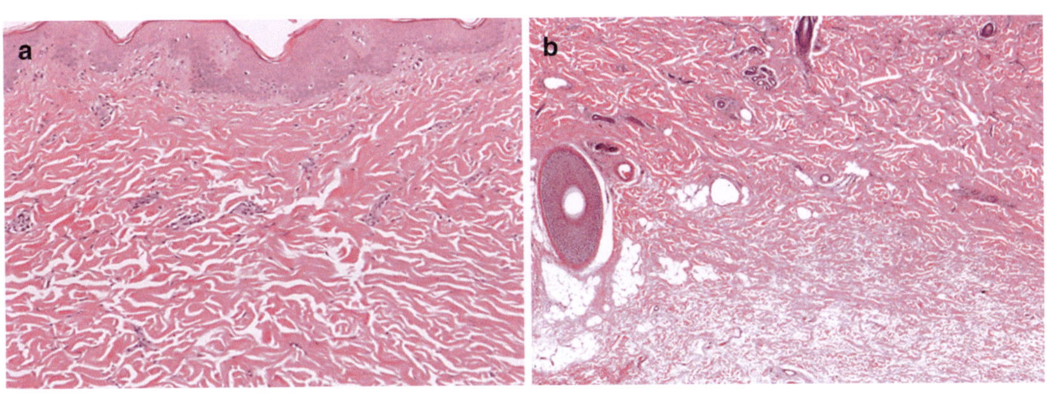

Fig. 1.218 (**a**, **b**) Dermal fibrosis and scarring

Apocrine Adenocarcinoma

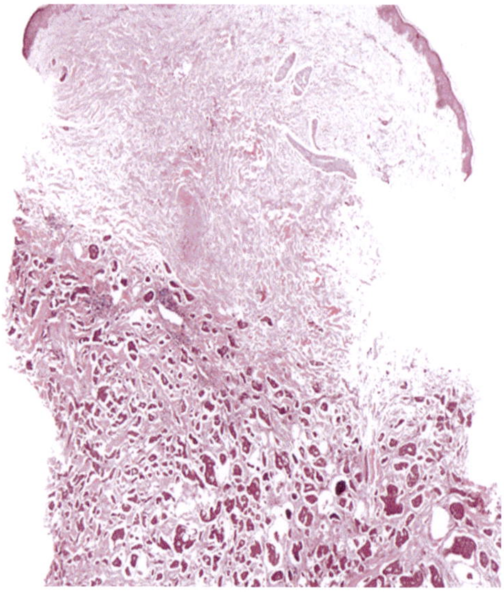

Fig. 1.219 Poorly circumscribed subcutaneous tumor

Histopathology (Figs. 1.219, 1.220, 1.221, and 1.222)

- Poorly circumscribed tumor
- Tumor consists of variable glandular/tubular structures in diffuse or solid pattern
- Cells have eosinophilic cytoplasm and apocrine snouts and round to oval nuclei
- Dense hyalinized stroma is common

P.S. rare tumor (GCDFP-15+, ER+) that occurs most commonly in axilla

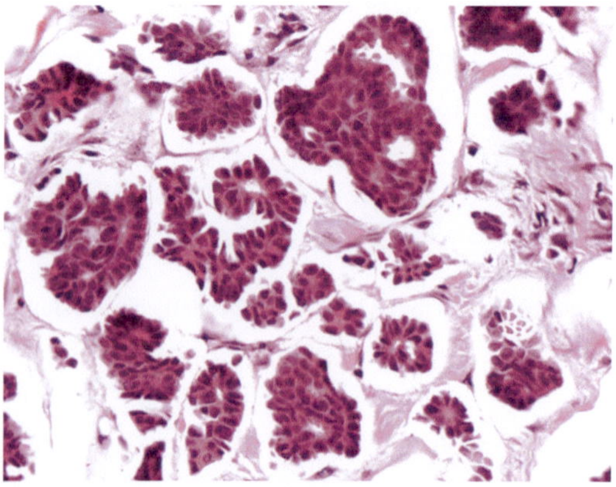

Fig. 1.220 Eosinophilic cytoplasm with apocrine snouts

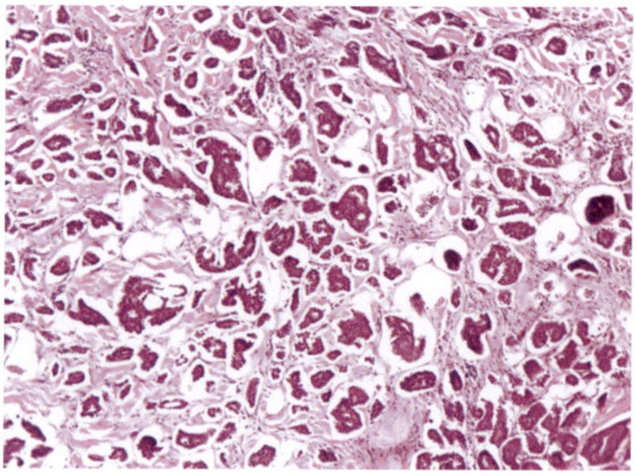

Fig. 1.221 Tumor consists of ducts and tubules

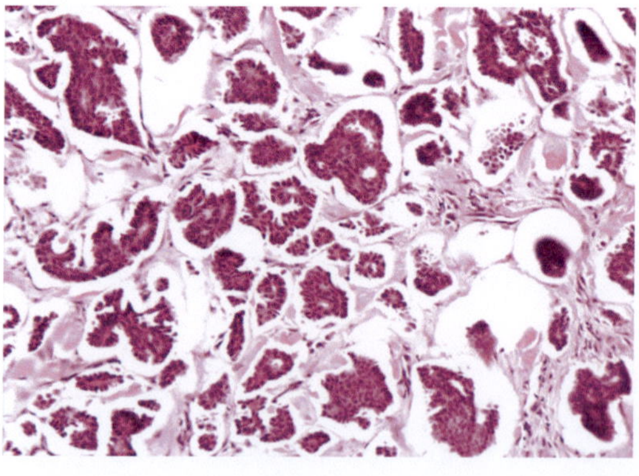

Fig. 1.222 Tumor embedded in hyalinized stroma

Apocrine Papillary Cystadenoma

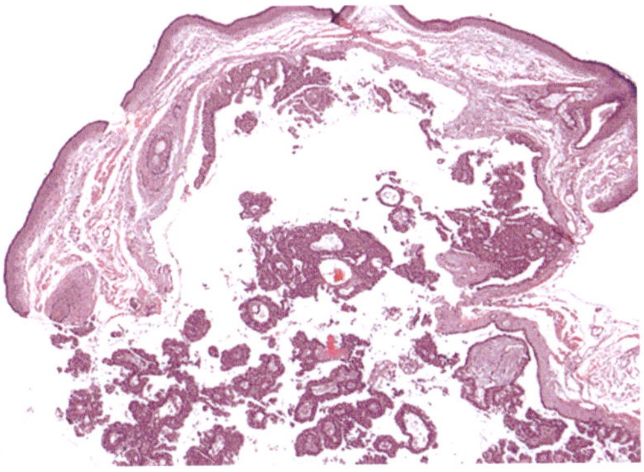

Fig. 1.223 Cystic tumor with numerous papillae

Histopathology (Figs. 1.223, 1.224, 1.225, 1.226, and 1.227)

- Cystic tumor with papillary and some solid areas
- Cystic areas are lined with stratified cuboidal cells with apocrine snouts
- Irregular papillae protruding into the cyst cavity
- Papillae have a delicate fibrovascular core and are lined with cuboidal cells with apocrine snouts
- Solid area has ductal structures lined with apocrine cuboidal cells

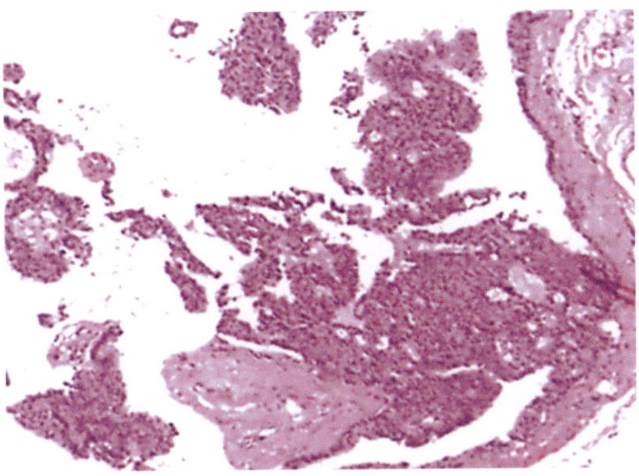

Fig. 1.224 Peripheral lining is identical to apocrine hidrocystoma

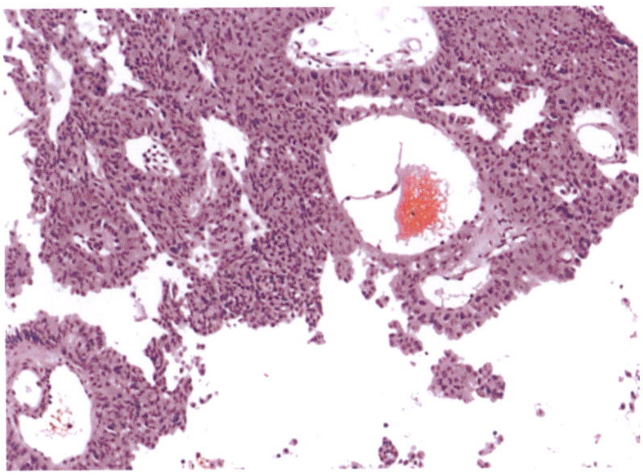

Fig. 1.225 Solid areas have ductal structures

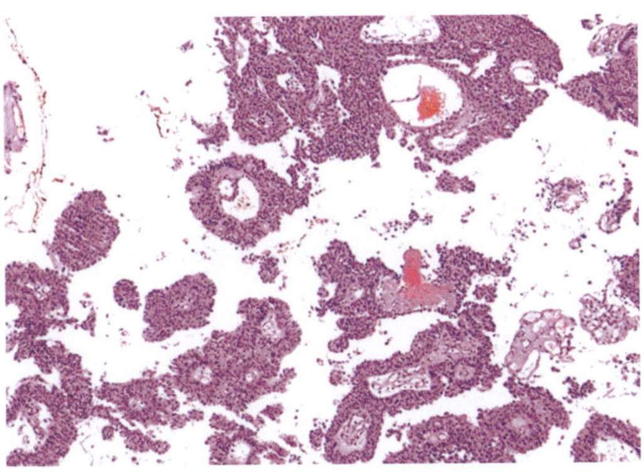

Fig. 1.226 Papillary and solid areas occupy the cavity

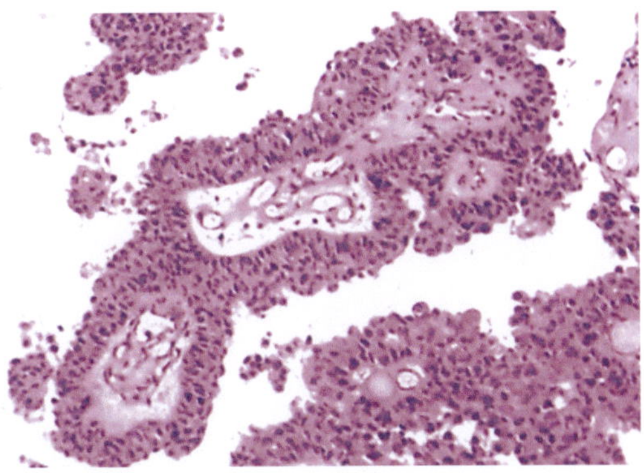

Fig. 1.227 Papillae have a fibrovascular core and are lined with stratified cuboidal cells with apocrine snouts

Argyria

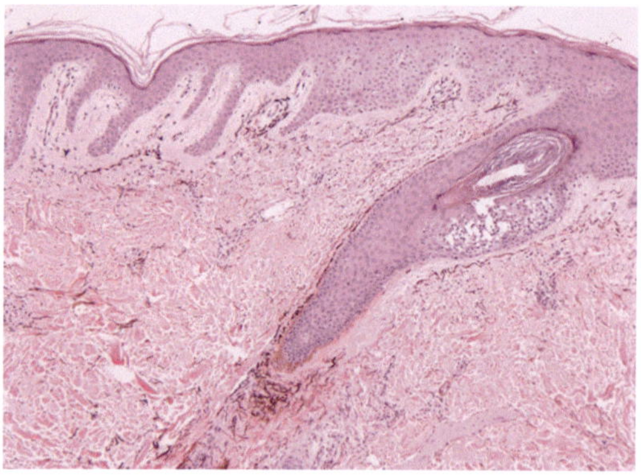

Fig. 1.228 Dermal foreign body deposits

Synonym: Silver Deposition

Histopathology (Figs. 1.228, 1.229, 1.230, 1.231, and 1.232)

- Brown/yellow strands ("pseudoochronosis") and granules distributed between collagen bundles, along elastic fibers, vessels, and adnexal structures
- Dark field microscopy demonstrates characteristic "starry sky" image

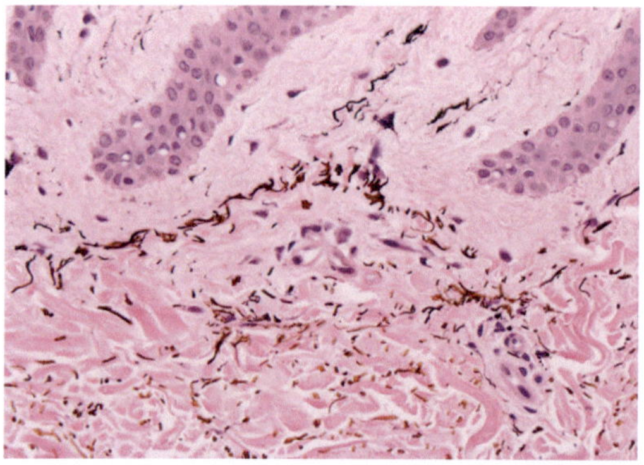

Fig. 1.229 Dermal brown/yellow granules and strands distributed between collagen bundles

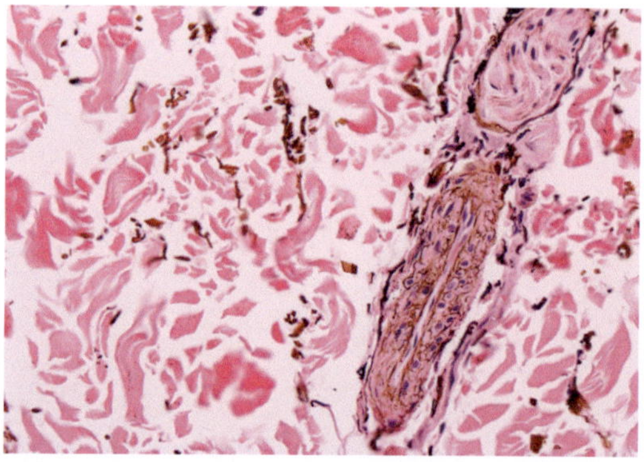

Fig. 1.230 Interstitial and perivascular/periadnexal pigment

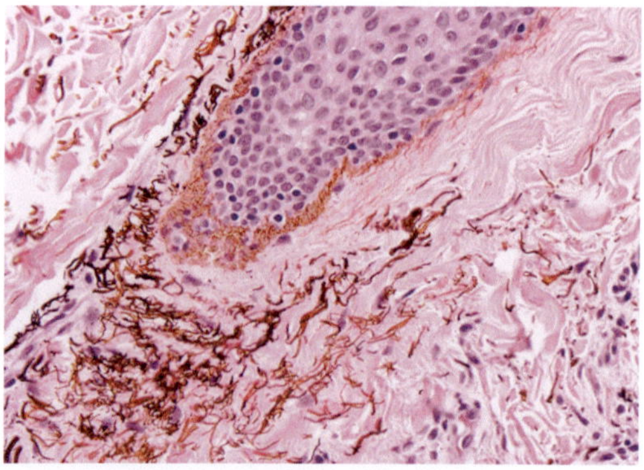

Fig. 1.231 Perifollicular pigment distribution

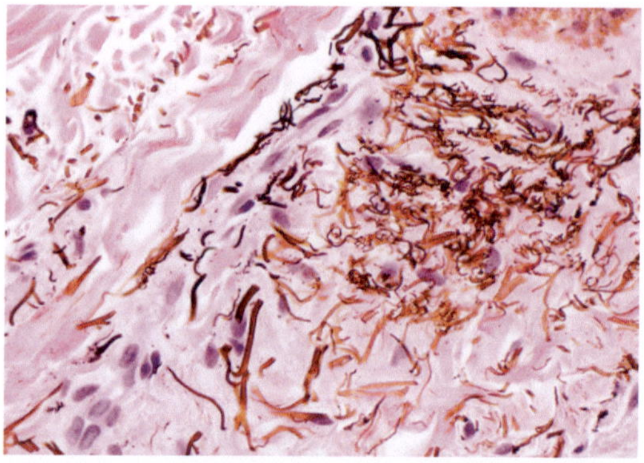

Fig. 1.232 "Pseudoochronosis" appearance of pigment strands

Arteriovenous Hemangioma

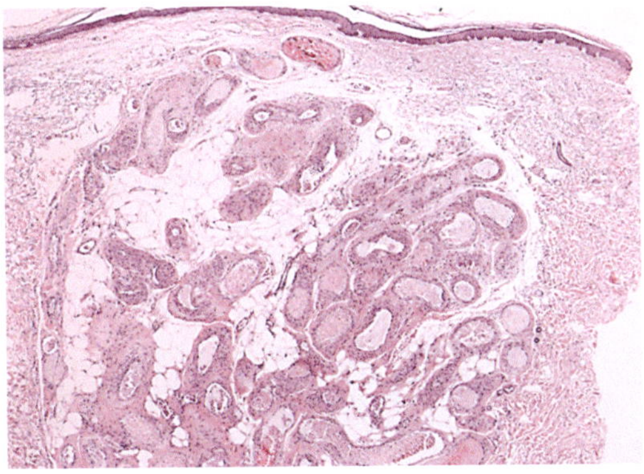

Fig. 1.233 Subcutaneous vascular nodule

Histopathology (Figs. 1.233, 1.234, and 1.235)

- Usually well circumscribed dermal and subcutaneous nodule
- Mixture of thick walled arterioles and thin walled venules
- Endothelial cells have bland appearance

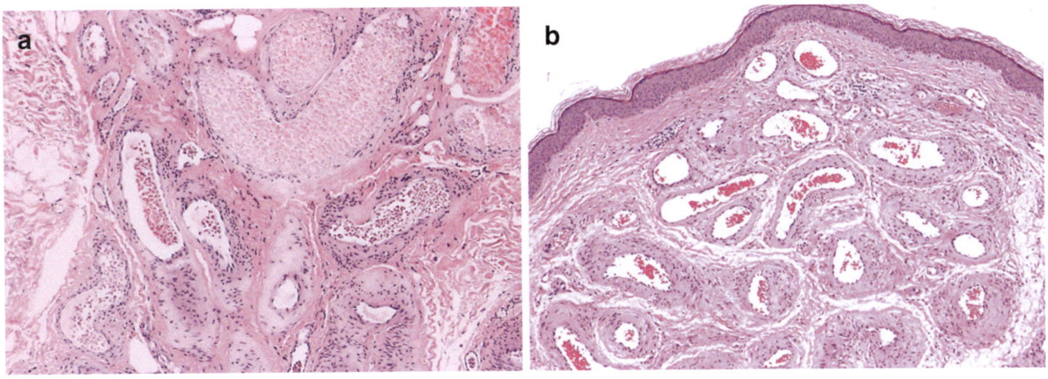

Fig. 1.234 (**a**, **b**) Numerous small arteries and veins forming dermal and subcutaneous nodule

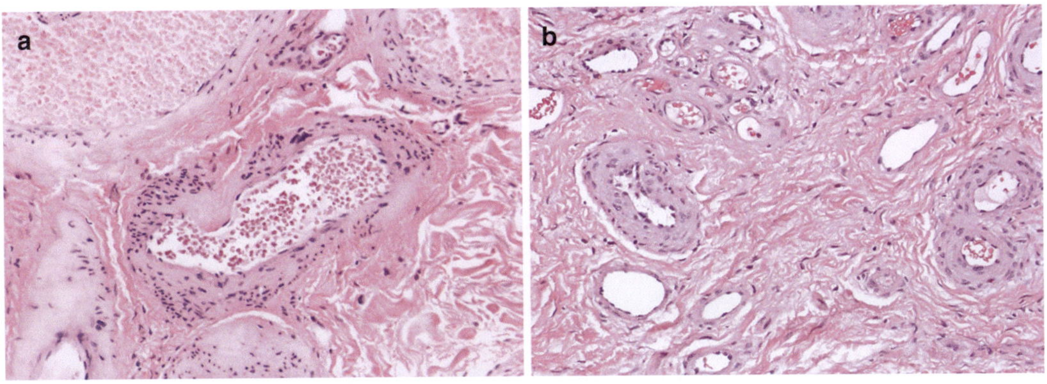

Fig. 1.235 (**a**, **b**) Admixture of vessels with thin and thick walls with endothelial cells looking unremarkable

Arteriovenous Malformation

Histopathology (Figs. 1.236, 1.237, 1.238, and 1.239)

- Subcutaneous poorly circumscribed vascular proliferation forming complex connected vascular structures
- Presence of medium to large size arteries and veins with absence of capillaries
- Nerve bundles are present in malformation and absent in arteriovenous hemangioma

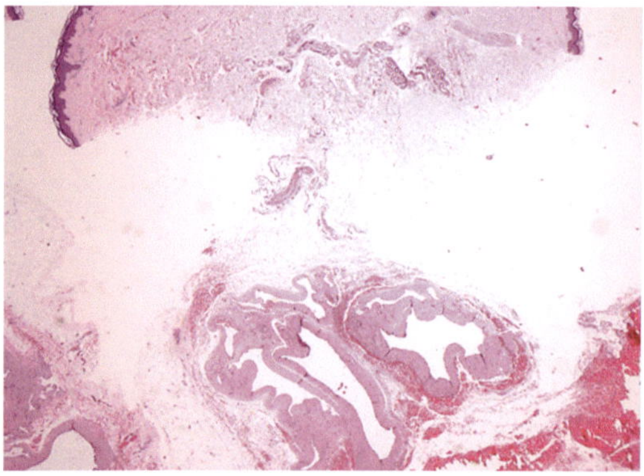

Fig. 1.236 Multiple subcutaneous, dilate, thick-walled vessels

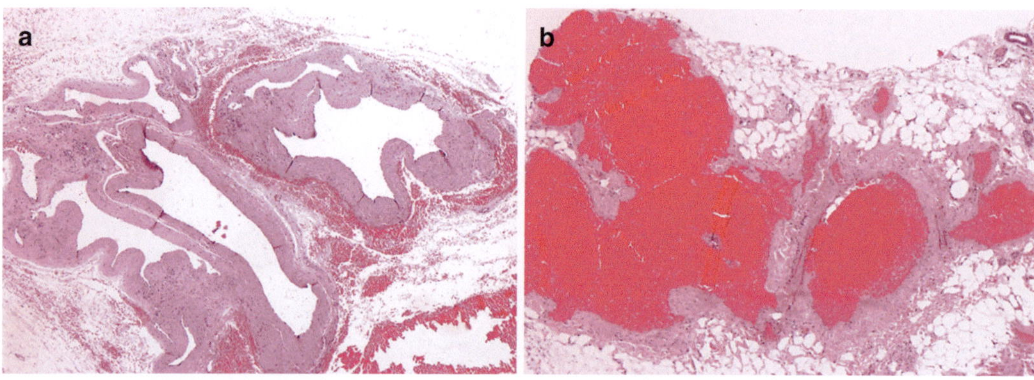

Fig. 1.237 (**a**, **b**) Irregular thick and thin walled vascular structures with absence of capillaries

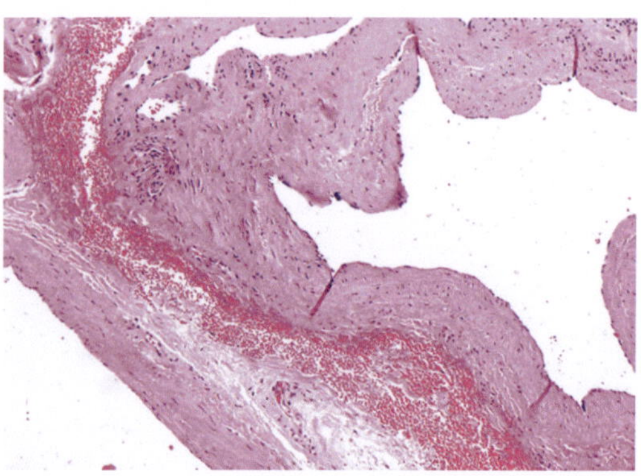

Fig. 1.238 Thick walled vessel with no endothelial atypia

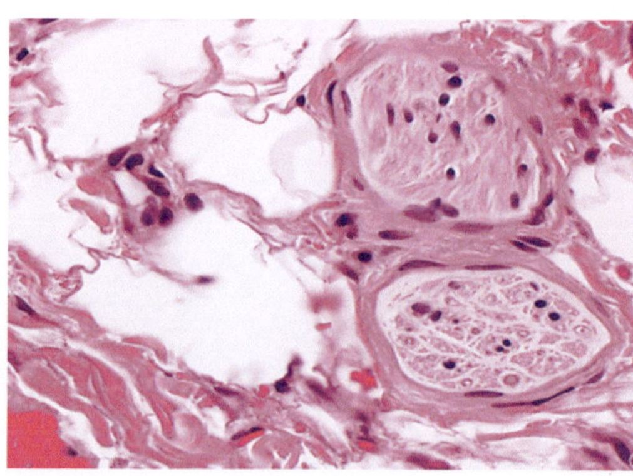

Fig. 1.239 Nerves are present

Arthropod Bite

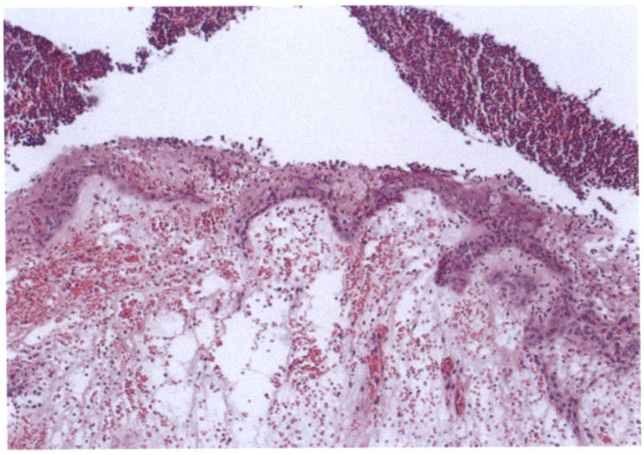

Fig. 1.240 Necrotic epidermis with acutely inflamed serum crust and extensive dermal edema and RBC extravasation

Histopathology (Figs. 1.240, 1.241, 1.242, 1.243, and 1.244)

- Spongiotic and commonly ulcerated epidermis with serum crust
- Wedge shaped, superficial and deep, perivascular and interstitial infiltrate composed of admixed lymphocytes, neutrophils, and eosinophils
- Papillary dermal edema with possible blister formation
- Sometimes foci of dermal necrosis or abscess formation

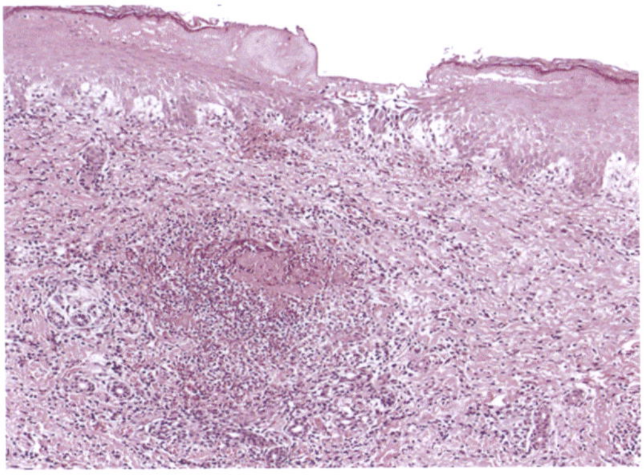

Fig. 1.241 Ulcerated epidermis with underlying necrosis

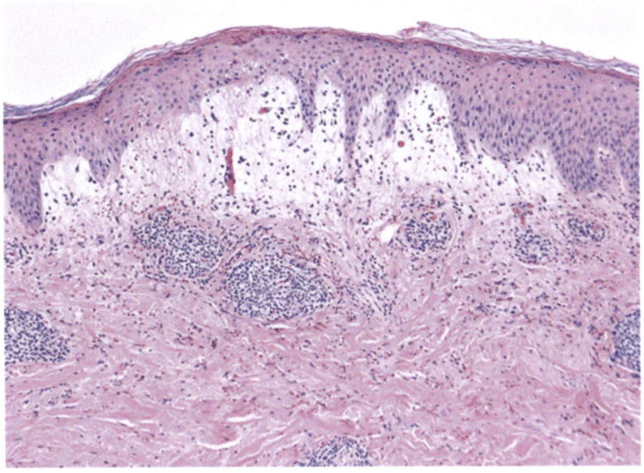

Fig. 1.242 Dermal edema and wedge shaped inflammation

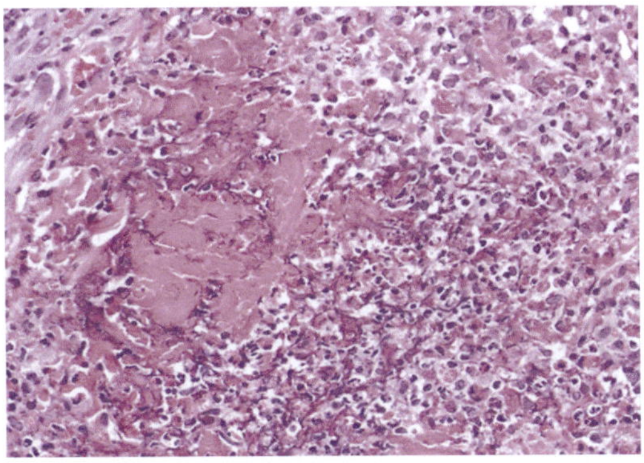

Fig. 1.243 Focal dermal necrosis and abscess surrounded by mixed inflammation

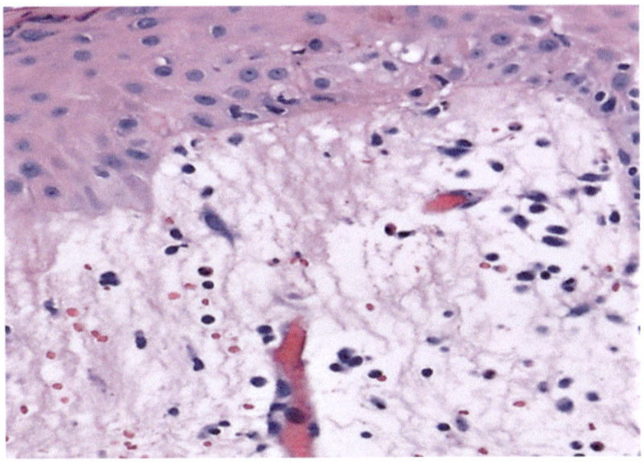

Fig. 1.244 Scattered epidermal necrotic keratinocytes with dermal edema and mixed inflammation with eosinophils

Aspergillosis

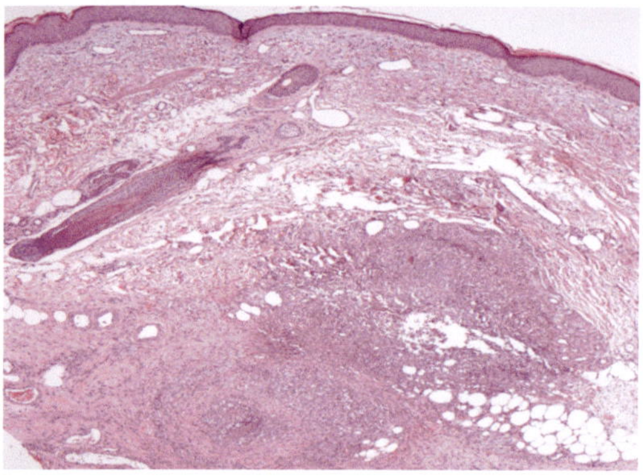

Fig. 1.245 Deep dermal and subcutaneous abscess

Histopathology (Figs. 1.245, 1.246, 1.247, 1.248, and 1.249)
- Dermal and subcutaneous neutrophilic infiltrate with abscess formation
- Common necrosis
- Septate hyphae that branch at 45° angle
- Common vascular invasion

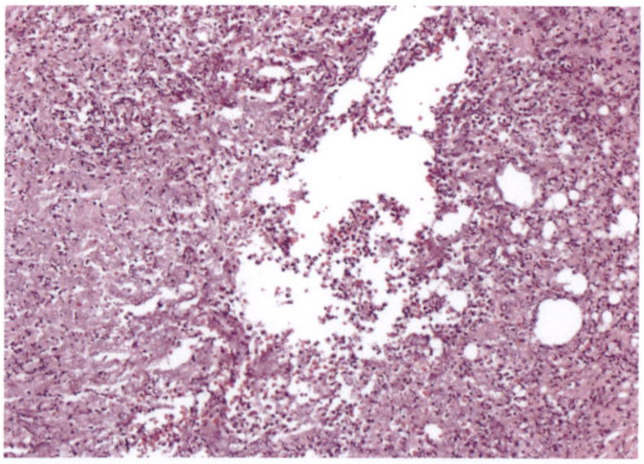

Fig. 1.246 Abscess with central necrosis

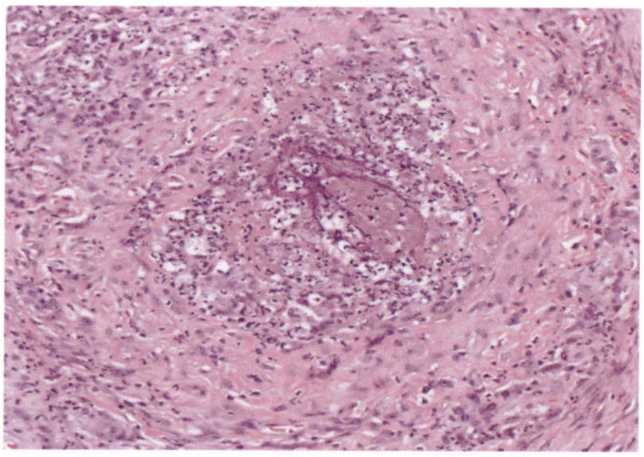

Fig. 1.247 Vessel necrosis and thrombosis

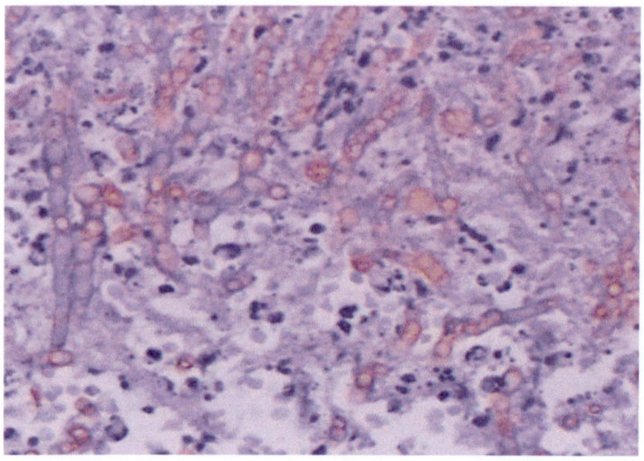

Fig. 1.248 Branching hyphae (PAS)

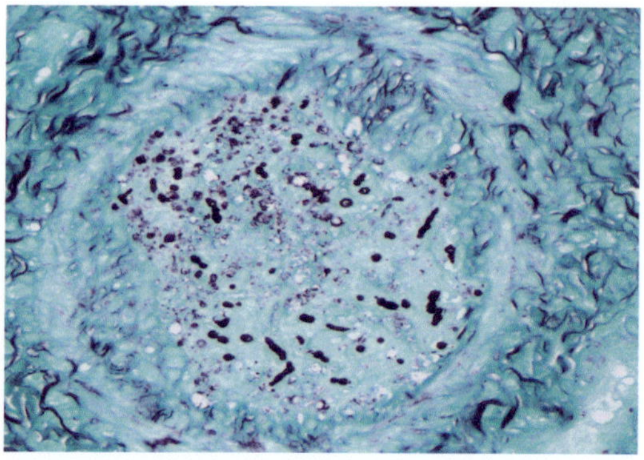

Fig. 1.249 Intravascular aspergillosis (GMS)

Asteatotic Dermatitis

Synonym: Eczema Craquelé

Histopathology is not specific (Figs. 1.250, 1.251, 1.252, 1.253, and 1.254)

- Presents as chronic spongiotic dermatitis
- Mildly spongiotic epidermis with hyperkeratosis and hypergranulosis
- Mild perivascular lymphocytic infiltrate
- Focal lymphocytic exocytosis

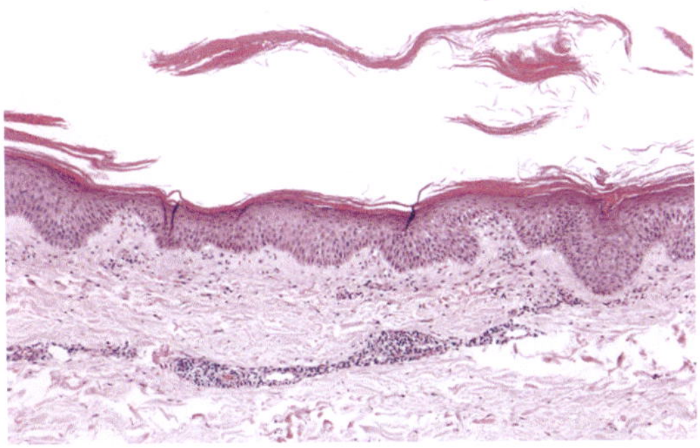

Fig. 1.250 Epidermis with extensive hyperkeratosis

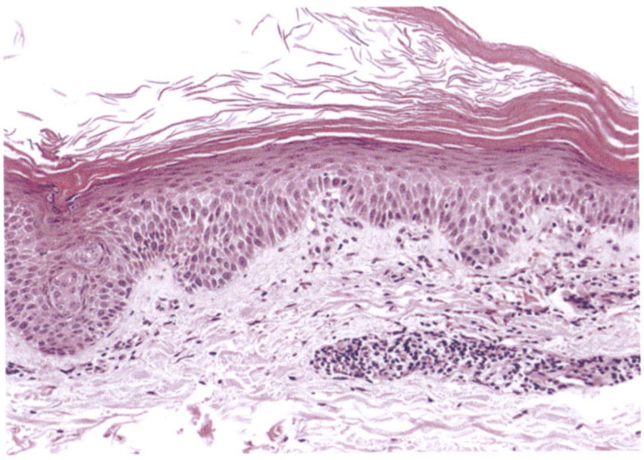

Fig. 1.251 Mild epidermal spongiosis

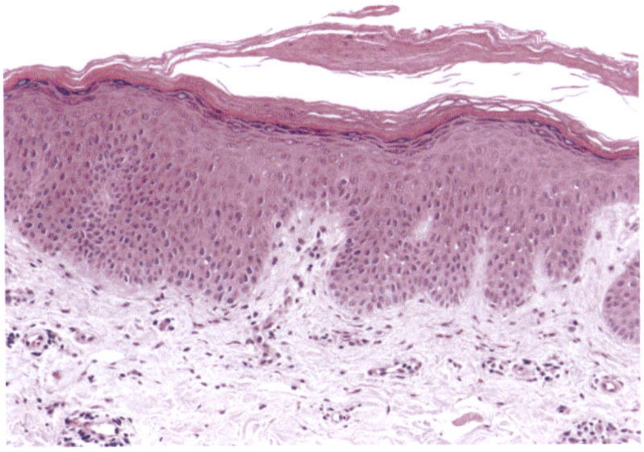

Fig. 1.252 Mild perivascular lymphocytic inflammation

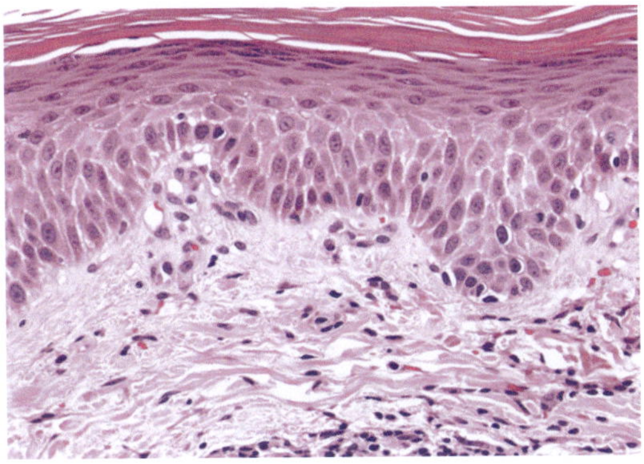

Fig. 1.253 Prominent desmosomes and focal epidermal lymphocytes

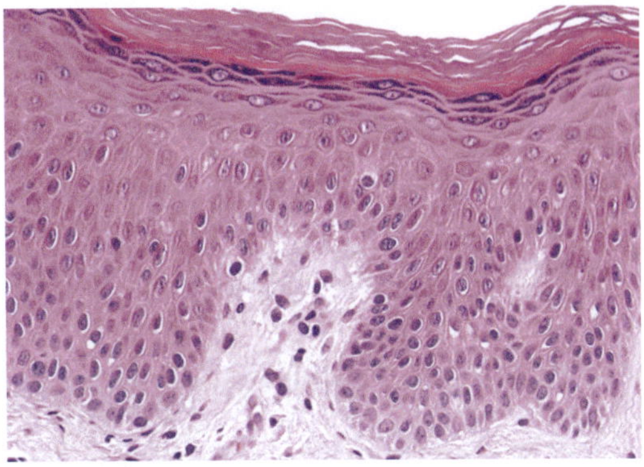

Fig. 1.254 Hyperkeratotic epidermis with hypergranulosis

Atopic Dermatitis

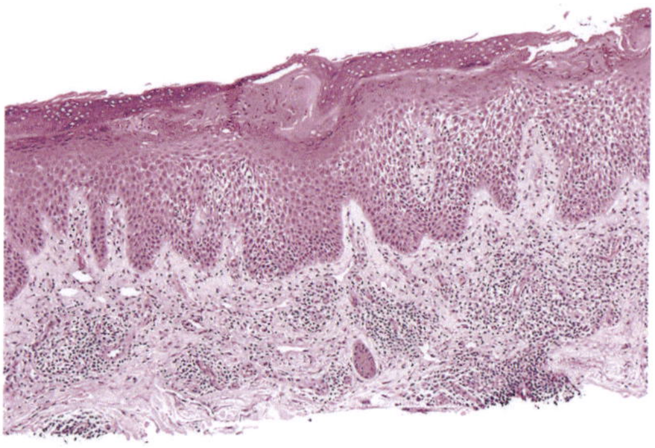

Fig. 1.255 **Subacute atopic dermatitis**

Synonyms: Eczema, Eczematous Dermatitis

Histopathology:

– Usually subacute or chronic spongiotic dermatitis with eosinophils

Subacute: moderate spongiosis, acanthosis, psoriasiform hyperplasia (Figs. 1.255, 1.256, and 1.257)

Chronic: acanthosis, hyperkeratosis, hypergranulosis (Figs. 1.258 and 1.259)

– Both types have perivascular lymphocytic infiltrates and scattered eosinophils but it is more pronounced in subacute stage

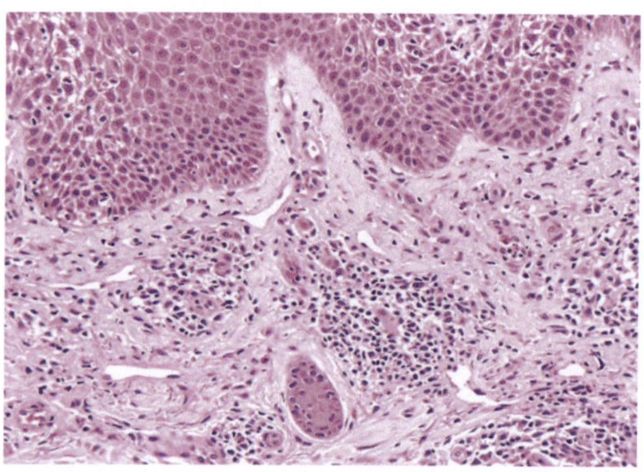

Fig. 1.256 Moderate spongiosis with perivascular inflammation

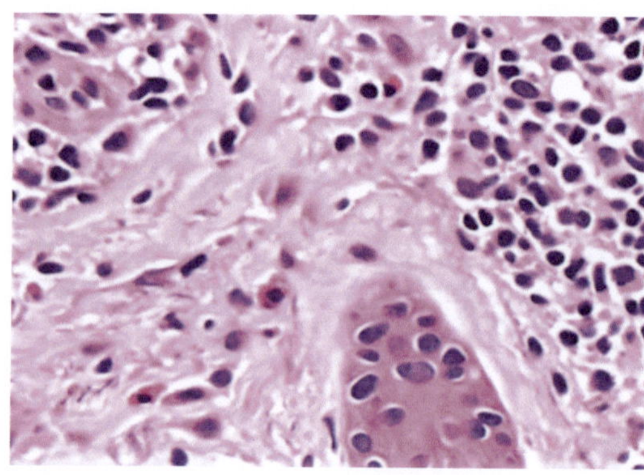

Fig. 1.257 Lymphocytic infiltrate with scattered eosinophils

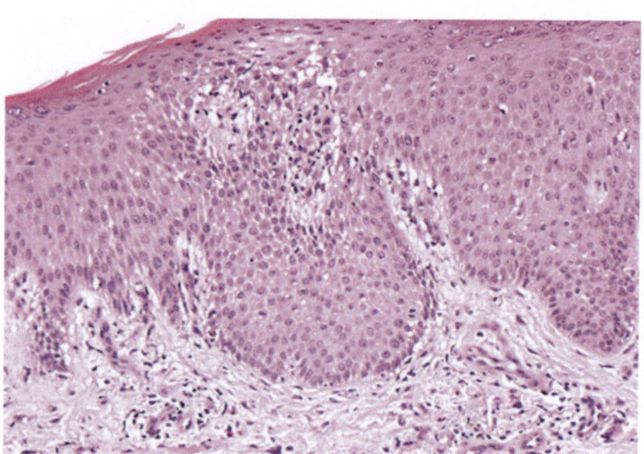

Fig. 1.258 **Chronic atopic dermatitis** with epidermal acanthosis and hyperkeratosis

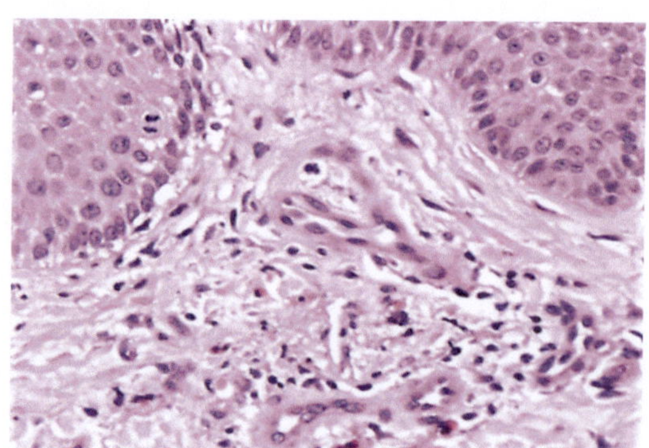

Fig. 1.259 Mild spongiosis with a few lymphocytes and eosinophils

Atrophie Blanche

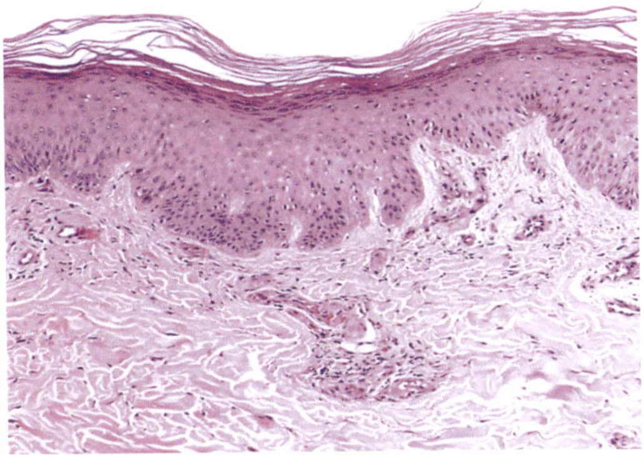

Fig. 1.260 Capillaries in the superficial dermis are affected

Synonyms: Livedo Vasculitis, Segmental Hyalinizing Vasculitis

Histopathology (Figs. 1.260, 1.261, 1.262, 1.263, and 1.264)

- Superficial dermal capillaries with endothelial proliferation and thickening of the wall
- Thrombi in the lumen
- Variable number of extravasated red blood cells
- Variable perivascular lymphocytic inflammation

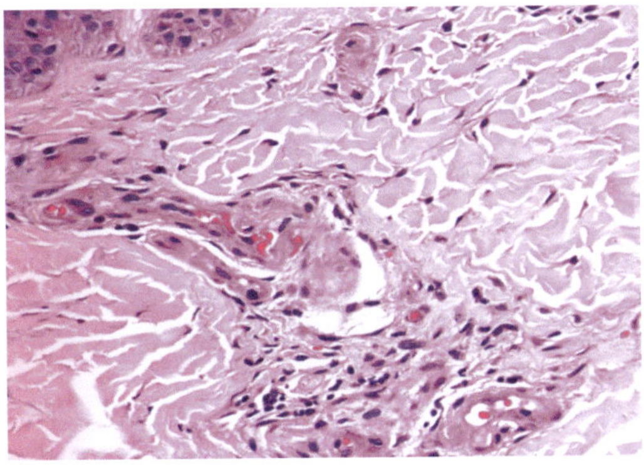

Fig. 1.261 Plump endothelial cells with capillary thrombi

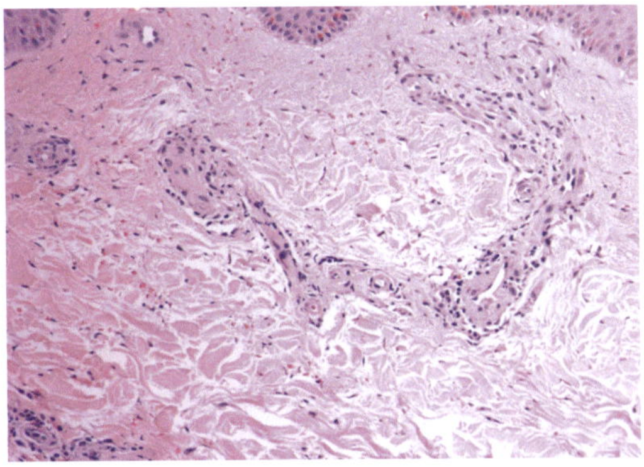

Fig. 1.262 Mild perivascular lymphocytic infiltrate and few extravasated RBCs

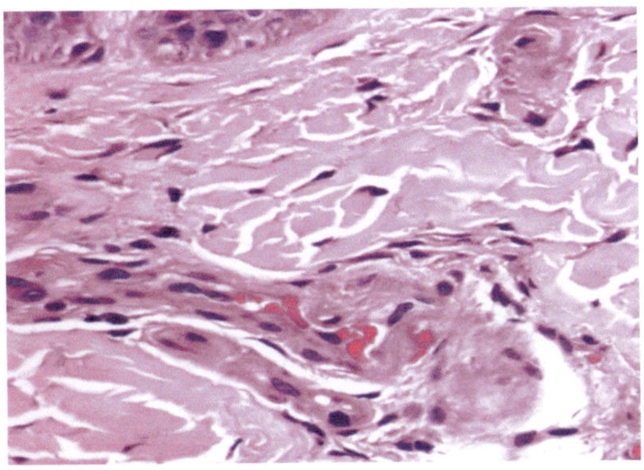

Fig. 1.263 Congested capillaries with thrombi

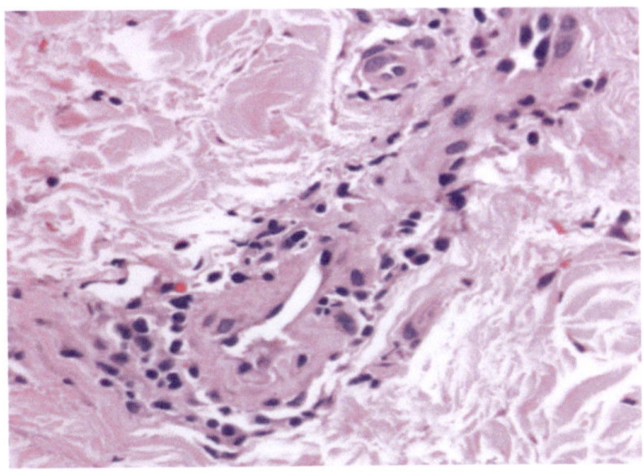

Fig. 1.264 Wall is thickened by fibrinoid material

Atrophoderma of Pasini and Pierini

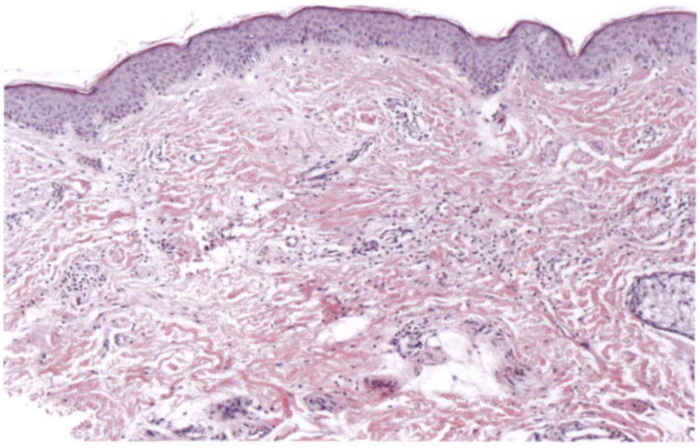

Fig. 1.265 Very subtle dermal changes

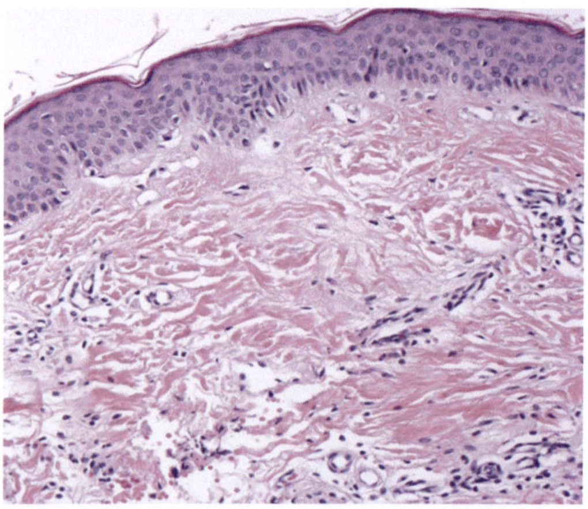

Fig. 1.266 Mild perivascular lymphocytic infiltrate with mildly thickened collagen bundles

Histopathology (Figs. 1.265 and 1.266)

- Findings are very subtle
- Normal or mildly atrophic epidermis
- Mild perivascular lymphocytic inflammation
- Slightly homogenized collagen bundles
- Elastic fibers usually show no changes

Atypical Fibroxanthoma

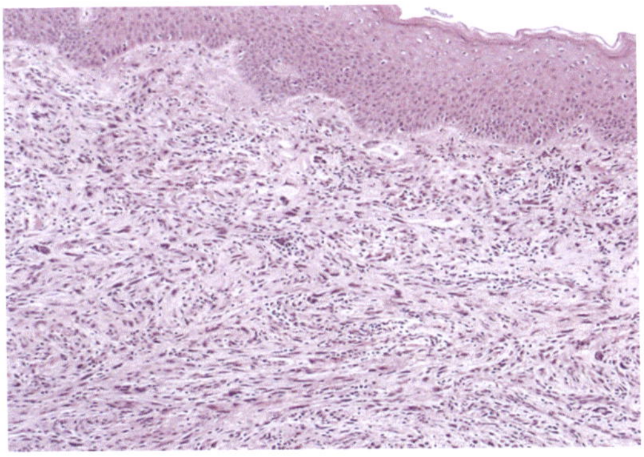

Fig. 1.267 Atypical dermal infiltrate in the background of solar elastosis

Histopathology (Figs. 1.267, 1.268, 1.269, and 1.270)

- Proliferation of atypical spindle cells in the dermis with significant background solar elastosis
- Tumor cells (CD10+, CD68+, factor XIII+) show prominent polymorphism with atypical, bizarre cells
- Mitoses can be numerous
- Tumor usually does not invade subcutis and invasion into subcutis should raise suspicion for pleomorphic sarcoma

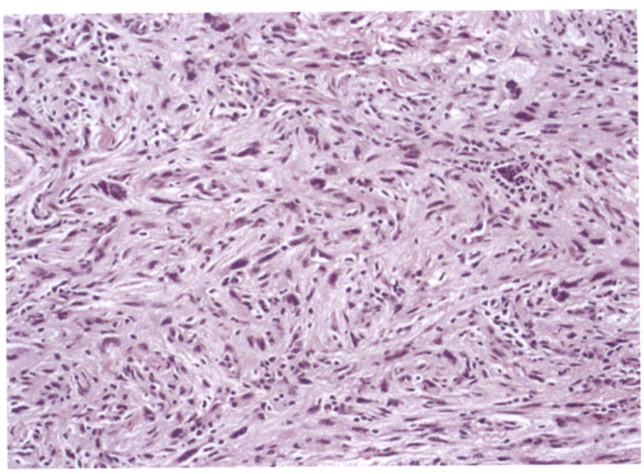

Fig. 1.268 Dermis with spindle cell proliferation

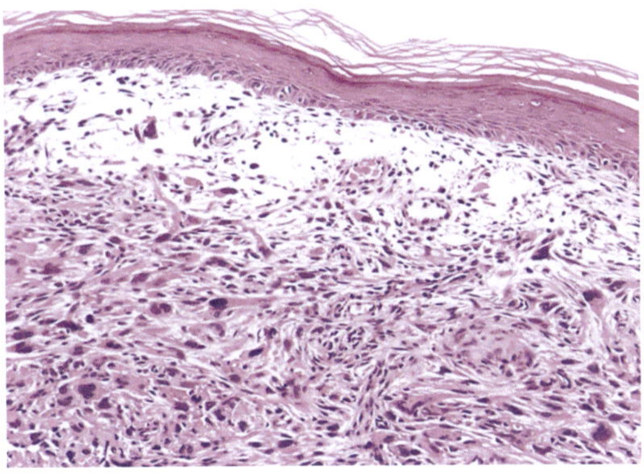

Fig. 1.269 Normal appearing epidermis with dermal atypical tumor

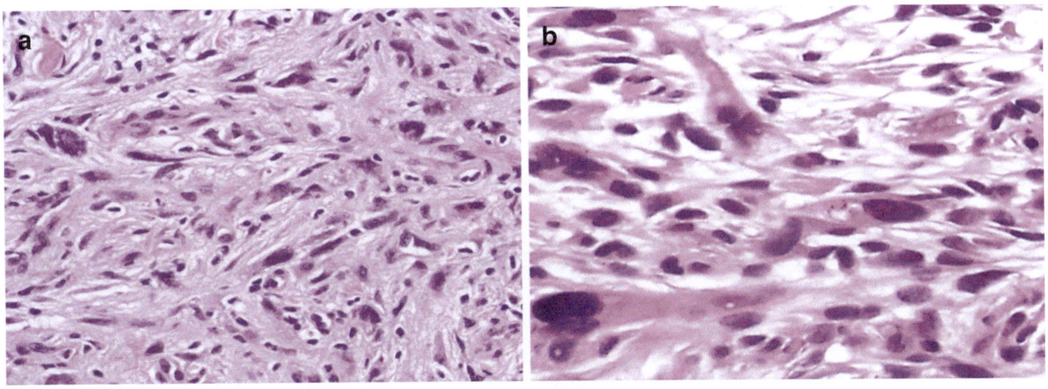

Fig. 1.270 (**a**, **b**) Polymorphic spindle cells with very irregular dark enlarged nuclei

Atypical Mycobacterial Infection

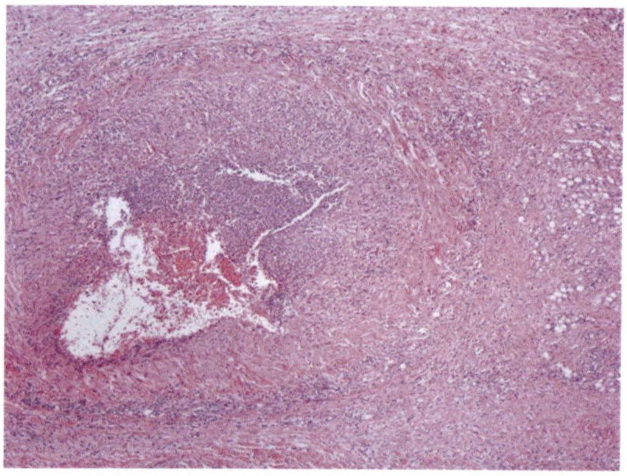

Fig. 1.271 Buruli ulcer

M.ulcerans (Buruli Ulcer) and M.marinum (Swimming Pool Granuloma) cause cutaneous infections.

Buruli ulcer (Figs. 1.271, 1.272, and 1.273)

- Epidermal ulceration
- Suppuration and necrosis of the subcutis
- Numerous mycobacteria in the necrotic area

Swimming Pool Granuloma (Figs. 1.274 and 1.275)

- Inflammation limited to the dermis
- Vague granulomas surrounded by lymphocytes
- No evidence of caseating necrosis
- Mycobacteria rarely found by AFB stain
- Tissue culture needed to confirm diagnosis

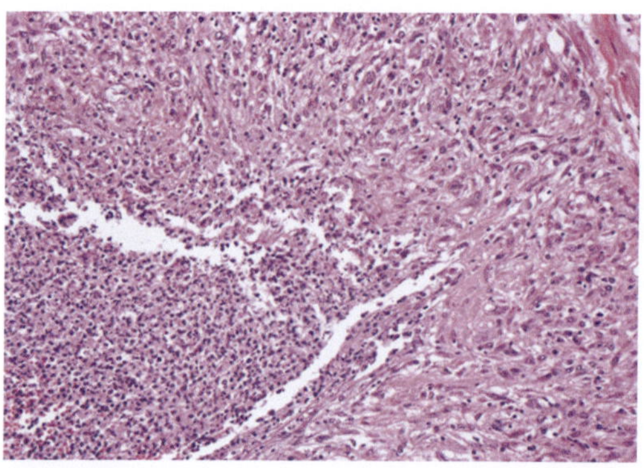

Fig. 1.272 Suppurative, necrotic subcutis with an abscess

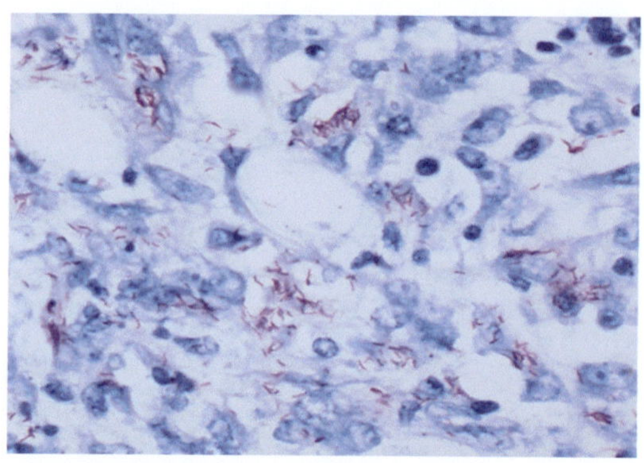

Fig. 1.273 AFB stain highlights mycobacteria

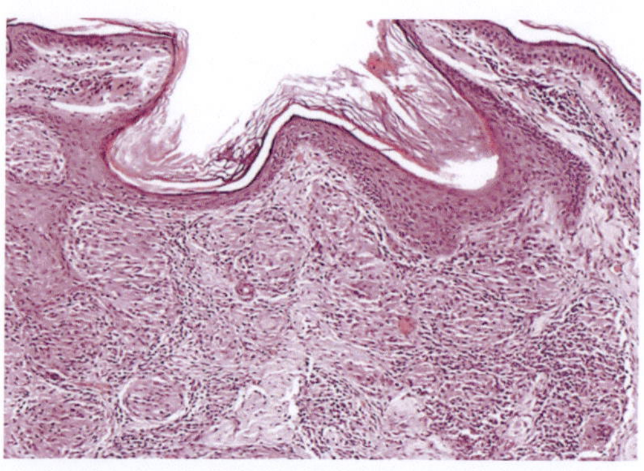

Fig. 1.274 **Swimming Pool Granuloma** with vague dermal epithelioid granulomas with no evidence of necrosis

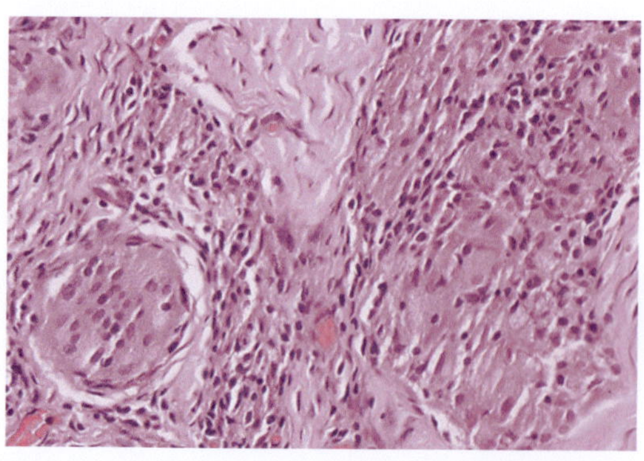

Fig. 1.275 Lymphocytes surround granulomas

Axillary Granular Parakeratosis

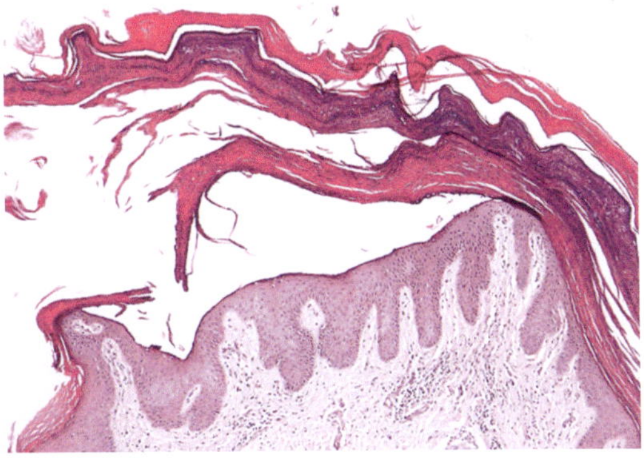

Fig. 1.276 Hyperkeratotic epidermis with irregular papillomatosis

Synonym: Granular Parakeratosis

Histopathology (Figs. 1.276, 1.277, and 1.278)

- Extensive hyperkeratosis with characteristic dark eosinophilic stratum corneum
- Parakeratosis with retention of keratohyaline granules

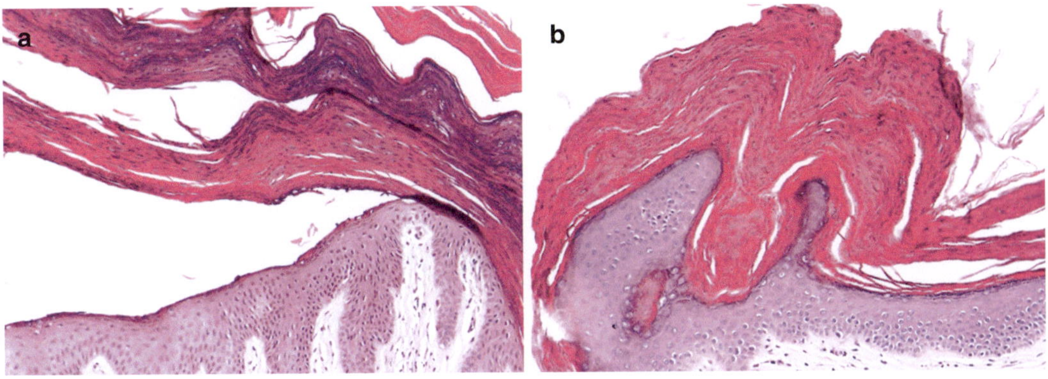

Fig. 1.277 (**a**, **b**) Characteristic darkly eosinophilic (pink) stratum corneum

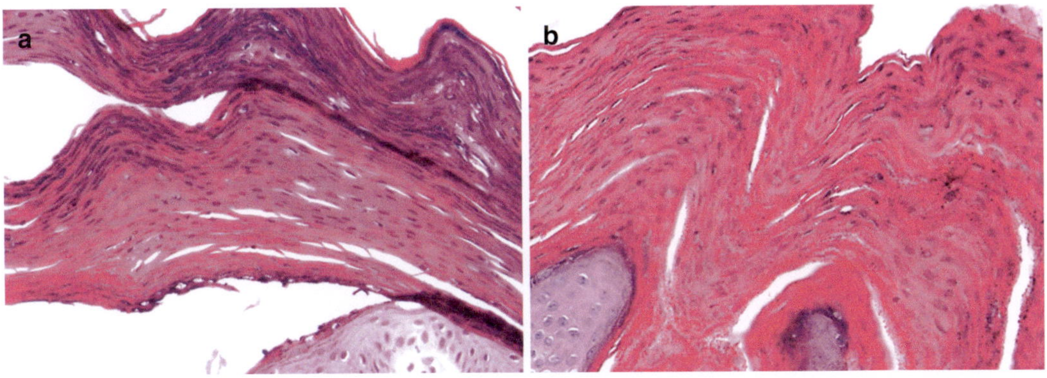

Fig. 1.278 (**a**, **b**) Stratum corneum with parakeratosis and retention of keratohyaline granules

2 Dermatopathology B

V. Vincek, *Dermatopathology A–Z*, https://doi.org/10.1007/978-3-319-89486-7_2

Bacillary Angiomatosis

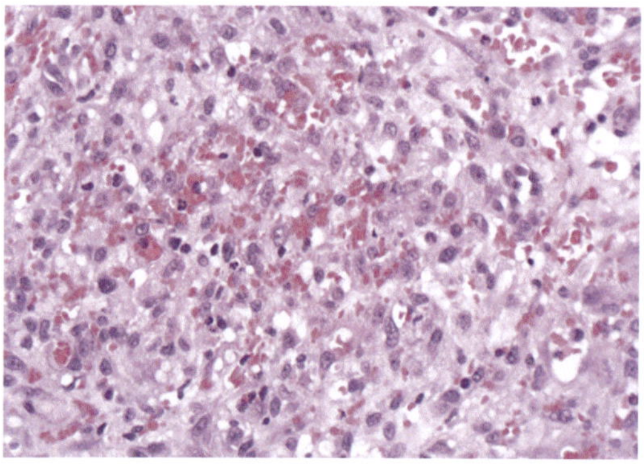

Fig. 2.1 Numerous tightly grouped small capillaries

Histopathology (Figs. 2.1, 2.2, 2.3, 2.4, and 2.5)

- Numerous small vascular channels
- Endothelial cells with epithelioid appearance and mild atypia
- Scattered mitoses are common
- Neutrophils in between vessels
- Red blood cell extravasation
- Silver stain outlines *Bartonella* in areas rich with neutrophils

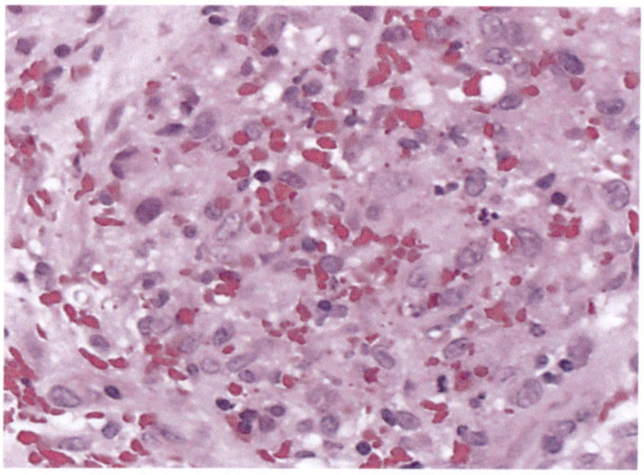

Fig. 2.2 Plump endothelial cells with scattered mitoses

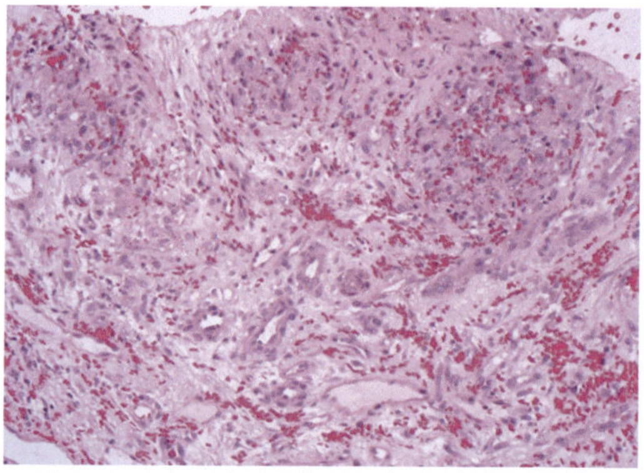

Fig. 2.3 Extensive red blood cell extravasation

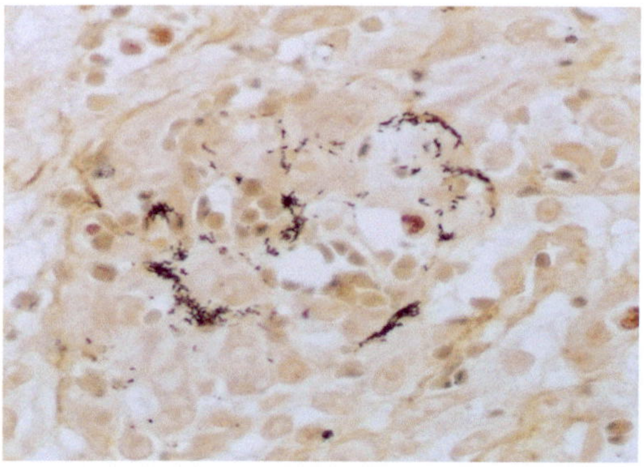

Fig. 2.4 Warthin Starry stain highlights *Bartonella*

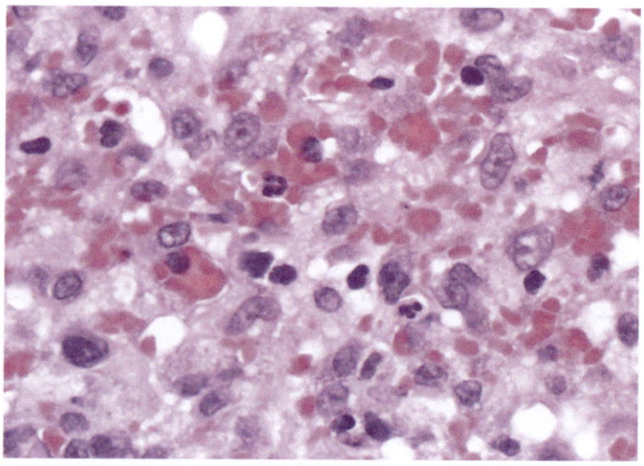

Fig. 2.5 Scattered neutrophils

Balloon Cell Nevus

Histopathology (Figs. 2.6, 2.7, and 2.8)

- Nevus made of 50% or more of pale, swollen, clear cell melanocytes ("balloon" cells)
- Remaining nevus cell are normal nevus cells
- Ordinary nevus cells and "balloon" nevus cells demonstrate maturation
- There is no evidence of mitosis or atypia

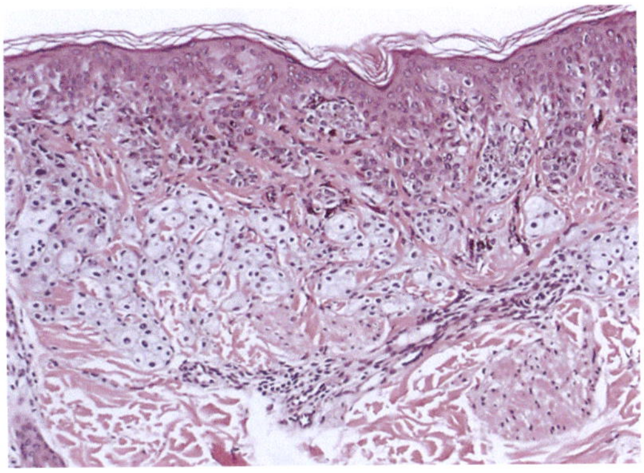

Fig. 2.6 Compound nevus with clear cell features

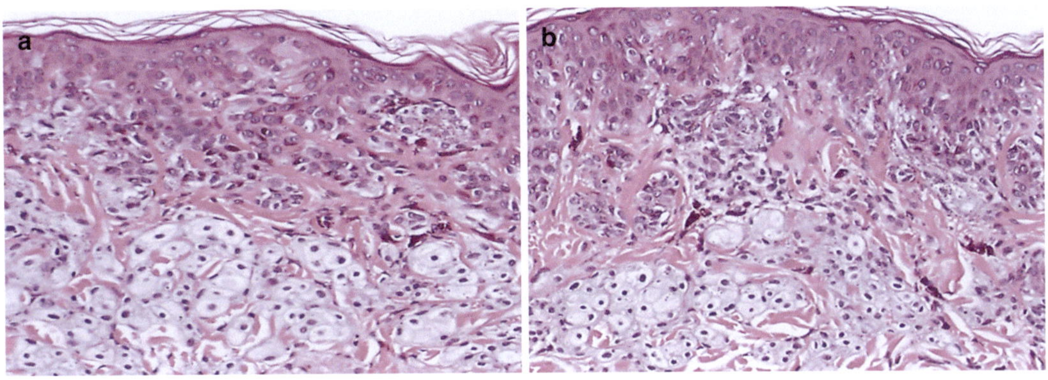

Fig. 2.7 (**a**, **b**) Nevus with more than 50% of cells with clear cell features; nevus cells demonstrate maturation with descent

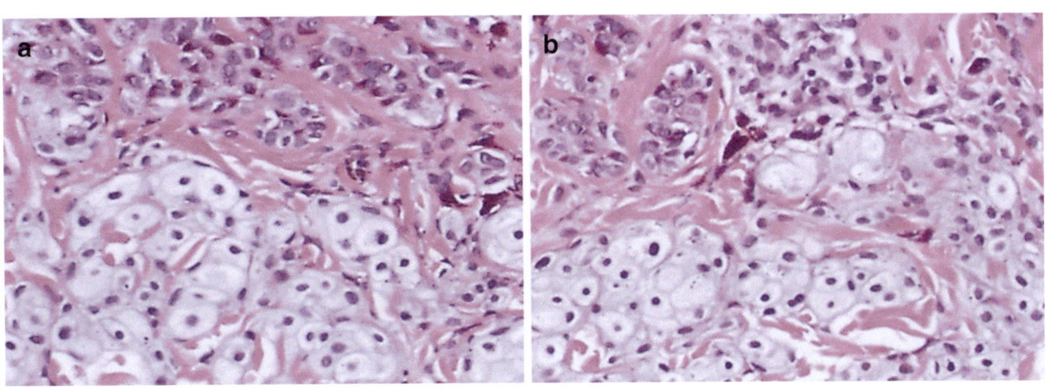

Fig. 2.8 (**a**, **b**) Cells have dark uniform nuclei and pale large cytoplasm and there is no evidence of atypia or mitosis

Basal Cell Carcinoma

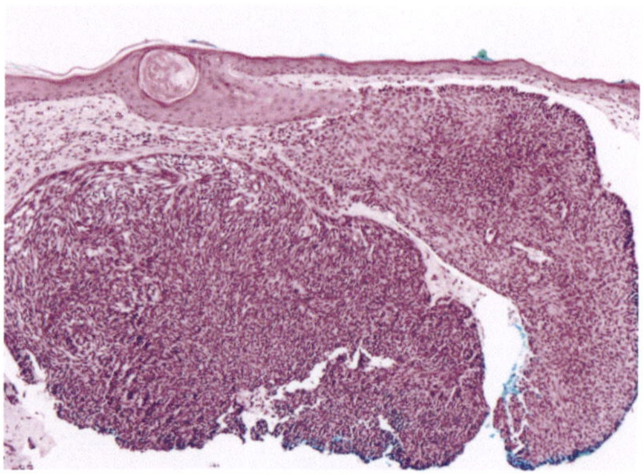

Fig. 2.9 **Nodular BCC** made of large basaloid dermal nodules

Variable **histopathology** with multiple variants but most of them demonstrate (Figs. 2.9, 2.10, 2.11, 2.12, 2.13, 2.14, 2.15, 2.16, 2.17, 2.18, and 2.19)

- Epidermal attachment of atypical basaloid dark cells (BerEP4+, EMA-, CEA-)
- Peripheral palisading of tumor cells
- Retraction of tumor from bluish myxoid stroma
- Variable number of mitoses or necrotic cells

P.S. associated with Gorlin's syndrome (*PTCH*)

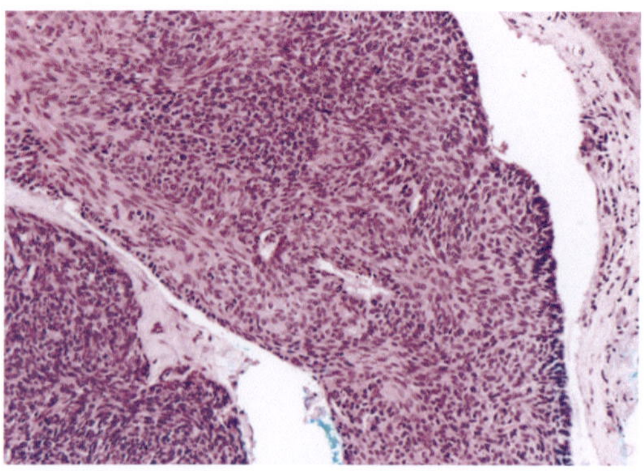

Fig. 2.10 Basaloid cells with retraction from surrounding myxoid stroma

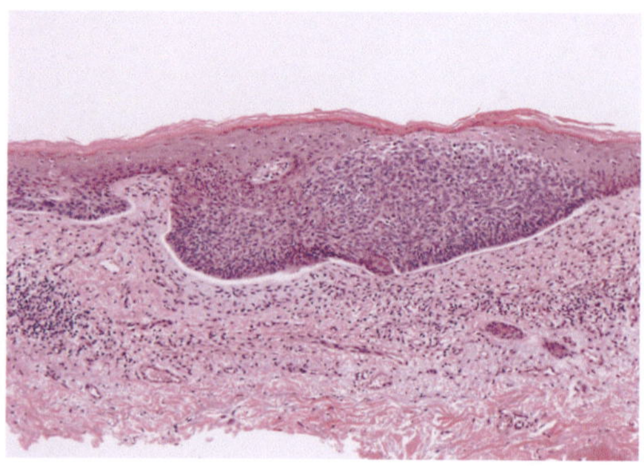

Fig. 2.11 **Superficial BCC** made of multiple small islands of basaloid cells confined to the upper dermis

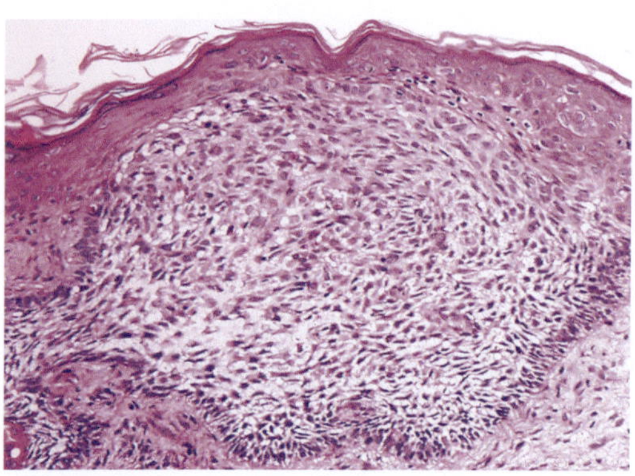

Fig. 2.12 **BCC with clear cell features**

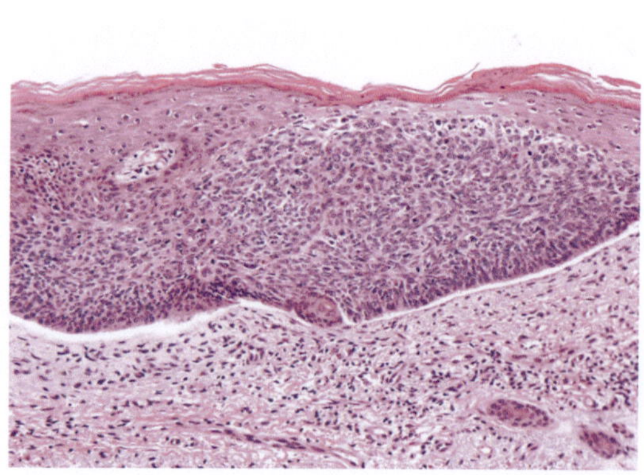

Fig. 2.13 Peripheral palisading and stromal retraction

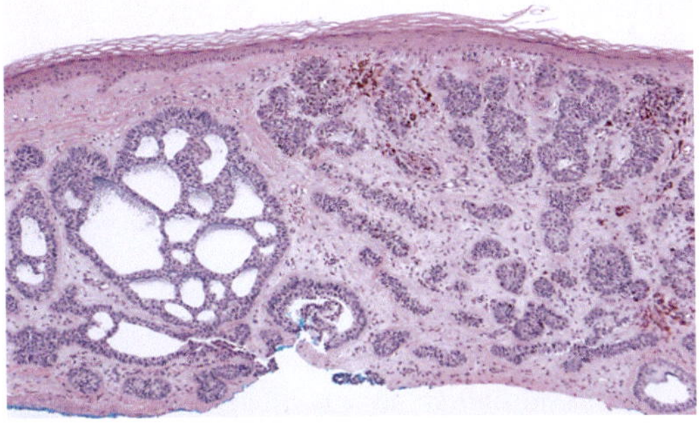

Fig. 2.14 **Adenoid cystic BCC** to the left and **pigmented BCC** with pigment in tumor cells and stroma to the right

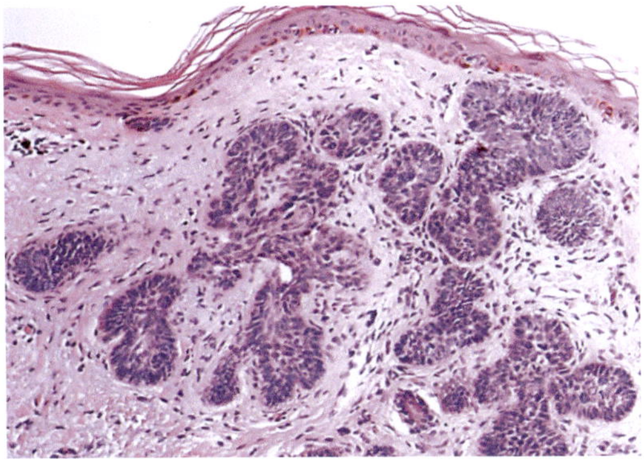

Fig. 2.15 **Micronodular BCC** with small basaloid nodules present in myxoid stroma

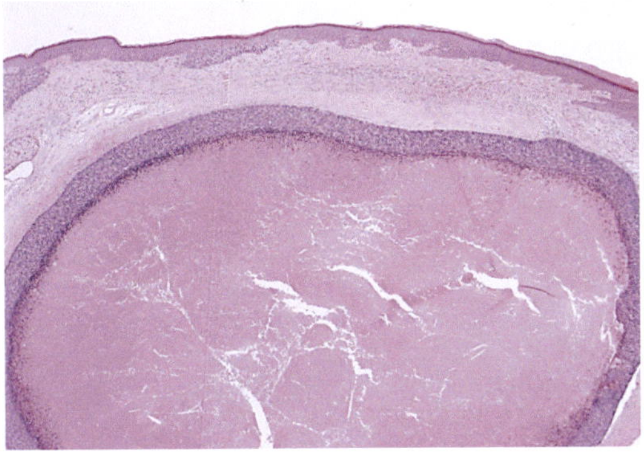

Fig. 2.16 **Cystic BCC** with large cyst lined with basaloid cells and the lumen filled with necrotic tissue

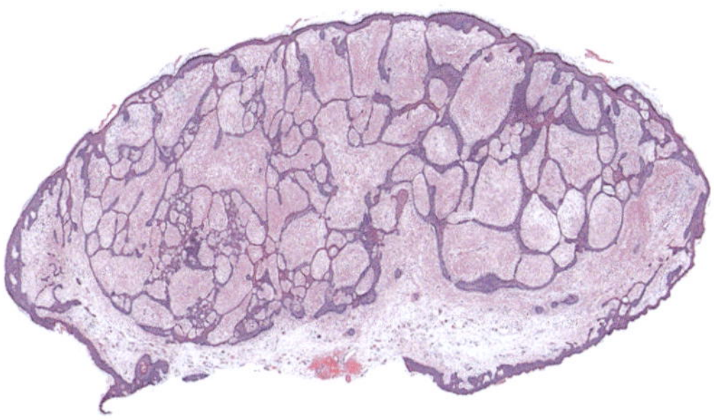

Fig. 2.17 Polypoid **Fibroepithelioma BCC** with basaloid cords attached to the epidermis at multiple points

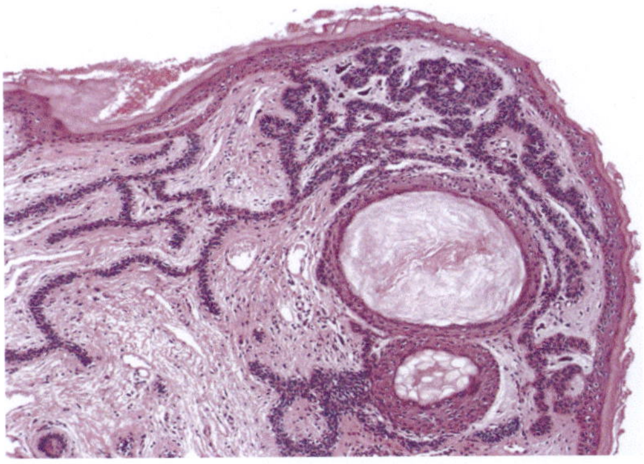

Fig. 2.18 **Infundibulocystic BCC** made of anastomosing strands of basaloid cells and small cysts

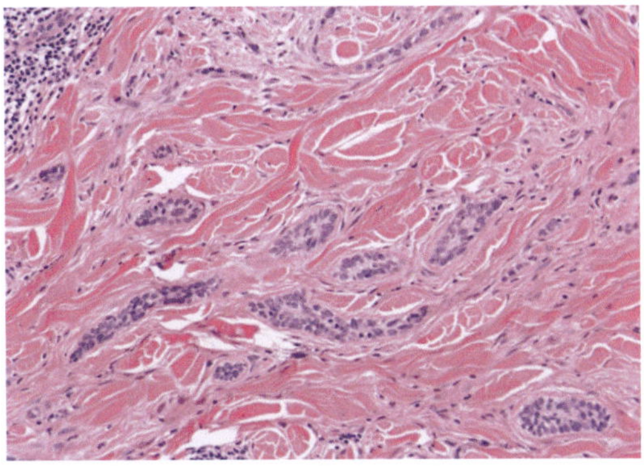

Fig. 2.19 **Morpheaform BCC** made of narrow bands of basaloid cells in dense stroma with minimal stromal retraction

Basaloid Follicular Hamartoma

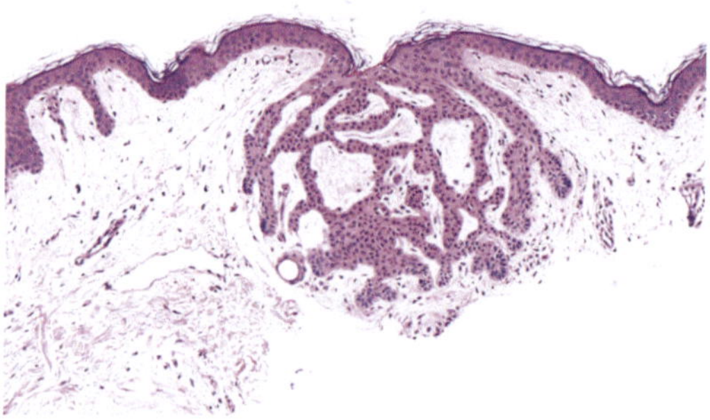

Fig. 2.20 Small reticulated tumor

Histopathology (Figs. 2.20, 2.21, and 2.22)

- Strands of basaloid cells in reticulated pattern
- Small trichillemal cysts are present
- No significant stromal retraction
- No significant atypia or mitoses

P.S. although many believe it is a hamartomatous lesion some believe it represents an incipient trichoepithelioma

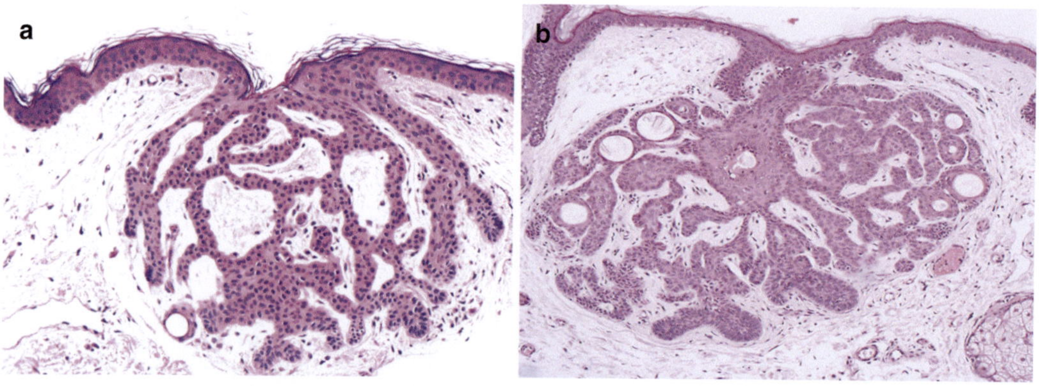

Fig. 2.21 (**a**, **b**) Strands of basaloid cells extending from central primitive follicle

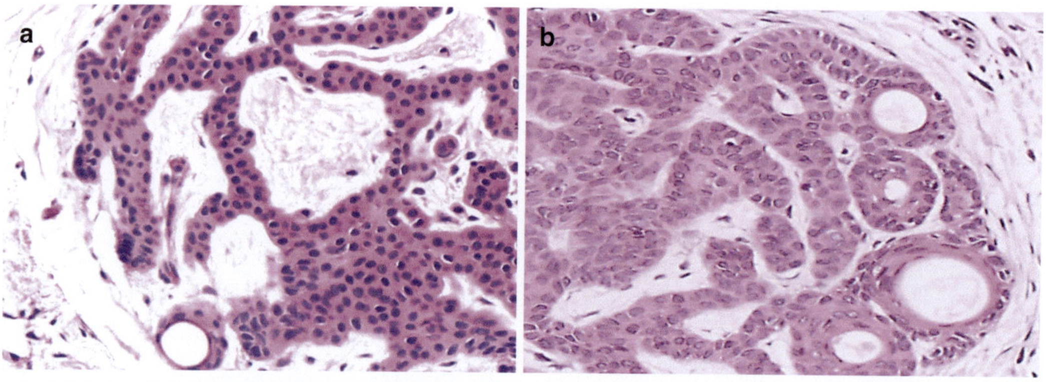

Fig. 2.22 (**a**, **b**) No stromal retraction or cytological atypia; small cysts are present

Becker's Nevus

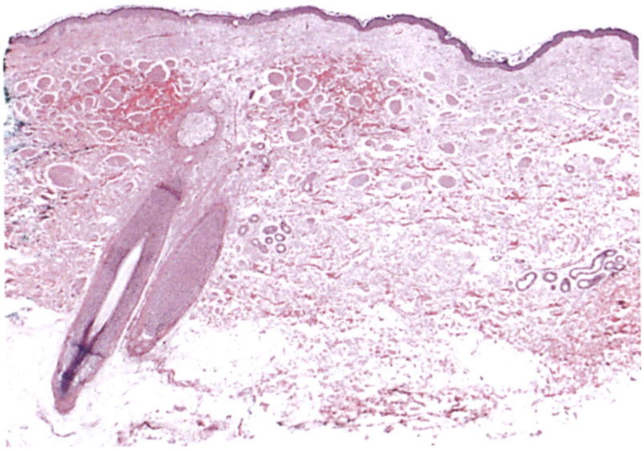

Fig. 2.23 Muscle fascicles scattered in the dermis

Synonym: Smooth Muscle Hamartoma

Histopathology (Figs. 2.23, 2.24, 2.25, and 2.26)

- Epidermal acanthosis and basal layer hyperpigmentation
- Increased number of smooth muscles arranged in the dermis in a haphazard manner usually around hair follicle
- Number of hair follicles sometimes increased

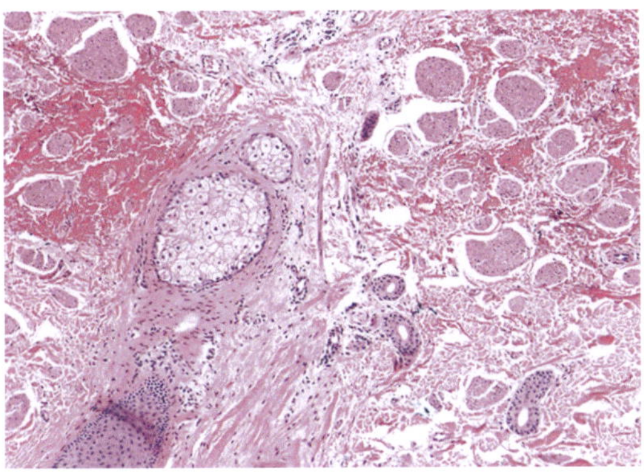

Fig. 2.24 Haphazardly arranged muscle bundles around the follicle

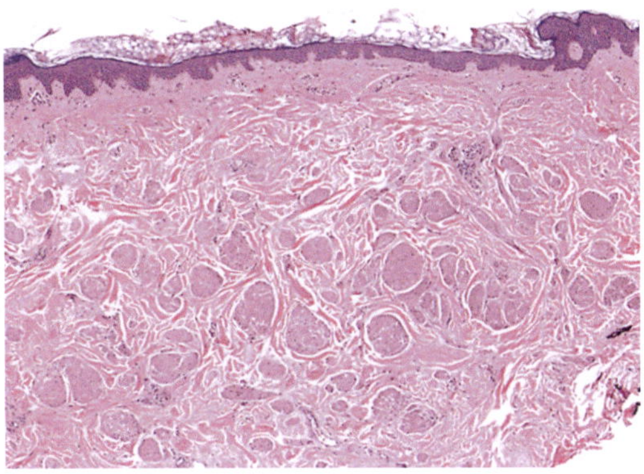

Fig. 2.25 Acanthotic epidermis with scattered dermal muscle bundles

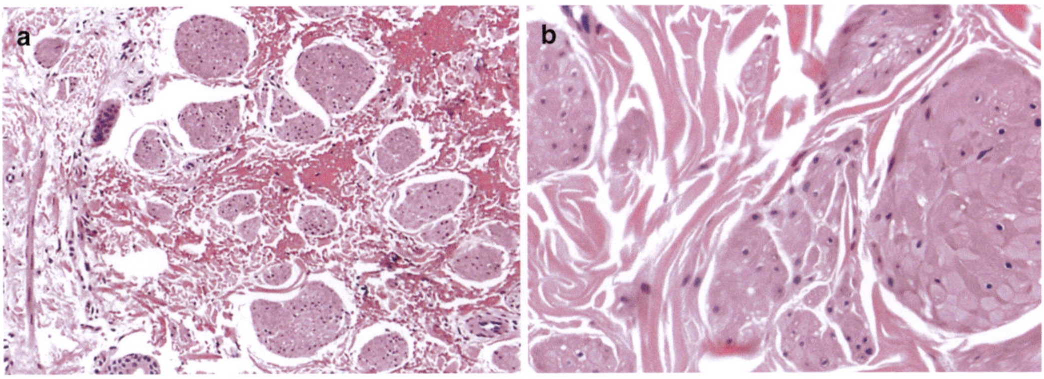

Fig. 2.26 (**a**, **b**) Muscle cells don't show any atypia and mitoses are absent

Bednar's Tumor

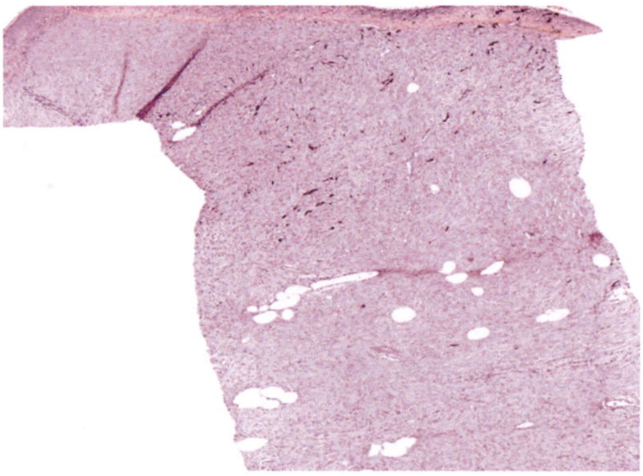

Fig. 2.27 Dermal and subcutaneous tumor

Synonym: Pigmented Dermatofibrosarcoma Protuberans

Histopathology (Figs. 2.27, 2.28, 2.29, and 2.30)

- Dermal and subcutaneous spindle cell tumor
- Storiform pattern
- Monotonous population of spindled fibroblasts (factor XIII+, CD34+)
- Diffuse infiltration of fat
- Scattered melanin within dendritic cells

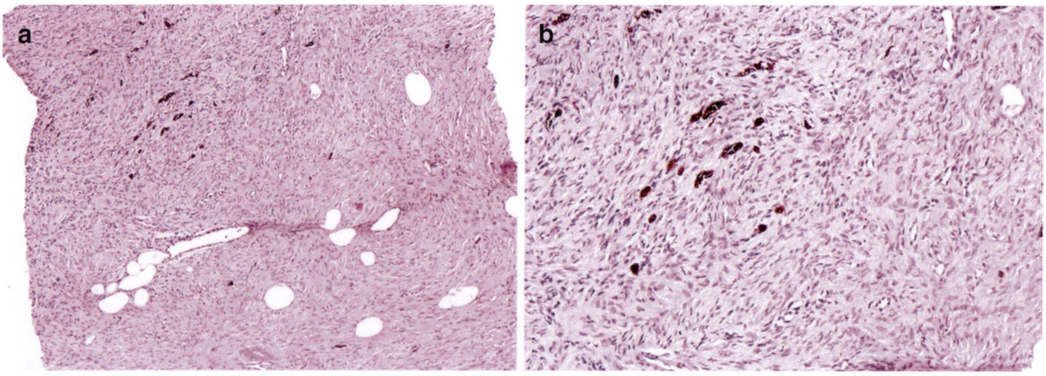

Fig. 2.28 (**a**, **b**) Uniform spindle cells organized in storiform pattern infiltrating into the adipose tissue

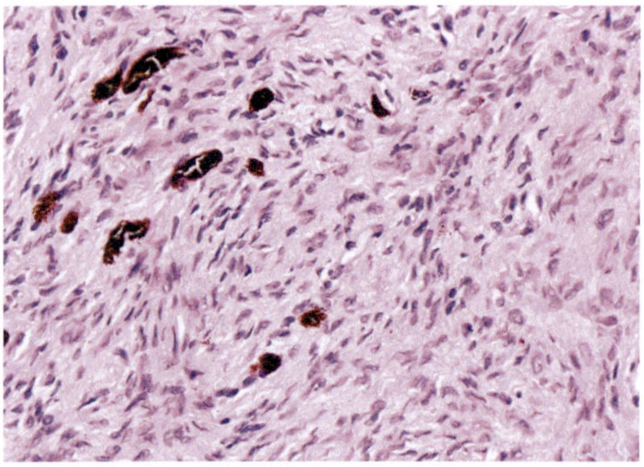

Fig. 2.29 Melanin filled dendrocytes are observed

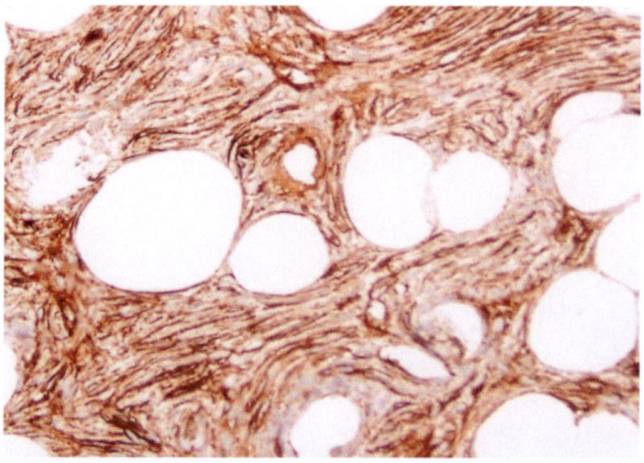

Fig. 2.30 Tumor cells are CD34 positive

Behçet's Disease

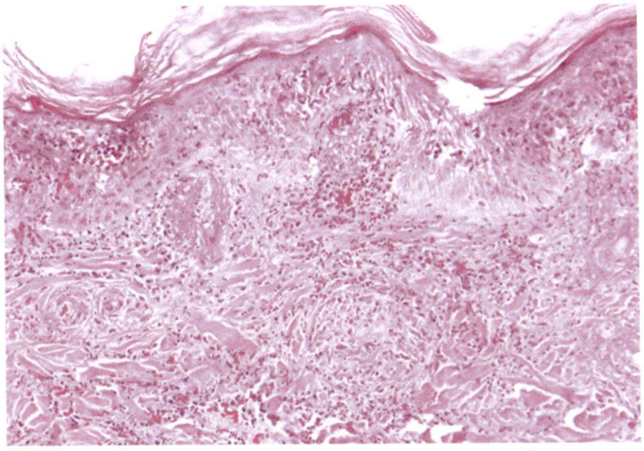

Fig. 2.31 Dermal leukocytoclasia and RBC extravasation

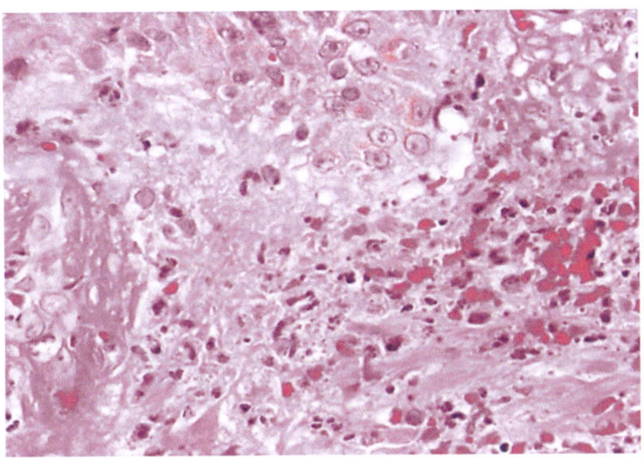

Fig. 2.32 Dermal neutrophilic inflammation

Histopathology is not specific and clinical correlation is necessary (Figs. 2.31, 2.32, 2.33, and 2.34).

Oral Aphthae and Genital Ulcers:

- Ulcer with lymphocytes, histiocytes and neutrophils at the ulcer base

Erythema Nodosum-like Lesions:

- Findings of erythema nodosum with necrobiosis and neutrophilic/lymphocytic vasculitis

Pathergy Reaction:

- Perivascular lymphocytic inflammation with variable neutrophilic vasculitis

Thrombophlebitis:

- Thrombi in larger veins with perivascular lymphocytic inflammation

Papulopustular Lesions (the most common cutaneous manifestation):

- Spongiosis with intraepidermal pustules
- Focal basal layer vacuolization
- Epidermal neutrophilic/lymphocytic exocytosis
- Dermal neutrophilic inflammation with admixed lymphocytes and histiocytes
- Variable leukocytoclastic vasculitis and fibrin deposition

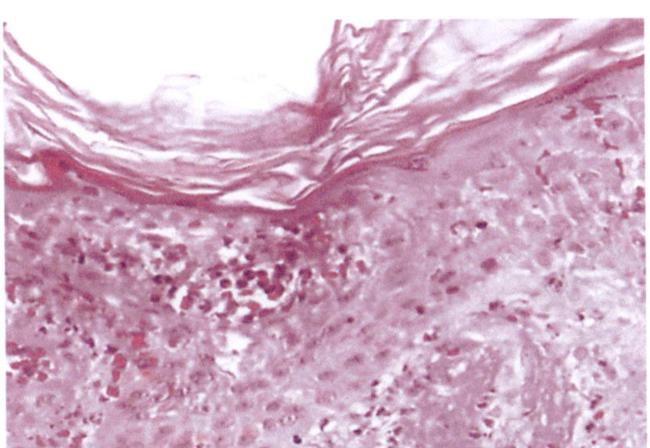

Fig. 2.33 Epidermal neutrophilic exocytosis and micropustule

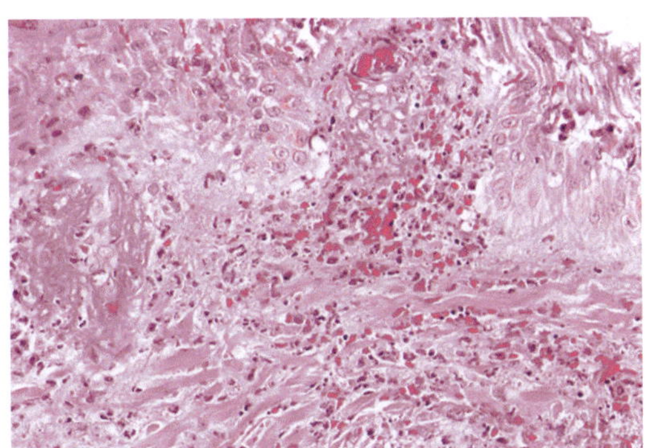

Fig. 2.34 Fibrin deposition within vessel wall

Blastomycosis

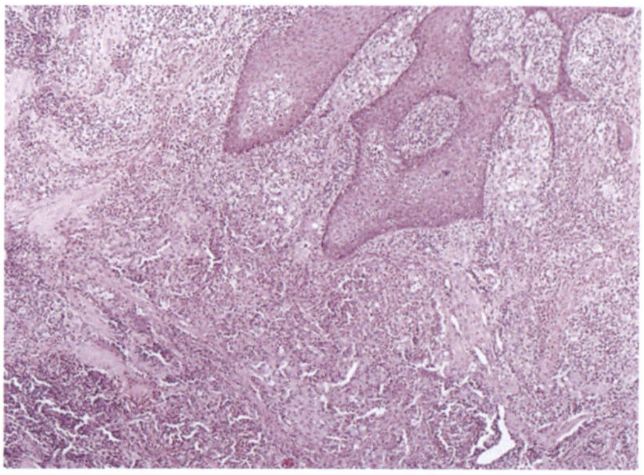

Fig. 2.35 Pseudoepitheliomatous hyperplasia with exuberant inflammation

Synonyms: North American Blastomycosis, Chicago Disease

Histopathology (Figs. 2.35, 2.36, 2.37, 2.38, and 2.39)

- Pseudoepitheliomatous hyperplasia
- Dermal neutrophilic infiltrate and microabscess
- Scattered giant cells
- Suppurative granulomas may be present
- Thick-walled spores that can have broad-based buds

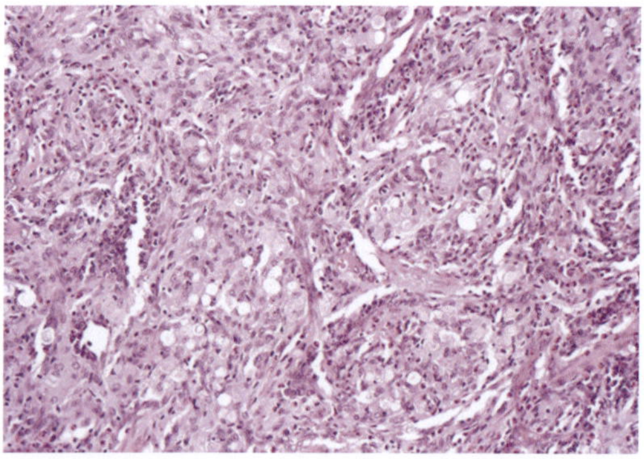

Fig. 2.36 Numerous neutrophils, histiocytes, and some giant cells

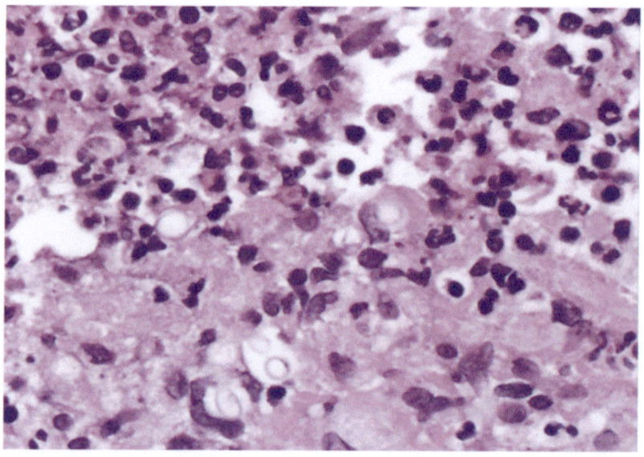

Fig. 2.37 Abscess with thick-walled fungus outside and within histiocytes

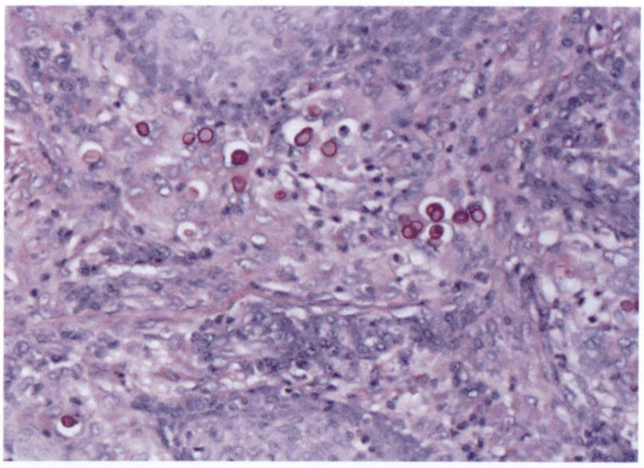

Fig. 2.38 PAS stain highlights spores within microabscesses

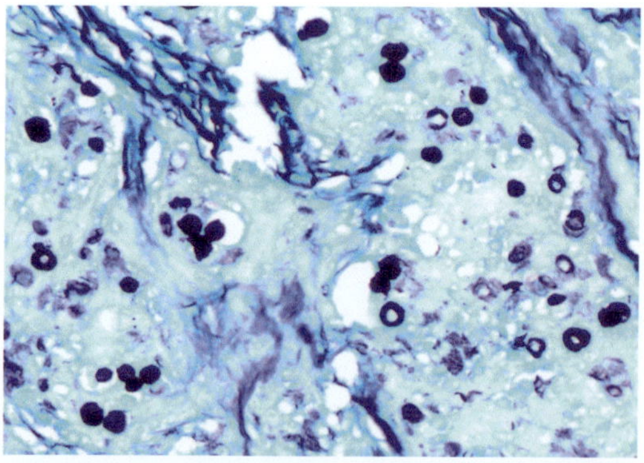

Fig. 2.39 Fungal elements with broad-based budding (GMS)

Blastomycosis-Like Pyoderma

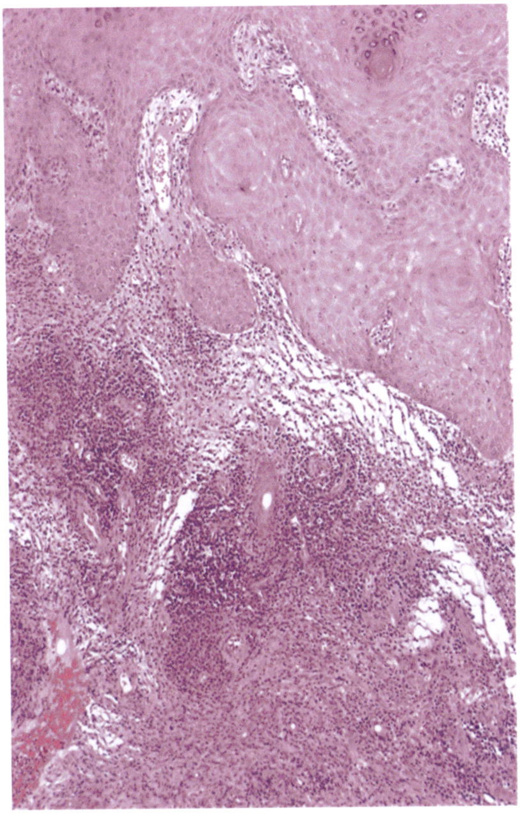

Fig. 2.40 Pseudoepitheliomatous hyperplasia with extensive inflammation

Synonym: Pyoderma Vegetans

Histopathology (Figs. 2.40, 2.41, and 2.42)

- Extensive pseudoepitheliomatous hyperplasia
- Epidermal and dermal microabscesses
- Exuberant dermal acute and chronic inflammation
- Bacterial colonies present particularly around areas rich in neutrophils

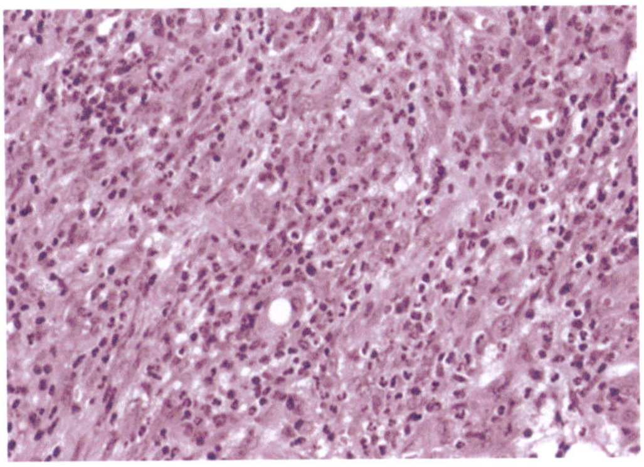

Fig. 2.41 Numerous neutrophils forming abscess

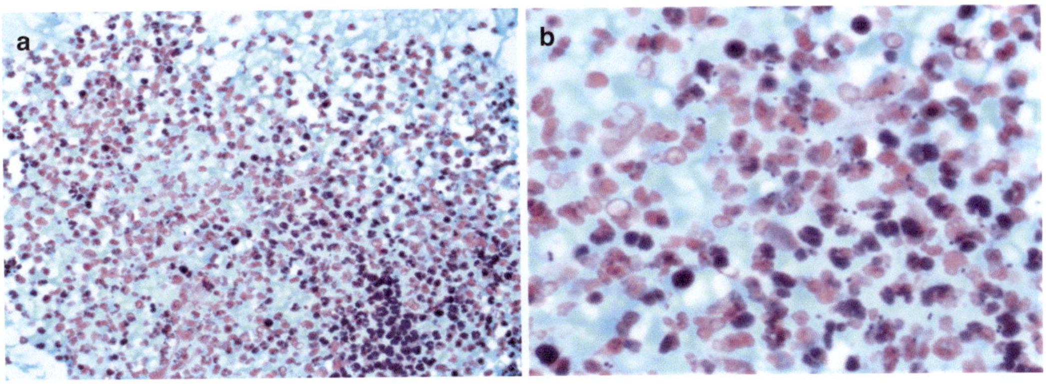

Fig. 2.42 (**a**, **b**) Gram stain identifies bacterial colonies within neutrophils rich area

Blue Nevus

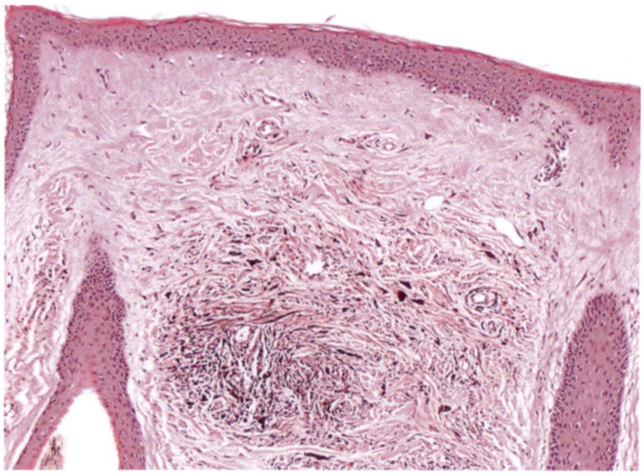

Fig. 2.43 Pigmented spindle lesion in the upper dermis

Synonym: Common Blue Nevus

Histopathology (Figs. 2.43, 2.44, and 2.45)

- Dermal elongated pigmented dendritic melanocytes
- Thickened hyalinized collagen bundles
- Spindle cells like to encircle adnexal and neurovascular structures
- Melanocytes respect adnexal structure (unlike melanoma)

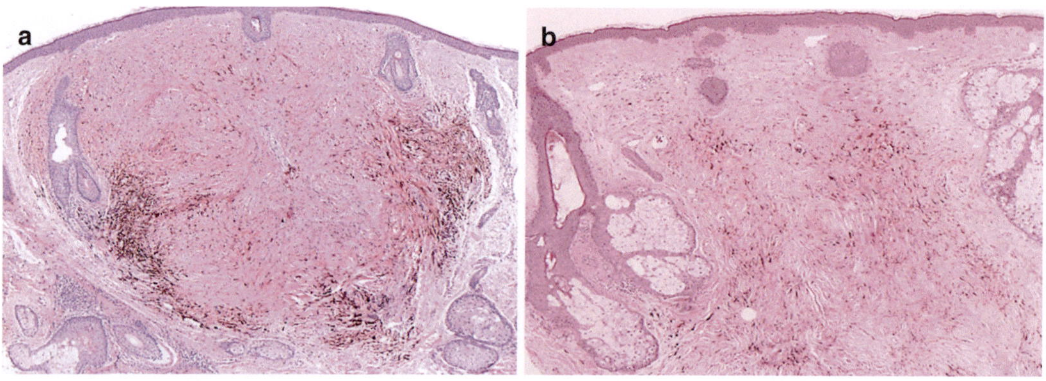

Fig. 2.44 (a, b) Melanocytic proliferation preserves adnexal structures while pink collagen and brown pigment stand out

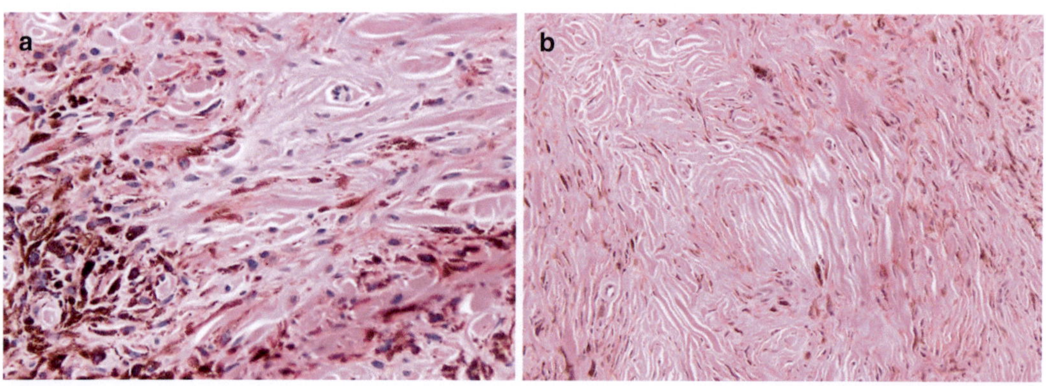

Fig. 2.45 (a, b) Pigmented elongated melanocytes with no atypia or mitoses are dispersed among thick hyalinized collagen bundles

Botryomycosis

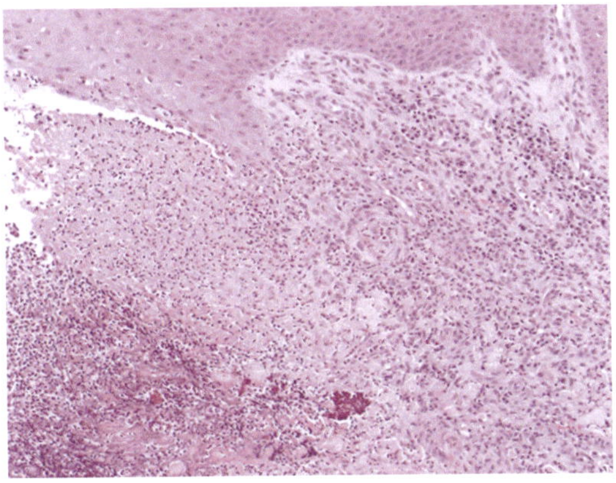

Fig. 2.46 Exuberant neutrophilic infiltrate forming abscess

Histopathology (Figs. 2.46, 2.47, 2.48, and 2.49)

- Large dermal/subcutaneous abscess
- Dark purple granules made of bacterial colonies admixed with neutrophils, so-called "sulfur granules", are pathognomonic
- *S. aureus* is the most common bacteria
- *Pseudomonas*, *E. coli*, *Proteus*, *Streptococci* can be also present

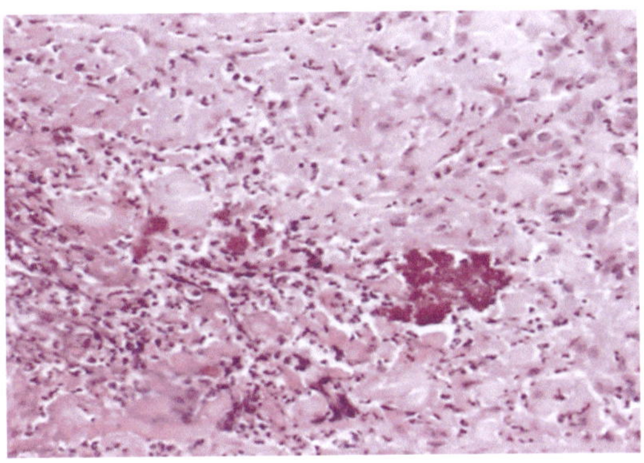

Fig. 2.47 "Sulfur granules" are present within an abscess

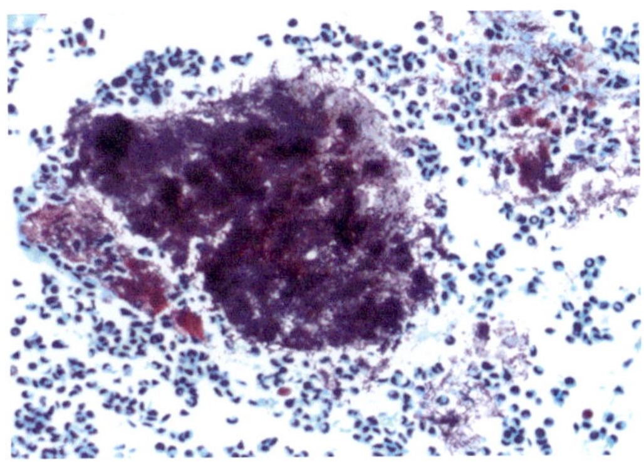

Fig. 2.48 Gram stain highlights bacterial colonies

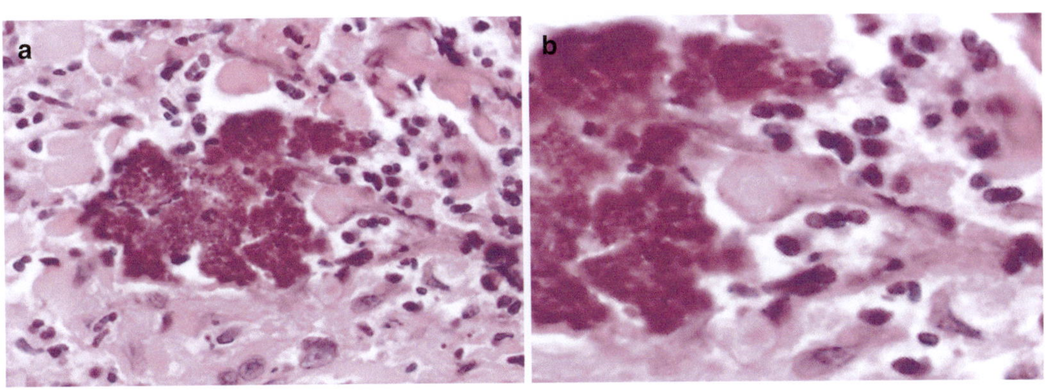

Fig. 2.49 (**a**, **b**) Dark purple bacteria form granule surrounded by neutrophils

Bowen's Disease

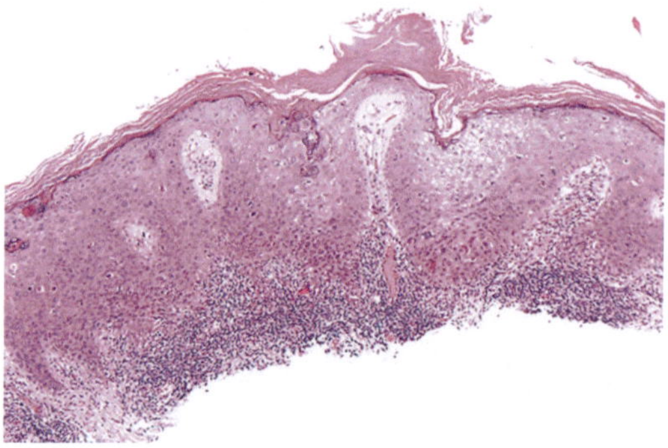

Fig. 2.50 Hypertrophic highly atypical epidermis

Synonym: In-Situ Squamous Cell Carcinoma

Histopathology (Figs. 2.50, 2.51, and 2.52)

- Full thickness atypia of the epidermis
- Keratinocytes do not mature
- Numerous apoptotic keratinocytes with scattered mitoses
- Epidermis is usually acanthotic and hyperkeratotic but can be also atrophic

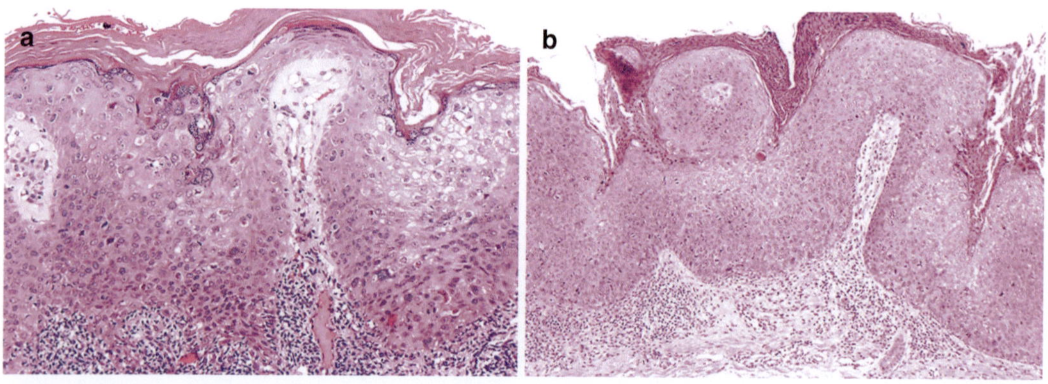

Fig. 2.51 (a, b) Hyperkeratotic acanthotic epidermis with full thickness epidermal atypia

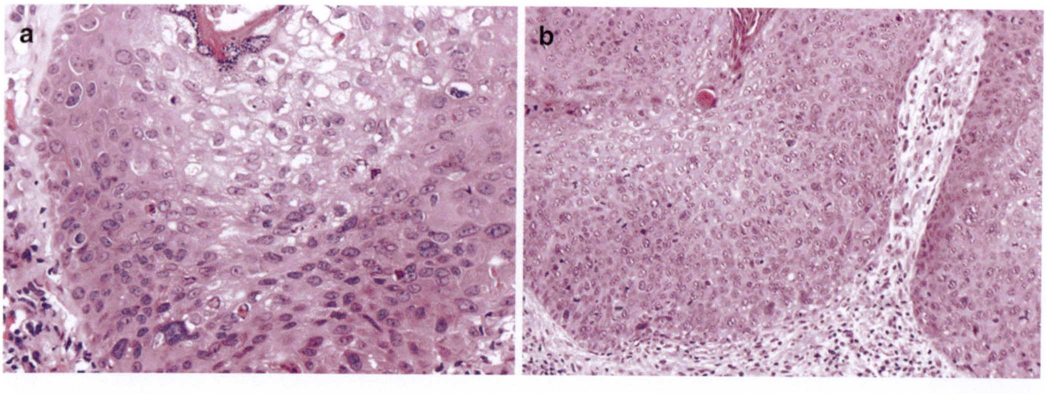

Fig. 2.52 (a, b) Numerous mitoses and apoptotic keratinocytes with cytological atypia and lack of keratinocytic maturation

Bowenoid Papulosis

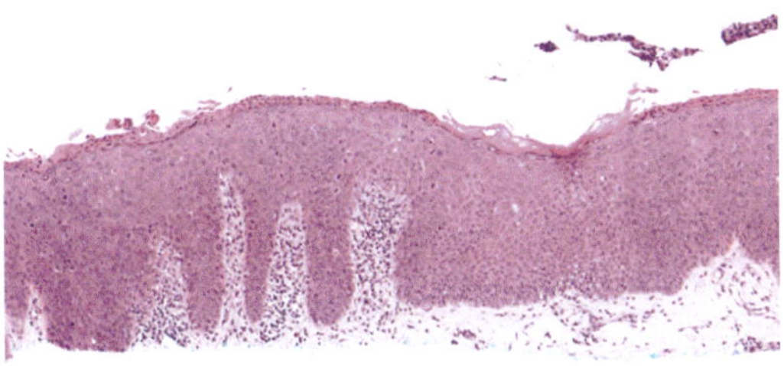

Fig. 2.53 Hypertrophic highly atypical epidermis

Histopathology (Figs. 2.53, 2.54, 2.55, 2.56, and 2.57)

- Full thickness epidermal atypia but not as prominent and irregular as in Bowen's disease
- Loss of maturation with frequent parakeratosis
- Numerous apoptotic keratinocyte and multiple mitoses

P.S. many believe that Bowenoid papulosis is Bowen's disease in genital area. In author's opinion "uniform" atypia of keratinocytes from the top to bottom of epidermis separates Bowenoid papulosis from Bowen's disease

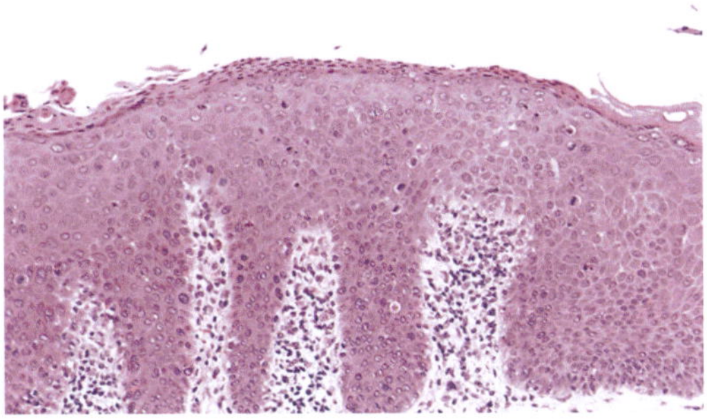

Fig. 2.54 Acanthosis with full thickness epidermal atypia

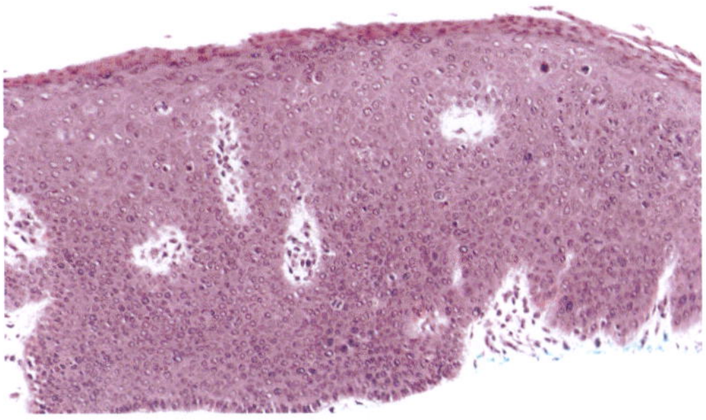

Fig. 2.55 Atypical epidermis with thin layer of parakeratosis

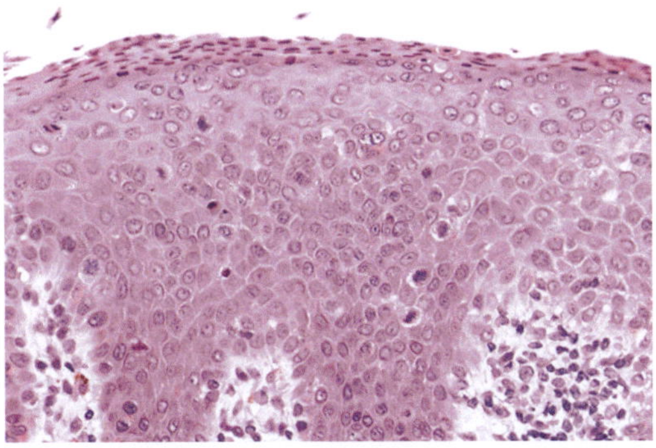

Fig. 2.56 Numerous scattered apoptotic keratinocytes

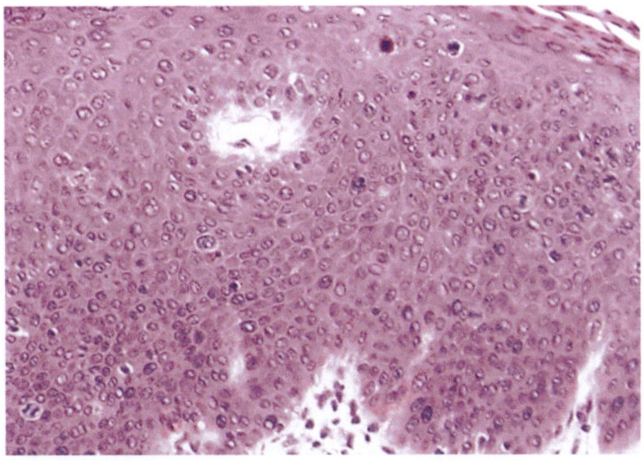

Fig. 2.57 Relatively uniform full thickness epidermal atypia

Branchial Cleft Cyst

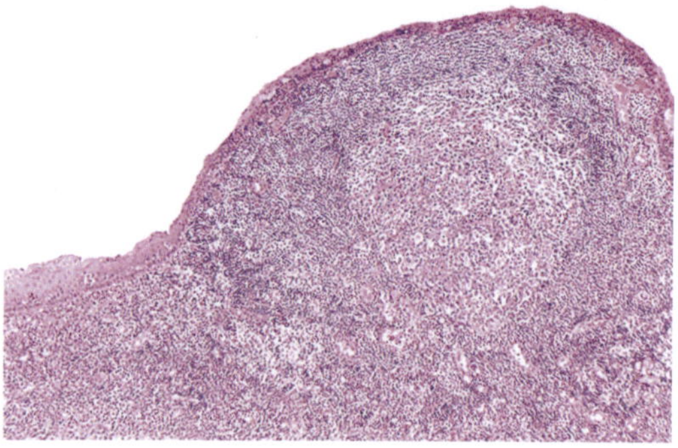

Fig. 2.58 Irregular cyst with lymphoid follicle in the wall

Histopathology (Figs. 2.58, 2.59, and 2.60)
- Irregular cyst lined with stratified ciliated columnar or stratified squamous epithelium
- Wall contains heavy lymphoid infiltrate
- Occasional lymphoid follicle
- Lack of goblet cells that are found in bronchogenic cyst

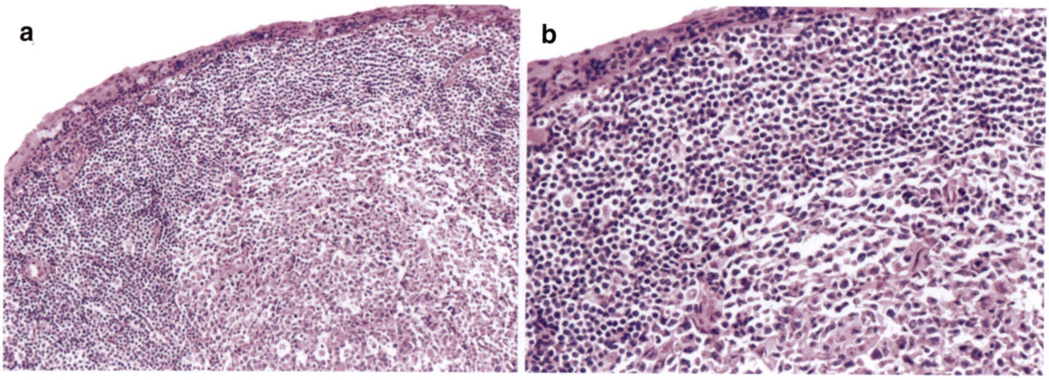

Fig. 2.59 (**a**, **b**) Cyst wall contains dense lymphocytic infiltrate forming vague germinal center

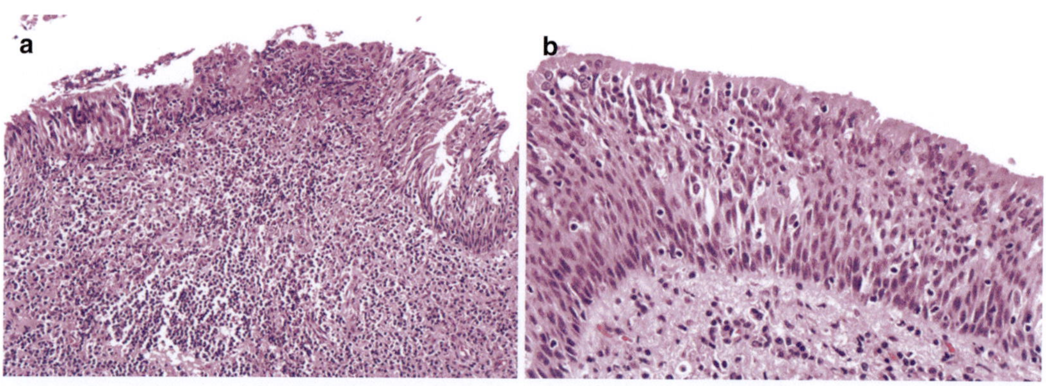

Fig. 2.60 (**a**, **b**) Cyst wall is lined with stratified squamous and columnar ciliated lining

Bronchogenic Cyst

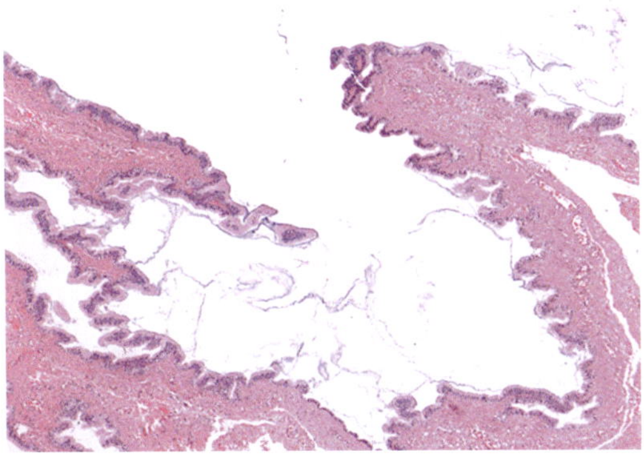

Fig. 2.61 Cyst filled with loose pink material

Histopathology (Figs. 2.61, 2.62, and 2.63)

- Cyst lined with ciliated and mucin producing pseudostratified columnar epithelium
- Smooth muscle and cartilage occasionally found in the wall
- Lumen contains serous pale acellular material
- Goblet cells can be present in wall lining

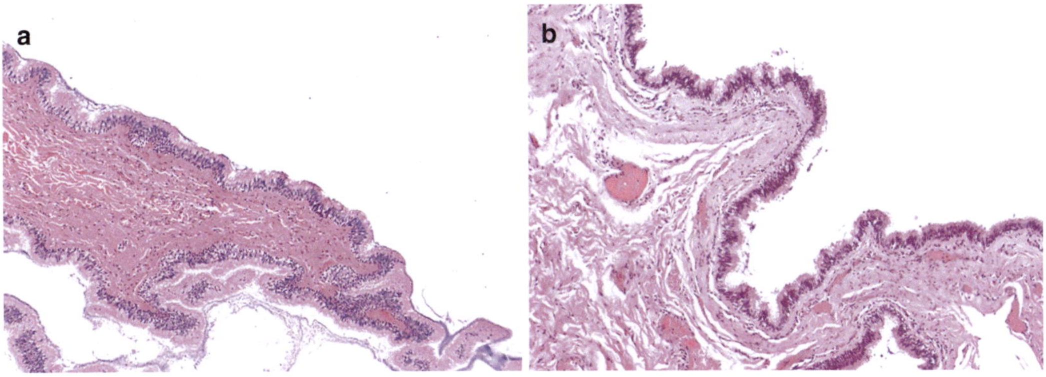

Fig. 2.62 (**a**, **b**) Wall is made of fibroconnective tissue without the presence of lymphocytes

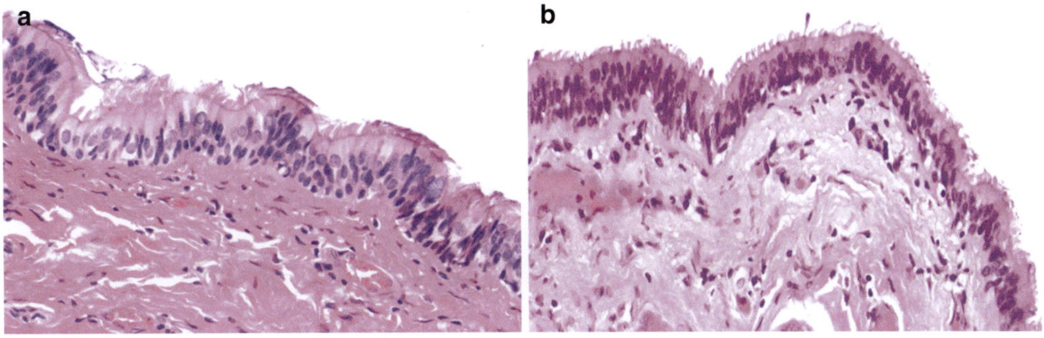

Fig. 2.63 (**a**, **b**) Pseudostratified ciliated lining of cyst wall

Bullosis Diabeticorum

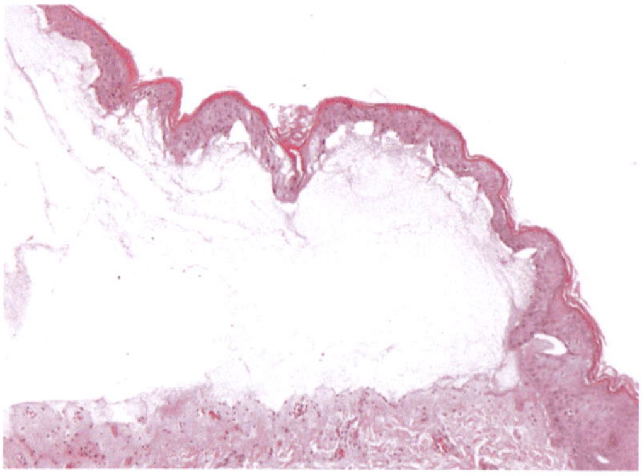

Fig. 2.64 Subepidermal fibrin filled blister

Histopathology (Figs. 2.64, 2.65, 2.66, and 2.67)

- Subepidermal, "cell-poor", fibrin filled blister
- Often necrotic blister roof
- Dermal festooning less pronounced comparing to porphyria
- Spare perivascular lymphocytic infiltrate and more prominent dermal vessels
- Sometimes the blister can be intraepidermal (believed as a result of epithelization) and have mild inflammatory content

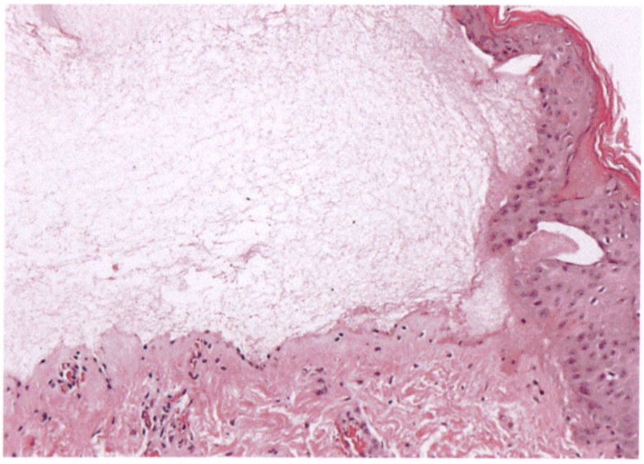

Fig. 2.65 Inflammatory cells are absent in the blister and mild dermal festooning is present

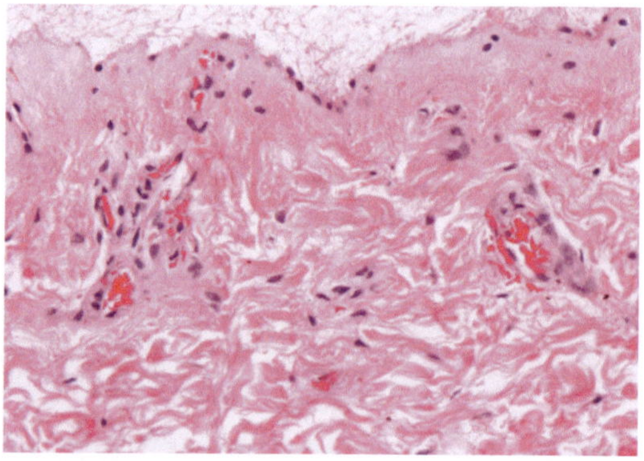

Fig. 2.66 Mild dermal perivascular lymphocytic infiltrate with more prominent blood vessels

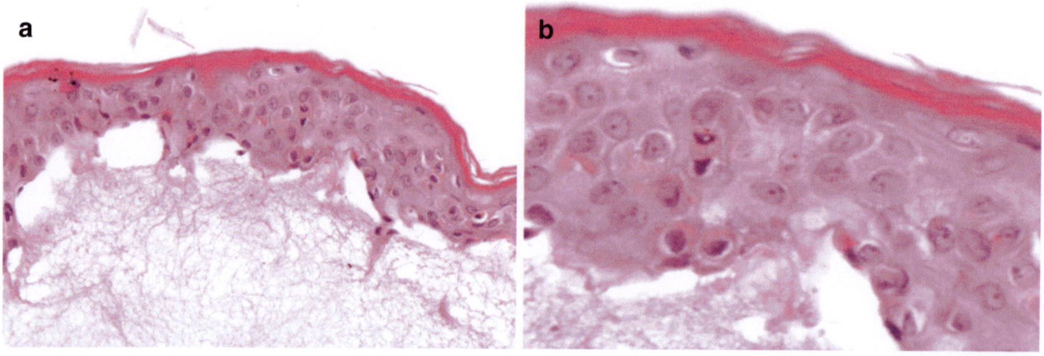

Fig. 2.67 (a, b) Scattered necrotic keratinocytes in the blister roof

Bullous Lupus Erythematosus

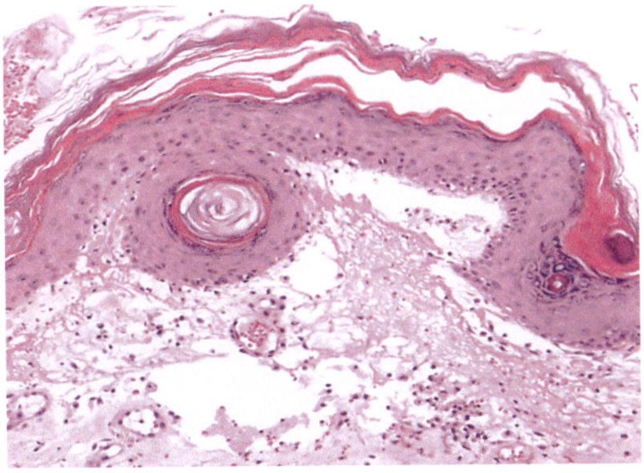

Fig. 2.68 Subepidermal blistering dermatosis

Histopathology (Figs. 2.68, 2.69, and 2.70)
- Subepidermal blistering dermatosis
- Neutrophils in the papillary dermis and in the dermis
- DIF is variable with mixed granular and linear patterns with IgG and commonly IgA and IgM

P.S. similar histology to dermatitis herpetiformis and linear IgA pemphigus

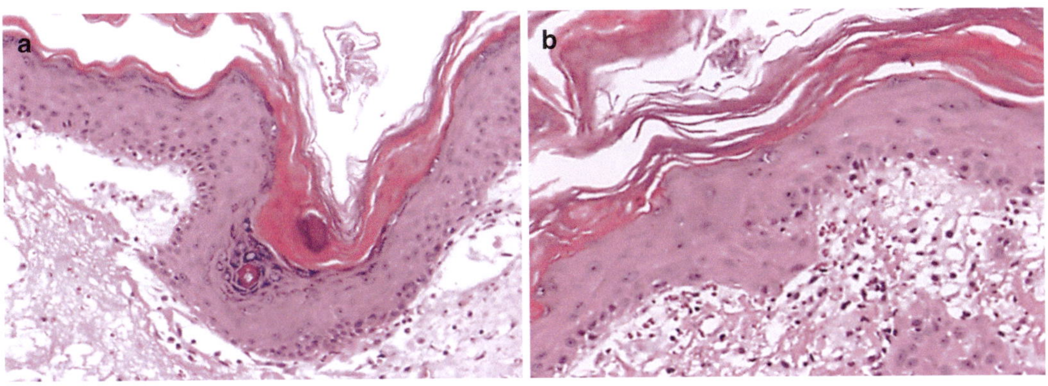

Fig. 2.69 (**a**, **b**) Subepidermal blister with neutrophils in the papillary dermis

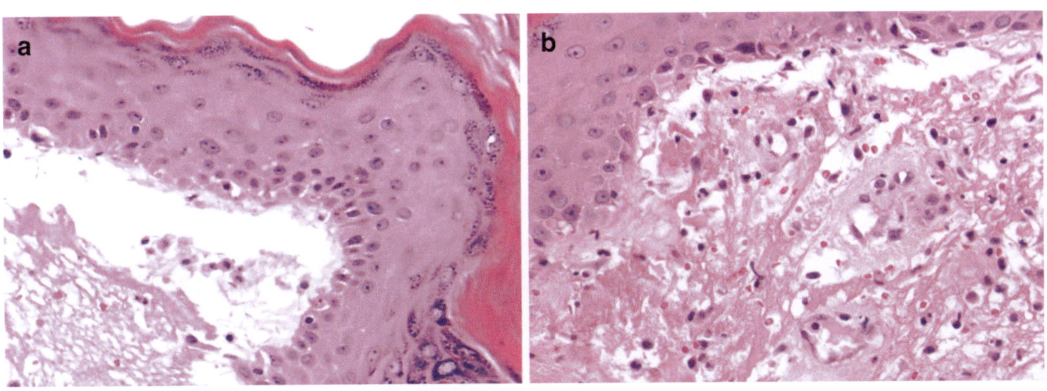

Fig. 2.70 (**a**, **b**) Neutrophils are also present in the reticular dermis and red blood cell extravasation is common

Bullous Pemphigoid

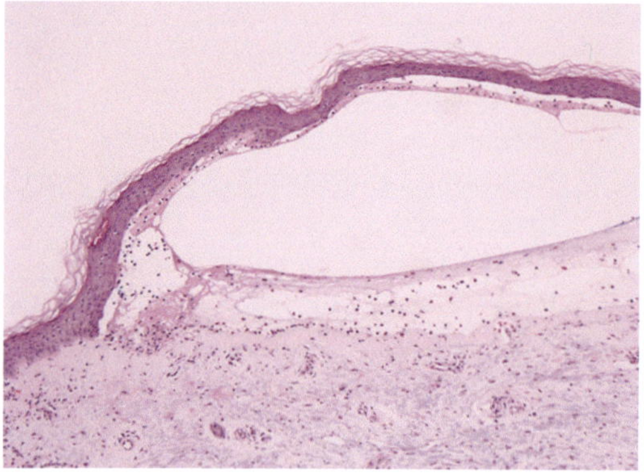

Fig. 2.71 Established lesion of BP

Histopathology (Figs. 2.71, 2.72, and 2.73)

- Subepidermal blister with linear IgG and C3 on DIF
- Lymphocytes with numerous eosinophils present in the blister and the dermis
- Rare variants may be neutrophilic or cell-poor

Histopathology of urticarial phase of BP (Figs. 2.74 and 2.75)

- Extensive papillary dermal edema with no blister formation
- Eosinophils and lymphocytes in the dermis and epidermis

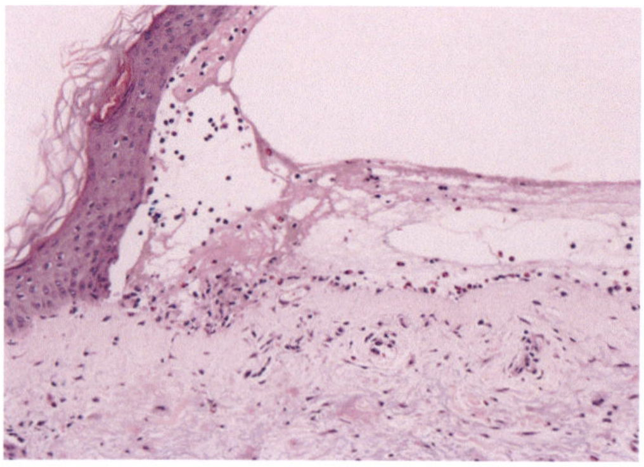

Fig. 2.72 Subepidermal blister

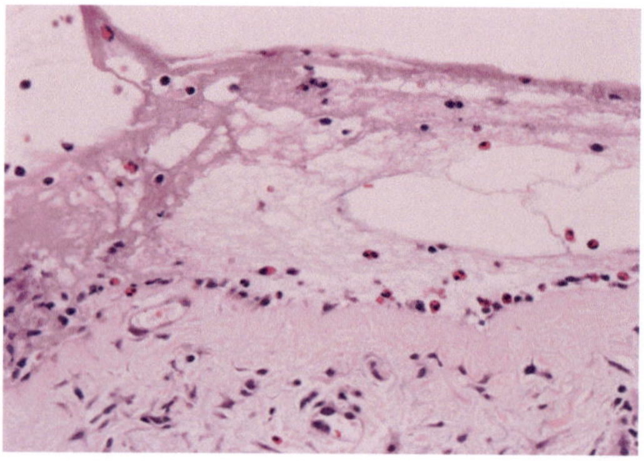

Fig. 2.73 Eosinophils and lymphocytes in the dermis and in the blister

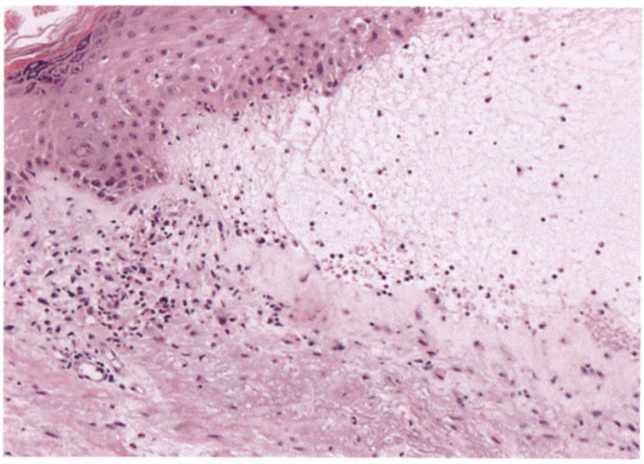

Fig. 2.74 Urticarial phase BP with papillary dermal edema

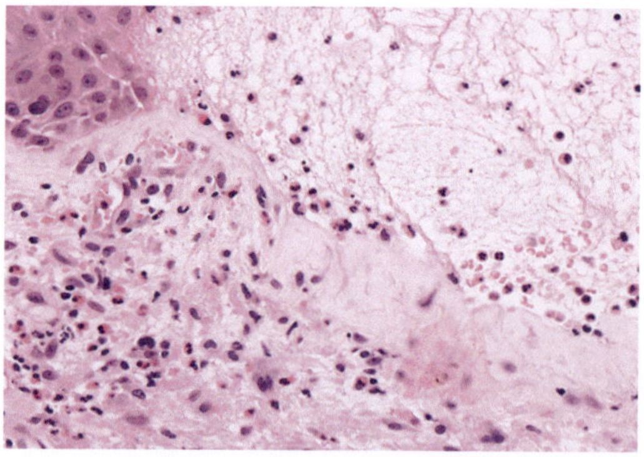

Fig. 2.75 Dermal eosinophils and lymphocytes

Burn

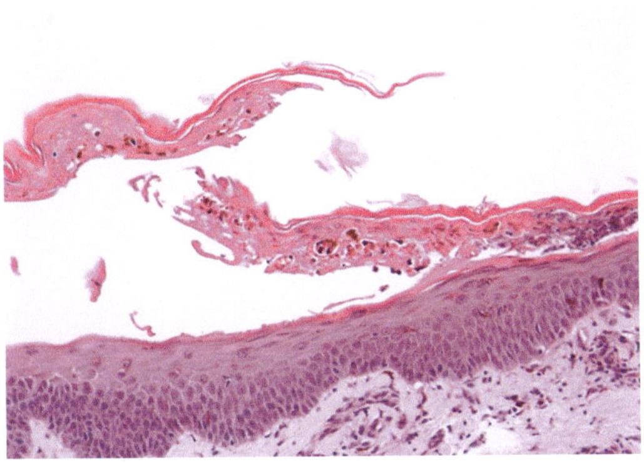

Fig. 2.76 **First** degree burn with necrosis of the superficial epidermis

Histopathology

First-degree burn: (Figs. 2.76 and 2.77) partial to full thickness necrosis involving upper part of the epidermis with no dermal damage

Second-degree burn: (Figs. 2.78 and 2.79) necrosis of the entire epidermis with mild to moderate dermal damage

Third-degree burn: necrosis involves the entire skin including subcutis and appendages

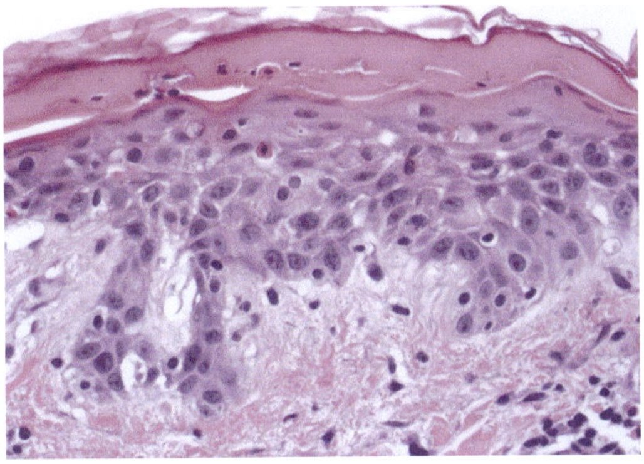

Fig. 2.77 **First** degree burn with superficial necrosis and serum crust

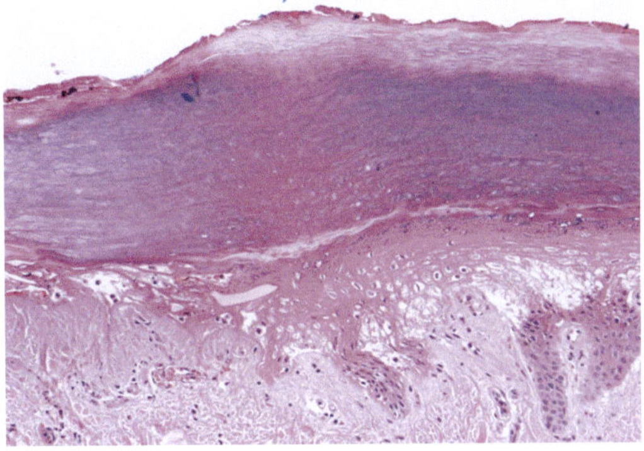

Fig. 2.78 **Second** degree burn

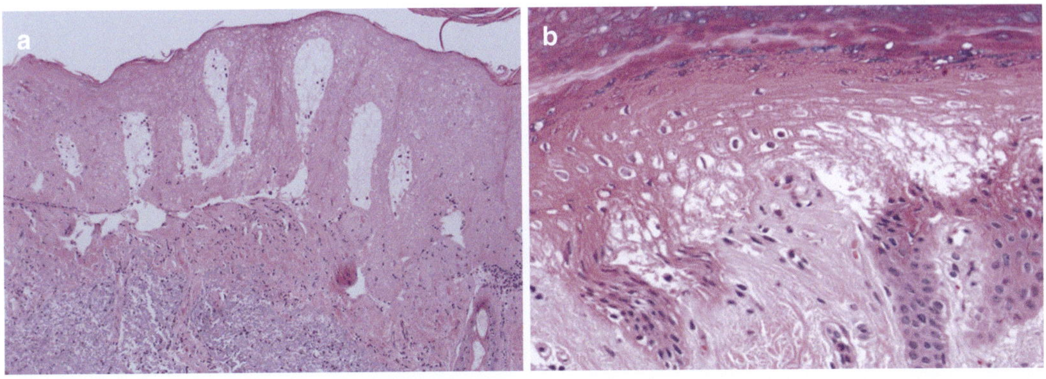

Fig. 2.79 (**a**, **b**) **Second** degree burn with focal full thickness epidermal necrosis and damage to the papillary dermis

3 Dermatopathology C

V. Vincek, *Dermatopathology A–Z*, https://doi.org/10.1007/978-3-319-89486-7_3

Café au Lait Macules

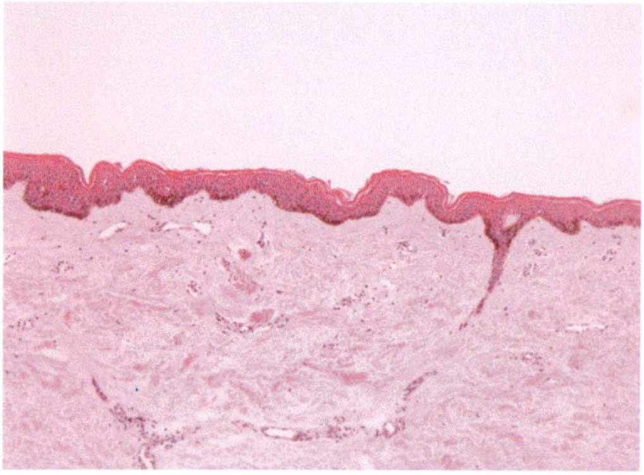

Fig. 3.1 Normal epidermis on low power magnification

Histopathology is similar to **freckles** (Figs. 3.1, 3.2, and 3.3)

- Architecturally normal appearing epidermis with some focally elongated rete
- Hyperpigmentation of basal layer keratinocytes
- Slight increase in number of melanocytes

P.S. found in **NF1** and **LEOPARD syndrome**. Macules of **Albright's syndrome** and **Peutz-Jeghers syndrome** show similar histopathology and clinical correlation is necessary to separate them

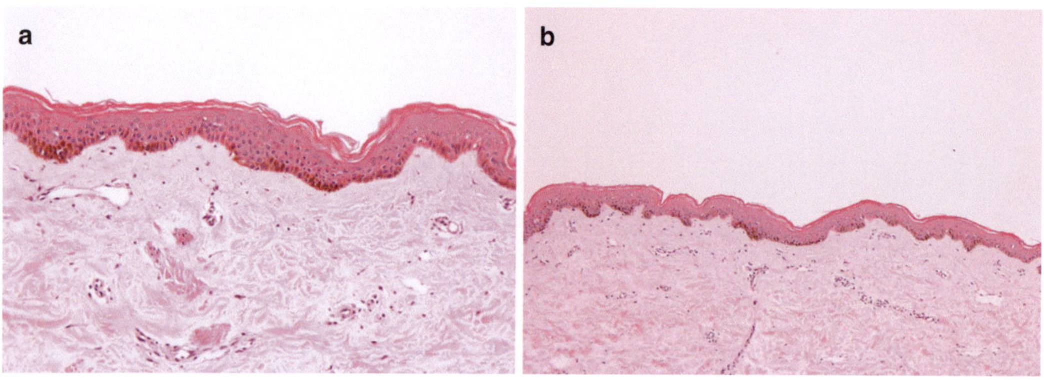

Fig. 3.2 (**a**, **b**) Normal appearing epidermis with focally elongated rete ridges

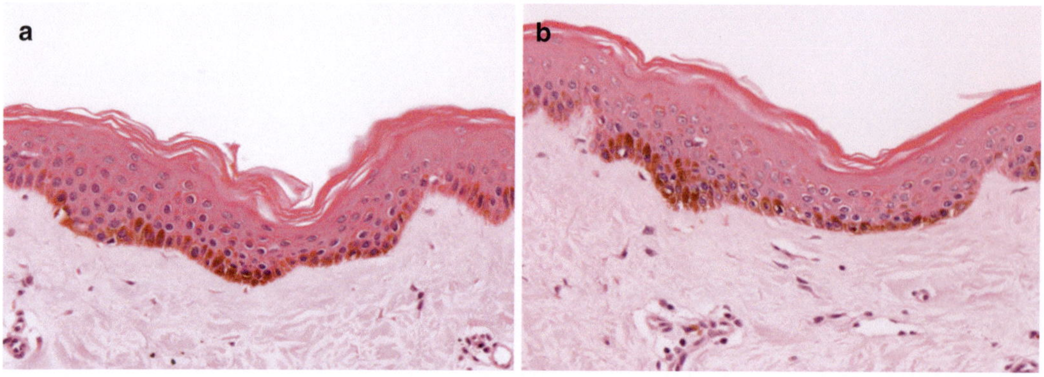

Fig. 3.3 (**a**, **b**) Hyperpigmentation of the basal layer keratinocytes

Calcifying (Juvenile) Aponeurotic Fibroma

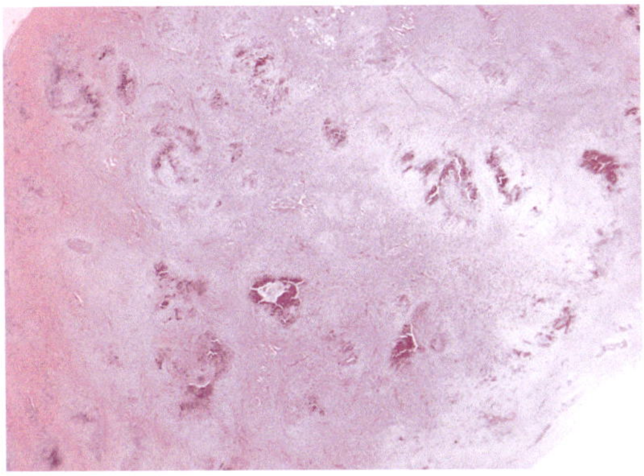

Fig. 3.4 Multiple areas of calcifications within fibrotic tumor

Histopathology (Figs. 3.4, 3.5, 3.6, 3.7, and 3.8)

- Deep subcutaneous tumor with infiltrative pattern
- Tumor is made of plump oval fibroblast/myofibroblasts
- Multiple foci of calcification with focal chondroid metaplasia
- Tumor cells are CD99+, CD68+, SMA variable+

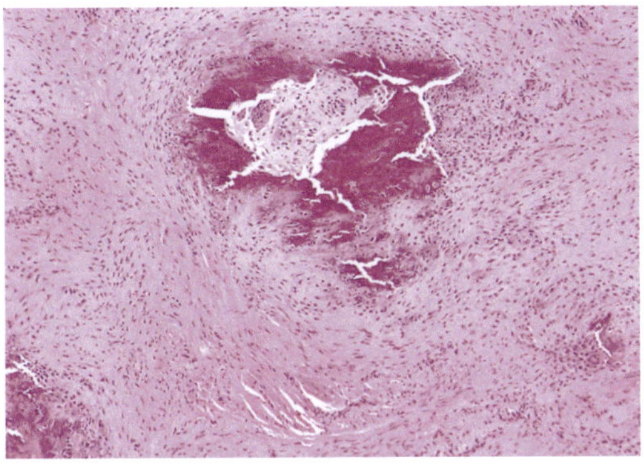

Fig. 3.5 Tumor cells in dense stroma surround calcified area

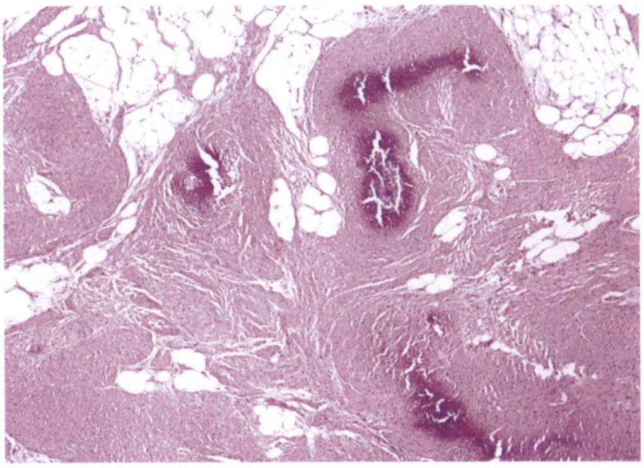

Fig. 3.6 Tumor infiltrates the subcutaneous fat

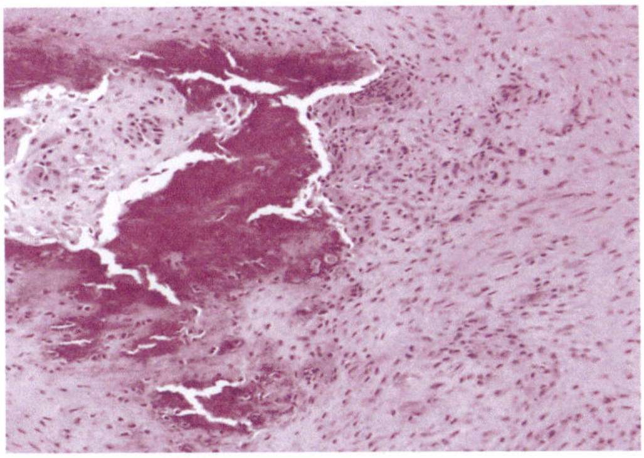

Fig. 3.7 Calcified area with chondroid metaplasia

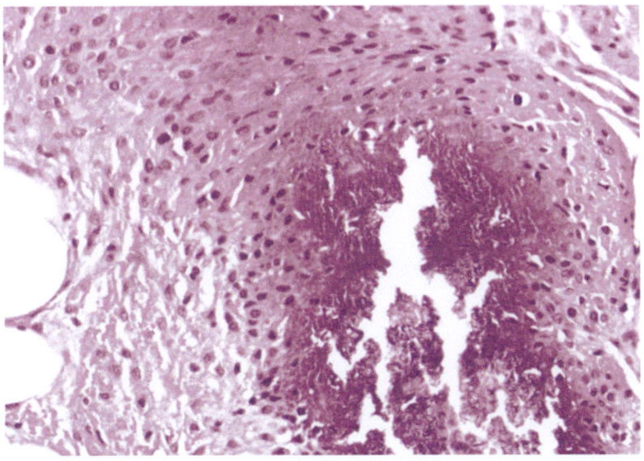

Fig. 3.8 Plump oval myofibroblast

Calcinosis Cutis

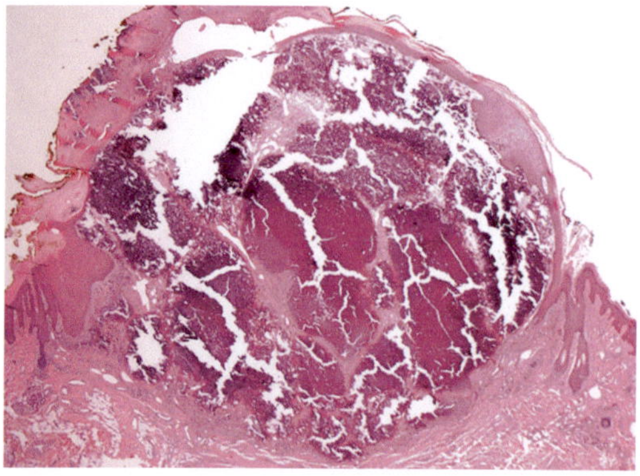

Fig. 3.9 Subepidermal calcified nodule

Histopathology (Figs. 3.9, 3.10, 3.11, 3.12, and 3.13)

- Calcium deposition in dermis and subcutis
- Deposits are amorphous and show intense dark purple color
- Von Kossa stain for calcium can be used if needed

P.S. before tissue processing the biopsy sometimes need to be decalcified and therefore morphology and staining of epidermis and dermis is altered

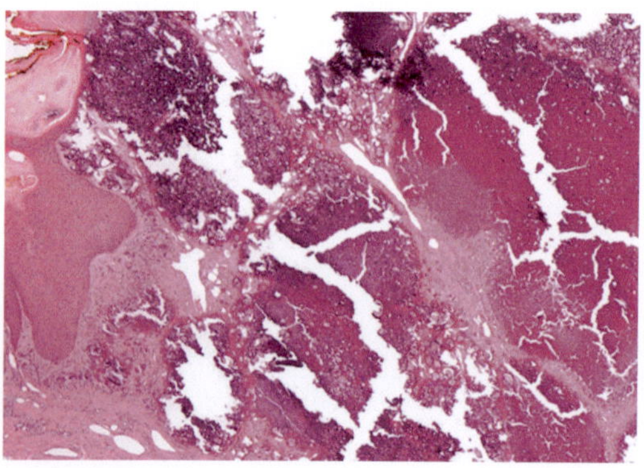

Fig. 3.10 Acellular calcium deposit in the specimen that was not decalcified

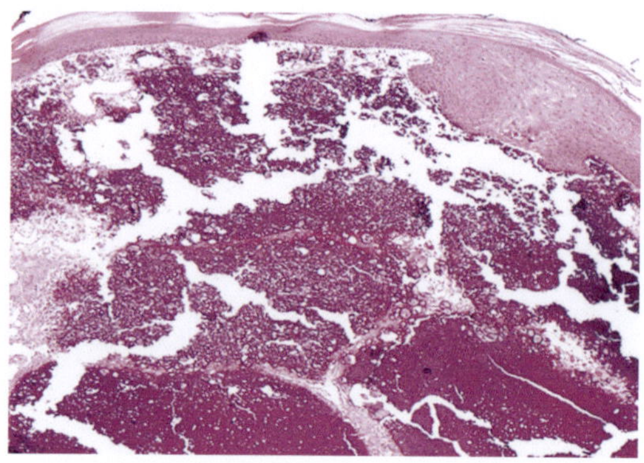

Fig. 3.11 Amorphous deposition of dark purple calcium in the specimen that was decalcified prior to processing

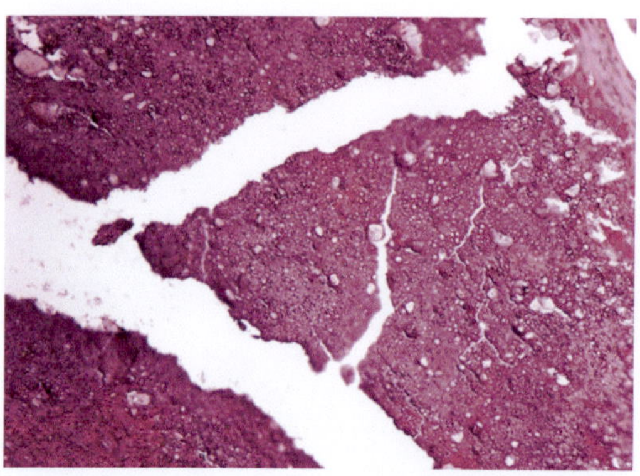

Fig. 3.12 Amorphous calcium deposition

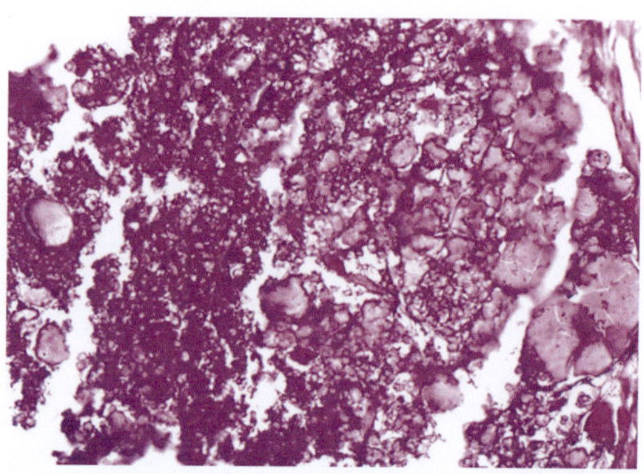

Fig. 3.13 Cracked appearing calcium globules

Calciphylaxis

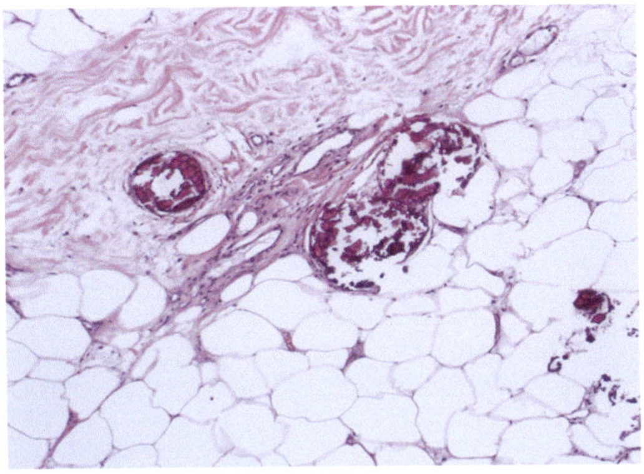

Fig. 3.14 Calcification of medium and small size vessels

Histopathology (Figs. 3.14, 3.15, 3.16, 3.17, and 3.18)

- Calcium deposits in the subcutis (von Kossa +)
- Deposits are mostly within the wall of small and medium size vessels
- Hemorrhage within adipose tissue can be seen
- Focal fat necrosis with lipophages

P.S. *Mönckeberg's* sclerosis differ by dystrophic calcification of media of larger muscular arteries and no clinical symptoms unlike calciphylaxis that is usually painful

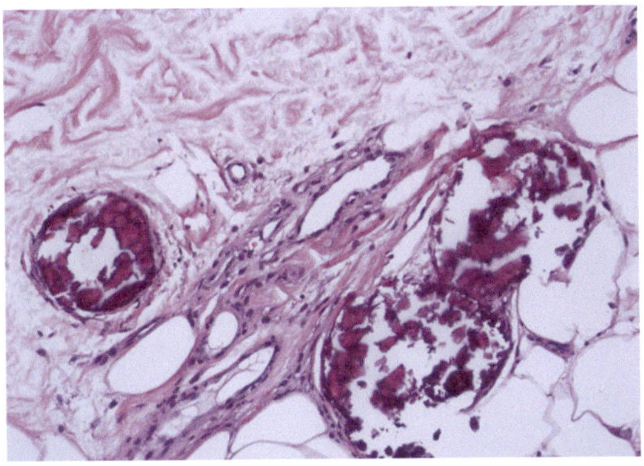

Fig. 3.15 Calcium deposition within the wall and the lumen of blood vessels

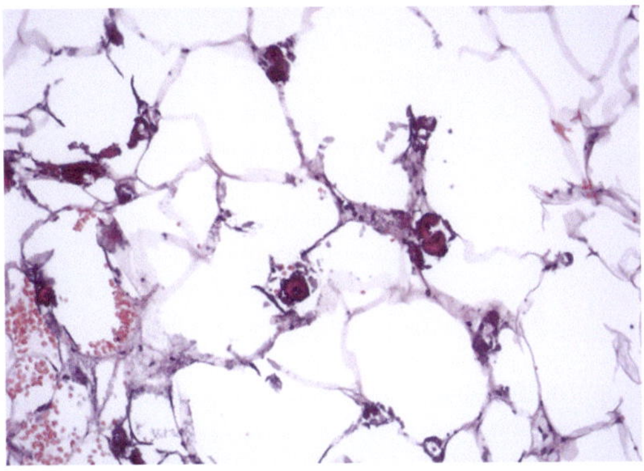

Fig. 3.16 Hemorrhage within adipose tissue

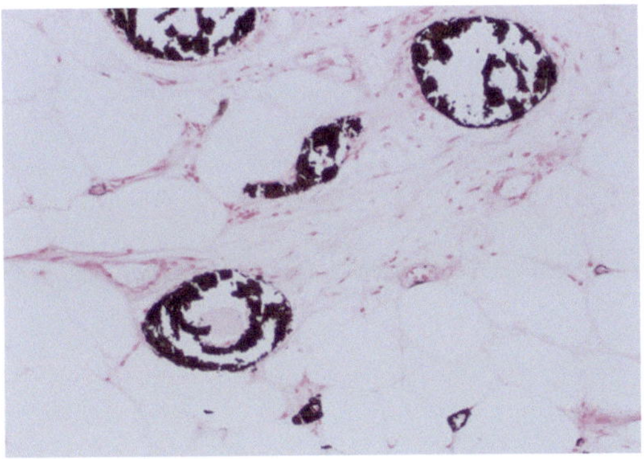

Fig. 3.17 Calcium is stained black with von Kossa stain

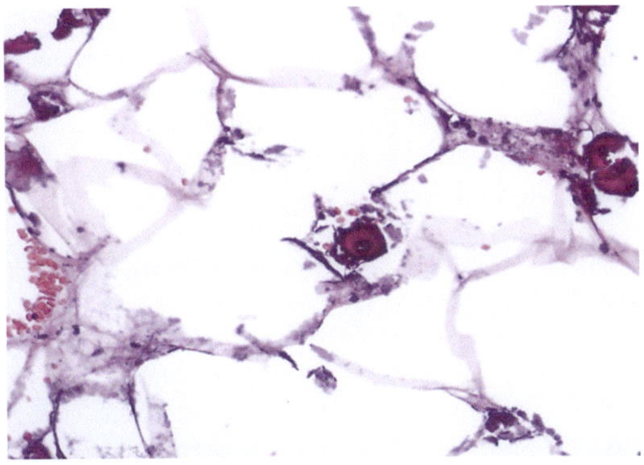

Fig. 3.18 Focal fat necrosis and calcification

Callus

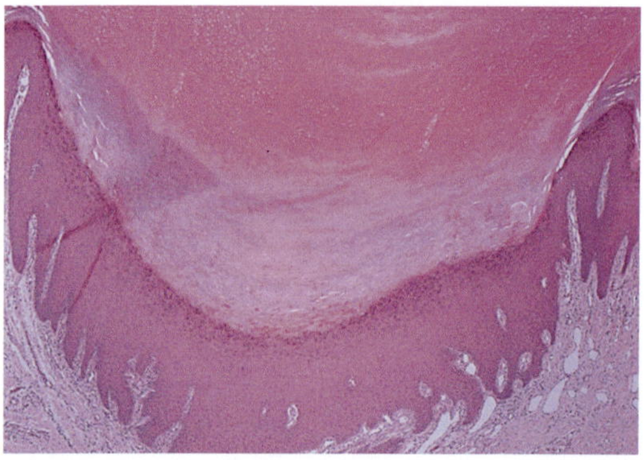

Fig. 3.19 Cup-shaped epidermal lesion

Histopathology (Figs. 3.19, 3.20, 3.21, and 3.22)

- Cup-shaped well circumscribed epidermal lesion
- Extensive epidermal hyperkeratosis with hypergranulosis
- Dermal telangiectasias and no inflammation

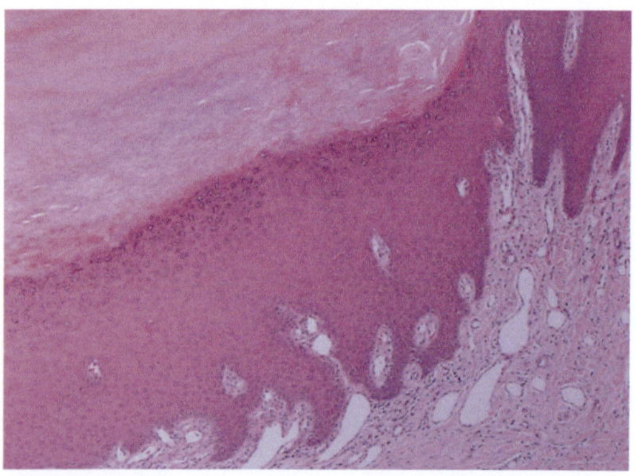

Fig. 3.20 Dilated dermal capillaries and no inflammation

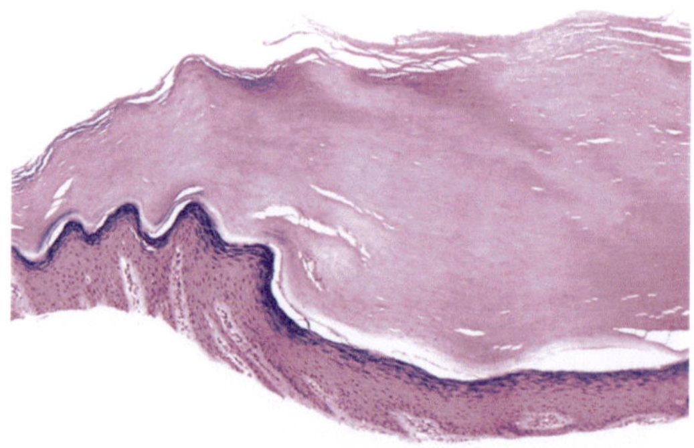

Fig. 3.21 Inverted, U-shaped epidermal lesion

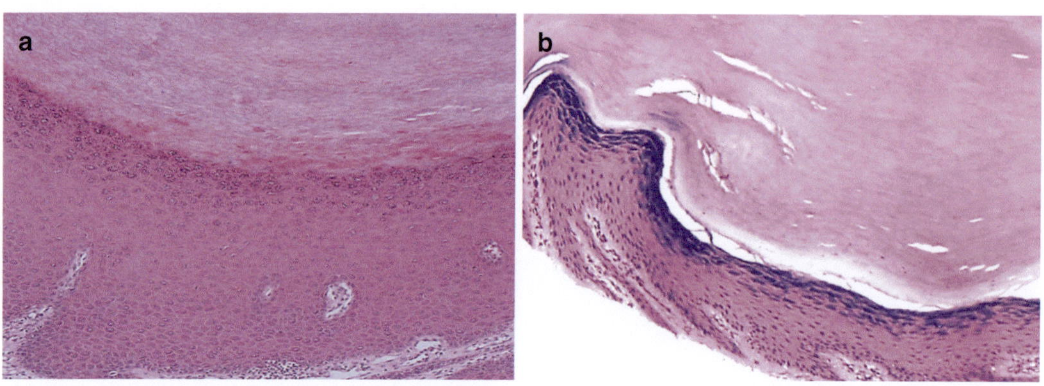

Fig. 3.22 (**a**, **b**) Extensive hyperkeratosis and hypergranulosis

Candidiasis

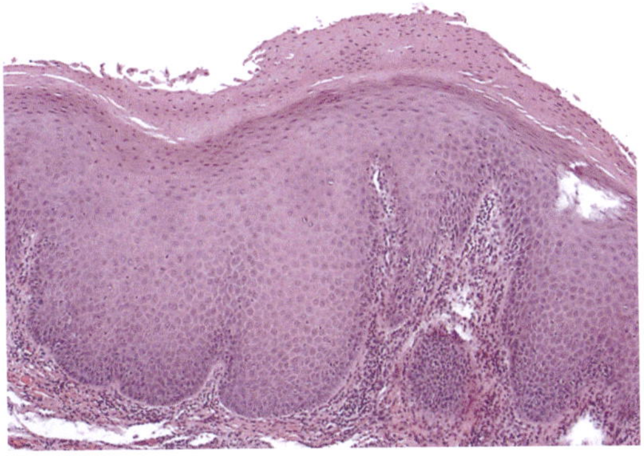

Fig. 3.23 Hyperkeratotic acanthotic epidermis with parakeratosis

Synonym: Moniliasis

Histopathology (Figs. 3.23, 3.24, and 3.25)

- Usually hyperkeratotic acanthotic epidermis
- Parakeratosis or neutrophils in the stratum corneum
- Spores, branching pseudohyphae, and hyphae in the stratum corneum
- Both dermatophytes and candida are oriented parallel but candida may also be oriented perpendicular to epidermis

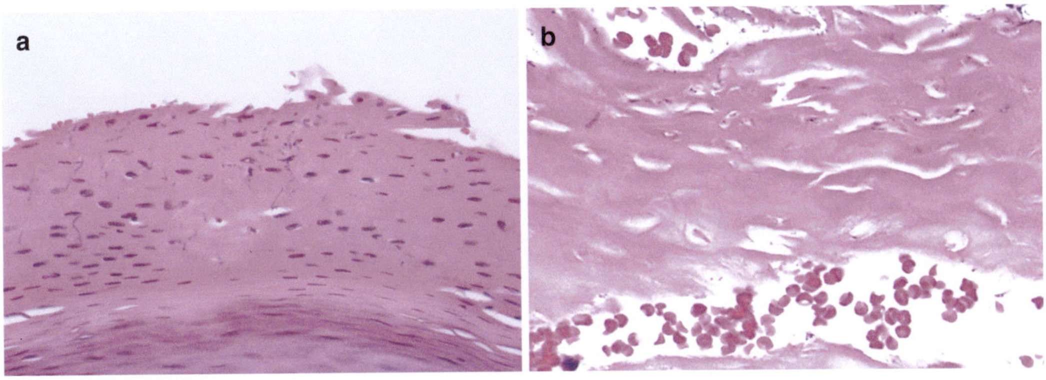

Fig. 3.24 (**a**, **b**) Fungal elements are barely visible on H&E stained slides

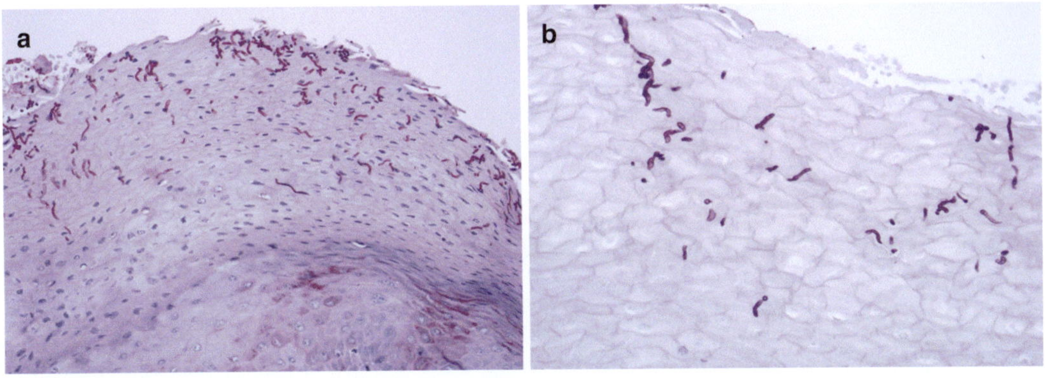

Fig. 3.25 (**a**, **b**) PAS stain highlights *Candida* in the stratum corneum with growth perpendicular to epidermis

Capillary Hemangioma

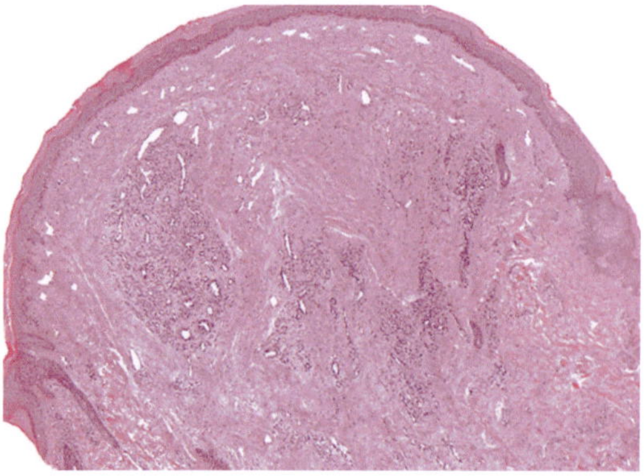

Fig. 3.26 Dermal vascular proliferation

Synonyms: Juvenile Capillary Hemangioma, Strawberry Hemangioma

Histopathology (Figs. 3.26, 3.27, and 3.28)

- Multilobular architecture
- Small vascular channels organized in the lobular pattern
- Inconspicuous vascular lumina in immature lesions and more prominent lumina in older lesions
- No cytological atypia

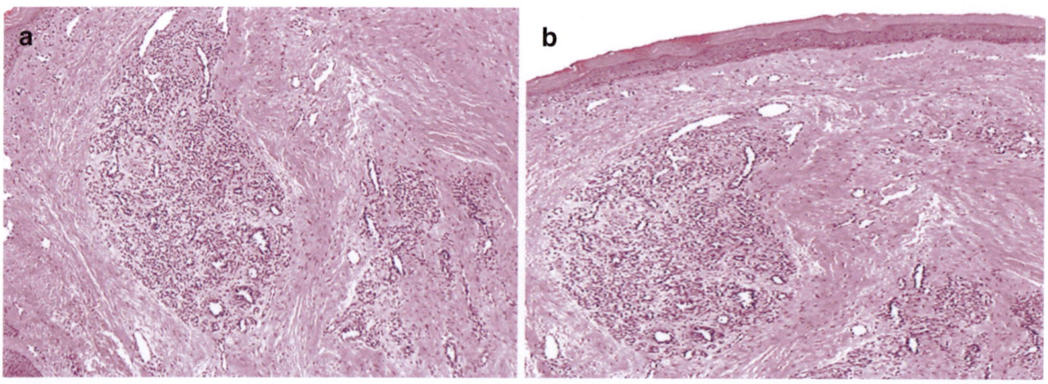

Fig. 3.27 (**a**, **b**) Multiple well-defined dermal vascular nodules

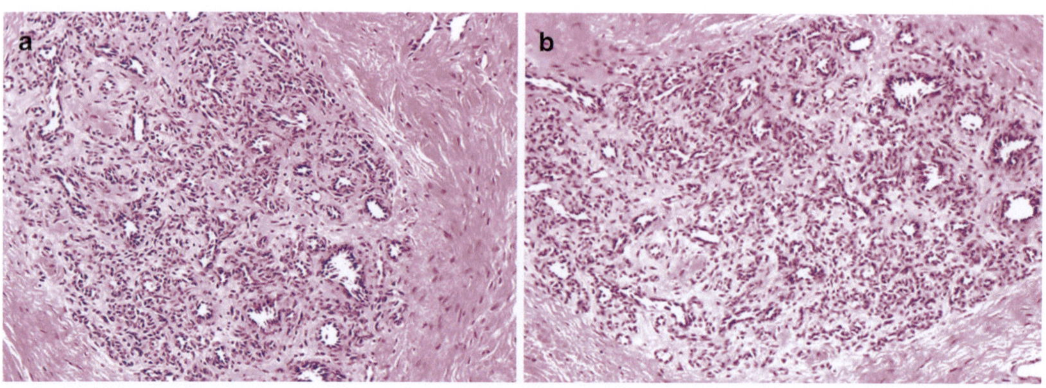

Fig. 3.28 (**a**, **b**) Proliferation of small vascular channels some with inconspicuous lumina; endothelial cells appears plump but with no cytological atypia

Carcinosarcoma

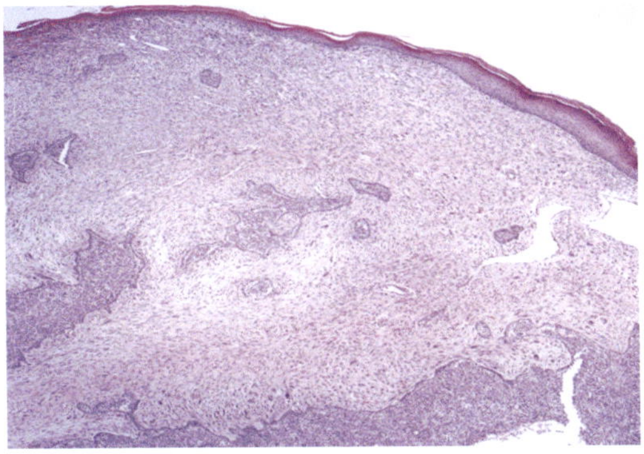

Fig. 3.29 Tumor made of epithelioid and spindle cell component

Synonym: Metaplastic Carcinoma

Histopathology (Figs. 3.29, 3.30, and 3.31)

- Tumor consists of epithelial and mesenchymal component
- Both components are malignant
- Epithelial component includes basal cell carcinoma or squamous cell carcinoma
- Mesenchymal component includes atypical fibrous histiocytoma, fibrosarcoma, chondrosarcoma, osteogenic sarcoma, or leiomyosarcoma

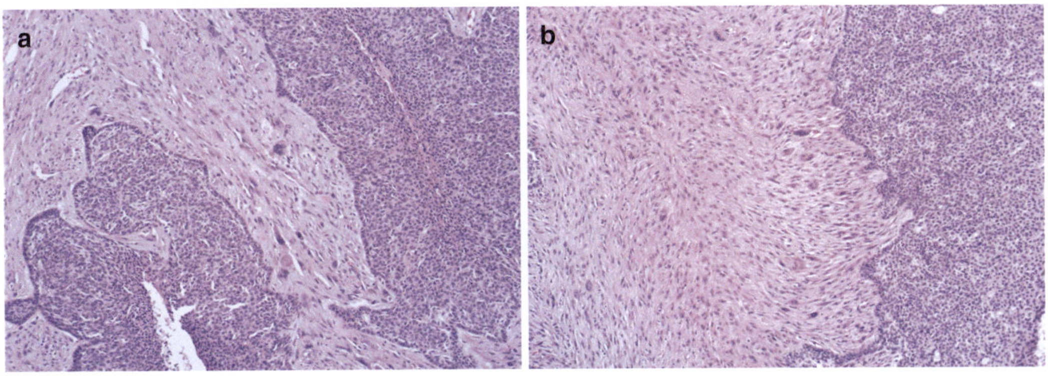

Fig. 3.30 (**a**, **b**) Combination of basal cell carcinoma and atypical fibrous histiocytoma

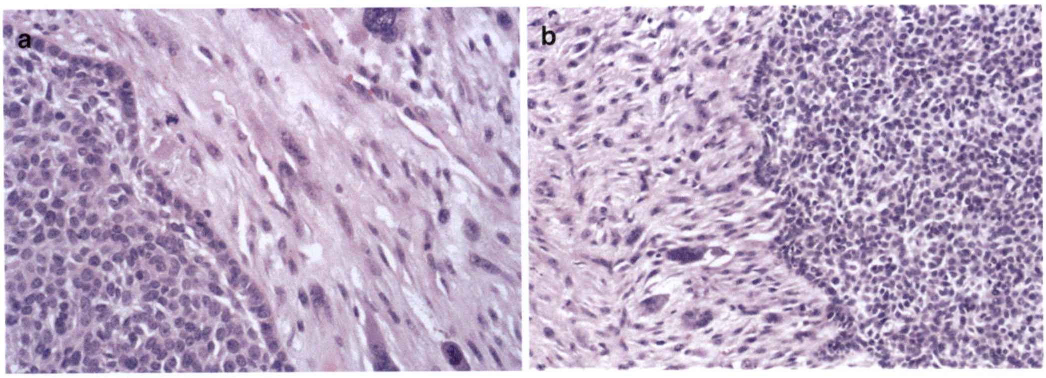

Fig. 3.31 (**a**, **b**) BCC with basaloid cells with peripheral palisading and adjacent AFX with highly atypical spindle cells

Cat Scratch Disease

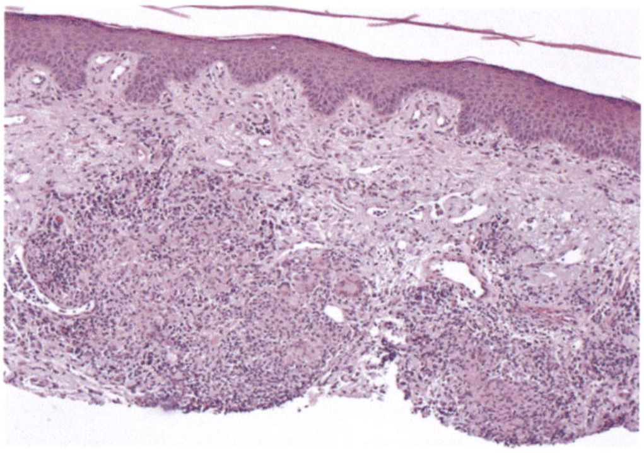

Fig. 3.32 Focal necrosis with plasma cells, lymphocytes, histiocytes, and some giant cells

Skin **histopathology** is variable and not specific (Figs. 3.32 and 3.33)
- Epidermal ulceration only in early lesion
- Focal dermal necrosis surrounded by lymphocytes, plasma cells, and histiocytes
- Granulomas may be present and thin *Bartonella henselae* rods can be sometimes detected

Histopathology of the lymph nodes is more specific (Figs. 3.34, 3.35, and 3.36)
- Lymph node with necrotic stellate shaped granulomas with neutrophils and peripheral epithelioid cells

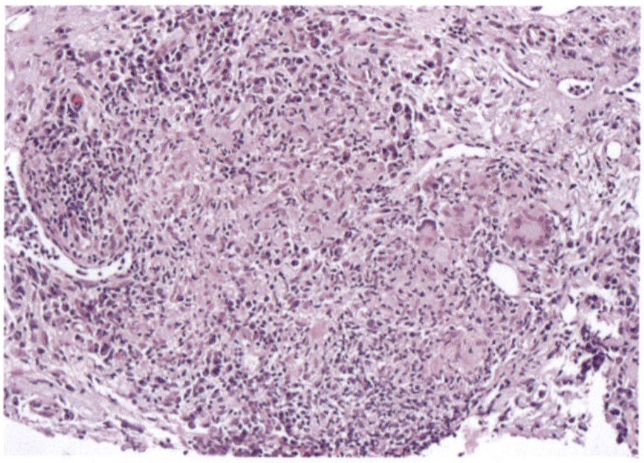

Fig. 3.33 Vague dermal granulomas with focal necrosis

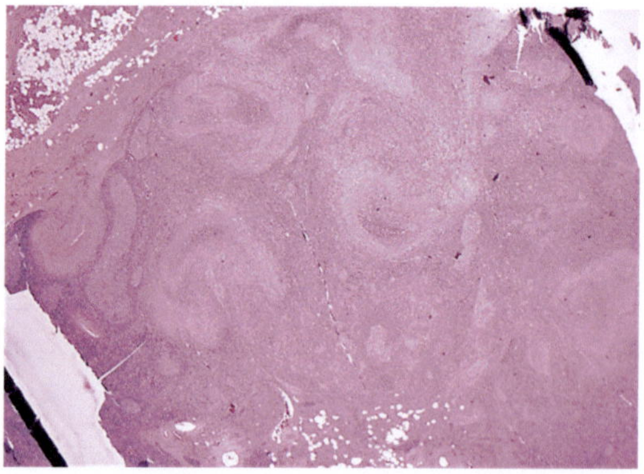

Fig. 3.34 Lymph node with multiple granulomas

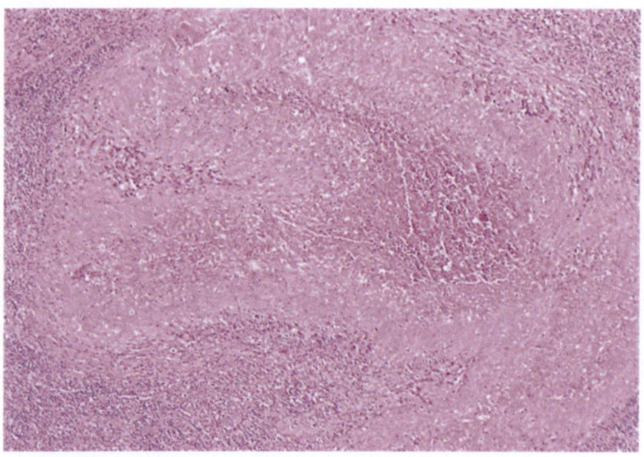

Fig. 3.35 Central irregularly shaped necrosis

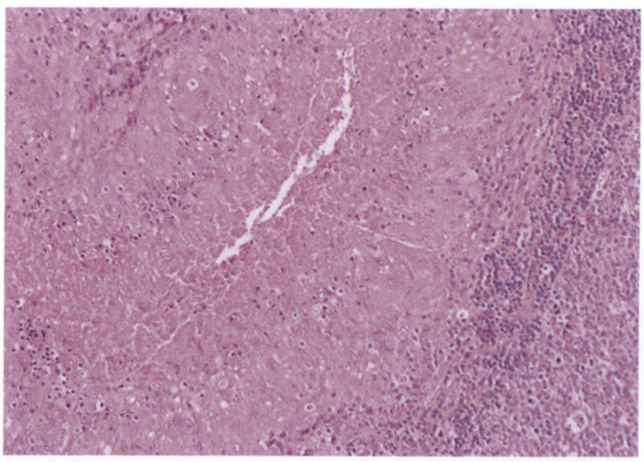

Fig. 3.36 Necrosis containing neutrophils is surrounded by palisaded histiocytes

Cavernous Hemangioma

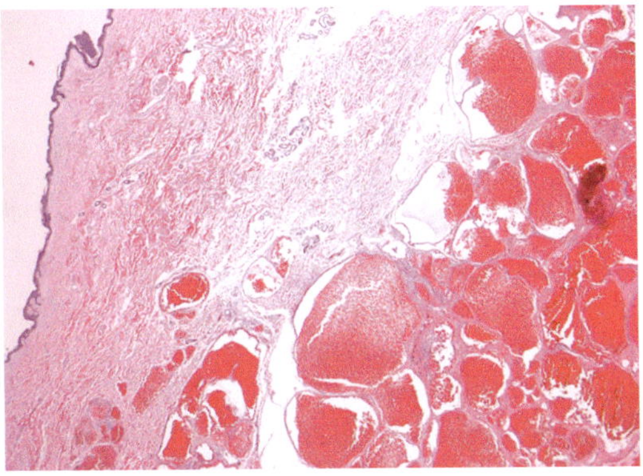

Fig. 3.37 Vascular lesion in dermis and subcutis

Histopathology (Figs. 3.37, 3.38, and 3.39)

- Vascular lesion with multinodular appearance
- Large dilated vascular channels with flat endothelial cells
- The vessel wall is thin
- Blood vessels are usually congested with red blood cells

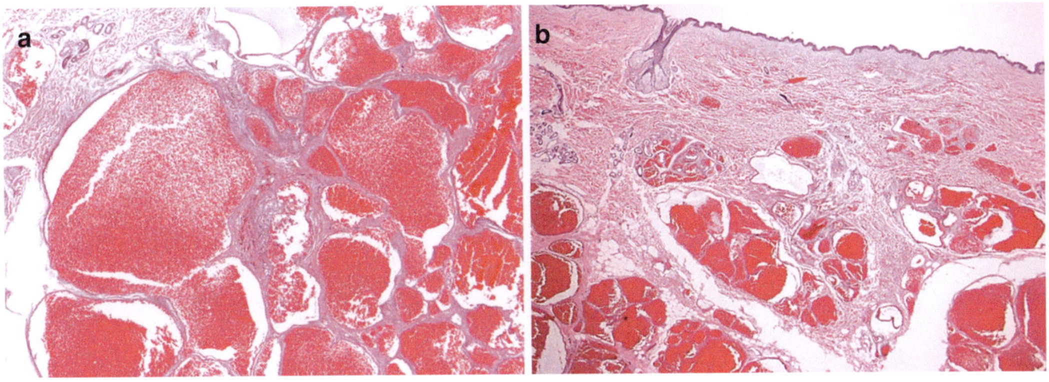

Fig. 3.38 (**a**, **b**) Large dilated vascular channels filled with red blood cells

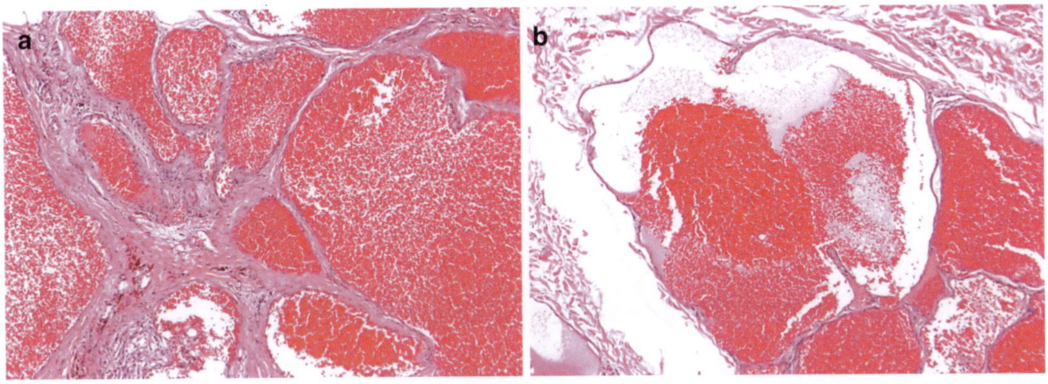

Fig. 3.39 (**a**, **b**) Vessel wall is thin and lined with flat endothelial cells

Cellular Blue Nevus

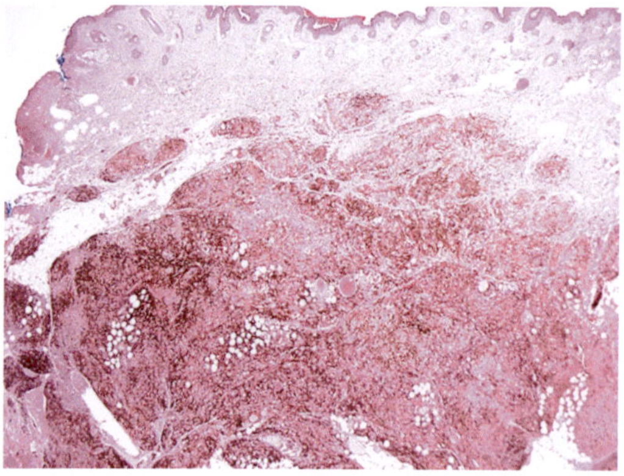

Fig. 3.40 "Dumbbell" shaped melanocytic lesion with pushing borders

Histopathology (Figs. 3.40, 3.41, 3.42, 3.43, and 3.44)

- Heavily pigmented lesion with a "dumb-bell' shape that start in dermis and extends into subcutis
- Dual cell population in variable ratio
  - (a) Heavily pigmented spindle dendritic melanocytes as in common blue nevus
  - (b) Islands of pale epithelioid cells with less pigment
- Necrosis and mitoses are not present
- Intertwining stroma is sclerotic

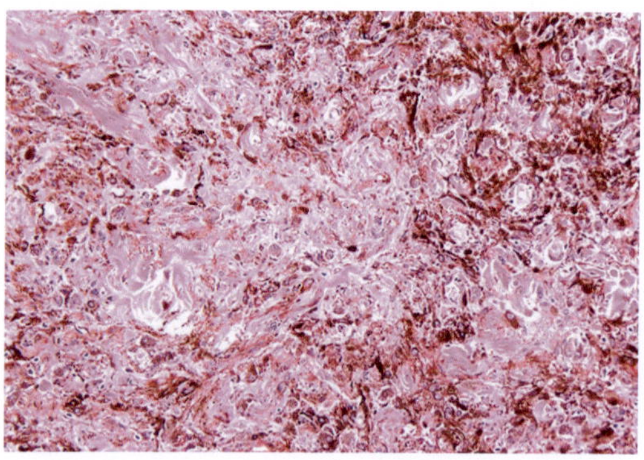

Fig. 3.41 Heavily pigmented dendritic melanocytes mixed with pale epithelioid cells with less pigment

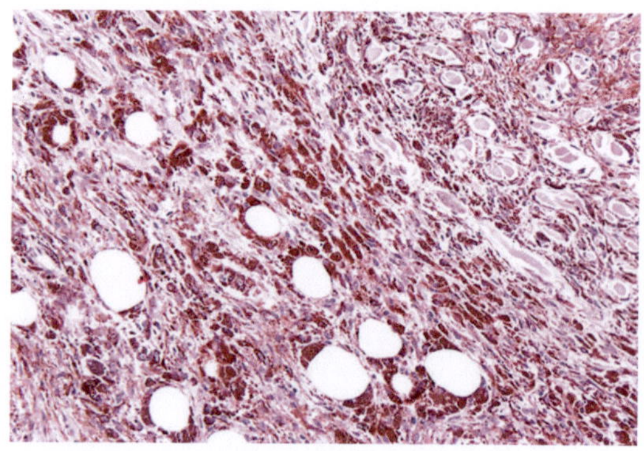

Fig. 3.42 The lesion is pushing into the adipose tissue

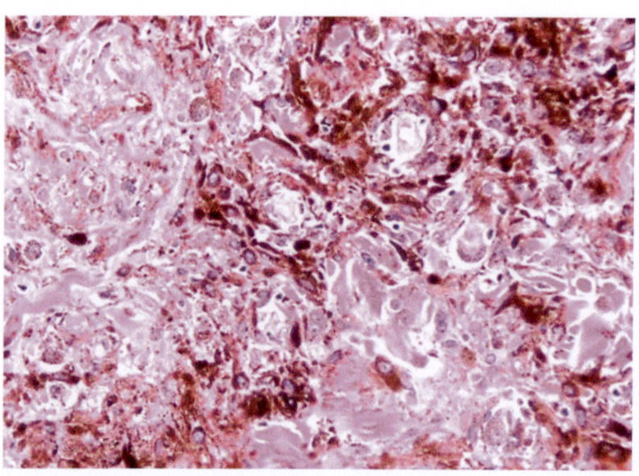

Fig. 3.43 There is no evidence of mitoses or necrosis

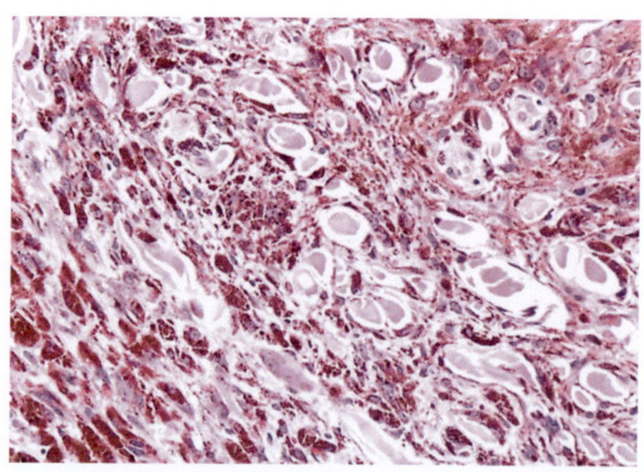

Fig. 3.44 Stroma is hyalinized

Cellular Digital Fibroma

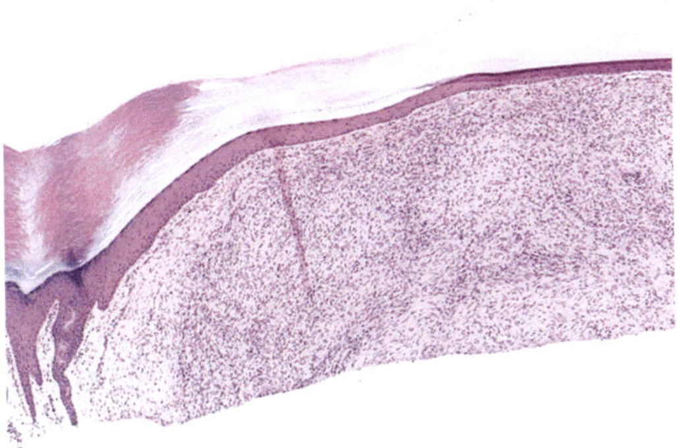

Fig. 3.45 Nodular dermal proliferation

Histopathology (Figs. 3.45, 3.46, and 3.47)
- Nodular tumor of reticular dermis
- Benign appearing spindle cells with no atypia or mitoses
- Spindle cells form short fascicles
- Somewhat myxoid appearing stroma

P.S. tumor cells are CD34 positive with minimal factor XIII staining

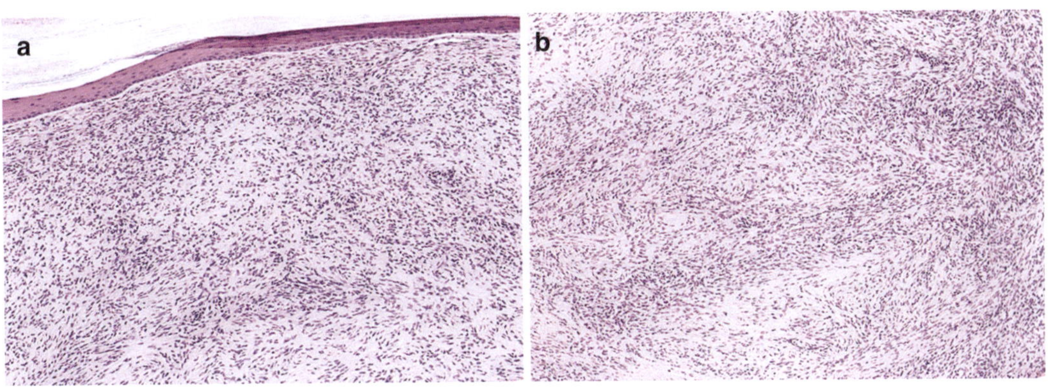

Fig. 3.46 (**a**, **b**) Spindle cells forming short fascicles ramifying in irregular manner

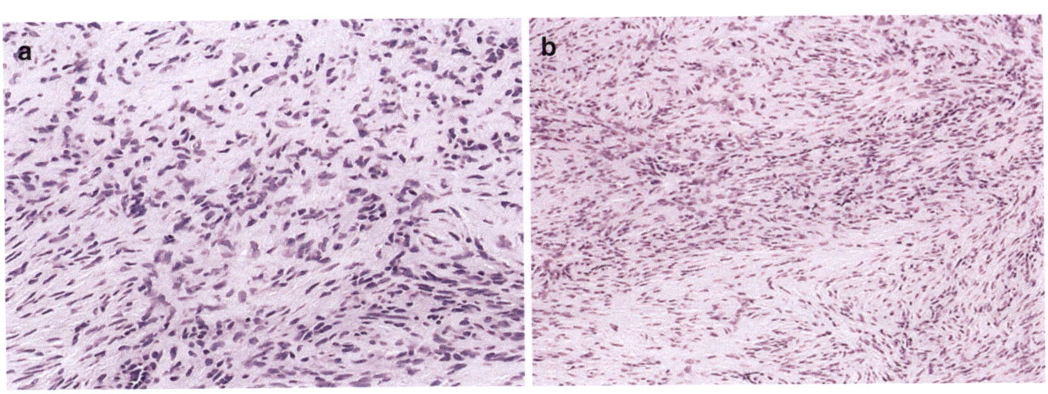

Fig. 3.47 (**a**, **b**) Spindle cells with no atypia or mitoses embedded in somewhat myxoid stroma without prominent vessels

Cellulitis

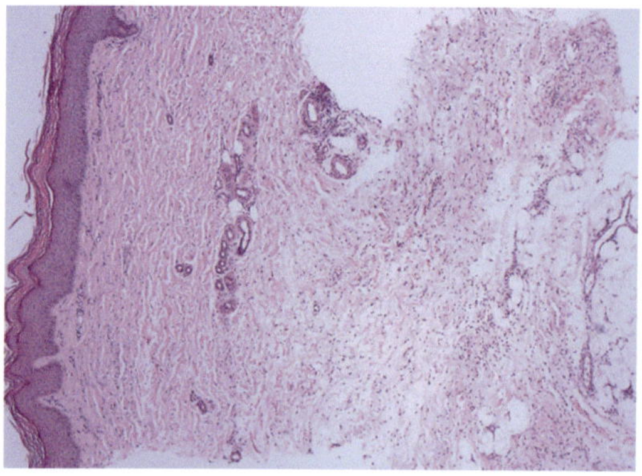

Fig. 3.48 Skin with pale dermis and subcutis

Histopathology (Figs. 3.48, 3.49, and 3.50)
- Variable dermal edema
- Superficial and deep dermal interstitial neutrophilic infiltrate
- Interstitial infiltrate predominate and there is only minimal neutrophilic infiltrate around the vessels
- Organisms are few or absent

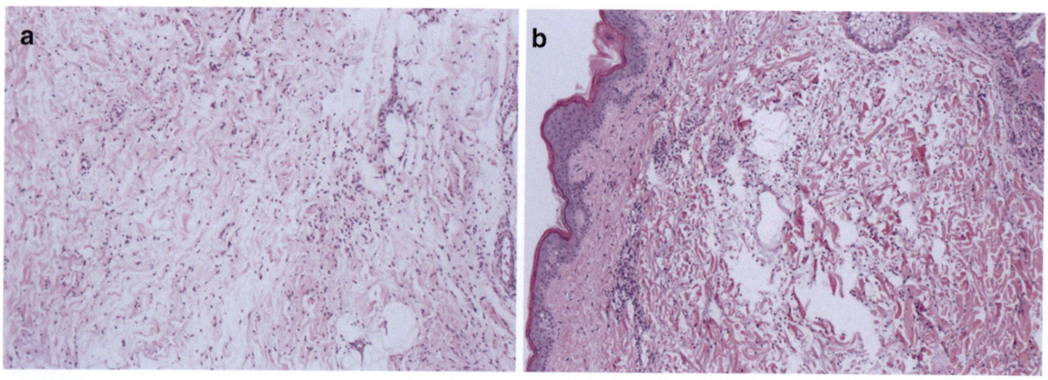

Fig. 3.49 (a, b) Superficial and deep dermal edema

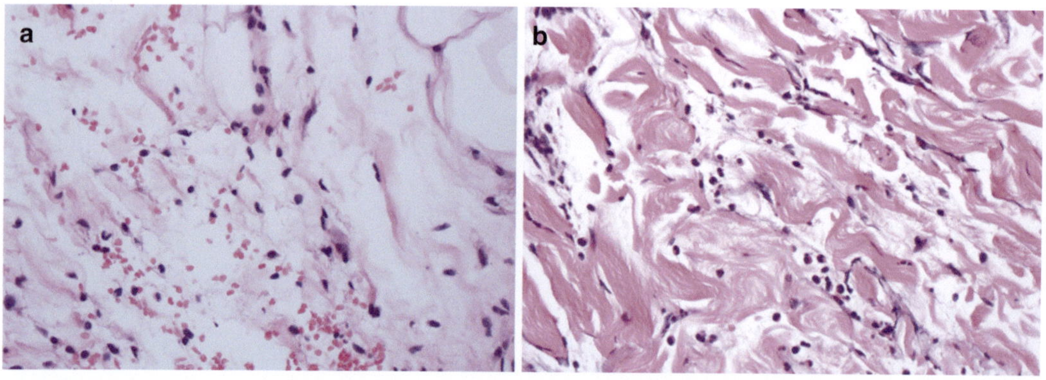

Fig. 3.50 (a, b) Collagen bundles are separated by edema and numerous scattered neutrophils are infiltrating the dermis

Chalazion

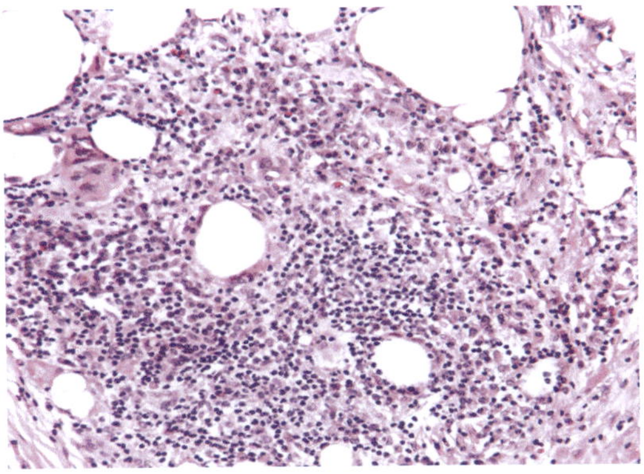

Fig. 3.51 Granulomatous dermatitis with empty vacuoles

Histopathology (Figs. 3.51, 3.52, 3.53, 3.54, and 3.55)

- Foreign body reaction to lipid from ruptured Meibomian glands
- Lymphocytic and histiocytic inflammation with occasional giant cells
- Empty holes of lipid vacuoles surrounded by non-caseating granulomas

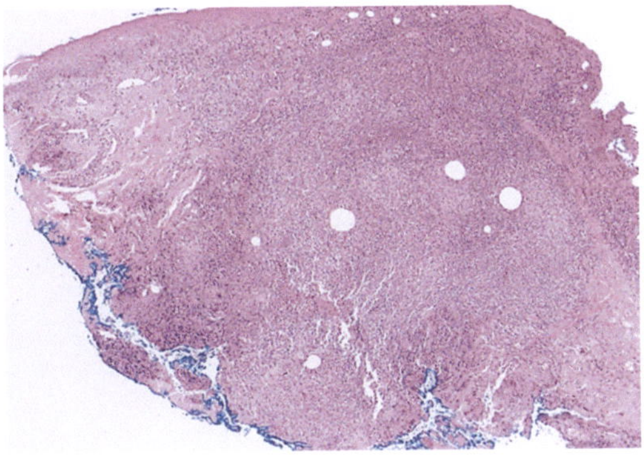

Fig. 3.52 Diffuse inflammation with empty round spaces

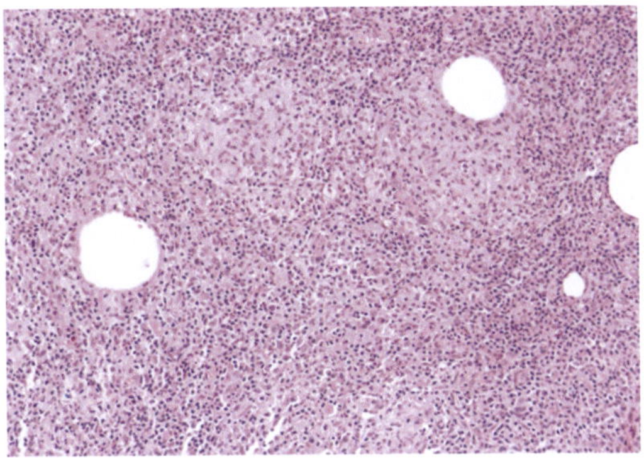

Fig. 3.53 Empty vacuoles surrounded by histiocytes forming non-caseating granulomas

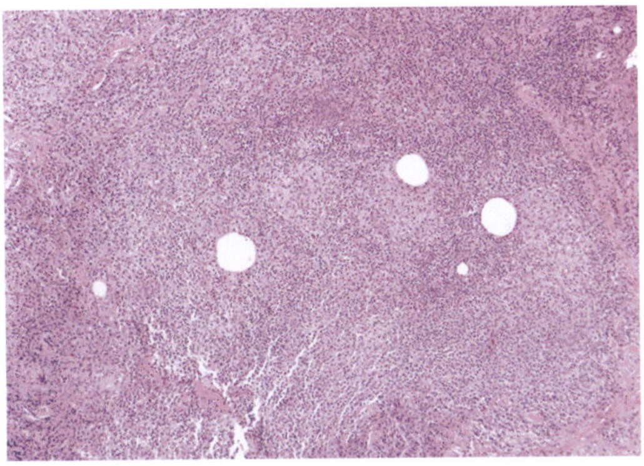

Fig. 3.54 Empty vacuoles of washed out lipids

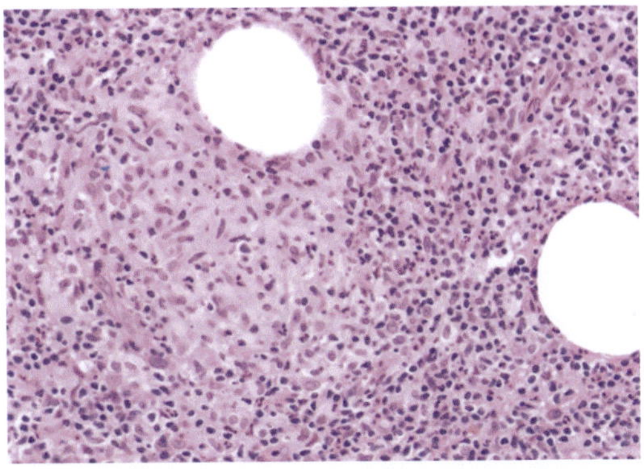

Fig. 3.55 Histiocytic aggregate surrounded by lymphocytes

Chancroid

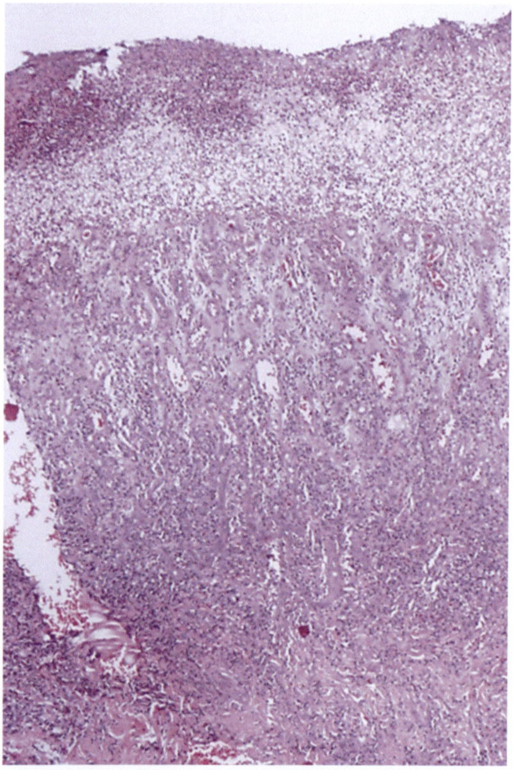

Fig. 3.56 Excoriated skin with three layers

Histopathology (Figs. 3.56, 3.57, and 3.58)

- Excoriated epidermis
- Consists of three layered zones
  (a) Upper serum crust with acute inflammation
  (b) Middle layer of granulation tissue
  (c) Lower dense plasmolymphocytic infiltrate
- Gram negative staining of *Haemophilus ducreyi*

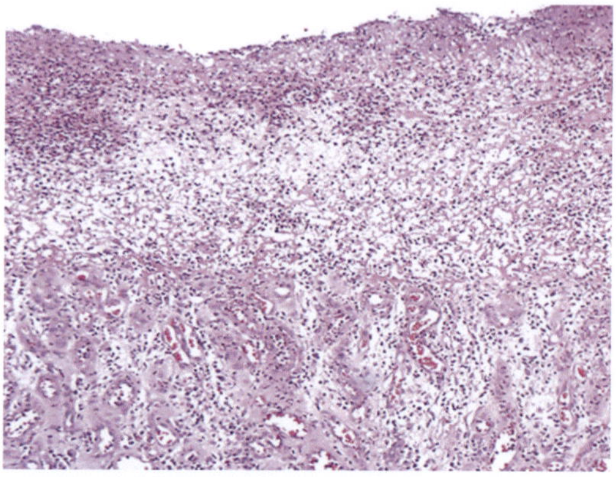

Fig. 3.57 Acutely inflamed serum crust and underlying granulation tissues

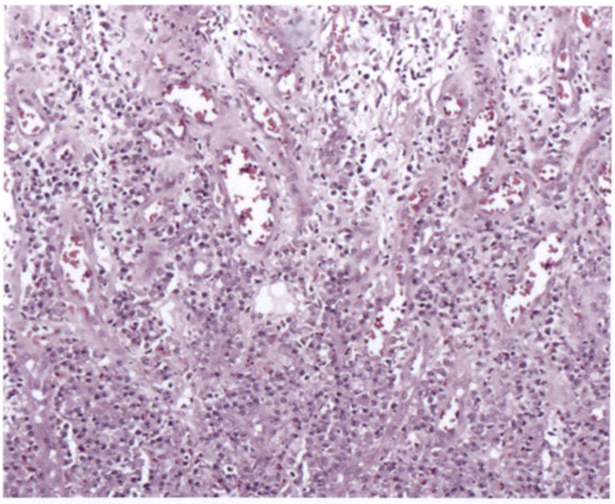

Fig. 3.58 Granulation tissue with underlying lymphoplasmocytic infiltrate

Cherry Angioma

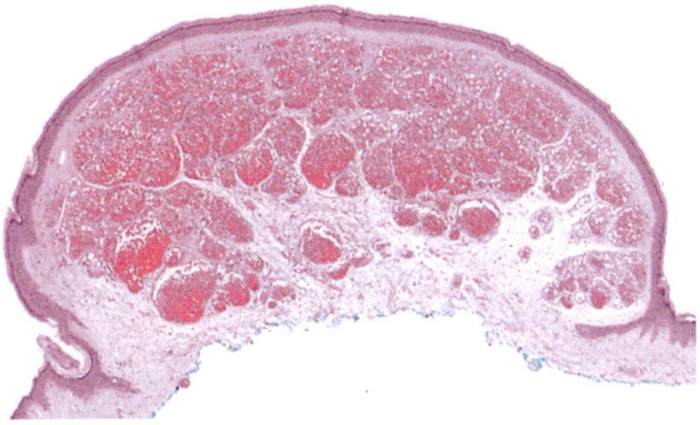

Fig. 3.59 Nodular dome-shaped vascular lesion

Histopathology (Figs. 3.59, 3.60, and 3.61)

- Polypoid dome-shaped lesion
- Epidermis is atrophic with epidermal collarettes
- Proliferation of medium size dermal vessels forming dermal nodule
- Vessels have thin wall with no atypia

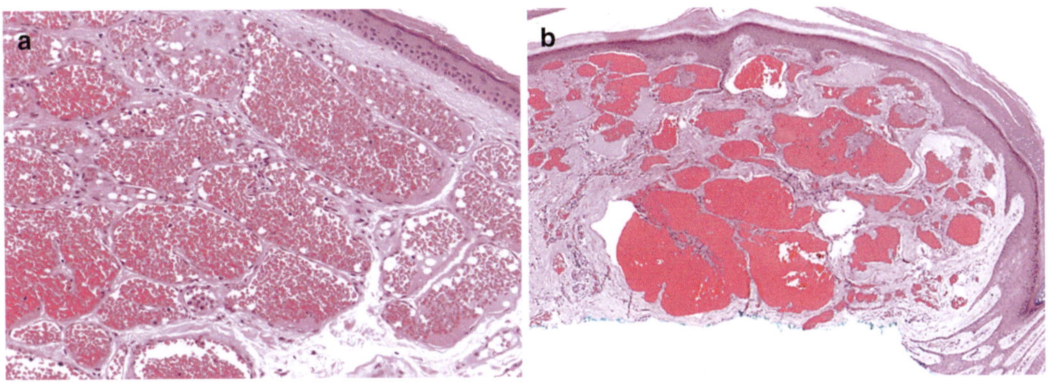

Fig. 3.60 (a, b) Atrophic epidermis with collarettes

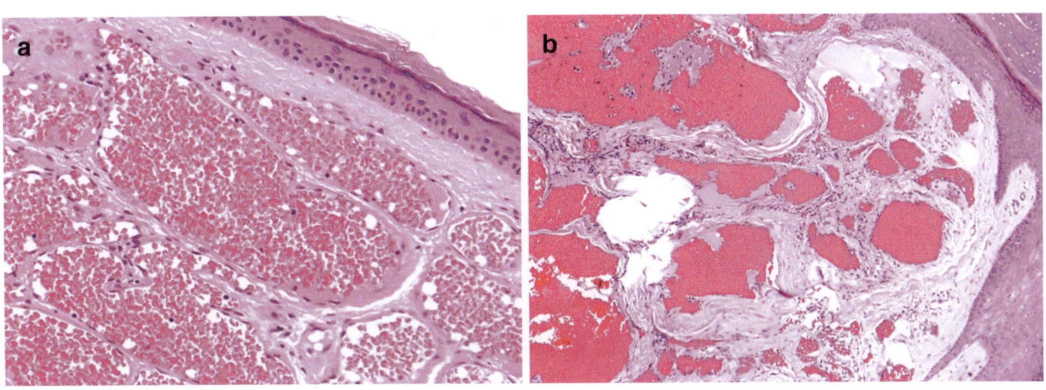

Fig. 3.61 (a, b) Medium size dilated congested vessels with thin walls

Chondroid Syringoma

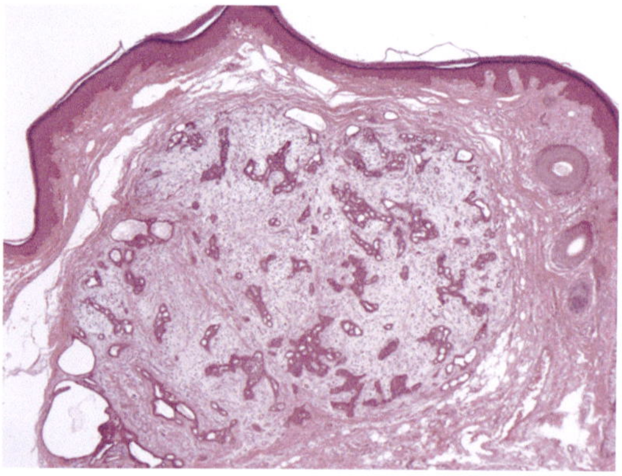

Fig. 3.62 Well circumscribed nodule

Synonym: Mixed Tumor of Skin

Histopathology can be quite variable: (Figs. 3.62, 3.63, 3.64, 3.65, and 3.66)

- Circumscribed dermal tumor with epithelioid component (EMA+, CEA+) in myxoid, chondroid stroma
- Epithelioid component consists of individual cells, smaller clusters and/or larger sheets of cells resembling sweat ducts
- Ductal structures have variable syringoid ("comma" like) shape and are lined by two cell layers

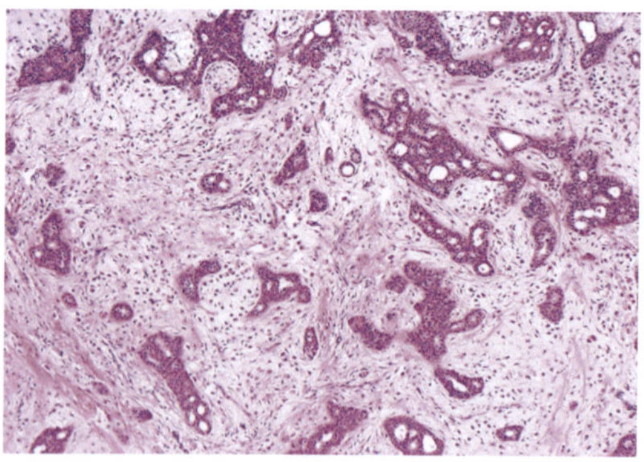

Fig. 3.63 Ductul structures with two cell layers

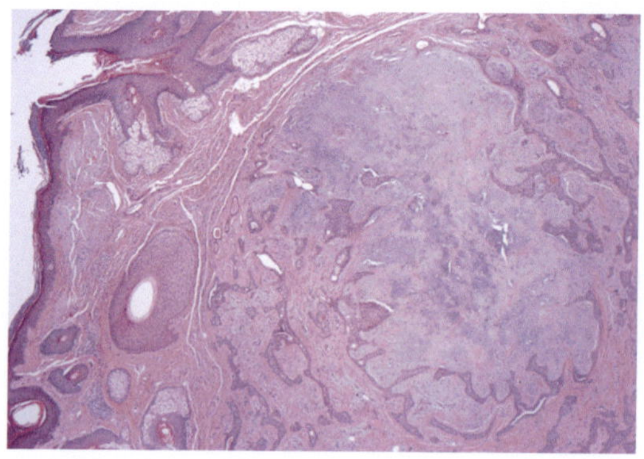

Fig. 3.64 Hyalinized stroma (pink) with chondroid changes (blue)

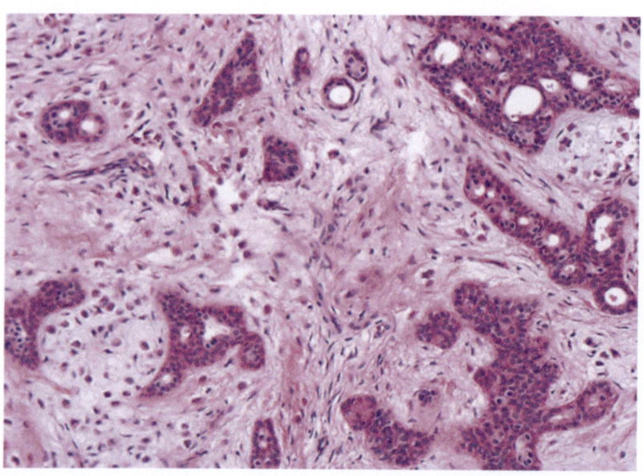

Fig. 3.65 Some ducts are "comma" shaped

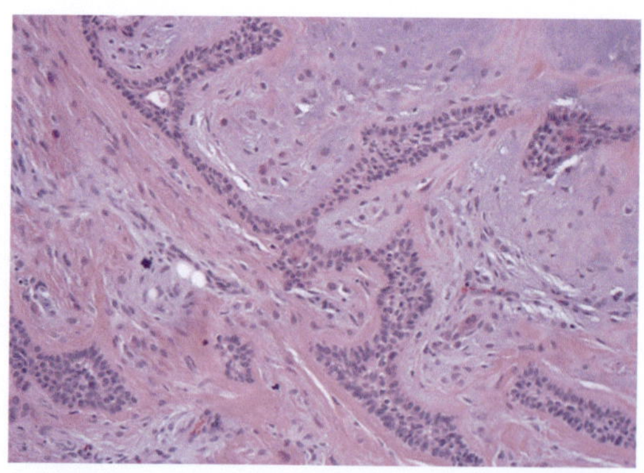

Fig. 3.66 Irregularly shaped ducts with no atypia or mitoses

Chondrodermatitis Nodularis Helicis

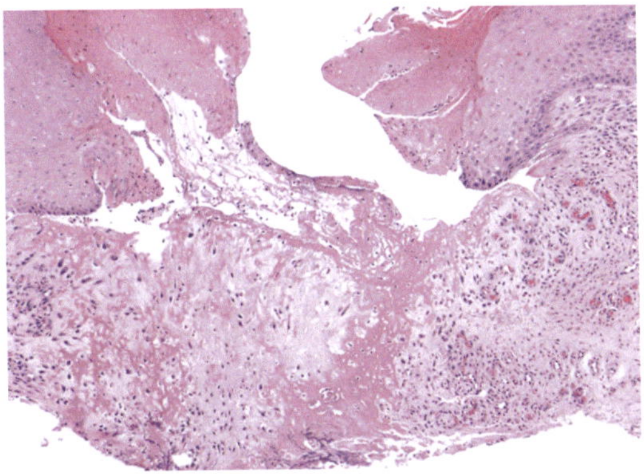

Fig. 3.67 Ulcerated hyperkeratotic acanthotic epidermis

Histopathology (Figs. 3.67, 3.68, 3.69, 3.70, and 3.71)

- Hyperkeratotic acanthotic epidermis
- Central area of ulceration with inflammation
- Prominent fibrin deposition at the base of the ulceration
- Dermis shows chondroid appearance
- Granulation tissue is present adjacent to the ulceration

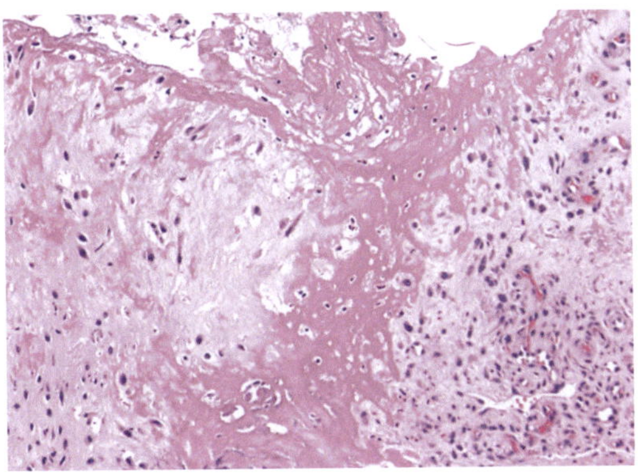

Fig. 3.68 Pink fibrin deposition and granulation tissue form the base of the ulcer

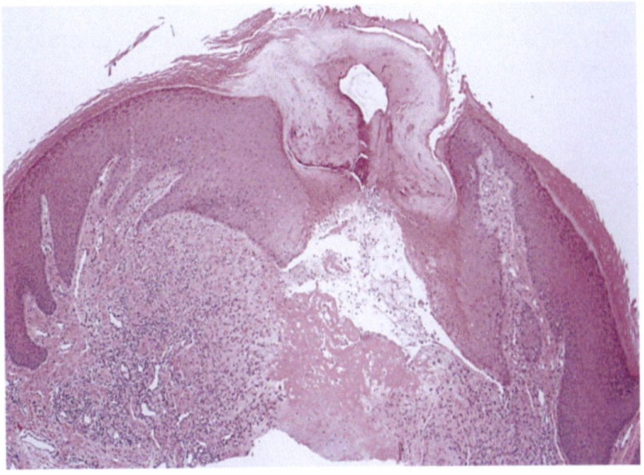

Fig. 3.69 Central ulceration with dermal chondroid changes

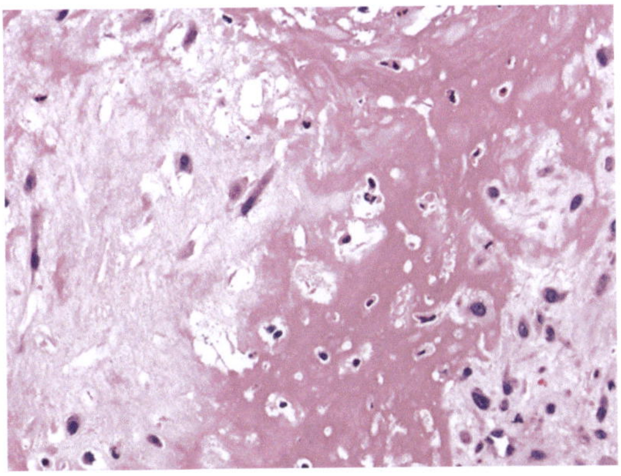

Fig. 3.70 Atypical fibroblasts are present within fibrin deposition

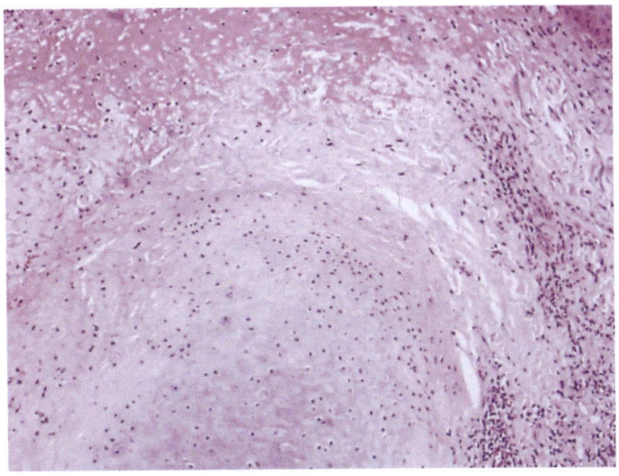

Fig. 3.71 Chondroid (bluish) changes are present underneath the granulation tissue and fibrin. Granulation tissue is present adjacent

Chondroma

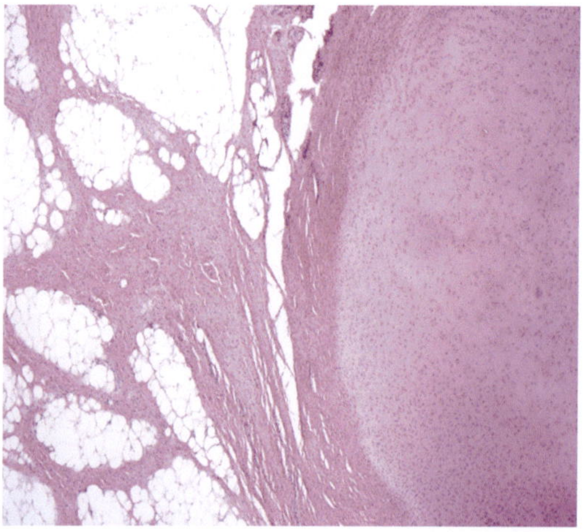

Fig. 3.72 Well circumscribed cartilaginous nodule in subcutaneous fibroadipose tissue

Synonym: Extraskeletal Chondroma, Soft Tissue Chondroma

Histopathology (Figs. 3.72, 3.73, and 3.74)

- Well circumscribed nodule
- Tumor is not encapsulated
- Tumor consists of mature hyalinized cartilage
- Chondrocytes are not atypical
- Some chondrocytes at the tumor periphery demonstrate some degenerative changes

P.S. 12q13-15 (HMGA2/HMGI-C) rearrangement

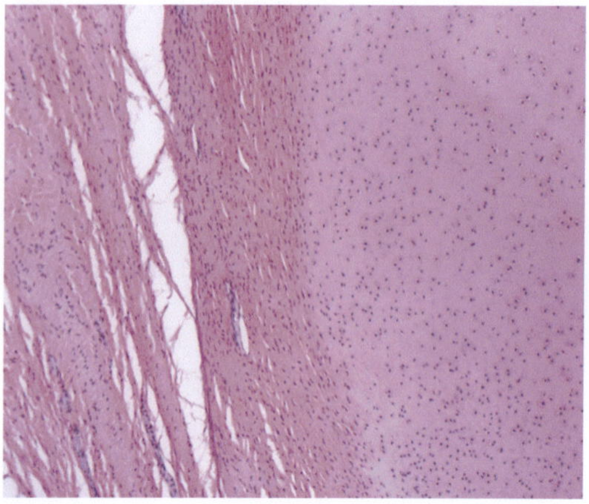

Fig. 3.73 Tumor has fibrous pseudocapsule

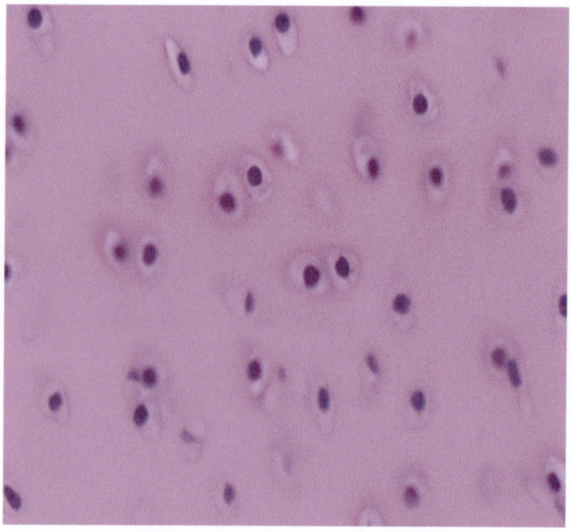

Fig. 3.74 Normal appearing chondrocytes

Chondrosarcoma

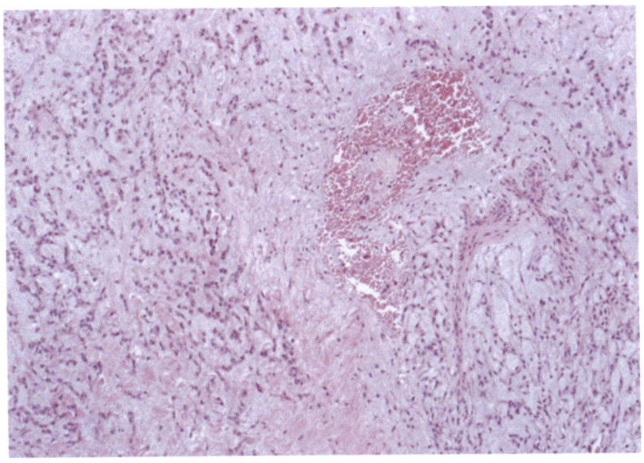

Fig. 3.75 Alternating hyper and hypocellular areas

Synonym: Extraskeletal Myxoid Chondrosarcoma

Histopathology (Figs. 3.75, 3.76, and 3.77)

- Irregular but well defined lobules
- Small round to oval chondroblasts in abundant myxoid stroma
- Periphery of the tumor is more cellular and center is more myxoid
- Variable number of mitoses and necrosis

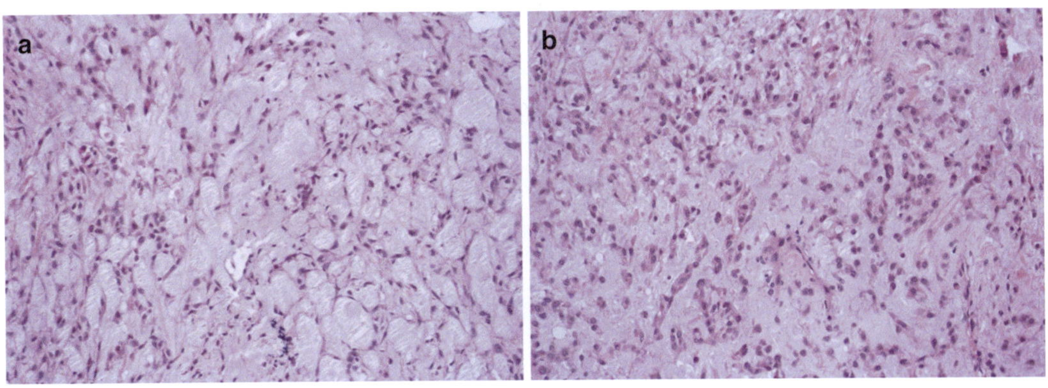

Fig. 3.76 (**a**, **b**) Round to oval irregular cells in bluish myxoid stroma

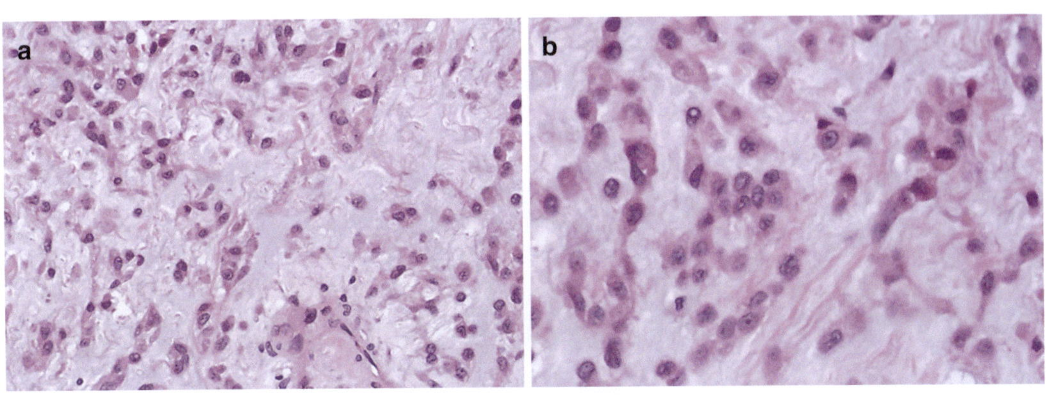

Fig. 3.77 (**a**, **b**) Tumor cells are pleomorphic and apoptosis are present

Chordoma

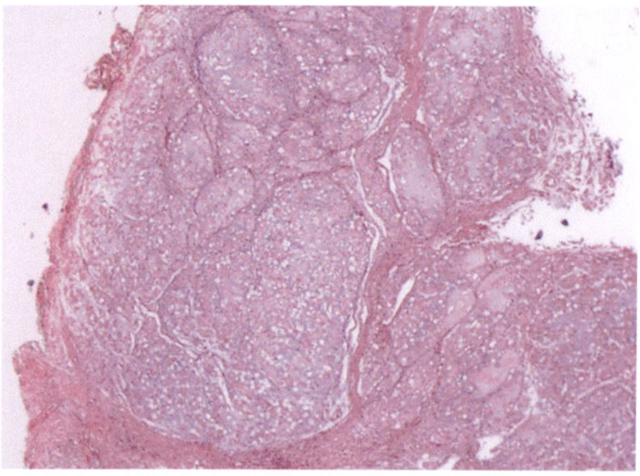

Fig. 3.78 Multiple irregular nodules separated by fibrous septa

Histopathology (Figs. 3.78, 3.79, and 3.80)
- Nodules and cords of "bubbly" cells in exuberant myxoid stroma
- Cells are large with vesicular nuclei and vacuolated cytoplasm
- Nuclear pleomorphism is present
- Tumor cells are S-100, cytokeratin AE1/AE3, EMA, and CEA positive

P.S. malignant midline tumor arising from fetal notochord

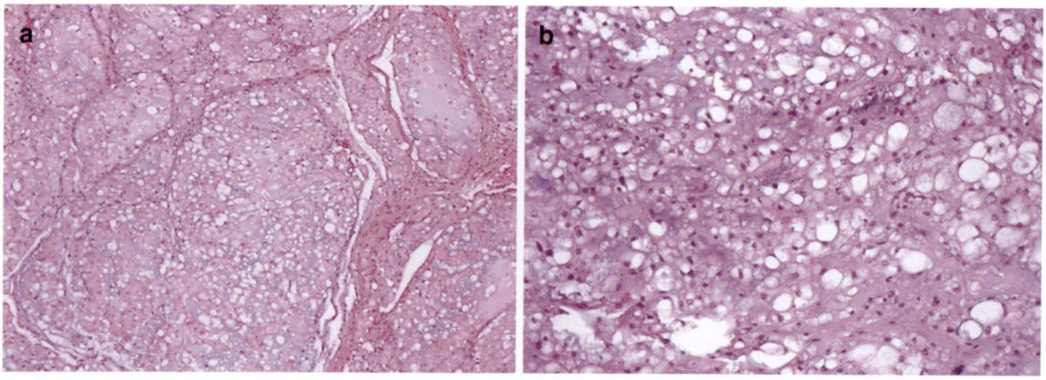

Fig. 3.79 (a, b) Loose atypical cells in myxoid stroma

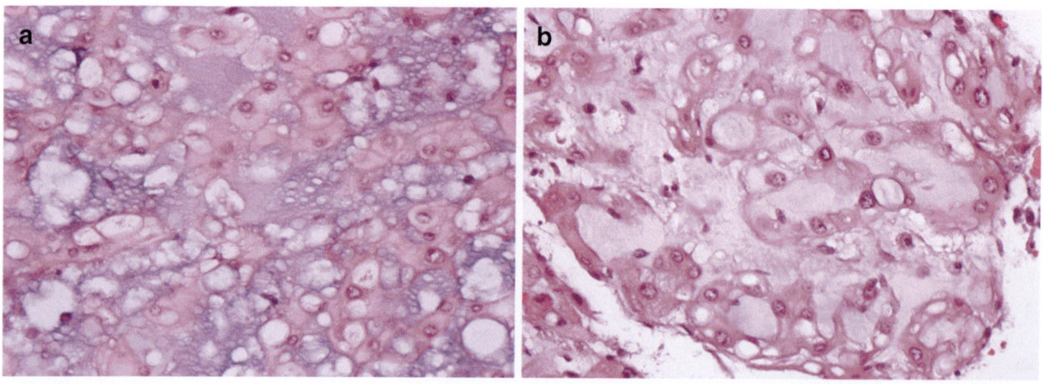

Fig. 3.80 (a, b) Pleomorphic oval cells with vesicular nuclei in bluish cartilage-like myxoid stroma

Chromoblastomycosis

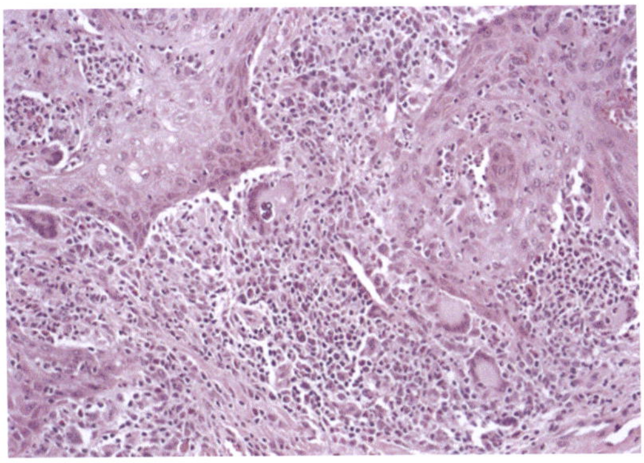

Fig. 3.81 Pseudoepitheliomatous hyperplasia with mixed dermal inflammation with giant cells

Histopathology (Figs. 3.81, 3.82, 3.83, 3.84, and 3.85)

- Epidermal pseudoepitheliomatous hyperplasia
- Dermal and subcutaneous acute inflammation with microabscesses
- Round, thick-walled brown sclerotic ("copper pennies") bodies
- Pigmented sclerotic bodies prefer to be within giant cells and microabscesses but can also be extracellularly

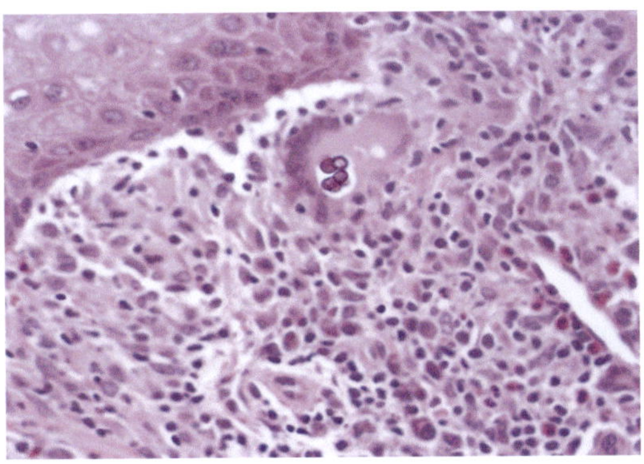

Fig. 3.82 Multiple "copper pennies" are present within giant cell

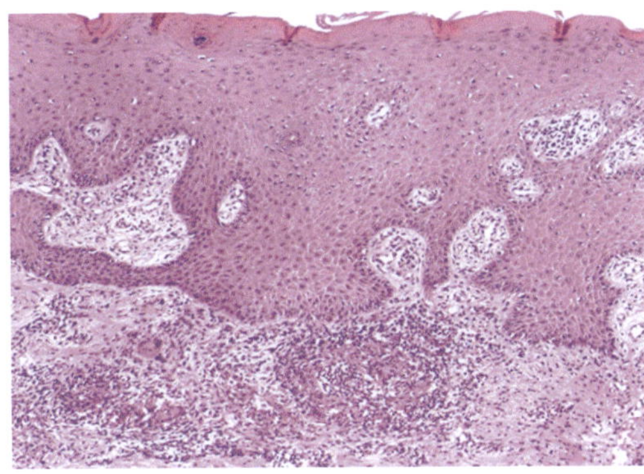

Fig. 3.83 Pseudoepitheliomatous hyperplasia with dermal microabscess

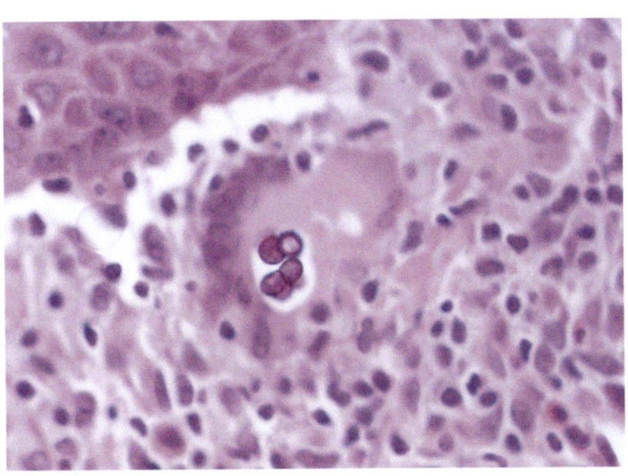

Fig. 3.84 "Copper pennies"

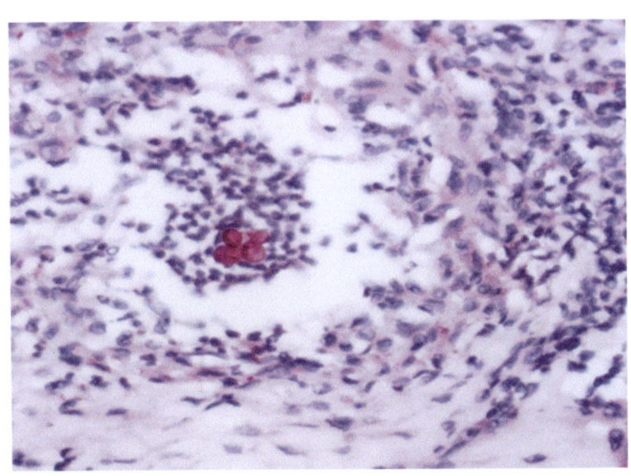

Fig. 3.85 Sclerotic bodies in the microabscess (PAS)

Chrysiasis

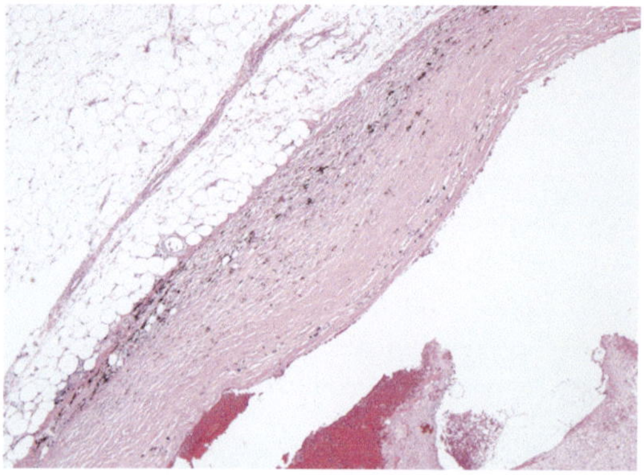

Fig. 3.86 A patient that underwent gold therapy for rheumatoid arthritis 10 years ago

Synonym: Gold Deposition

Histopathology (Figs. 3.86, 3.87, 3.88, 3.89, and 3.90)

- In an early lesion, deep granulomatous reaction within deep subcutis is present
- In an older lesion, there are subcutaneous sclerotic nodules within deep subcutis and subcutaneous fat
- Finely refractile, yellow-brown granules of gold are present
- Granules are birefringent and present between thick collagen

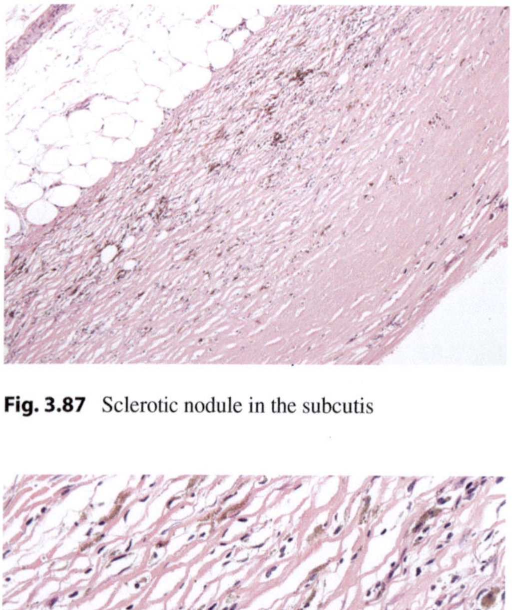

Fig. 3.87 Sclerotic nodule in the subcutis

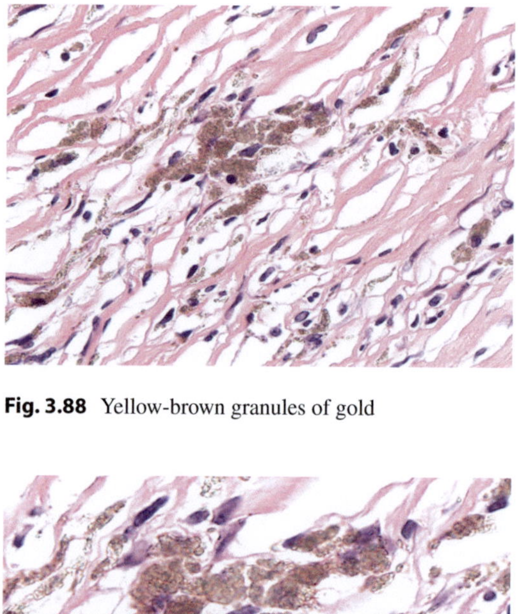

Fig. 3.88 Yellow-brown granules of gold

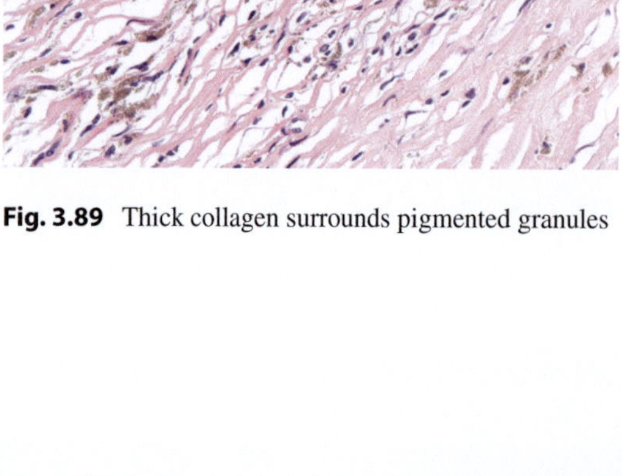

Fig. 3.89 Thick collagen surrounds pigmented granules

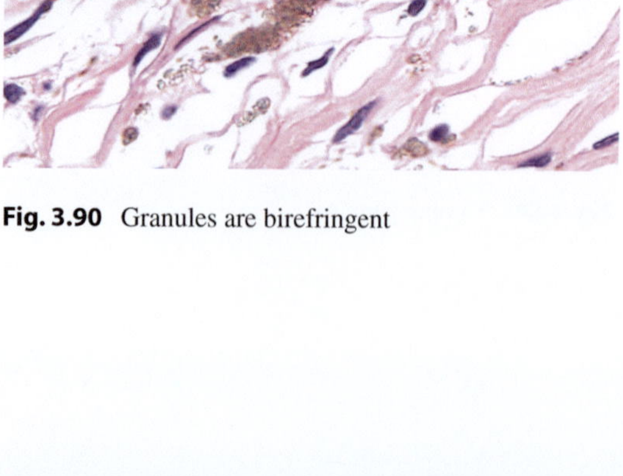

Fig. 3.90 Granules are birefringent

Churg Strauss Disease

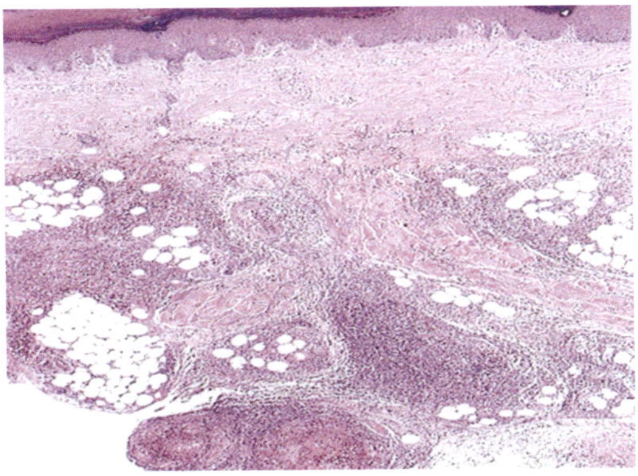

Fig. 3.91 Subcutaneous angiocentric inflammation

Synonym: Allergic Granulomatosis with Polyangiitis

Histopathology of cutaneous lesion is variable (Figs. 3.91, 3.92, 3.93, 3.94, and 3.95)

- Mixed angiocentric inflammation with vague granulomas and variable eosinophils
- Some cases have significant leukocytoclastic vasculitis with eosinophils
- Necrosis of medium and large vessels with eosinophilic infiltrate is a common systemic feature but is actually rarely found in the skin

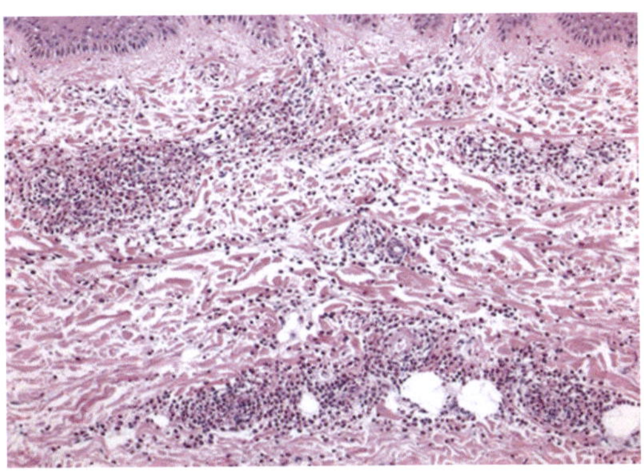

Fig. 3.92 Early lesion with vague granulomatous appearance

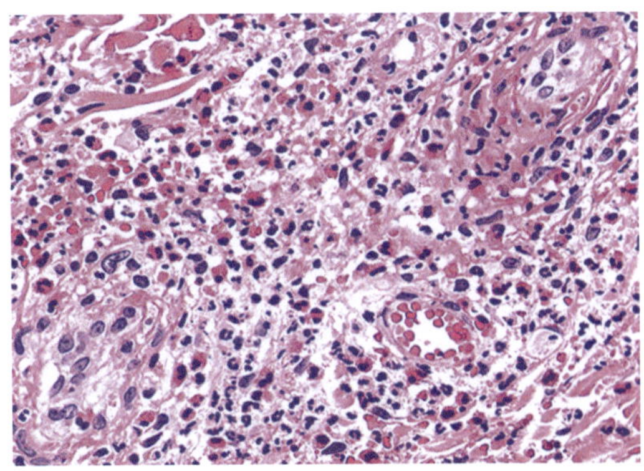

Fig. 3.93 Leukocytoclastic vasculitis with eosinophils

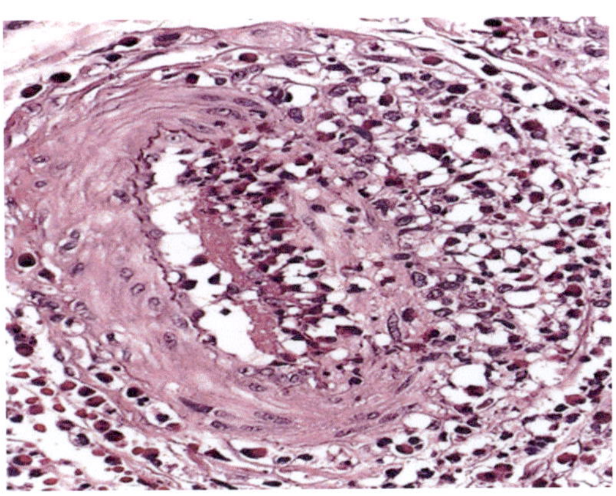

Fig. 3.94 Medium size vessel with partial wall necrosis

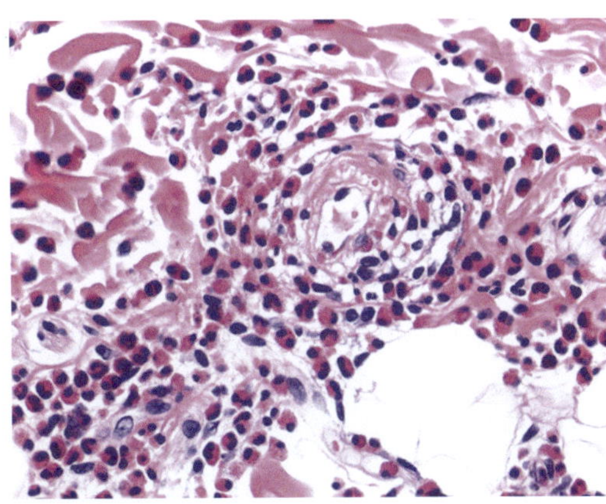

Fig. 3.95 Small vessel surrounded by numerous eosinophils

Cicatricial Pemphigoid

Synonym: Mucous Membrane Pemphigoid
Despite the name about a third of the cases have concomitant skin lesions. Histologically lesion are indistinguishable from bullous pemphigoid.

Histopathology (Figs. 3.96, 3.97, 3.98, and 3.99)
- Subepithelial/subepidermal blister
- Submucosal/dermal fibrosis and scarring
- Mixed inflammatory infiltrate with a variable number of eosinophils

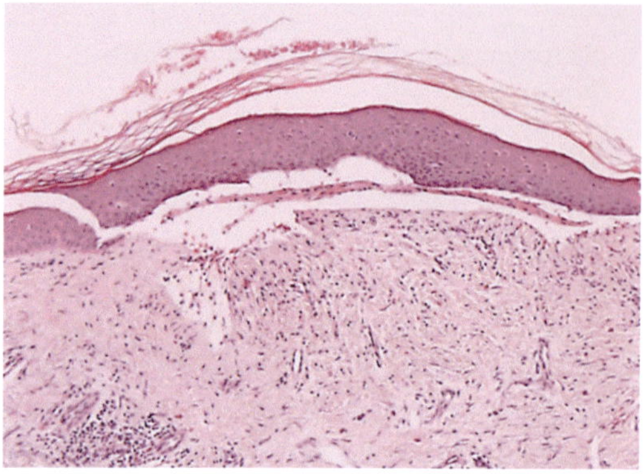

Fig. 3.96 Lip lesion with subepidermal blister

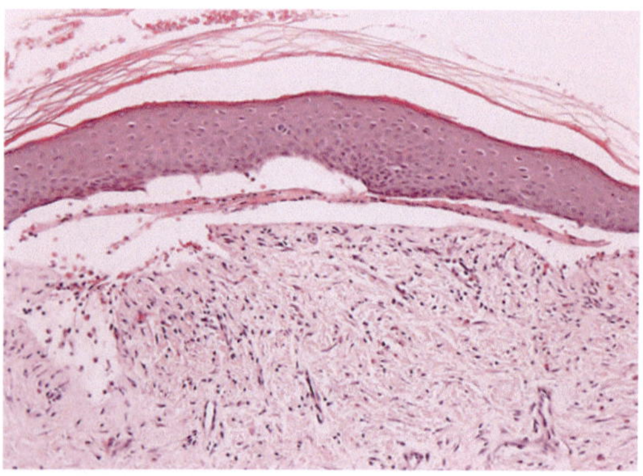

Fig. 3.97 Submucosal scarring

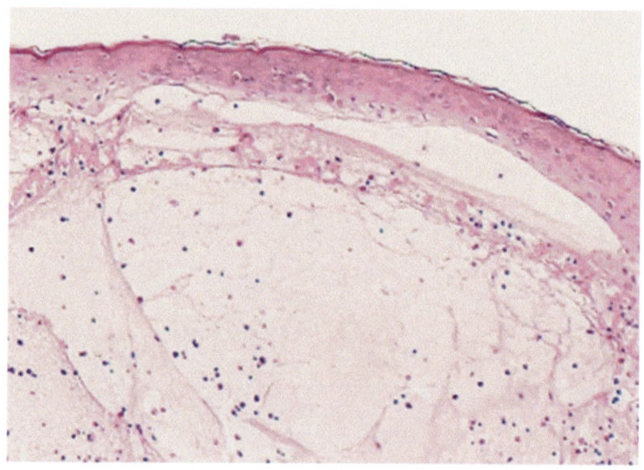

Fig. 3.98 Submucosal blister with mixed inflammation

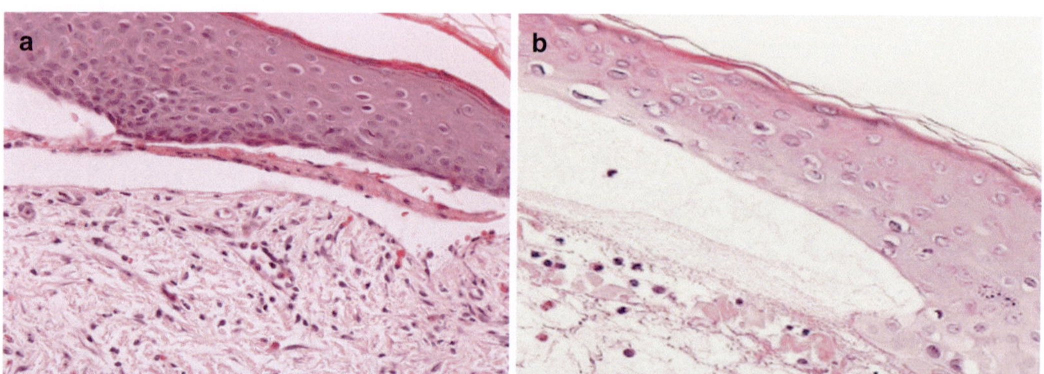

Fig. 3.99 (**a**, **b**) Mixed inflammation with eosinophils

Ciliated Cyst

Synonym: Cutaneous Ciliated Cyst

Histopathology (Figs. 3.100, 3.101, and 3.102)

- Cyst located in the deep dermis or subcutis
- Irregular cyst with cuboidal or/and columnar ciliated lining with mucinous changes
- Small intraluminar papillary projections
- Foci of squamous metaplasia can be seen

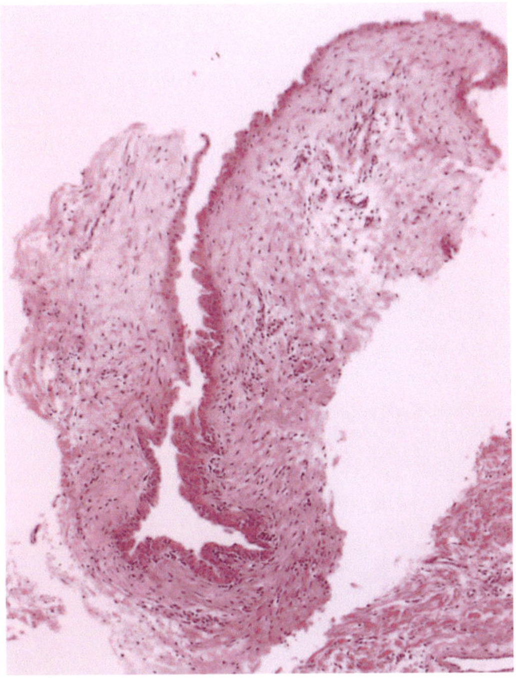

Fig. 3.100 Irregular cyst with small papillary projections

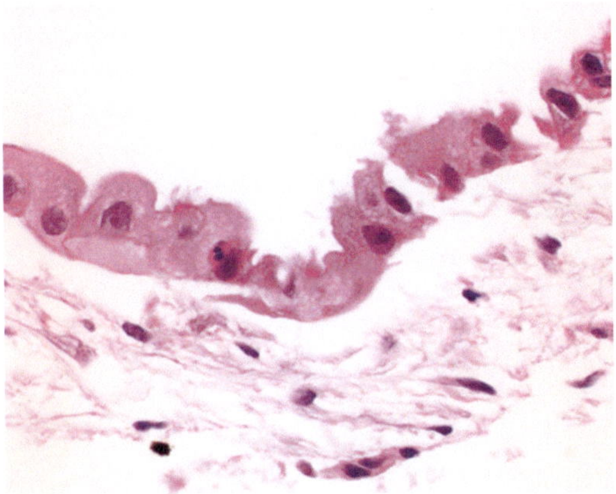

Fig. 3.101 Cilia are evident in the central cuboidal cells

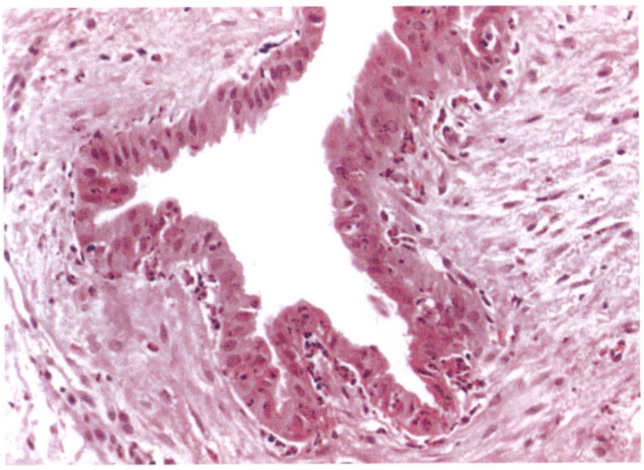

Fig. 3.102 Cyst is lined by cuboidal cells

Circumscribed Acral Hypokeratosis

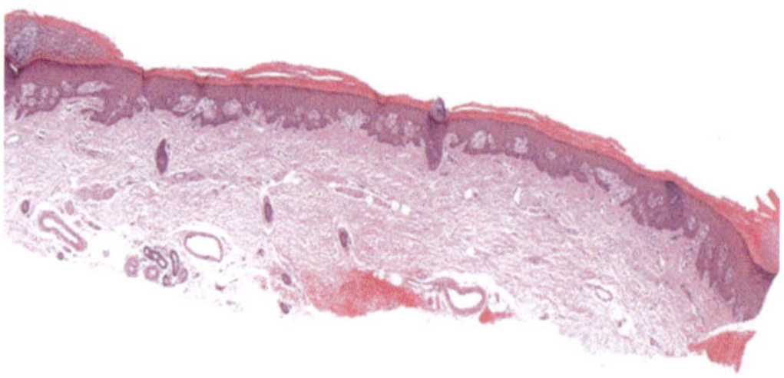

Fig. 3.103 Acral skin with sharply delineated hypokeratotic patch

Histopathology (Figs. 3.103, 3.104, and 3.105)
- Acral skin with a predilection for the thenar or hypothenar
- Abrupt decrease in the thickness of the stratum corneum
- Sharp delineation between normal and involved skin
- Absence of atypia, parakeratosis, or koilocytes allows separation from Bowen disease, porokeratosis, and/or wart

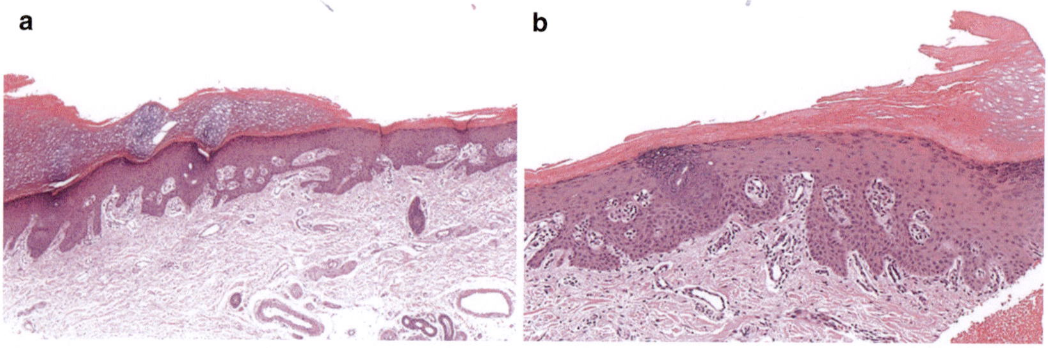

Fig. 3.104 (**a**, **b**) Abrupt decrease in the thickness of the stratum corneum

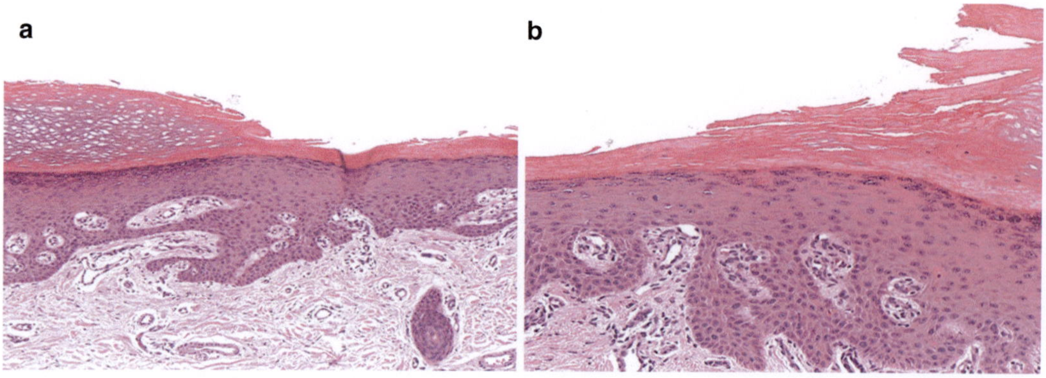

Fig. 3.105 (**a**, **b**) No evidence of atypia, parakeratosis, or koilocytes

Clavus

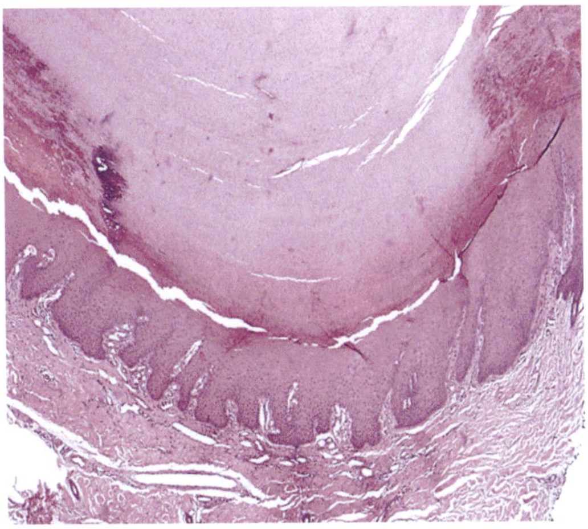

Fig. 3.106 Cup-shaped acral epidermal lesion

Synonym: Corn

Histopathology (Figs. 3.106, 3.107, and 3.108)

- Cup-shaped well circumscribed epidermal lesion
- Extensive epidermal hyperkeratosis with an absence of the granular layer
- Mild parakeratosis is present
- Dermal dilated vessels and no inflammation

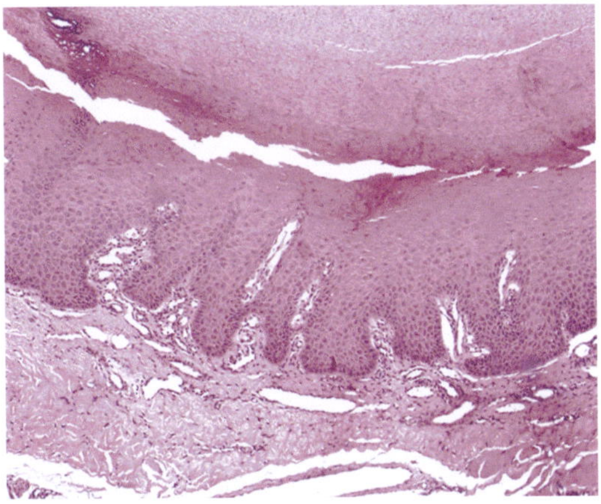

Fig. 3.107 Dilated dermal capillaries and no inflammation

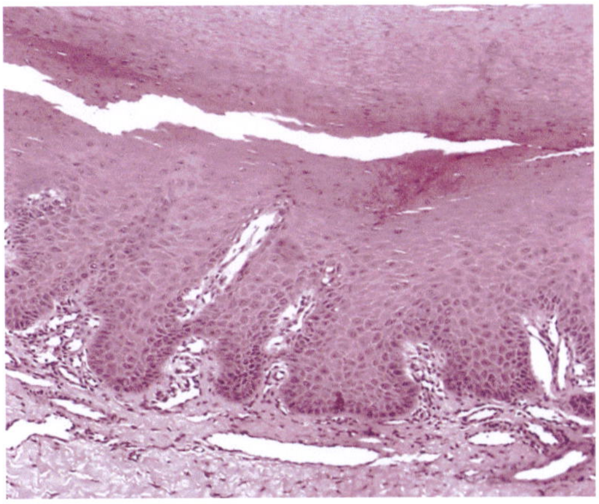

Fig. 3.108 Hyperkeratosis, parakeratosis and absence of the granular layer

Clear Cell Acanthoma

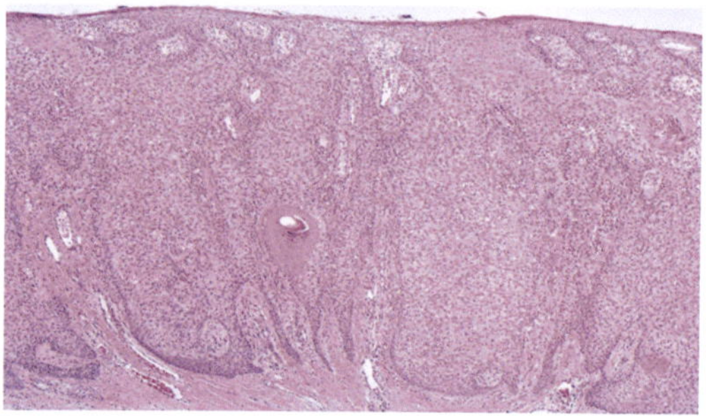

Fig. 3.109 Pale acanthotic psoriasiform epidermis

Synonym: Degos Acanthoma, Pale Cell Acanthoma

Histopathology (Figs. 3.109, 3.110, 3.111, 3.112, and 3.113)

- Laterally well demarcated lesion
- Acanthotic psoriasiform epidermis with thin suprapapillary plates
- Uniformed pale keratinocytes rimmed with darker peripheral keratinocytes (EMA+, CEA-)
- Neutrophils are scattered over the epidermis

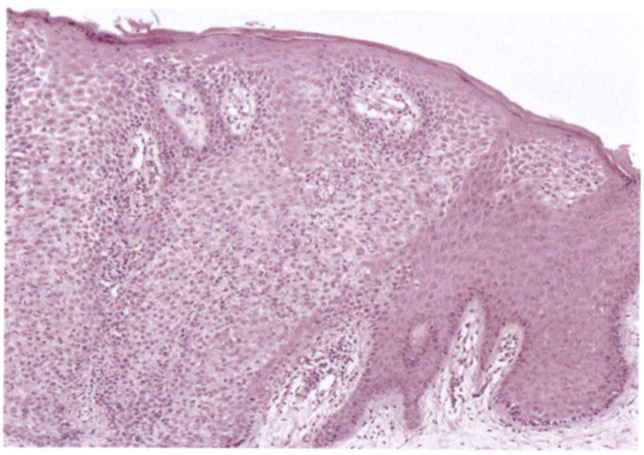

Fig. 3.110 Lateral border is clearly demarcated

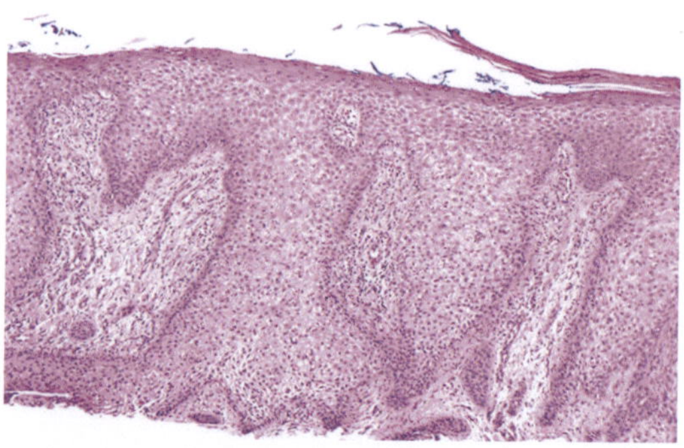

Fig. 3.111 Thin suprapapillary plates with interconnected retes

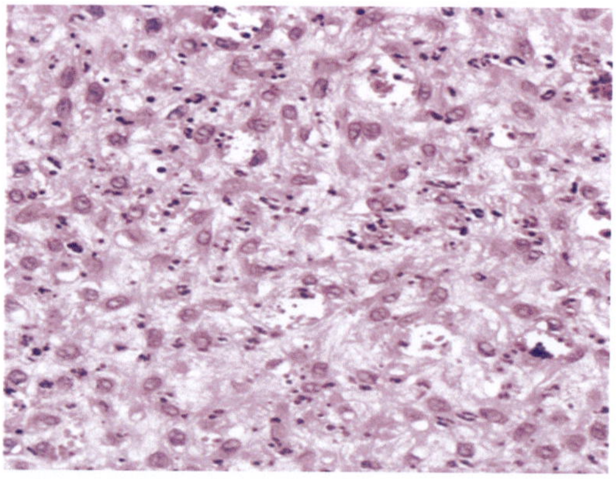

Fig. 3.112 Neutrophils are "peppered" over the keratinocytes

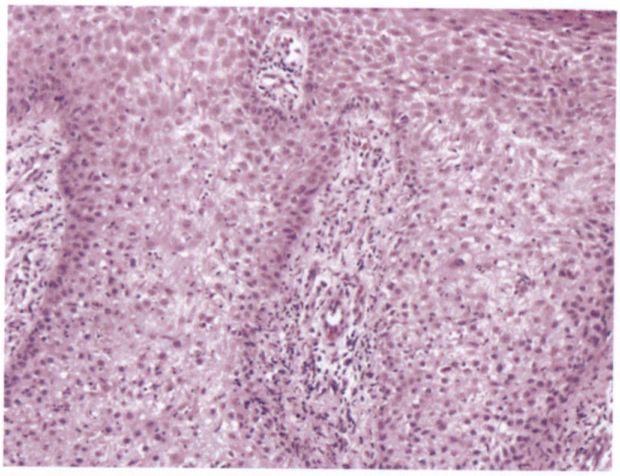

Fig. 3.113 Pale glycogen filled keratinocytes surrounded with darker basal layer keratinocytes

Clear Cell Sarcoma

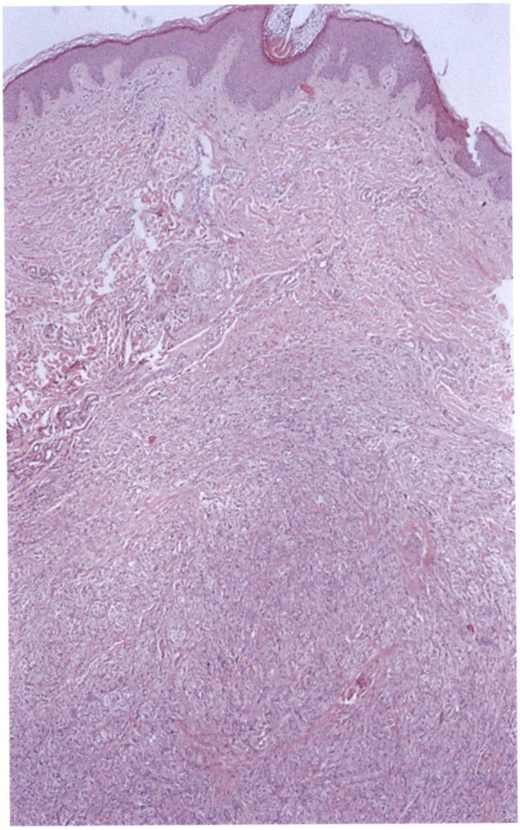

Fig. 3.114 Subcutaneous tumor infiltrating dermis

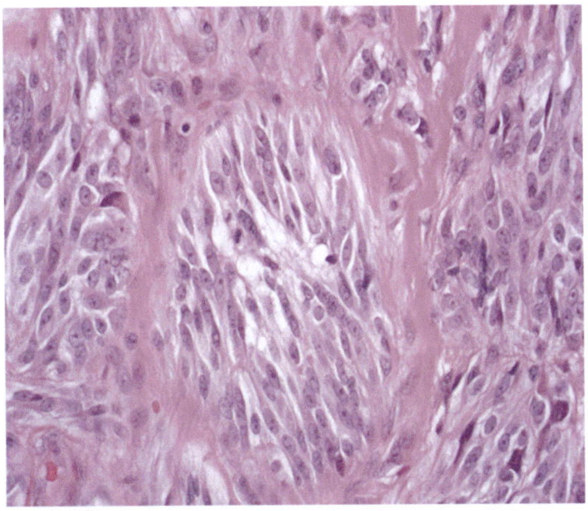

Fig. 3.115 Within prominent fibrous stroma there are elongated cells with pale cytoplasm and vesicular nuclei resembling cytology of melanoma cells

Synonym: Malignant Melanoma of Soft Parts

Histopathology (Figs. 3.114, 3.115, and 3.116)

- Occur in the soft tissue and dermis
- Relatively uniform but atypical cells with clear to eosinophilic cytoplasm forming fascicles
- Round to oval nuclei with vesicular chromatin
- Fibrous septa separate aggregates
- Melanin pigment found in about half of the cases
- Tumor cells are S-100, Melan-A, HMB45 positive
- Specific t(12;22) (q13;q12) translocation

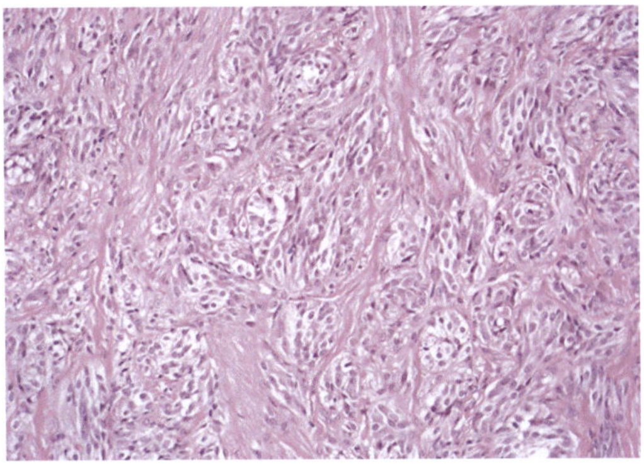

Fig. 3.116 Fascicles of clear cells separated by fibrous septa

Coccidioidomycosis

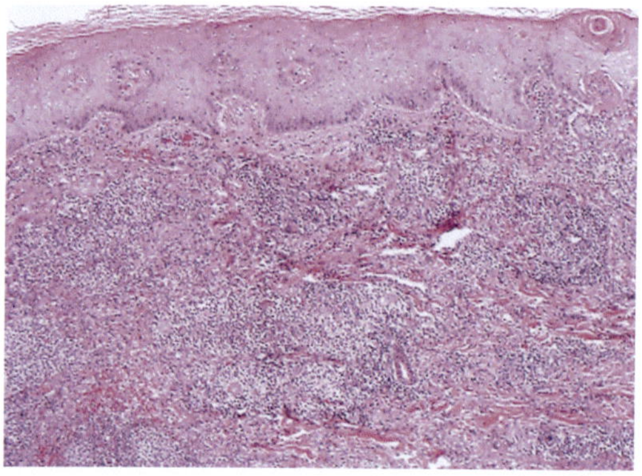

Fig. 3.117 Pseudoepitheliomatous hyperplasia with exuberant granulomatous inflammation

Histopathology (Figs. 3.117, 3.118, 3.119, and 3.120)
- Pseudoepitheliomatous hyperplasia
- Granulomatous dermatitis with mixed inflammation
- Spherules (up to 100 μm) contain numerous endospores (up to 5 μm)
- Spherules have thick wall and increase in the size till they burst and release endospores

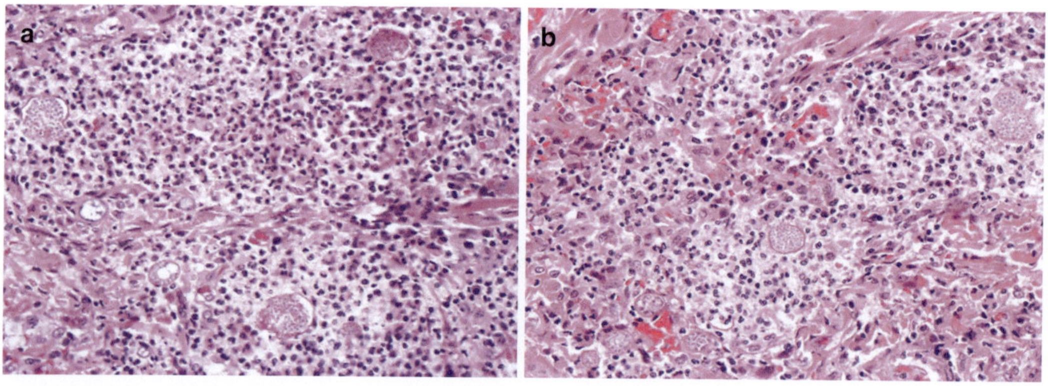

Fig. 3.118 (**a**, **b**) Mixed inflammation with giant cells and scattered spherules

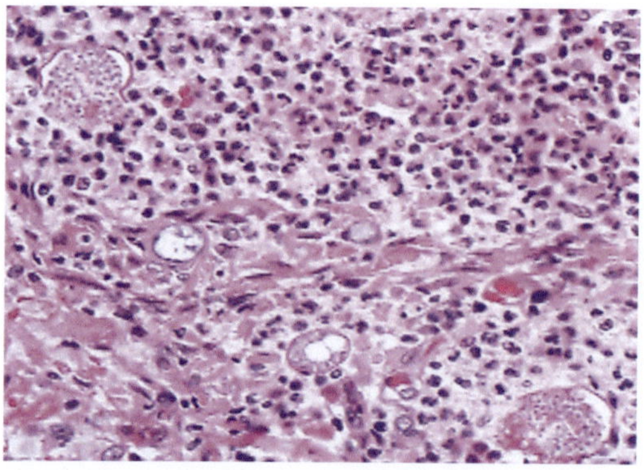

Fig. 3.119 Neutrophilic inflammation with admixed lymphocytes and histiocytes

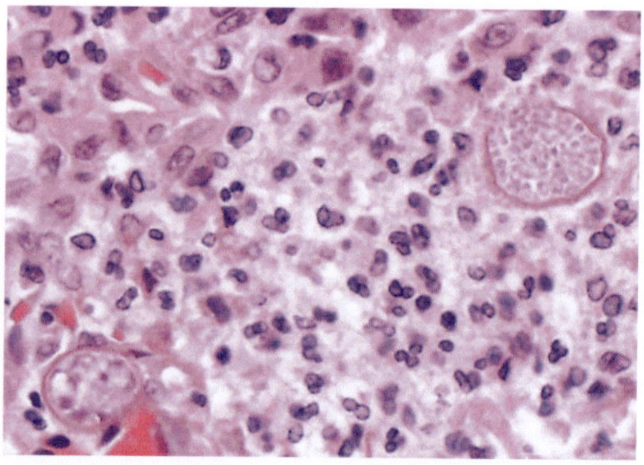

Fig. 3.120 Spherules vary in size and have thick pink wall; bluish endospores fill the spherules

Cold Panniculitis

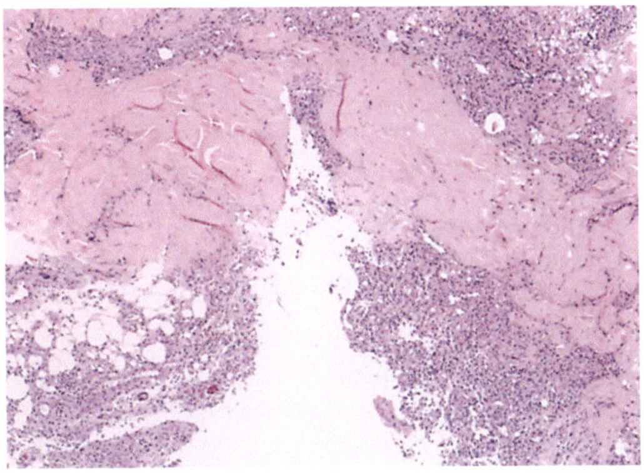

Fig. 3.121 Inflammation at the junction of the dermis and subcutis

Histopathology (Figs. 3.121, 3.122, 3.123, 3.124, and 3.125)

- Lobular panniculitis with mixed inflammation made of lymphocytes, histiocytes, neutrophils, and occasional giant cells
- Intense inflammation at the junction of the dermis and subcutaneous fat
- Variable fat necrosis
- Focal endothelial swelling and thickening of blood vessel wall

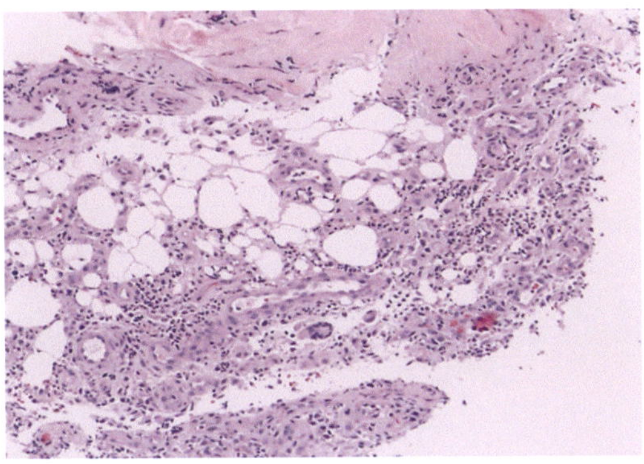

Fig. 3.122 Focal fat necrosis with mixed inflammation

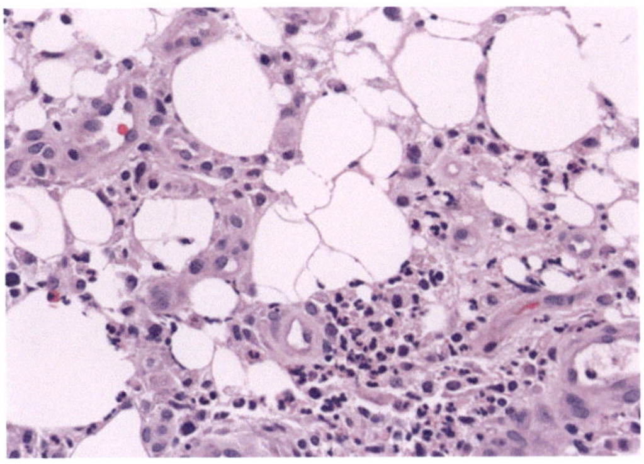

Fig. 3.123 Mixed inflammation of lymphocytes, histiocytes, and neutrophils

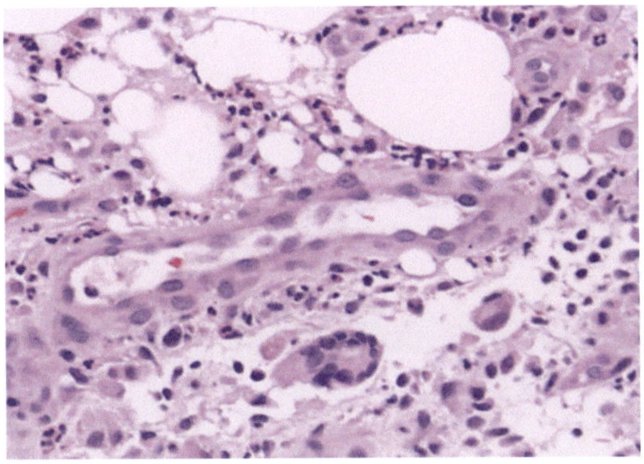

Fig. 3.124 Plump endothelial cells and a giant cell

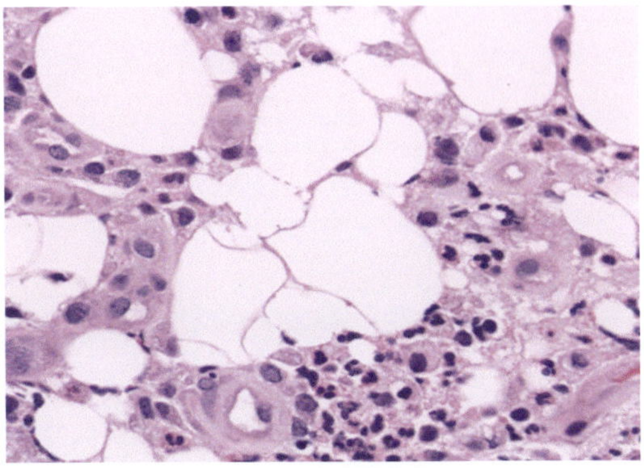

Fig. 3.125 Irregular damaged adipocytes

Collagenoma

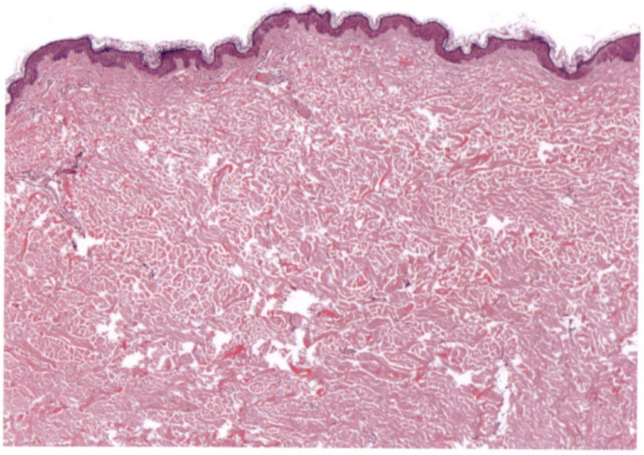

Fig. 3.126 Thickened homogenized dermis

Synonym: Collagenous Connective Tissue Nevus, Shagreen Patch

Histopathology (Figs. 3.126, 3.127, 3.128, 3.129, and 3.130)
- Significantly thickened dermis
- Broad bundles of haphazardly arranged homogenized collagen fibers
- Elastic fibers are normal or decreased in number
- Adnexal structures are missing

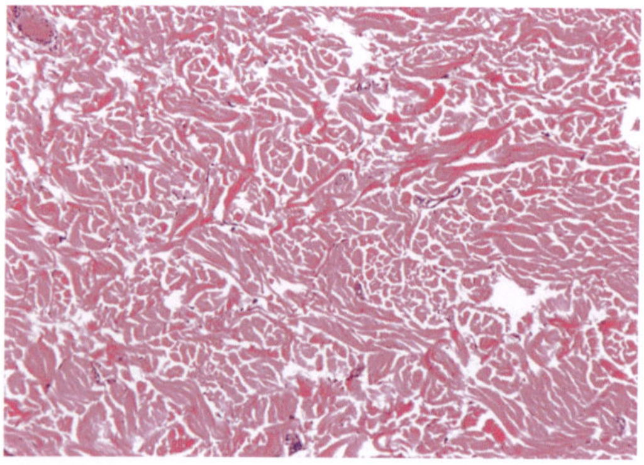

Fig. 3.127 Haphazardly arranged collagen bundles

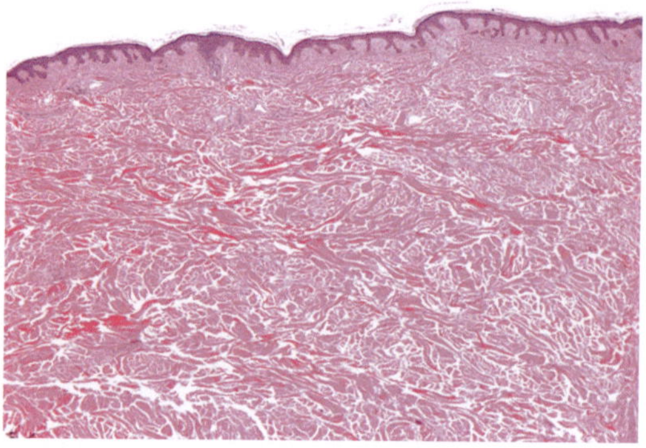

Fig. 3.128 Adnexal structures are absent

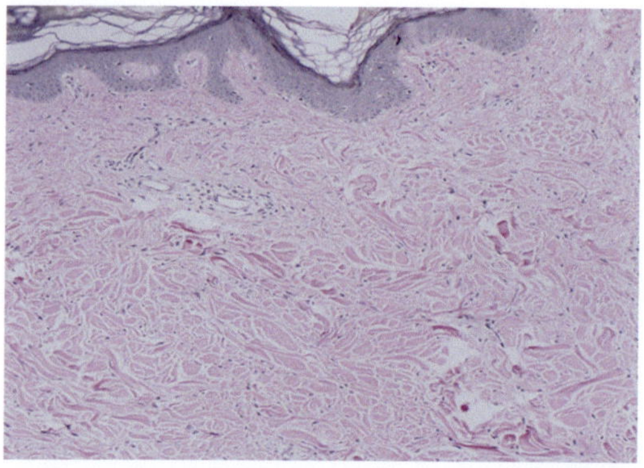

Fig. 3.129 VVG stains demonstrates decreased dermal elastic fibers

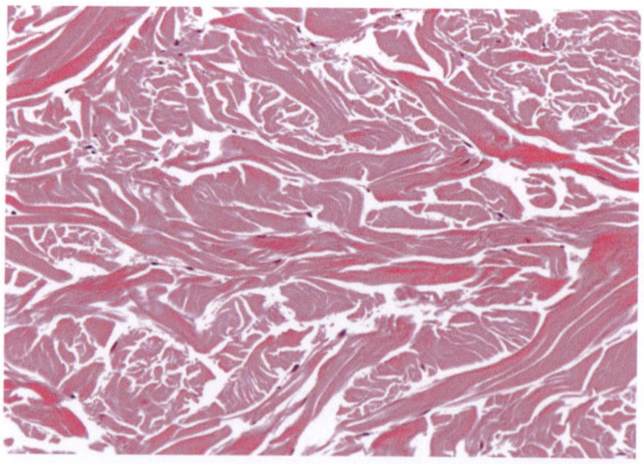

Fig. 3.130 Broad bundles made of homogenized collagen fibers

Collagenous and Elastotic Plaques of the Hands

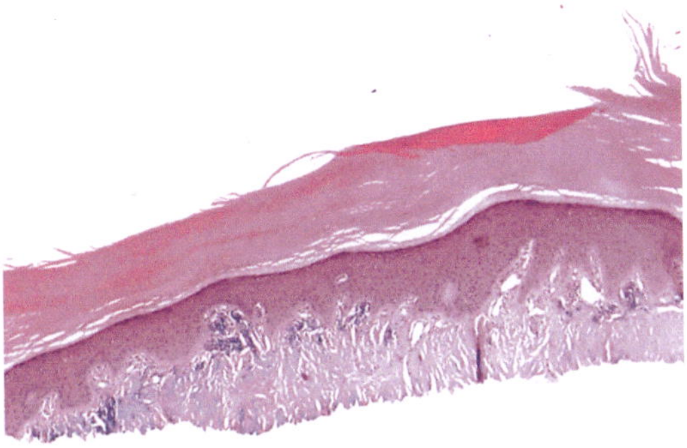

Fig. 3.131 Acral skin with abnormal dermal stroma

Synonym: Degenerative Collagenous Plaques of the Hand

Histopathology (Figs. 3.131, 3.132, and 3.133)

- Acral skin with epidermal hyperkeratosis and acanthosis
- Thick collagen in the upper portion of the dermis
- Fragmented degenerated elastic fibers
- Elastic fibers form amorphous masses that can calcify

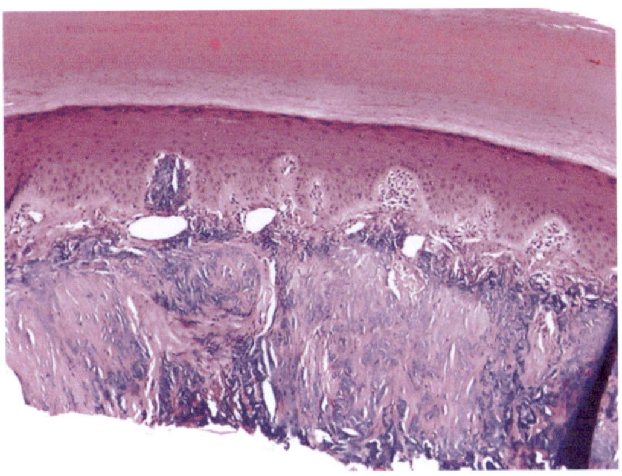

Fig. 3.132 Hyalinized papillary dermis

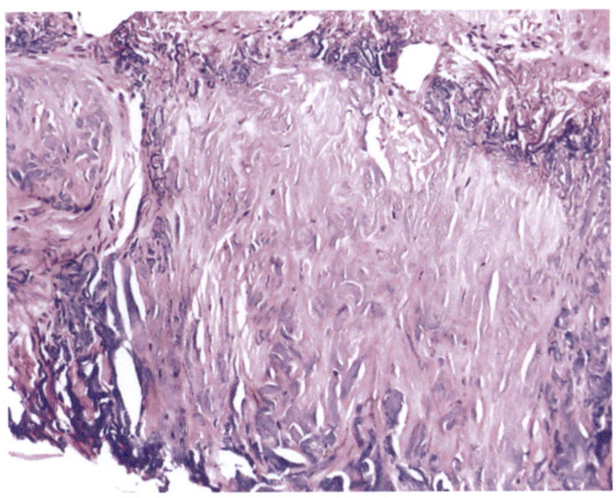

Fig. 3.133 Thickened collagen bundles with irregular mass of degenerated elastic fibers

Collision Tumor

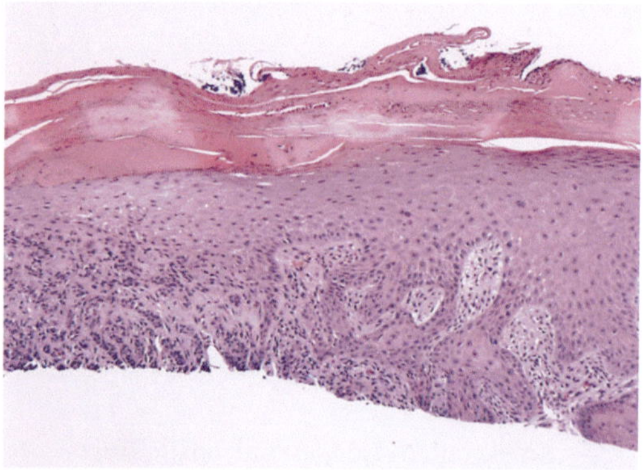

Fig. 3.134 Collision of two different tumors

Histopathology (Figs. 3.134, 3.135, 3.136, 3.137, and 3.138)

- Two histologically distinct tumors collide
- Most commonly, basal cell carcinoma collides with squamous cell carcinoma
- Tumors do not infiltrate each other

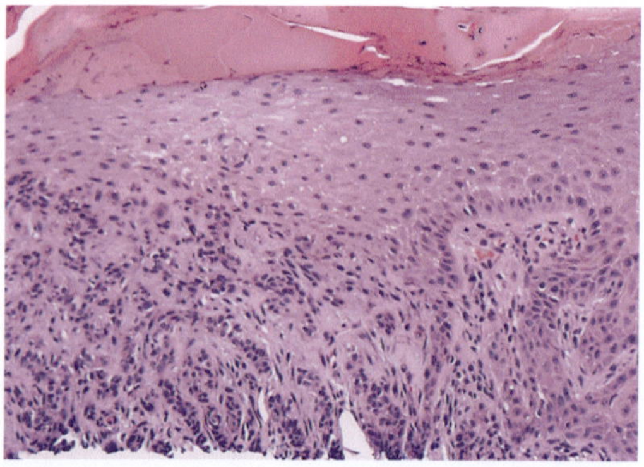

Fig. 3.135 Collision between basal cell carcinoma (left) and squamous cell carcinoma (right)

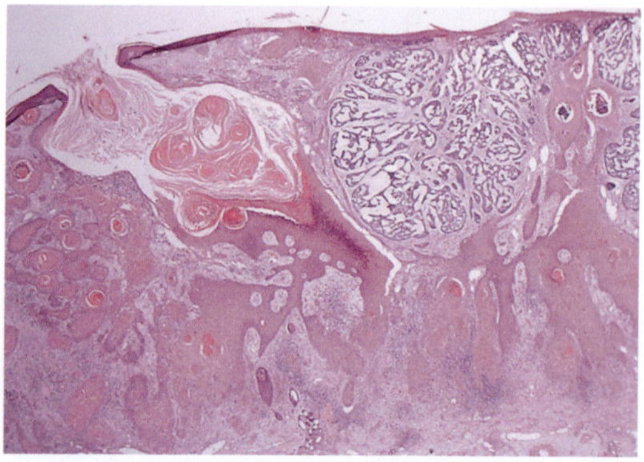

Fig. 3.136 Collision between squamous cell carcinoma on the left and basal cell carcinoma on the right

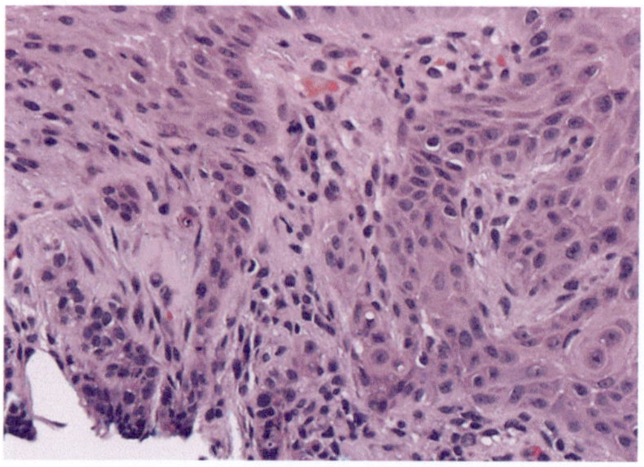

Fig. 3.137 Atypical basaloid cells (left) and squamoid cells (right)

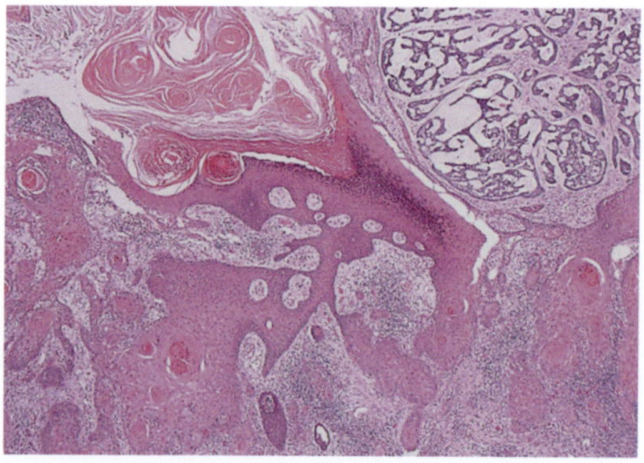

Fig. 3.138 Infiltrating squamous cell carcinoma (left) and nodular basal cell carcinoma (right)

Colloid Milium

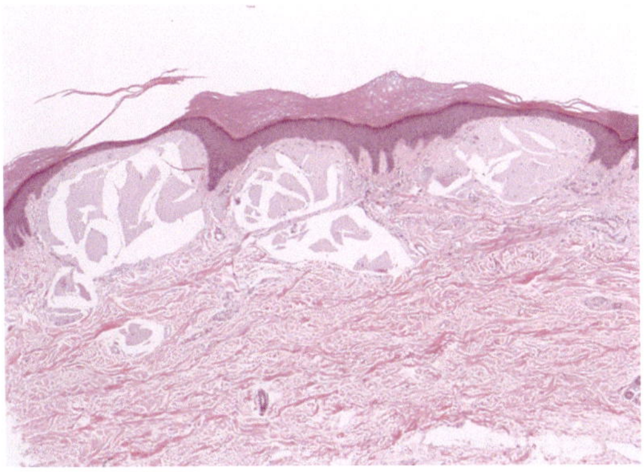

Fig. 3.139 Dermal aggregates of pink cleaved material

Histopathology (Figs. 3.139, 3.140, and 3.141)

Adult type:

- Homogenous, eosinophilic material (derived from degenerated elastic fibers) in the papillary dermis
- Fissures and clefts divide deposits that stain same as amyloid (PAS, thioflavin T, Congo red, crystal violet +)

Juvenile type:

- Pinkish homogenous material (derived from and positive with keratin) in the papillary dermis
- Less clefts in colloid

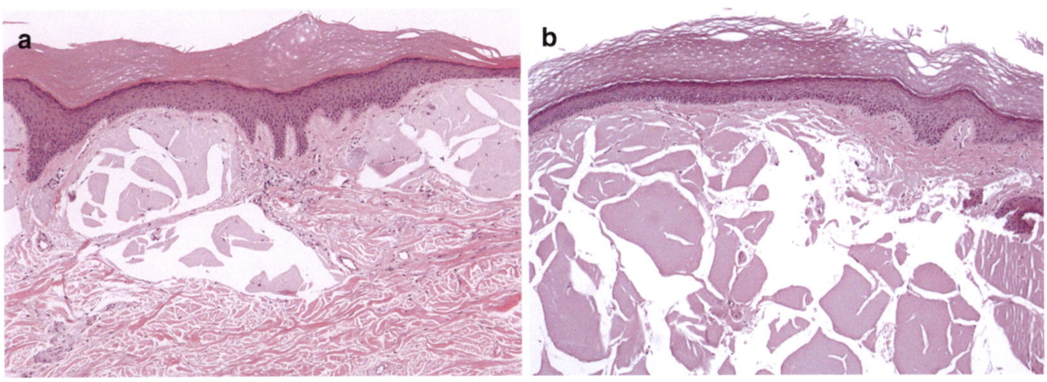

Fig. 3.140 (**a**, **b**) Homogeneous eosinophilic deposits in the papillary dermis separated from the epidermis by narrow Grenz zone

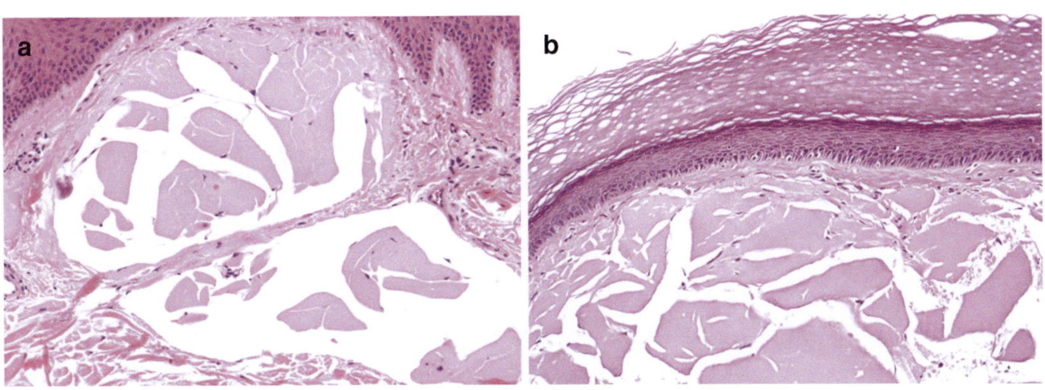

Fig. 3.141 (**a**, **b**) Fractured appearance of dermal deposits with numerous clefts and fissures

Coma Blister

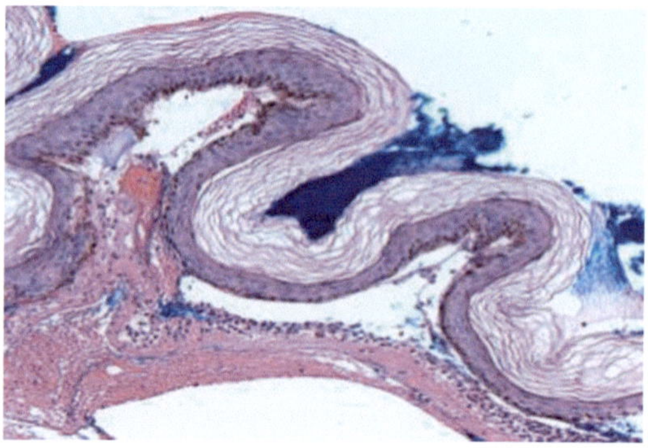

Fig. 3.142 Subepidermal blister

Histopathology (Figs. 3.142, 3.143, 3.144, 3.145, and 3.146)

- Subepidermal or suprabasal blister with mild dermal inflammation
- Usually partial necrosis of the overlying epidermis
- Dermal hemorrhage and sweat gland necrosis

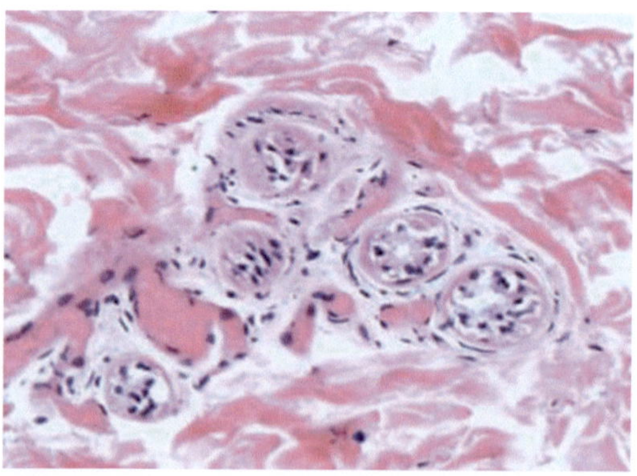

Fig. 3.143 Partial necrosis of eccrine glands

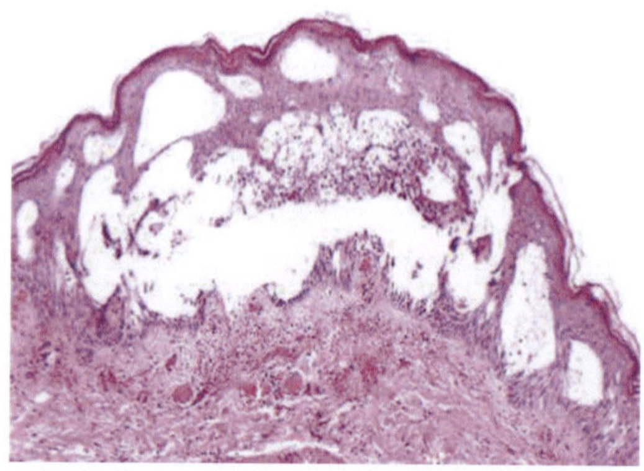

Fig. 3.144 Suprabasal blister with dermal hemorrhage

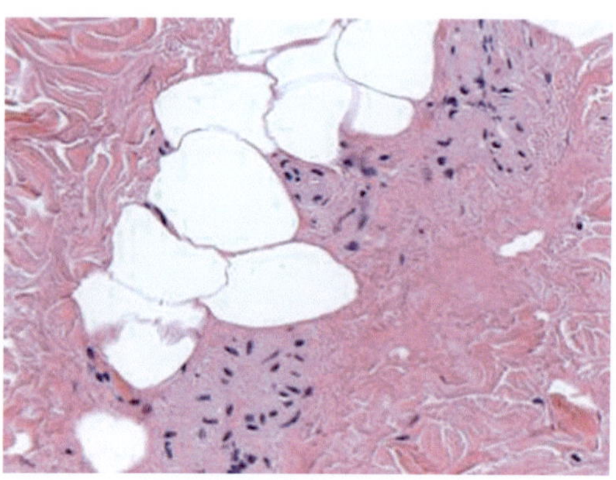

Fig. 3.145 Complete necrosis of eccrine glands

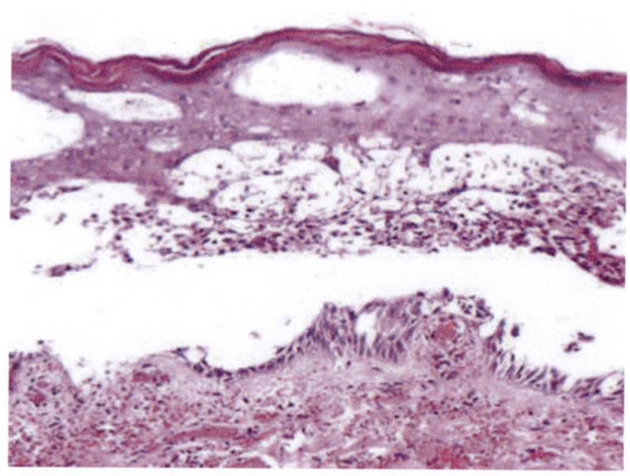

Fig. 3.146 Partial necrosis of smudgy epidermis above the blister

Combined Nevus

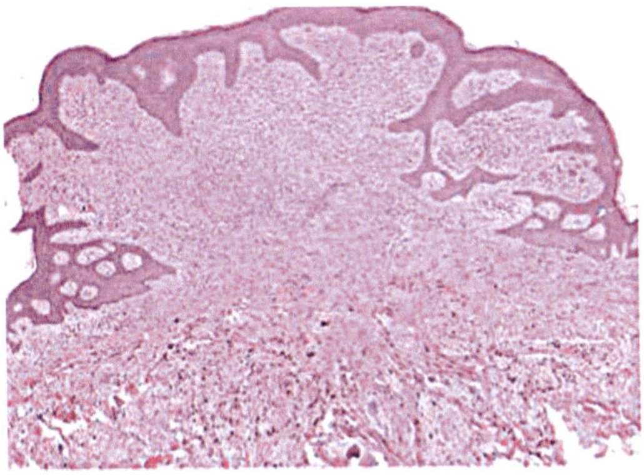

Fig. 3.147 Combined dermal and blue nevus

Histopathology (Figs. 3.147, 3.148, and 3.149)
- Composed of a mixture of junctional, dermal, or compound nevus with blue nevus
- Less common is a combination of Spitz nevus and blue nevus

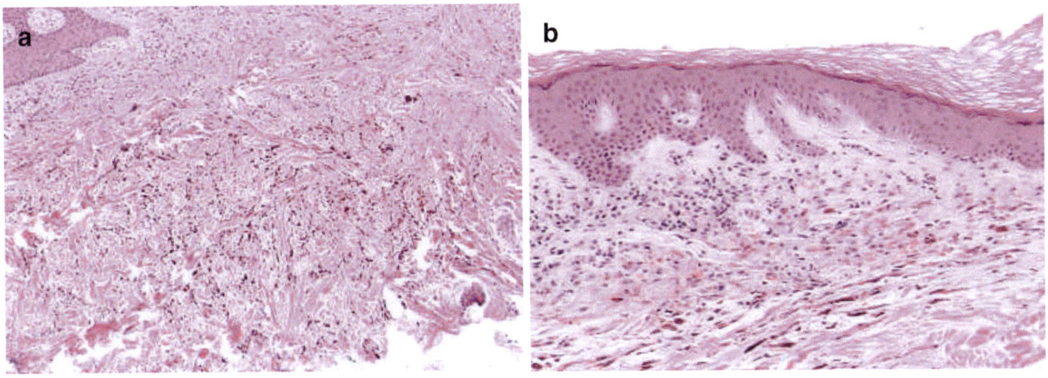

Fig. 3.148 (a, b) Dermal nevus with maturing melanocytes combined with pigmented spindle melanocytes of the blue nevus

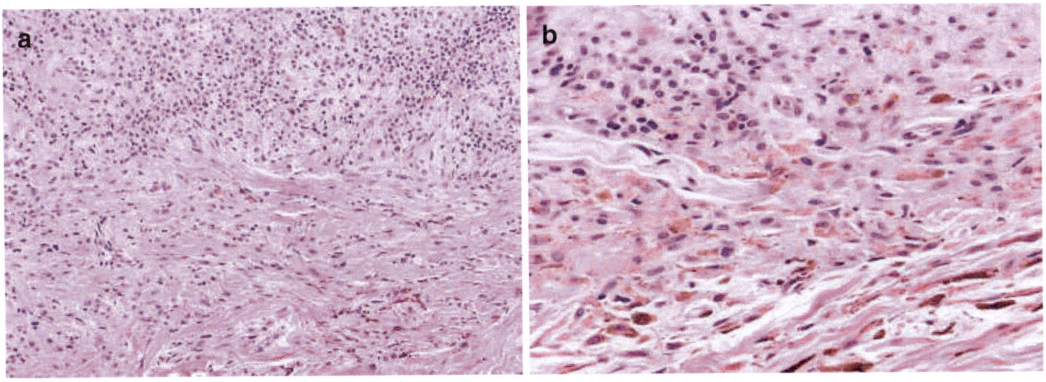

Fig. 3.149 (a, b) Interface between dermal nevus (above) and blue nevus (below)

Compound Nevus

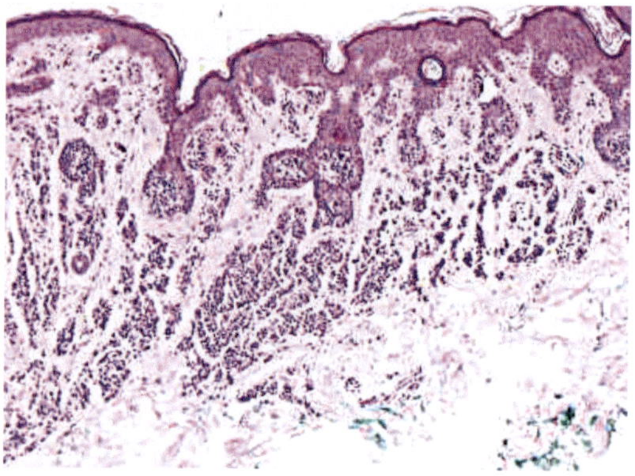

Fig. 3.150 Junctional and dermal melanocytic proliferation

Histopathology (Figs. 3.150, 3.151, 3.152, 3.153, and 3.154)

- Junctional melanocytic nests at the tip of the rete ridges
- Nests have regular arrangement and no atypia
- No significant lateral extension of junctional nests over dermal melanocytic component
- Dermal component makes nests in the papillary dermis that become smaller and end up as single cells with descent (maturation)
- Pigment distribution follows melanocytic maturation

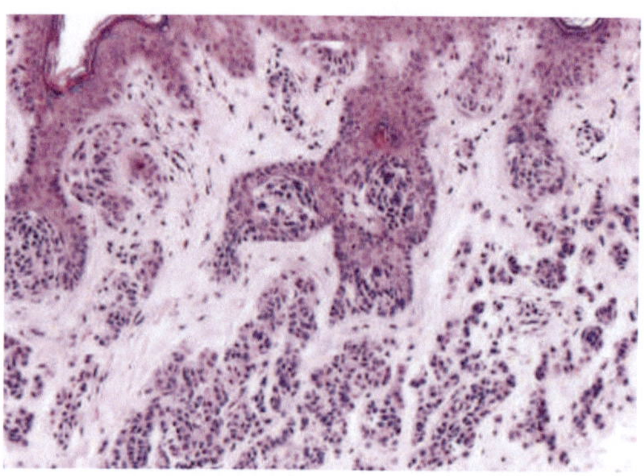

Fig. 3.151 Dermal melanocytes mature with descent

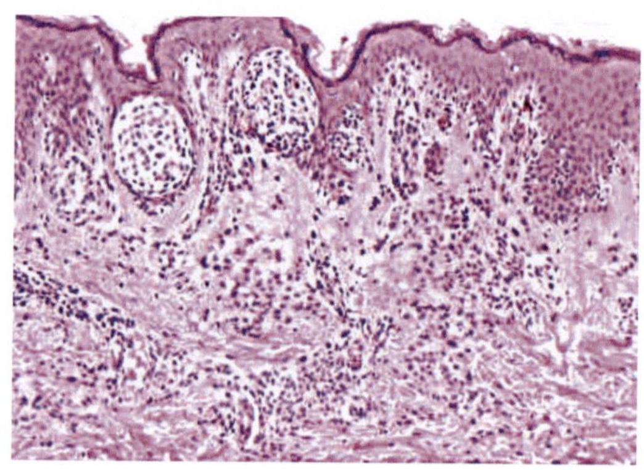

Fig. 3.152 Regular junctional nests present at the rete ridges tips with melanin pigment in the upper part of the nevus

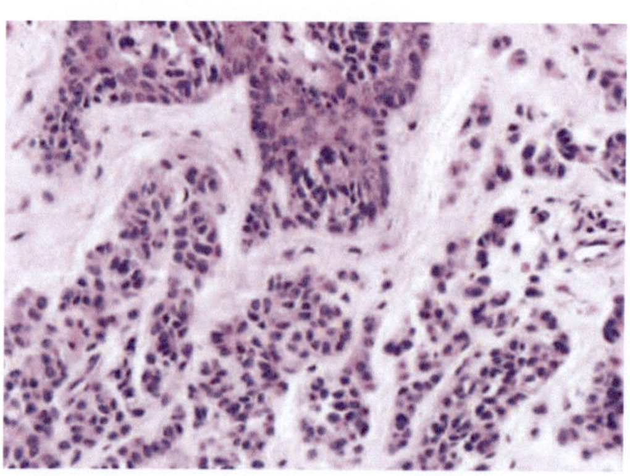

Fig. 3.153 No cytological atypia or mitoses

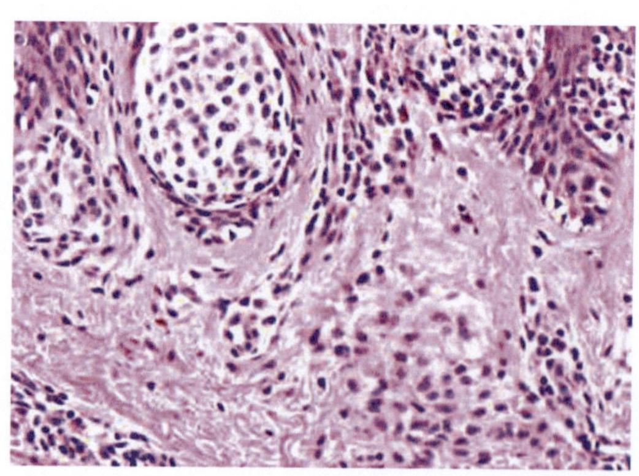

Fig. 3.154 Melanocytes within the nest appear uniform

Condyloma Accuminatum

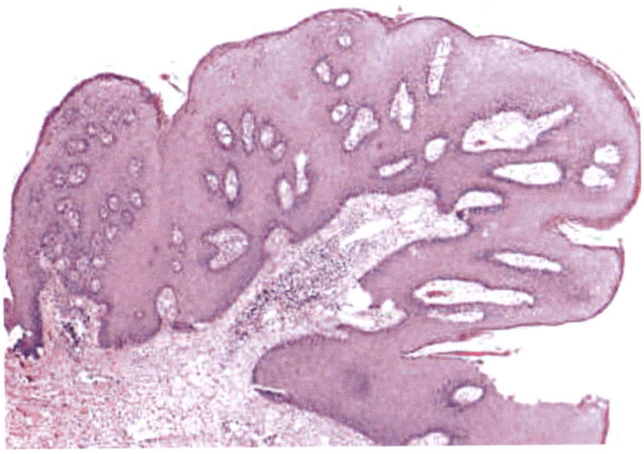

Fig. 3.155 Acanthotic epidermis with moderate papillomatosis

Synonym: Genital Wart

Histopathology:

- Thick epidermis with hyperkeratosis, parakeratosis, and papillomatosis that varies from mild to florid
- Keratinocytes with dark nuclei and pale cytoplasm, so called koilocytes (keratinocytes infected by HPV), are present but less than in verruca vulgaris
- There is well demarcated pushing deep margin

P.S. two lesions from the penis. The lesion on the top (Figs. 3.155, 3.156, and 3.157) is prototypical *condyloma acuminatum*, whereas the lesion on the bottom resembles *verruca vulgaris.* (Figs. 3.158 and 3.159)

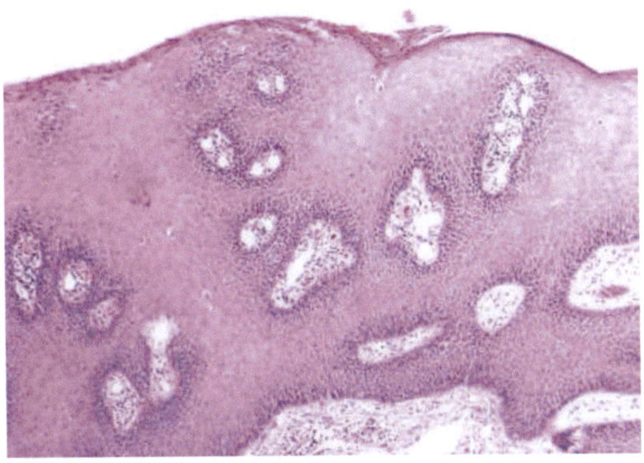

Fig. 3.156 Deep margin is well defined

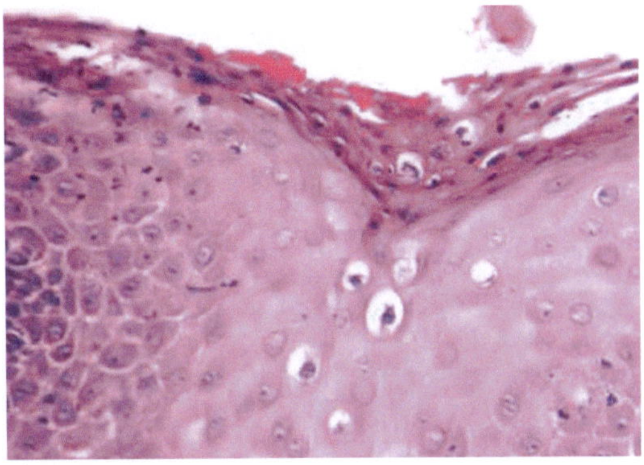

Fig. 3.157 Epidermal parakeratosis with few koilocytes

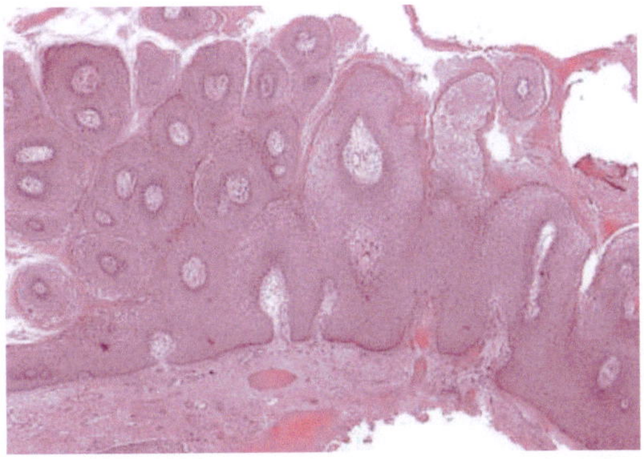

Fig. 3.158 Verruciform epidermis with pushing deep border

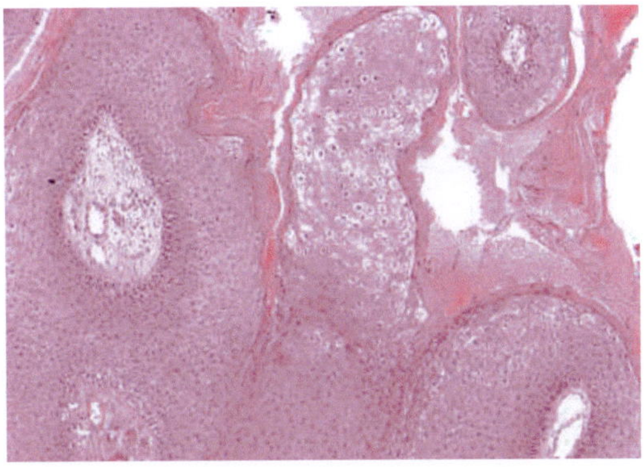

Fig. 3.159 Numerous koilocytes with dark nuclei and pale cytoplasm

Condyloma Lata

Histopathology (Figs. 3.160, 3.161, and 3.162)
- Marked irregular psoriasiform hyperplasia
- Intraepidermal neutrophilic aggregates
- Dermal lymphocytic infiltrate with numerous plasma cells

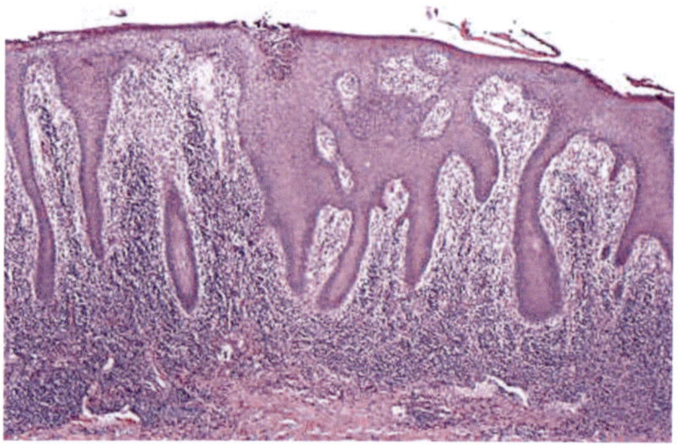

Fig. 3.160 Irregular psoriasiform epidermis with dense dermal inflammation

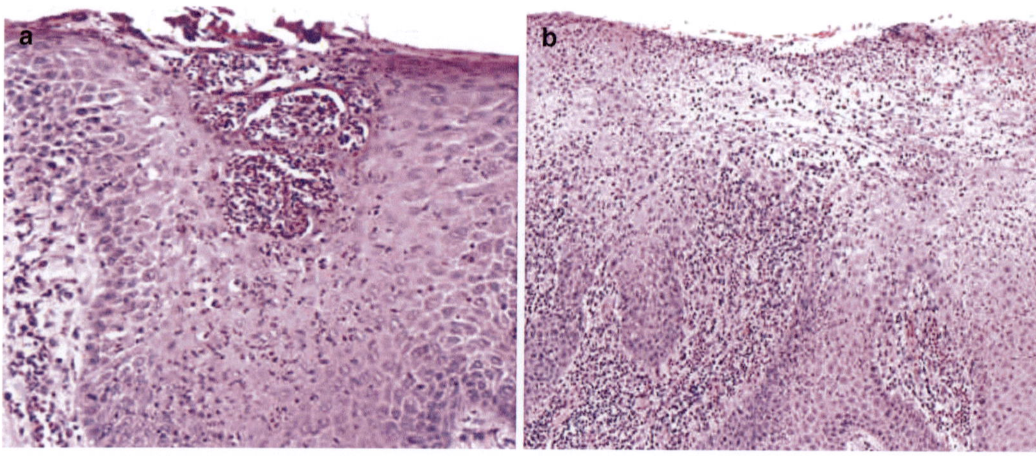

Fig. 3.161 (**a**, **b**) Pseudoepitheliomatous hyperplasia with intraepidermal microabscess

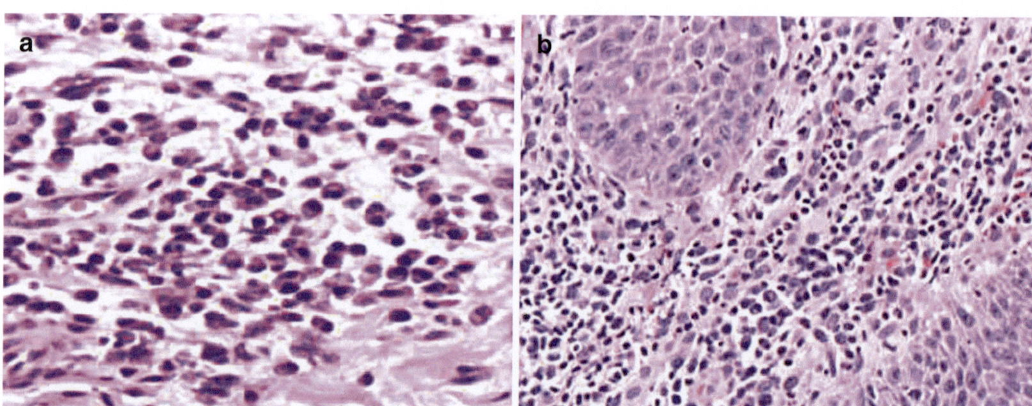

Fig. 3.162 (**a**, **b**) Numerous plasma cells in the dermis

Confluent and Reticulated Papillomatosis of Gourgerout and Cartoud

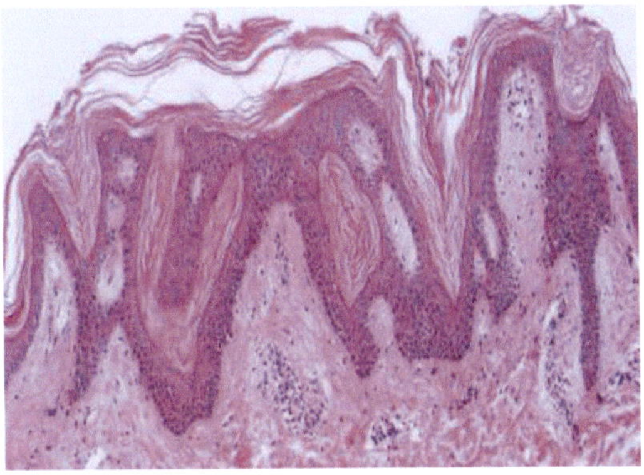

Fig. 3.163 Hyperkeratotic papillomatous epidermis

Synonym: CARP

Histopathology (Figs. 3.163, 3.164, and 3.165)

- Hyperkeratotic epidermis with papillomatosis and acanthosis
- Some downgrowth of epidermal retes
- Mild hyperpigmentation of basal layer

P.S. histologically and clinically there is similarity to acanthosis nigricans and many believe that *CARP* is a variant of *acanthosis nigricans*

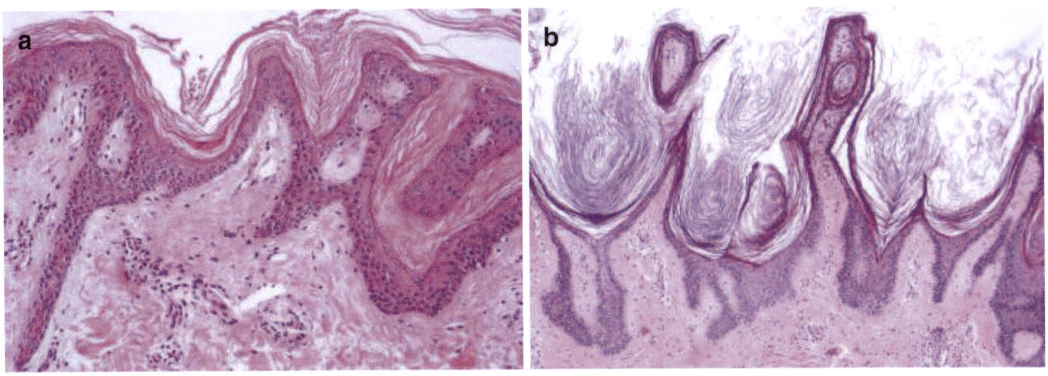

Fig. 3.164 (**a**, **b**) Undulated epidermis with hyperkeratosis and mild downgrowth of the epidermis

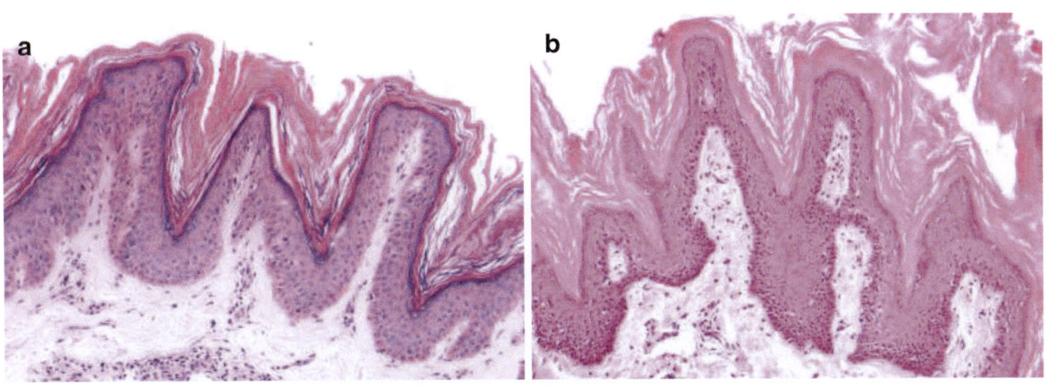

Fig. 3.165 (**a**, **b**) Hyperpigmentation of basal layer keratinocytes

Congenital Nevus

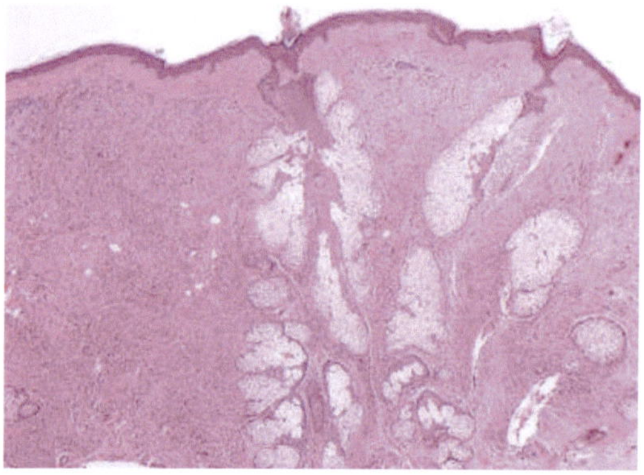

Fig. 3.166 Melanocytic proliferation surrounding adnexal structures

Histopathology (Figs. 3.166, 3.167, and 3.168)
- Dermal or compound nevus
- Periadnexal, perivascular, and perineural nevoid infiltrate in single cell pattern
- Nevus cells can be found within pilar muscle, hair follicle, sebaceous and/or sweat glands
- No evidence of atypia

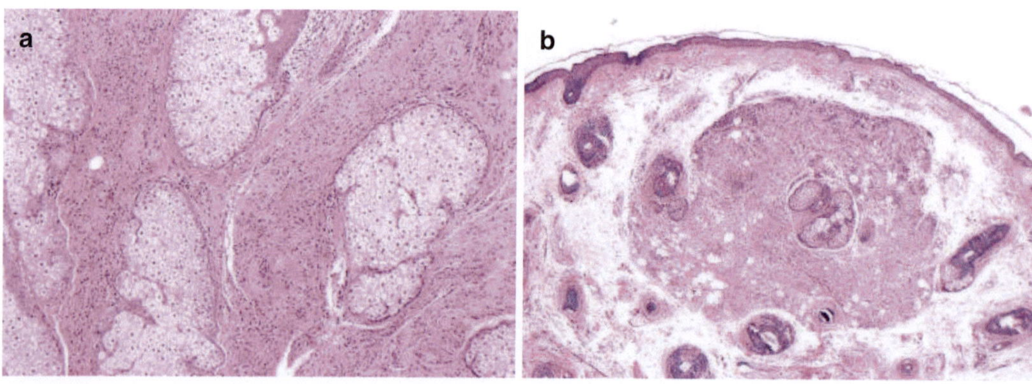

Fig. 3.167 (**a**, **b**) Periadnexal accumulation of benign nevus cells

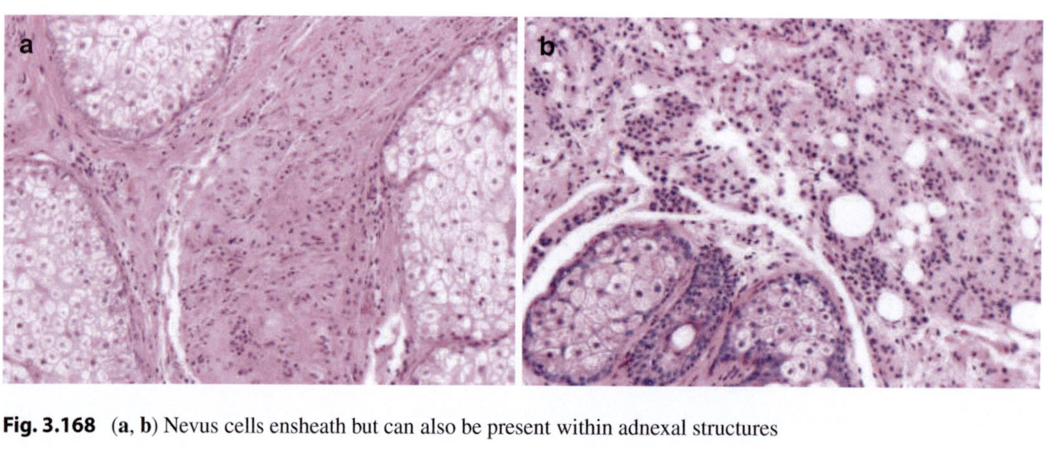

Fig. 3.168 (**a**, **b**) Nevus cells ensheath but can also be present within adnexal structures

Connective Tissue Nevus

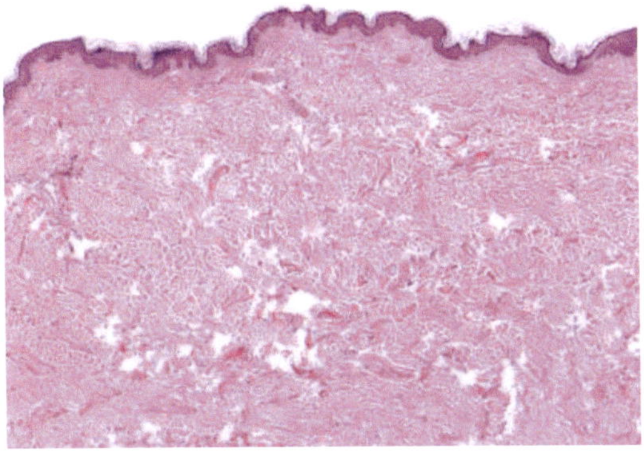

Fig. 3.169 Collagenoma

Histopathology
- Cutaneous hamartoma
- One component of the connective tissue predominates
- **Collagenoma**: thickened dermis with increase in homogenized dermal collagen and normal or decreased number of elastic fibers (Figs. 3.169, 3.170, and 3.171)
- **Elastoma**: normal appearance on H&E slides but increased elastic fibers on elastic special stain (Figs. 3.172 and 3.173)

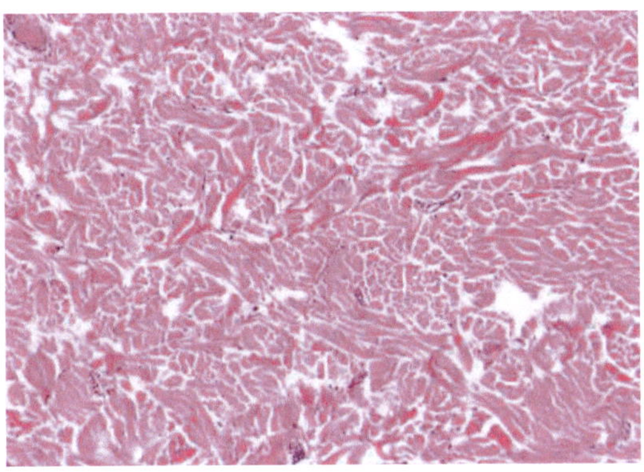

Fig. 3.170 Thickened dermis with broad hyalinized collagen bundles

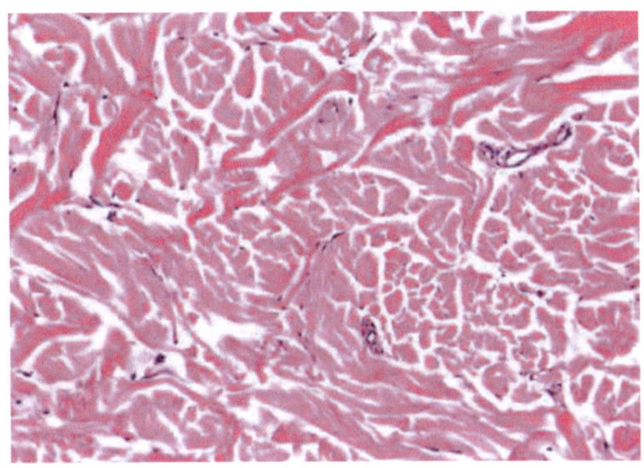

Fig. 3.171 Thickened eosinophilic collagen

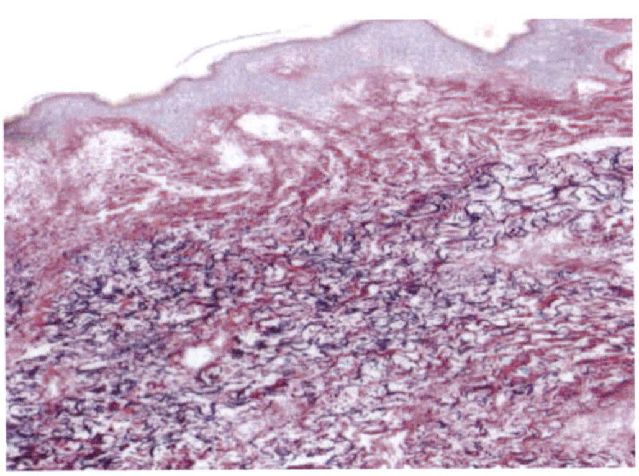

Fig. 3.172 **Elastoma**: increased number of elastic fibers (VVG)

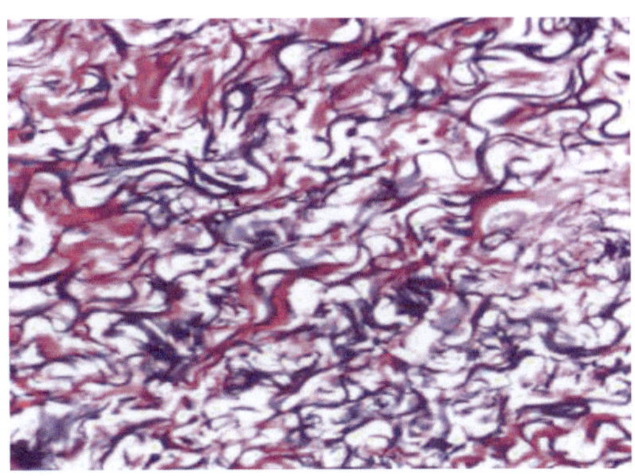

Fig. 3.173 Increased dermal wavy elastic fibers

Cranial Fasciitis

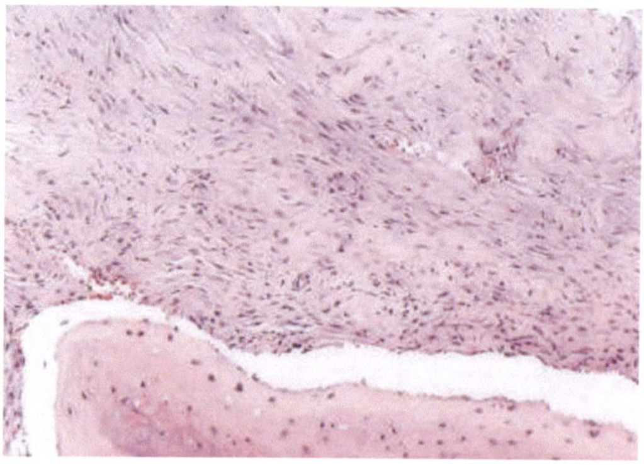

Fig. 3.174 Spindle cell lesion involving bone

Histopathology (Figs. 3.174, 3.175, 3.176, and 3.177)

- Subcutaneous ill-defined tumor of the scalp with bony involvement in majority of the cases
- Hyper and hypocellular areas of spindle-shaped myofibroblasts in myxoid stromal background forming tissue culture appearance
- Osseous metaplasia, hemorrhage, keloidal collagen changes can be present
- Cells are SMA positive

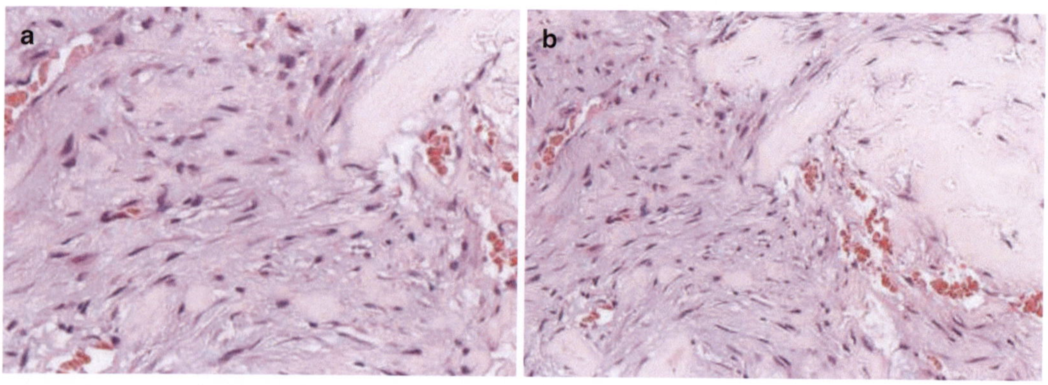

Fig. 3.175 (**a**, **b**) Spindle cell proliferation with osseous metaplasia

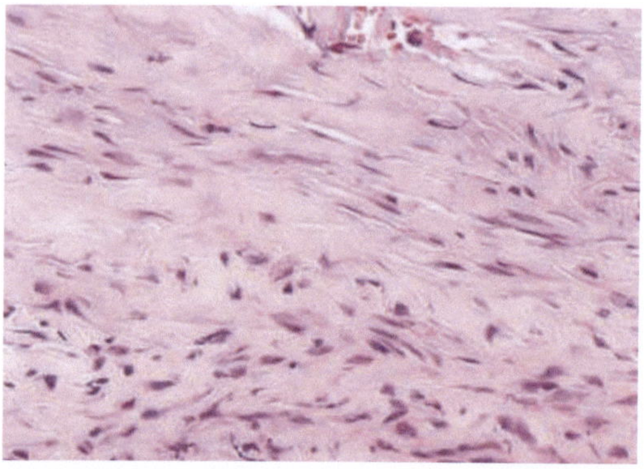

Fig. 3.176 Alternating hyper and hypo cellular area

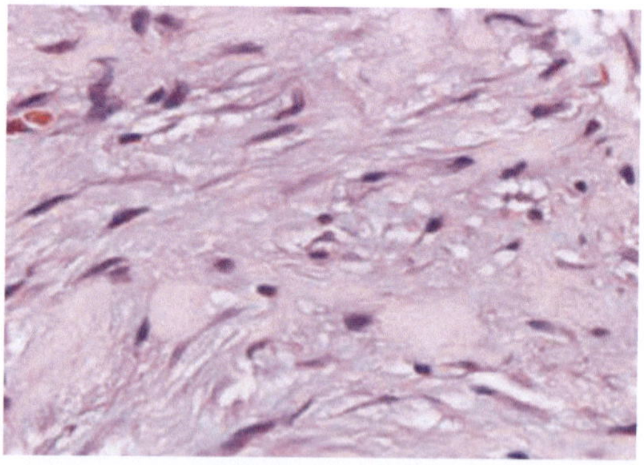

Fig. 3.177 Elongated plumped fibroblasts

Crohn's Disease

Histopathology (Figs. 3.178, 3.179, 3.180, 3.181, and 3.182)

- Dermal mixed inflammation
- Small subtle non-caseating granulomas
- Granulomas are usually present in the superficial dermis
- As with any granuloma, an infection should be excluded

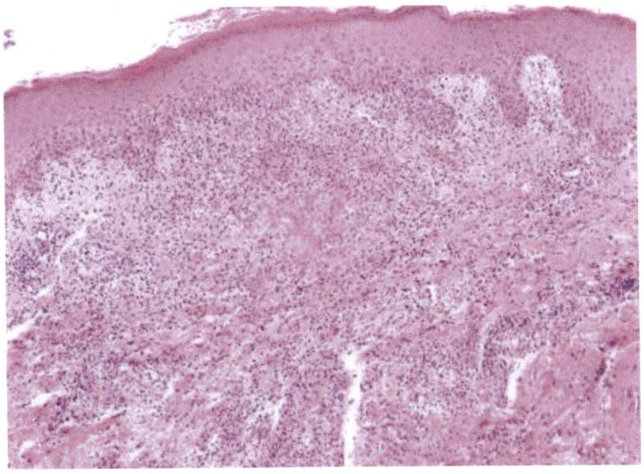

Fig. 3.178 Subtle granuloma in the papillary dermis

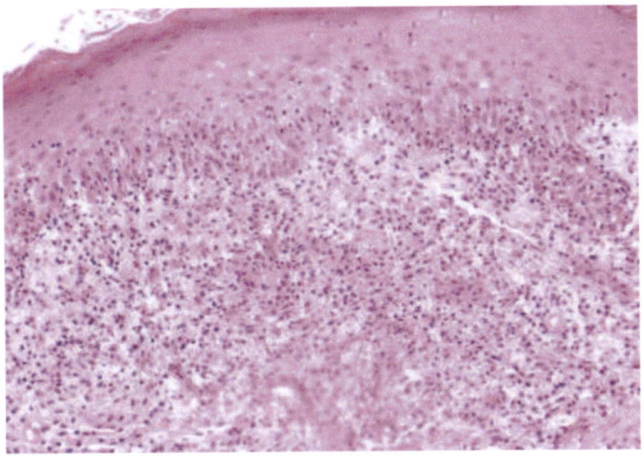

Fig. 3.179 Small granuloma without evidence of necrosis

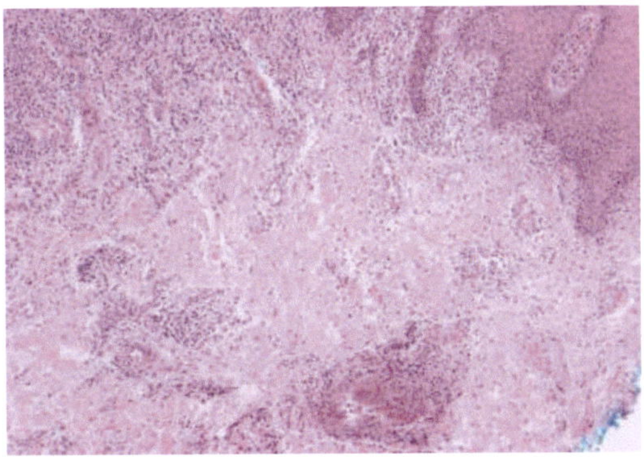

Fig. 3.180 In this patient this was the only granuloma present

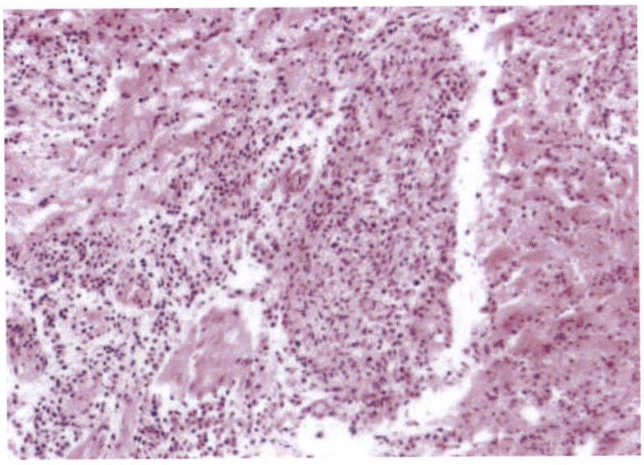

Fig. 3.181 Mixed inflammation in between granulomas

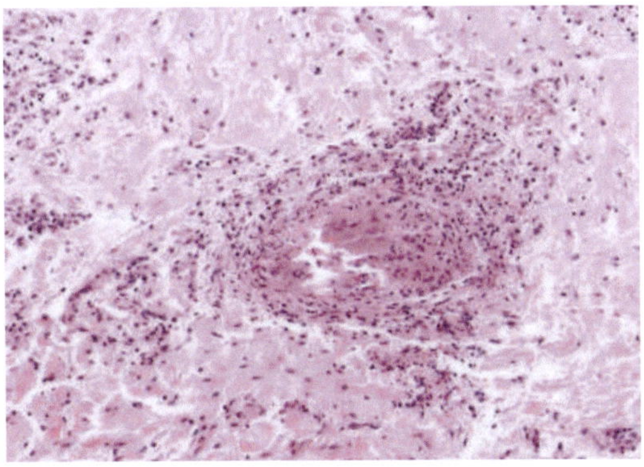

Fig. 3.182 Giant cell is present within granuloma

Cryoglobulinemia

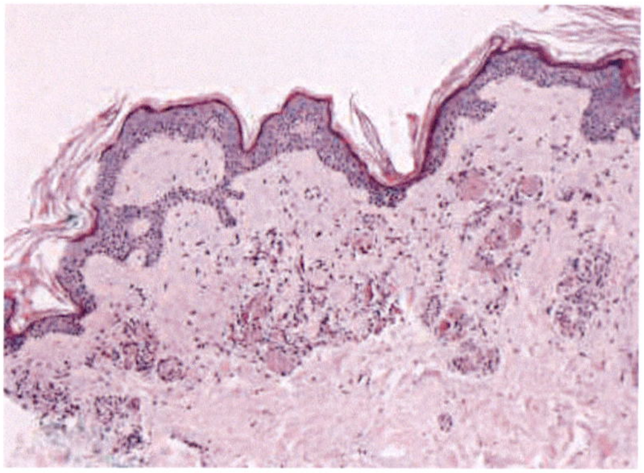

Fig. 3.183 **Type I** cryoglobulinemia

Histopathology

Type I (Figs. 3.183, 3.184, and 3.185)
- Small dermal vessels filled with homogeneous, eosinophilic material (PAS/D+)
- Perivascular RBCs extravasation
- Mild perivascular lymphocytic inflammation

Type II/III (10L Figs. 12.35 and 12.36)
- Presents as leukocytoclastic vasculitis

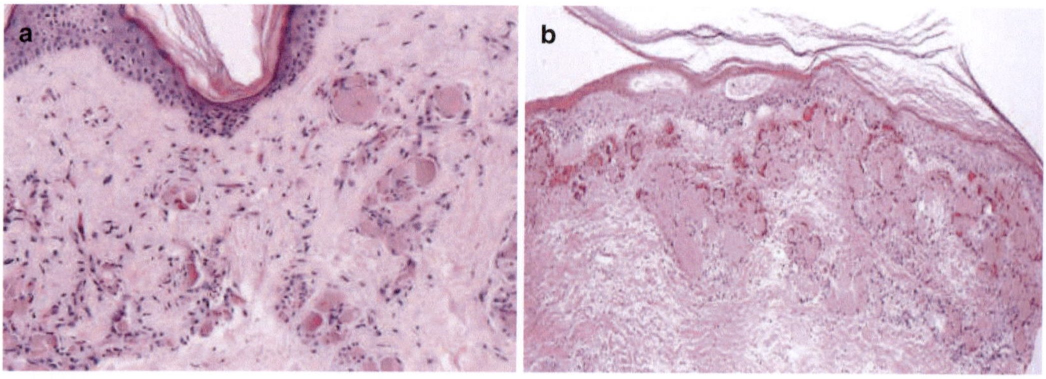

Fig. 3.184 (**a**, **b**) Dilated occluded dermal vessels with perivascular hemorrhage and mild lymphocytic inflammation

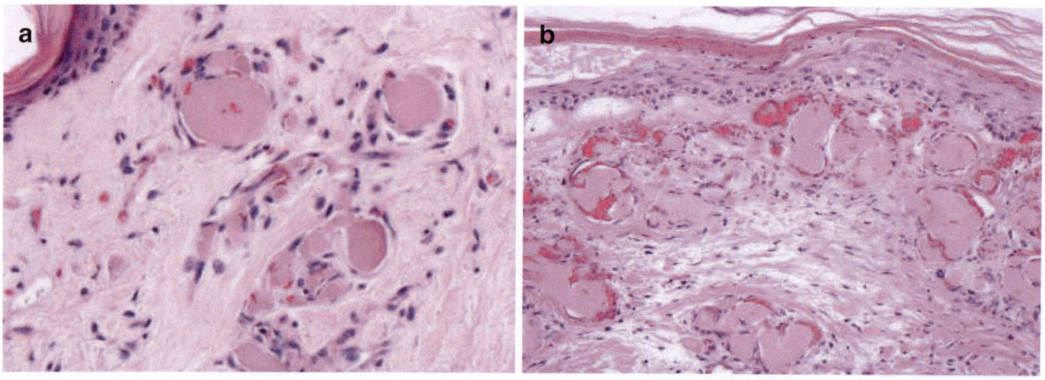

Fig. 3.185 (**a**, **b**) Smooth homogeneous pink material fills small dermal capillaries

Cryptococcus

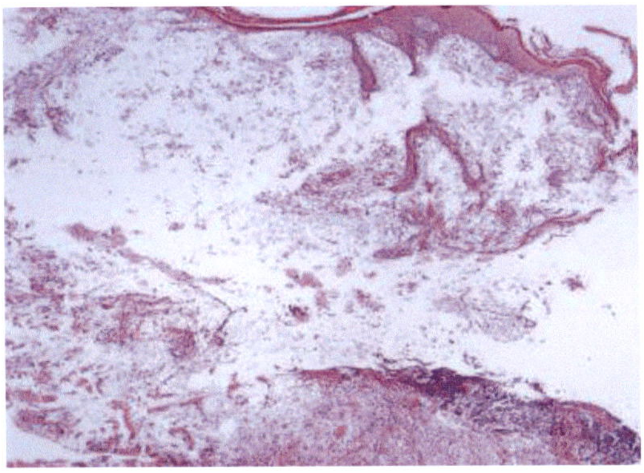

Fig. 3.186 Gelatinous dermal reaction with minimal inflammation

Histopathology (Figs. 3.186, 3.187, 3.188, 3.189, and 3.190)

- Inflammatory response to *Cryptococcus* varies depending on the immunological status
- Gelatinous dermal reaction with minimal inflammation at one end of the spectrum to exuberant mixed inflammation with abscesses and granulomas at the other part of the spectrum
- Encapsulated yeasts with polysaccharide rich capsule which stain with mucin stains

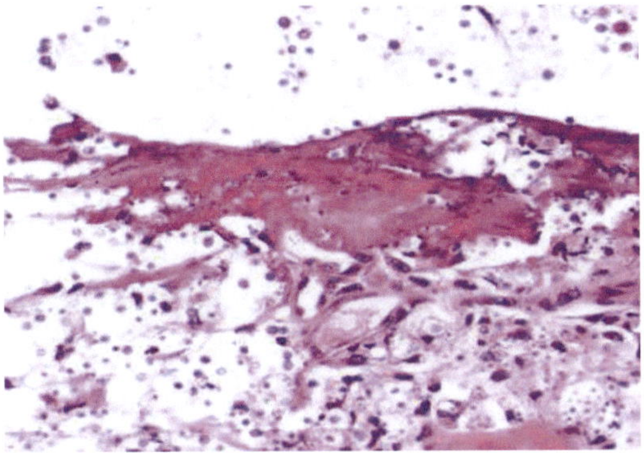

Fig. 3.187 Numerous gelatin producing encapsulated yeasts

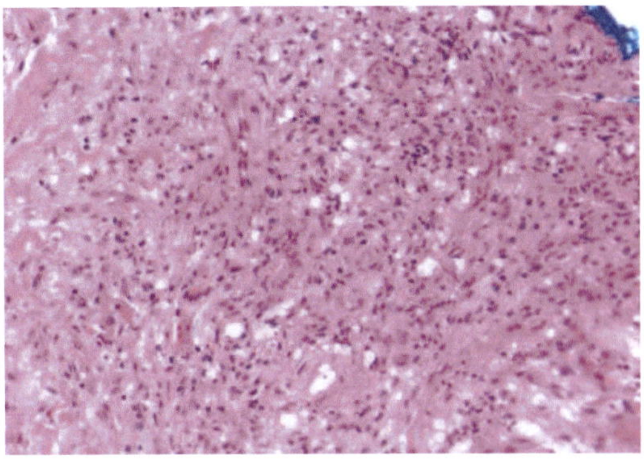

Fig. 3.188 Exuberant mixed inflammation with lymphocytes, histiocytes, and giant cells

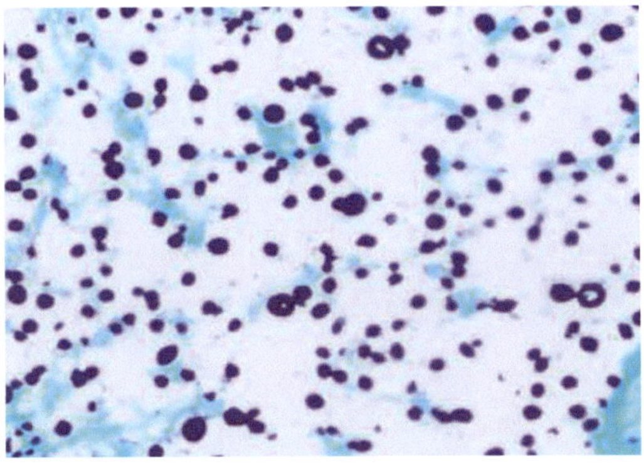

Fig. 3.189 Budding yeasts are present (GMS)

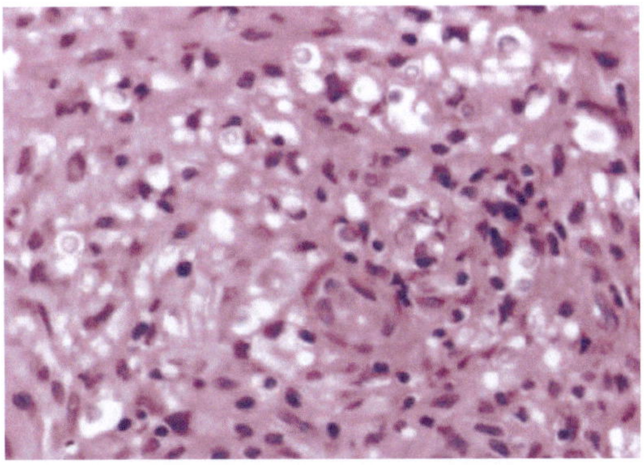

Fig. 3.190 Yeasts can be seen within the histiocytes

Cutaneous B-Cell Lymphoma

These four types are the most common:

Primary Cutaneous Diffuse Large B-Cell Lymphoma, Leg Type (Figs. 3.191 and 3.192)
- Dense dermal and subcutaneous infiltrate
- Made of large cells with irregular nuclei and very few reactive lymphocytes
- Mitoses are easily identified
- Cells are CD20+, CD79a+, Bcl-2+, MUM1+, FOX-P1+, Bcl-6+/−, CD10−

Primary Cutaneous Follicle Center Lymphoma (Fig. 3.193)
- Follicular pattern with follicles missing the mantle zone and tingible body macrophages
- The diffuse pattern also exists but is less common
- Composed of two cell types normally found in the follicular center: small to medium cells (centrocytes) and large lymphocytes (centroblasts) admixed with some normal small lymphocytes
- Tumor cells are CD20+, CD79a+, Bcl-6+/−, CD10+/−, CD5−, CD43−, Bcl-2−, cyclin D1−

Primary Cutaneous Mantle Cell Lymphoma (Fig. 3.194)
- Diffuse dermal/subcutaneous infiltrate
- Small to medium sized lymphocytes with irregular nuclei
- Lymphocytes are CD5+, CD20+, cyclin D1+, Bcl-2+, Bcl-6+/−, CD10−, CD23−

P.S. primary cutaneous mantle cell lymphomas are extremely rare and most cases represent cutaneous manifestation of the systemic disease

Primary Cutaneous Marginal Zone Lymphoma (Fig. 3.195)
- Dense nodular infiltrate with vague pale germinal centers surrounded by dark small lymphocytes and more peripherally, with pale neoplastic marginal zone lymphocytes
- Germinal center can be present within the nodule
- The marginal zone cells are CD20+, CD79a+, Bcl-2−, Bcl-6−, CD5−, CD10−

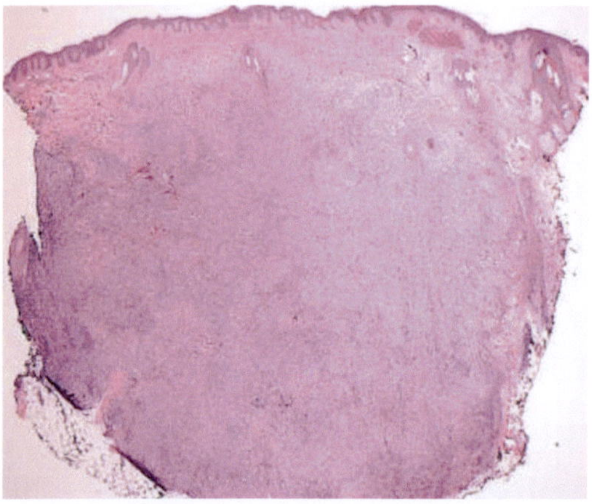

Fig. 3.191 **Primary cutaneous diffuse large B-cell lymphoma, leg type**

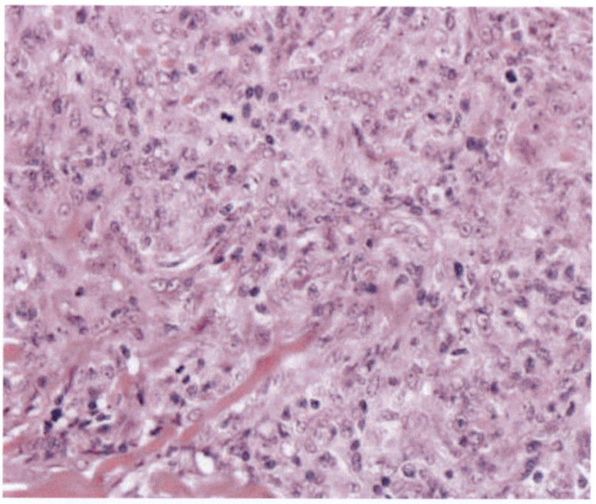

Fig. 3.192 Dense infiltrate of atypical large lymphocytes with numerous mitoses

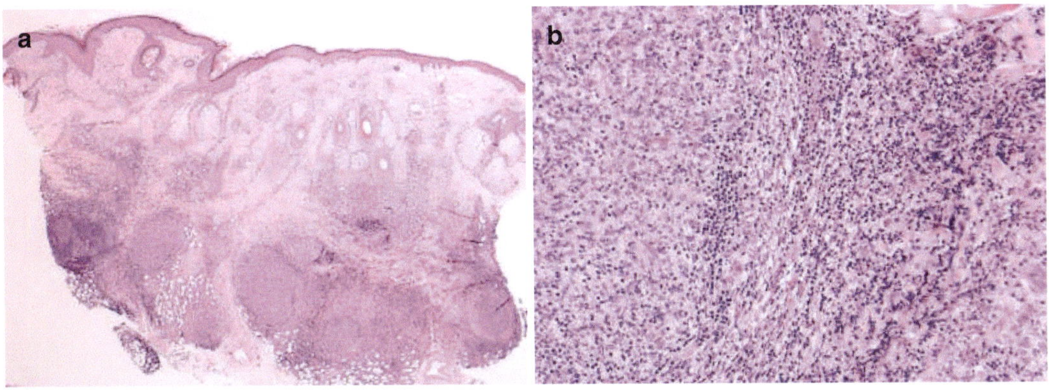

Fig. 3.193 (**a**, **b**) **Cutaneous follicle center lymphoma**: follicles have reduced mantle zone. Centers are made of monomorphic cells with no tangible body macrophages. These are all atypical findings that are not seen in reactive lymphoid follicles

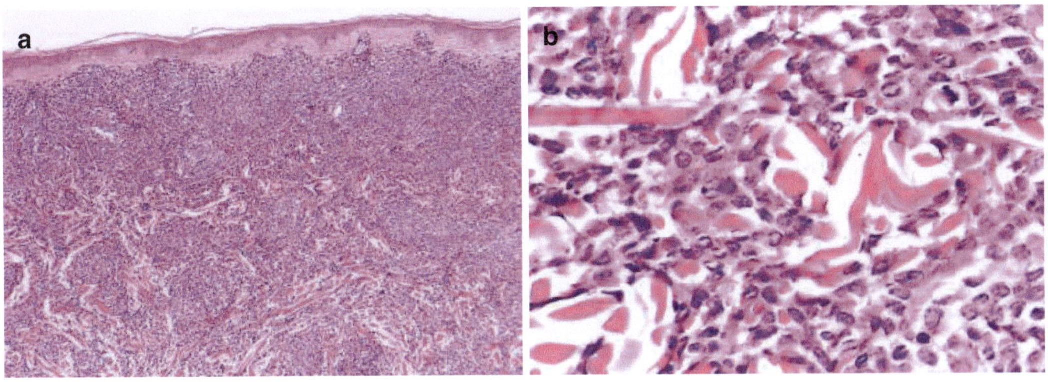

Fig. 3.194 (**a**, **b**) **Cutaneous mantle cell lymphoma**: monotonous diffuse infiltrate of small to medium sized atypical lymphocytes

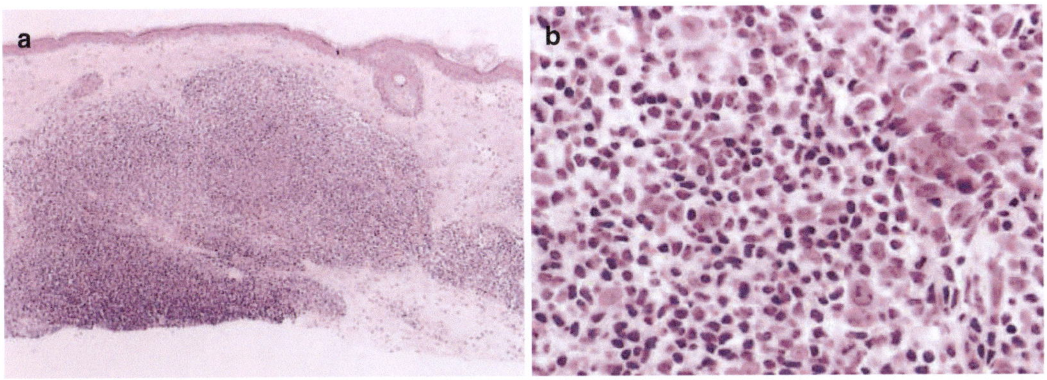

Fig. 3.195 (**a**, **b**) **Cutaneous marginal zone lymphoma**: vague germinal center is present in the nodule. Dark cells of the follicular mantle surrounded with neoplastic large pale marginal zone cells

Cutaneous Horn

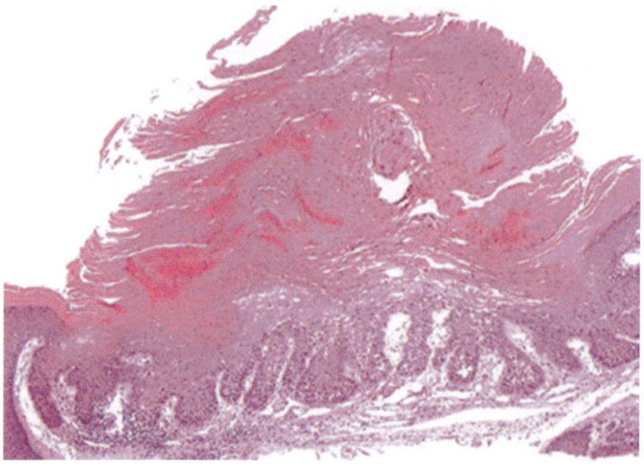

Fig. 3.196 Cutaneous horn with underlying **actinic keratosis**

Histopathology
- Horn-shaped amorphous or laminated hyperkeratosis
- Underlying epidermis can demonstrate actinic keratosis (Fig. 3.196), squamous cell carcinoma (Fig. 3.197), seborrheic keratosis (Fig. 3.198), or verruca vulgaris (Figs. 3.199)

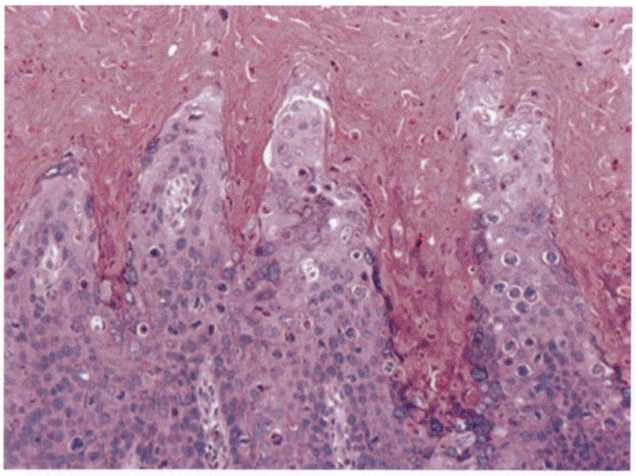

Fig. 3.197 Cutaneous horn with underlying **in situ squamous cell carcinoma**

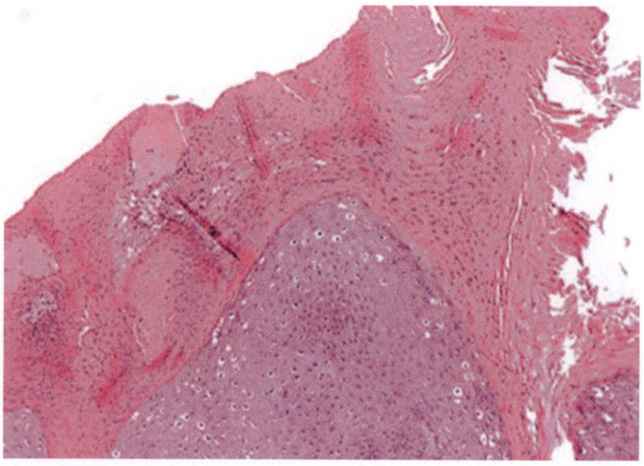

Fig. 3.199 Cutaneous horn with underlying **verruca vulgaris**

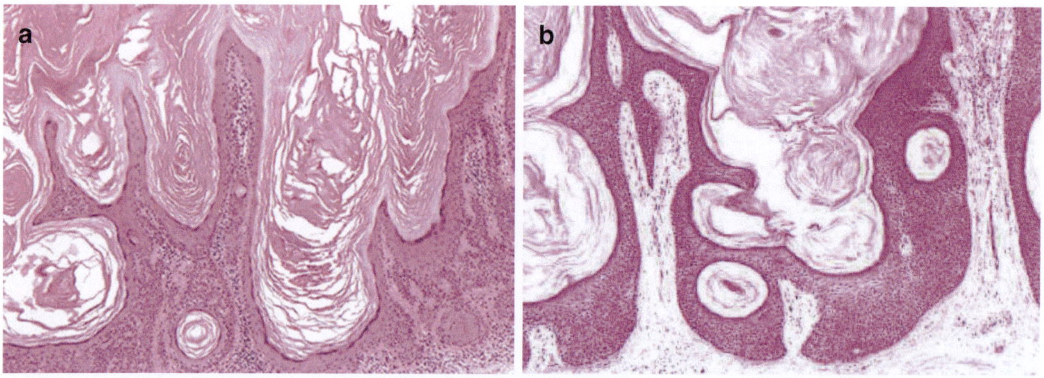

Fig. 3.198 (**a**, **b**) Cutaneous horn with underlying **seborrheic keratosis**

Cutaneous Metastasis

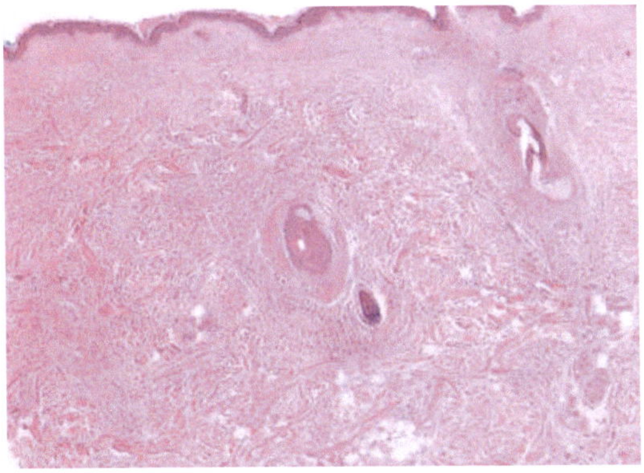

Fig. 3.200 Metastatic **breast** carcinoma can be subtle on low magnification

Histopathology

- Dermal and subcutaneous infiltrate of frankly malignant cells that do not belong to the skin
- Histology depends on the origin of metastasis (Figs. 3.200, 3.201, 3.202, 3.203, 3.204, 3.205, 3.206, 3.207, 3.208, 3.209, 3.210, 3.211, and 3.212)

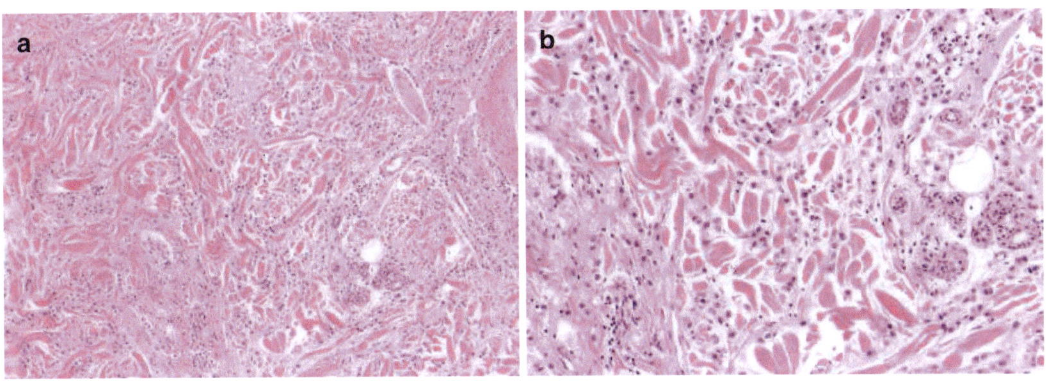

Fig. 3.201 (**a**, **b**) Metastatic **breast** lobular carcinoma

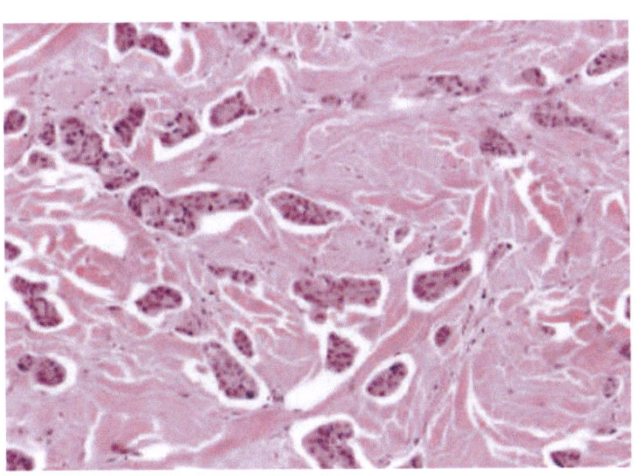

Fig. 3.202 Metastatic invasive ductal carcinoma of the **breast**

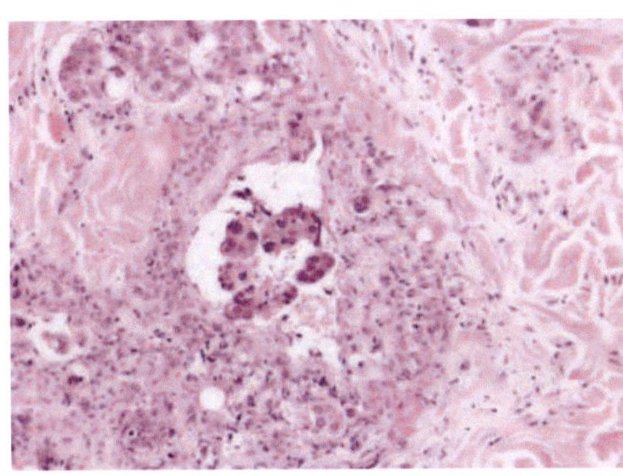

Fig. 3.203 Inflammatory **breast** carcinoma within the vessel

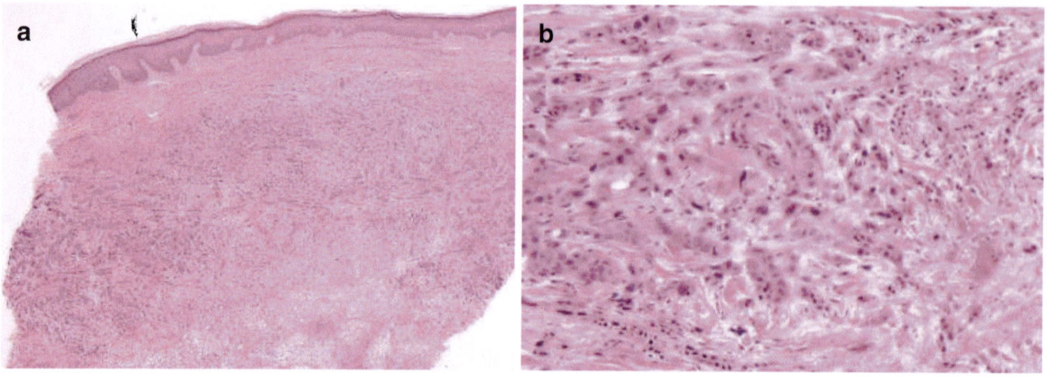

Fig. 3.204 (**a**, **b**) Metastatic adenocarcinoma of the **colon**

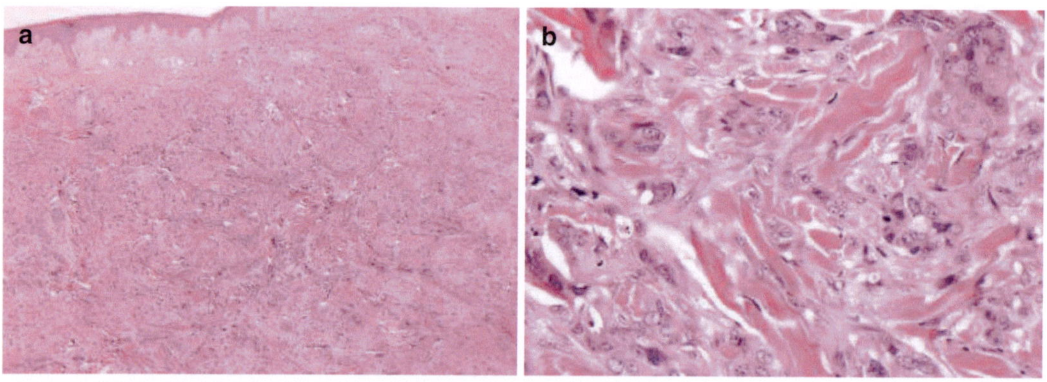

Fig. 3.205 (**a**, **b**) Metastatic squamous cell carcinoma of the **esophagus**

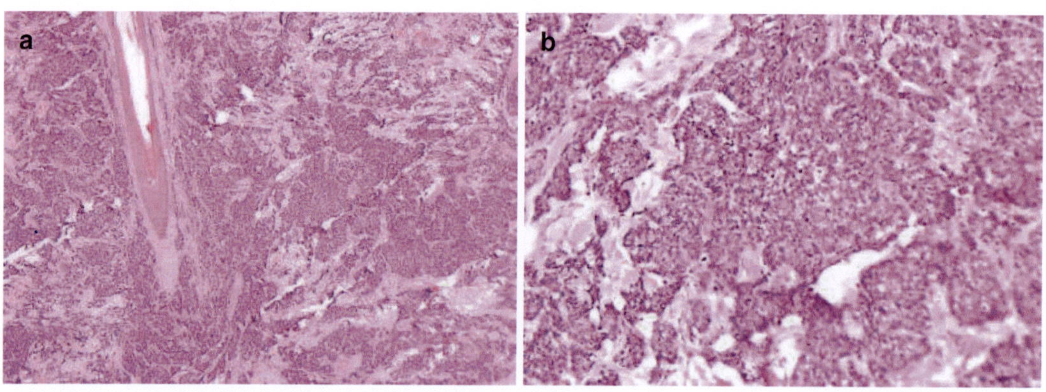

Fig. 3.206 (**a**, **b**) Metastatic small cell carcinoma of the **lung**

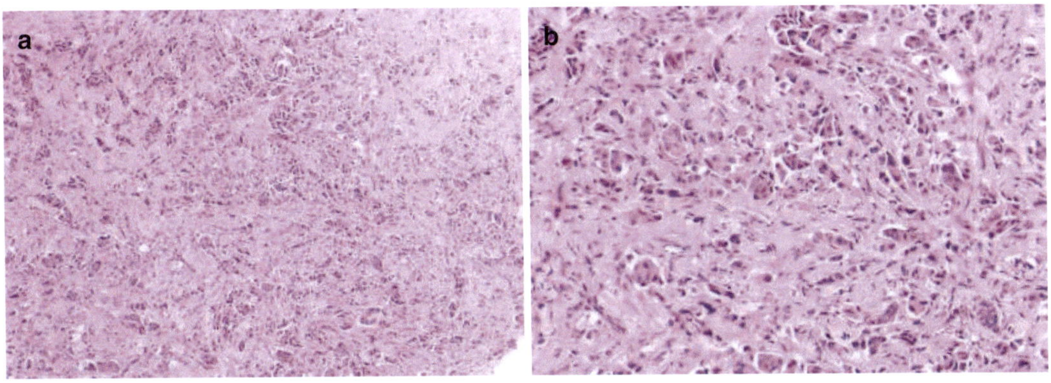

Fig. 3.207 (**a**, **b**) Metastatic squamous cell carcinoma of the **lung**

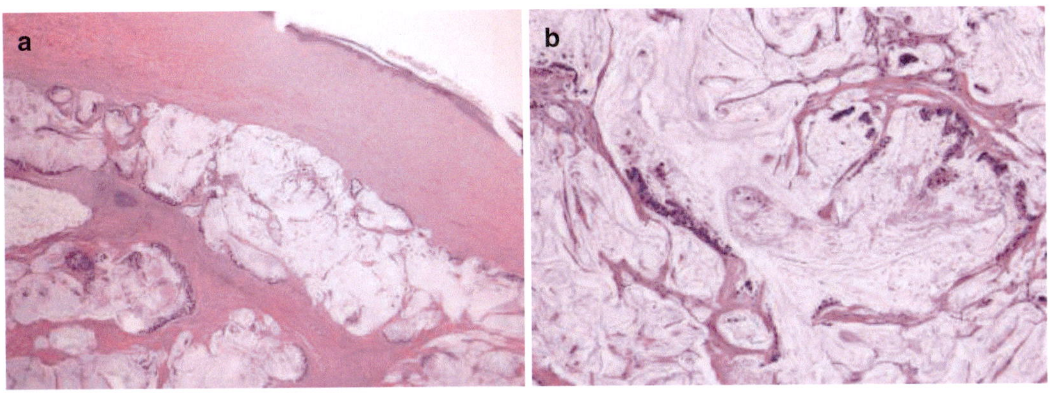

Fig. 3.208 (**a**, **b**) Metastatic mucinous carcinoma of the **stomach**

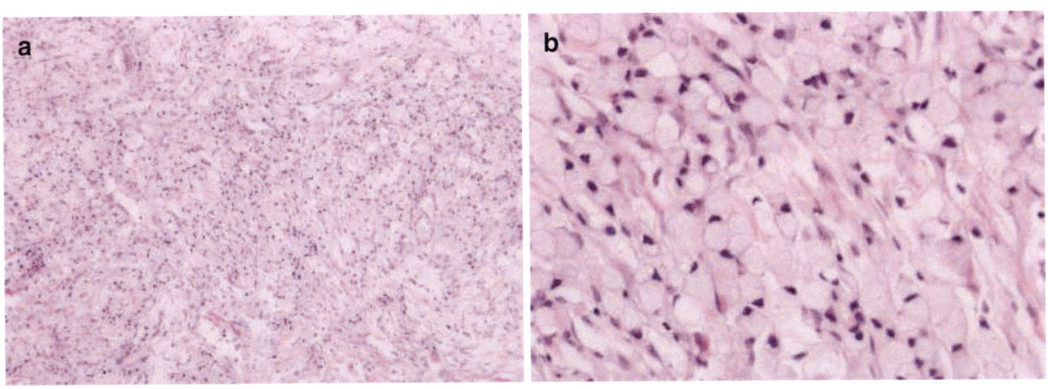

Fig. 3.209 (**a**, **b**) Metastatic signet ring carcinoma of the **stomach**

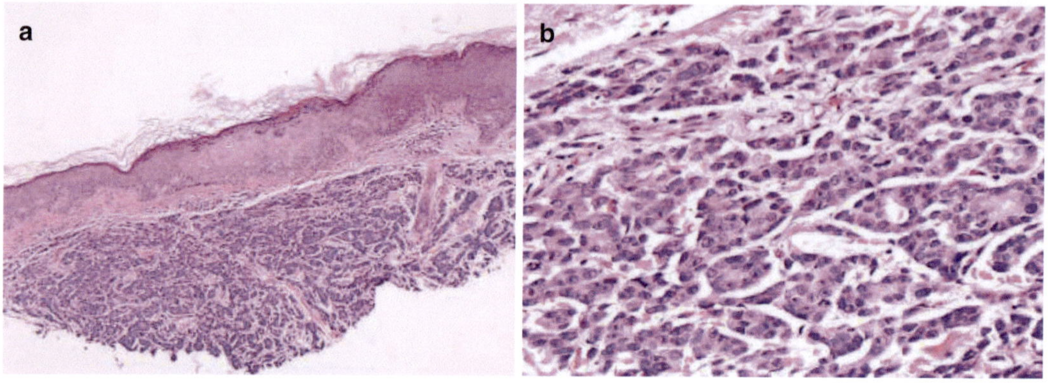

Fig. 3.210 (**a**, **b**) Metastatic adenocarcinoma of the **prostate**

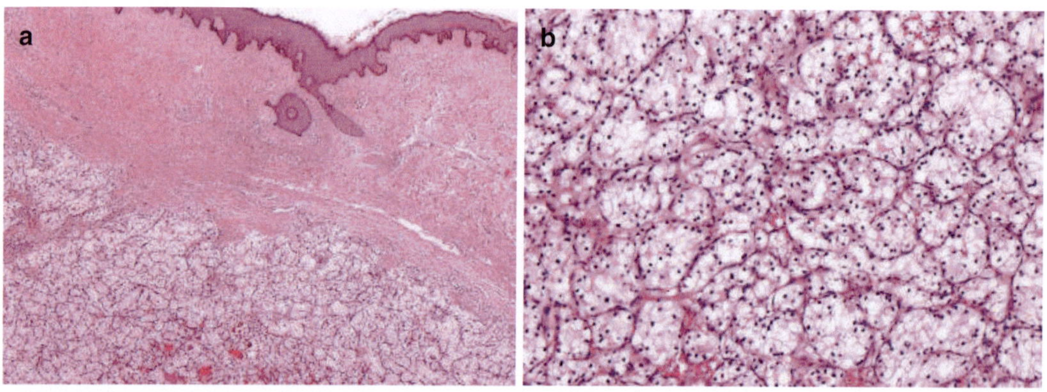

Fig. 3.211 (**a**, **b**) Metastatic **renal** adenocarcinoma

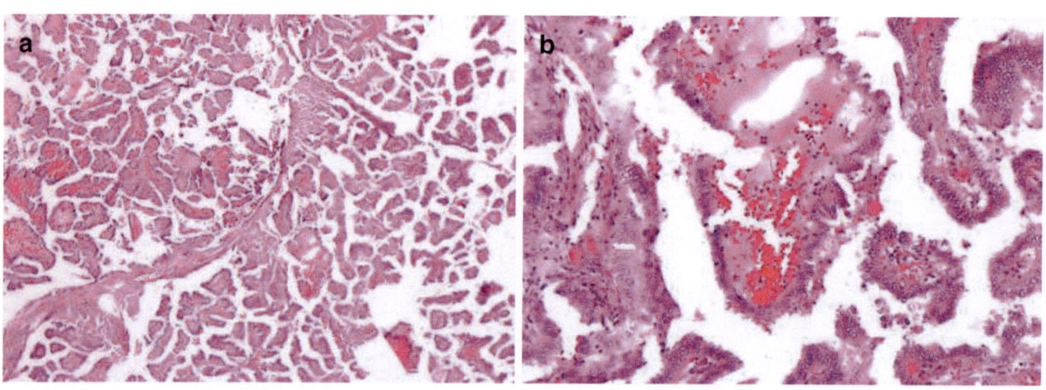

Fig. 3.212 (**a**, **b**) Metastatic **thyroid** papillary carcinoma

Cutaneous NK/T Cell Lymphomas

There are several types, but these five are the most common:

Mycosis Fungoides (Figs. 3.213 and 3.214)
- Scattered epidermal lymphocytes forming microabscesses and with tendency to line up at the base of the epidermis
- Dermal infiltrate enlarges with disease progression
- Cells are CD2+, CD3+, CD4+, CD5+, CD8–

Adult T-cell Leukemia/Lymphoma (Fig. 3.215)
- Perivascular (most common), nodular, or diffuse dermal infiltrate with variable epidermotropism
- Cells are CD3+, CD4+, CD8–, CD25+
- HTLV-1 is integrated in the lymphocytes

Extranodular NK/T cell Lymphoma, Nasal Type (Angiocentric Lymphoma) (Figs. 3.216 and 3.217)
- diffuse infiltrate of CD2+, granzyme B+, perforin+, CD56+ and CD3–, CD4–, CD5–, CD7–, CD8– cells
- Prominent angiocentricity and/or angiodestruction

Primary Cutaneous Anaplastic Large Cell Lymphoma (Fig. 3.218)
- Nodular or diffuse dermal infiltrate of large anaplastic cells that are usually not epidermotropic
- Cells are CD2+, CD3+, CD4+, CD8–
- Majority of cells are CD30 positive

Subcutaneous Panniculitis-like T-Cell Lymphoma (Fig. 3.219)
- Dense infiltrate involving the subcutaneous fat
- Cells are CD2+, CD3+, CD5+, CD8+, perforin+, granzyme B+, CD4–, CD30–

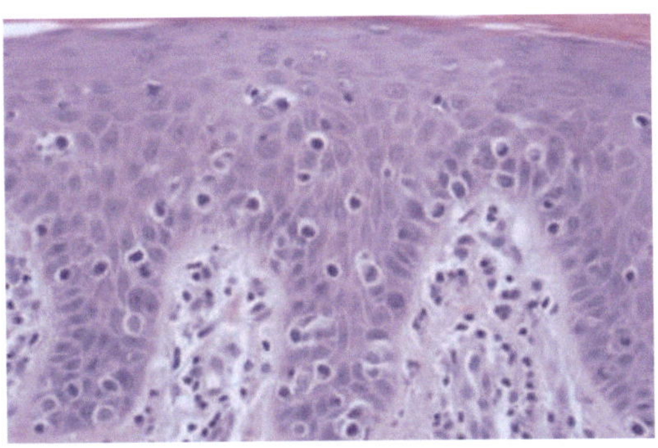

Fig. 3.213 Patch stage MF with lymphocytic epidermotropism

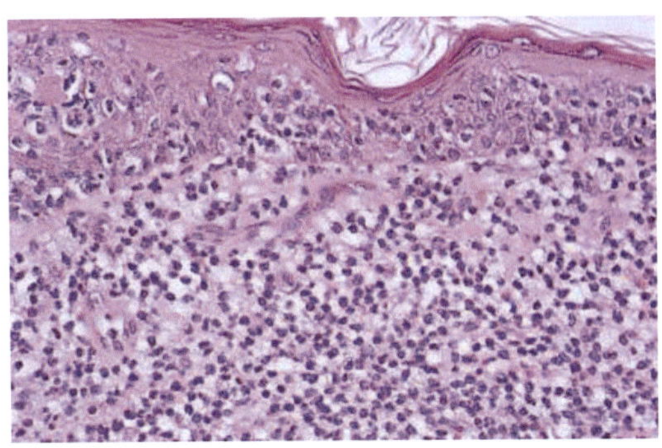

Fig. 3.214 Tumor stage MF with epidermal lymphocytes and extensive dermal lymphocytic infiltrate

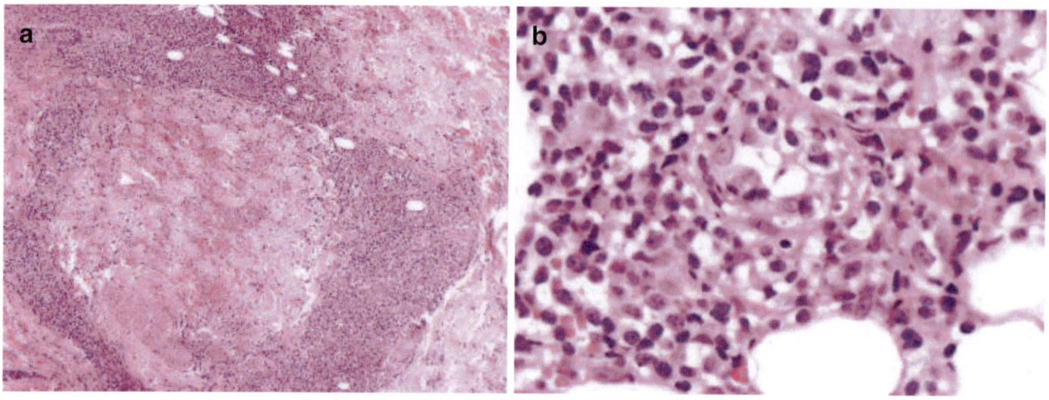

Fig. 3.215 (a, b) **Adult T-cell leukemia/lymphoma** with nodular perivascular infiltrate of atypical lymphocytes

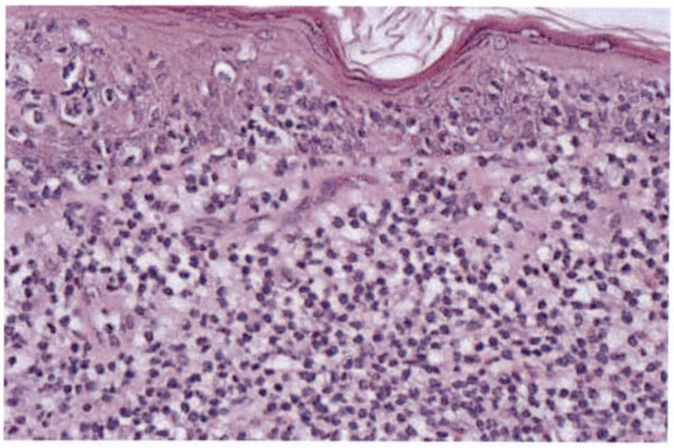

Fig. 3.216 **Extranodular NK/T cell lymphoma**

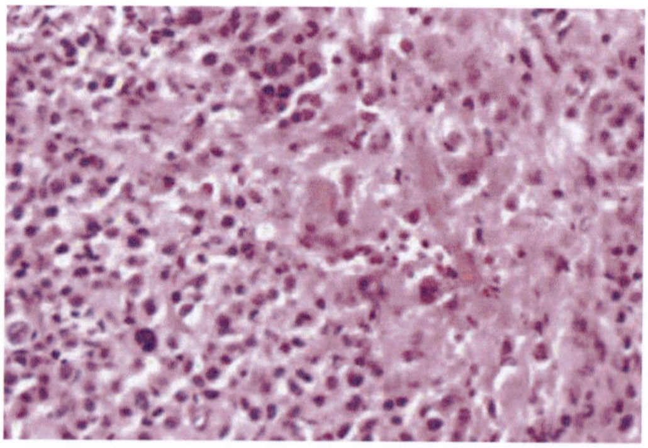

Fig. 3.217 Diffuse infiltrate of atypical lymphocytes with vascular destruction

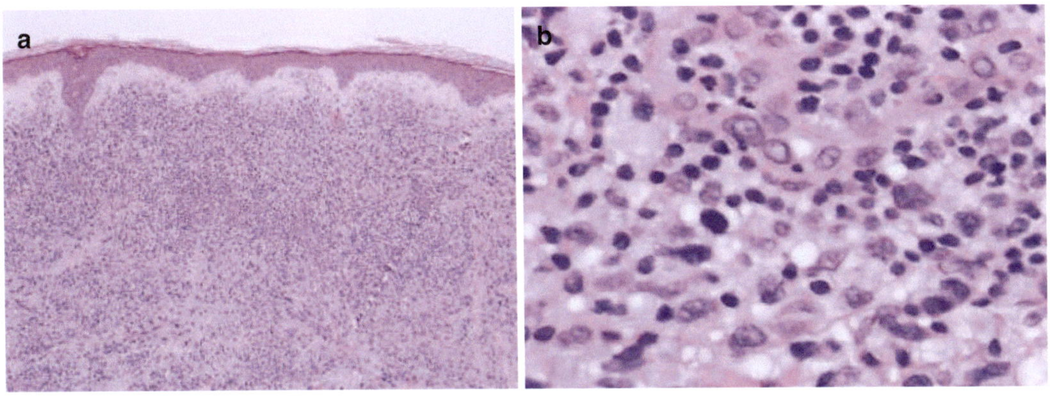

Fig. 3.218 (a, b) **Primary cutaneous anaplastic large cell lymphoma** with diffuse infiltrate of large atypical cells (CD30+)

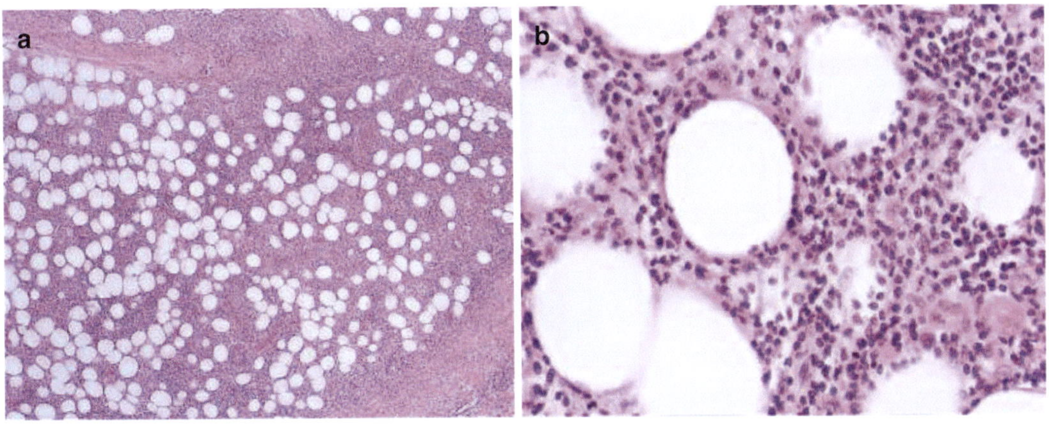

Fig. 3.219 (a, b) **Subcutaneous Panniculitis-like T-cell lymphoma** with malignant lymphocytes infiltrating subcutaneous tissue forming a "Swiss cheese" pattern

Cutis Laxa

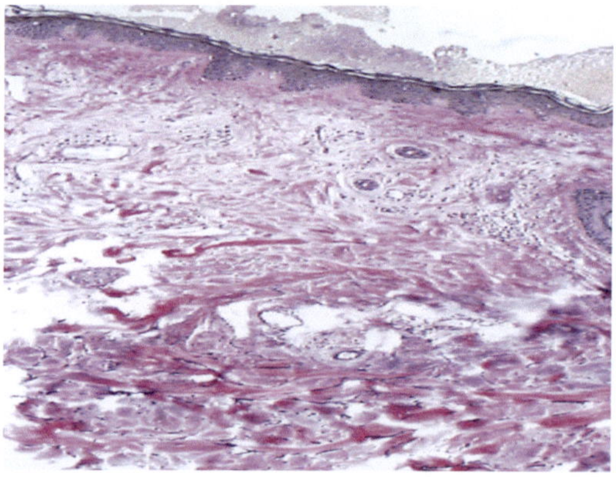

Fig. 3.220 Dermis with a few elastic fibers (VVG)

Histopathology (Figs. 3.220, 3.221, and 3.222)
- Absent dermal elastic fibers in papillary dermis and diminished elastic fibers in reticular dermis
- Residual elastic fibers are short and fragmented

P.S. changes are difficult to appreciate on the H&E stained slides and the elastic fibers special stain (Verhoeff Van Gieson) is recommended

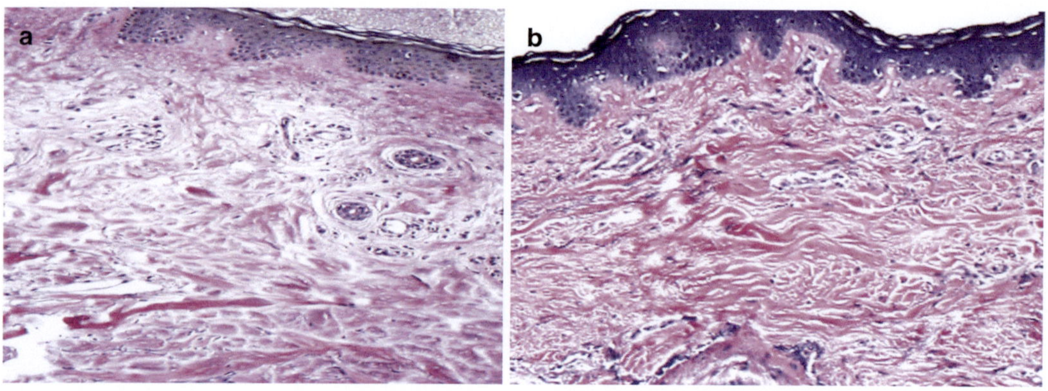

Fig. 3.221 (**a**, **b**) VVG stain demonstrates decreased dermal elastic fibers (black)

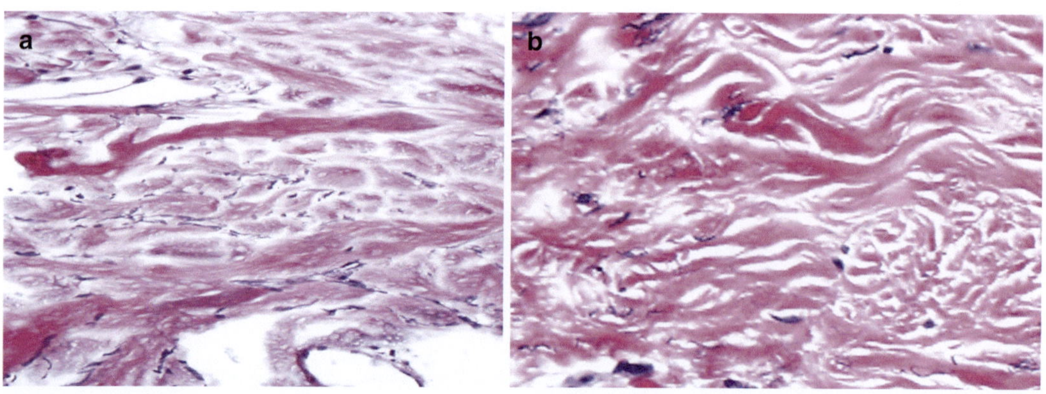

Fig. 3.222 (**a**, **b**) Remaining elastic fibers are short and fragmented (VVG)

Cylindroma

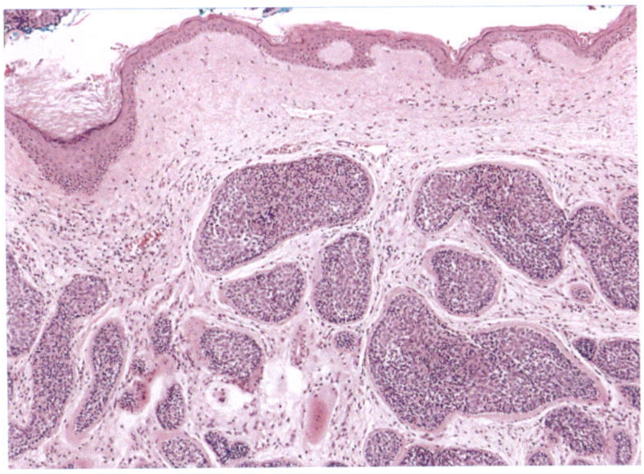

Fig. 3.223 Irregular tumor made of multiple variable nodules

Synonym: Eccrine Cylindroma

Histopathology (Figs. 3.223, 3.224, and 3.225)

- Irregularly shaped tumor islands forming mosaic "jigsaw" puzzle appearance in eosinophilic hyaline stroma
- Islands made of two cell types: peripheral palisading cells with dark nuclei and scant cytoplasm and centrally located larger cells with vesicular nuclei and more cytoplasm

P.S. associated with Brooke-Spiegler syndrome (*CYLD*)

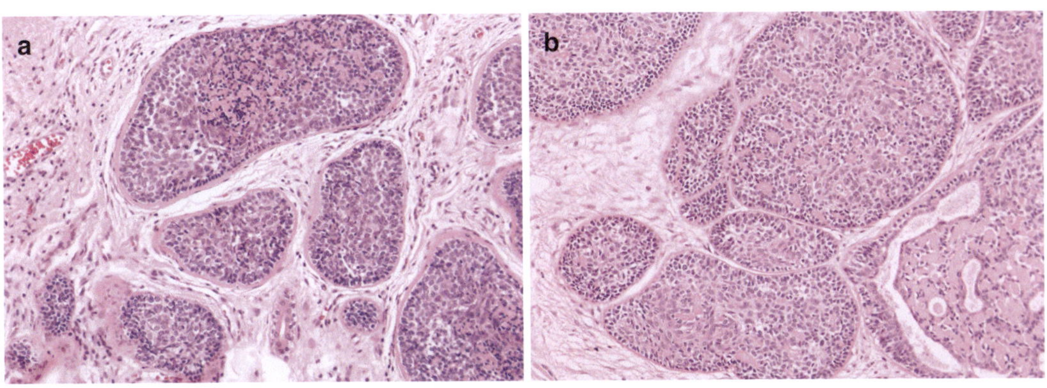

Fig. 3.224 (**a**, **b**) Tumor island forming "jigsaw" puzzle

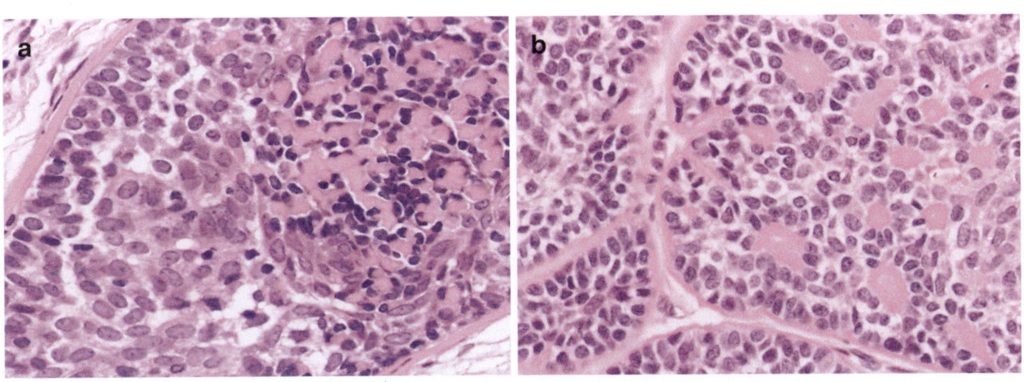

Fig. 3.225 (**a**, **b**) Two cell population (dark and pale) with hyalinized stroma between and within the island

Cylindroma Malignant

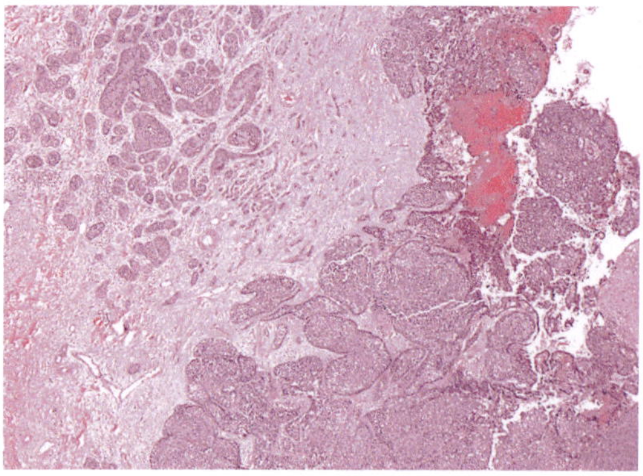

Fig. 3.226 Multinodular tumor with benign cylindroma top left and malignant portion on the right

Synonym: Carcinoma Ex Dermal Cylindroma

Histopathology (Figs. 3.226, 3.227, 3.228, 3.229, and 3.230)

- Large tumor with remnant of benign cylindroma
- Loss of "jigsaw" pattern and loss of hyalinized stroma
- Atypical tumor cells form tumor sheets with scattered mitoses and necrosis

P.S. tumor develops in long standing cylindroma. Associated with Brooke-Spiegler syndrome (*CYLD1*).

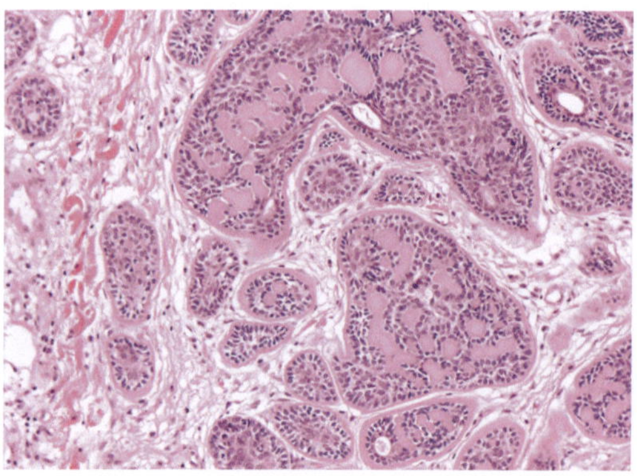

Fig. 3.227 Benign islands of cylindroma with hyalinized stroma forming "jigsaw" pattern

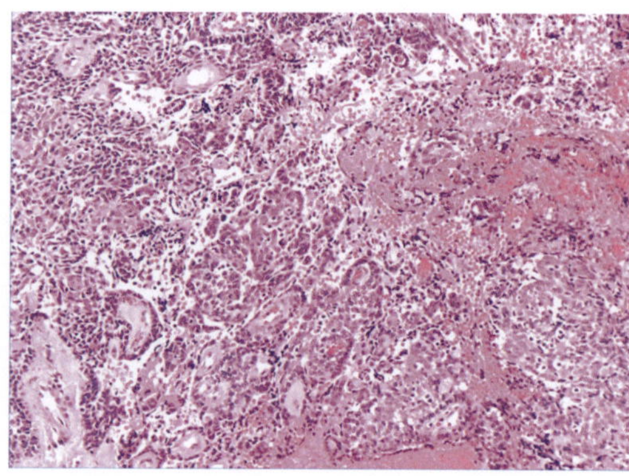

Fig. 3.228 Malignant cells with hemorrhage and necrosis

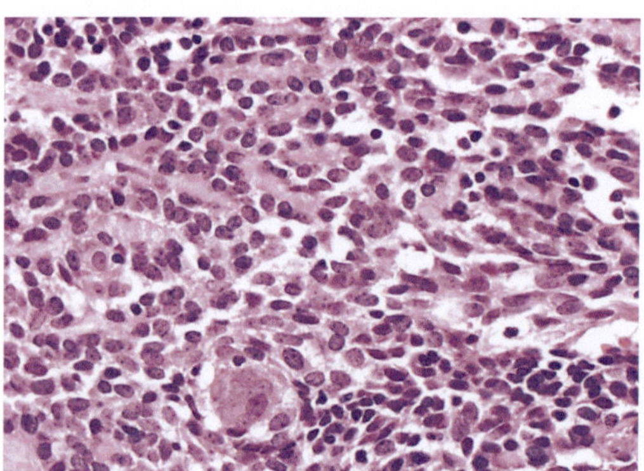

Fig. 3.229 Sheet of atypical tumor cells with cytological atypia

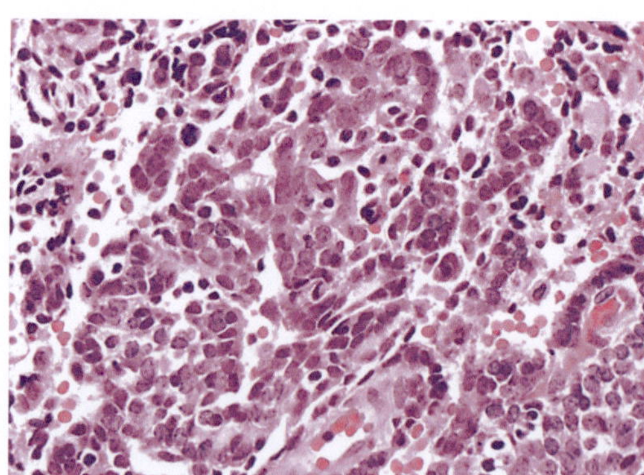

Fig. 3.230 Scattered necrotic cells are present

Cytomegalovirus

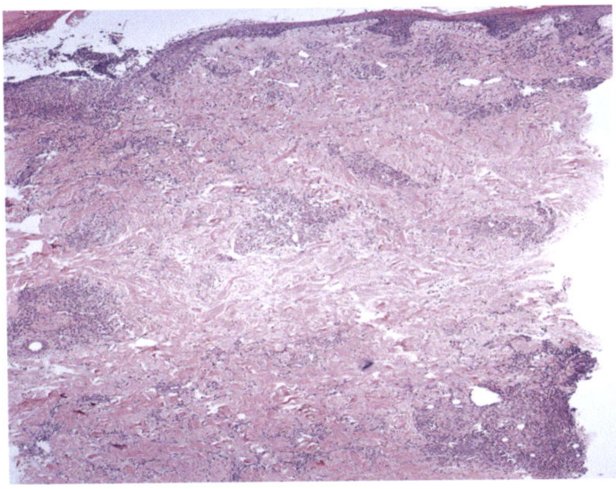

Fig. 3.231 Patchy dermal/subcutaneous perivascular inflammation

Histopathology (Figs. 3.231, 3.232, 3.233, and 3.234)

- Mixed dermal inflammation
- Dermal blood vessels have enlarged endothelial cells
- Large viral eosinophilic inclusions in nuclei of endothelial cells

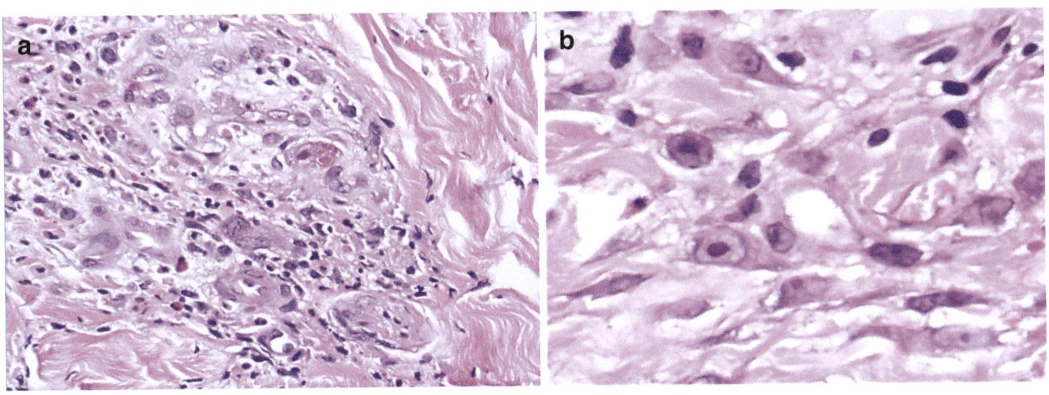

Fig. 3.232 (**a**, **b**) Mixed inflammation with plump endothelial cells with intranuclear inclusions

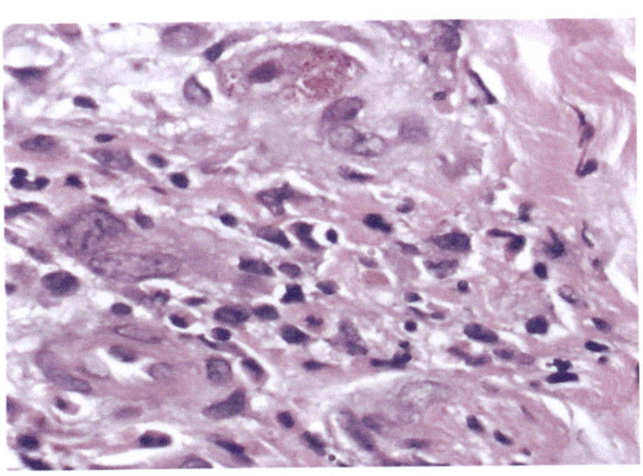

Fig. 3.233 Eosinophilic inclusion within endothelial cells

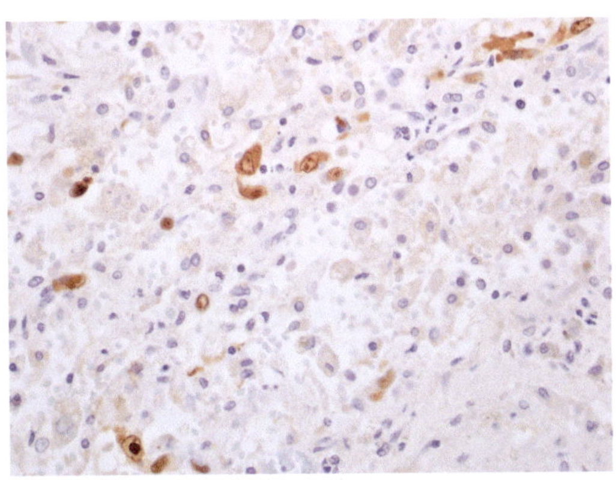

Fig. 3.234 IHC CMV stain highlights CMV inclusions

Cytophagic Histiocytic Panniculitis

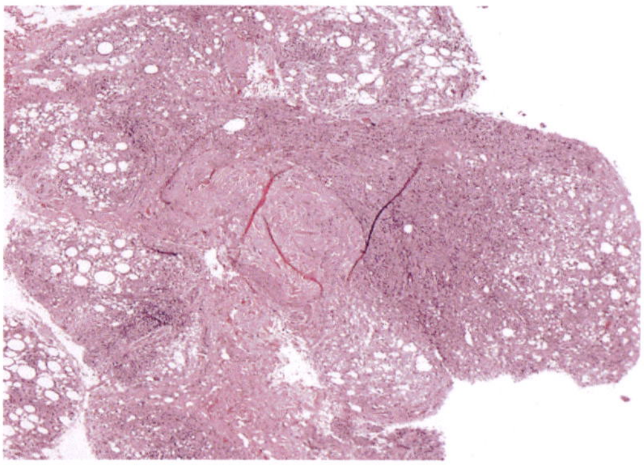

Fig. 3.235 Mostly lobular panniculitis

Histopathology (Figs. 3.235, 3.236, 3.237, 3.238, and 3.239)

- Lobular panniculitis with mixed inflammation
- Pronounced red blood extravasation
- Main characteristic is the presence of histiocytes with phagocytosed red blood cells (erythrophagocytes)
- Phagocytosis of lymphocytes, neutrophils, and nuclear debris is also common, forming so called "bean-bag" cells

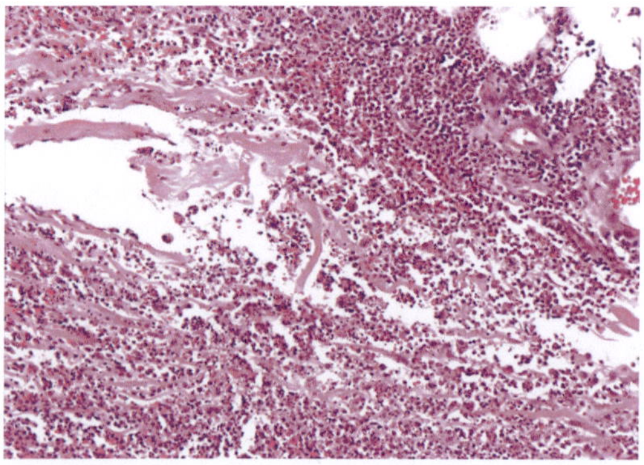

Fig. 3.236 Exuberant mixed inflammation with RBC extravasation

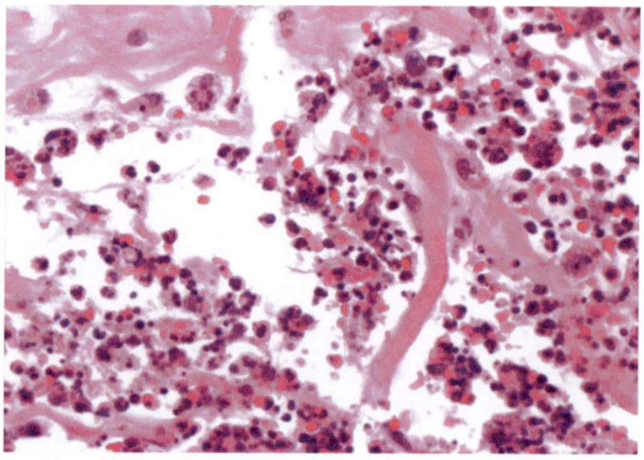

Fig. 3.237 Histiocytes with engulfed red blood cells, neutrophils, and lymphocytes

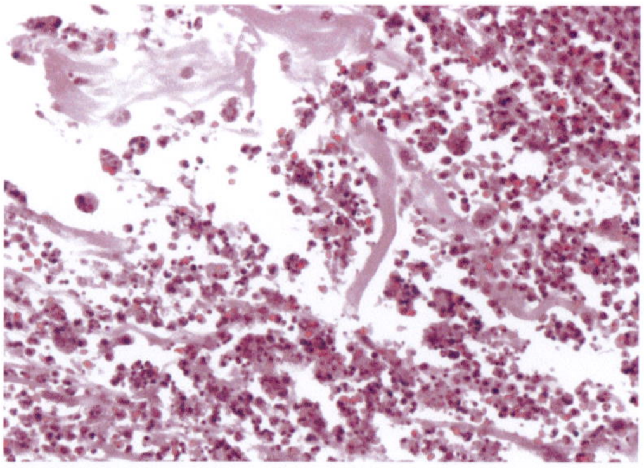

Fig. 3.238 Inflammation made of histiocytes, neutrophils, and lymphocytes

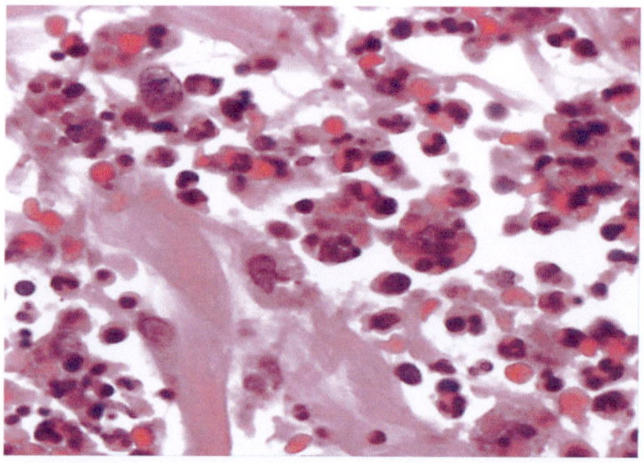

Fig. 3.239 Erythrophagocytosis is pathognomonic

4 Dermatopathology D

V. Vincek, *Dermatopathology A–Z*, https://doi.org/10.1007/978-3-319-89486-7_4

Darier's Disease

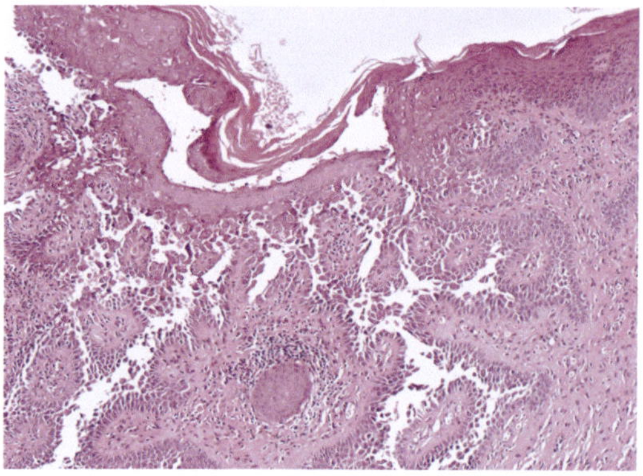

Fig. 4.1 Hyperkeratotic epidermis with suprabasal split

Synonym: Keratosis Follicularis

Histopathology (Figs. 4.1, 4.2, 4.3, and 4.4)
- Hyperkeratotic epidermis
- Suprabasal acantholysis with small clefts
- Dyskeratotic cells form corp ronds and corp grains
- Corp ronds are cells with dark, shrunken nuclei, a clear halo, and eosinophilic cytoplasm
- Corp grains are smaller cells with elongated nuclei and scant cytoplasm

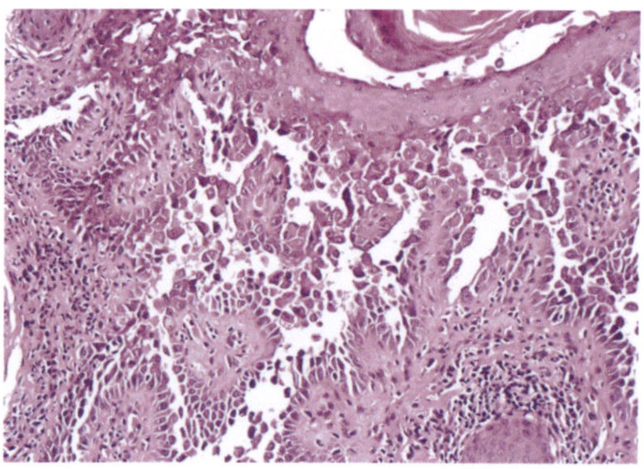

Fig. 4.2 Acantholysis results in multiple small clefts within the epidermis

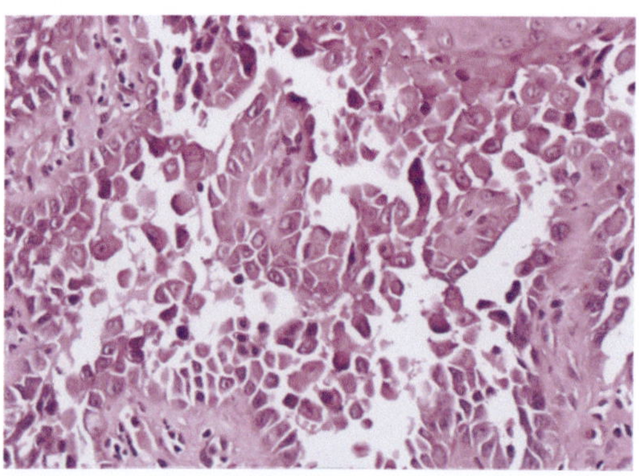

Fig. 4.3 Epidermal basal layer is preserved

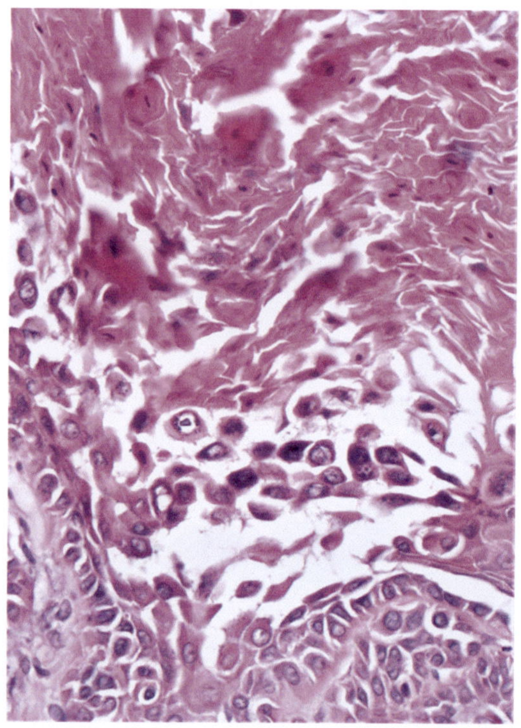

Fig. 4.4 Dyskeratotic cells forming corp ronds and corp grains

Deep Penetrating Nevus

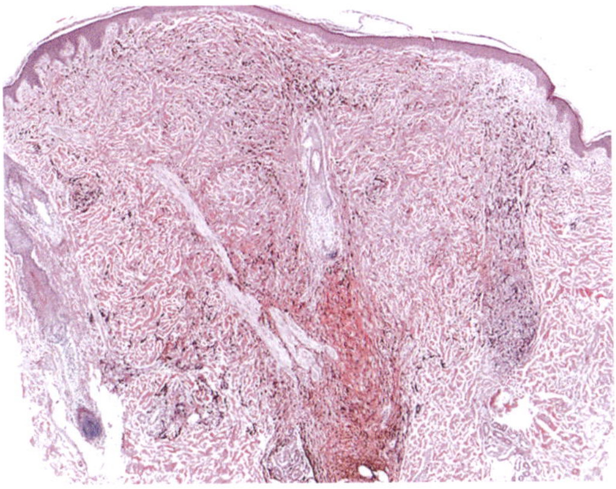

Fig. 4.5 V-shaped pigmented lesion surrounds the hair follicle

Histopathology (Figs. 4.5, 4.6, 4.7, 4.8, and 4.9)

- Wedge shaped symmetrical lesion surrounding the hair follicle, sweat glands, and nerves that extends into the deep reticular dermis and subcutis
- Variable ratio of vertically oriented pigmented spindle cells and/or pale epithelioid cells admixed with melanophages and prominent collagen
- Slight maturation is present and mitoses are rare

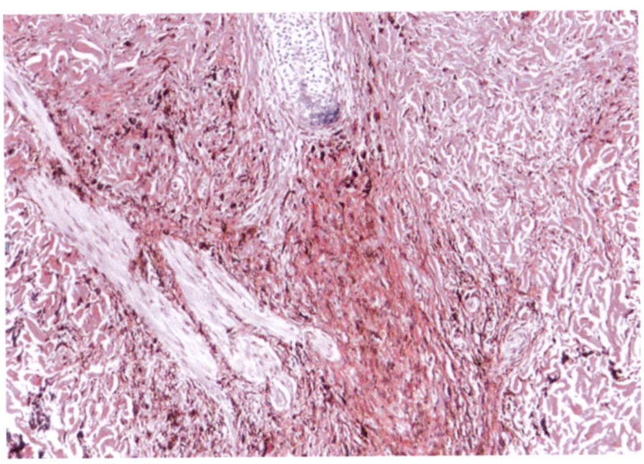

Fig. 4.6 Heavily pigmented spindle cells predominate and pale epithelioid cells are in minority

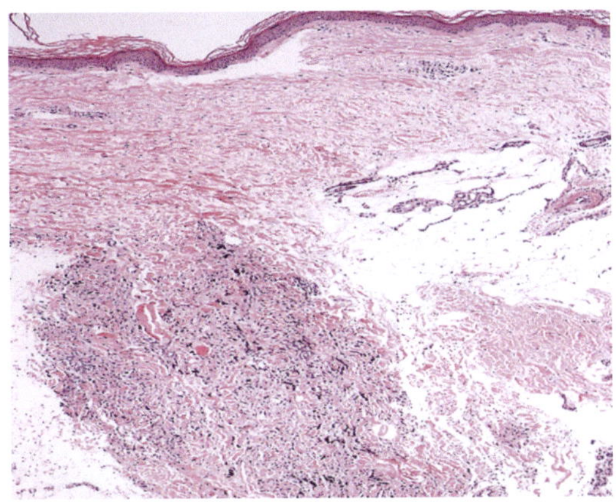

Fig. 4.7 Melanocytic cells vertically surround adnexal structures

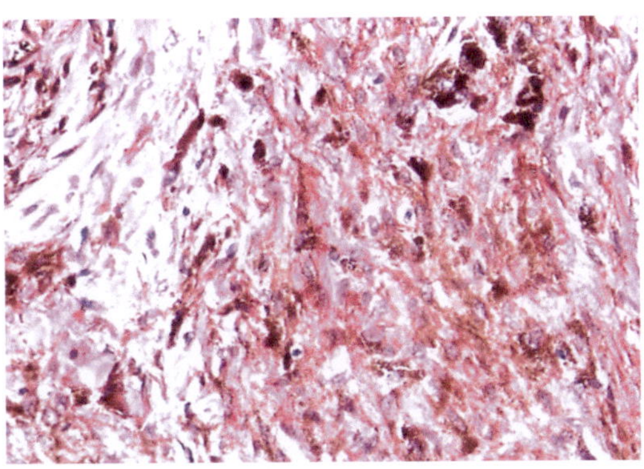

Fig. 4.8 No evidence of mitoses

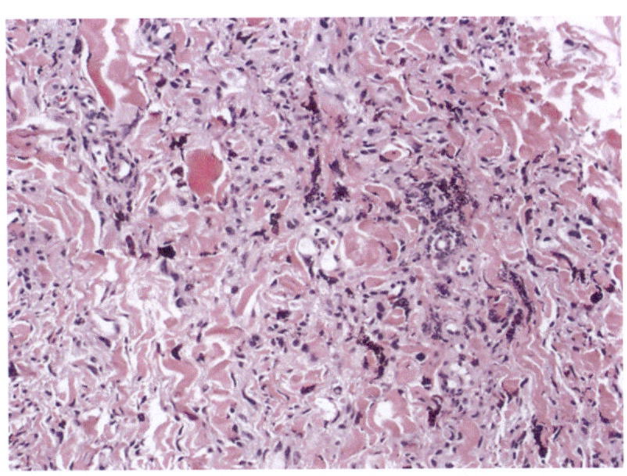

Fig. 4.9 Epitheliod cells with scattered spindle cells and pigment

Degos Disease

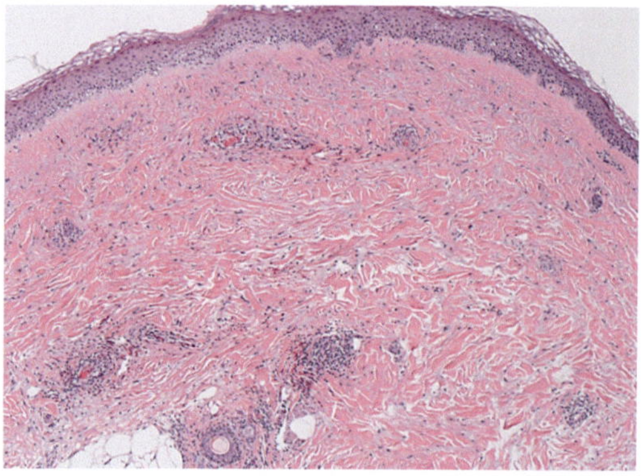

Fig. 4.10 Wedge-shaped lesion with small vessel vasculitis

Synonym: Malignant Atrophic Papulosis

Histopathology (Figs. 4.10, 4.11, and 4.12)

- Hyperkeratotic flattened epidermis
- Wedge-shaped dermal ischemia and edema
- Endothelial swelling with fibrin thrombi
- Perivascular lymphocytic inflammation with red blood cell extravasation
- Increased dermal mucin

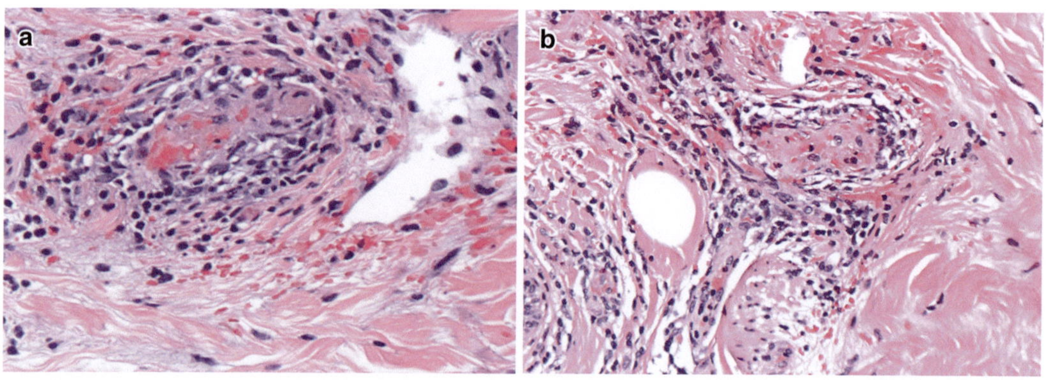

Fig. 4.11 (**a**, **b**) Blood vessels at the apex of the lesion have reactive endothelial cells with hyalinized wall and thromboses; perivascular lymphocytic inflammation with extensive red blood cell extravasation

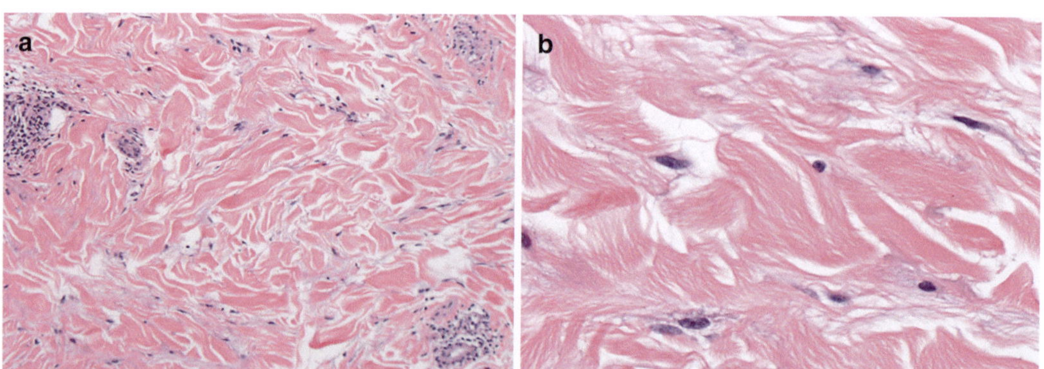

Fig. 4.12 (**a**, **b**) Prominent dermal mucin separates collagen bundles

Dermal Duct Tumor

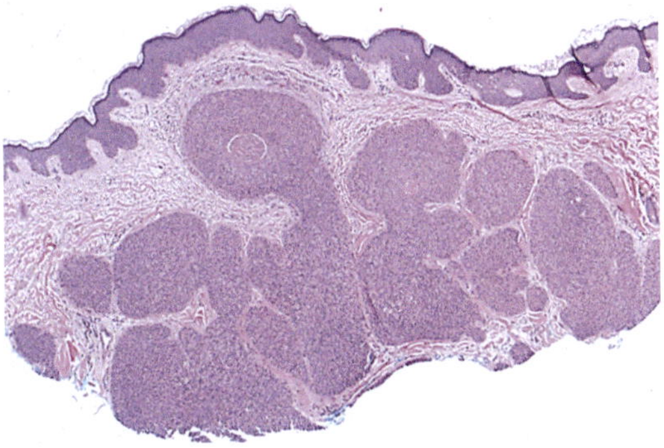

Fig. 4.13 Islands of tumor within the dermis

Histopathology

- Islands of uniform basaloid cells within the dermis
- No evidence of peripheral palisading
- No epidermal connection
- No evidence of stromal retraction
- Duct-like structures within the tumor islands highlighted with CEA stain

P.S. "poroma-like" tumor with no epidermal connection (Figs. 4.13, 4.14, 4.15, 4.16, and 4.17)

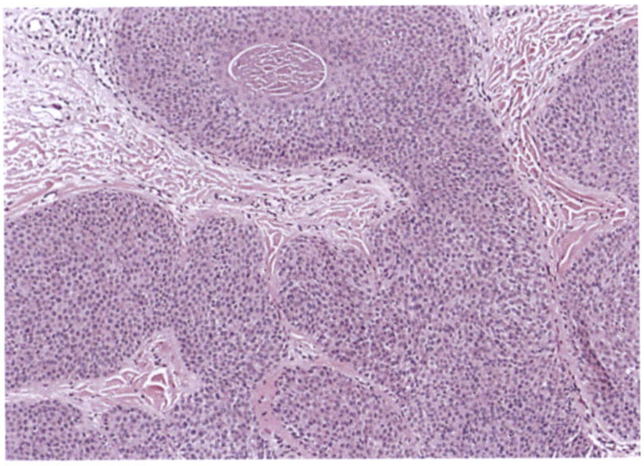

Fig. 4.14 Uniform basaloid cells with no atypia

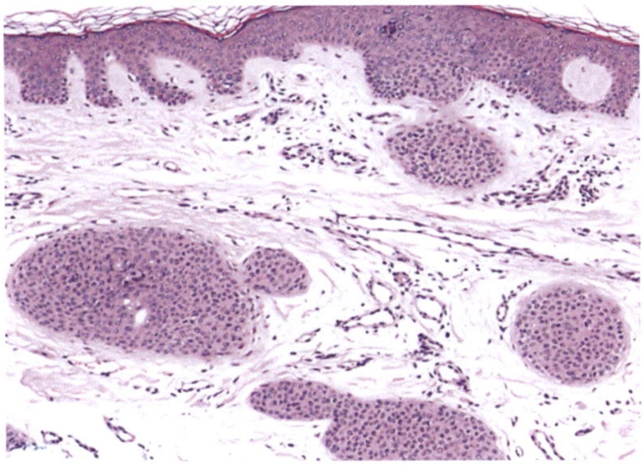

Fig. 4.15 Stromal retraction is absent

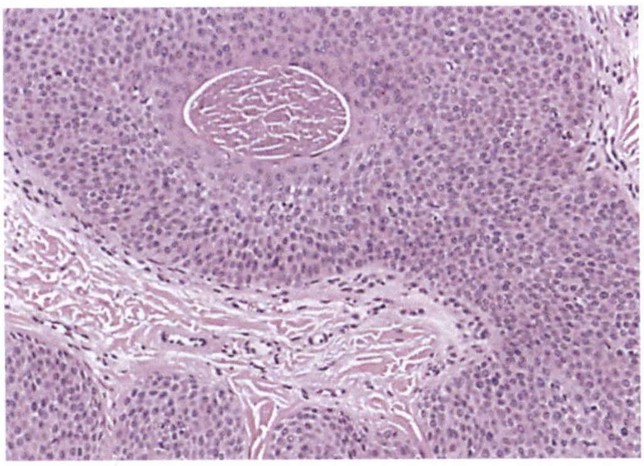

Fig. 4.16 Larger duct-like structure is present within the tumor

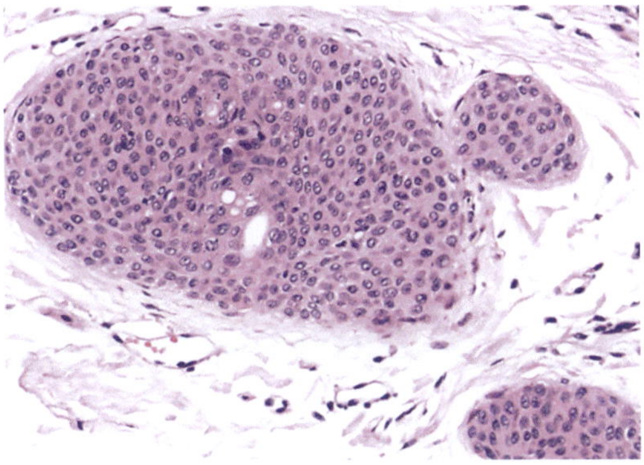

Fig. 4.17 Small ducts within the tumor island

Dermal Melanocytosis

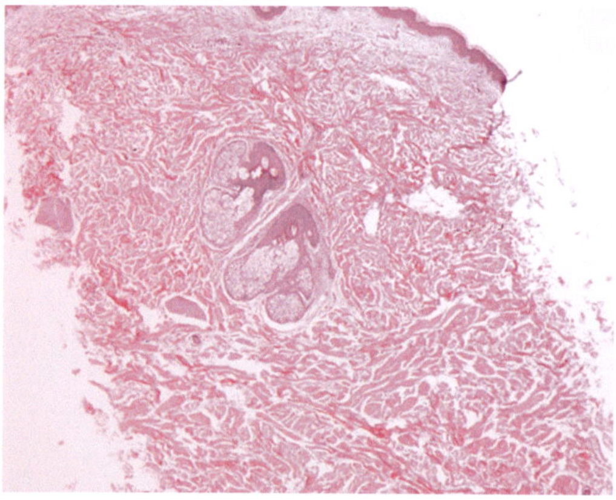

Fig. 4.18 On low magnification skin looks unremarkable

It includes Nevus of **Ito, Nevus of Ota, Nevus of Sun, and Mongolian Spot**.

Histopathology (Figs. 4.18, 4.19, 4.20, and 4.21)

- Heavily pigmented spindle dendritic melanocytes
- Pigmented cells tend to be oriented parallel to the surface or circular around appendages
- In **Nevus of Ota/Ito/Hori/Sun** dendritic melanocytes are located in the upper and mid dermis
- In **Mongolian Spot** dendritic melanocytes are mostly in the deeper reticular dermis

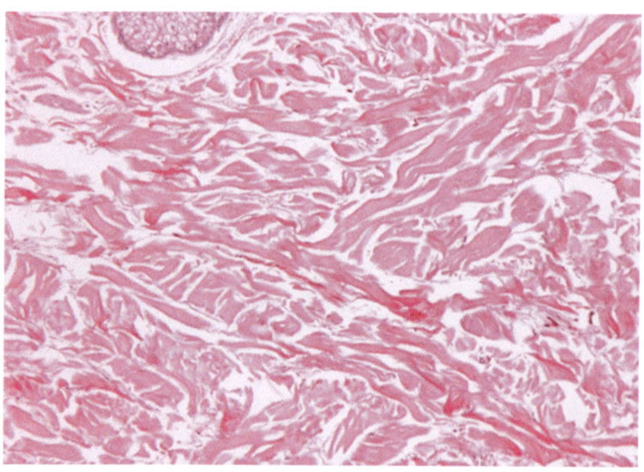

Fig. 4.19 Pigmented dendritic melanocytes in the deeper dermis

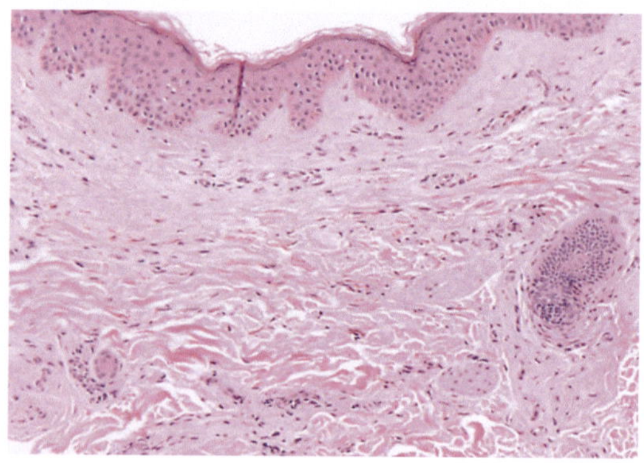

Fig. 4.20 Upper and mid dermis contains scattered pigmented dendritic melanocytes

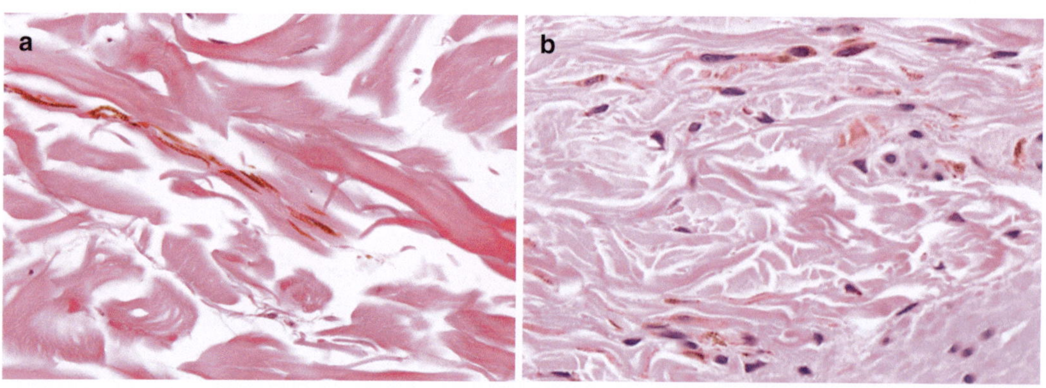

Fig. 4.21 (**a**, **b**) Pigmented dendritic melanocytes are oriented parallel with the collagen

Dermal Nevus

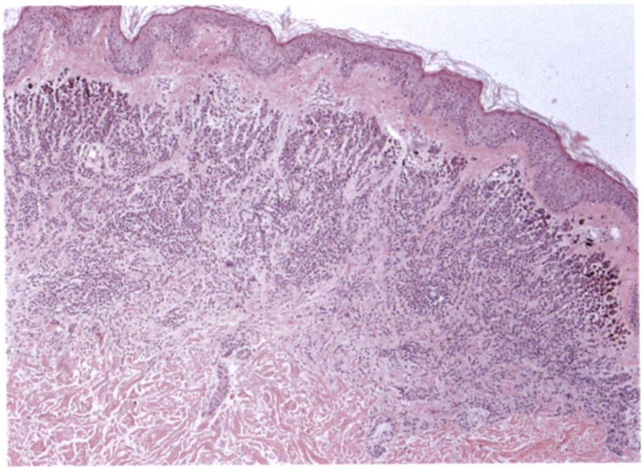

Fig. 4.22 Symmetrical dermal melanocytic lesion

Synonym: Intradermal Nevus

Histopathology (Figs. 4.22, 4.23, and 4.24)

- No intra-epidermal melanocytic nests
- Nests of nevus cells are present in the dermis
- Superficial cells are larger and form nests
- Deeper cells are smaller forming smaller nests and eventually become single (maturation)
- Pigment is present in the upper part of the nevus

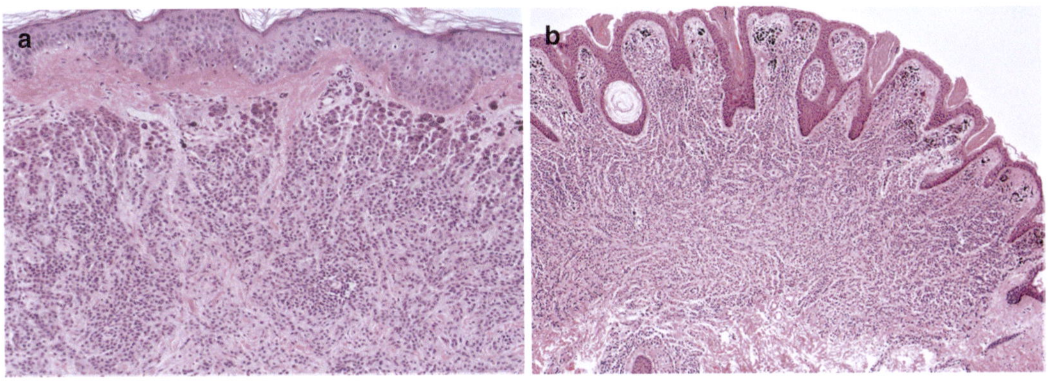

Fig. 4.23 (**a**, **b**) Nevus cells are maturing with descent. Nests and larger cells are more superior and smaller individual cells are inferior. Pigmented cells are present only in the superficial portion

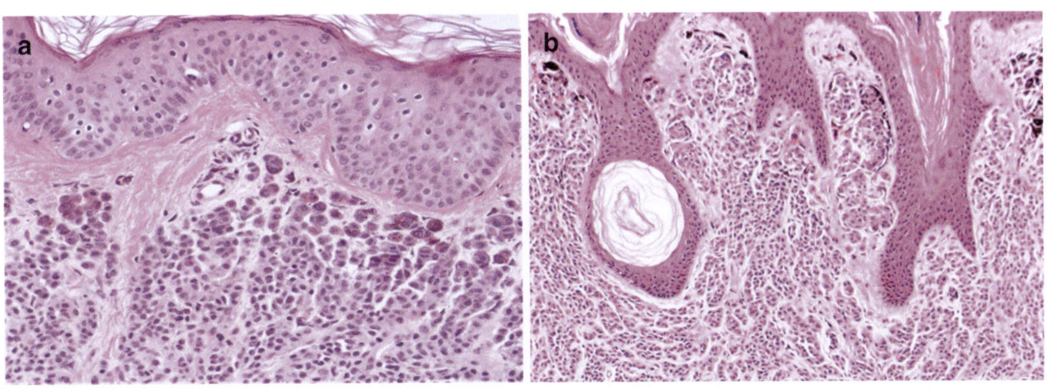

Fig. 4.24 (**a**, **b**) Nevus cells don't show any cytological atypia and mitoses are absent

Dermatitis Herpetiformis

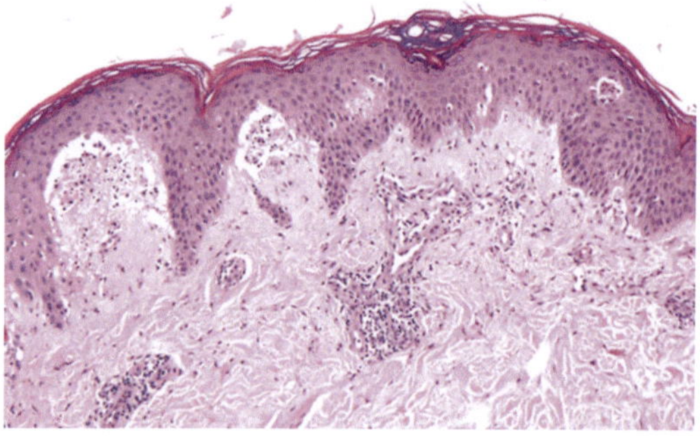

Fig. 4.25 Subepidermal blister with dermal inflammation

Histopathology (Figs. 4.25, 4.26, and 4.27)

- Subepidermal blister
- Neutrophils in dermal papillae forming microabscesses
- In older lesions eosinophils can appear and there is mild leukocytoclasia
- Mild perivascular lymphocytic infiltrate

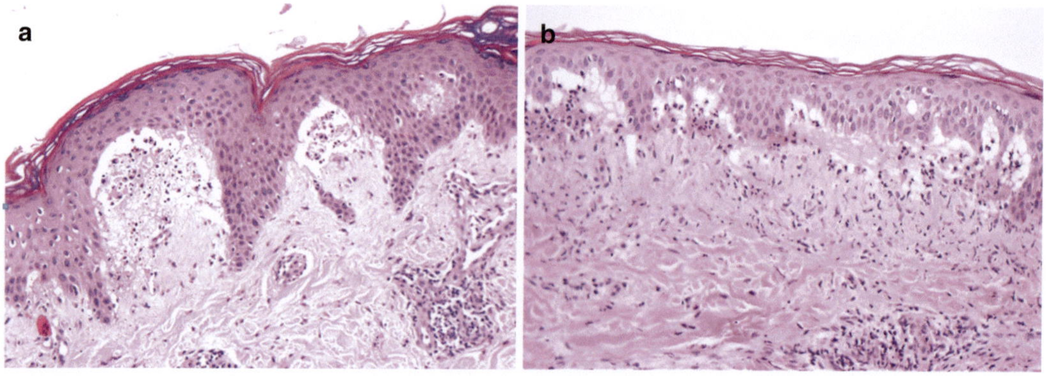

Fig. 4.26 (**a**, **b**) Subepidermal blister with neutrophils within papillae and perivascular lymphocytes

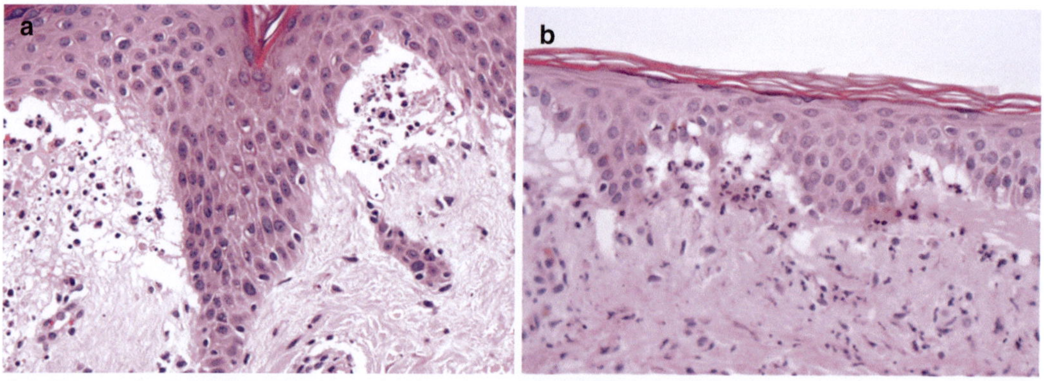

Fig. 4.27 (**a**, **b**) Neutrophilic aggregates in the dermal papillae form microabscesses

Dermatofibroma

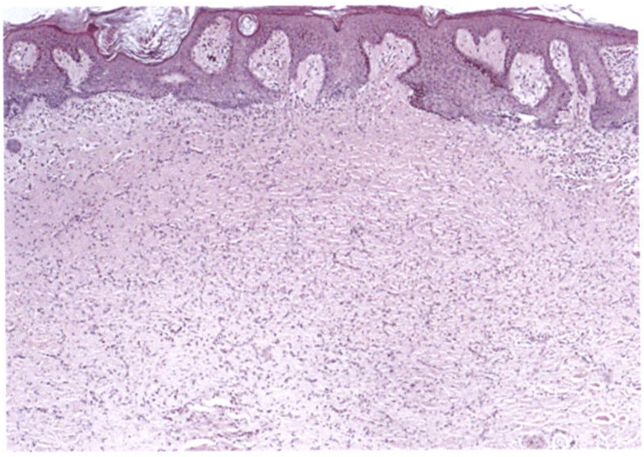

Fig. 4.28 **Common DF** with dermal tumor abutting papillomatous and hyperpigmented epidermis

Synonym: Benign Fibrous Histiocytoma
Many variants but most common **histopathology** (Figs. 4.28, 4.29, 4.30, 4.31, 4.32, 4.33, 4.34, 4.35, 4.36, 4.37, and 4.38) is featured by:

- Acanthotic epidermis with irregular papillomatosis and hyperpigmentation of the basal layer ("dirty feet")
- Storiform pattern of spindle/oval fibroblasts (factor XIII+) and round/oval histiocytic cells (focally CD68+) without Grenz zone
- Stoma between tumor cells is hyalinized with few giant cells and xanthoma cells

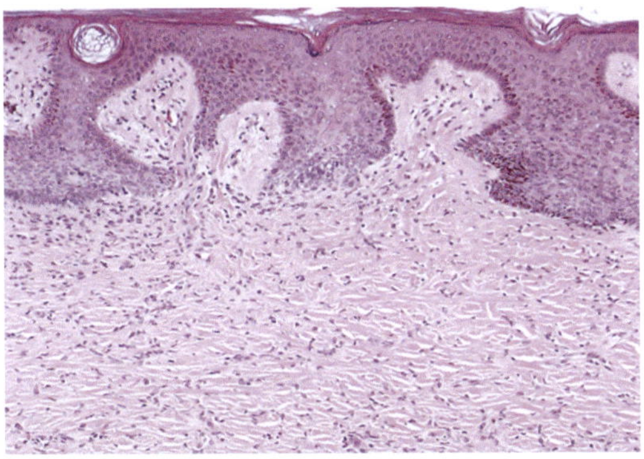

Fig. 4.29 Spindle and oval fibroblasts in hyalinized stroma

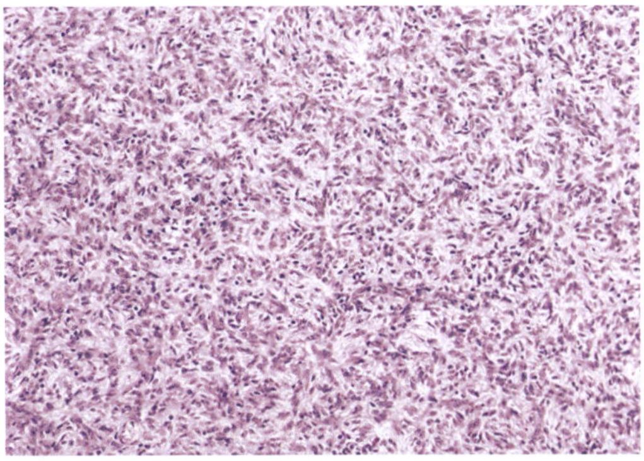

Fig. 4.30 **Cellular DF** with increased cellularity and more round, epithelioid cells

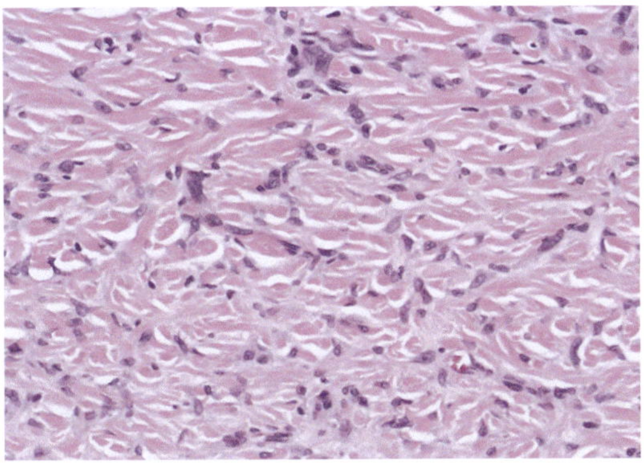

Fig. 4.31 Prominent entrapped collagen

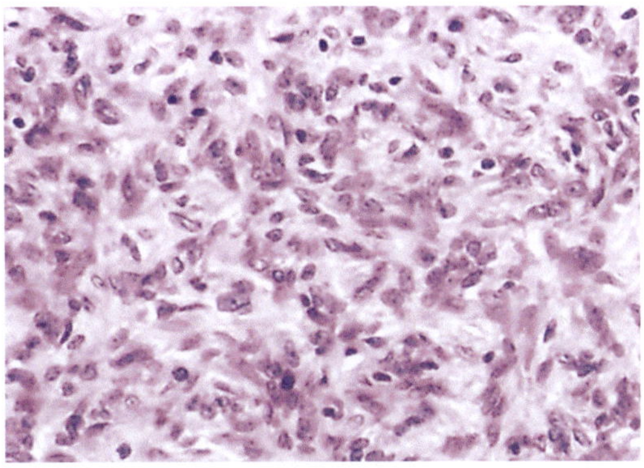

Fig. 4.32 No atypia or mitoses

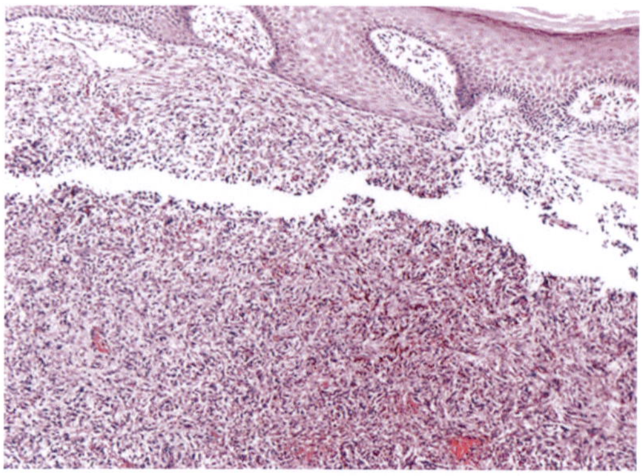

Fig. 4.33 Aneurysmal (hemosiderotic) DF

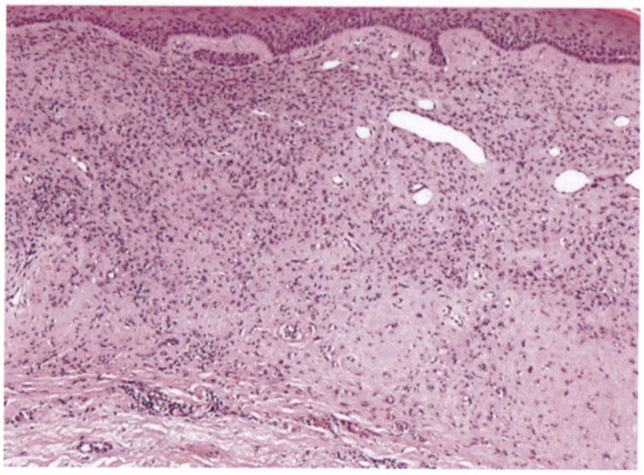

Fig. 4.34 Sclerotic DF

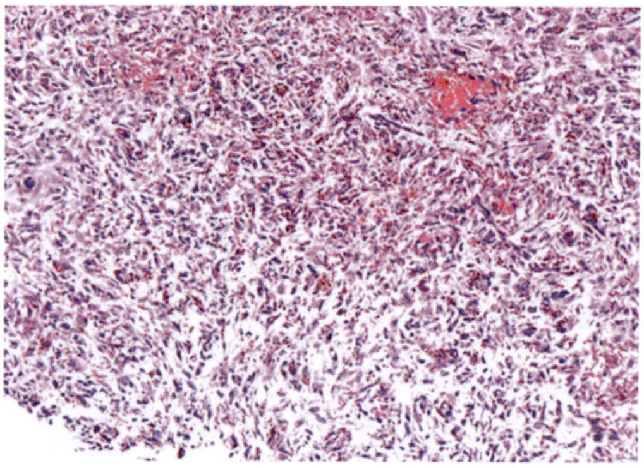

Fig. 4.35 Tumor is very cellular with spindle and epithelioid cells with some cytological atypia

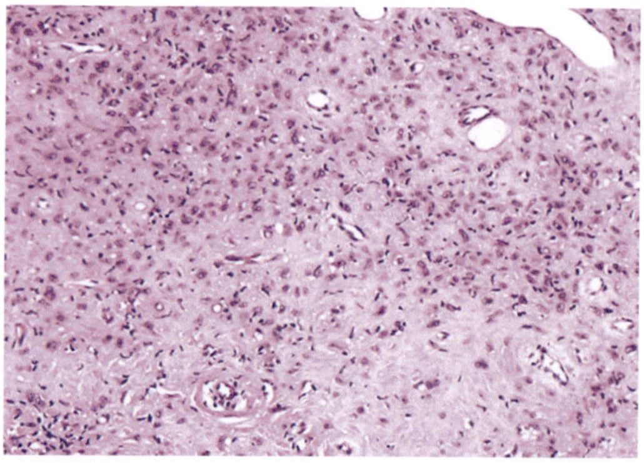

Fig. 4.36 Tumor consists of rounded epithelioid cells

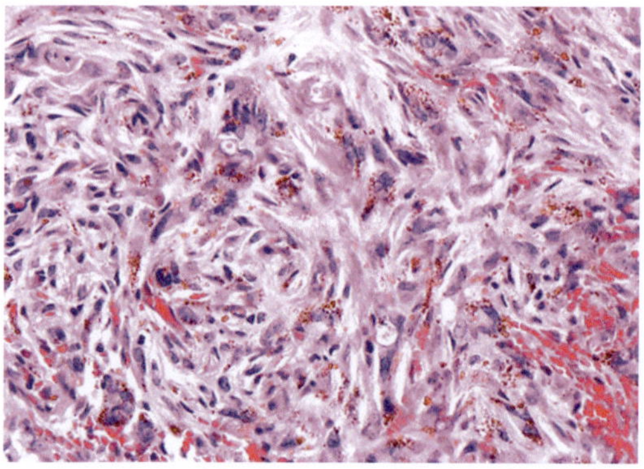

Fig. 4.37 Extensive red blood cell extravasation and hemosiderin

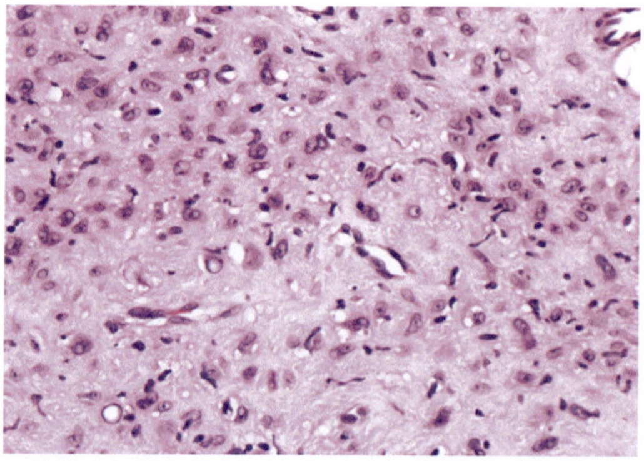

Fig. 4.38 Cells are separated by thick hyalinized stroma

Dermatofibrosarcoma Protuberans

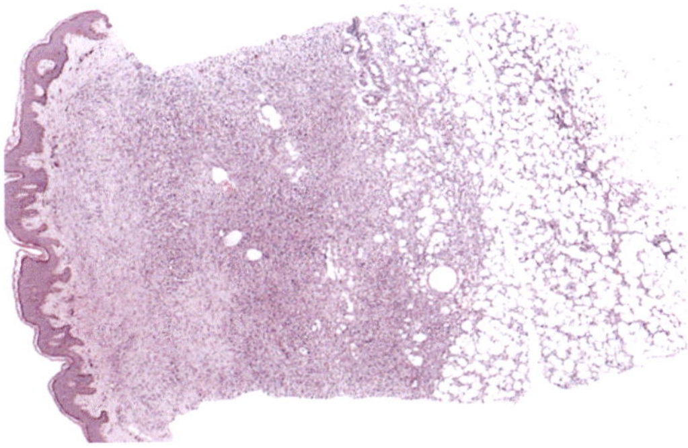

Fig. 4.39 Dermal tumor infiltrating into subcutis

Synonym: DFSP

Histopathology (Figs. 4.39, 4.40, 4.41, 4.42, and 4.43)

- Dermal tumor that always invades subcutaneous tissue
- Monotonous storiform pattern
- Homogenous population of spindled fibroblasts
- Diffuse infiltration of fat in "Swiss cheese" pattern
- Spindle cells are CD34 positive, factor XIII-

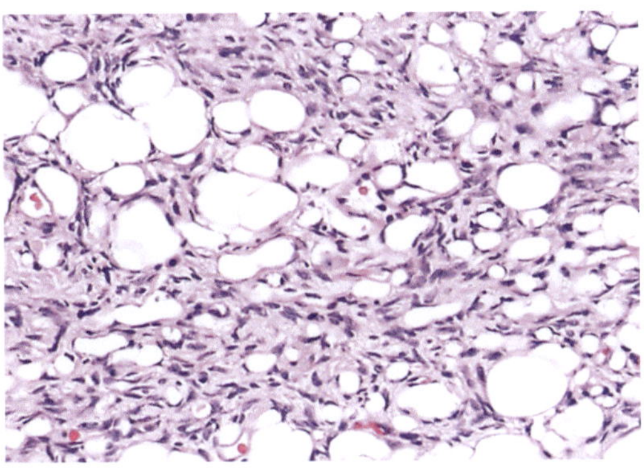

Fig. 4.40 Spindle cells infiltrate in between adipocytes

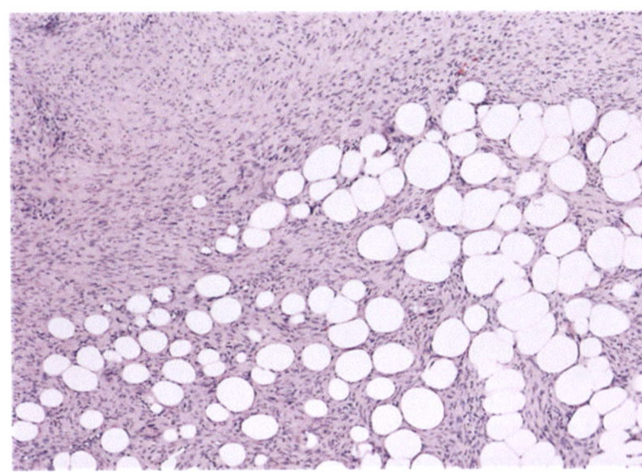

Fig. 4.41 Tumor infiltrates adipose tissue and form "Swiss cheese" pattern

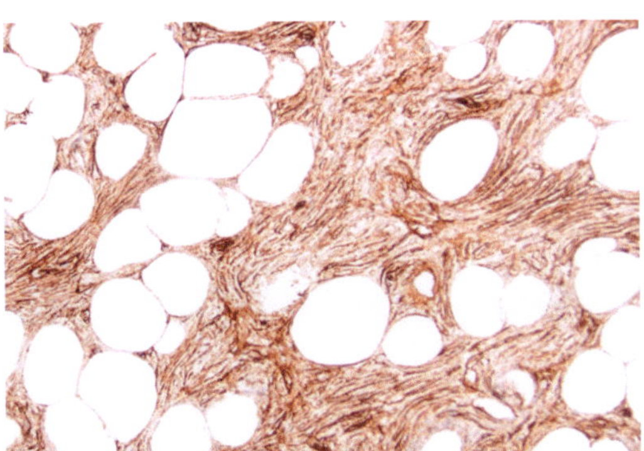

Fig. 4.42 CD34 stains tumor cells

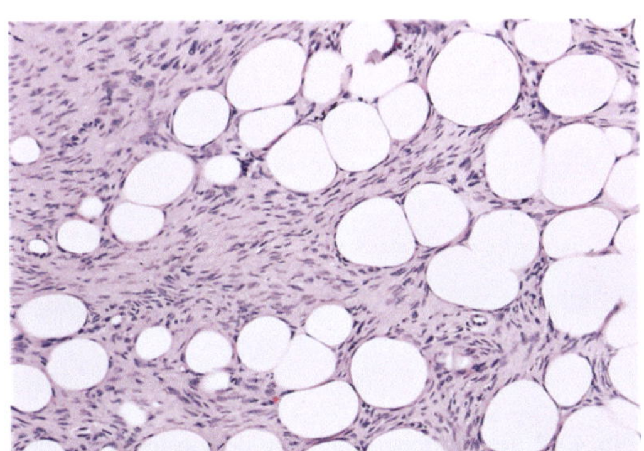

Fig. 4.43 Spindled fibroblasts in storiform pattern

Dermatomyositis

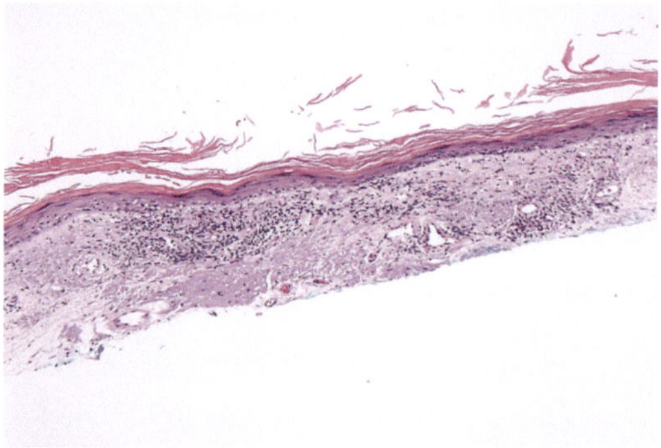

Fig. 4.44 Atrophic epidermis

Histopathology (Figs. 4.44, 4.45, 4.46, and 4.47)

- Atrophic epidermis
- Mild subtle interface vacuolar changes with occasional apoptotic keratinocytes
- Minimal to moderate dermal lymphocytic infiltrate
- Increased dermal mucin
- Variable dermal edema

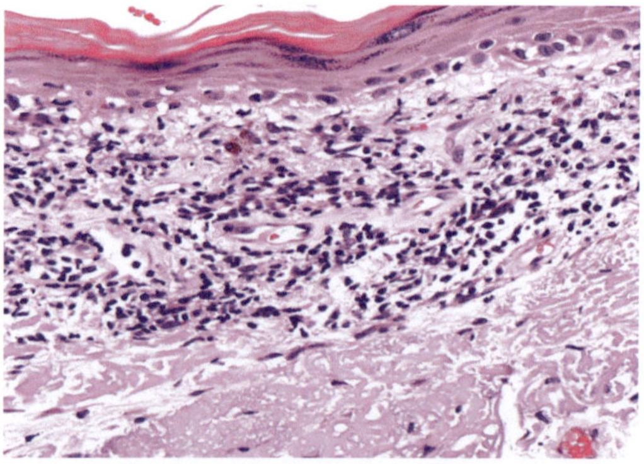

Fig. 4.45 Interface vacuolar changes with dermal lymphocytic infiltrate and pigment incontinence

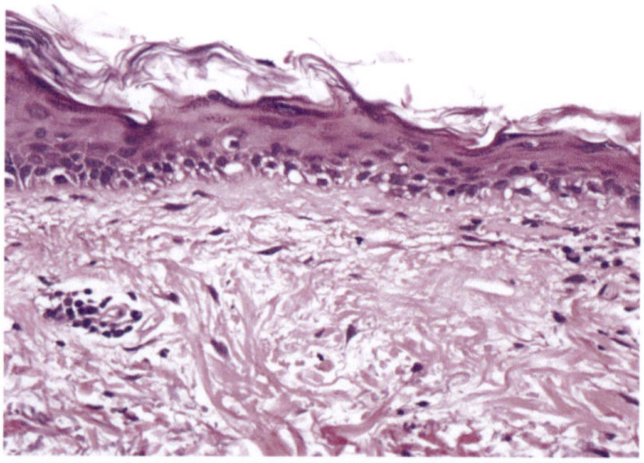

Fig. 4.46 Interface changes with increased dermal mucin

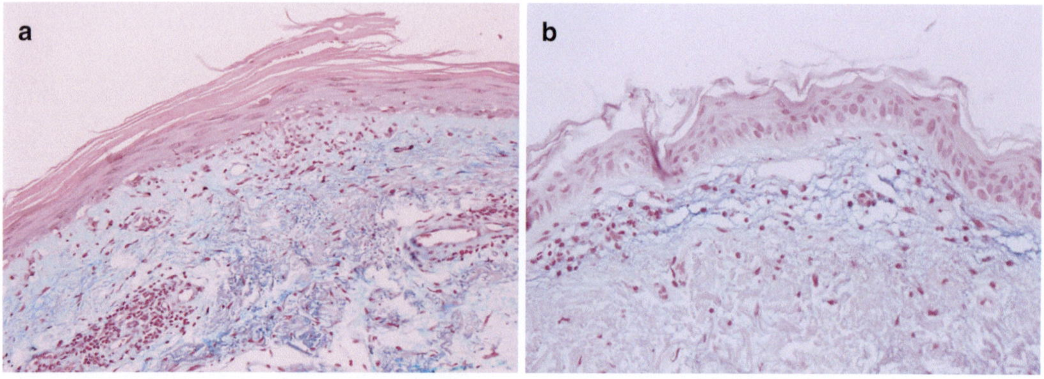

Fig. 4.47 (a, b) Alcian Blue stain demonstrates increased dermal mucin (blue)

Dermatomyofibroma

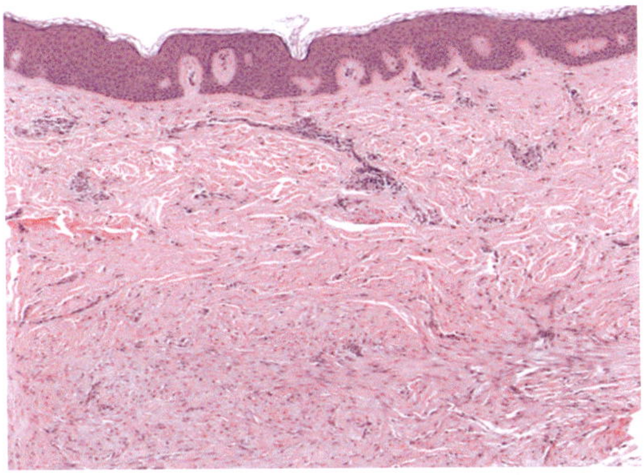

Fig. 4.48 Plaque-like dermal tumor

Histopathology (Figs. 4.48, 4.49, 4.50, 4.51, and 4.52)

- Plaque-like dermal tumor
- Composed of spindle cells with eosinophilic cytoplasm
- Cells form fascicles that tend to be parallel to the epidermis
- No cytological atypia or mitoses
- Papillary dermis is usually spared
- Cells are SMA+, desmin-, factor XIII-

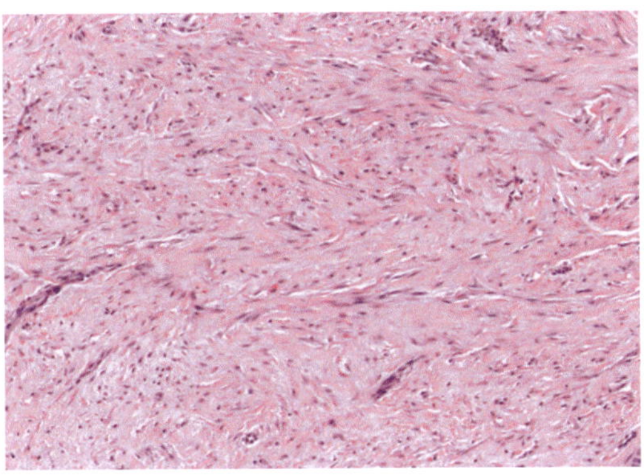

Fig. 4.49 Fascicles tend to be parallel to the epidermis

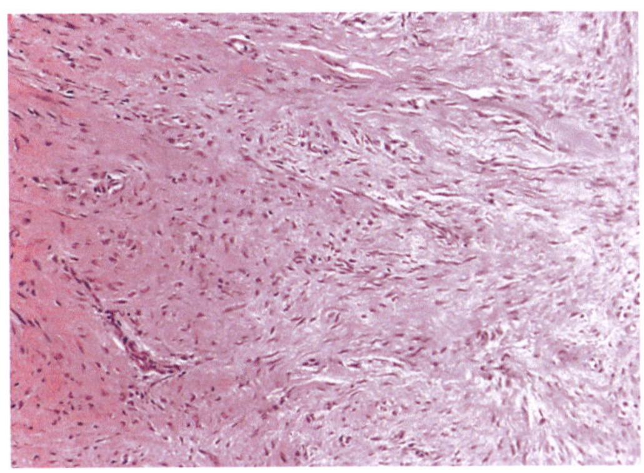

Fig. 4.50 Cells form subtle fascicles in thickened stroma

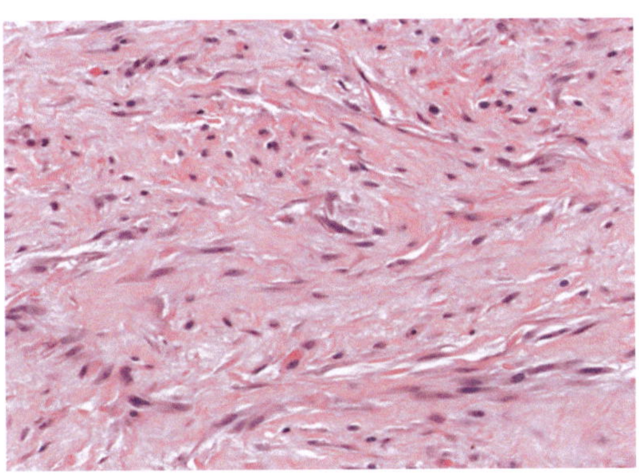

Fig. 4.51 Elongated nuclei and abundant eosinophilic cytoplasm

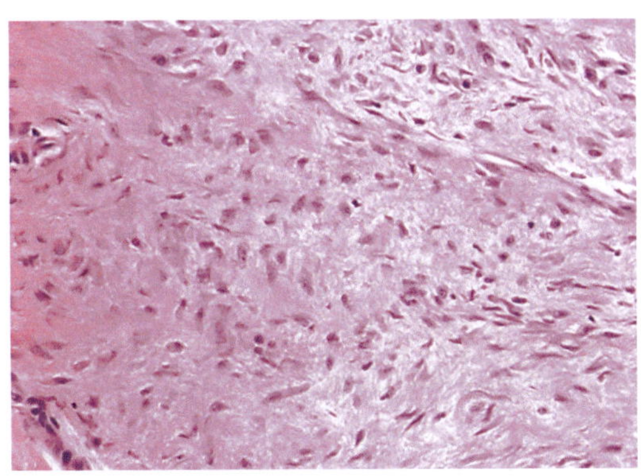

Fig. 4.52 Ovoid/spindle cells with muscle like appearance

Dermatosis Papulosa Nigra

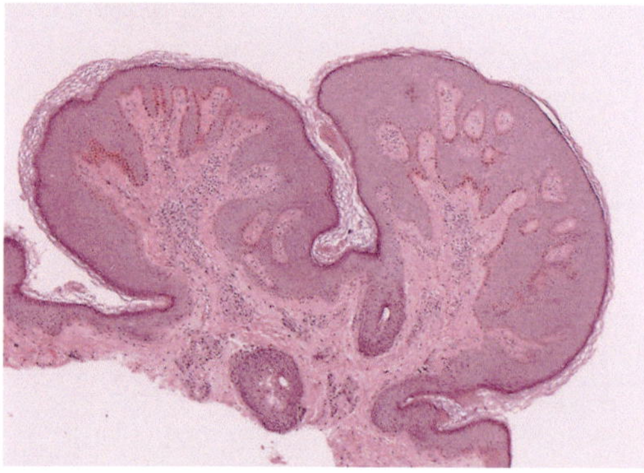

Fig. 4.53 Polypoid epidermal lesion

Histopathology (Figs. 4.53, 4.54, 4.55, 4.56, and 4.57)

- Polypoid architecture
- Hyperkeratosis and irregular acanthosis with uniform keratinocytes
- Horn cysts within epidermis
- Hyperpigmentation of the epidermal basal layer

P.S. histological appearance of seborrheic keratosis in darkly pigmented individuals

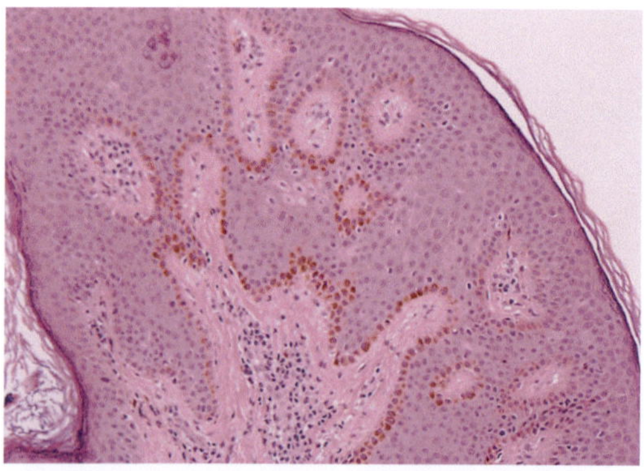

Fig. 4.54 Uniform proliferation of keratinocytes

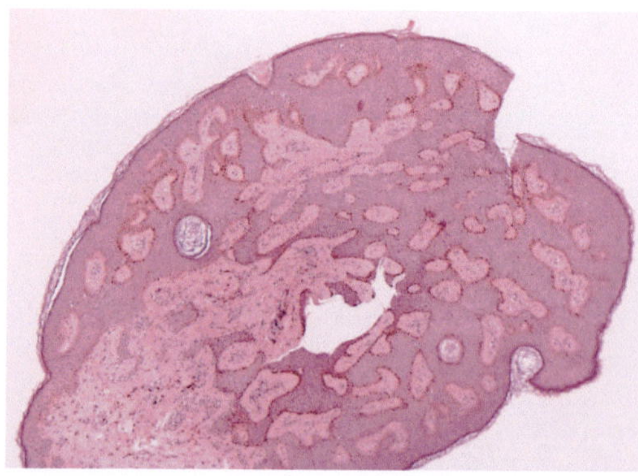

Fig. 4.55 Interwoven tracts of epidermal cells in a reticulated pattern

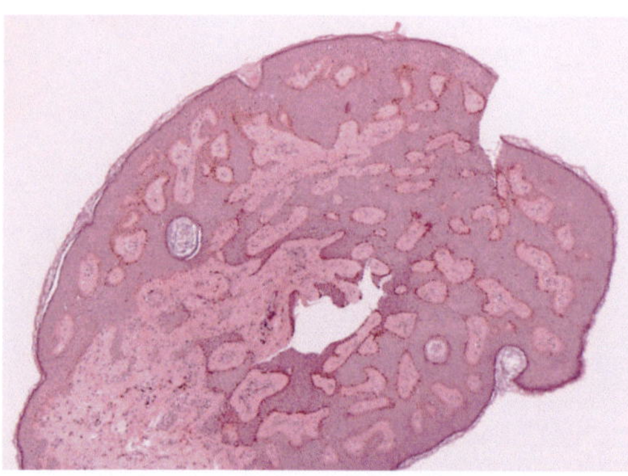

Fig. 4.56 Hyperpigmentation of the basal layer

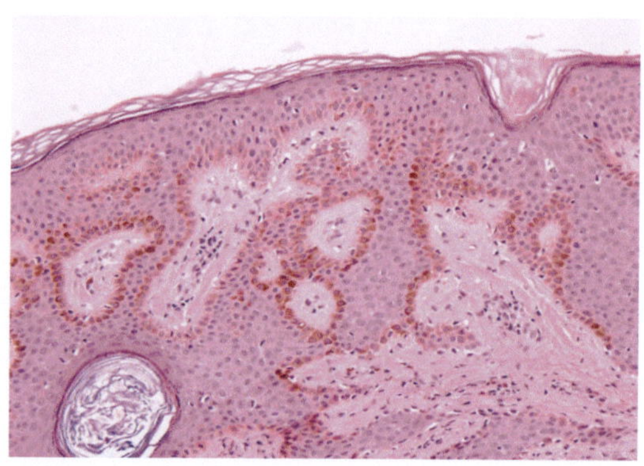

Fig. 4.57 Keratin-filled epidermal invagination (horn cyst)

Dermoid Cyst

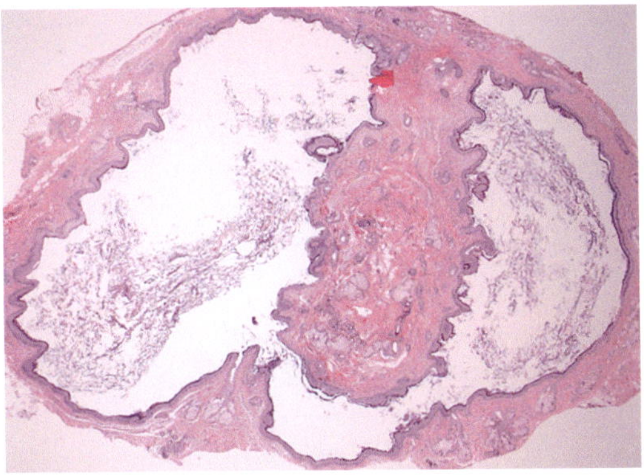

Fig. 4.58 Irregular cyst with corrugated wall

Histopathology (Figs. 4.58, 4.59, and 4.60)
- Cyst lined with stratified squamous epithelium
- Adnexal structures (such as hair follicles and sebaceous glands) are attached to the cyst wall
- Eccrine glands, apocrine glands, and pilar muscle can be present close to the wall

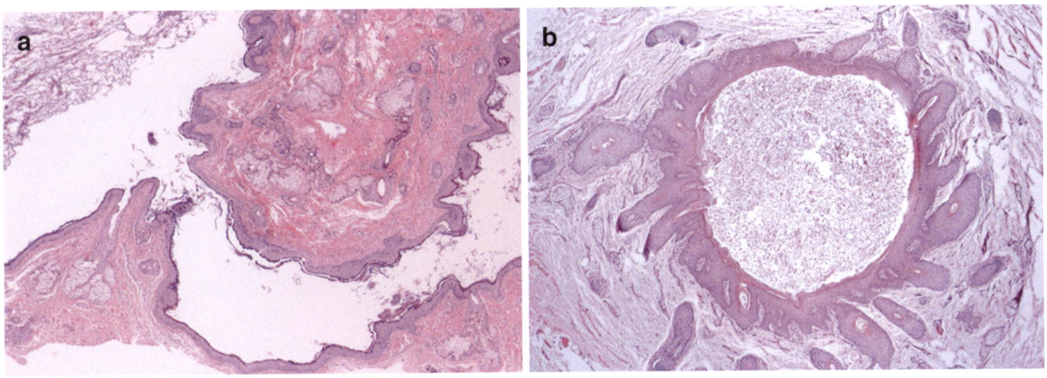

Fig. 4.59 (**a**, **b**) Cyst lined with stratified squamous epithelium and filled with keratin and sebaceous secretion

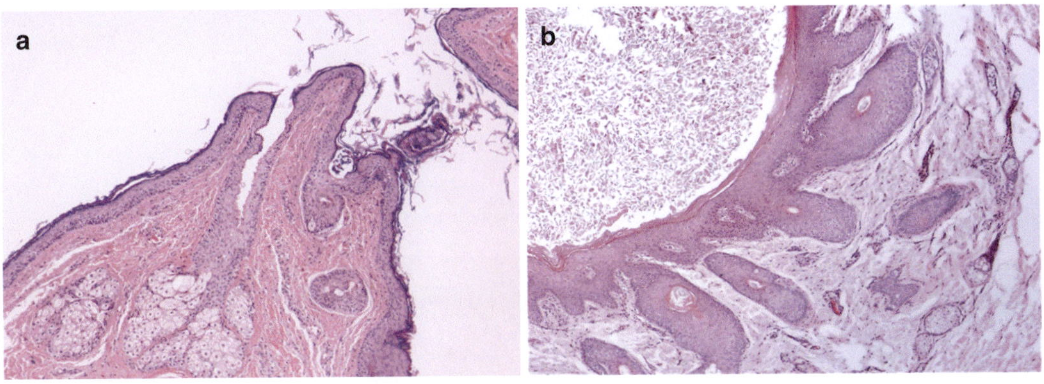

Fig. 4.60 (**a**, **b**) Pilosebaceous units attached to the cyst wall

Digital Mucous Cyst

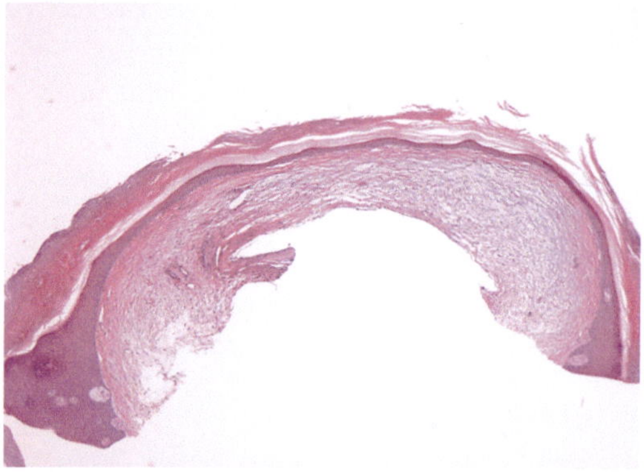

Fig. 4.61 Acral skin with atrophic epidermis and dermal mucin

Synonym: Digital Myxoid Cyst

Histopathology (Figs. 4.61, 4.62, 4.63, and 4.64)

- Acral skin with well-circumscribed dermal accumulation of mucin
- Despite the name it is a pseudocyst as there is no real epithelial lining
- Pseudowall is made of dense fibrous tissue
- There is epidermal collarette trying to embrace the mucin

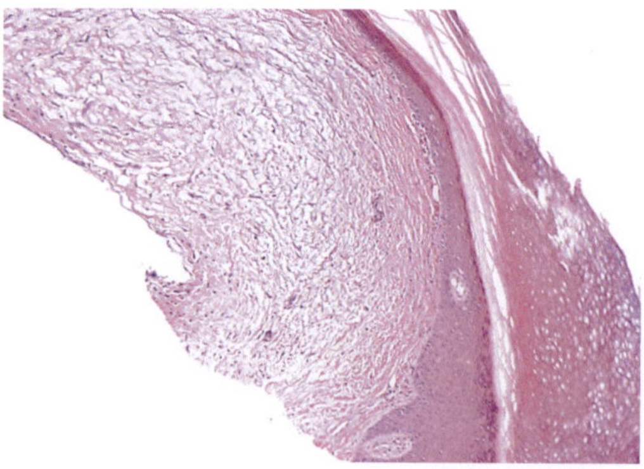

Fig. 4.62 Dense fibrous tissue encircle dermal mucin

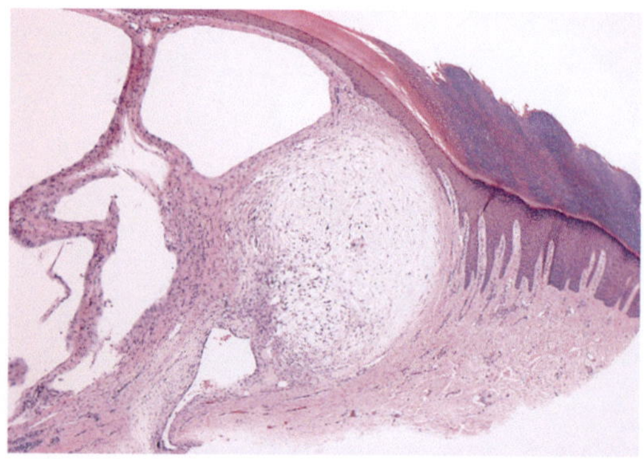

Fig. 4.63 Epidermal collarette around dermal mucin

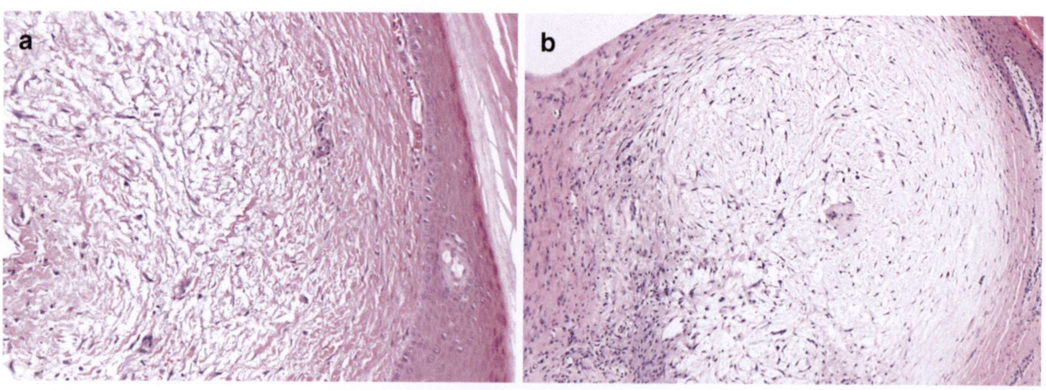

Fig. 4.64 (a, b) Scattered fibroblasts are present within a pool of mucin

Dilated Pore of Winer

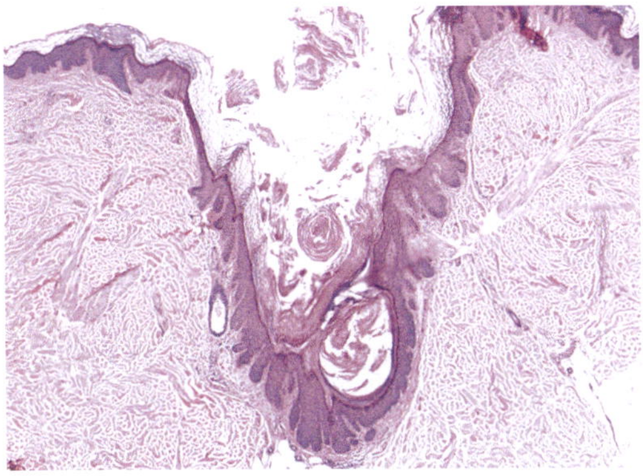

Fig. 4.65 Dilated hair follicle with keratin plugging

Histopathology (Figs. 4.65, 4.66, and 4.67)

- Dilated follicle with keratin plugging
- Acanthotic epithelium with "finger-like" budding and thick stratum corneum
- No epithelial atypia
- No inflammation

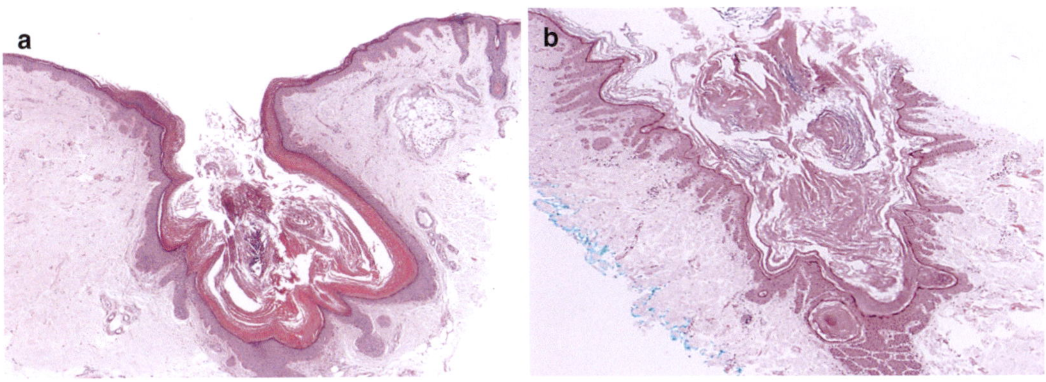

Fig. 4.66 (a, b) Dilated hair follicle lined with hyperkeratotic wavy epidermis with no atypia

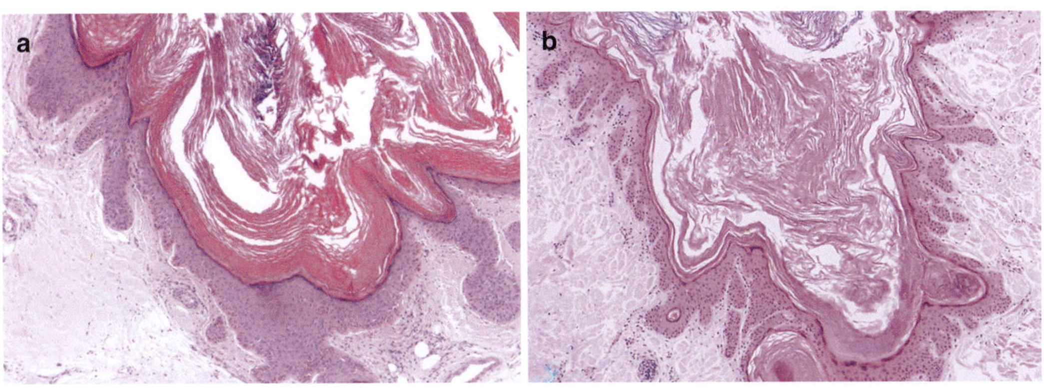

Fig. 4.67 (a, b) "Finger-like" epithelial budding from the lining of the pore

Discoid Lupus Erythematosus

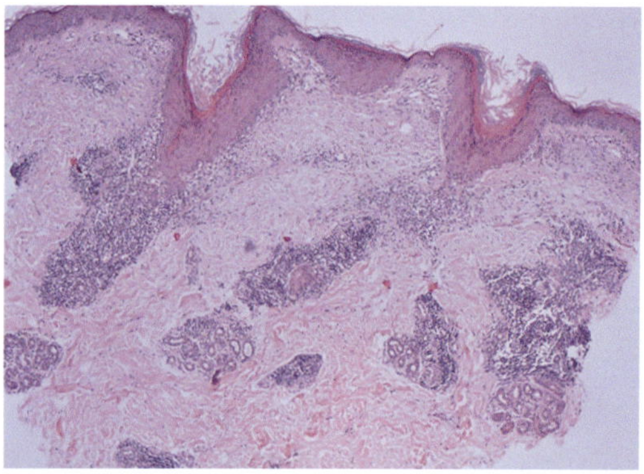

Fig. 4.68 Dilated hair follicles with follicular plugging and perifollicular and perivascular inflammation

Histopathology (Figs. 4.68, 4.69, 4.70, and 4.71)

- Atrophic epidermis with hyperkeratosis and follicular plugging
- Interface changes with vacuolar degeneration of the basal layer keratinocytes that are focally necrotic
- Dermal mucin, pigment incontinence, and thickening of the basement membrane in the older lesions
- Perifollicular and perivascular lymphocytes

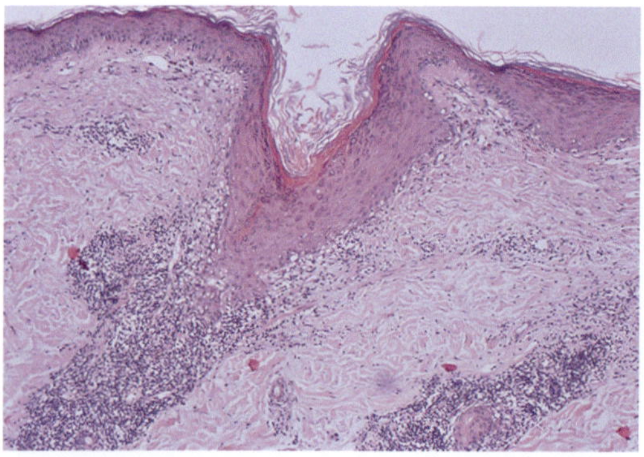

Fig. 4.69 Perifollicular and perivascular lymphocytic infiltrate

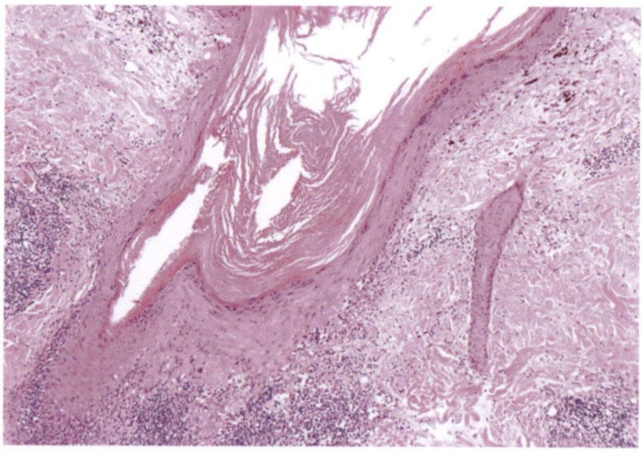

Fig. 4.70 Interface vacuolar changes and pigment incontinence

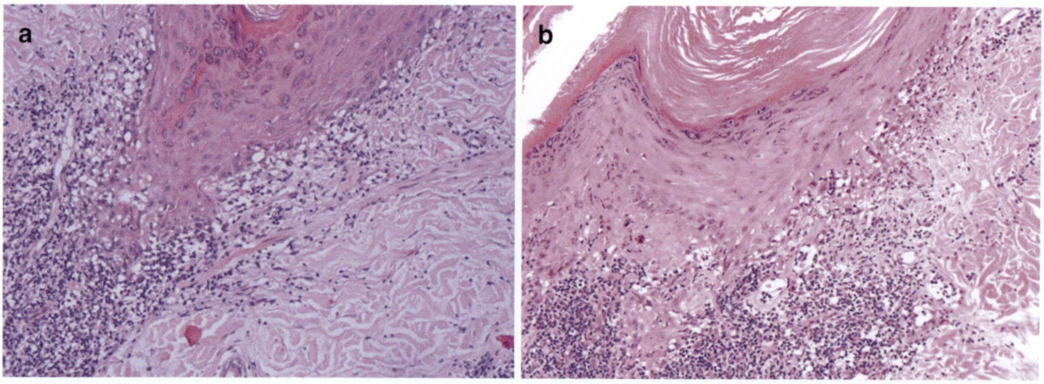

Fig. 4.71 (**a**, **b**) Perifollicular lymphocytic infiltrate with interface vacuolar changes, focal necrotic keratinocytes, and pigment incontinence

Dissecting Cellulitis

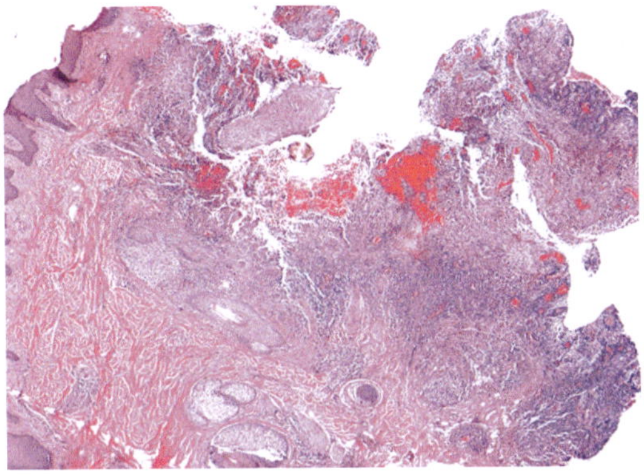

Fig. 4.72 Ruptured follicle with deep abscess formation

Histopathology (Figs. 4.72, 4.73, and 4.74)
- Neutrophilic folliculitis
- Destroyed hair follicle
- Dermal/subcutaneous abscess with sinus formation
- Hair fragments within the abscess

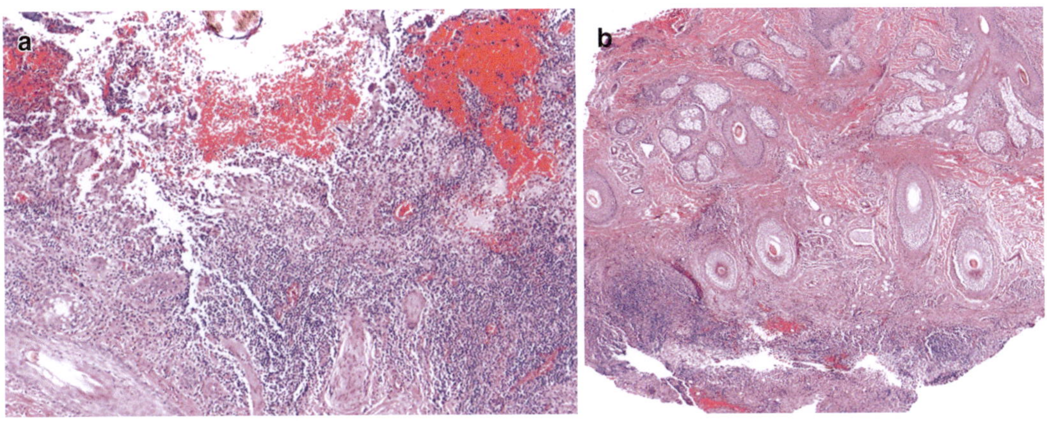

Fig. 4.73 (**a**, **b**) Follicle is completely destroyed and neutrophilic aggregates form large abscess

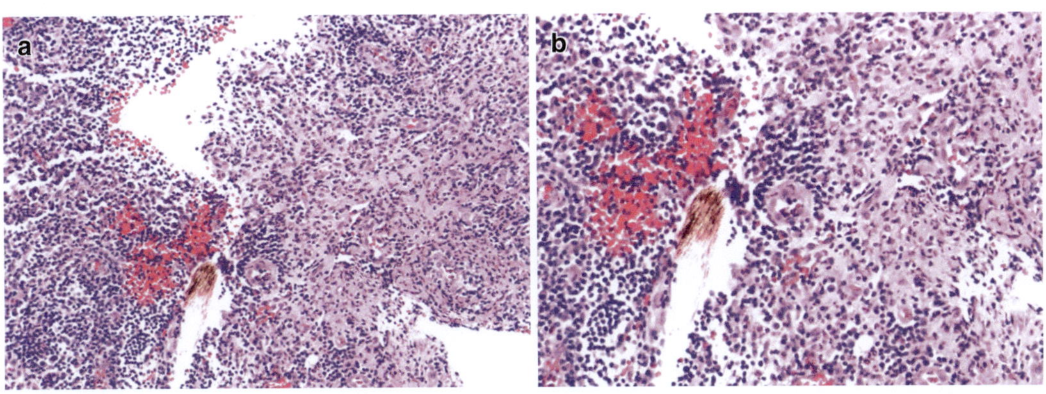

Fig. 4.74 (**a**, **b**) Pigmented hair shaft fragment is present within the abscess

Dowling Degos Disease

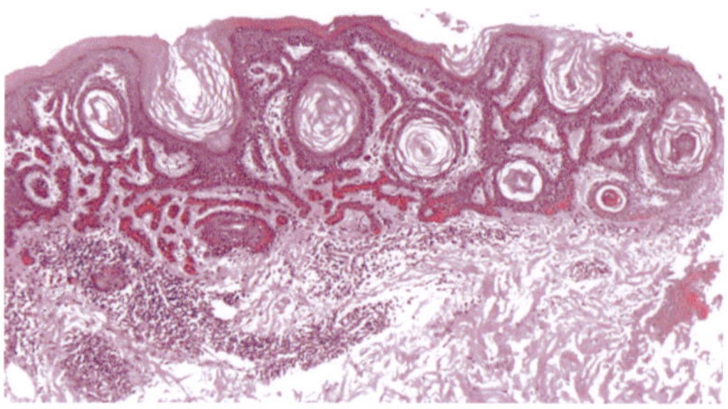

Fig. 4.75 Downgrowth of interconnected rete ridges

Synonym: Reticulate Pigmented Anomaly of the Flexures

Histopathology is similar to adenoid seborrheic keratosis (Figs. 4.75, 4.76, 4.77, 4.78, and 4.79) and clinical correlation is necessary

- Downgrowth of the epidermis in the retiform interconnected pattern
- Horn cysts and "comedo-like" structures are present
- Hyperpigmentation at the tips of the rete ridges

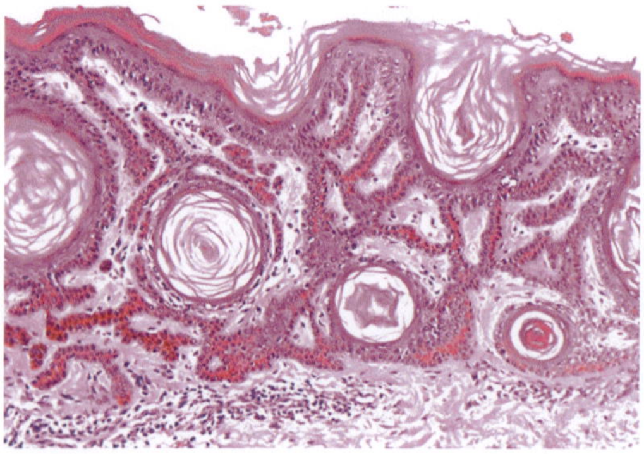

Fig. 4.76 Horn cysts and "comedo-like" structures are present

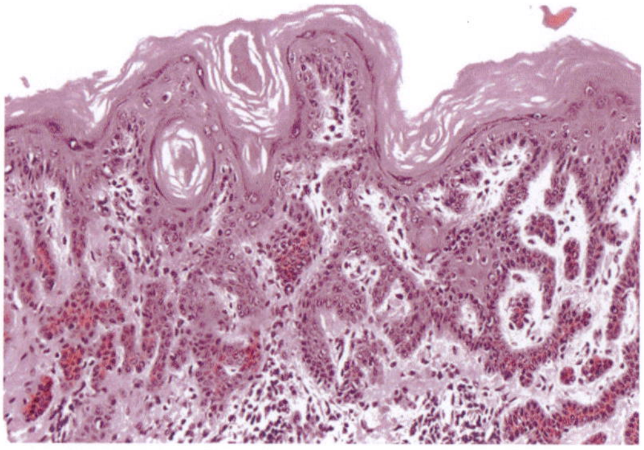

Fig. 4.77 Tips of rete ridges are hyperpigmented

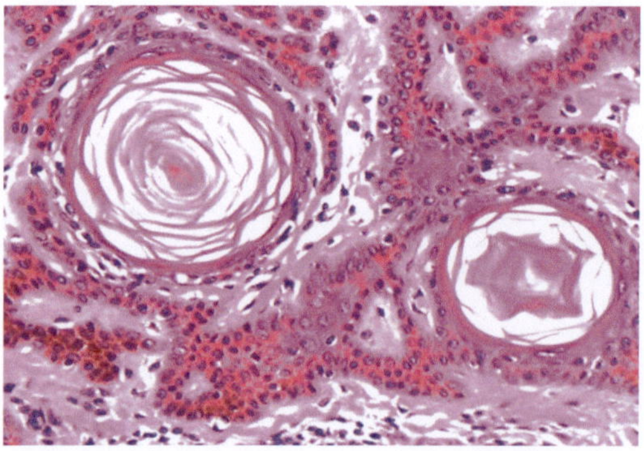

Fig. 4.78 Rete ridges are two to three cells thick

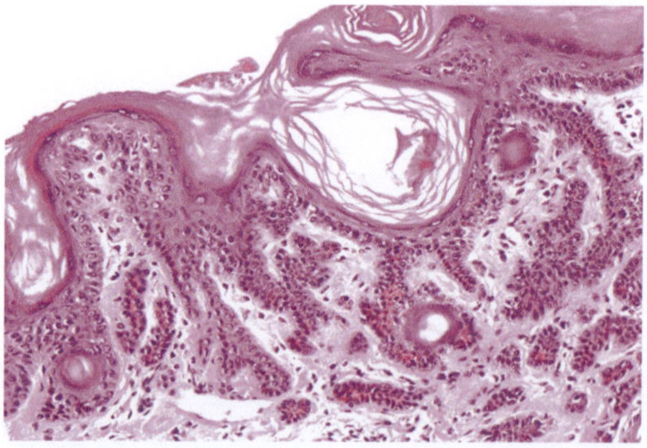

Fig. 4.79 There is no evidence of epithelial atypia

Drug Reaction

Histopathology of drug reaction can resemble any inflammatory disease with an addition of eosinophils:

Bullous reaction: appears as linear IgA disease with subepidermal blister with neutrophils and occasional eosinophils or as pemphigus with intraepidermal vesicle

Exanthematous reaction (the most common): spongiotic dermatitis with perivascular lymphocytic infiltrate and perivascular and interstitial eosinophils (Figs. 4.80 and 4.81)

Erythema Multiforme-like: interface dermatitis with scattered necrotic keratinocytes and dermal eosinophils (Fig. 4.82)

Erythema Annular Centrifugum-like: tightly cuffed perivascular lymphocytes with scattered eosinophils (Fig. 4.83)

Granulomatous reaction: granuloma annulare-like appearance with eosinophils

Lichenoid reaction: lichenoid dermatitis with conspicuous eosinophils (Fig. 4.84)

Photoallergic and phototoxic: appears as allergic or irritant contact dermatitis with necrotic keratinocytes in the upper part of the epidermis

Pseudolymphoma reaction: dense lymphocytic infiltrate with eosinophils

Psoriasiform reaction: psoriasiform dermatitis with eosinophils (Fig. 4.85)

Pustular reaction: presents as acute generalized exanthematous pustulosis (Fig. 4.86)

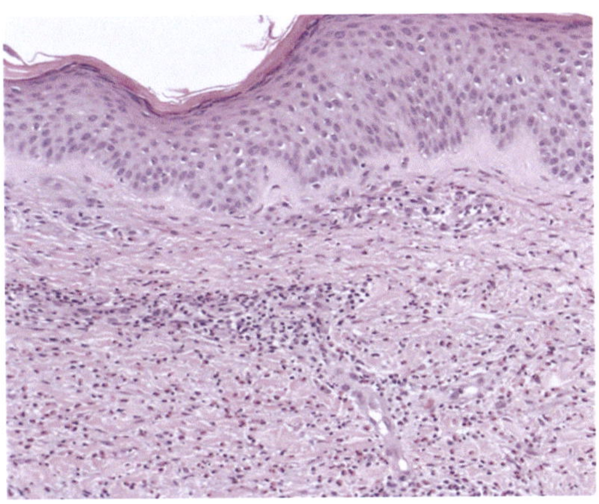

Fig. 4.80 **Exanthematous** drug reaction with mild spongiosis

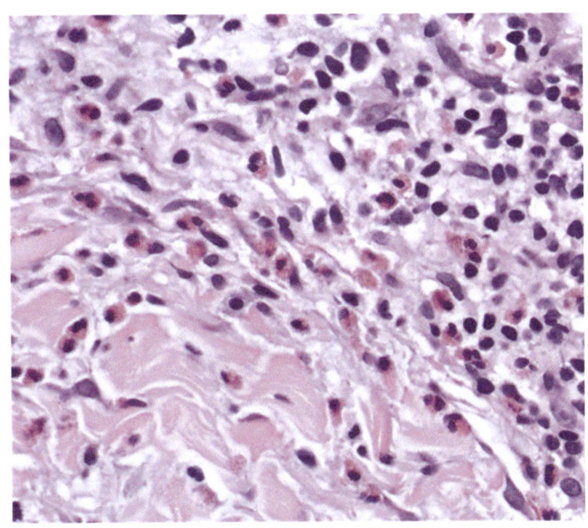

Fig. 4.81 Dermal perivascular lymphocytic inflammation with perivascular and interstitial eosinophils

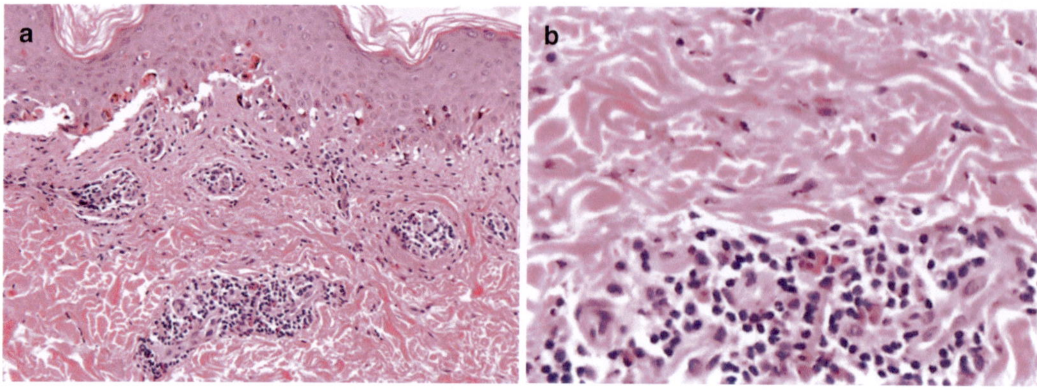

Fig. 4.82 (**a**, **b**) **Erythema multiforme-like** drug reaction with necrotic keratinocytes and perivascular lymphocytes and few eosinophils

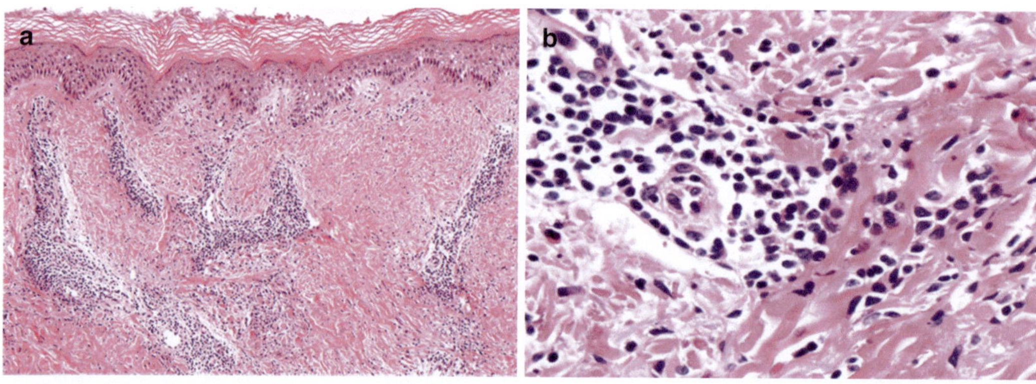

Fig. 4.83 (**a**, **b**) **Erythema annulare centrifugum-like** drug reaction with tightly cuffed perivascular lymphocytes and few eosinophils

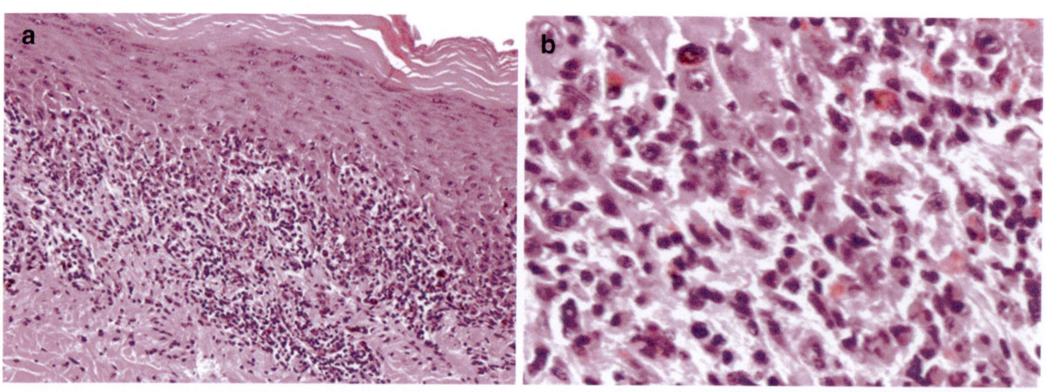

Fig. 4.84 (**a**, **b**) **Lichen planus-like** drug reaction with wedge shaped epidermis, apoptotic keratinocytes and lichenoid lymphocytic infiltrate with eosinophils

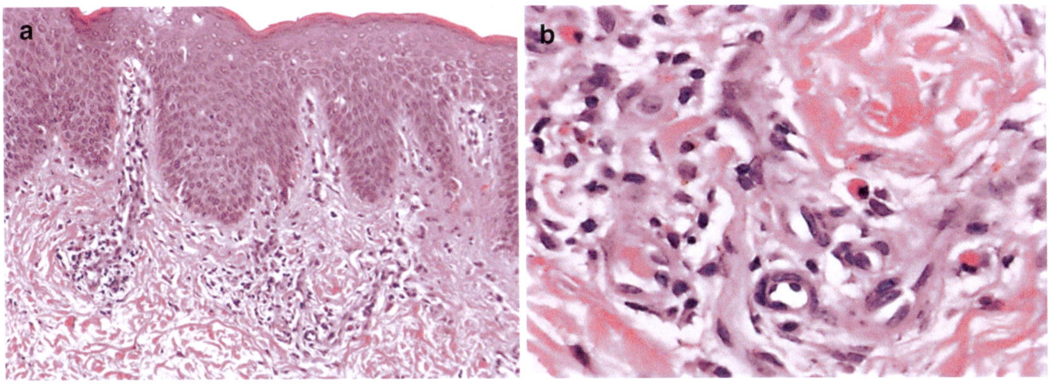

Fig. 4.85 (**a**, **b**) **Psoriasiform drug reaction** with wavy psoriasiform epidermis and dermal lymphocytic inflammation with eosinophils

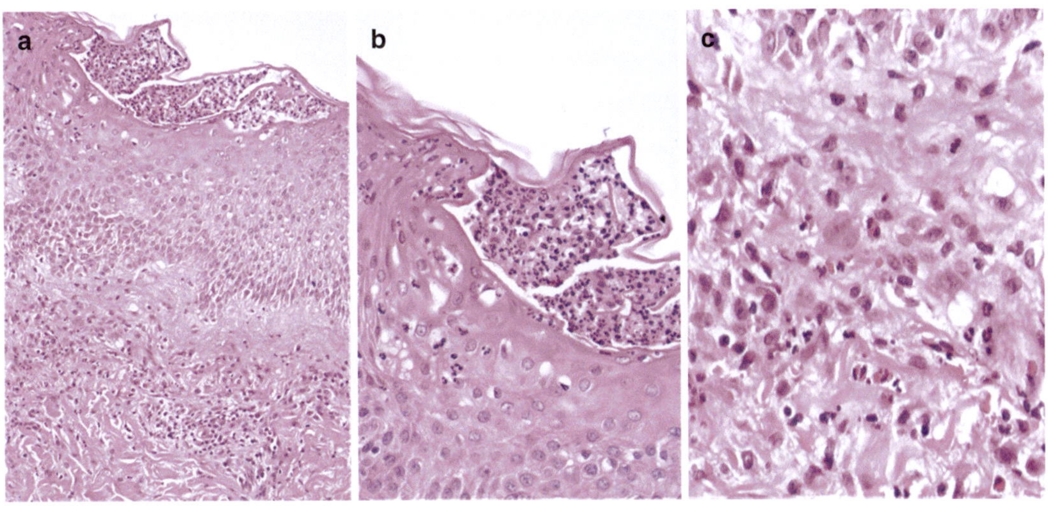

Fig. 4.86 (**a**–**c**) **Pustular drug reaction** with intracorneal neutrophilic pustules and dermal mixed inflammation with eosinophils

Ductal Eccrine Adenocarcinoma

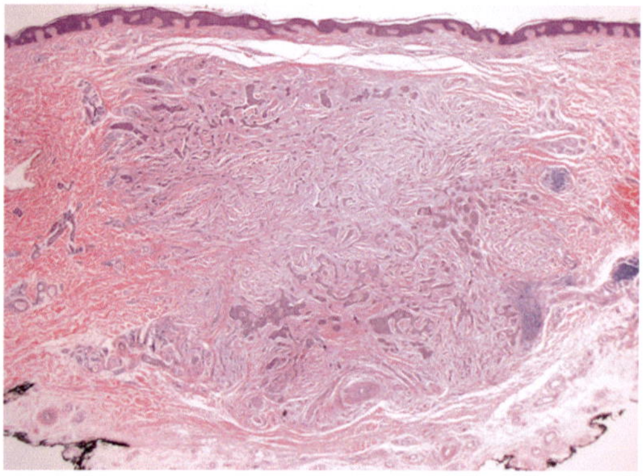

Fig. 4.87 Infiltrating dermal and subcutaneous tumor

Histopathology is identical to *invasive carcinoma of the breast* (Figs. 4.87, 4.88, 4.89, 4.90, and 4.91) and therefore clinical correlation is necessary:

- Infiltrating dermal and subcutaneous tumor
- Infiltrating dermal tubules, strands, and ducts
- Cytological atypia
- Variable desmoplastic stroma

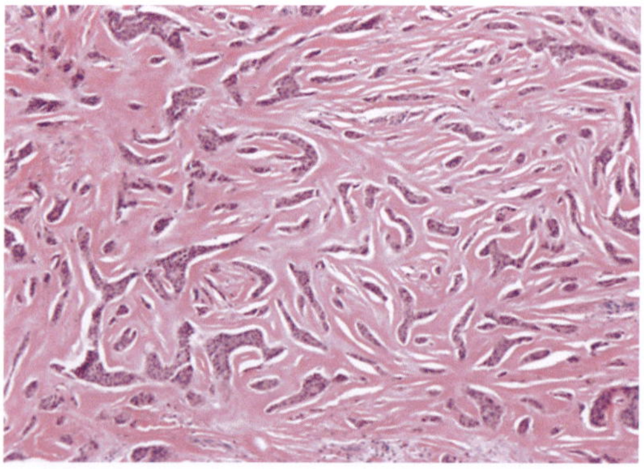

Fig. 4.88 Tumor strands infiltrating subcutis

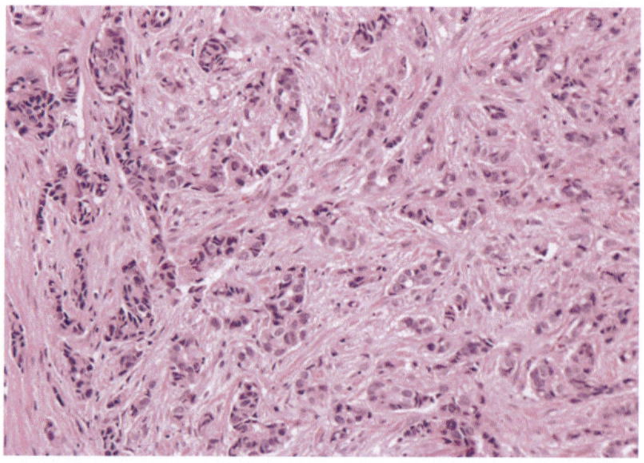

Fig. 4.89 Infiltrating ducts lined with atypical epithelioid cells

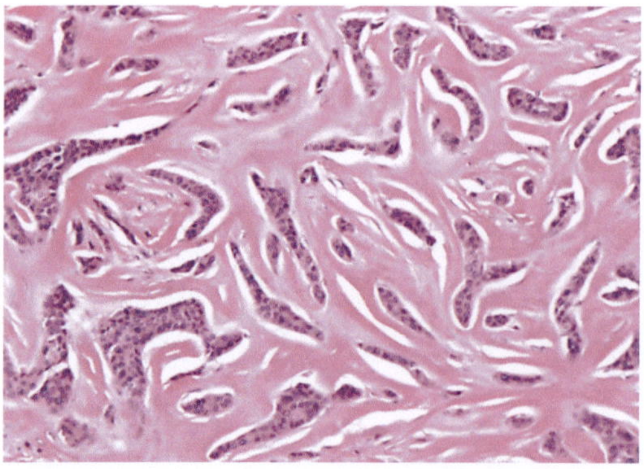

Fig. 4.90 Tumor cells embedded in desmoplastic stroma

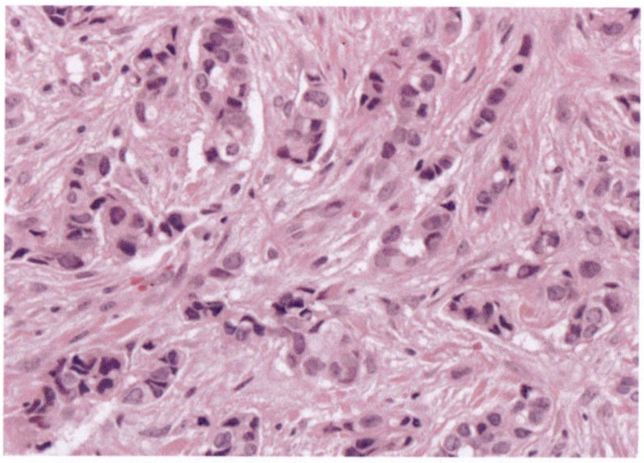

Fig. 4.91 Numerous necrotic cells and scattered mitoses

Dyshidrotic Dermatitis

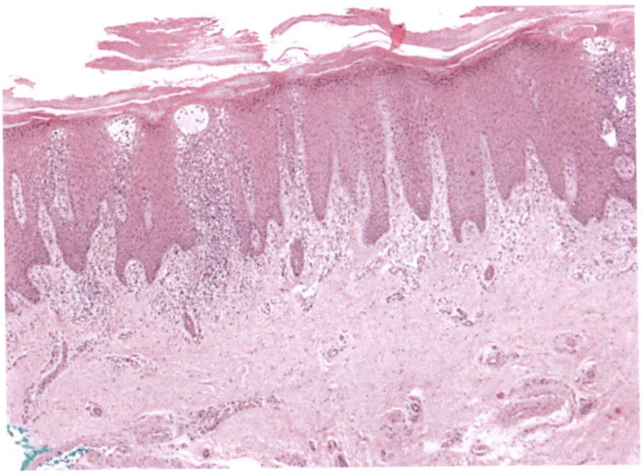

Fig. 4.92 Acral skin with epidermal vesicles

Synonyms: Acral Vesicular Dermatitis, Pompholyx

Histopathology (Figs. 4.92, 4.93, and 4.94)

- Thick stratum corneum consistent with acral skin
- Epidermal spongiosis with intraepidermal vesicles
- Vesicles contain lymphocytes and occasionally few neutrophils
- Mild to moderate perivascular lymphocytic infiltrate

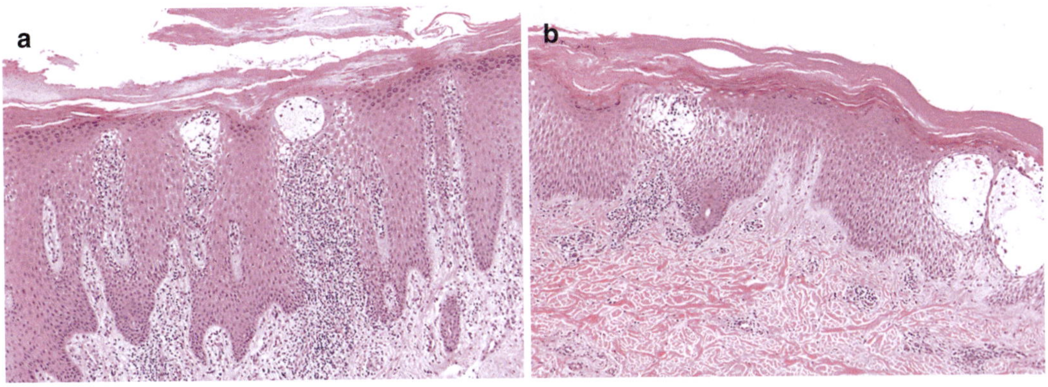

Fig. 4.93 (**a**, **b**) Acral skin with thick stratum corneum; epidermis demonstrates irregular acanthosis, papillomatosis, spongiosis and intraepidermal vesicles

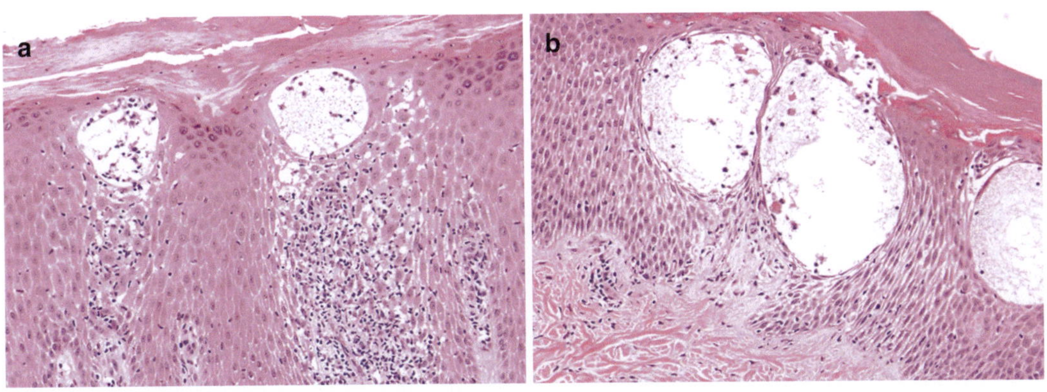

Fig. 4.94 (**a**, **b**) Sparse lymphocytes are in the vesicles and dermal lymphocytic inflammation is present

Dysplastic Nevus

Synonyms: Atypical Nevus, Clark's Nevus

Histopathology (Figs. 4.95, 4.96, and 4.97)

- Lentiginous epidermal hyperplasia with nevus cells present in nests and as single cells along the junction
- Nests of various sizes and shapes with bridging between nests
- If the nevus is compound, junctional component extends beyond the dermal part, so called "shoulder" phenomenon

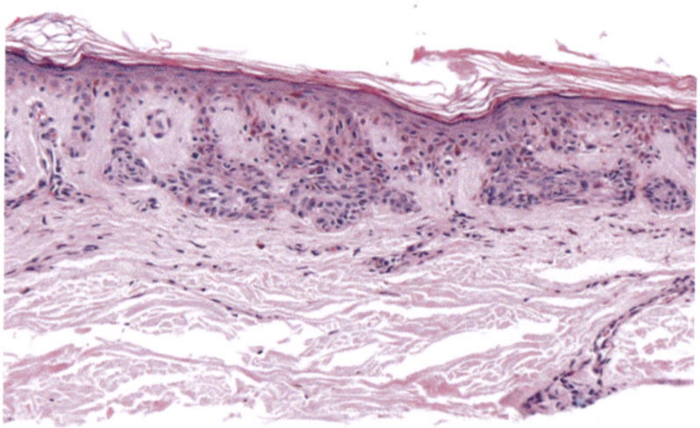

Fig. 4.95 Irregular melanocytic nests with the "bridging"

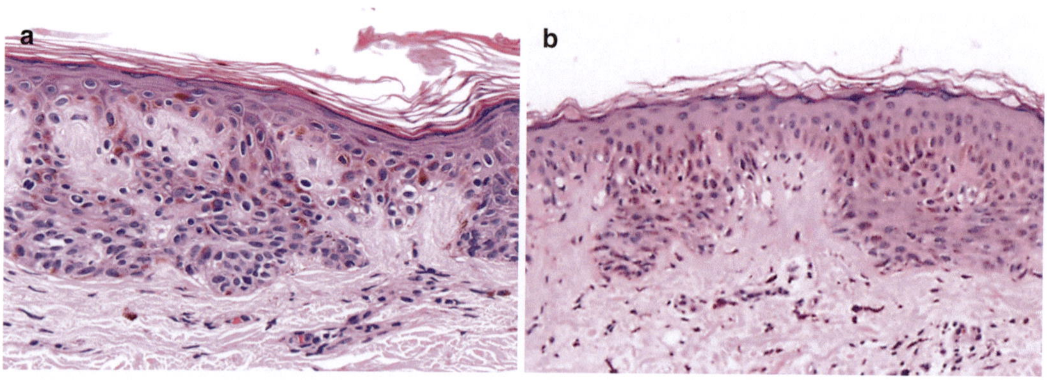

Fig. 4.96 (**a**, **b**) Melanocytic cells demonstrate variable cytological atypia with increased nuclear size, nuclear pleomorphism, prominent nucleoli, and abundant cytoplasm; level of dysplasia depends on the extent of these changes

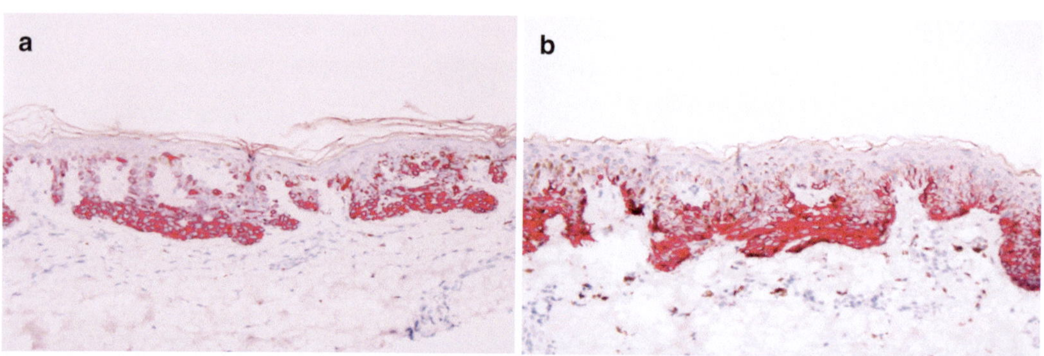

Fig. 4.97 (**a**, **b**) MART-1 stain demonstrates architectural atypia characterized by melanocytic bridging and individual single nevus cells with focal pagetoid nevus cells

5 Dermatopathology E

V. Vincek, *Dermatopathology A–Z*, https://doi.org/10.1007/978-3-319-89486-7_5

Ecthyma

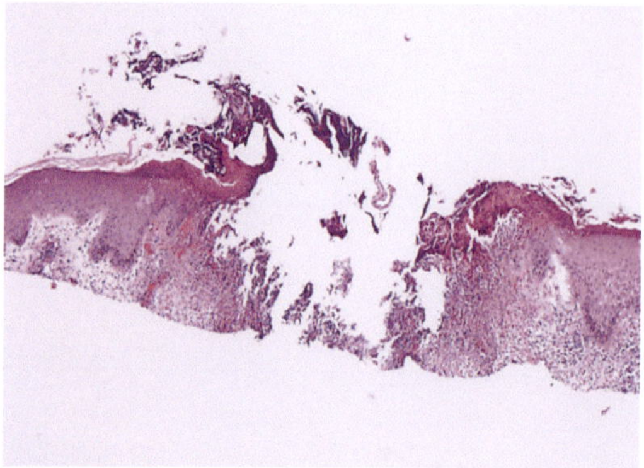

Fig. 5.1 Ulcerated inflamed epidermis

Histopathology (Figs. 5.1, 5.2, 5.3, 5.4, and 5.5)

- Ulcerated skin
- Acutely inflamed serum crust
- Heavy neutrophilic infiltrate in the dermis
- Gram positive bacterial colonies are present

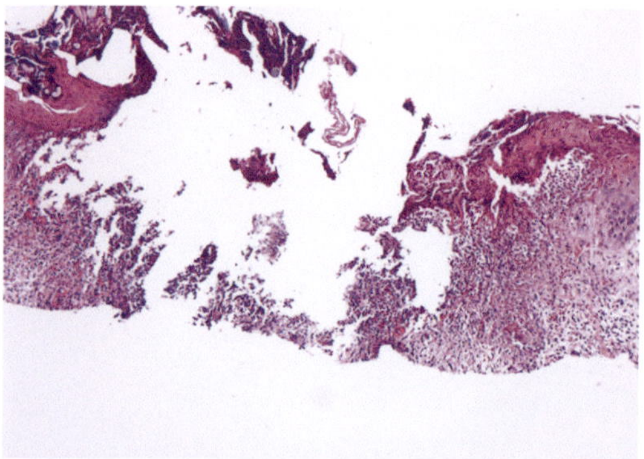

Fig. 5.2 Ulceration covered with serum crust

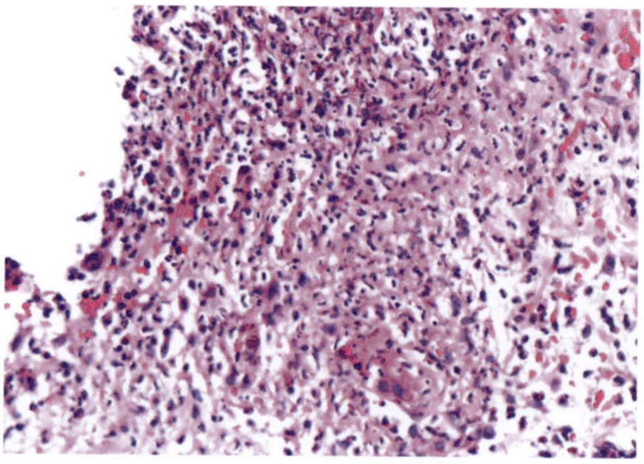

Fig. 5.3 Neutrophilic infiltrate in the dermis

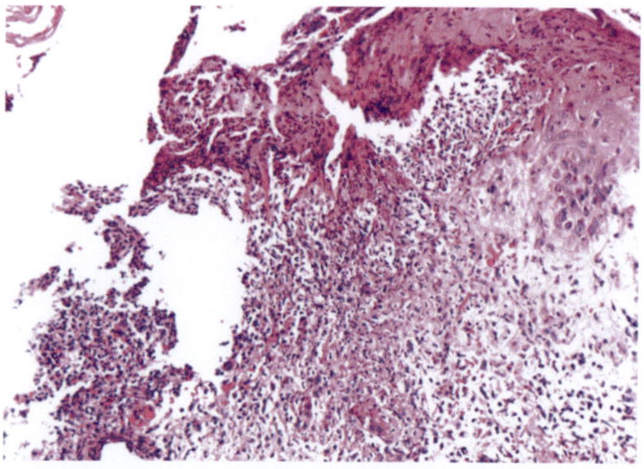

Fig. 5.4 Serum crust with numerous neutrophils

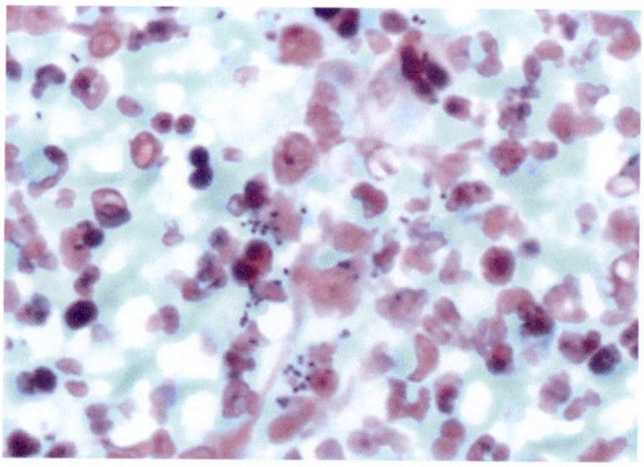

Fig. 5.5 Gram stain detects gram positive bacteria

Ecthyma Gangrenosum

Histopathology (Figs. 5.6, 5.7, and 5.8)

- Necrotic epidermis, dermis, and subcutis
- Lymphocytic and neutrophilic inflammation
- Hemorrhage is commonly present
- Special stains detect *Pseudomonas aeruginosa*
- Bacterial colonies mostly present in necrotic areas and wall of blood vessels
- Necrotizing vasculitis with thrombosis is common

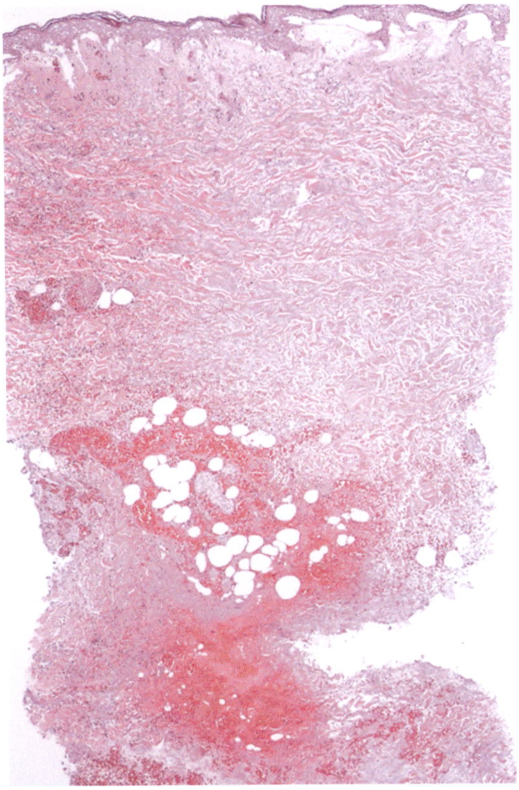

Fig. 5.6 Diffuse superficial and deep necrosis with extensive hemorrhage

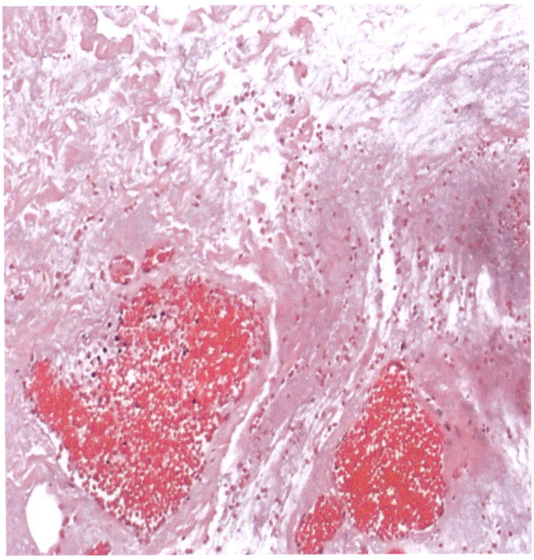

Fig. 5.7 Congested blood vessels with necrotic wall

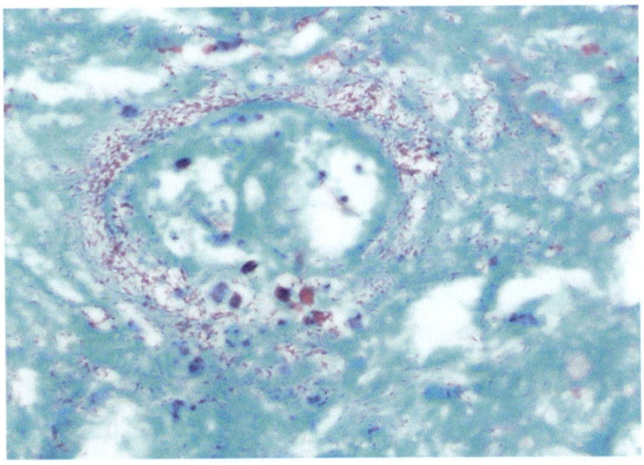

Fig. 5.8 Gram stain detects bacteria in and around the wall of blood vessel

Elastofibroma

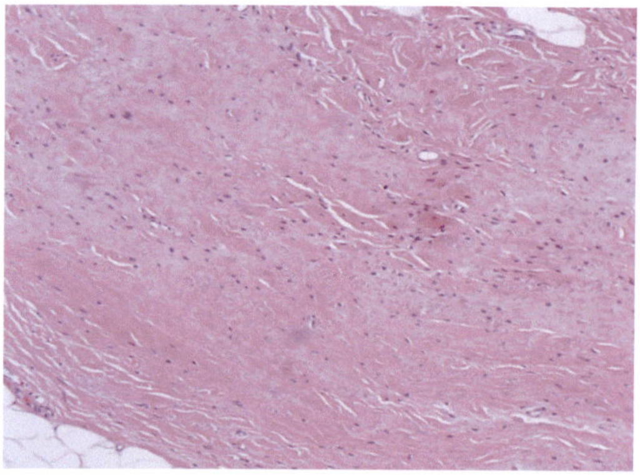

Fig. 5.9 Deep ill-defined eosinophilic tumor

Histopathology (Figs. 5.9, 5.10, 5.11, 5.12, and 5.13)

- Ill-defined lesion
- Usually adherent to underlying periosteum
- Hyalinized collagen admixed with increased number of "beaded" coarse elastic fibers
- Thickened, serrated "pipe cleaner" like elastic fibers
- Xq12-q22 or #19 gains in 30% cases

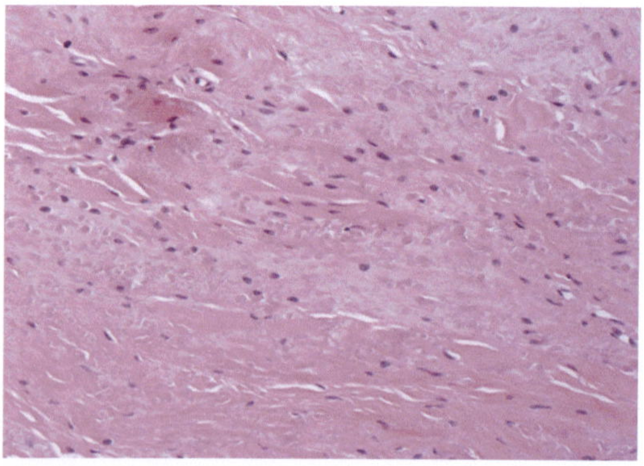

Fig. 5.10 Increased number of elastic fibers

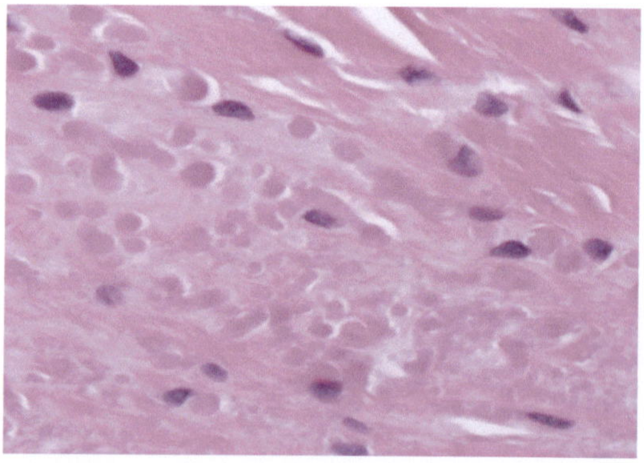

Fig. 5.11 Fragmented elastic fragments in "beaded" pattern

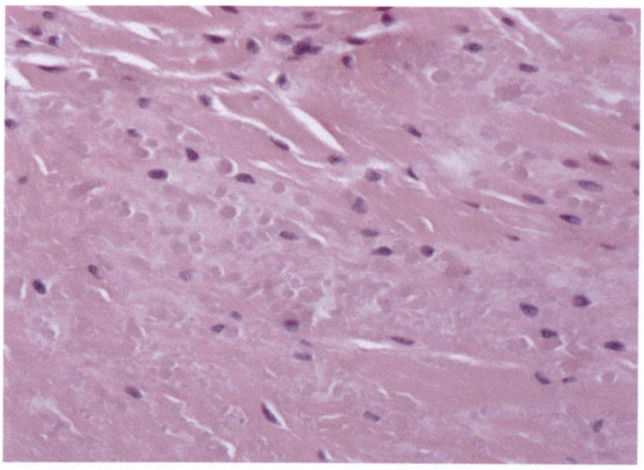

Fig. 5.12 Elastic fibers admixed with hyalinized collagen

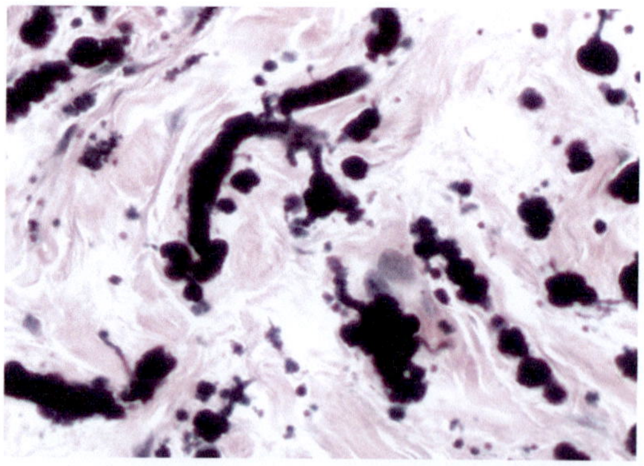

Fig. 5.13 Increased number of elastic fibers many of which have beaded "pipe cleaner" appearance (VVG)

Elastoma

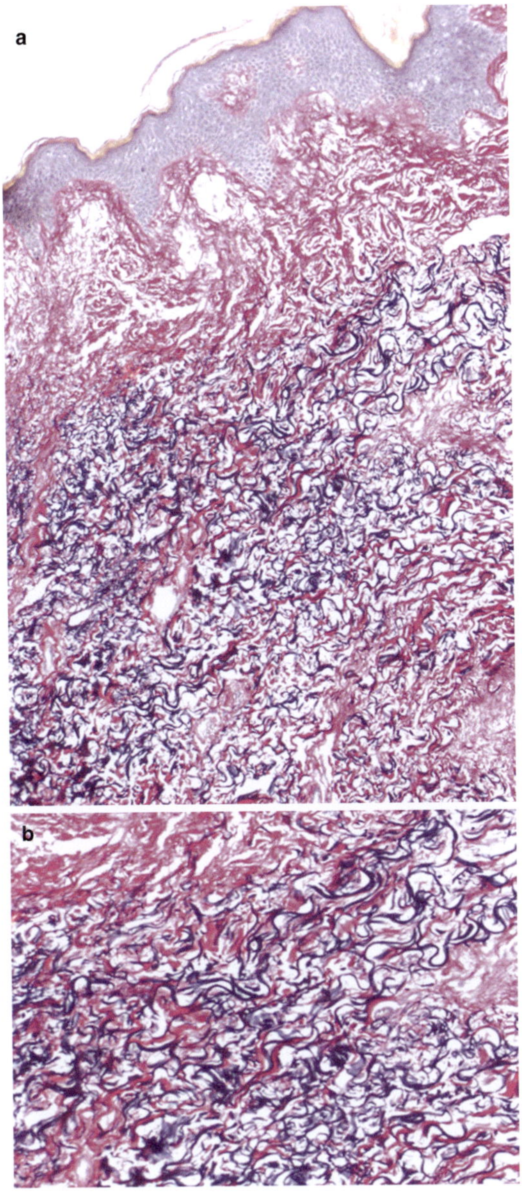

Fig. 5.14 (a, b) Verhoeff-Van Gieson (VVG) elastin stain highlights an increased number of dermal elastic fibers

Synonyms: Nevus Elasticus, Elastic Connective Tissue Nevus

Histopathology (Figs. 5.14 and 5.15)

- Usually normal appearing dermis on H&E stain
- Elastic special stain shows accumulation of branching, interlacing elastic fibers

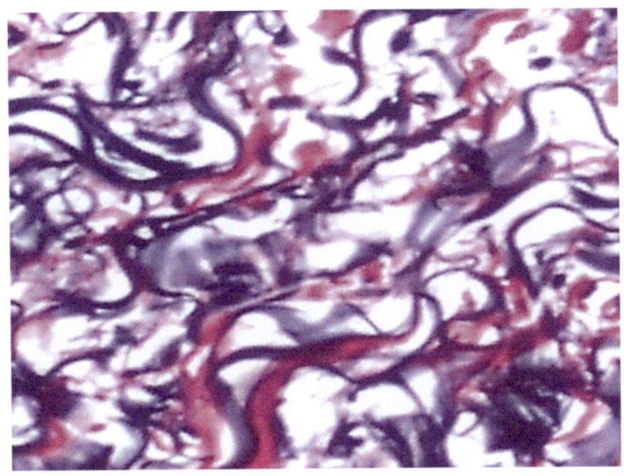

Fig. 5.15 Branching, interlacing elastic fibers (VVG)

Elastosis Perforans Serpiginosa

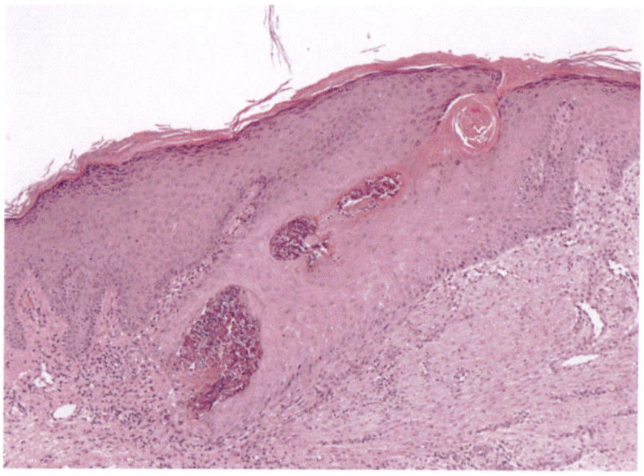

Fig. 5.16 Hyperplastic epidermis with the central channel filled with keratin in the upper portion

Histopathology (Figs. 5.16, 5.17, 5.18, and 5.19)

- Epidermal hyperplasia with epidermal channel through which elastic fibers are eliminated
- Superficial part of the channel is filled with keratin
- The lower portion of the channel is filled with degenerated elastic fibers and inflammatory cells

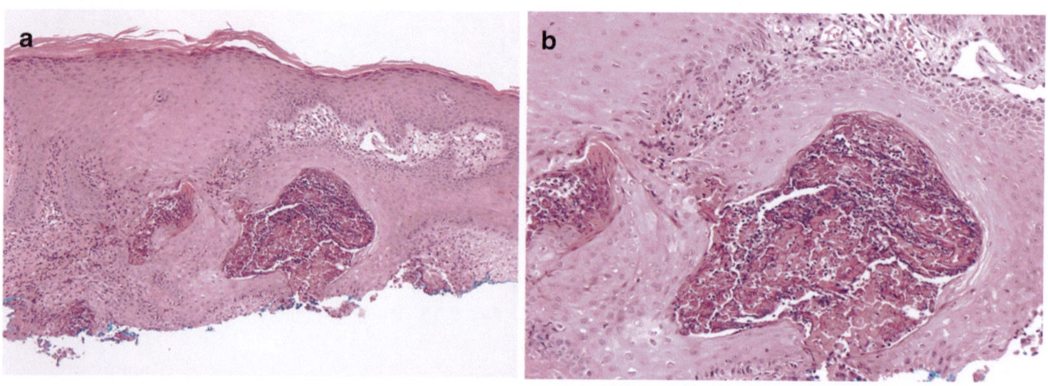

Fig. 5.17 (**a**, **b**) The lower portion of the channel is filled with degenerated elastic fibers

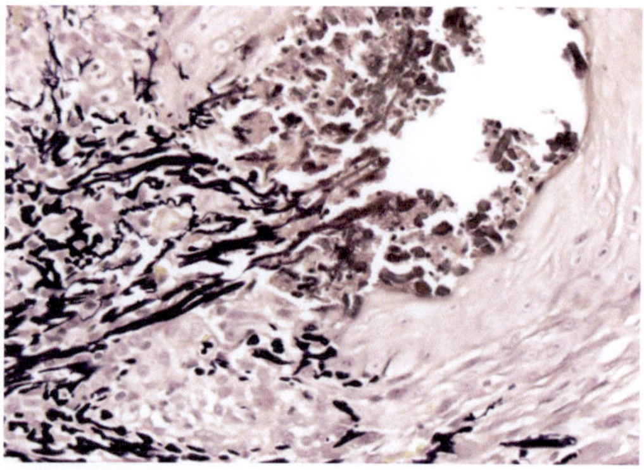

Fig. 5.18 VVG stain outlines elastic fibers

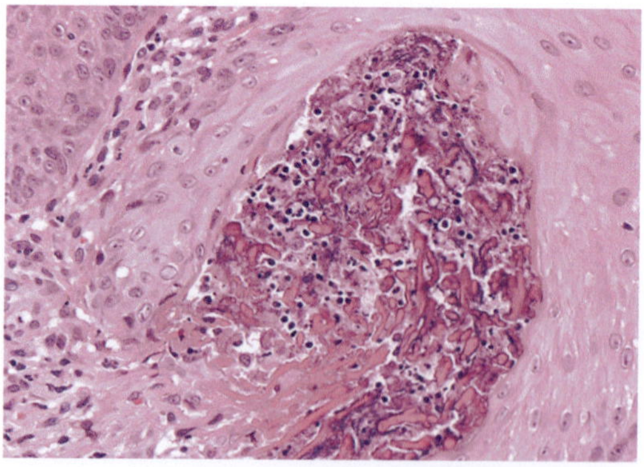

Fig. 5.19 Inflammatory cells are admixed with elastic fibers

Electrocautery/Electrodessication Artifact

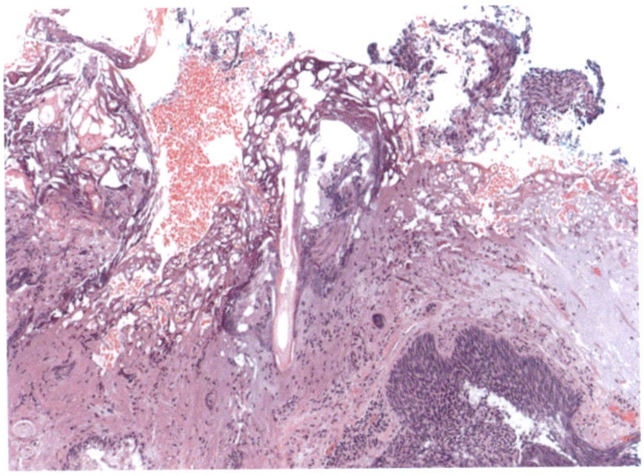

Fig. 5.20 Necrotic appearing tissue

Histopathology (Figs. 5.20, 5.21, 5.22, and 5.23)

- Severe artifact leads to coagulative "smudgy" tissue necrosis
- Milder artifact leads to elongation of cell nuclei and increased eosinophilic cytoplasm

P.S. dehydration after electrocautery can also cause cytoplasmic vacuolization

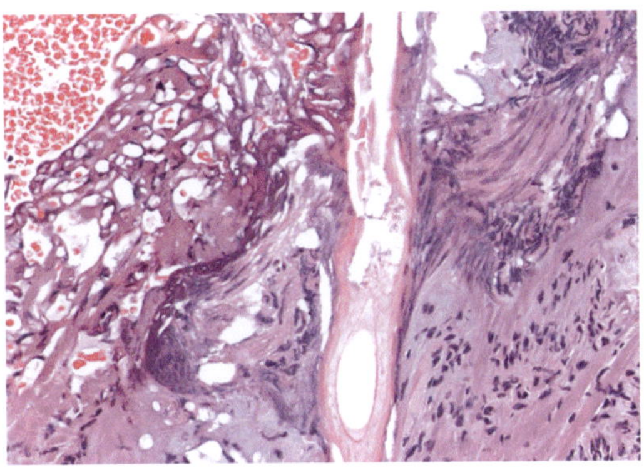

Fig. 5.21 Smudgy dermal necrosis

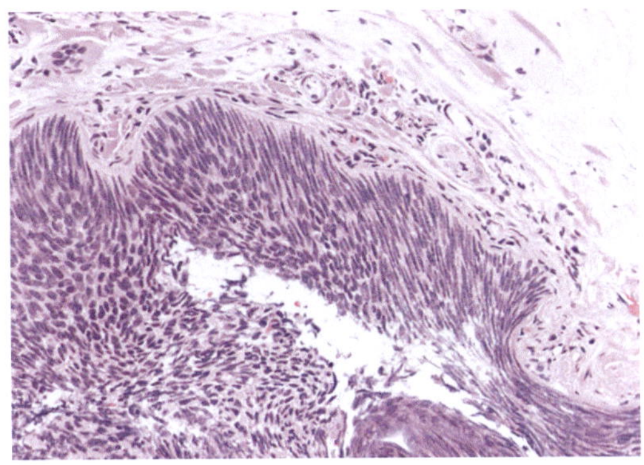

Fig. 5.22 Spindle elongation of keratinocytes

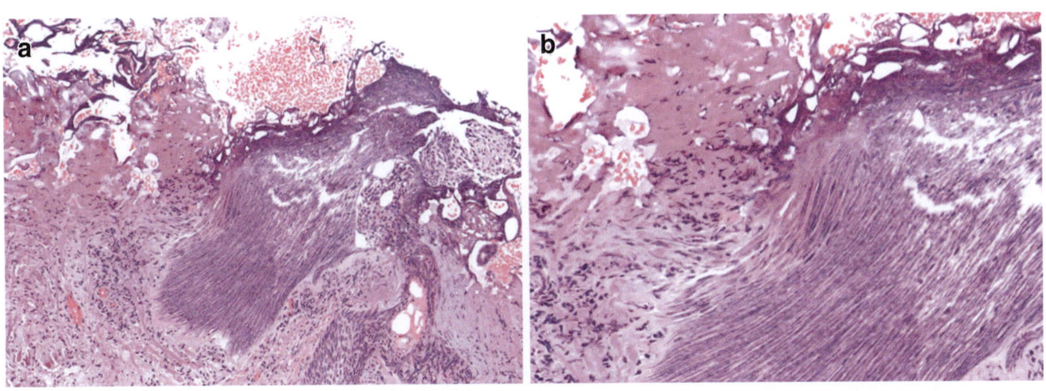

Fig. 5.23 (**a**, **b**) Necrosis of dermis with "pencil-like" distortion of keratinocytes

Encapsulated and Palisaded Neuroma

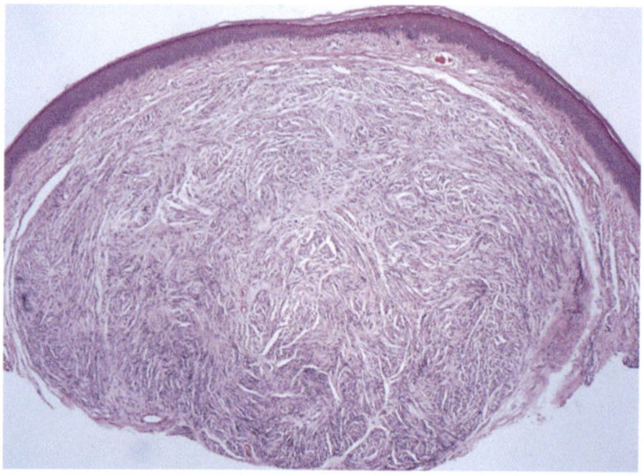

Fig. 5.24 Well-circumscribed dermal nodule

Synonyms: Solitary Encapsulated Neuroma, Palisaded Encapsulated Neuroma

Histopathology (Figs. 5.24, 5.25, 5.26, 5.27, and 5.28)

- Well-circumscribed dermal nodule
- Despite the name it is not encapsulated; instead pseudocapsule is present
- Made of fascicles of spindle cells (S-100+) resembling the endoneurium
- Vague palisading is present

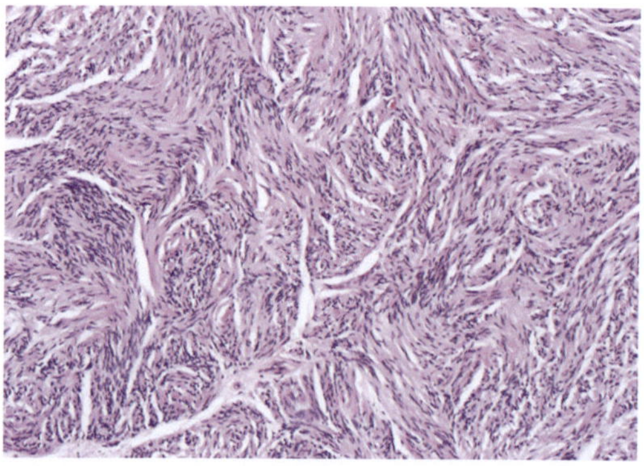

Fig. 5.25 Elongated spindle cells are forming fascicles

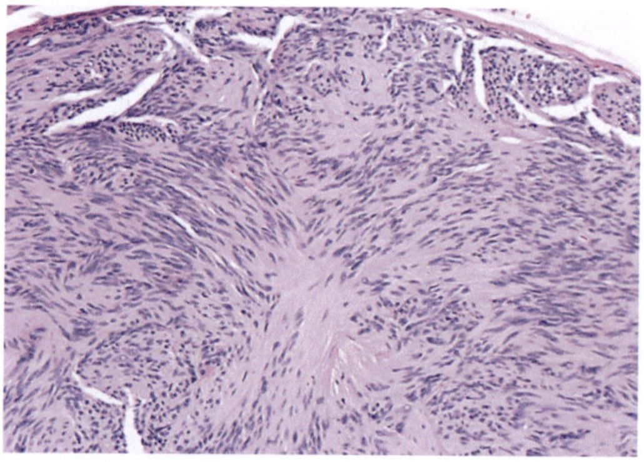

Fig. 5.26 Hyalinized stroma separates fascicles

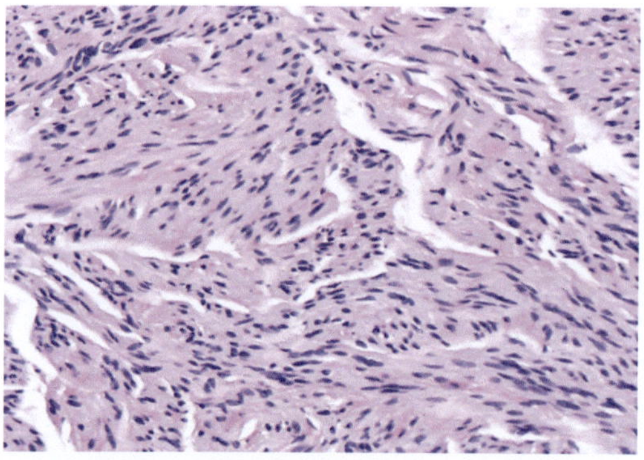

Fig. 5.27 Wavy nuclei with no evidence of atypia or mitoses

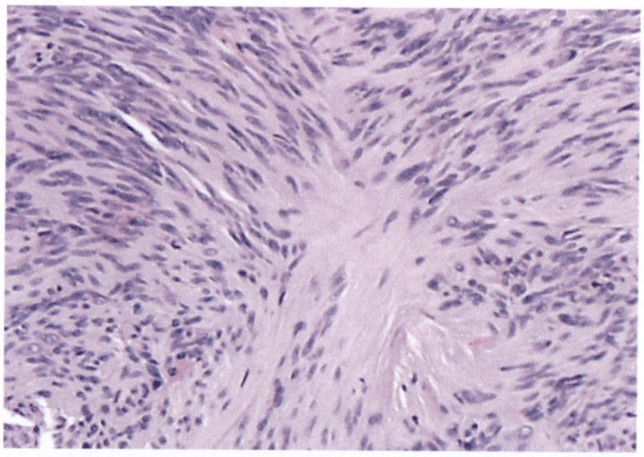

Fig. 5.28 Vague palisading of nuclei is present

Endometriosis

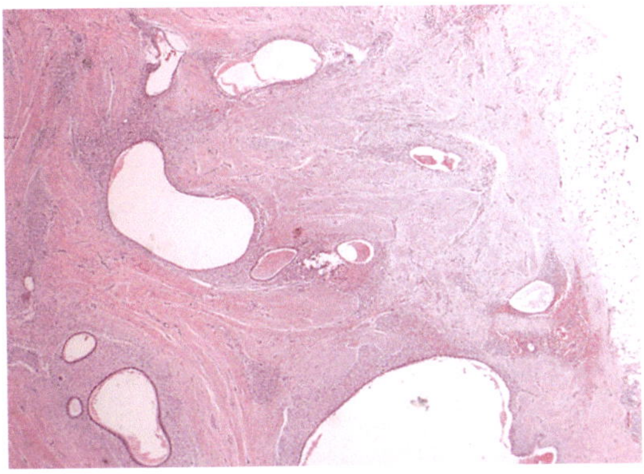

Fig. 5.29 Multiple cystically dilated glands

Histopathology (Figs. 5.29, 5.30, 5.31, 5.32, and 5.33)

- Endometrial glands (CK7+, ER+, PR+) embedded in deep subcutis
- Gland lining changes as glands show cyclical changes of endometrium
- Glands are functional so there are frequently red blood cells in the lumen and stroma
- Uterine like stroma (CD10+) surrounds glands and decidualization can be present
- Hemosiderin is commonly present in the stroma

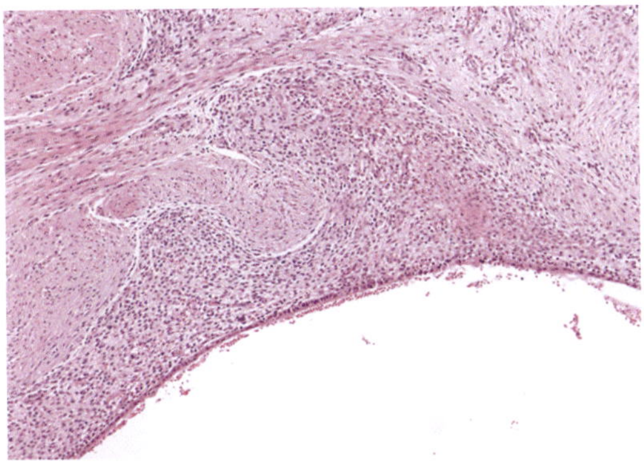

Fig. 5.30 Endometrial gland lined with columnar cells

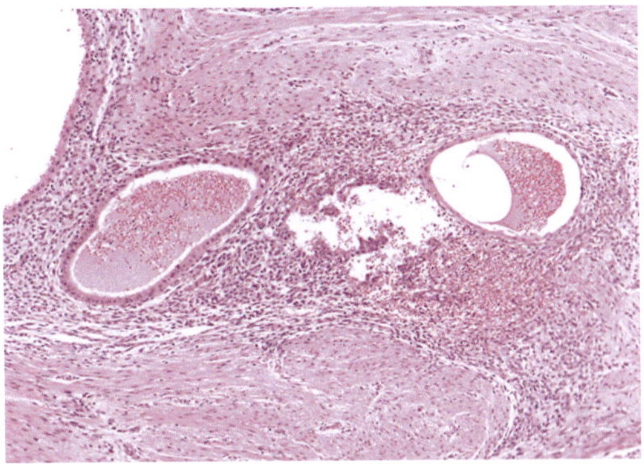

Fig. 5.31 Erythrocytes fill the glands

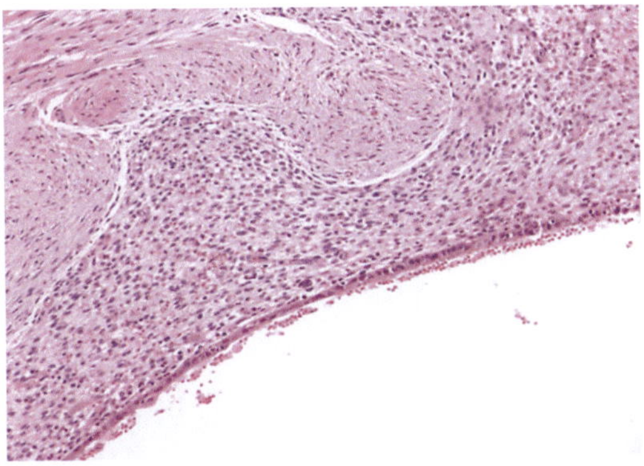

Fig. 5.32 Plump spindle stromal cells surround gland

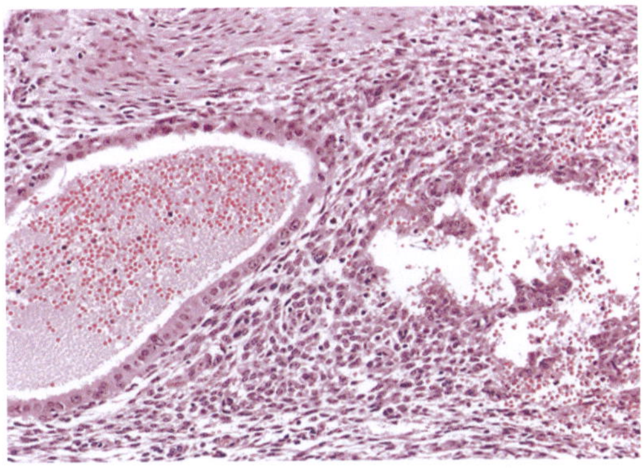

Fig. 5.33 Hemorrhage is also present in the stroma

Enterobiasis

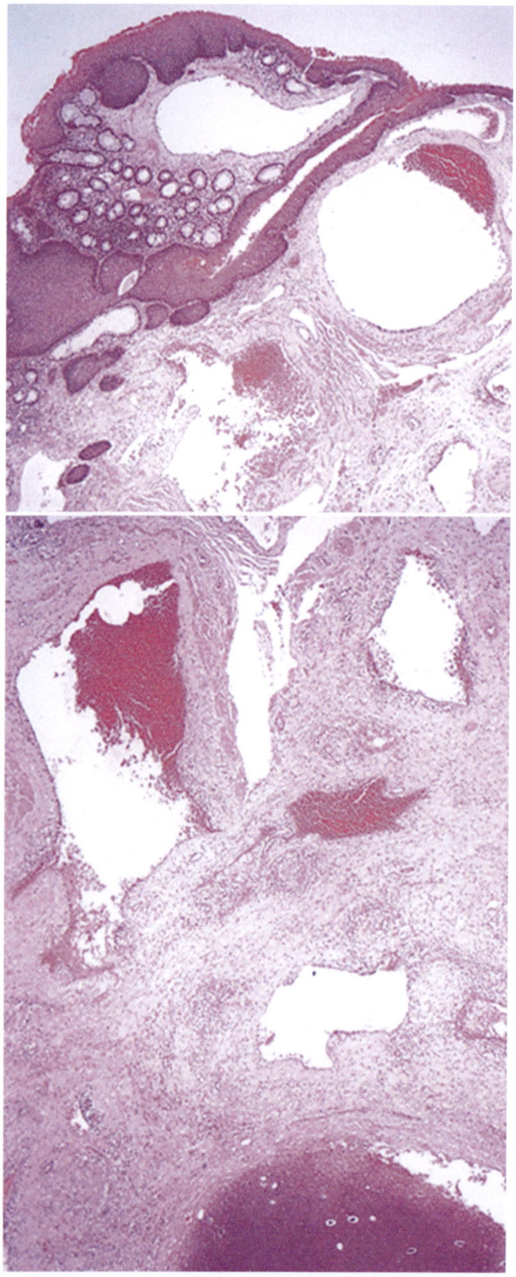

Fig. 5.34 Composite photo of perianal mucosa with dilated channels consistent with hemorrhoids; at the bottom there is an area of necrosis surrounding pinworm eggs

Synonym: Pinworm

Histopathology (Figs. 5.34, 5.35, and 5.36)

- Pinworm eggs in perianal skin and mucosa
- Extensive surrounding acute inflammation and necrosis with abscess formation

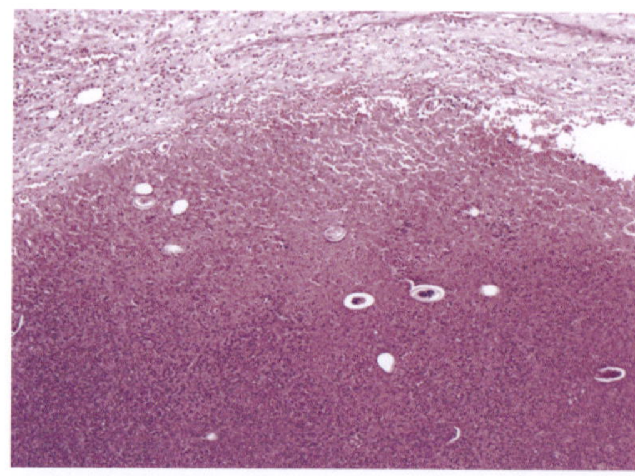

Fig. 5.35 Necrotic tissue with eggs

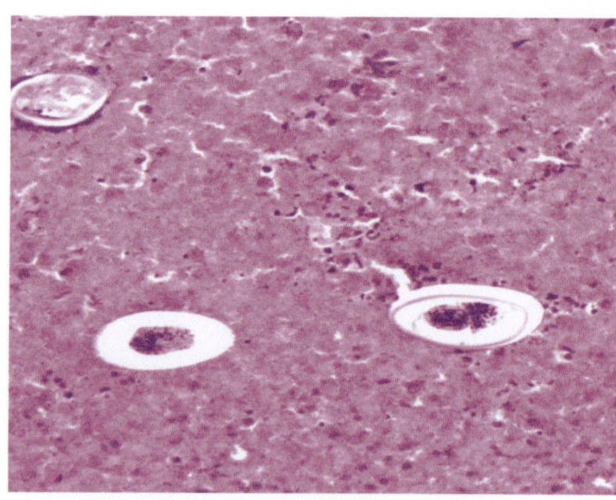

Fig. 5.36 Pinworm eggs in the necrotic abscess

Eosinophilic Fasciitis

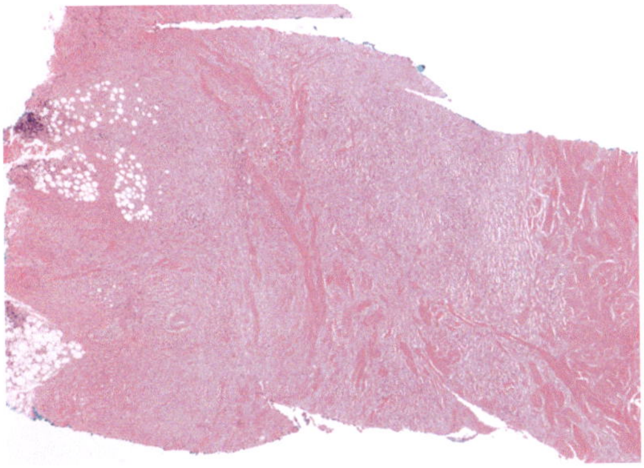

Fig. 5.37 Sclerosis of subcutis and fascia

Synonym: Morphea Profunda, Shulman Syndrome

Histopathology (Figs. 5.37, 5.38, and 5.39)
- Deep variant of morphea/scleroderma
- Thickening of the deep fascia and subcutis
- Fibrosis and hyalinization of collagen
- Lymphoplasmocytic infiltrate with a variable number of eosinophils in subcutis and fascia

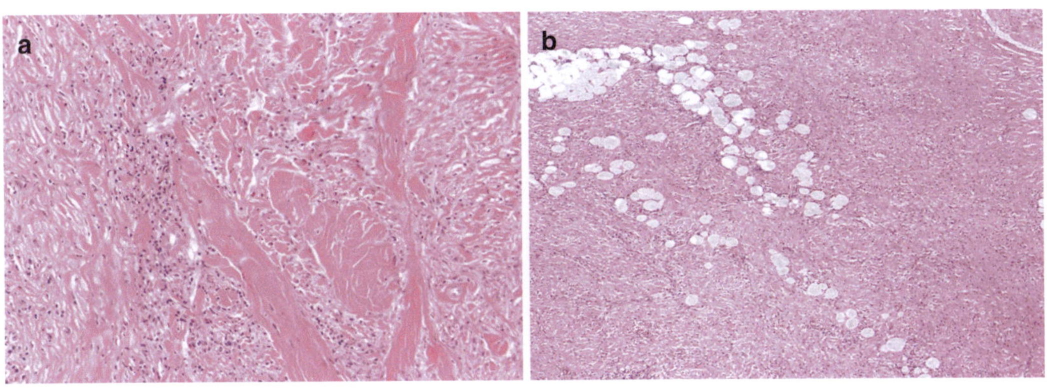

Fig. 5.38 (**a**, **b**) Inflammatory cells are scattered in the hyalinized stroma

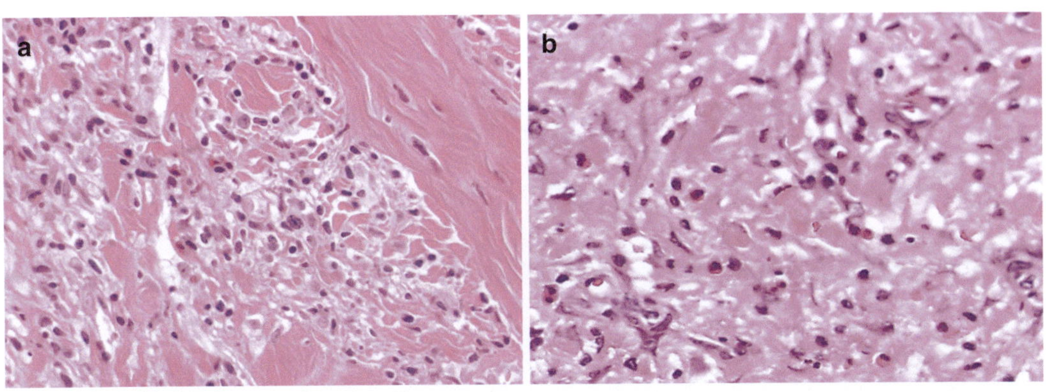

Fig. 5.39 (**a**, **b**) Inflammation consists of lymphocytes, histiocytes, plasma cells, and eosinophils

Eosinophilic Folliculitis

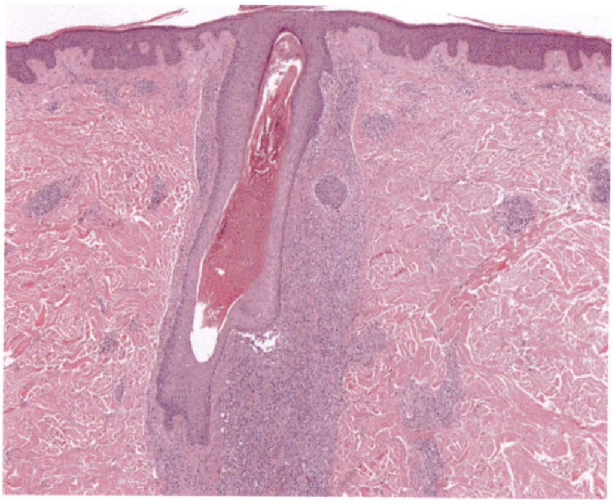

Fig. 5.40 Periinfundibular inflammation

Synonym: Ofuji's Disease

Histopathology (Figs. 5.40, 5.41, and 5.42)

- Follicular spongiosis with perifollicular and intrafollicular eosinophilic infiltrate particularly involving follicular infundibulum
- Mild to moderate perivascular lymphocytic infiltrate with eosinophils

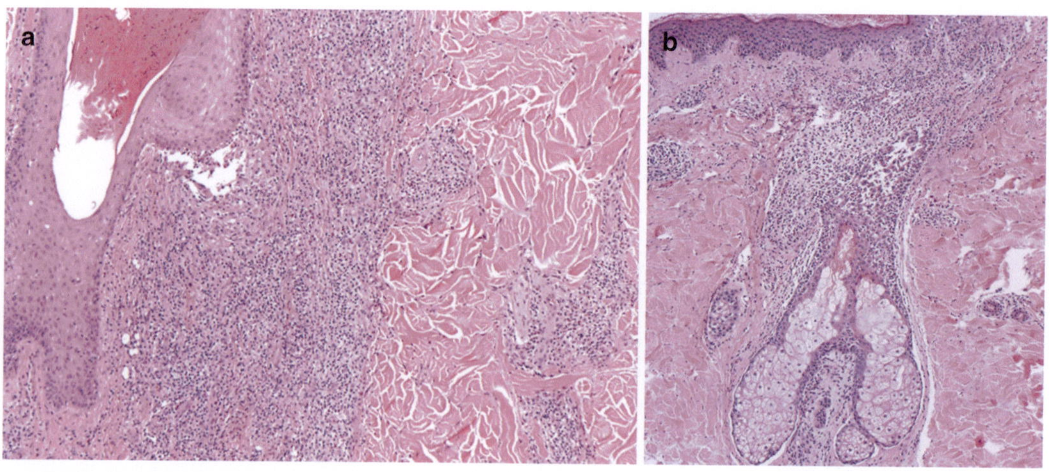

Fig. 5.41 (**a**, **b**) Perifollicular mixed inflammation with numerous eosinophils

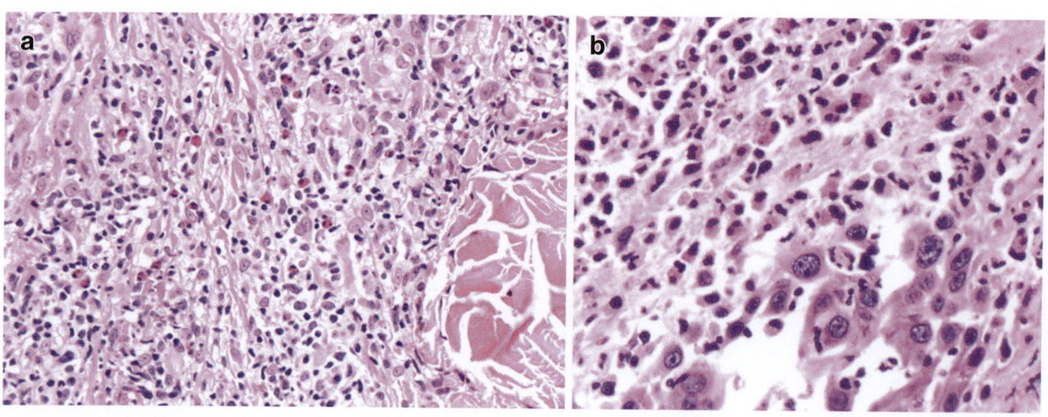

Fig. 5.42 (**a**, **b**) Eosinophilic and neutrophilic inflammation invades and destroys the hair follicle

Eosinophilic Panniculitis

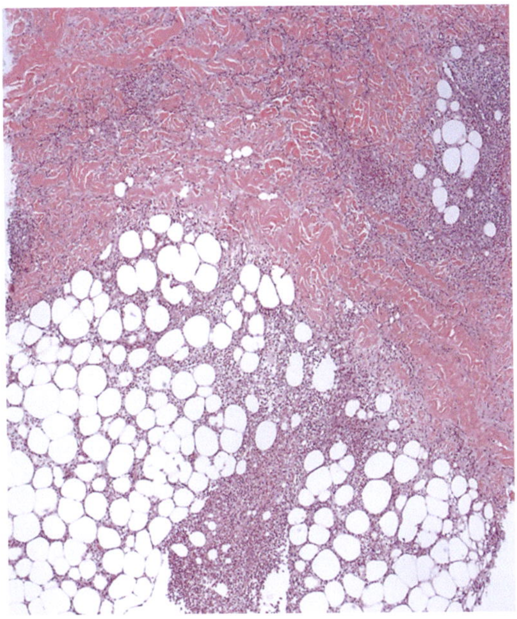

Fig. 5.43 Lobular and septal panniculitis

Histopathology (Figs. 5.43, 5.44, 5.45, and 5.46)

- Mixed lobular and septal panniculitis
- Mixed inflammation with numerous eosinophils
- Occasional "flame" figures

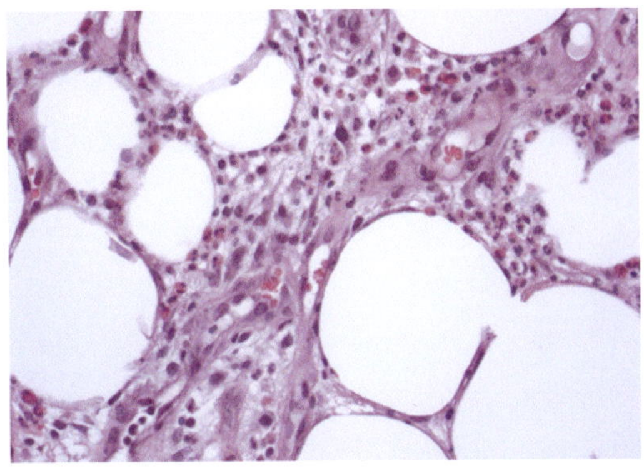

Fig. 5.44 Lymphocytes, histiocytes, neutrophils, and numerous eosinophils

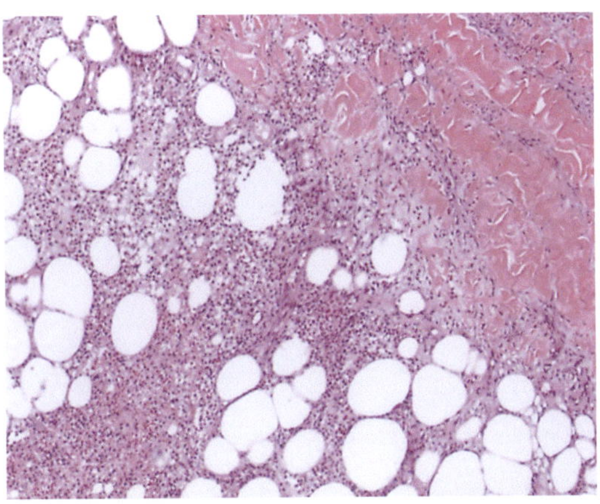

Fig. 5.45 Mixed inflammation in between adipocytes

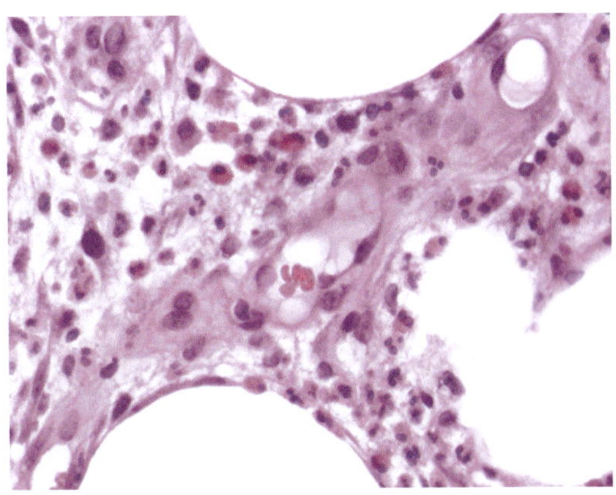

Fig. 5.46 Numerous eosinophils

Ephelis

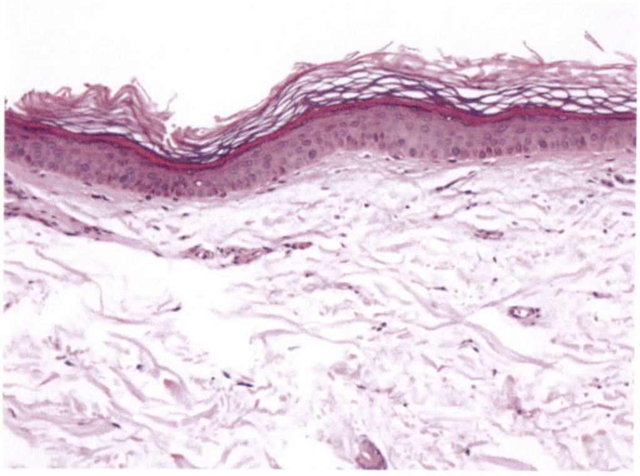

Fig. 5.47 Unremarkable skin on low magnification

Synonym: Freckle

Histopathology (Figs. 5.47, 5.48, 5.49, and 5.50)
- Epidermal architecture is normal
- Hyperpigmentation of basal layer keratinocytes
- Number of melanocytes is normal
- No significant solar elastosis or dermal pigment incontinence

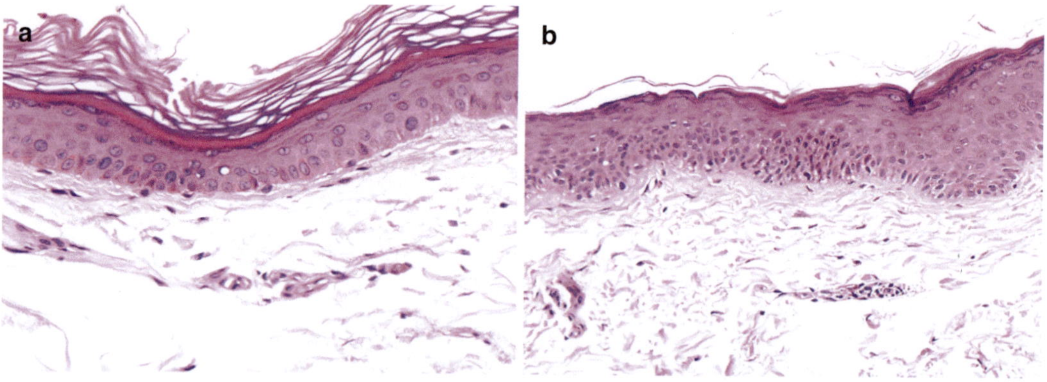

Fig. 5.48 (**a**, **b**) Normal epidermal architecture with no increase in number of melanocytes

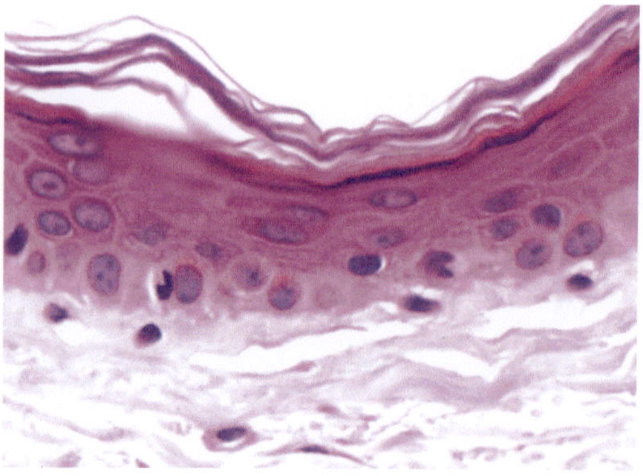

Fig. 5.49 Increased pigment amount within keratinocytes

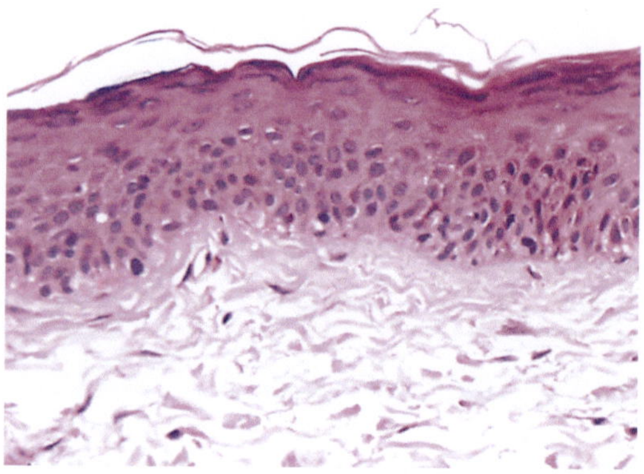

Fig. 5.50 Minimal solar elastosis and no dermal pigment incontinence

Epidermal Inclusion Cyst

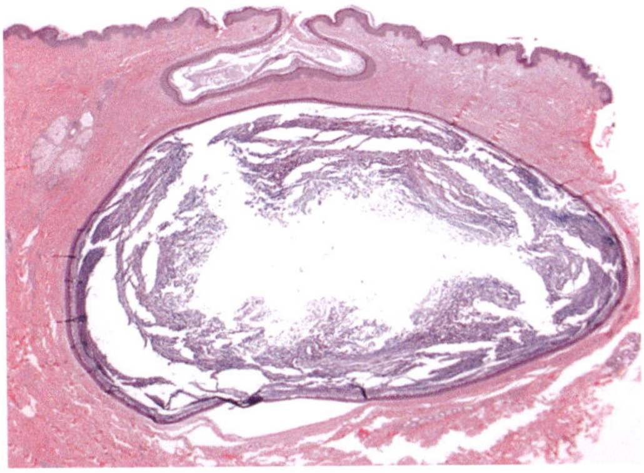

Fig. 5.51 Cyst with an epidermal opening

Synonym: Epidermoid Cyst

Histopathology (Figs. 5.51, 5.52, 5.53, 5.54, and 5.55)

- Dermal/subcutaneous cyst lined with stratified squamous epithelium with epidermal keratinization
- Lumen is filled with laminated orthokeratin
- Connection to the epidermis is commonly seen
- Cyst frequently ruptures causing keratin foreign body giant cell reaction

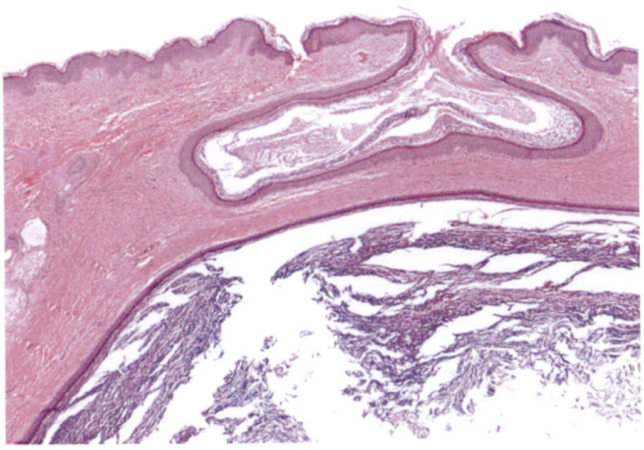

Fig. 5.52 Stratified squamous epithelium forms the cyst wall

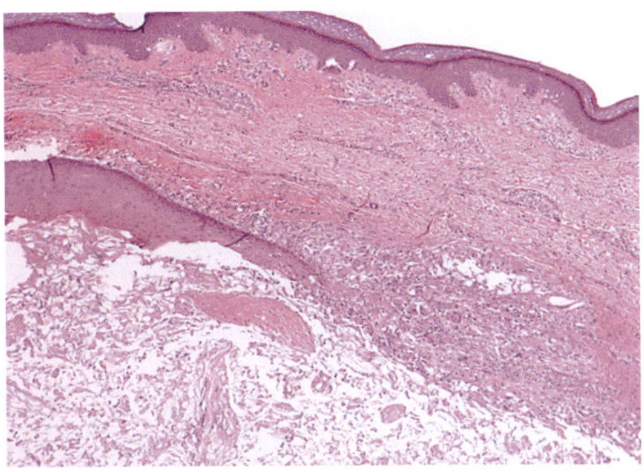

Fig. 5.53 Inflamed ruptured cyst

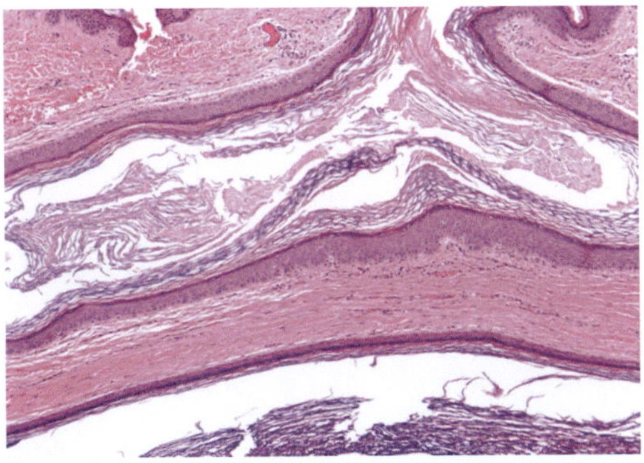

Fig. 5.54 The cyst lumen is filled with laminated keratin

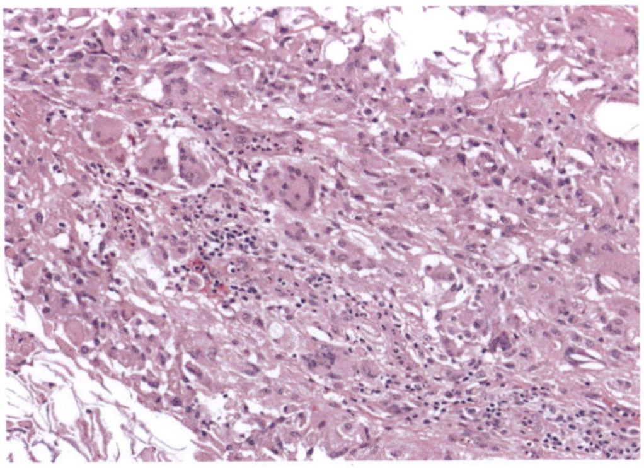

Fig. 5.55 Loose keratin and numerous giant cells forming keratin granuloma

Epidermal Nevus

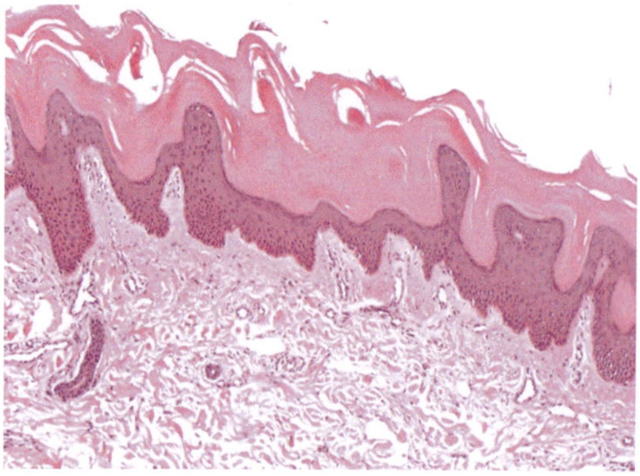

Fig. 5.56 Irregular hyperkeratotic epidermis

Epidermal nevus has over ten different **histopathological** presentations reported (Figs. 5.56, 5.57, and 5.58) but the most commonly reported features are:

- Papillomatosis, hyperkeratosis, hypergranulosis
- Hyperpigmentation of stratum basale
- No or mild dermal inflammation

P.S. clinical correlation is required to confirm diagnosis as there is a lot of similarity with *acanthosis nigricans*

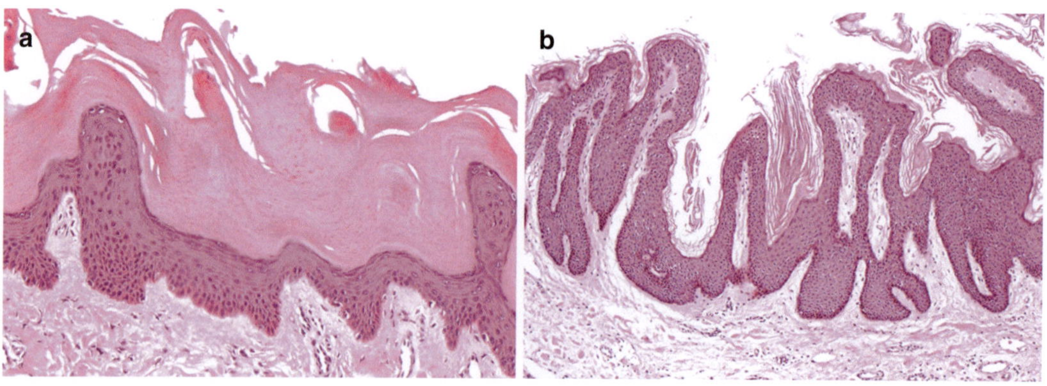

Fig. 5.57 (**a**, **b**) Hyperkeratotic epidermis with irregular papillomatosis

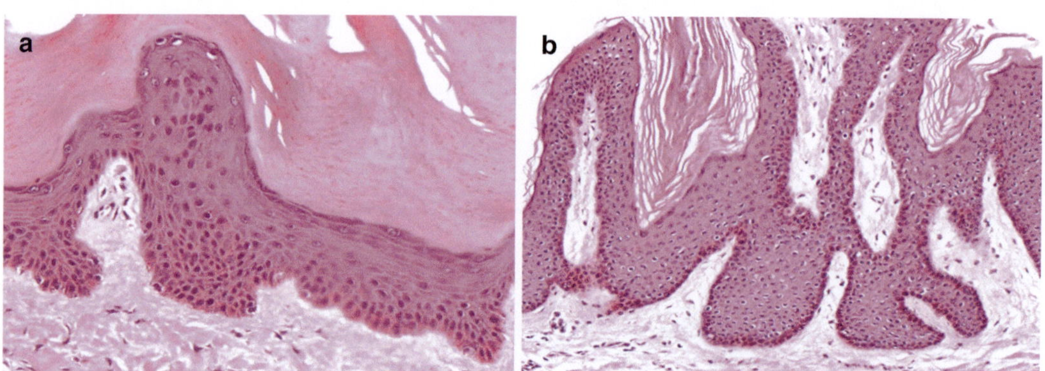

Fig. 5.58 (**a**, **b**) Basal layer is hyperpigmented

Epidermodysplasia Verruciformis

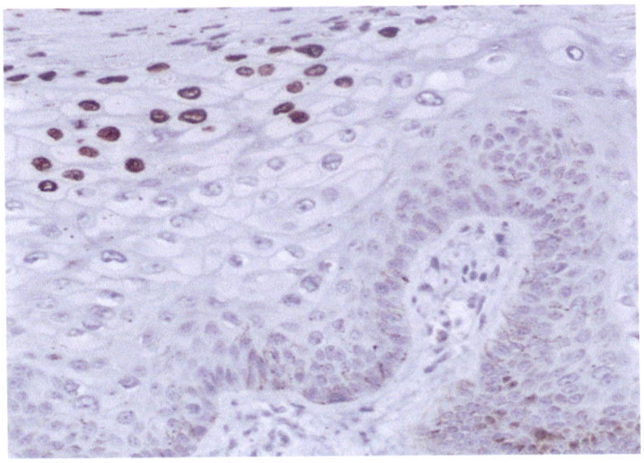

Fig. 5.59 IHS stain for HPV 3 outlines infected keratinocytes

Synonym: Lewandowsky-Lutz Dysplasia

Histopathology resembles wart (Figs. 5.59, 5.60, and 5.61)

- Epidermis varies from papillomatous epidermis, like in verruca vulgaris, to more undulated epidermis, like in verruca plana
- Large swollen cells usually in clusters present in stratum spinosum and granulosum
- Nucleus appears clear and there is perinuclear halo
- Cytoplasm contains coarse keratohyaline granules

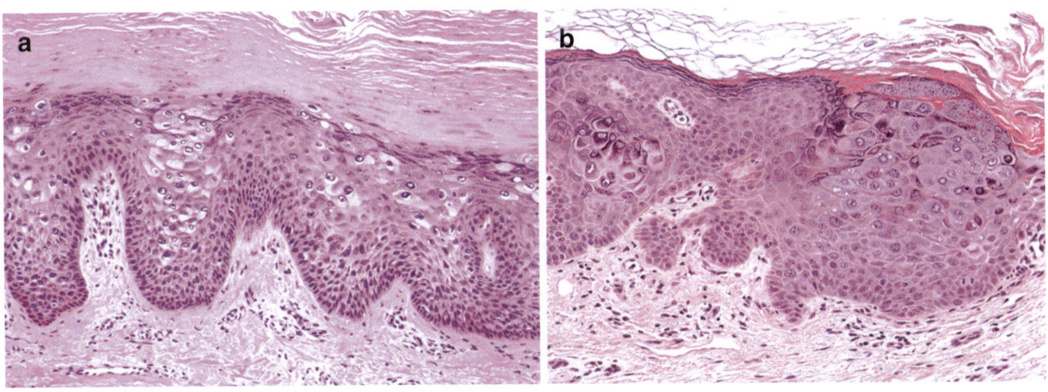

Fig. 5.60 (**a**, **b**) Hyperkeratotic acanthotic epidermis with viral changes in the stratum spinosum and granulosum

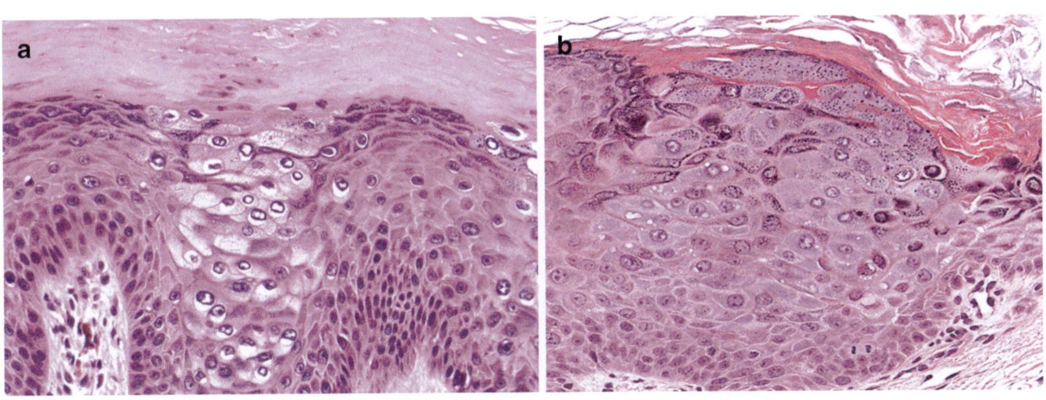

Fig. 5.61 (**a**, **b**) Swollen keratinocytes with nuclei pale in the center and dark thick nuclear membrane. Perinuclear halo is present. Keratohyaline granules are seen in the cytoplasm

Epidermolysis Bullosa Acquisita/Simplex

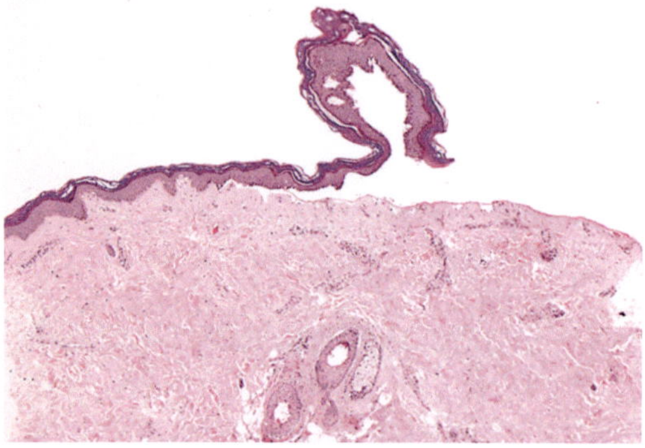

Fig. 5.62 Epidermis is separating from the dermis

EB acquisita and **EB simplex** have the same histopathology (Figs. 5.62, 5.63, and 5.64)

- Subepidermal blister filled with serum
- Minimal or no inflammation within the blister, so called "cell poor" blister
- Minimal "festooning" of dermal papillae
- Minimal dermal perivascular lymphocytic inflammation

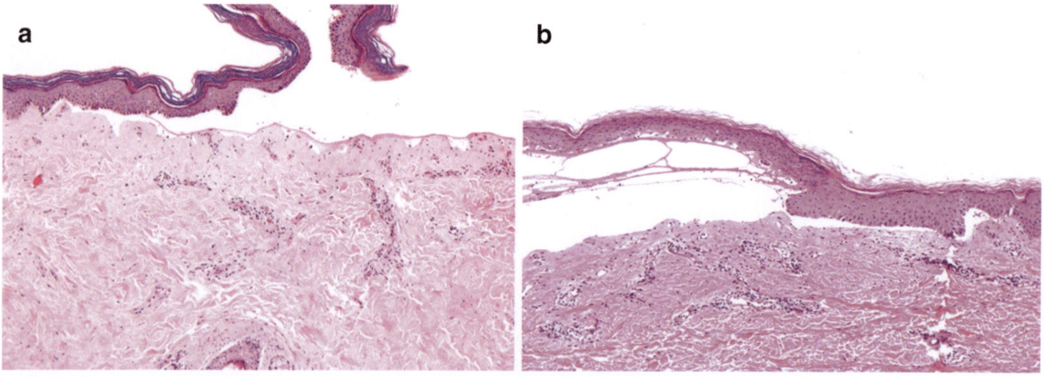

Fig. 5.63 (a, b) Subepidermal blister filled with serum and fibrin without inflammatory cells

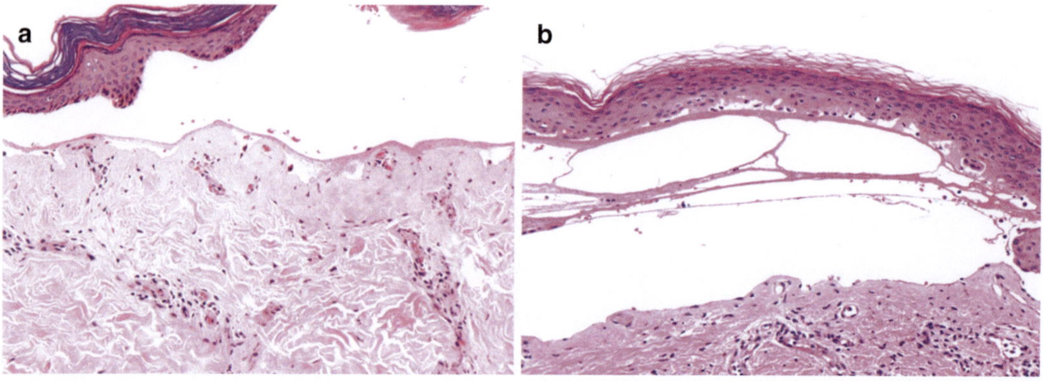

Fig. 5.64 (a, b) Dermal papillae are wavy with minimal "festooning"; minimal dermal perivascular inflammation is present

Epidermolytic Acanthoma/Hyperkeratosis

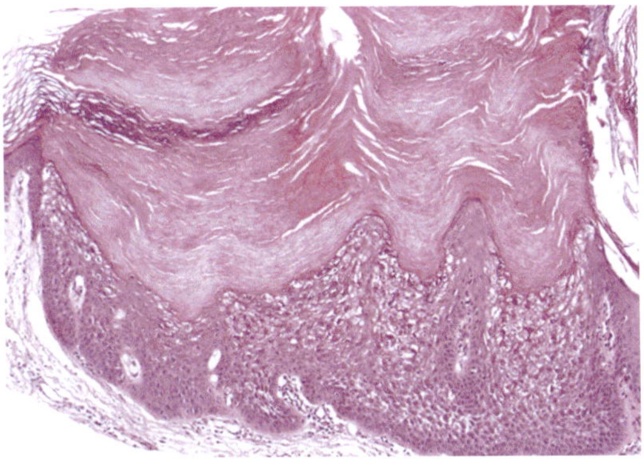

Fig. 5.65 Wart-like hyperkeratotic acanthotic epidermis

Histopathology (Figs. 5.65, 5.66, 5.67, 5.68, and 5.69)

- Wart-like hyperkeratotic acanthotic epidermis
- Vacuolated keratinocytes in the granular layer
- Coarse eosinophilic granules in the granular layer and upper part of spinous layer
- Some basophilic granules in the granular layer

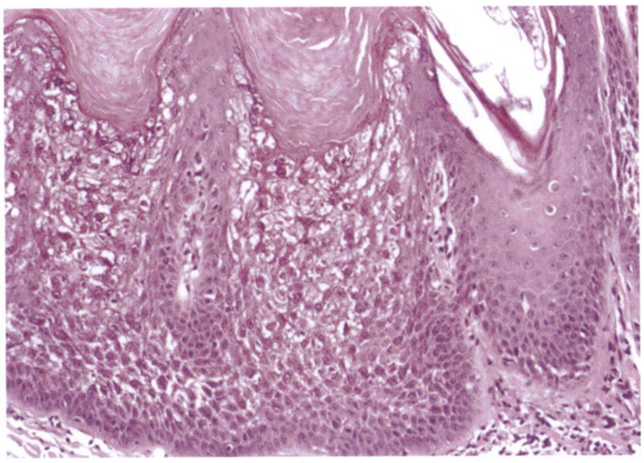

Fig. 5.66 Coarse eosinophilic granules in the upper portion of stratum spinosum

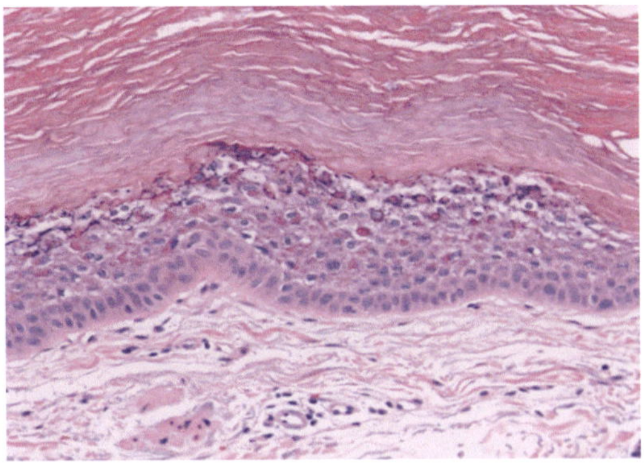

Fig. 5.67 Flat wart-like appearance with vacuolated keratinocytes in the upper part of the epidermis

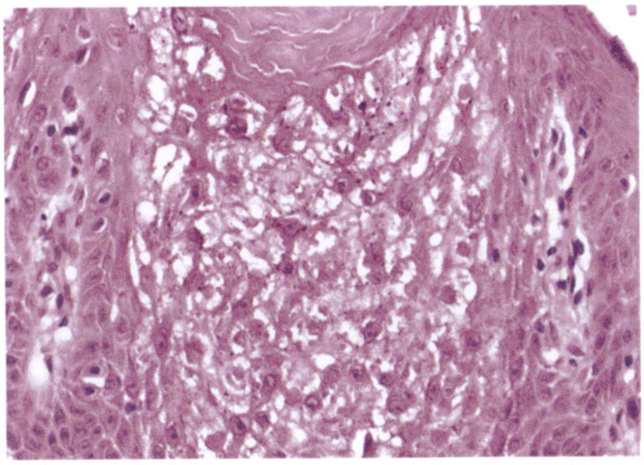

Fig. 5.68 Vacuolated keratinocytes with eosinophilic granules

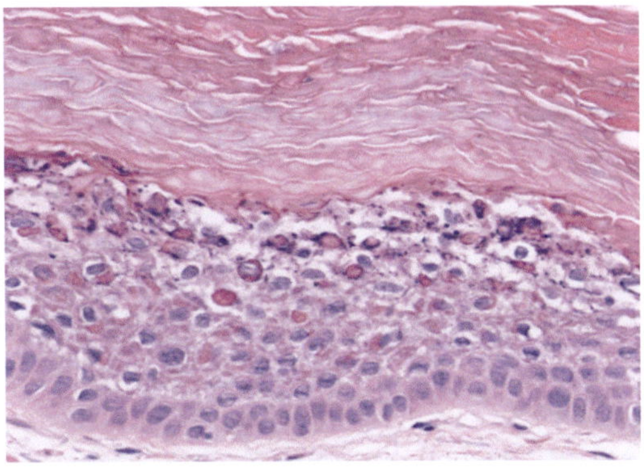

Fig. 5.69 Superficial keratinocytes with eosinophilic and basophilic granules

Epulis Fissuratum

Granuloma fissuratum (acanthoma fissuratum) develops on the skin at the site of pressure from eye glasses. **Epulis fissuratum** develops in the mouth at the site of poorly fitted dentures.

Histopathology (Figs. 5.70 and 5.71)

- Acanthotic epidermis (**granuloma fissuratum**) or squamous mucosa (**epulis fissuratum**) with pseudoepitheliomatous hyperplasia
- Central epidermal ulceration with granulation tissue and inflammation

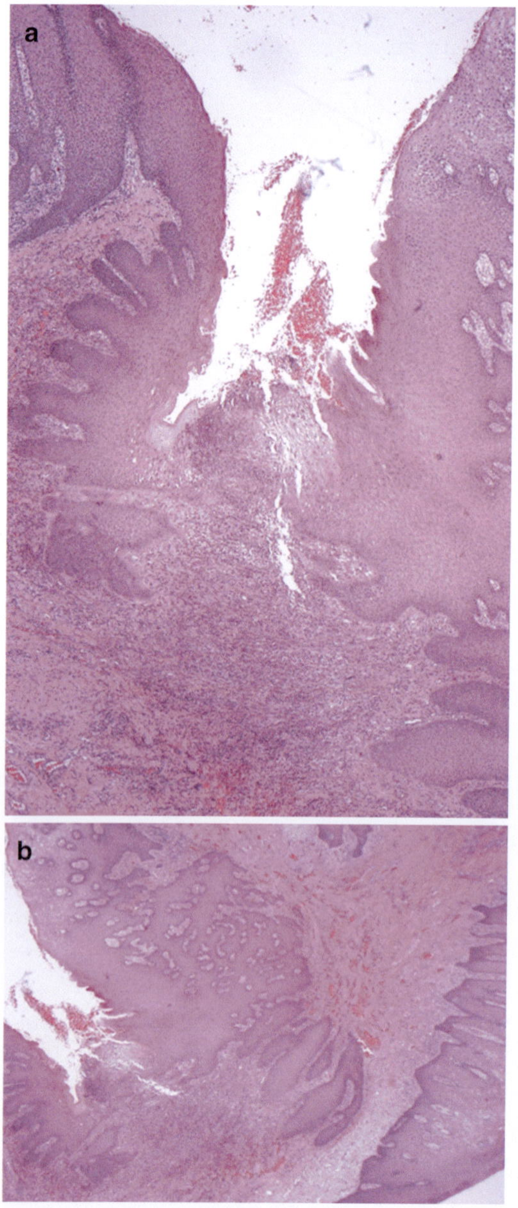

Fig. 5.70 (**a**, **b**) Pseudoepitheliomatous epidermal hyperplasia with central ulceration

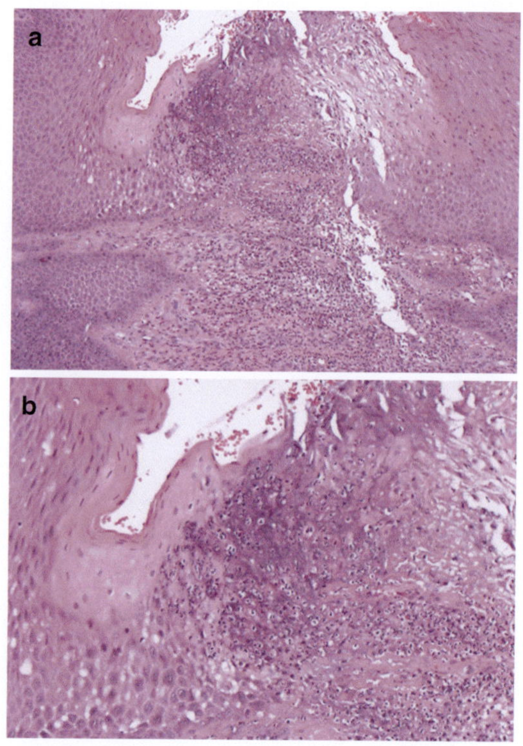

Fig. 5.71 (**a**, **b**) Necrotic tissue with acute inflammation and granulation tissue are forming ulcer bed

Erysipelas

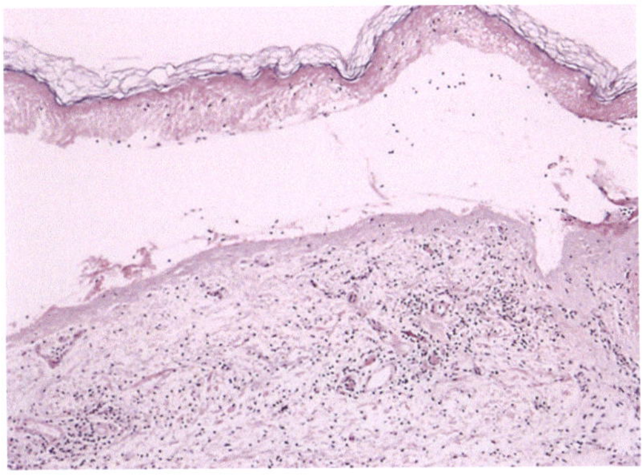

Fig. 5.72 Subepidermal blister

Histopathology (Figs. 5.72, 5.73, 5.74, and 5.75)

- Extensive dermal edema making biopsy tissue looking pale
- Formation of subepidermal vesicle/bullae
- Extensive neutrophilic infiltrate in the dermis

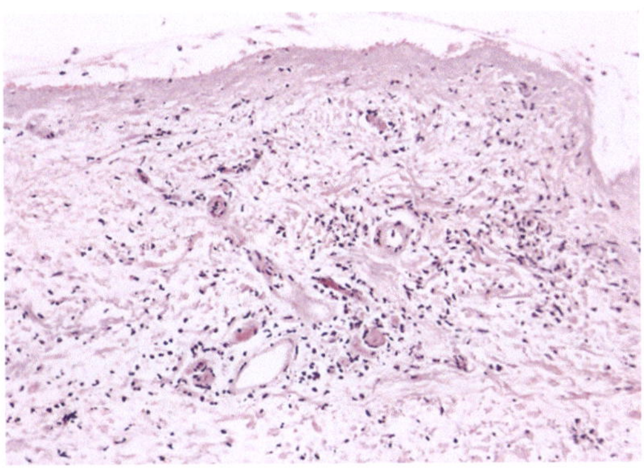

Fig. 5.73 Extensive dermal edema and numerous neutrophils

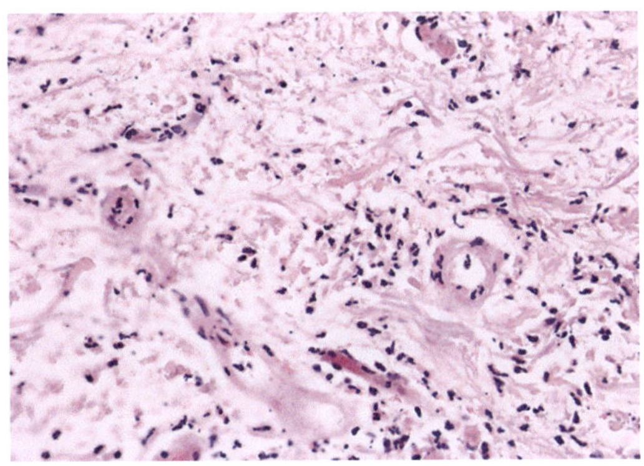

Fig. 5.74 Perivascular and interstitial neutrophils

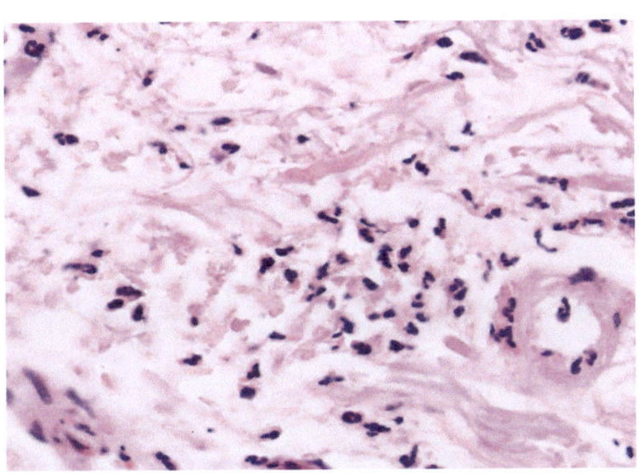

Fig. 5.75 No significant leukocytoclasia

Erythema Ab Igne

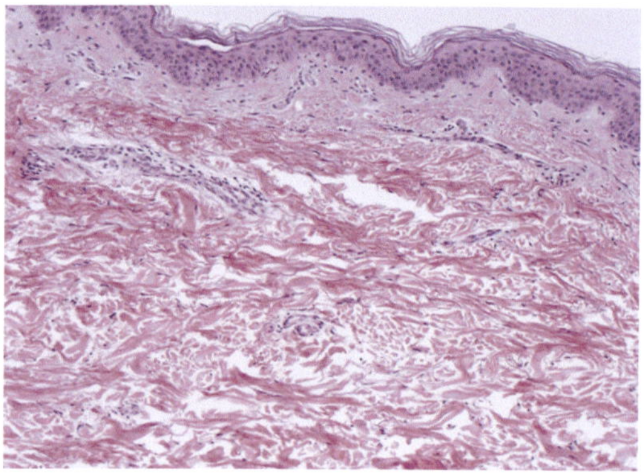

Fig. 5.76 Normal appearing skin with "smudgy" collagen

Histopathology (Figs. 5.76, 5.77, 5.78, 5.79, and 5.80)

- Changes are very subtle
- Atrophic epidermis
- Mild epithelial atypia akin to actinic keratosis with more prominent dermal capillaries
- Mild pigment incontinence in older lesions
- Prominent elastic material in the mid dermis
- "Smudgy" dermal collagen

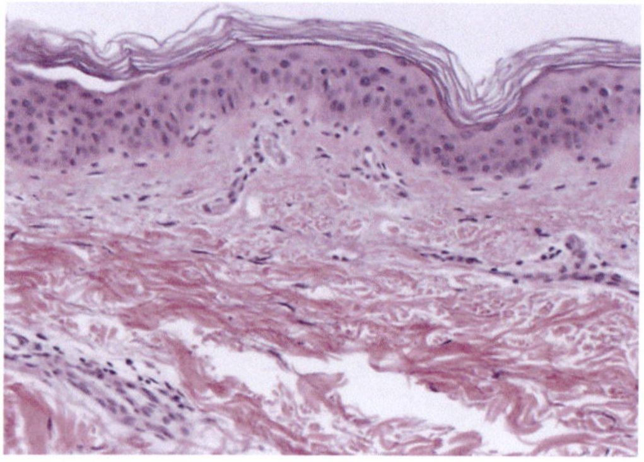

Fig. 5.77 Flattened epidermis with atypia of keratinocytes

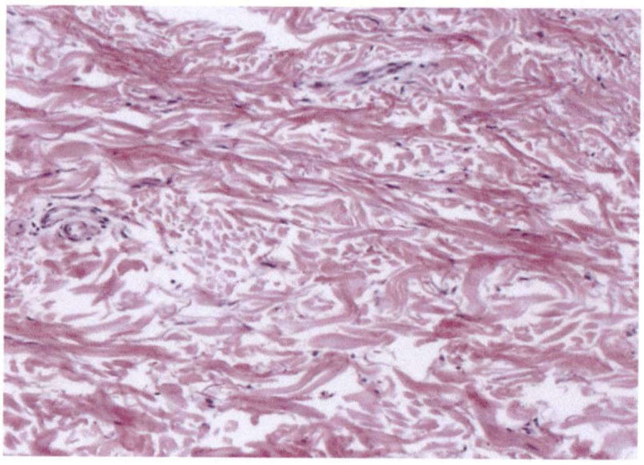

Fig. 5.78 Increased elastic material in the mid dermis

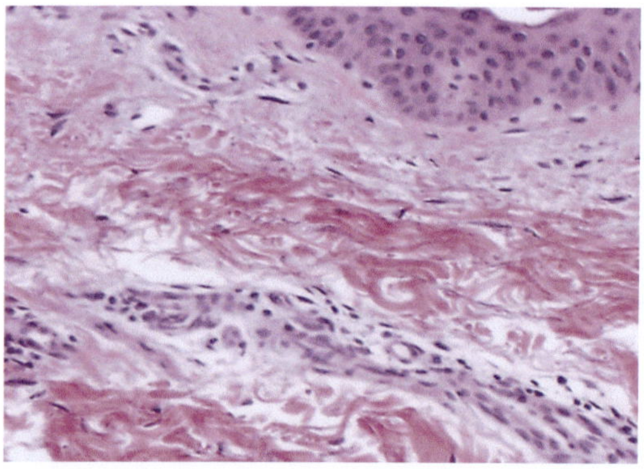

Fig. 5.79 Dermal capillaries are more prominent

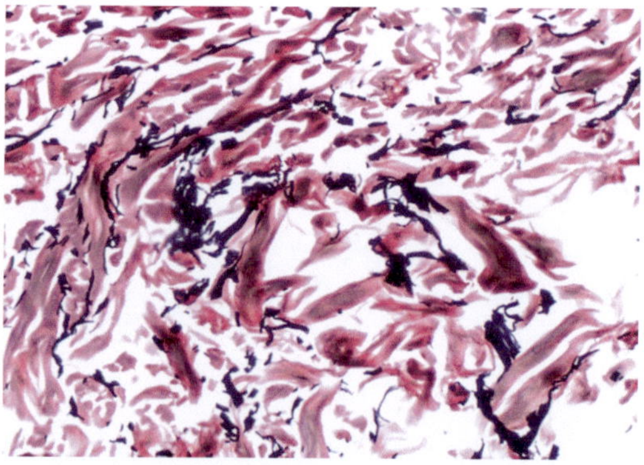

Fig. 5.80 VVG highlights increased elastic fibers

Erythema Annulare Centrifugum

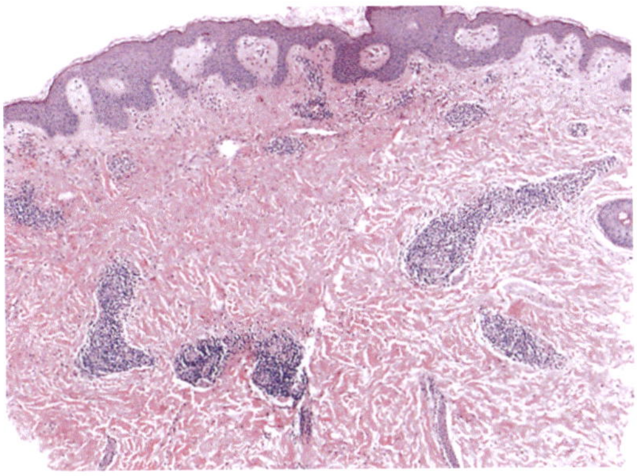

Fig. 5.81 Superficial and deep perivascular inflammation

Synonyms: Annular Erythema, Gyrate Erythema (Erythema Gyratum)

Histopathology (Figs. 5.81, 5.82, and 5.83)

- Epidermis is unremarkable
- Superficial or superficial/deep perivascular lymphocytic infiltrate
- Lymphocytic infiltrate is tightly "cuffed" around capillaries
- Interstitial infiltrate is minimal

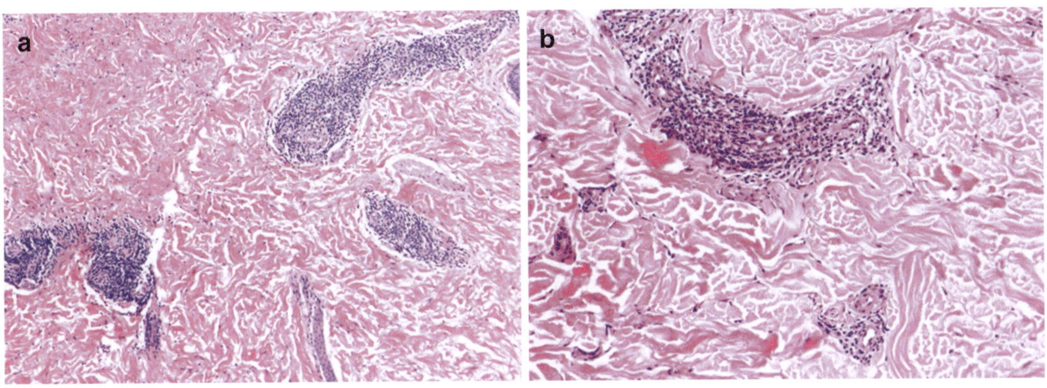

Fig. 5.82 (**a**, **b**) Lymphocytes are "tightly cuffed" around the capillaries and there are very few lymphocytes in between vessels

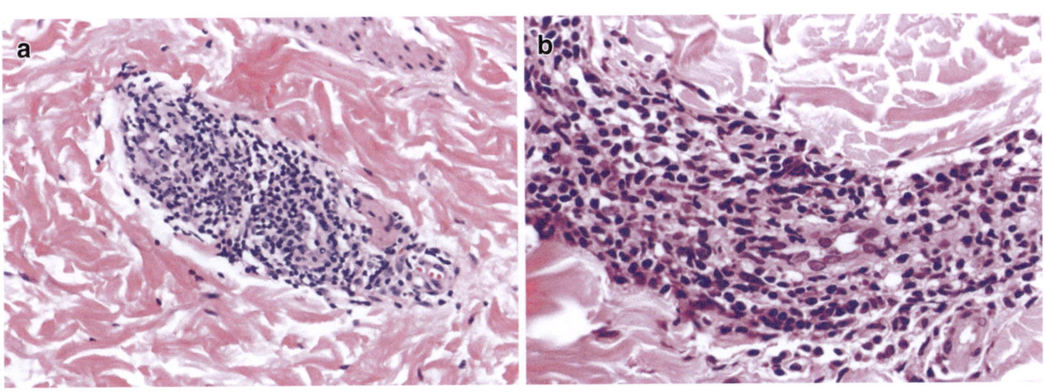

Fig. 5.83 (**a**, **b**) Perivascular lymphocytes are relatively uniform with no atypia

Erythema Chronicum Migrans

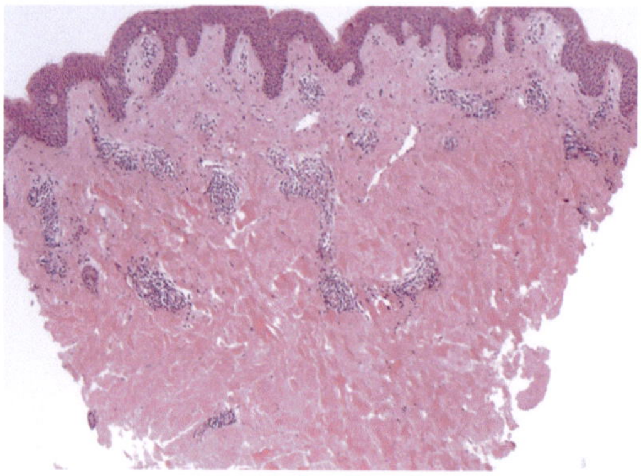

Fig. 5.84 Superficial and deep perivascular lymphocytic infiltrate

Synonym: Stage I Lyme Disease

Histopathology is not specific as it resembles *erythema annulare centrifugum*: (Figs. 5.84, 5.85, 5.86, and 5.87)

- Superficial and deep perivascular inflammation consisting of lymphocytes and plasma cells
- Endothelial swelling and mild mucin can be detected

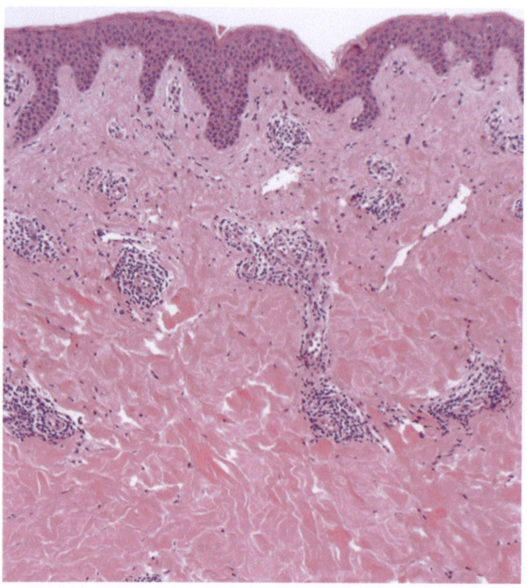

Fig. 5.85 Erythema annulare centrifugum-like pattern

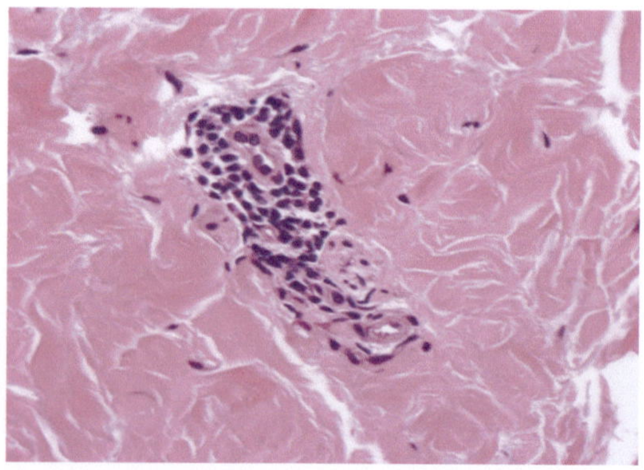

Fig. 5.86 Perivascular lymphocytes and plasma cell

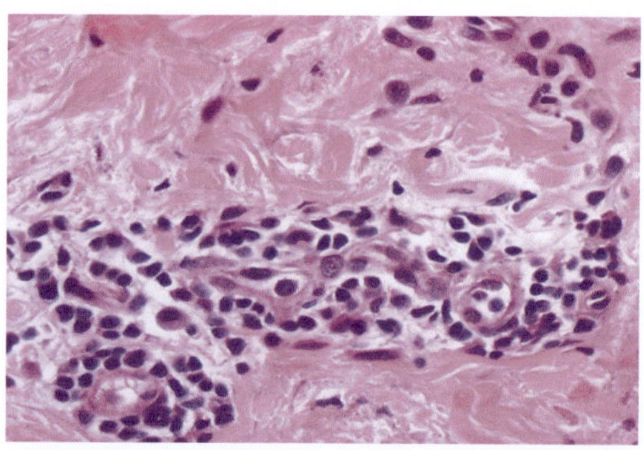

Fig. 5.87 Endothelial swelling and mildly increased perivascular mucin

Erythema Dischromicum Perstans

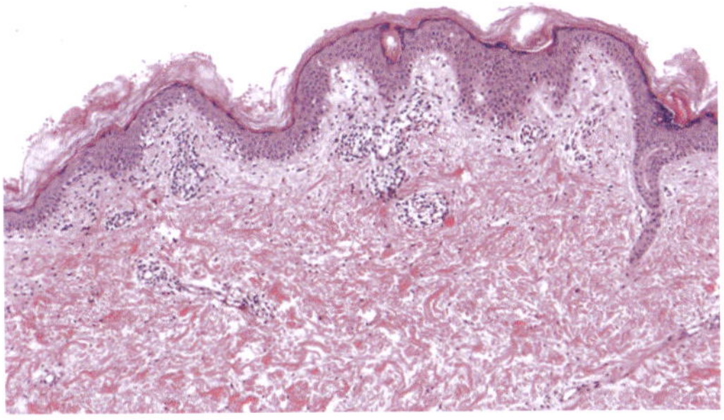

Fig. 5.88 Pathology is limited to the papillary dermis

Synonym: Ashy Dermatosis

Histopathology (Figs. 5.88, 5.89, 5.90, 5.91, and 5.92)
- Focal vacuolar interface changes
- Variable dermal pigment incontinence with melanophages
- Mild perivascular lymphocytic infiltrate

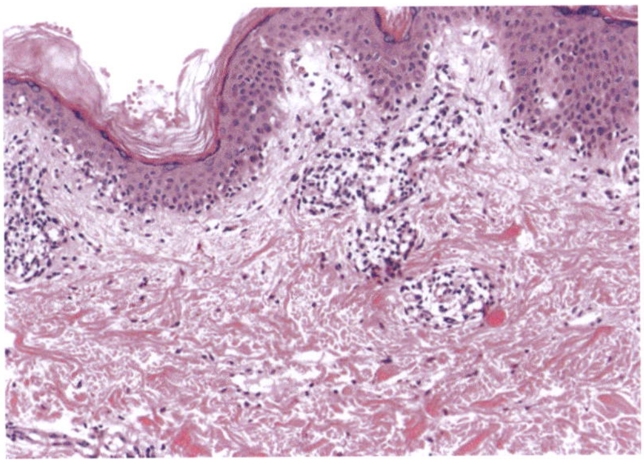

Fig. 5.89 Mild perivascular and interstitial lymphocytic infiltrate

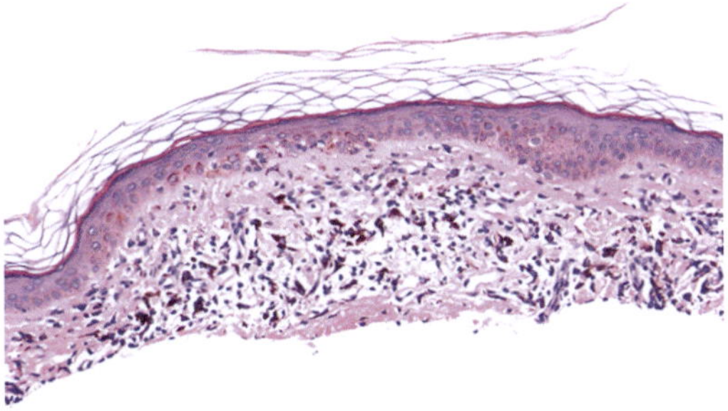

Fig. 5.90 Dermal pigment incontinence with dermal melanophages

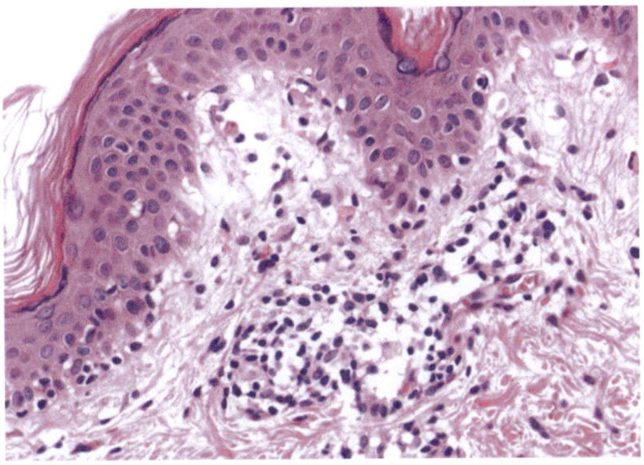

Fig. 5.91 Interface vacuolar changes and mild pigment incontinence

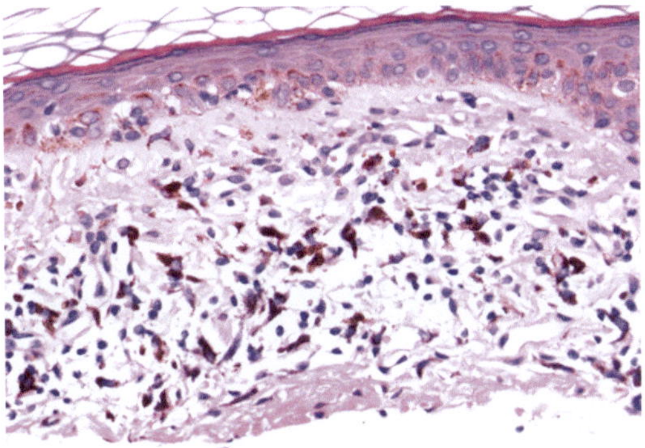

Fig. 5.92 Significant dermal pigment incontinence

Erythema Elevatum Diutinum

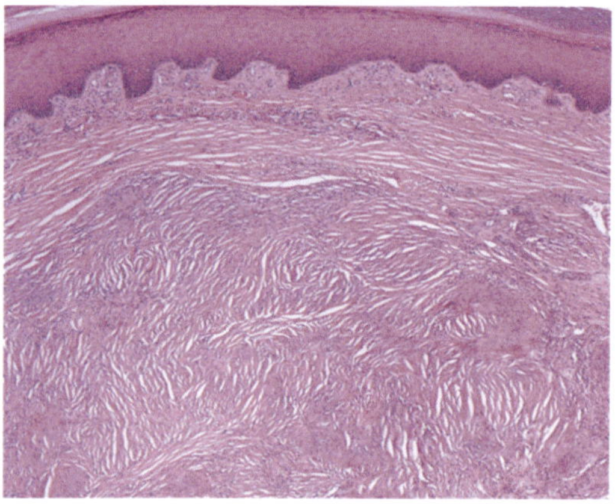

Fig. 5.93 Sclerotic collagenoma-like appearance

Histopathology

Early lesion:

- leukocytoclastic vasculitis in sclerotic dermis (Figs. 5.95 and 5.97)

Older lesion:

- Dermal and subcutaneous sclerosis with "onion skin" appearance resembling *sclerotic collagenoma* (Figs. 5.93 and 5.94)
- Nuclear debris is present between collagen bundles (Fig. 5.96)

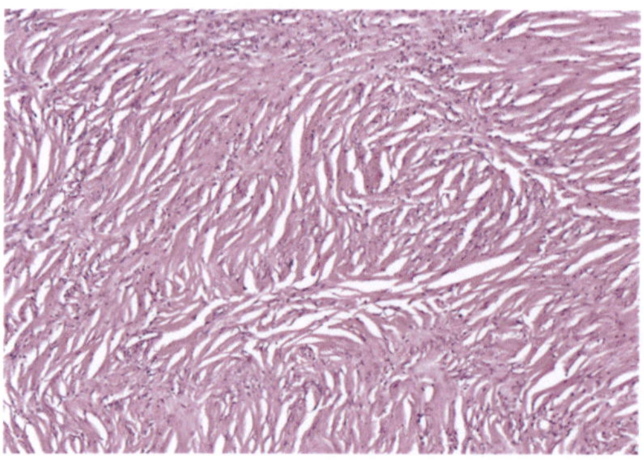

Fig. 5.94 Old lesion with extensive fibrosis forming clefts

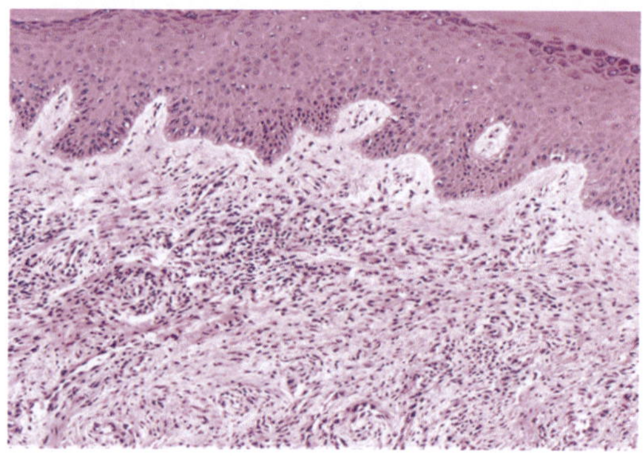

Fig. 5.95 Leukocytoclastic vasculitis-like lesiona

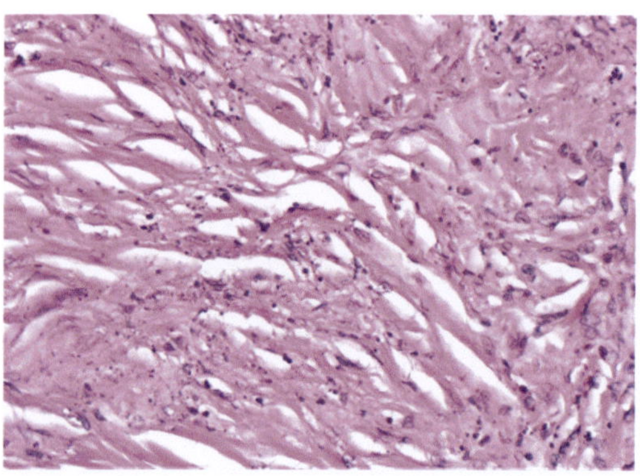

Fig. 5.96 Scattered subtle neutrophilic debris

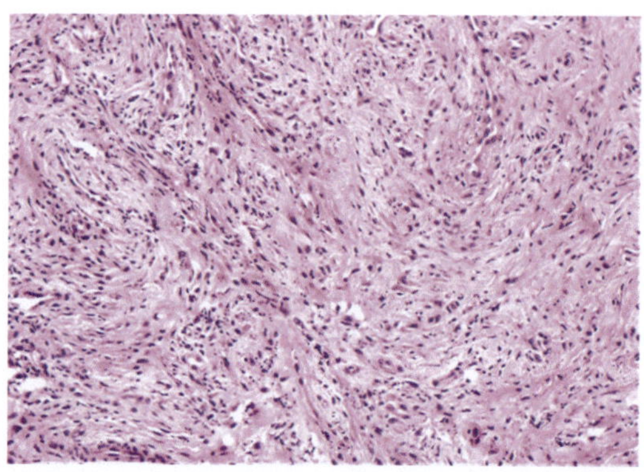

Fig. 5.97 Prominent neutrophilic debris in sclerotic stroma

Erythema Induratum

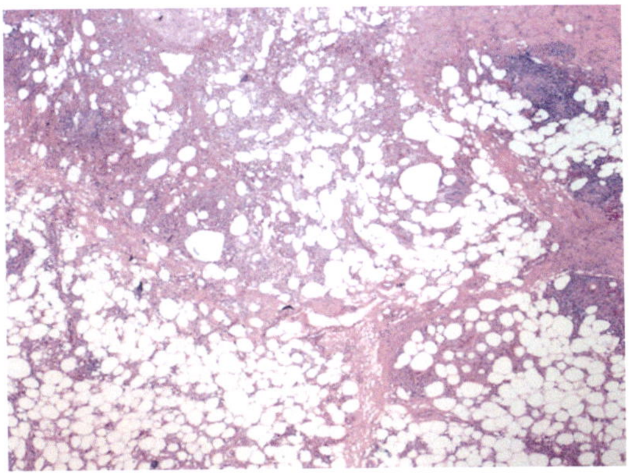

Fig. 5.98 Mixed panniculitis

Synonyms: Bazin's Disease, Nodular Vasculitis

Histopathology (Figs. 5.98, 5.99, 5.100, 5.101, and 5.102)

- Mixed septal and lobular panniculitis with mixed inflammation
- As the lesion progresses there is less inflammation and more fibrosis
- Epithelioid granulomas with giant cells are present and fat necrosis is common
- Vasculitis with mixed inflammatory cells is present in the majority of cases

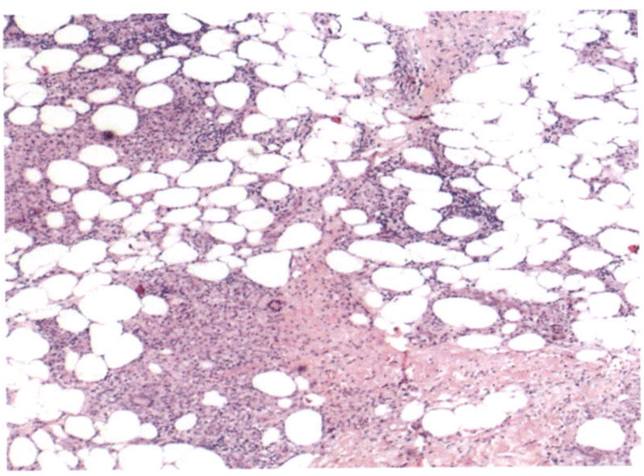

Fig. 5.99 Septal and lobular panniculitis with mixed inflammation

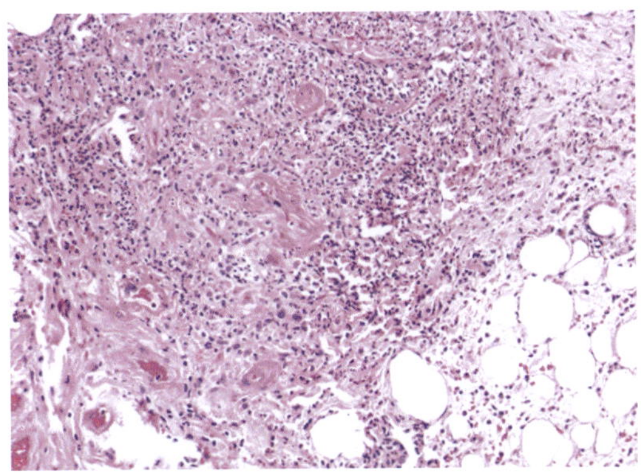

Fig. 5.100 Vasculitis is present in septa

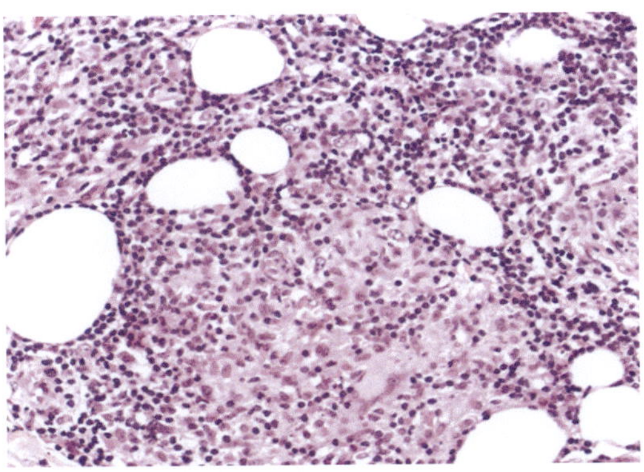

Fig. 5.101 Epithelioid granuloma with giant cells

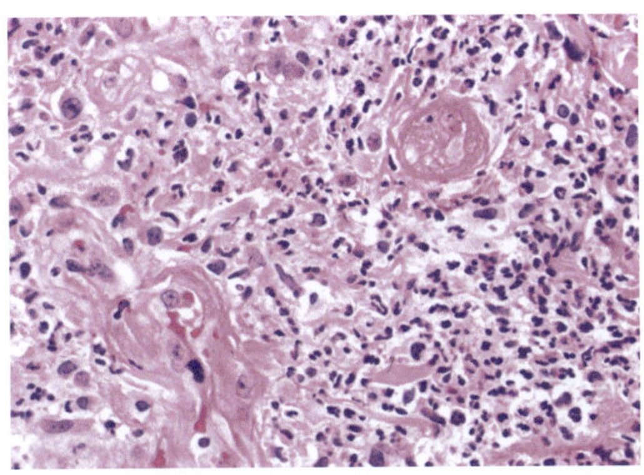

Fig. 5.102 Small blood vessels with fibrinoid changes

Erythema Marginatum

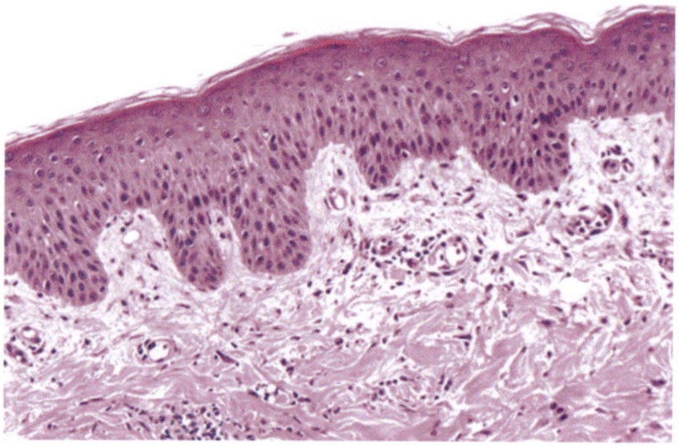

Fig. 5.103 Dermal neutrophilic inflammation

Synonyms: Erythema Marginatum Rheumaticum, Erythema Annulare Rheumaticum

Histopathology (Figs. 5.103, 5.104, 5.105, and 5.106)

- Variable number of perivascular neutrophils with few lymphocytes and eosinophils
- Sometimes associated mild leukocytoclasia
- No evidence of vasculitis (no thrombi or vascular fibrin deposition)
- Dermal papillary neutrophils and scattered dyskeratotic keratinocytes occasionally present

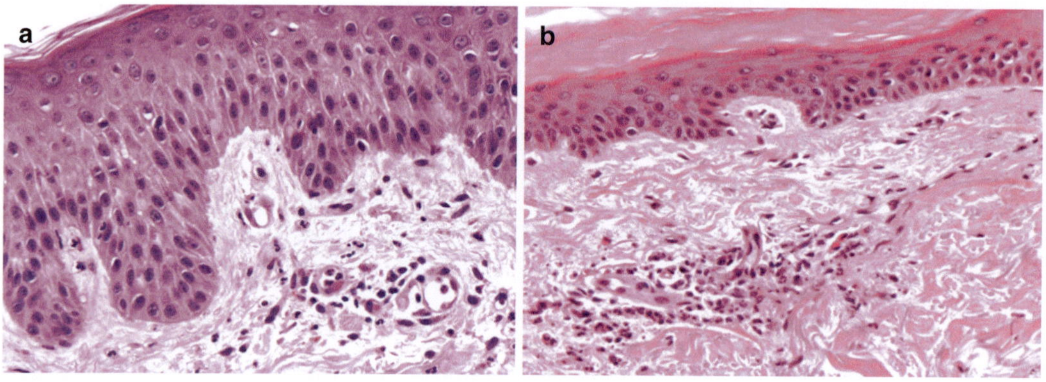

Fig. 5.104 (**a**, **b**) Dermal perivascular and interstitial neutrophils without obvious leukocytoclasia

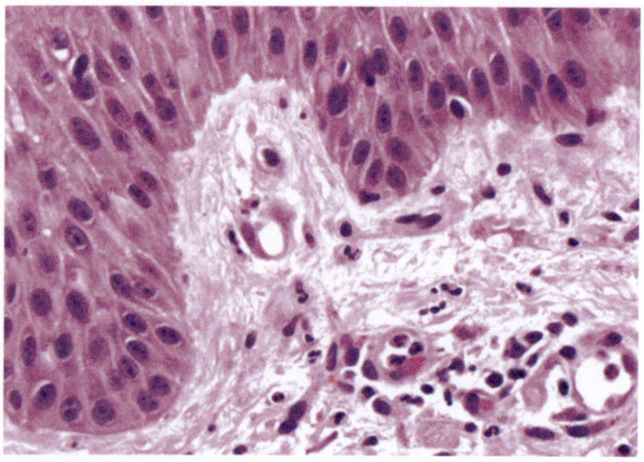

Fig. 5.105 Few neutrophils are present in dermal papilla

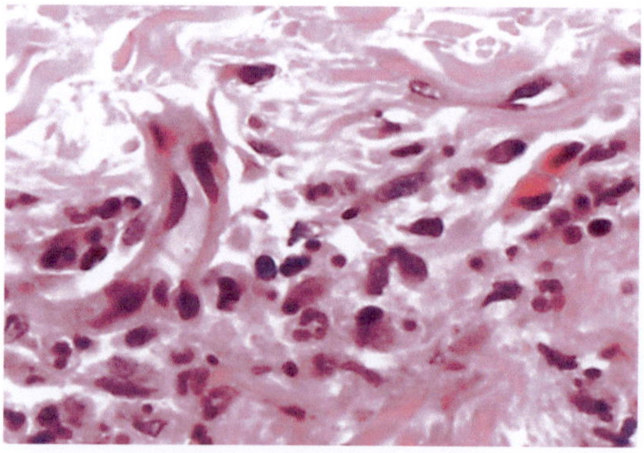

Fig. 5.106 Perivascular neutrophils and few lymphocytes and eosinophils with no thrombi or fibrin deposition

Erythema Multiforme

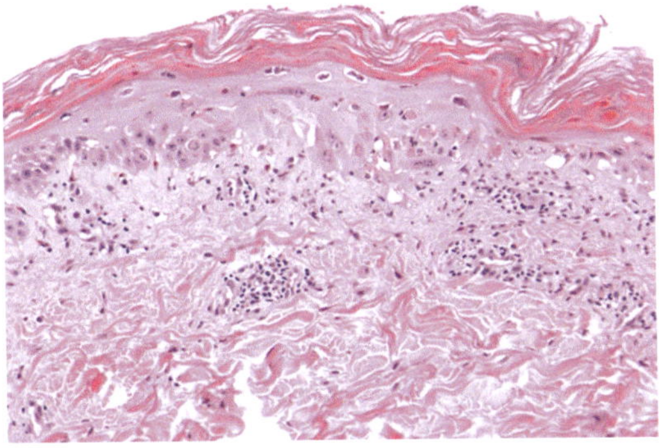

Fig. 5.107 Smudgy epidermis with mild dermal inflammation

Histopathology (Figs. 5.107, 5.108, 5.109, and 5.110)

- Interface vacuolar changes with mild epidermal spongiosis
- Variable number of individual necrotic keratinocytes within and above basal layer
- Mild to moderate perivascular lymphocytic infiltrate and pigment incontinence
- Dermal edema with formation of subepidermal blister is common

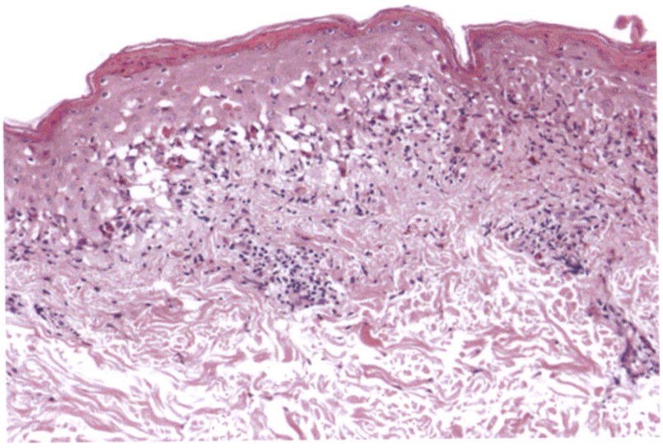

Fig. 5.108 Interface vacuolar changes with necrotic keratinocytes

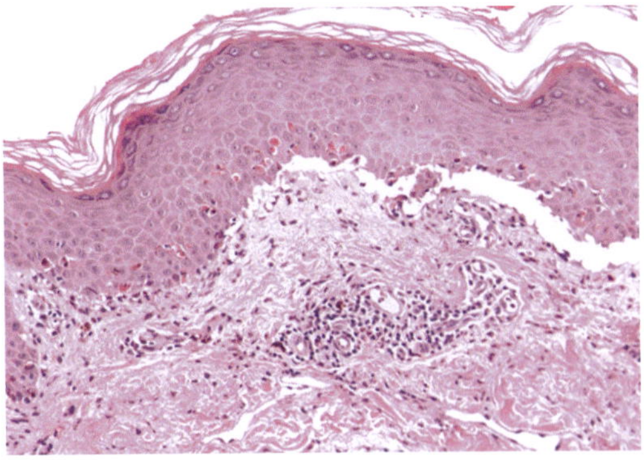

Fig. 5.109 Subepidermal split with dermal lymphocytic inflammation

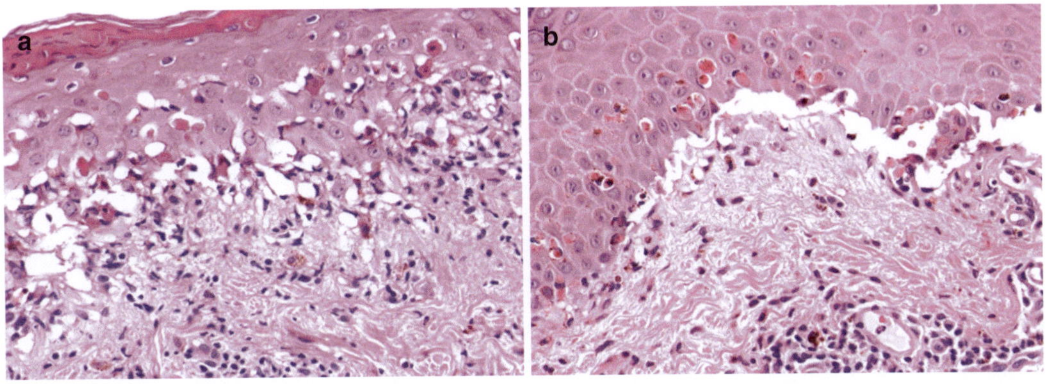

Fig. 5.110 (**a**, **b**) Scattered necrotic keratinocytes in the lower epidermis with dermal pigment incontinence and mild lymphocytic inflammation

Erythema Nodosum

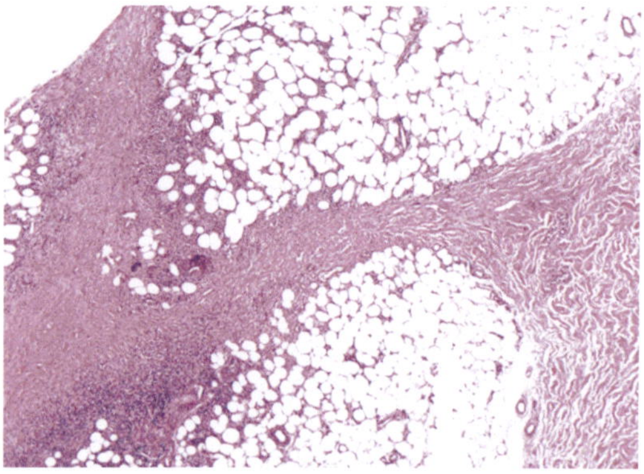

Fig. 5.111 Septal panniculitis with some periseptal "spillover"

Histopathology (Figs. 5.111, 5.112, and 5.113)

- Septal panniculitis with some "spill-over" into lobules in which the type of inflammatory cells changes with the aging of the lesion
- Early lesion contains neutrophils
- In an established lesion there are lymphocytes, histiocytes, and giant cells that form Miescher's granuloma
- In an old lesion septa are fibrotic and inflammation spills over into lobular adipose tissue

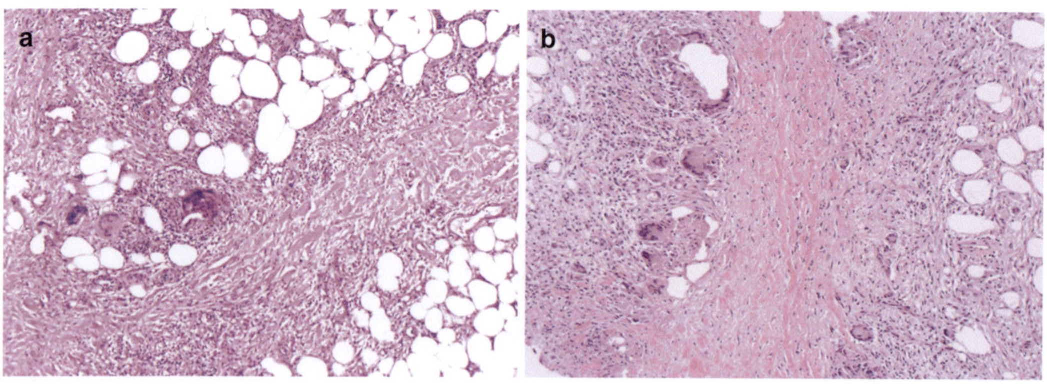

Fig. 5.112 (**a**, **b**) Septal fibrosis with lymphocytes, histiocytes, and focal giant cells. Neutrophils are absent in the established lesions

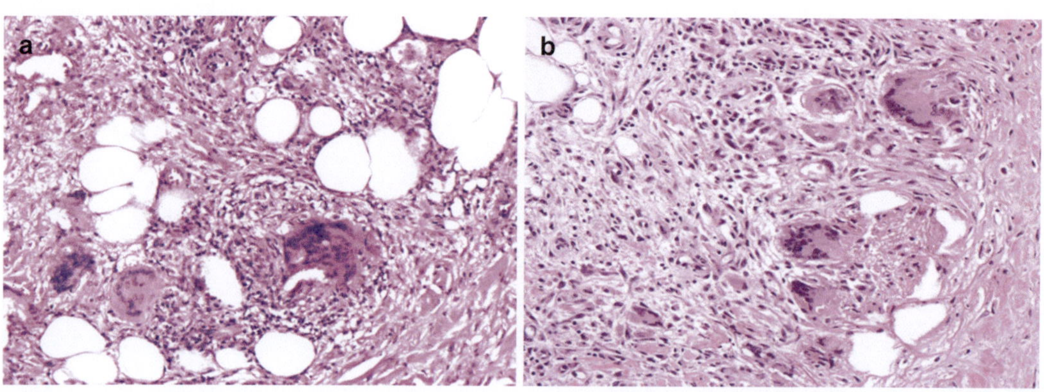

Fig. 5.113 (**a**, **b**) Giant cells and histiocytes form Miescher's granulomas

Erythema Nodosum Leprosum

It represents *type II reactional state of leprosy*.

Histopathology (Figs. 5.114, 5.115, and 5.116)

- Dermal edema with superficial and deep mixed perivascular, periadnexal, and perineural inflammation
- Mixed lobular and septal panniculitis with lymphocytes and histiocytes

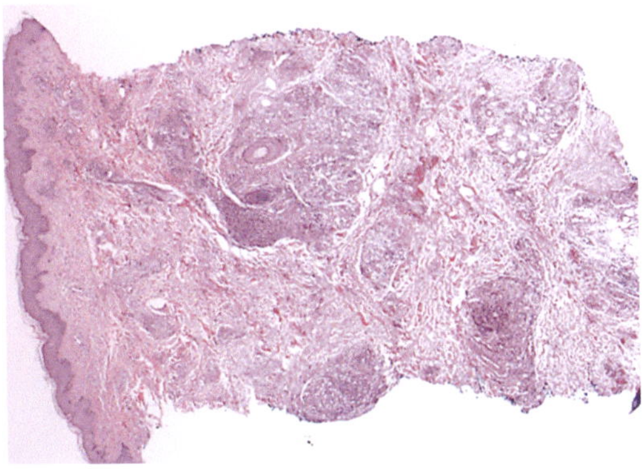

Fig. 5.114 Dense periadnexal lymphohistiocytic inflammation

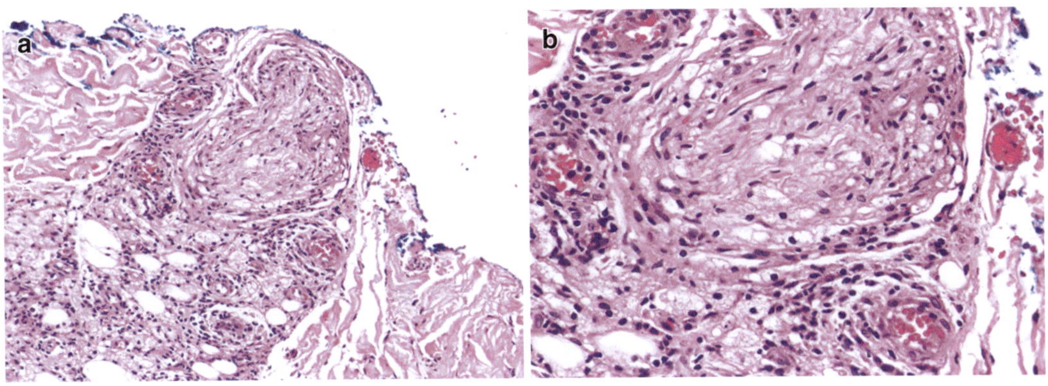

Fig. 5.115 (**a**, **b**) Periadnexal and perivascular lymphohistiocytic inflammation is seen but perineural inflammation is characteristic

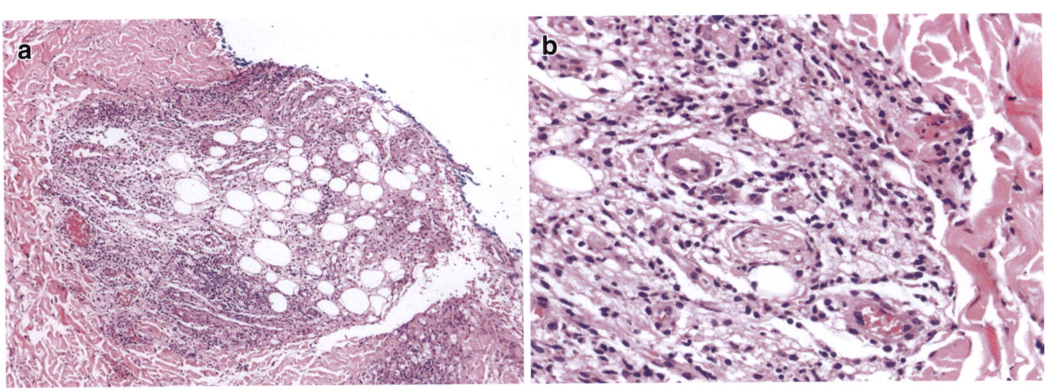

Fig. 5.116 (**a**, **b**) Lymphocytic and histiocytic inflammation in the panniculum with foamy histiocytes

Erythema Toxicum Neonatorum

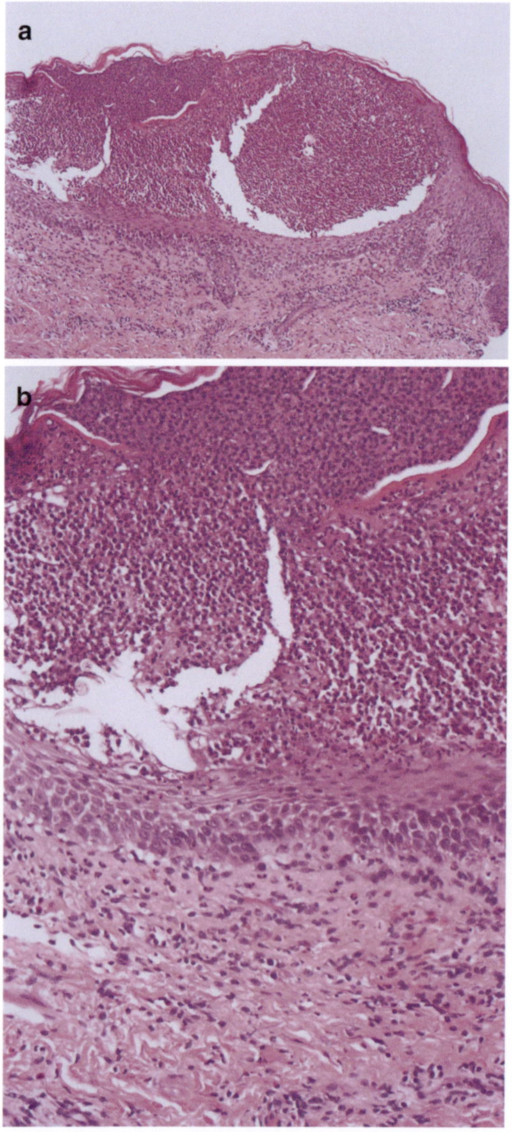

Fig. 5.117 (**a**, **b**) Eosinophilic intraepidermal pustule with dermal eosinophilic inflammation

Synonyms: Erythema Neonatorum, Toxic Erythema of Newborn

Histopathology (Figs. 5.117, 5.118, and 5.119)

- Intraepidermal pustule related to the opening of the follicular infundibulum
- Pustule contains eosinophils and scattered neutrophils
- Eosinophils ae present in the dermis underneath the pustule

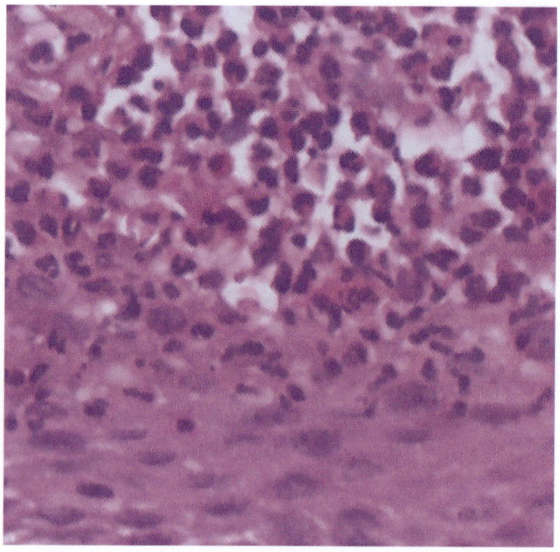

Fig. 5.118 Eosinophils and neutrophils are present in the pustule

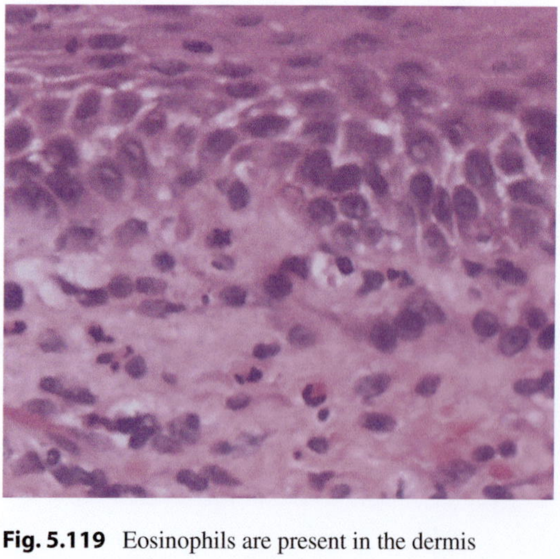

Fig. 5.119 Eosinophils are present in the dermis

Erythrasma

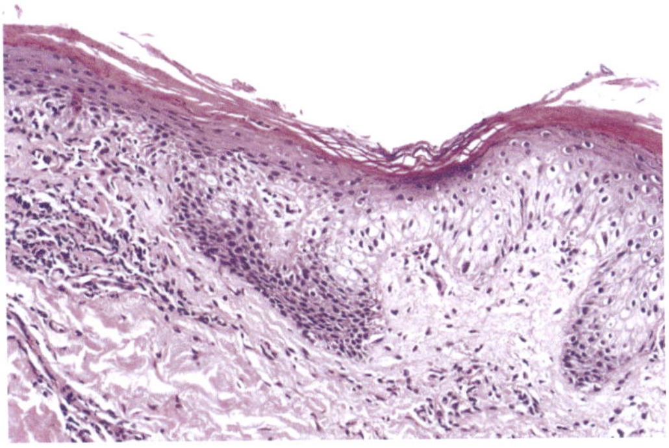

Fig. 5.120 Orthokeratotic epidermis with mild spongiosis and mild dermal perivascular lymphocytic infiltrate

Histopathology (Figs. 5.120, 5.121, 5.122, and 5.123)

- Thickened compact stratum corneum
- Mild epidermal spongiosis
- Mild perivascular lymphocytic infiltrate
- Coccobacilli of *C. minutissimus* in the stratum corneum

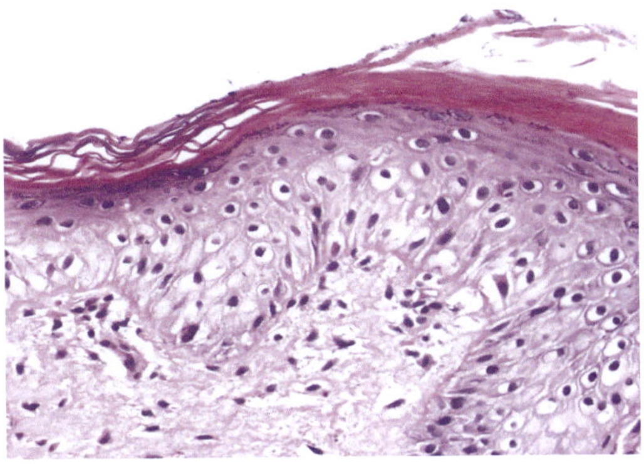

Fig. 5.121 Epidermis with compact stratum corneum

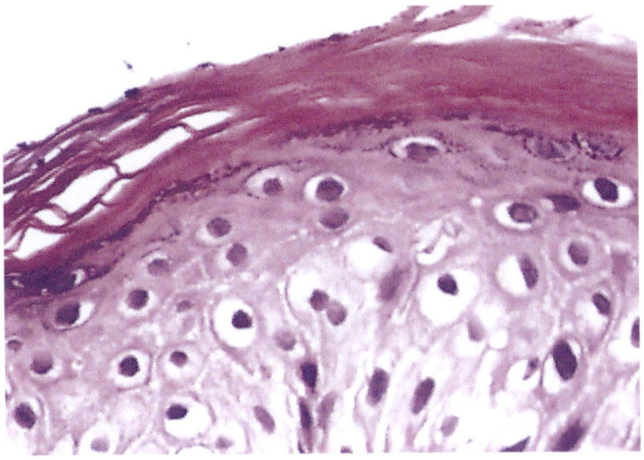

Fig. 5.122 Suggestion of bacteria in the top of stratum corneum

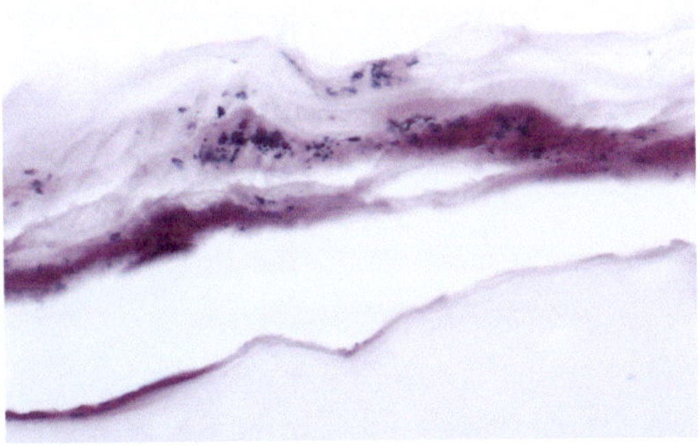

Fig. 5.123 Gram stain highlights coccobacilli in the stratum corneum

Extramammary Fibroadenoma

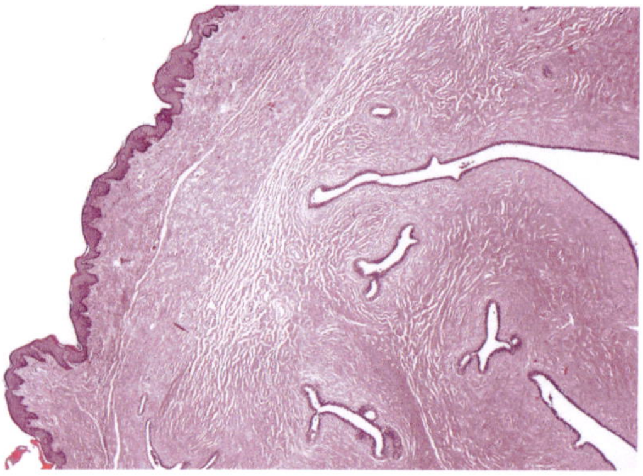

Fig. 5.124 Subcutaneous stroma rich tumor

Rare benign tumor arising in vulva or ectopic mammary tissue.

Histopathology (Figs. 5.124, 5.125, and 5.126)

- Well circumscribed subcutaneous tumor
- Stromal overgrowth (PR+, CD34+) with embedded epithelial elements (CK7+, EMA+)
- Epithelial part of tumor has two layers, inner epithelial and outer myoepithelial
- Apocrine secretion can be seen

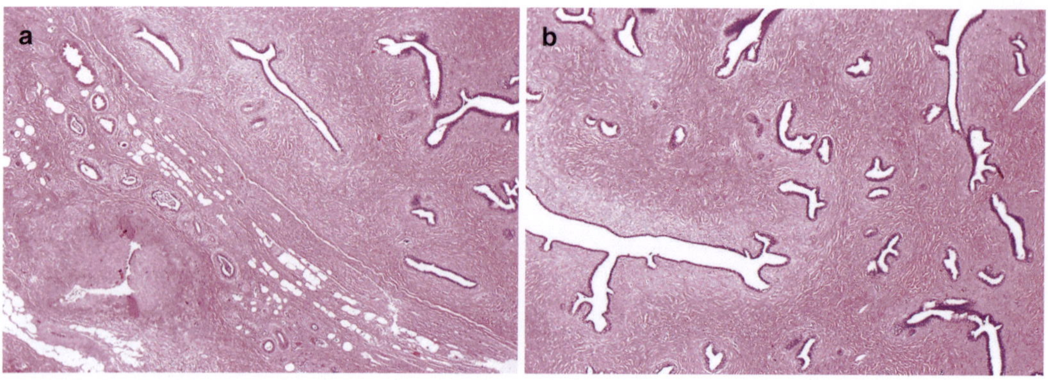

Fig. 5.125 (**a**, **b**) Breast like appearing glands are embedded in dense stroma

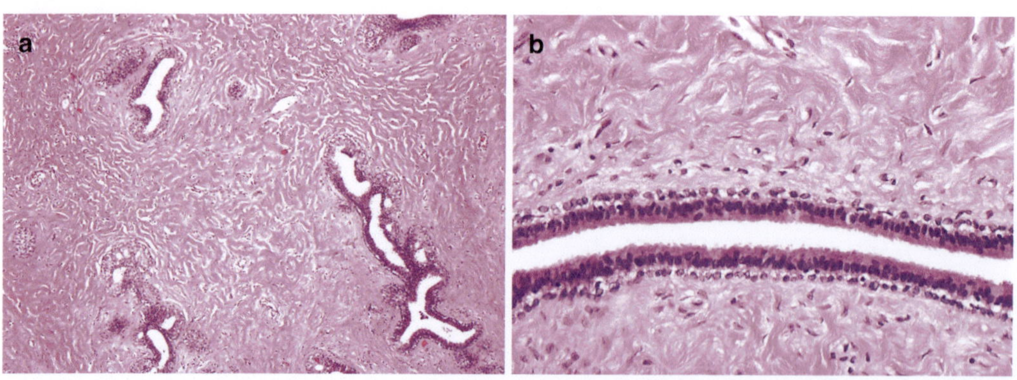

Fig. 5.126 (**a**, **b**) Glands are made of two layers, inner epithelial, with apocrine secretion, and outer myoepithelial

Extranodal NK/T-Cell Lymphoma, Nasal Type

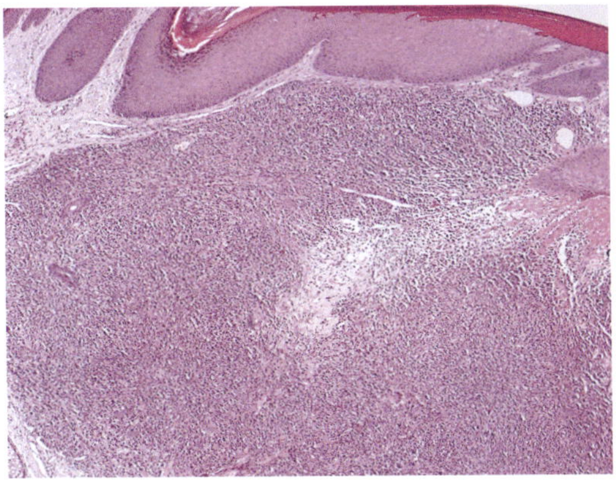

Fig. 5.127 Diffuse dermal and subcutaneous infiltrate

Synonym: Angiocentric Lymphoma

Histopathology (Figs. 5.127, 5.128, 5.129, 5.130, and 5.131)

- Diffuse dermal and subcutaneous atypical lymphocytic infiltrate that is CD2+, granzyme B+, perforin+, CD56+ and CD3−, CD4−, CD5−, CD7−, CD8−
- Prominent angiocentricity and/or angiodestruction with common necrosis
- Lymphocytes can have variable cytology from small to large cell size
- Strong EBV association

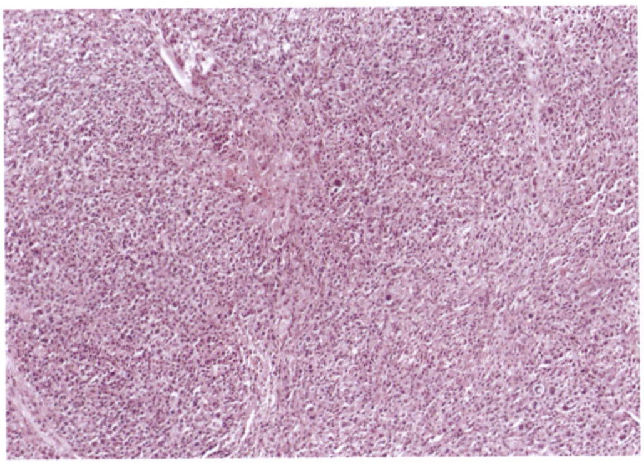

Fig. 5.128 Focal necrosis

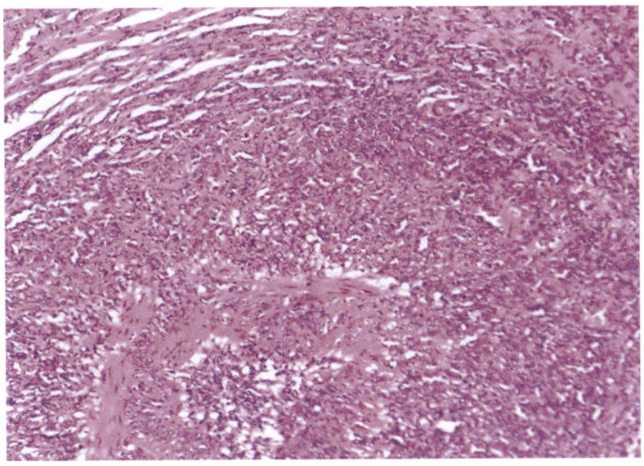

Fig. 5.129 Destruction of medium size vessel with necrosis

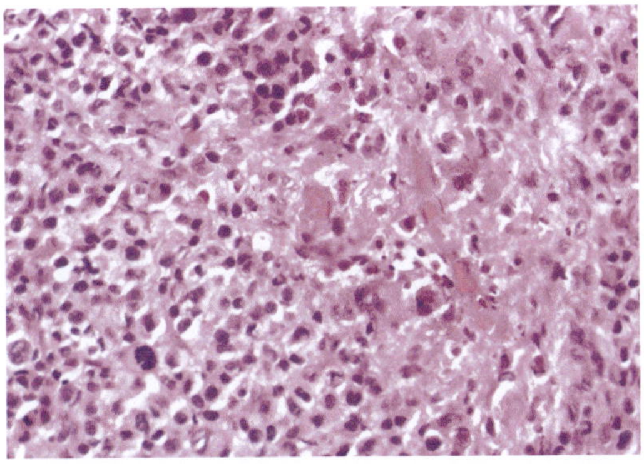

Fig. 5.130 Large atypical lymphocytes with vascular destruction

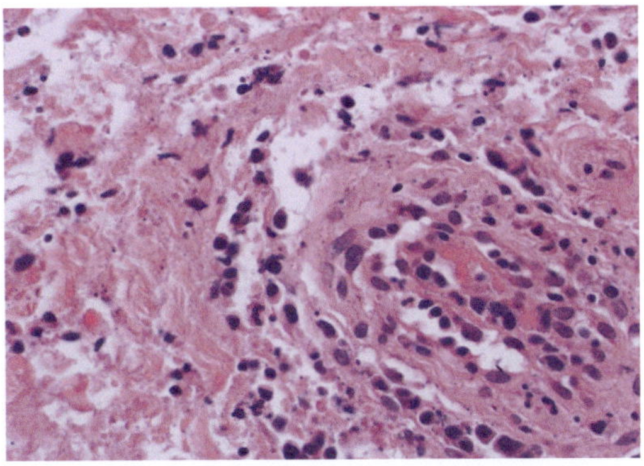

Fig. 5.131 Infiltrate demonstrates angiocentricity

Extrarenal Malignant Rhabdoid Tumor

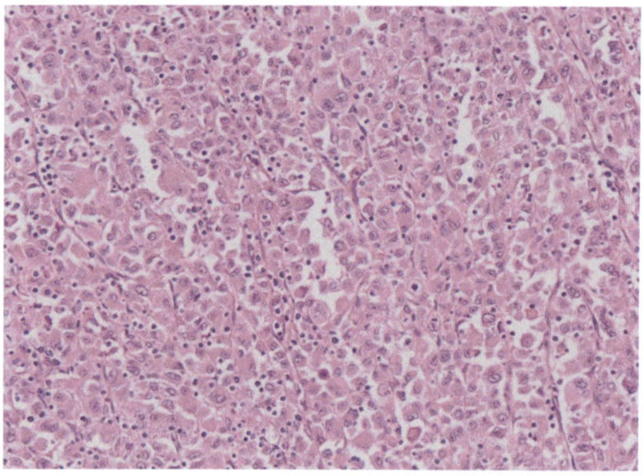

Fig. 5.132 Sheet of large polygonal cells

Histopathology (Figs. 5.132, 5.133, and 5.134)

- Very rare tumor of young children made of subcutaneous sheets of large polygonal cells
- Large round or bean shaped eccentric vesicular nuclei
- Eosinophilic cytoplasm with paranuclear eosinophilic inclusions
- Mitoses and apoptotic cells are frequent
- Tumor cells are keratin positive and negative for muscle markers

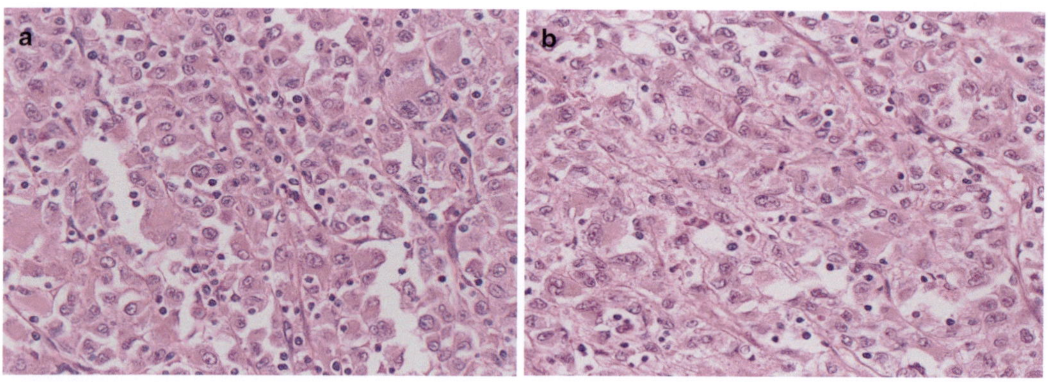

Fig. 5.133 (**a**, **b**) Loosely cohesive cells with prominent eosinophilic cytoplasm; scattered apoptotic cells and mitoses are present

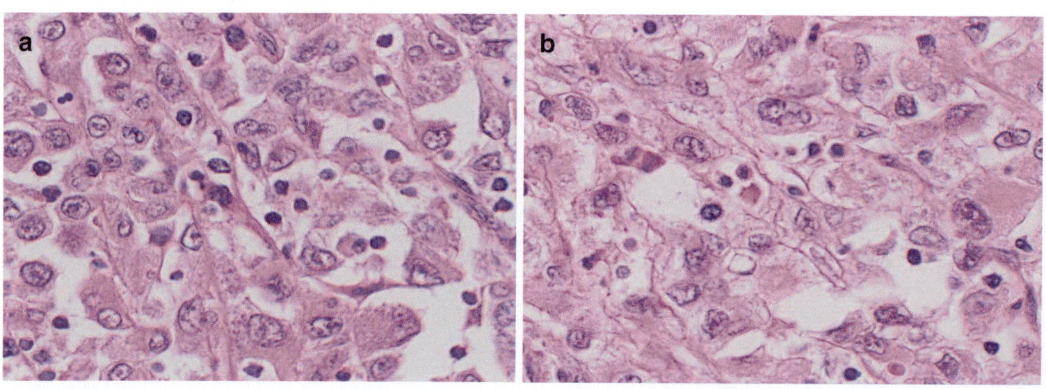

Fig. 5.134 (**a**, **b**) Irregular bean shaped vesicular nuclei, some with prominent nucleoli and eosinophilic cytoplasmic inclusions

6 Dermatopathology F

V. Vincek, *Dermatopathology A–Z*, https://doi.org/10.1007/978-3-319-89486-7_6

Factitial Dermatititis/Panniculitis

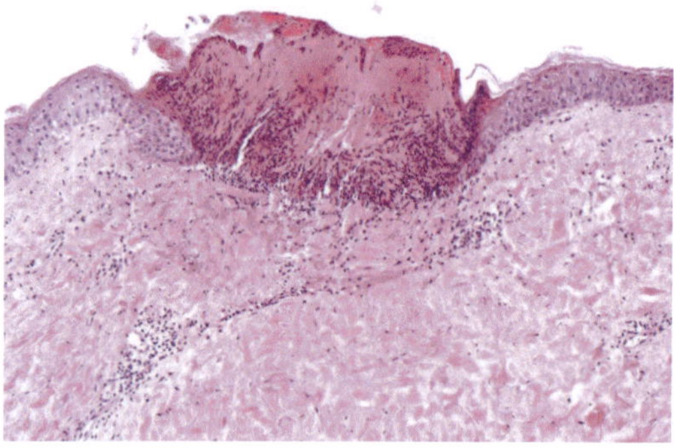

Fig. 6.1 Excoriated epidermis with acutely inflamed serum crust

Histopathology

Dermatitis (Figs. 6.1 and 6.2)

- Excoriated epidermis
- Serum crust with numerous neutrophils
- Mixed inflammation limited to the dermis underneath the excoriation

Panniculitis (Figs. 6.3, 6.4, and 6.5)

- Septal and lobular mixed inflammation
- Fat necrosis with lipogranulomas and "Swiss cheese" pattern
- Necrosis, microcysts and abscess can be present

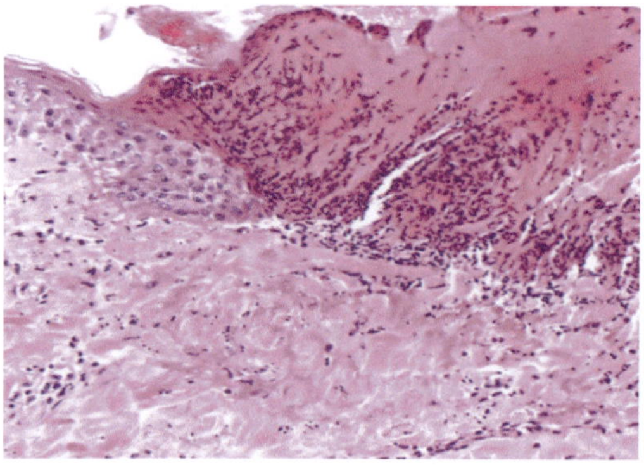

Fig. 6.2 Mixed dermal inflammation limited to the dermis underneath the excoriation

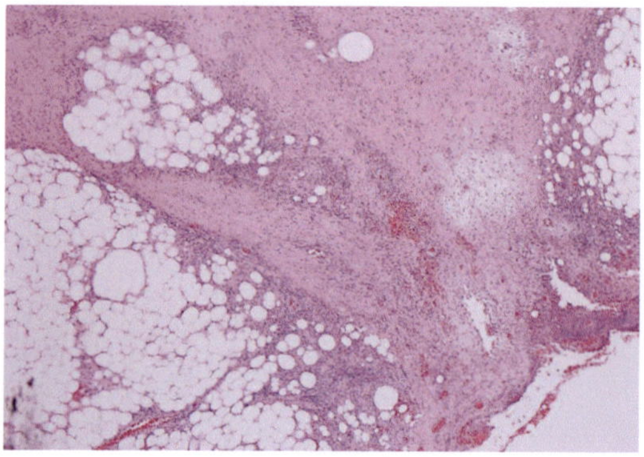

Fig. 6.3 Septal and lobular panniculitis

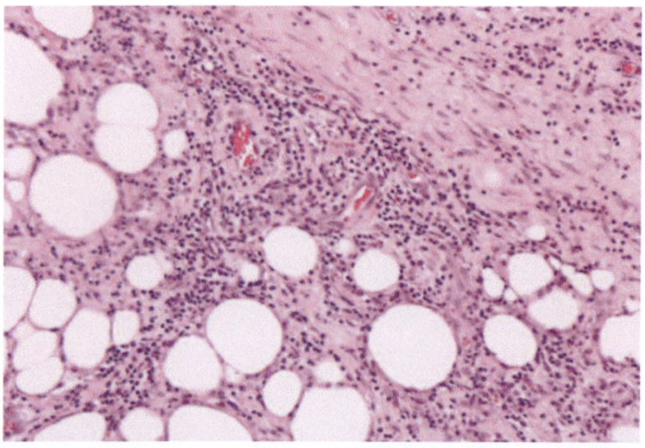

Fig. 6.4 "Swiss cheese" pattern with microcysts and mixed septal and lobular inflammation

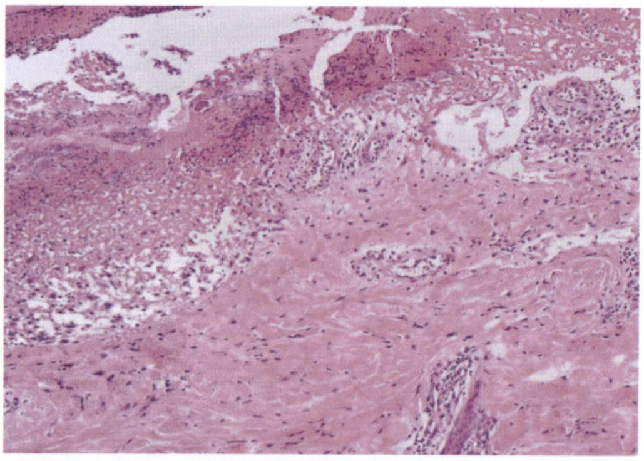

Fig. 6.5 Abscess with surrounding necrosis and scarring

Fibroblastic Connective Tissue Nevus

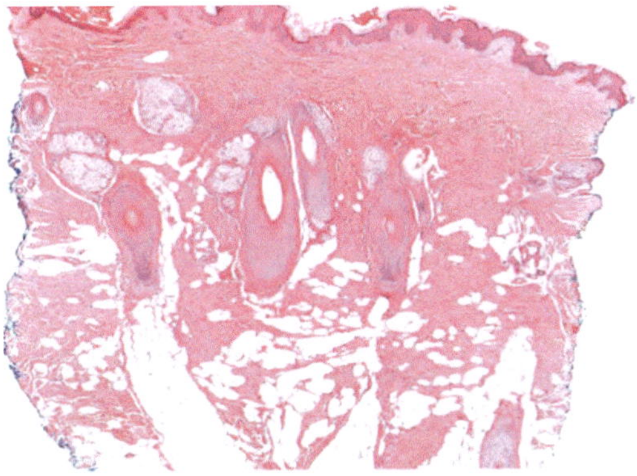

Fig. 6.6 Poorly defined subcutaneous tumor

Histopathology (Figs. 6.6, 6.7, and 6.8)

- Ill-defined proliferation of spindle cells
- Lesion involves deeper dermis and subcutaneous adipose tissue
- Cells have bland appearance with elongated fibroblast-like nuclei and eosinophilic cytoplasm
- No mitoses or cytological atypia
- Focal cells are CD34 positive

P.S. DFSP is in differential diagnosis but DFSP is more cellular and more diffusely CD34 positive

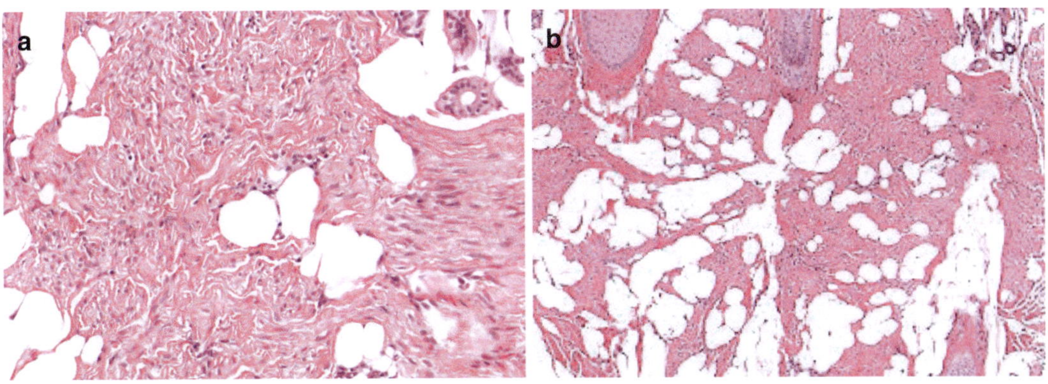

Fig. 6.7 (**a**, **b**) Bland appearing infiltrate in deeper dermis and subcutaneous adipose tissue

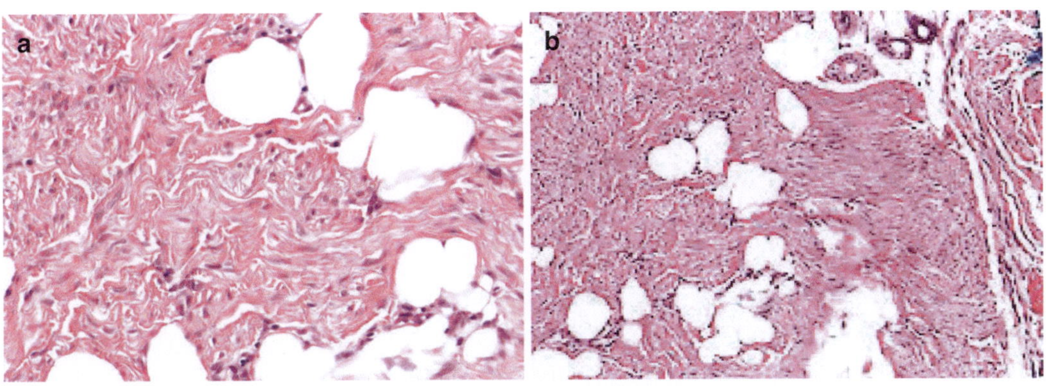

Fig. 6.8 (**a**, **b**) Fibroblast-like cells with elongated nuclei and eosinophilic cytoplasm

Fibroepithelioma of Pinkus

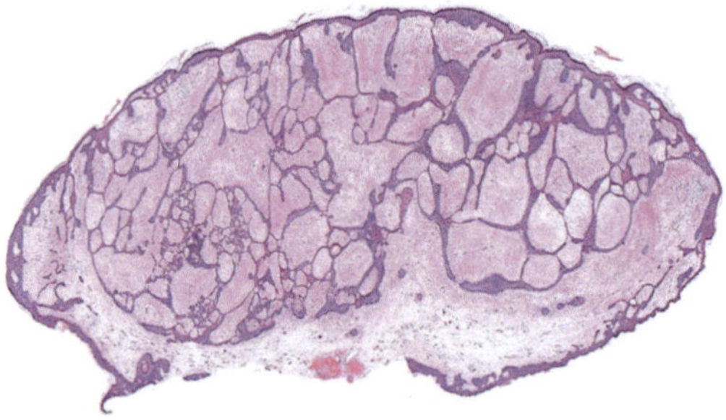

Fig. 6.9 Polypoid tumor originates from multiple epidermal points

A variant of basal cell carcinoma.

Histopathology (Figs. 6.9, 6.10, and 6.11)

- Polypoid tumor with thin cords of anastomosing basaloid cells forming complex "net-like" reticulate pattern
- The cords originate from multiple epidermal points and there is no evidence of well-defined peripheral palisading
- Tumor is surrounded by fibrous stroma without evidence of stromal retraction

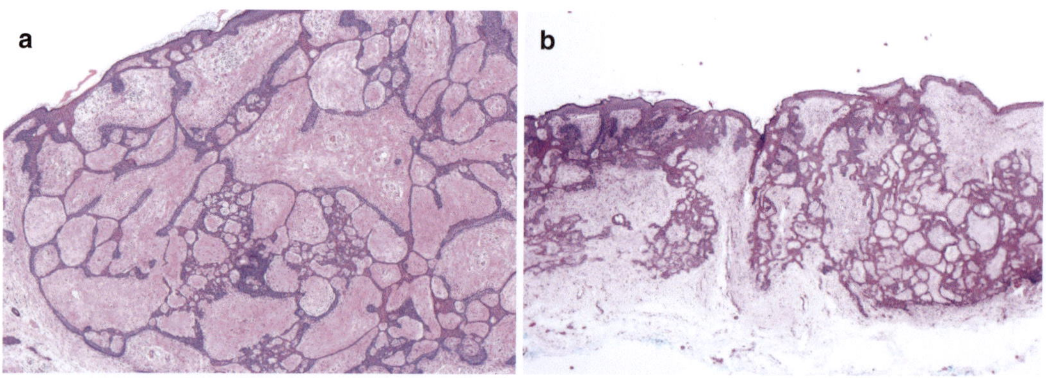

Fig. 6.10 (**a**, **b**) Basaloid cells form "net-like" pattern in fibrous stroma

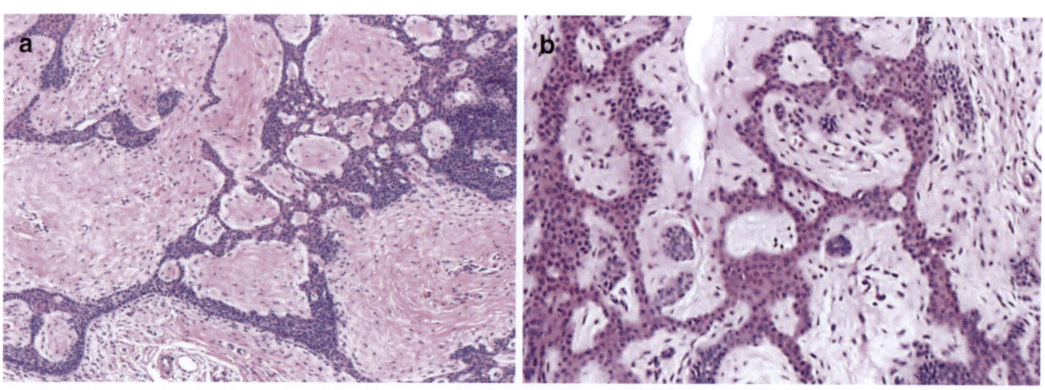

Fig. 6.11 (**a**, **b**) Tumor cords are made of two to three cells without peripheral palisading. Stroma is sclerotic and not retracted from the tumor

Fibrofolliculoma

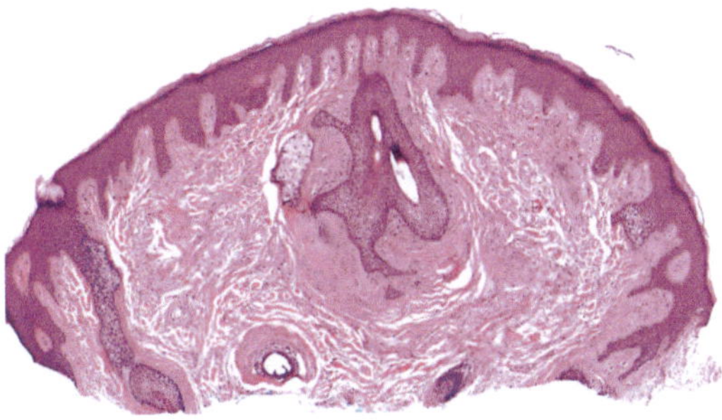

Fig. 6.12 Skin nodule with central follicular structure

Histopathology (Figs. 6.12, 6.13, and 6.14)

- Dilated distorted hair follicle
- Epithelioid strands arise from the infundibulum of the hair follicle and swirl around the central follicle
- Follicle is surrounded by sclerotic fibrous tissue in a circular pattern

P.S. associated with Birt-Hogg-Dubé syndrome (*FLCN*)

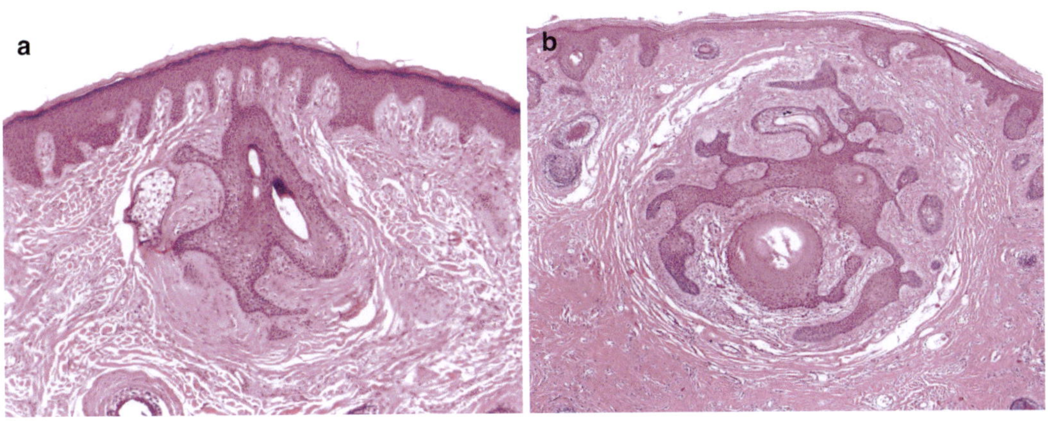

Fig. 6.13 (**a**, **b**) Dilated follicle with epithelial strands arising from the infundibulum

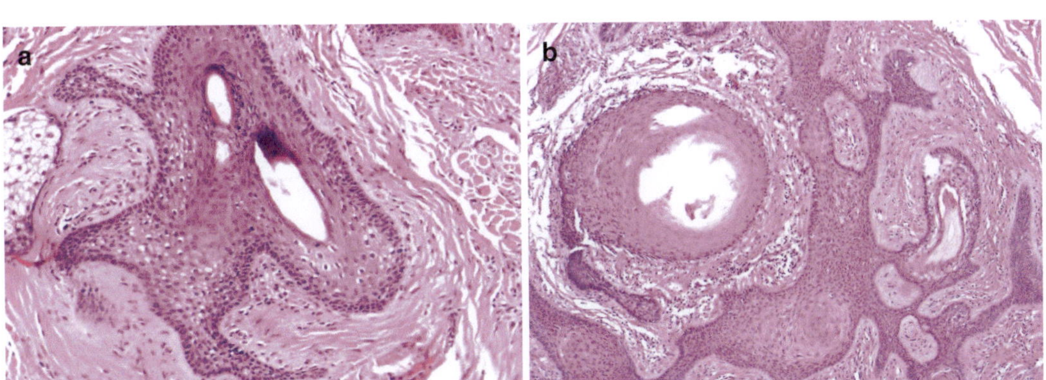

Fig. 6.14 (**a**, **b**) Fibrous stroma encircles the follicle

Fibroma of Tendon Sheath

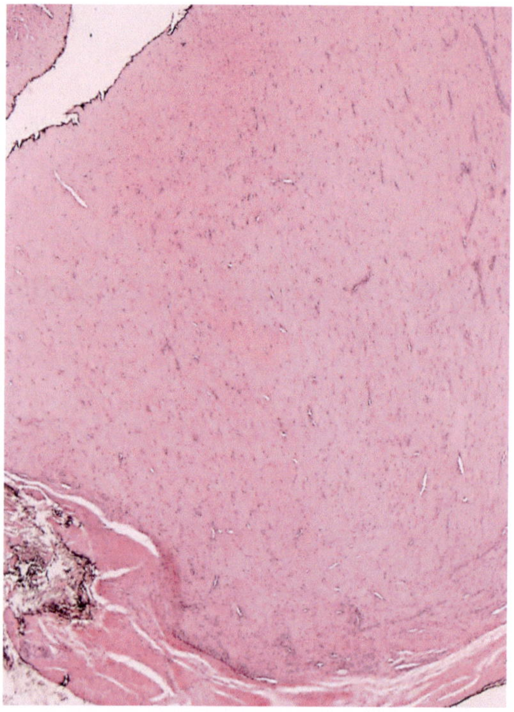

Fig. 6.15 Subcutaneous hypocellular sclerotic nodule

Histopathology (Figs. 6.15, 6.16, and 6.17)

- Well-circumscribed subcutaneous round or oval tumor nodule
- Sclerotic hyalinized eosinophilic stroma
- Spindle shaped tumor cells (SMA+, vimentin+) are few and scattered
- There are no mitoses or atypia
- Capillaries are compressed by the stroma

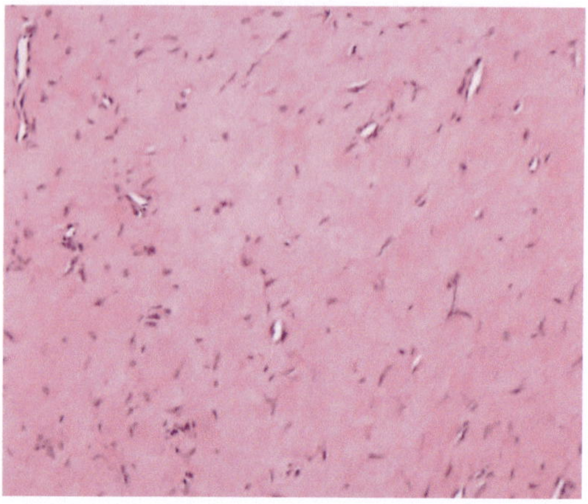

Fig. 6.16 Elongated spindle shape tumor cells in hyalinized stroma. Capillaries have "slit-like" appearance

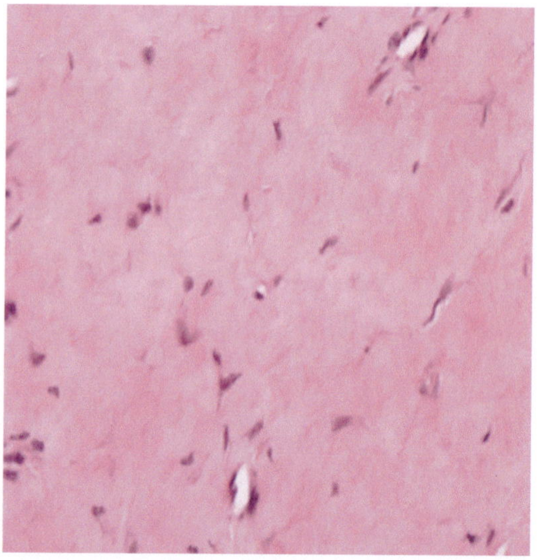

Fig. 6.17 Hypocellular tumor with no mitoses or significant atypia

Fibromatosis

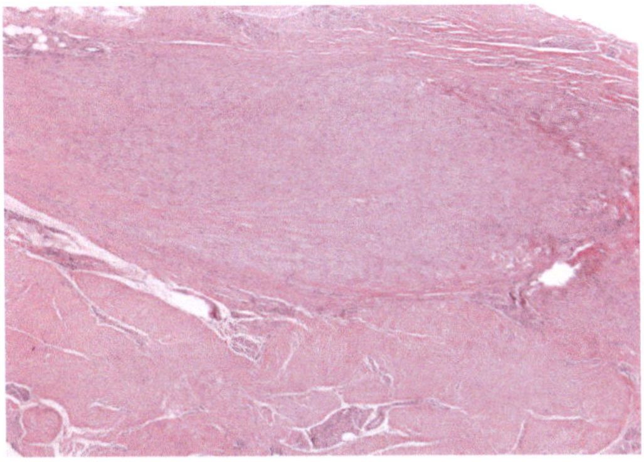

Fig. 6.18 Deep-seated tumor nodule

Synonyms: Desmoid Fibromatosis, Palmoplantar Fibromatosis

Histopathology (Figs. 6.18, 6.19, and 6.20)

- Subcutaneous deep-seated fibrous proliferation
- Growth along fascia, aponeurosis, and tendons
- Fascicles of spindle shaped, wavy fibroblasts with variable cellularity and fibrotic stroma
- 85% of cases have mutation in beta-catenin
- Cells are vimentin+, nuclear beta-catenin+

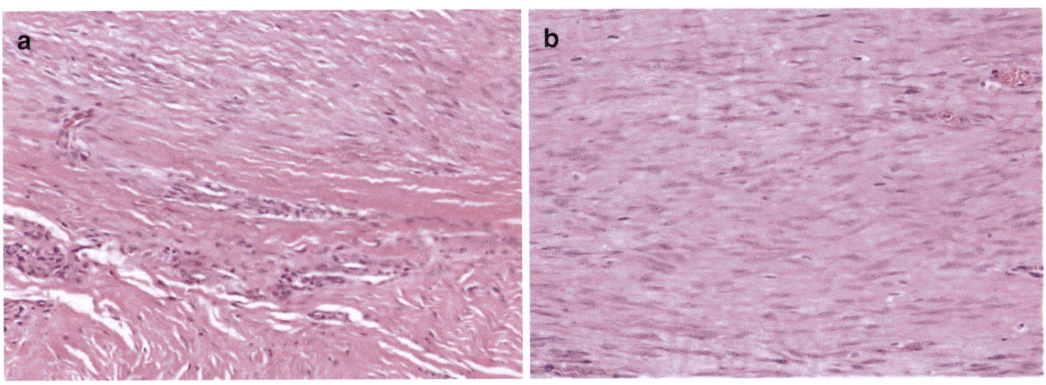

Fig. 6.19 (**a**, **b**) Spindle cells form fascicle with variable cellularity in fibrous stroma

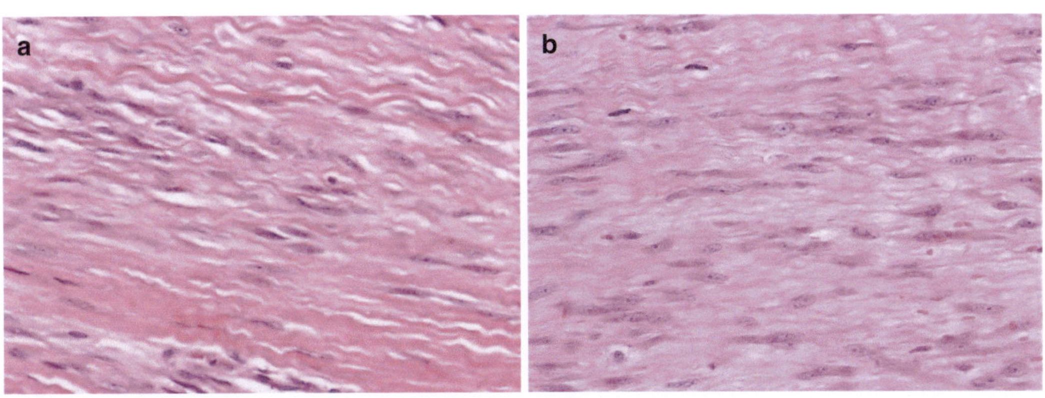

Fig. 6.20 (**a**, **b**) Elongated, wavy fibroblasts with vesicular nuclei

Fibro-osseous Pseudotumor of the Digits

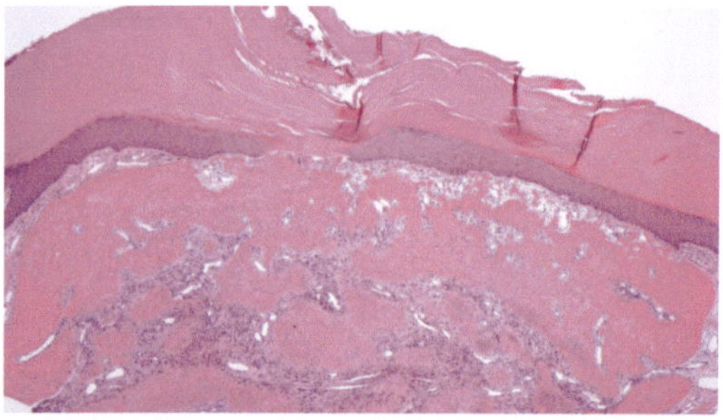

Fig. 6.21 Acral skin with ossified dermal tumor

Histopathology (Figs. 6.21, 6.22, and 6.23)

- Acral epidermis with thick stratum corneum
- Dermal ill-defined nodule
- Osteoid and mature bone in myxoid stroma
- Stroma contains spindle shaped myofibroblasts
- Mitotic figures can be seen
- Cells are calponin+, SMA+

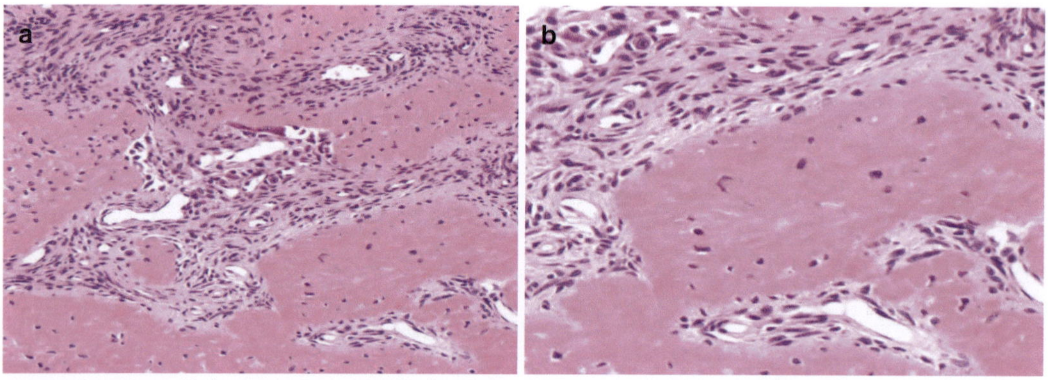

Fig. 6.22 (**a**, **b**) Spindle cells in myxoid stroma surround osteoid

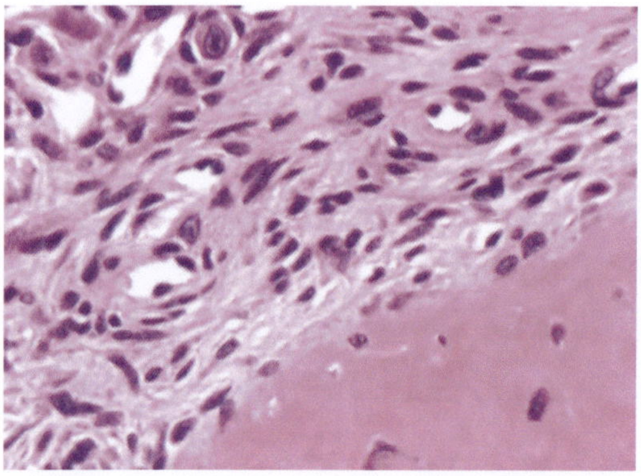

Fig. 6.23 Spindle cells show moderate atypia

Fibrosarcoma

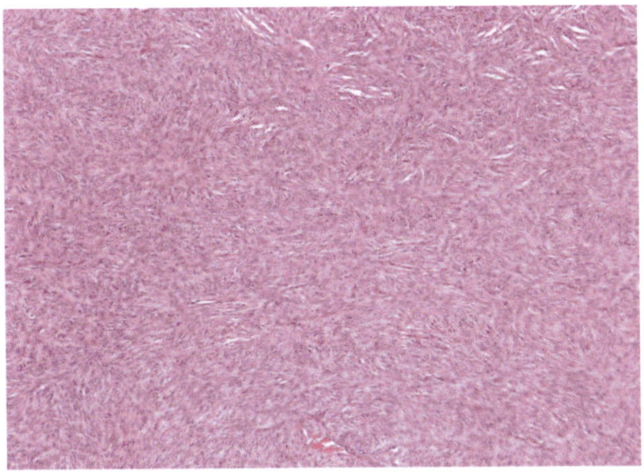

Fig. 6.24 Deeply seated hypercellular tumor

Diagnosis of fibrosarcoma is a diagnosis of exclusion as there are no specific IHC markers.

Histopathology (Figs. 6.24, 6.25, and 6.26)

- Deeply seated subcutaneous tumor made of spindled fibroblasts with elongated nuclei, thin tapered ends, and scant cytoplasm
- Cells form fascicles arranged in "herringbone" pattern with minimal intervening collagenous stroma
- Mild pleomorphism and increased mitotic activity

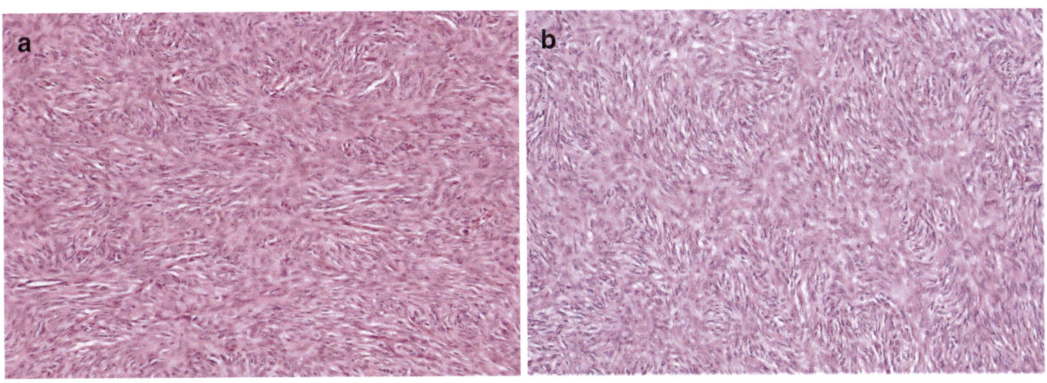

Fig. 6.25 (**a**, **b**) Fascicles arranged in acute angles to each other ("herringbone" pattern)

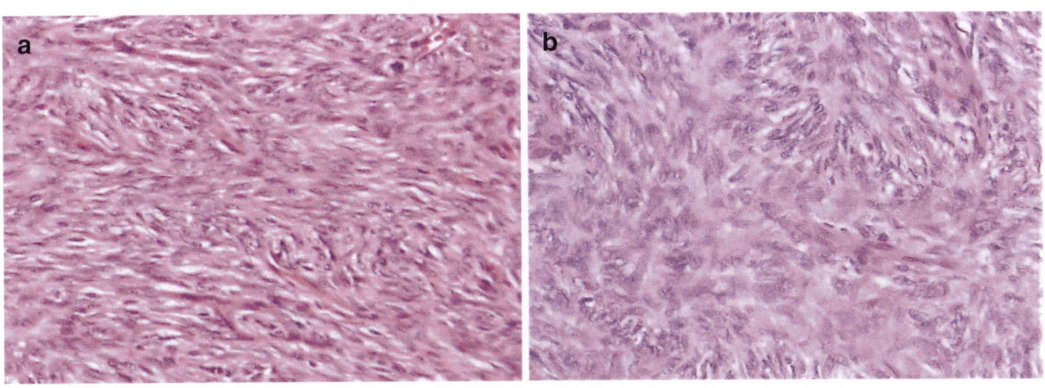

Fig. 6.26 (**a**, **b**) Cells are oval to spindle shaped with elongated nuclei and mild atypia; minimal stroma is present

Fibrous Hamartoma of Infancy

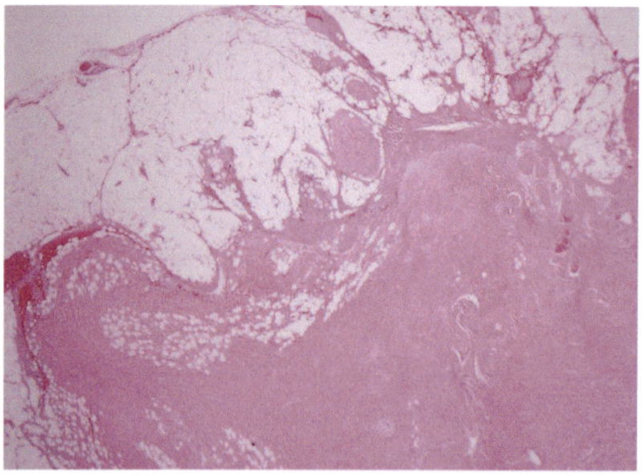

Fig. 6.27 Irregular subcutaneous lesion

Histopathology (Figs. 6.27, 6.28, 6.29, and 6.30)

- Poorly defined lesion in the deep subcutis
- The lesion consists of three components
  - a) Fibrous trabeculae
  - b) Mesenchymal myxoid foci with oval to spindle cells
  - c) Mature adipose tissue
- Fibrous and mesenchymal areas are vimentin+

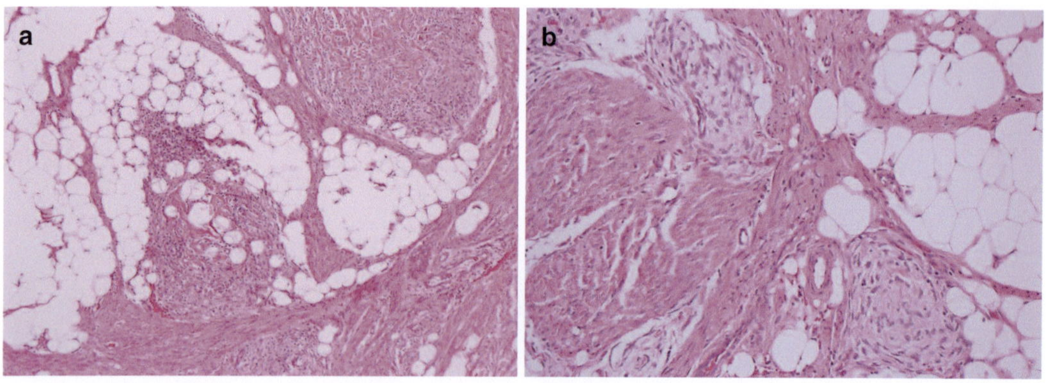

Fig. 6.28 (**a**, **b**) Fibrous fascicles with adipose tissue and myxoid islands

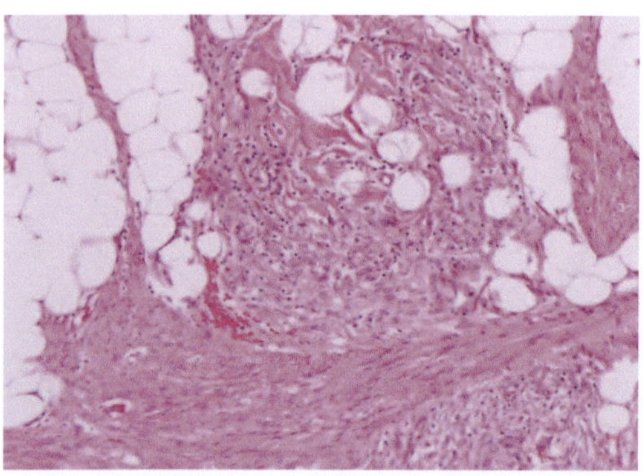

Fig. 6.29 Fascicles are made of delicate myofibroblasts in sclerotic stroma

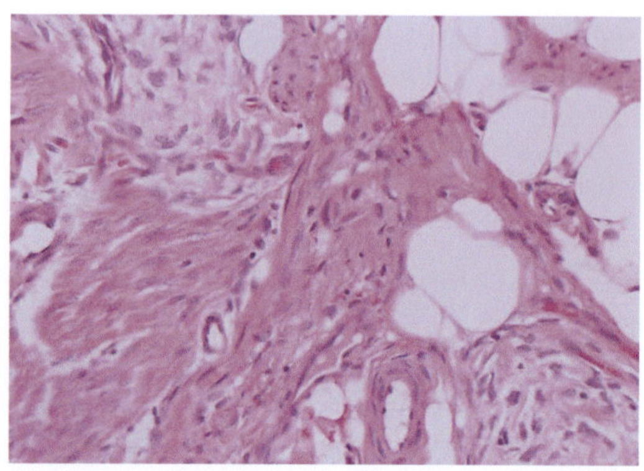

Fig. 6.30 Myxoid islands contain pale cells with vesicular nuclei

Fixed Drug Reaction

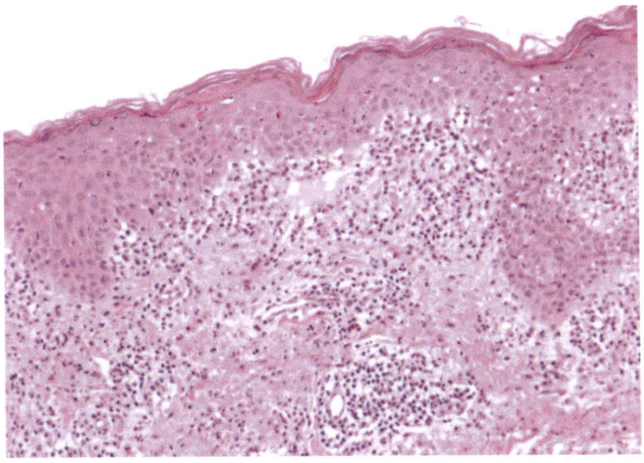

Fig. 6.31 Interface dermatitis

Histopathology (Figs. 6.31, 6.32, 6.33, 6.34, and 6.35)

- Epidermal interface vacuolar changes
- Focal necrotic keratinocytes
- Variable perivascular and lichenoid dermal lymphocytic infiltrate
- Number of dermal eosinophils and neutrophils vary from few to many
- Dermal pigment incontinence can be the only finding in late lesions with few or no eosinophils

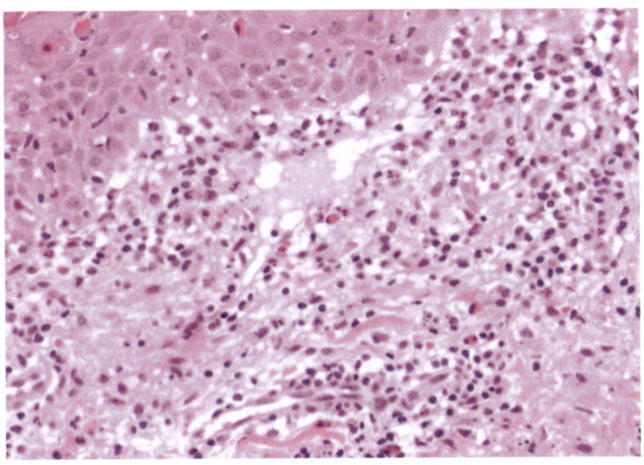

Fig. 6.32 Interface vacuolar changes with necrotic keratinocytes

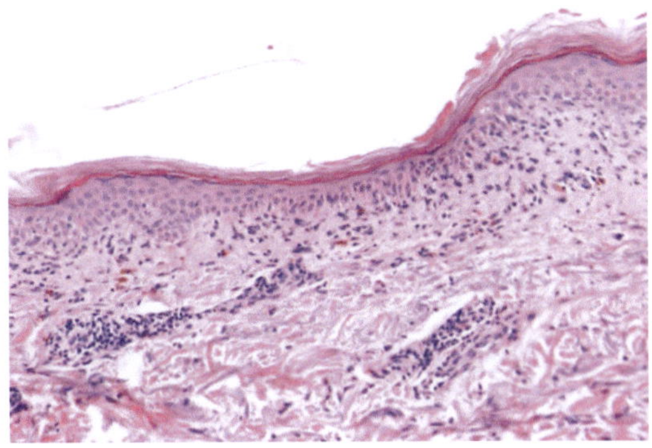

Fig. 6.33 In a late lesion, the epidermis is atrophic with subtle interface changes

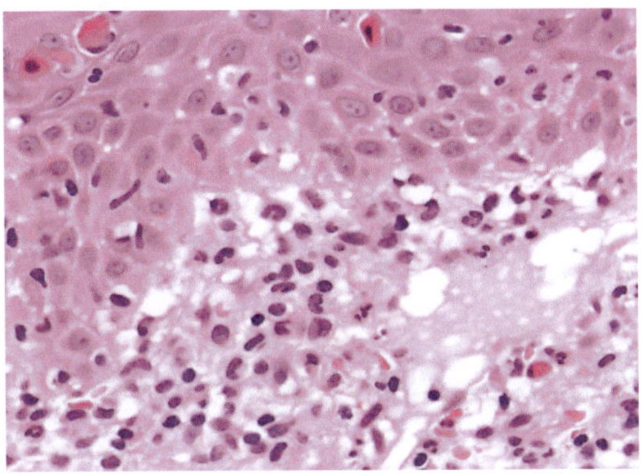

Fig. 6.34 Dermal mixed inflammation with eosinophils

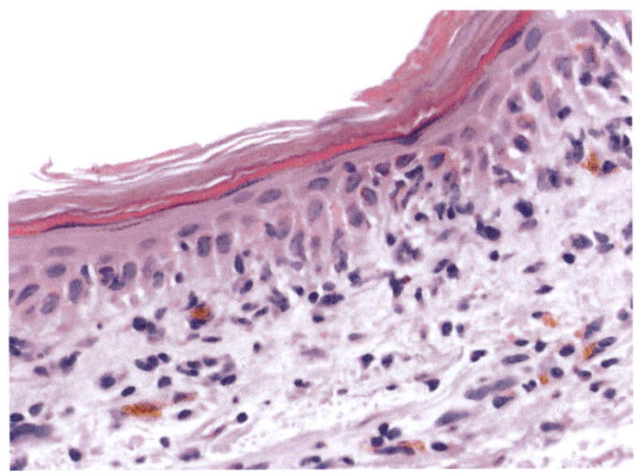

Fig. 6.35 Prominent dermal pigment incontinence with mild inflammation and no eosinophils

Focal Dermal Mucinosis

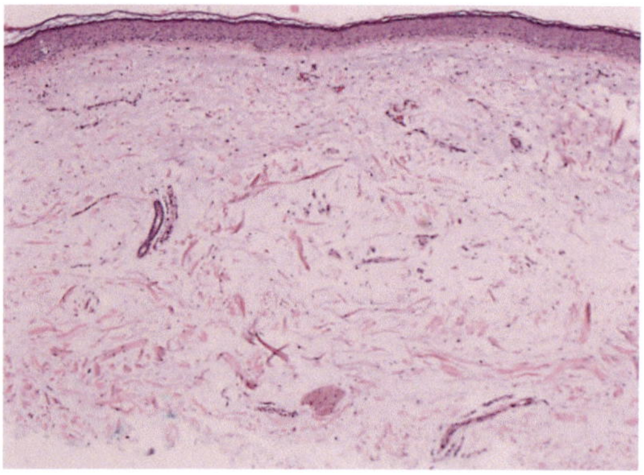

Fig. 6.36 Pale, bluish dermal deposition

Synonym: Focal Mucinosis

Histopathology (Figs. 6.36, 6.37, 6.38, and 6.39)

- Slightly elevated nodule
- Atrophic epidermis
- Replacement of dermal collagen with mucin
- Lesion is hypocellular with no inflammation

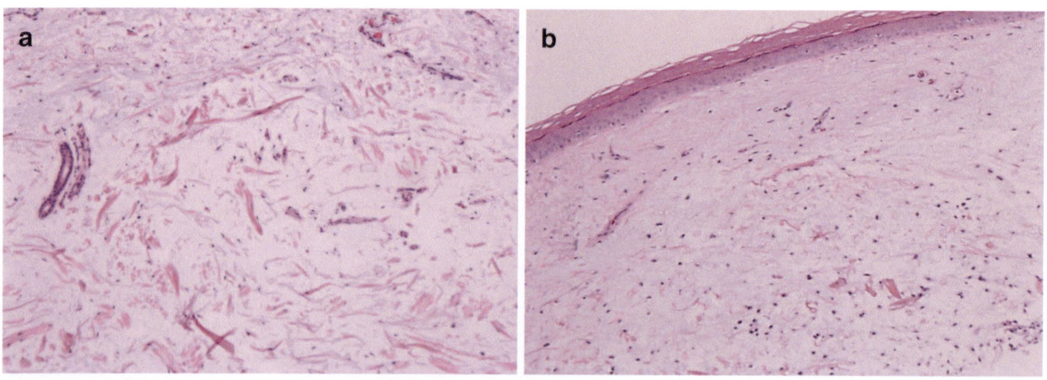

Fig. 6.37 (**a**, **b**) Dermal collagen is separated and replaced by bluish mucin

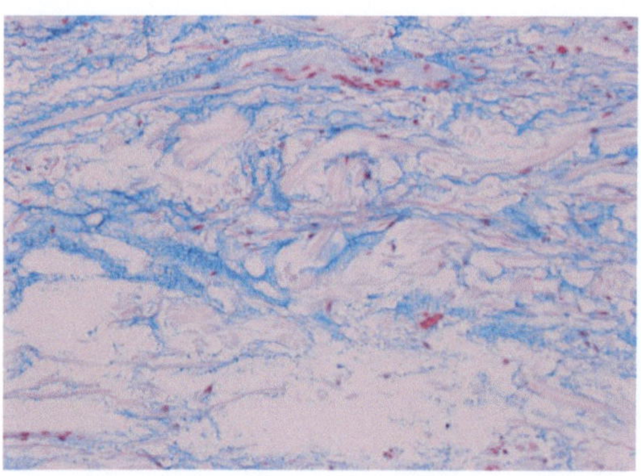

Fig. 6.38 Alcian Blue stains dermal mucin

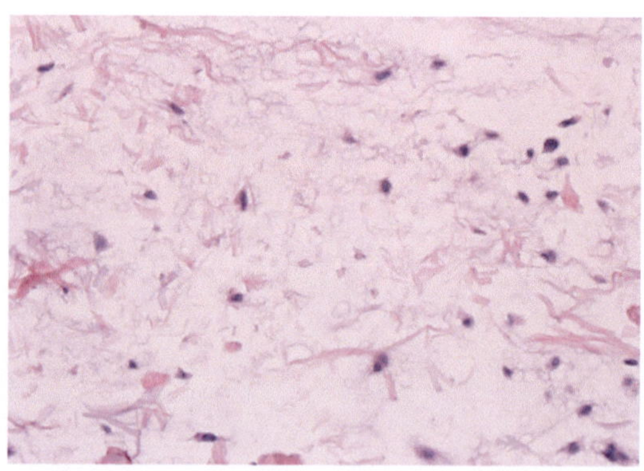

Fig. 6.39 Fibroblasts are scattered

Focal Dermal Hypoplasia

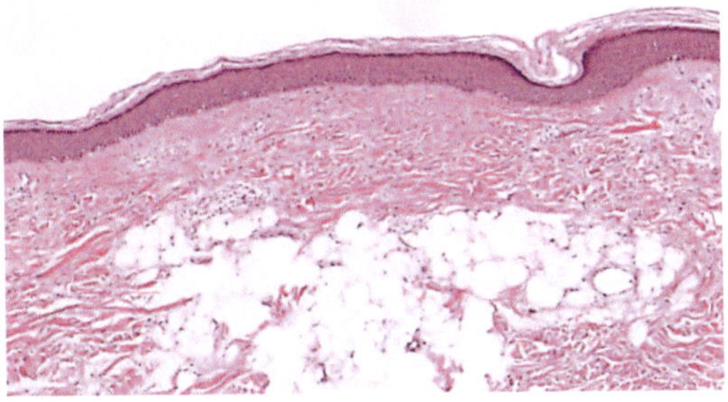

Fig. 6.40 Flattened epidermis with superficial extension of fat

Synonym: Goltz Gorlin Syndrome

Histopathology (Figs. 6.40, 6.41, and 6.42)
- Flattened epidermis
- Reduction in dermal thickness
- Attenuation of dermal collagen
- Absence of adnexal structures
- Extension of adipose tissue into the papillary dermis

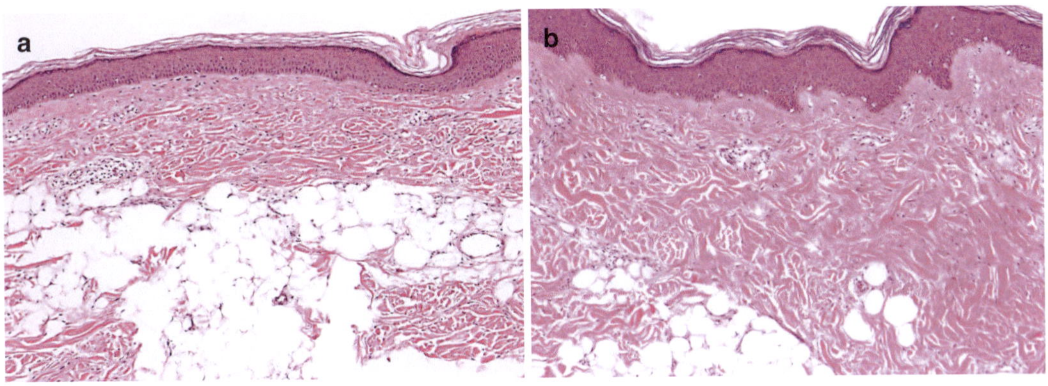

Fig. 6.41 (**a**, **b**) Reduced dermal thickness with extension of adipocytes into dermis

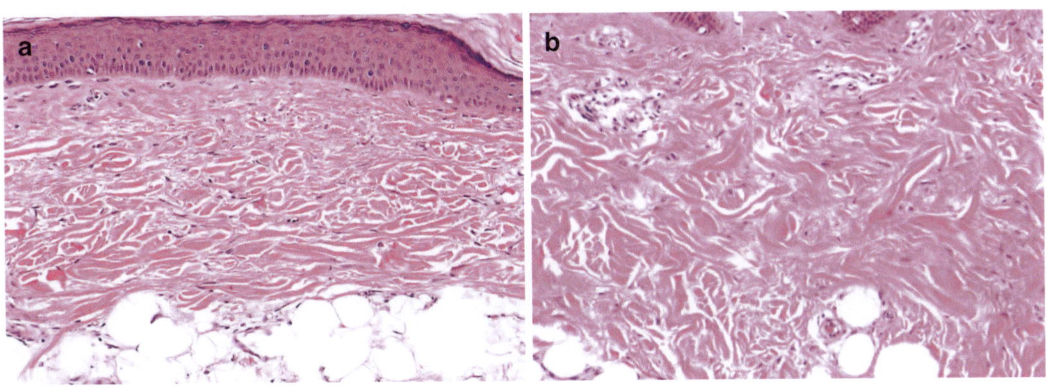

Fig. 6.42 (**a**, **b**) Absence of adnexal structures in the dermis

Follicular Eczema

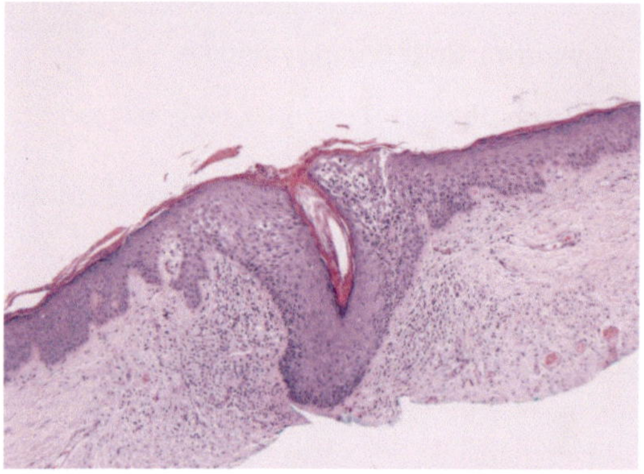

Fig. 6.43 Dilated hair follicle with spongiosis

Histopathology (Figs. 6.43, 6.44, and 6.45)
- Spongiosis of follicular infundibulum
- Lymphocytic exocytosis of infundibulum
- Adjacent epidermis is normal or can show mild spongiosis

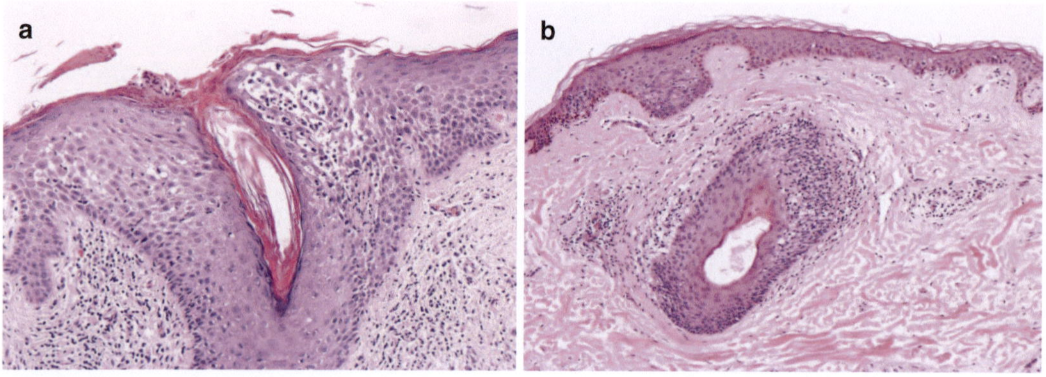

Fig. 6.44 (**a**, **b**) Spongiosis of the upper portion of the follicle while adjacent epidermis is unremarkable

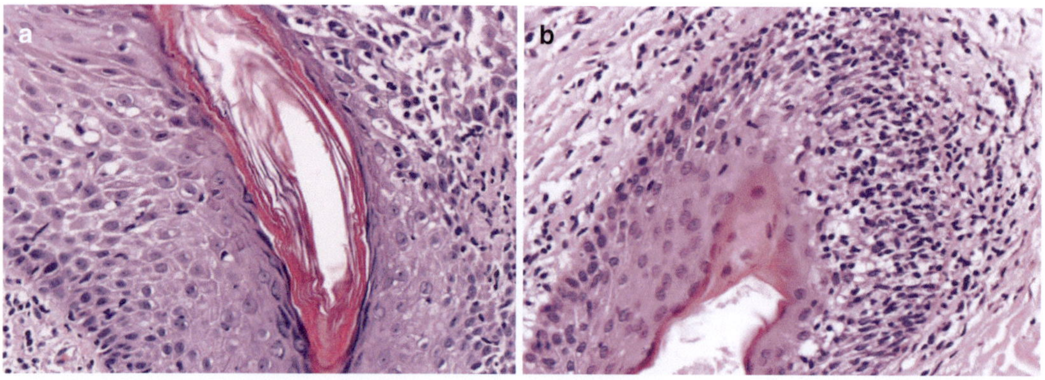

Fig. 6.45 (**a**, **b**) Lymphocytes are present in the follicular infundibulum

Follicular Mucinosis

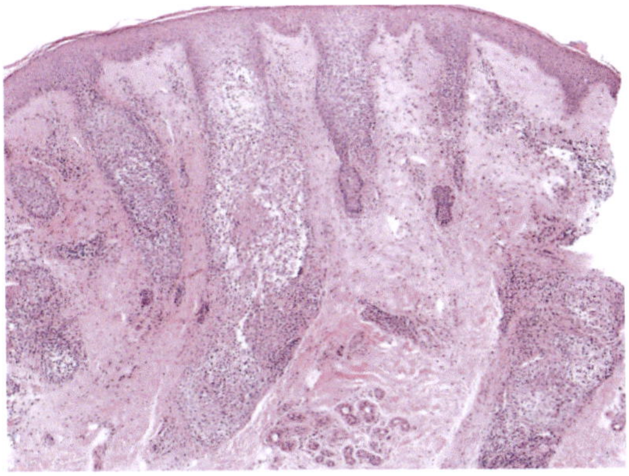

Fig. 6.46 Follicles with mucin and perifollicular inflammation

Synonym: Alopecia Mucinosa

Histopathology (Figs. 6.46, 6.47, 6.48, and 6.49)

- Accumulation of mucin within the hair follicles
- Perifollicular lymphocytic infiltrate
- Variable follicular lymphocytic and eosinophilic exocytosis
- Variable number of perifollicular eosinophils

P.S. cases with follicular lymphocytes and less eosinophils are more likely to represent follicular mycosis fungoides

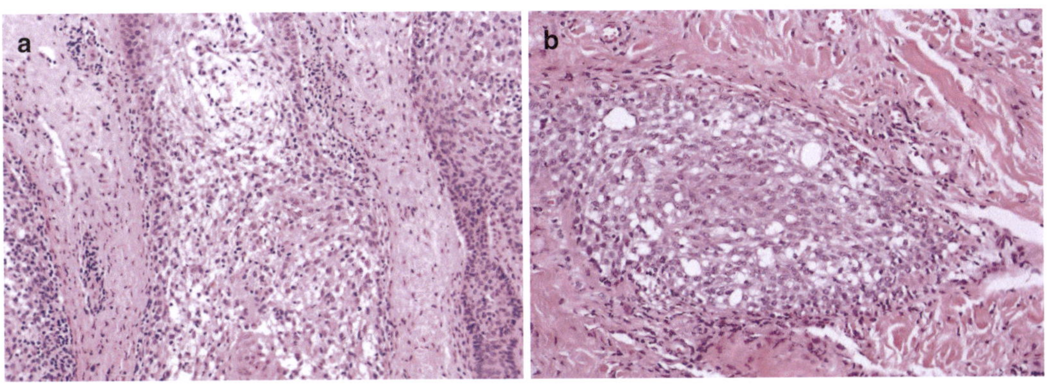

Fig. 6.47 (**a**, **b**) Follicles filled with mucin and lymphocytes

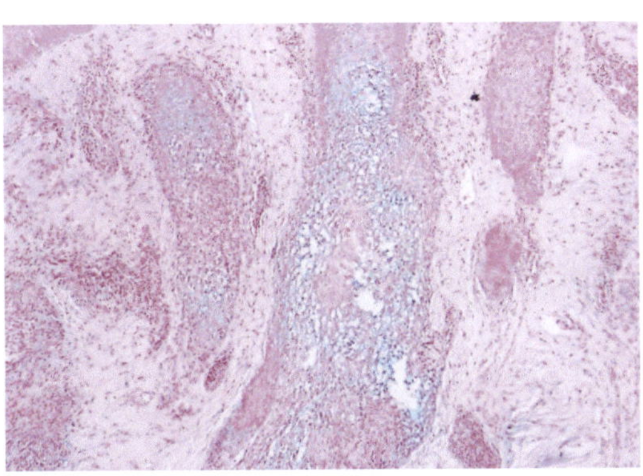

Fig. 6.48 Alcian Blue stain (blue) highlights follicular mucin

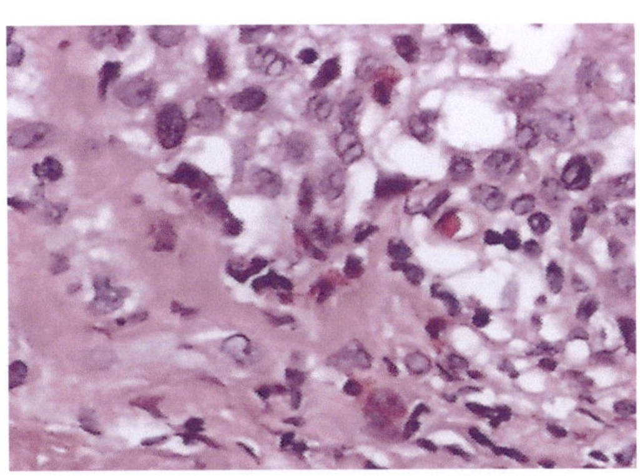

Fig. 6.49 Eosinophils are present in the follicle and in the dermis

Folliculosebaceous Cystic Hamartoma

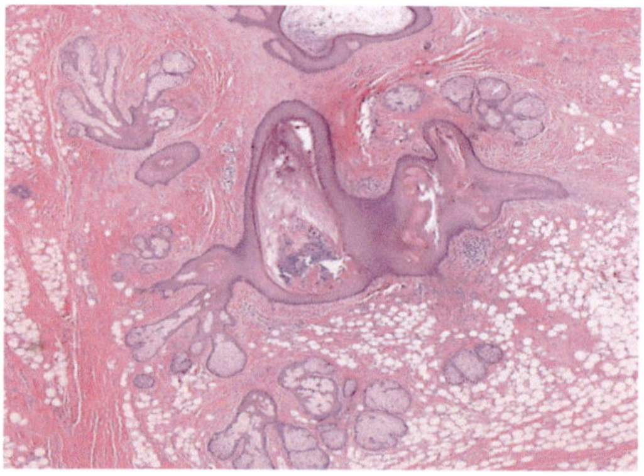

Fig. 6.50 Cystically dilated hair follicle

Hamartoma composed of follicular, sebaceous, and mesenchymal component.

Histopathology (Figs. 6.50, 6.51, 6.52, 6.53, and 6.54)
- Cystically dilated infundibulum
- Mature sebaceous lobules of various sizes are attached or surround the central follicle
- Mature adipocytes and collagen surround the follicle

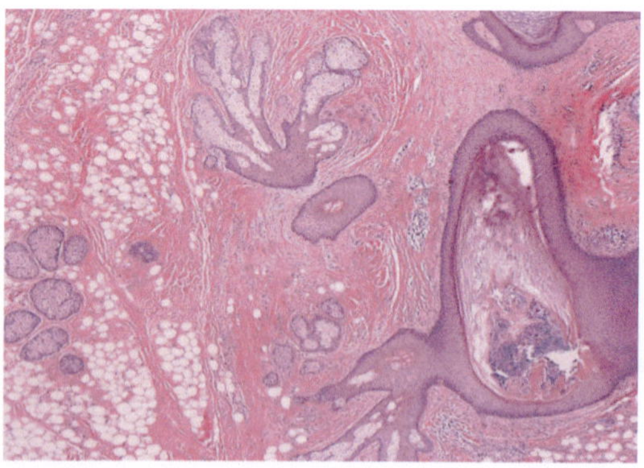

Fig. 6.51 Adipose tissue, follicle, and sebaceous glands

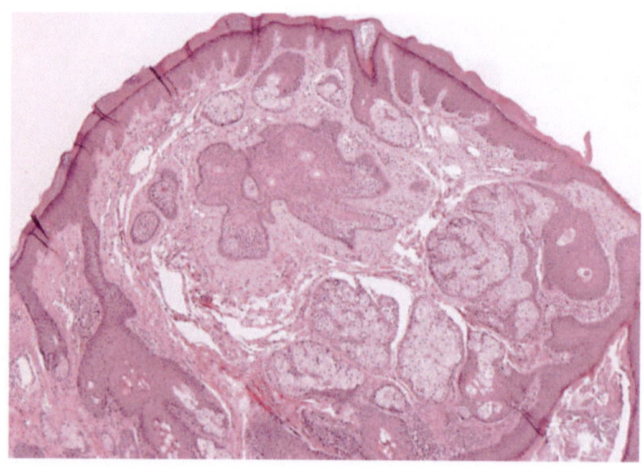

Fig. 6.52 Multiple sebaceous lobules of various sizes are attached to the follicle or standing alone

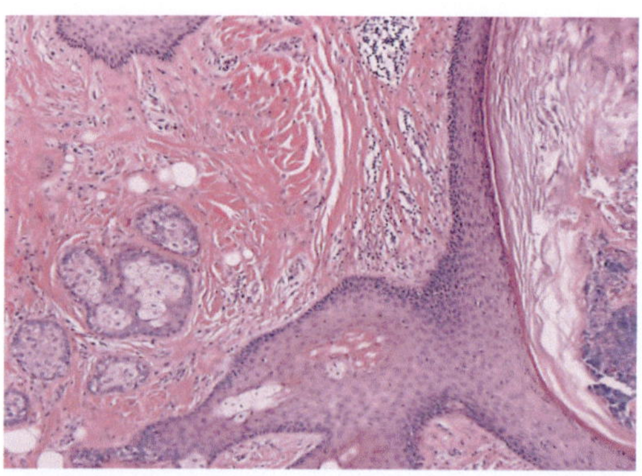

Fig. 6.53 Thick fibrous tissue surrounds adnexal structures

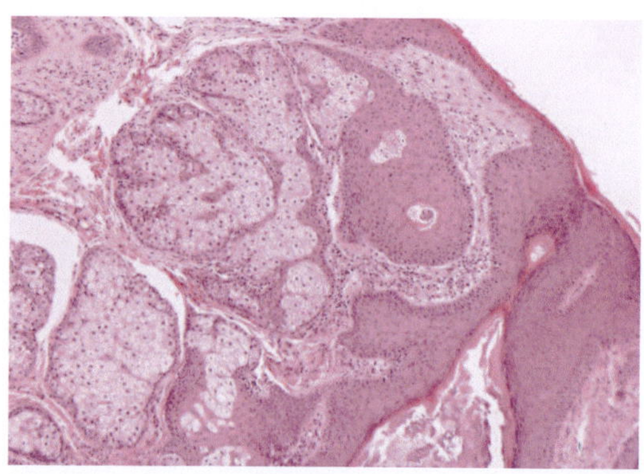

Fig. 6.54 Hair follicle, sebaceous glands, and dense stroma

Folliculitis: Acute

Histopathology (Figs. 6.55, 6.56, 6.57, and 6.58)

- Dilated ruptured follicle
- Intrafollicular and perifollicular neutrophilic inflammation

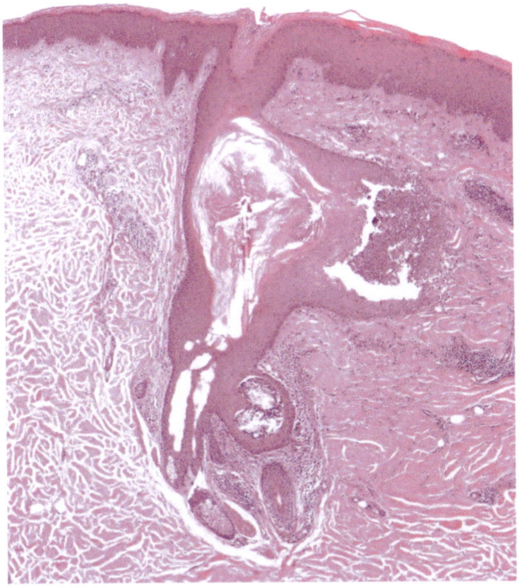

Fig. 6.55 Distorted dilated hair follicle with acute inflammation

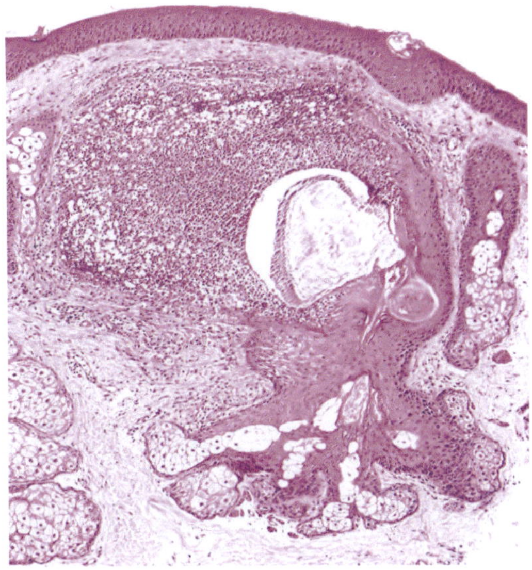

Fig. 6.56 Perifollicular abscess

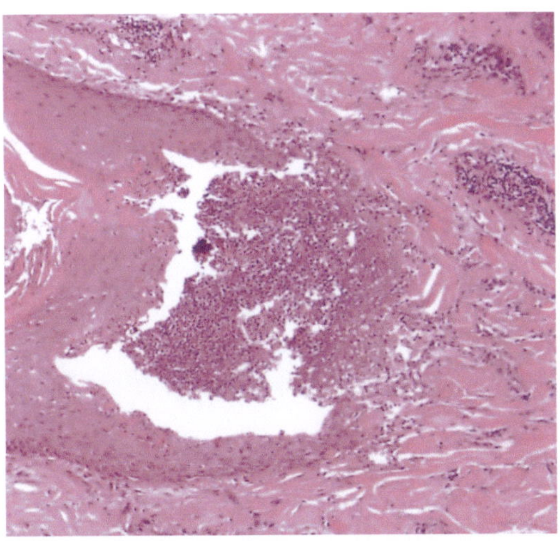

Fig. 6.57 Neutrophilic infiltrate within hair follicle

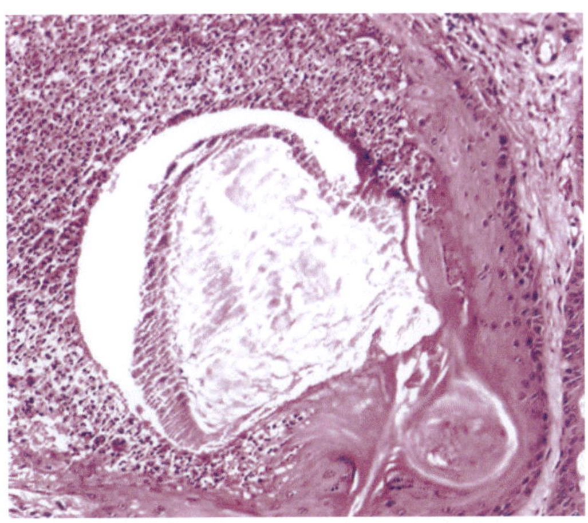

Fig. 6.58 Central necrosis

Folliculitis: Bacterial

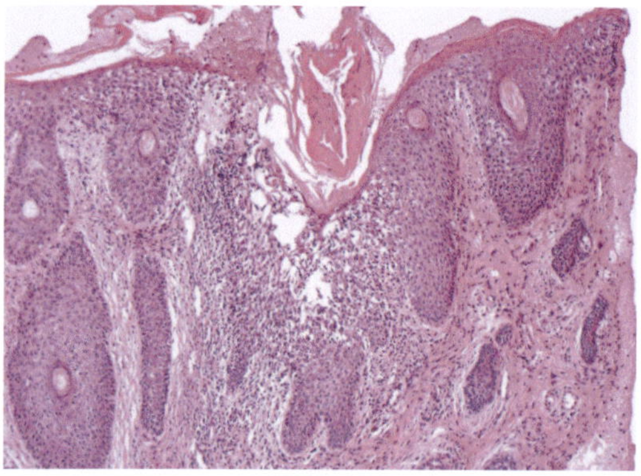

Fig. 6.59 Distorted hair follicle filled with keratin plugging

Histopathology (Figs. 6.59, 6.60, 6.61, 6.62, and 6.63)
- Distorted hair follicle
- Spongiosis of the hair follicle
- Follicle is filled with thick keratin
- Bacterial colonies are present within the follicle
- Perifollicular mixed inflammation
- Neutrophils and lymphocytes within the follicle

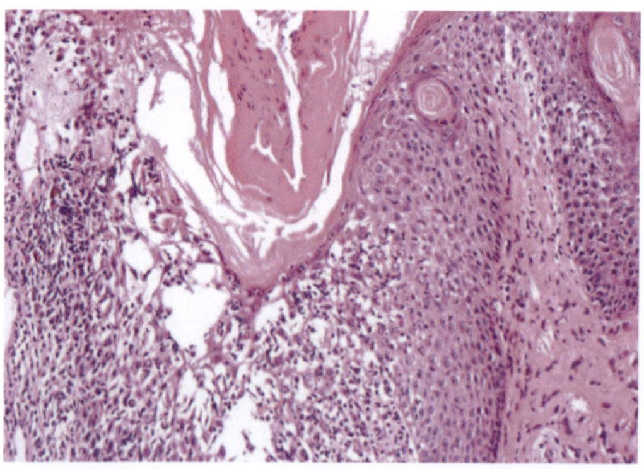

Fig. 6.60 Spongiosis of hair follicle with lymphocytes and neutrophils within the follicle

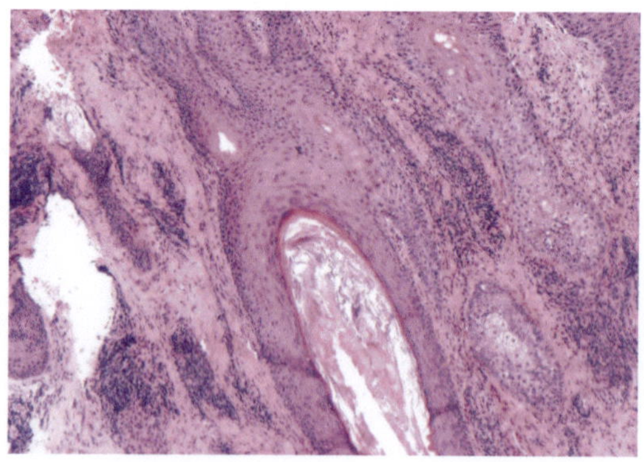

Fig. 6.61 Perifollicular scarring and inflammation

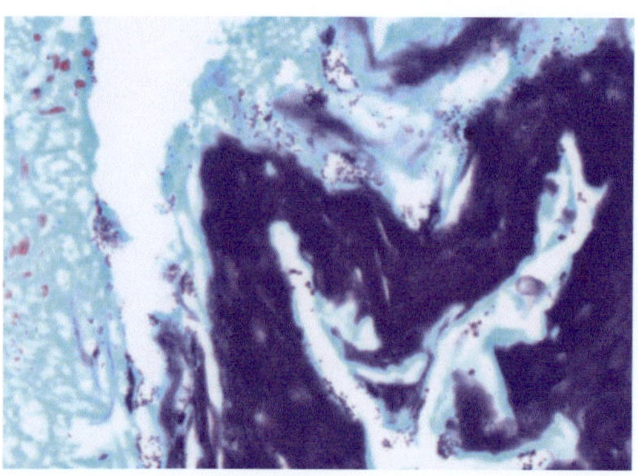

Fig. 6.62 Gram stain highlights bacterial colonies

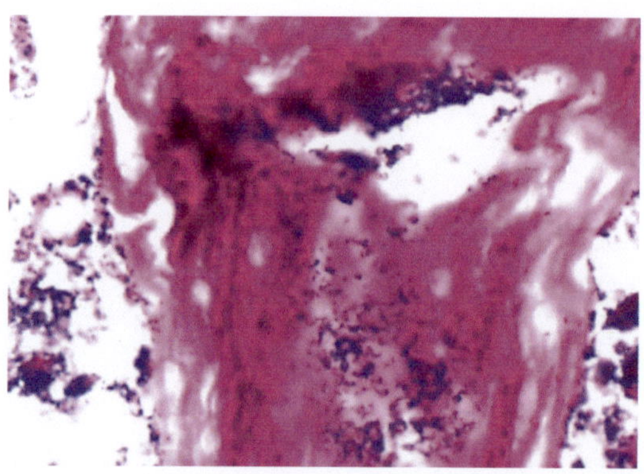

Fig. 6.63 PAS stain also demonstrates bacteria

Folliculitis Decalvans

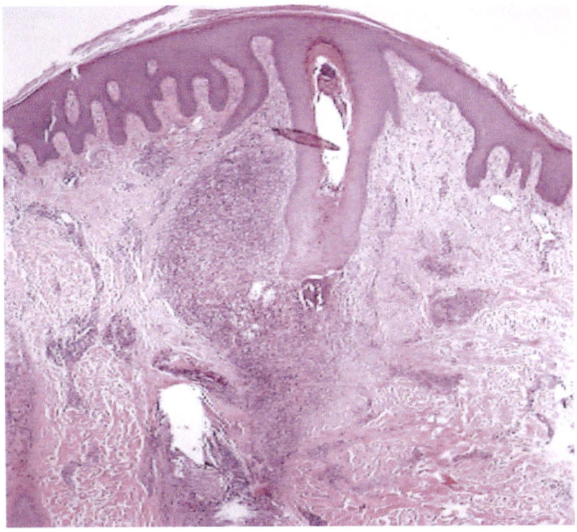

Fig. 6.64 Distorted hair follicle

Histopathology (Figs. 6.64, 6.65, 6.66, 6.67, and 6.68)

- Distorted, ruptured follicle
- Neutrophilic folliculitis with abscess formation
- Foreign body giant cell reaction against hair shaft
- Variable dermal scarring

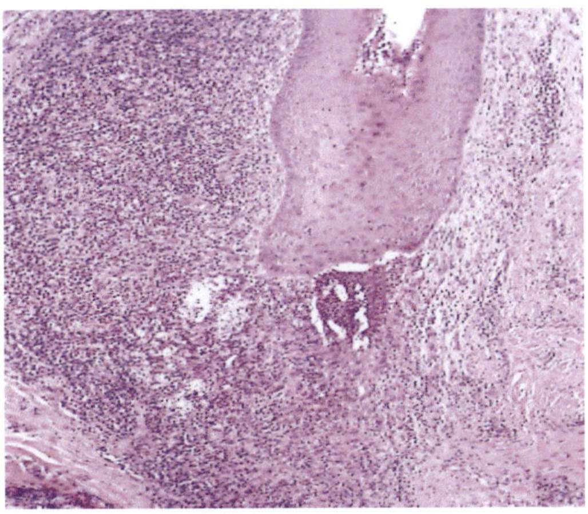

Fig. 6.65 Ruptured follicle with acute inflammation

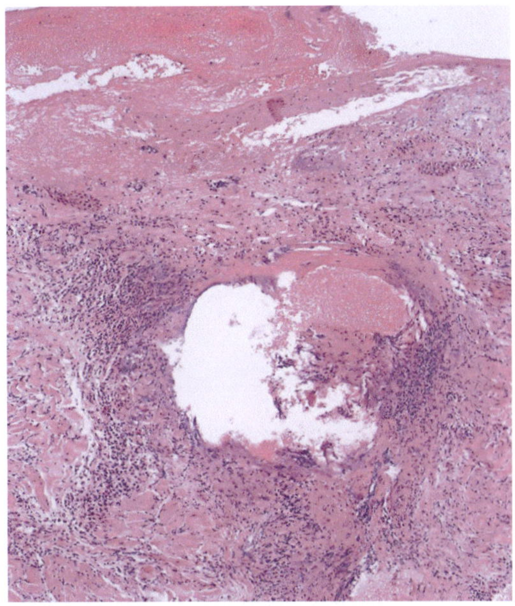

Fig. 6.66 Abscess formation with surrounding scarring

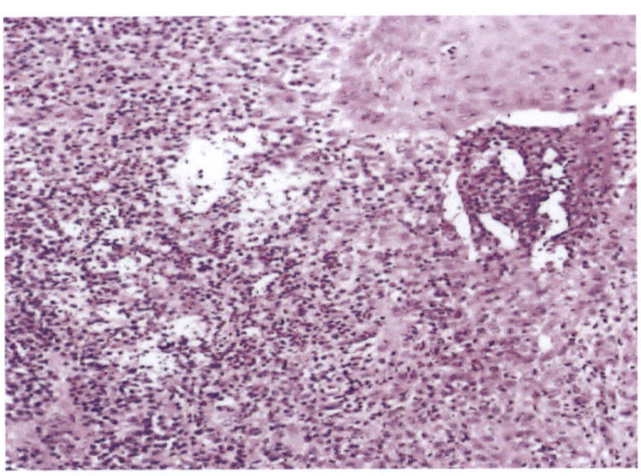

Fig. 6.67 Abscess and giant cell reaction

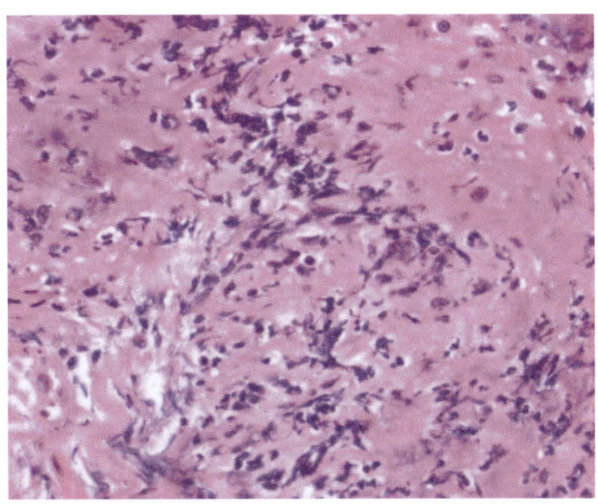

Fig. 6.68 Perifollicular scar

Folliculitis: Demodex

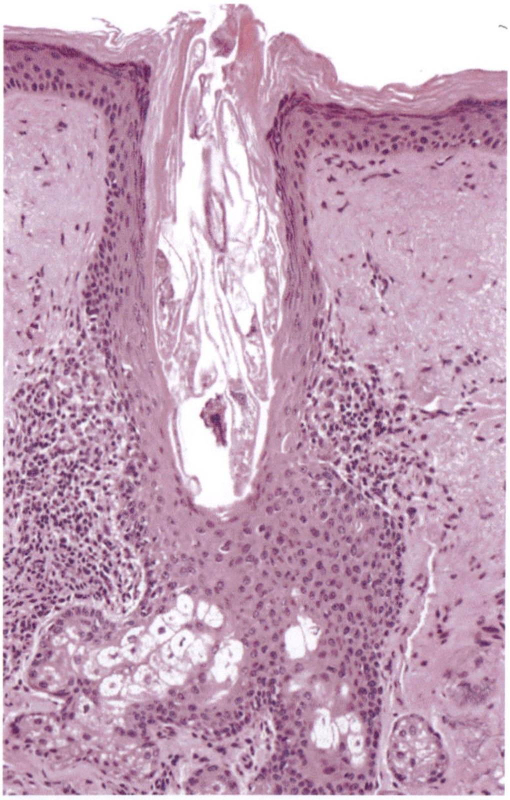

Fig. 6.69 Dilated follicle with *Demodex* mite

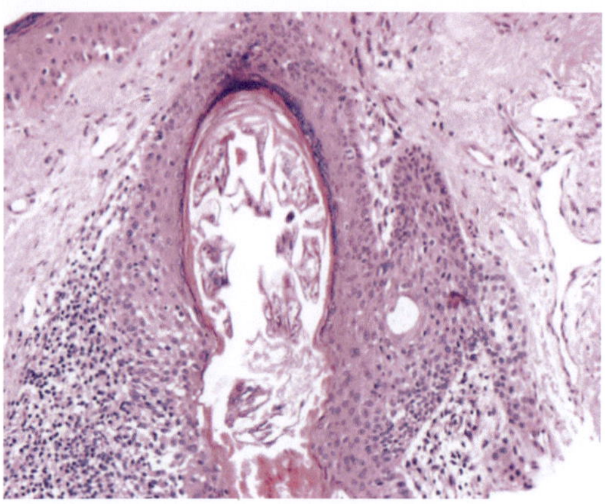

Fig. 6.71 Perifollicular lymphocytic inflammation

Histopathology (Figs. 6.69, 6.70, and 6.71)
- Dilated hair follicle
- The follicle is filled with loose keratin and *Demodex* mite
- Perifollicular lymphocytic infiltrate

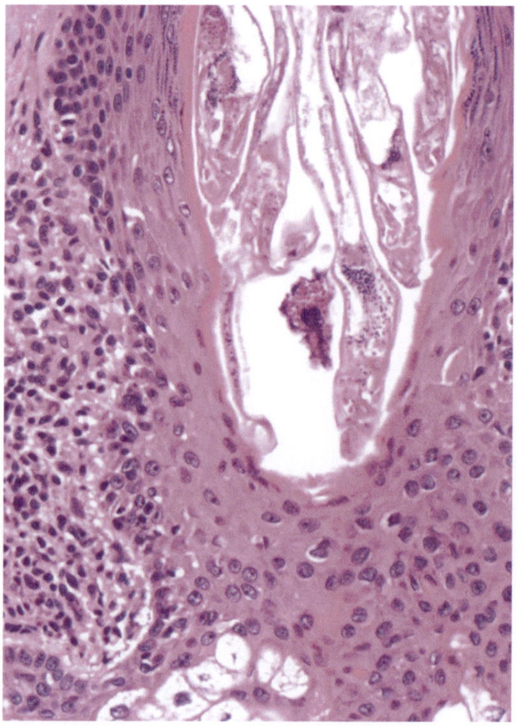

Fig. 6.70 Chitin exoskeleton and internal organs of *Demodex* mite

Folliculitis: Fungal

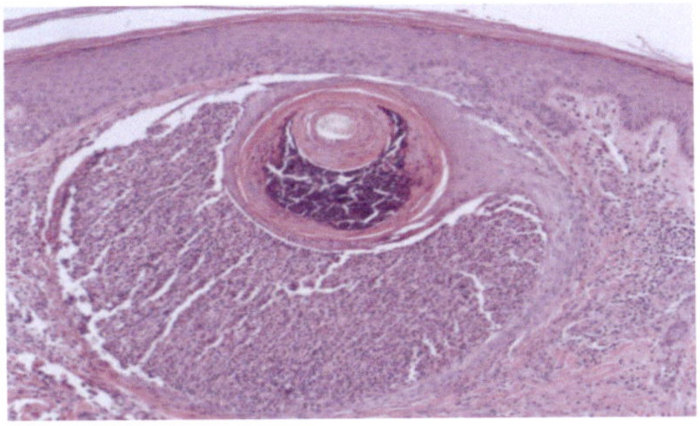

Fig. 6.72 Perifollicular abscess

Synonym: Majocchi's Granuloma

Histopathology (Figs. 6.72, 6.73, 6.74, 6.75, and 6.76)

- Distorted hair follicle
- Hyphae are infiltrating hair shaft
- Extensive perifollicular neutrophilic infiltrate
- Neutrophils and necrosis of the hair shaft

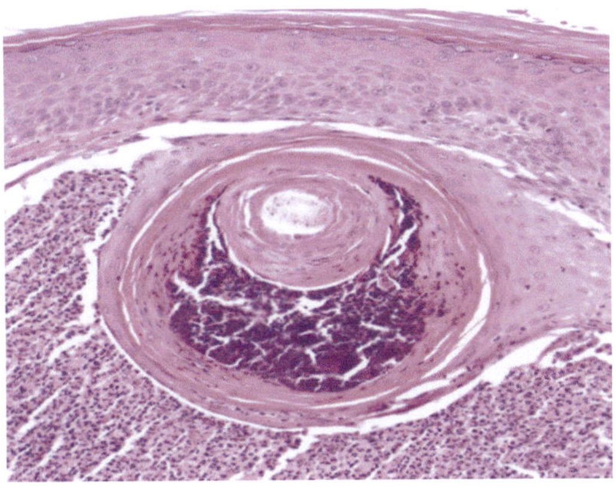

Fig. 6.73 Intrafollicular neutrophils with necrosis

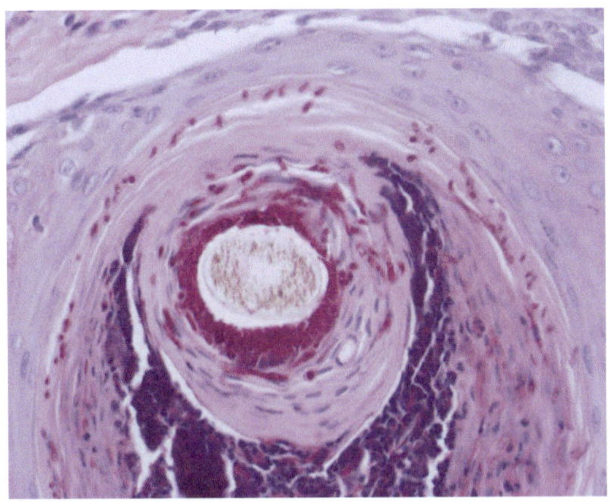

Fig. 6.74 PAS stain highlights dermatophyte hyphae within the hair shaft

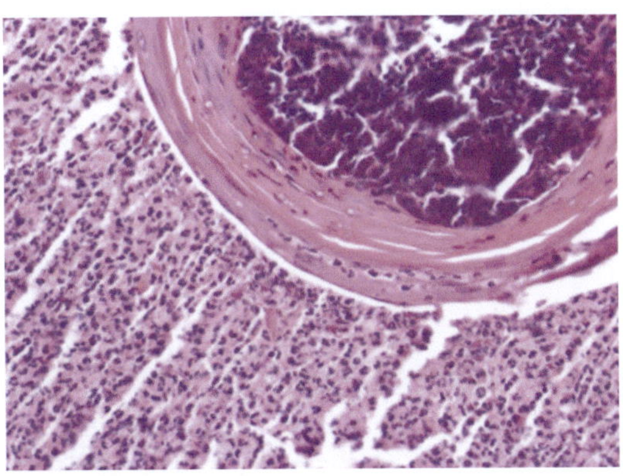

Fig. 6.75 Septate hyphae in outer layer of hair follicle (H&E)

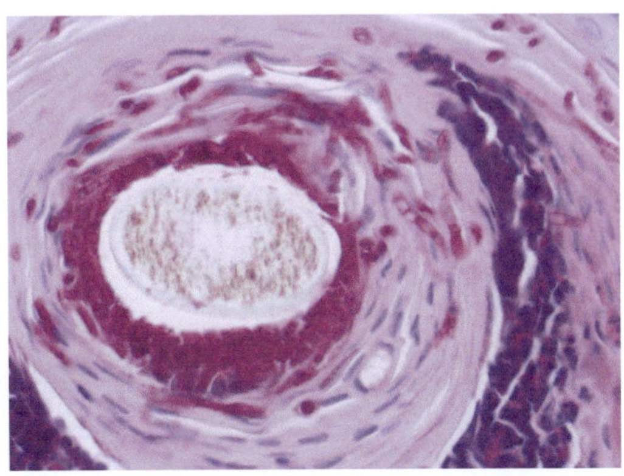

Fig. 6.76 Septate hyphae highlighted by PAS stain

Folliculitis: Herpetic

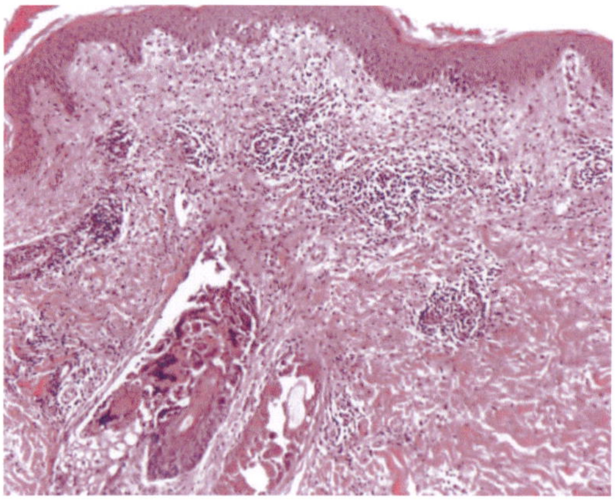

Fig. 6.77 Distorted hair follicles

Histopathology (Figs. 6.77, 6.78, and 6.79)
- Distorted inflamed hair follicle with background inflammation
- Acute perifollicular inflammation
- Intrafollicular herpetic inclusions
- Multinucleated keratinocytes with intranuclear inclusions

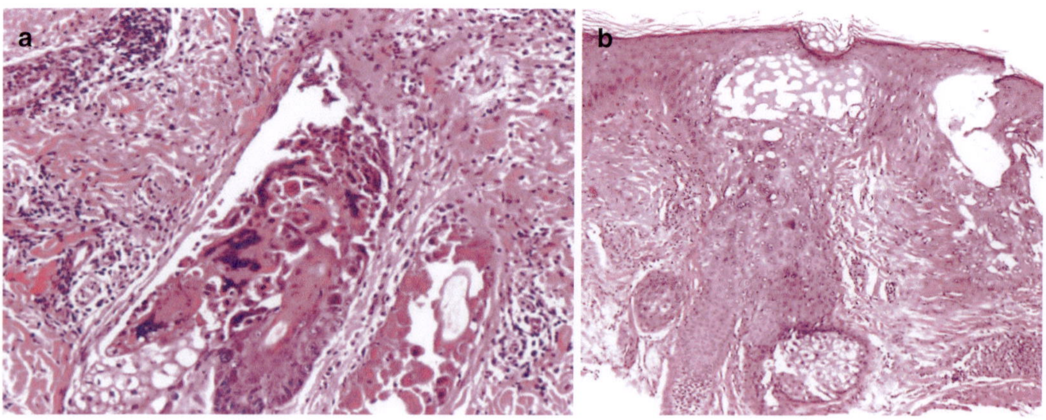

Fig. 6.78 (a, b) Necrotic hair follicles with perifollicular acute inflammation

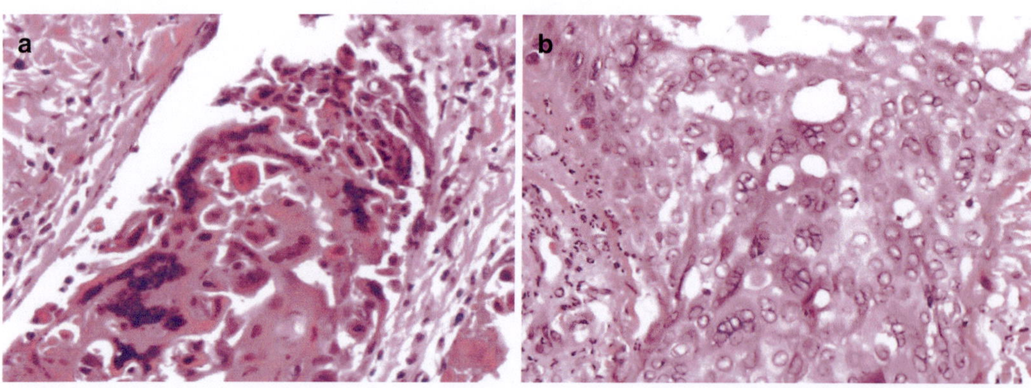

Fig. 6.79 (a, b) Multinucleated keratinocytes with nuclear molding and intranuclear inclusions

Folliculitis: Pityrosporum

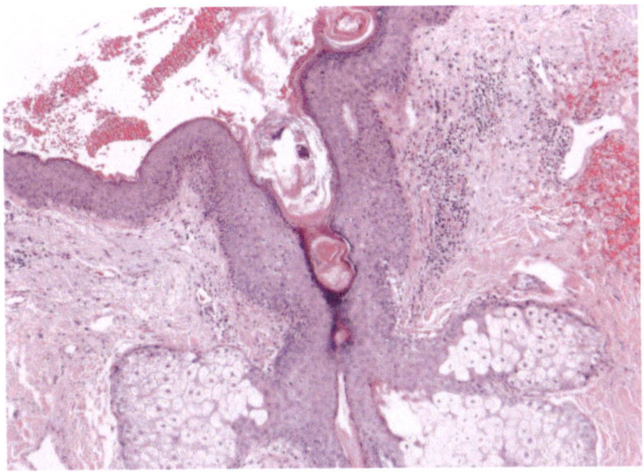

Fig. 6.80 Dilated hair follicle with follicular plugging

Histopathology (Figs. 6.80, 6.81, and 6.82)

- Dilated hair follicle
- Follicle filled with laminated keratin
- Round yeast and few short hyphae are present within the follicle or within an abscess if the follicle ruptures
- Perifollicular lymphocytic infiltrate with some histiocytes
- Occasionally the hair follicle ruptures and a neutrophilic abscess form

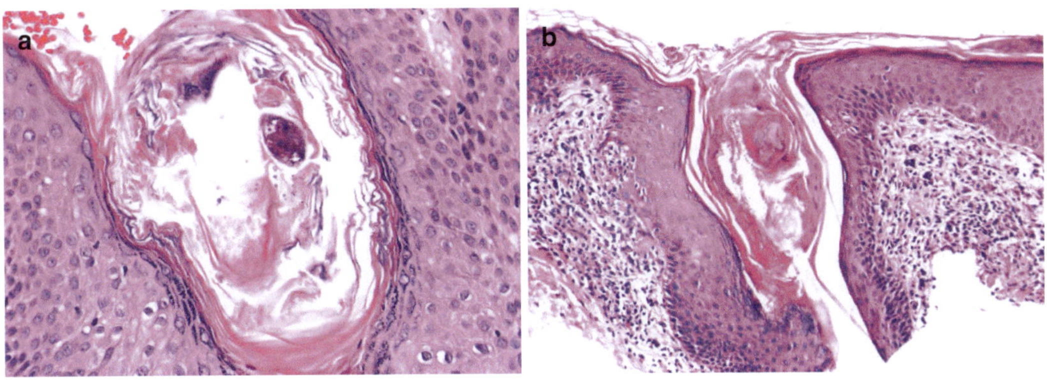

Fig. 6.81 (**a**, **b**) Dilated hair follicle filled with keratin and perifollicular moderate inflammation

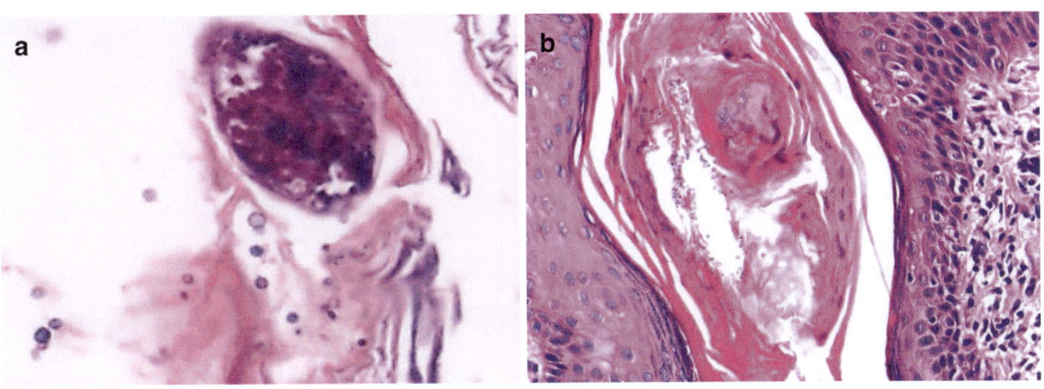

Fig. 6.82 (**a**, **b**) Round spores of *Masassezia furfur* can be seen without special stains. *Demodex* mite is also present in (**a**)

Foreign Body Reaction

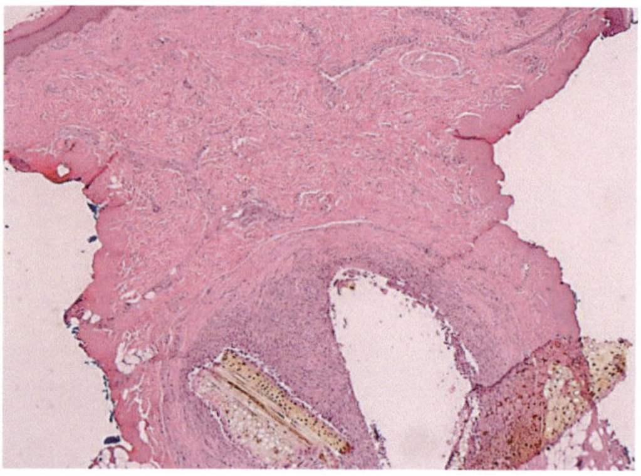

Fig. 6.83 **Splinter** embedded in the deep dermis

Histopathology (Figs. 6.83, 6.84, 6.85, 6.86, 6.87, 6.88, 6.89, and 6.90)
- Most foreign substances cause granulomatous reaction with histiocytes and giant cells
- Silicon and some tattoos cause only mild lymphohistiocytic inflammation
- Some foreign bodies (ex. plant material) can cause strong neutrophilic inflammation

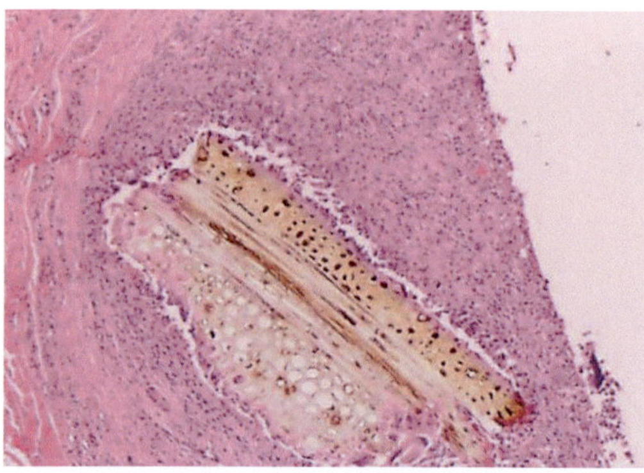

Fig. 6.84 Plant material is darkly pigmented

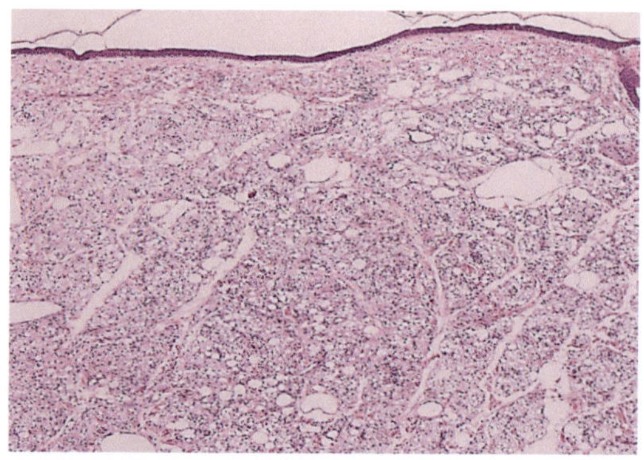

Fig. 6.85 **Silicon** form "Swiss cheese" appearance

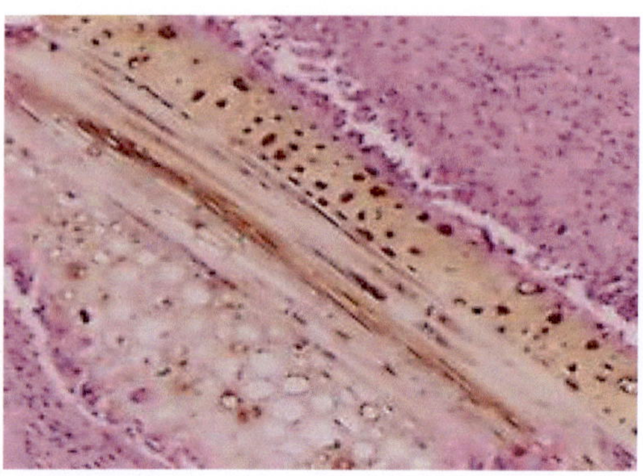

Fig. 6.86 Rectangular plant cells surrounding by acute inflammation

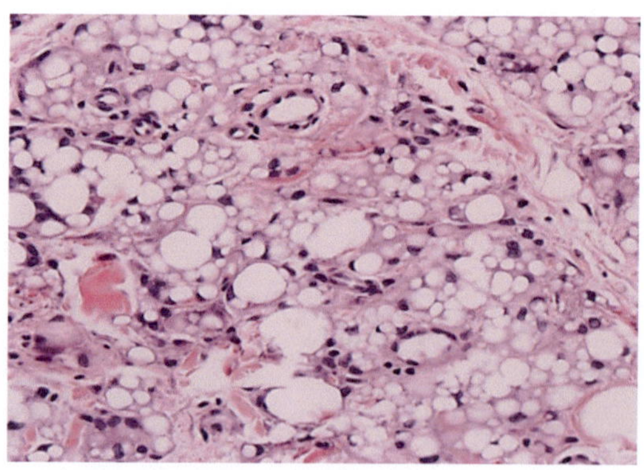

Fig. 6.87 Mild lymphocytic infiltrate and rare giant cells

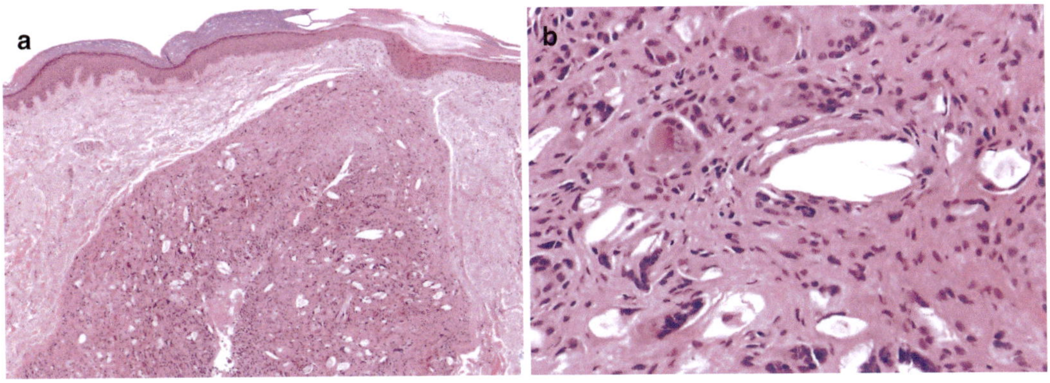

Fig. 6.88 (**a**, **b**) **Keratin granuloma** with foreign body giant cell reaction

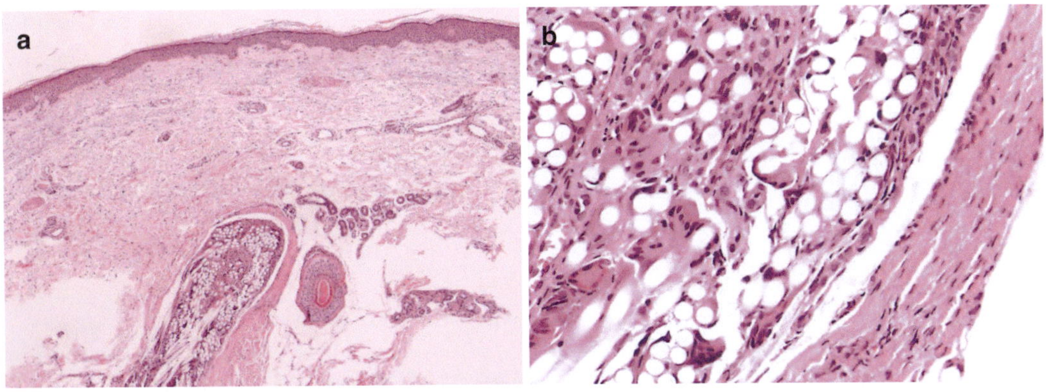

Fig. 6.89 (**a**, **b**) **Suture granuloma** with giant cell reaction

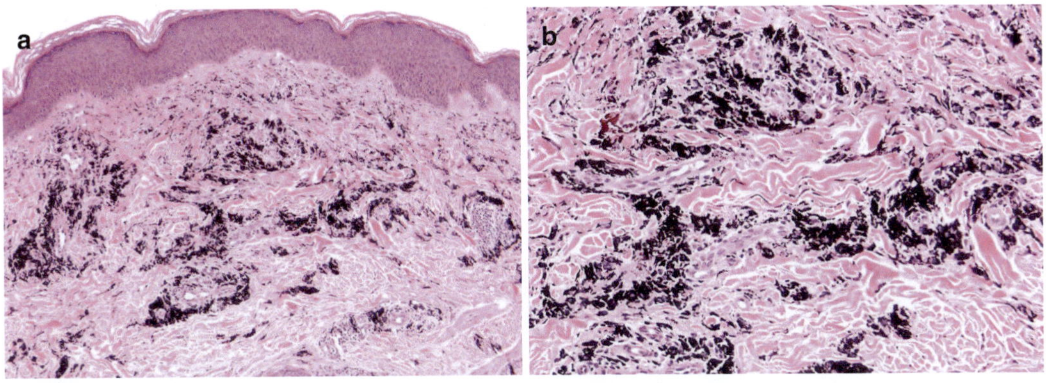

Fig. 6.90 (**a**, **b**) **Tattoo** material with minimal lymphocytic infiltrate

Fox-Fordyce Disease

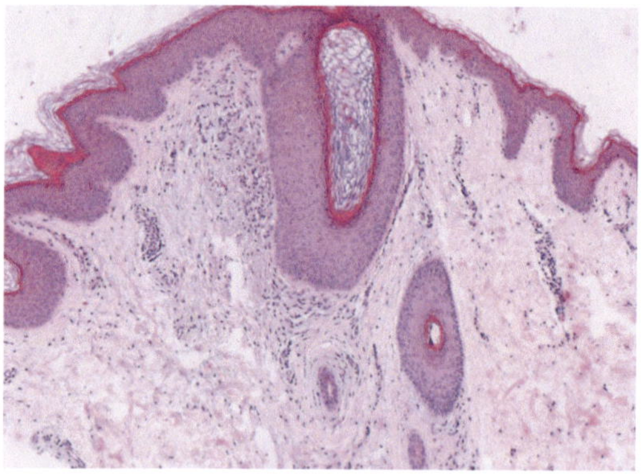

Fig. 6.91 Dome shaped papule with dilated follicle filled with keratin

Synonym: Apocrine Miliaria

Histopathology (Figs. 6.91, 6.92, and 6.93)

- Dome shaped papule
- Dilated follicle filled with keratin
- Focal follicular spongiosis
- Perifollicular lymphocytic inflammation with foamy histiocytes adjacent to entry of apocrine ducts to hair follicle

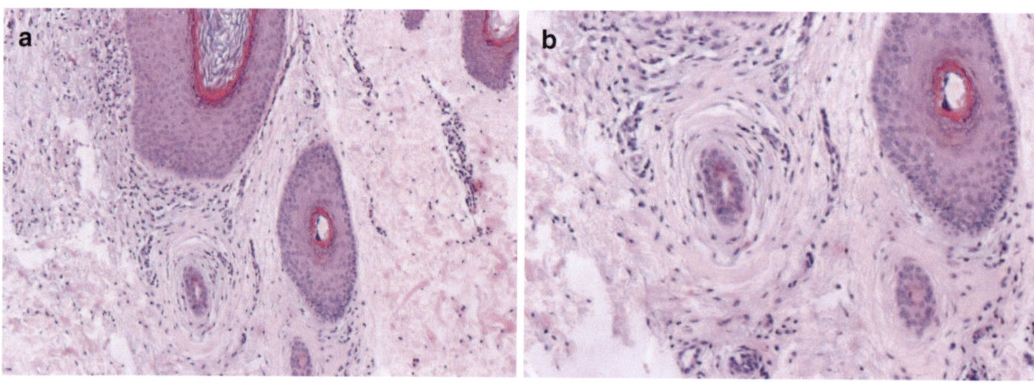

Fig. 6.92 (**a**, **b**) Apocrine ducts are seen in the vicinity of hair follicle

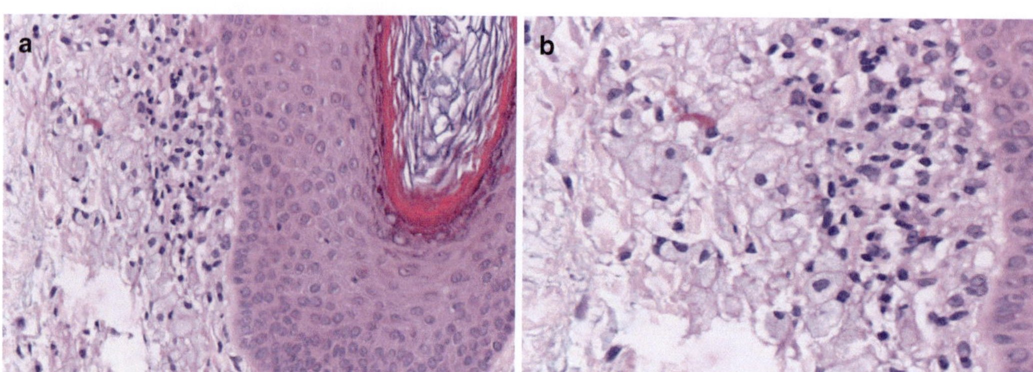

Fig. 6.93 (**a**, **b**) Perifollicular lymphocytic infiltrate with foamy histiocytes

Freeze Artifact

Freeze artifact can appear in tissue fixed in 10% formaldehyde and stored at temperature close to 0 °C or in tissue frozen with liquid nitrogen prior to the biopsy.

Histopathology (Figs. 6.94, 6.95, 6.96, and 6.97)

- Ice crystals form in the tissue
- Histologically crystals present as cellular "ballooning" (intracellular vacuoles)

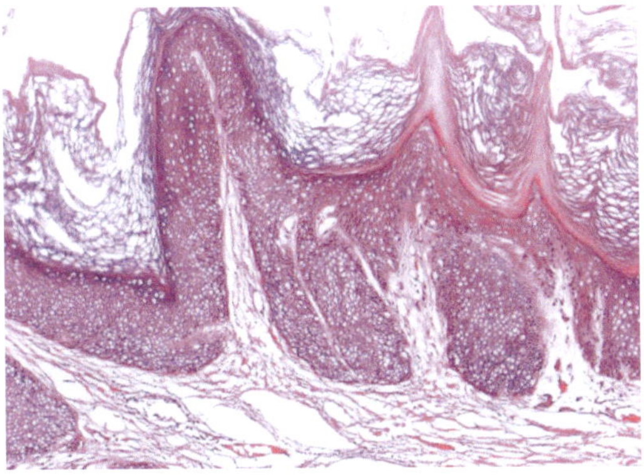

Fig. 6.94 Seborrheic keratosis frozen with LN2 prior to the biopsy

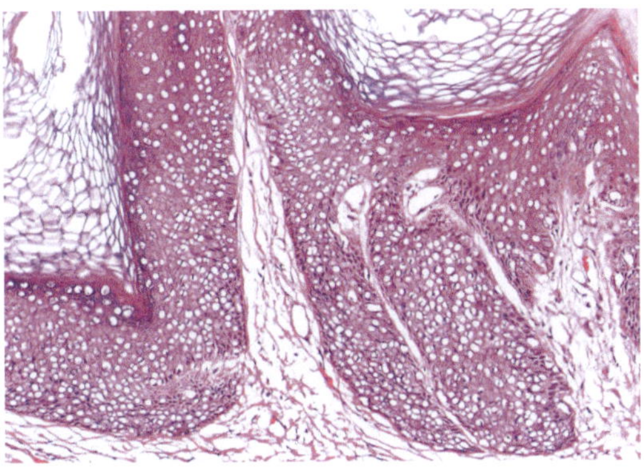

Fig. 6.95 Numerous pale vacuoles within epidermal keratinocytes

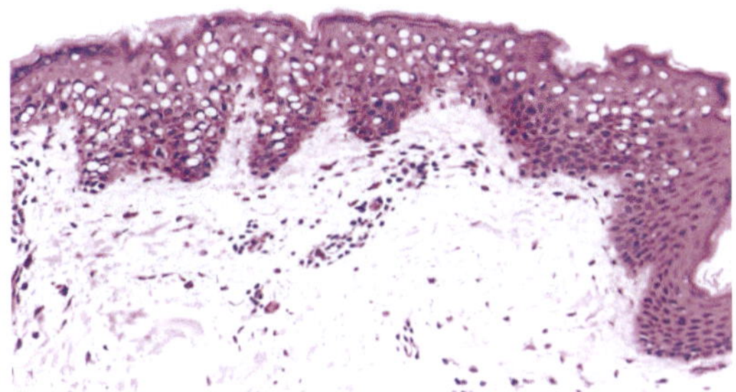

Fig. 6.96 Solar lentigo fixed in formalin and stored in refrigerator

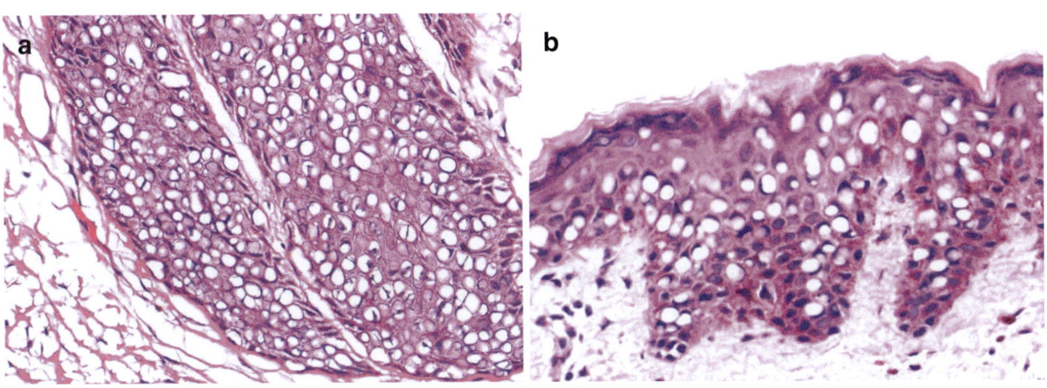

Fig. 6.97 (**a**, **b**) "Ballooning" of epidermal keratinocytes

Friction Blister

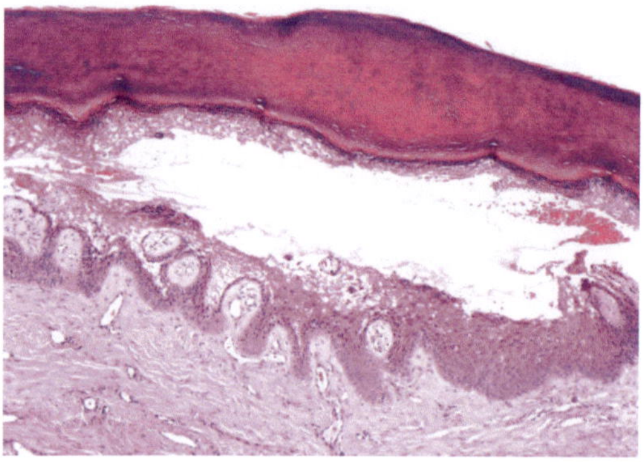

Fig. 6.98 Intraepidermal blister at the level below stratum granulosum

Histopathology (Figs. 6.98, 6.99, and 6.100)
- Usually acral skin
- Intraepidermal blister with split usually below stratum granulosum
- No evidence of dyskeratosis
- Lumen is filled with serum and some red blood cells
- Dermal inflammation is mild

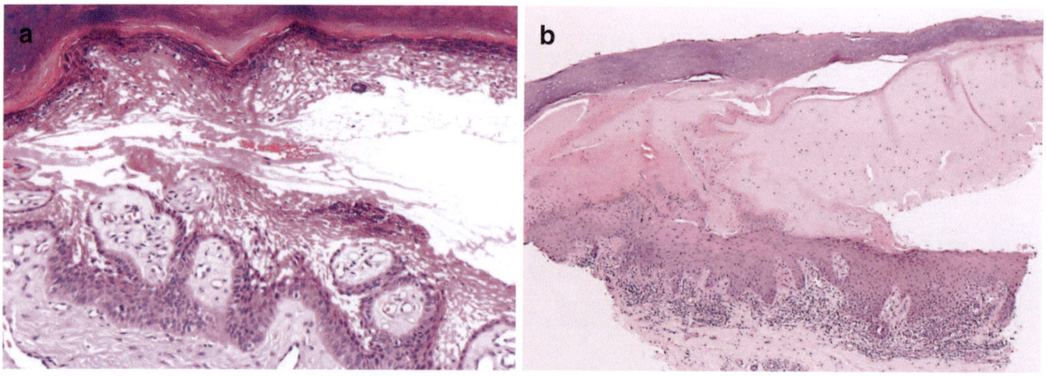

Fig. 6.99 (a, b) Blister is filled with serum and some red blood cells

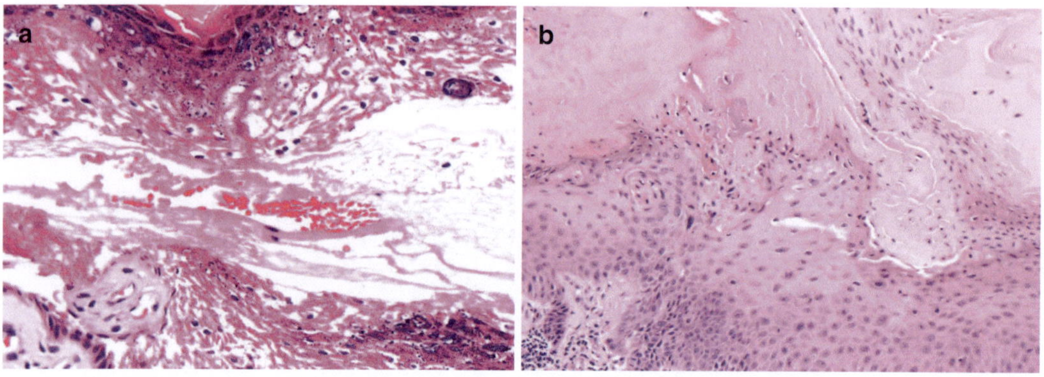

Fig. 6.100 (a, b) Keratinocytes appear elongated in shear plane with no evidence of dyskeratosis

Fusariosis

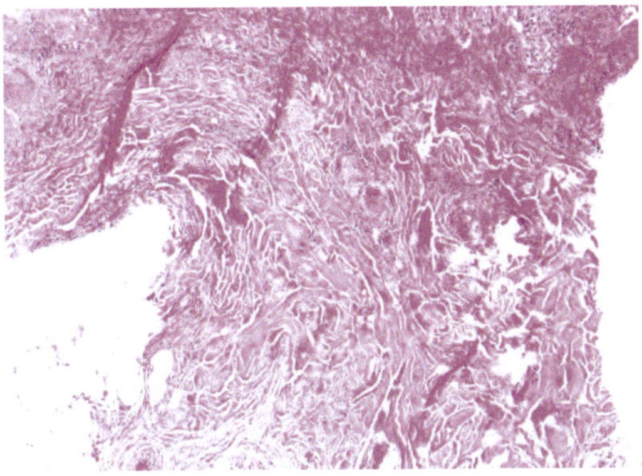

Fig. 6.101 Microvascular thrombi

Synonym: Plant Mold

Histopathology (Figs. 6.101, 6.102, 6.103, and 6.104)

- Vary from suppurative to granulomatous inflammation in immunosuppressed individuals
- In disseminated disease *Fusarium* demonstrates septic thrombi with vascular involvement similar to *Aspergillosis*
- Branching, septate hyphae
- Unlike in *Aspergillosis*, the hyphae branch irregularly under deferent angles

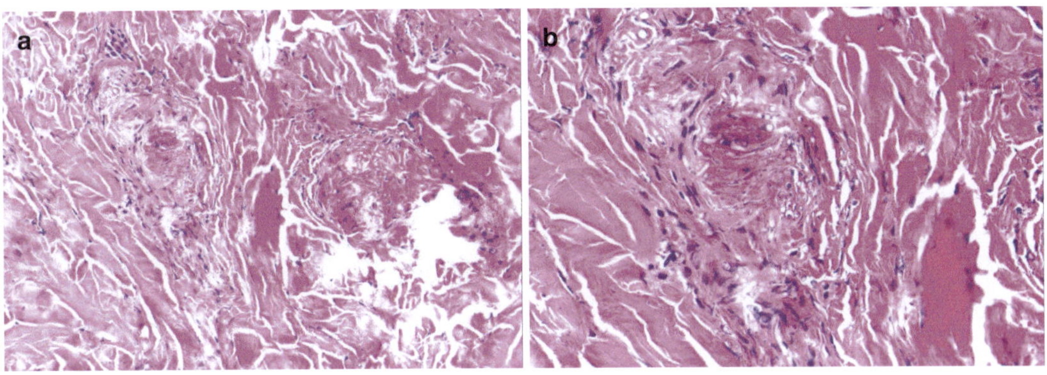

Fig. 6.102 (**a**, **b**) Septic thrombi and perivascular necrosis

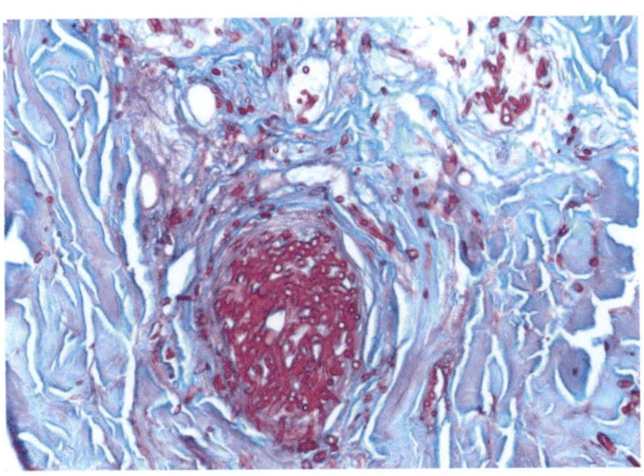

Fig. 6.103 Intravascular *Fusarium* ball (PAS stain)

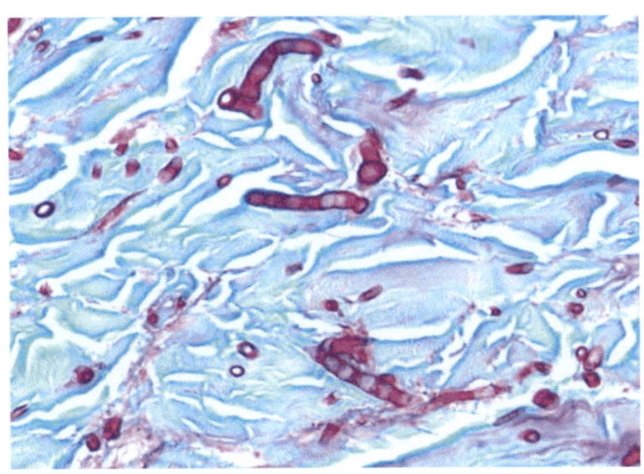

Fig. 6.104 Branching septate hypae (PAS stain)

7 Dermatopathology G

V. Vincek, *Dermatopathology A–Z*, https://doi.org/10.1007/978-3-319-89486-7_7

Galli-Galli Disease

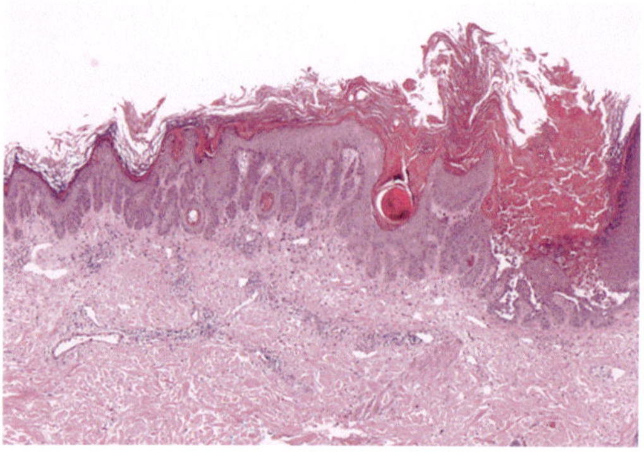

Fig. 7.1 Hyperkeratotic, acanthotic epidermis with focal acantholysis

Synonym: Dowling-Degos with Acantholysis

Histopathology (Figs. 7.1, 7.2, 7.3, 7.4, and 7.5)

- Epidermal acanthosis and hyperkeratosis
- Filiform projection of epidermal rete ridges
- Increased pigmentation of the basal layer
- Focal suprabasal acantholysis
- Preserved basal layer
- Mild dermal inflammation

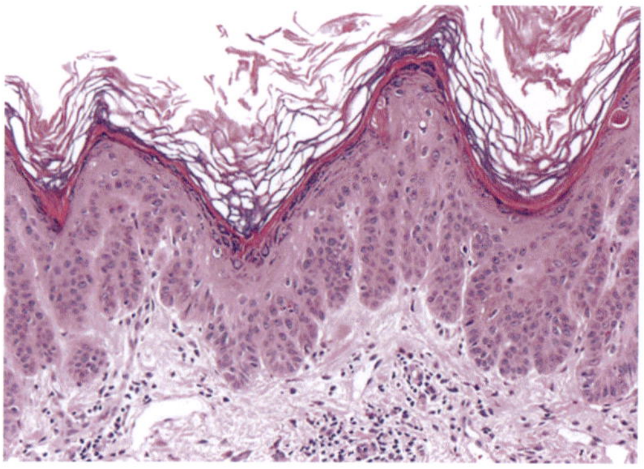

Fig. 7.2 Mild dermal lymphocytic inflammation

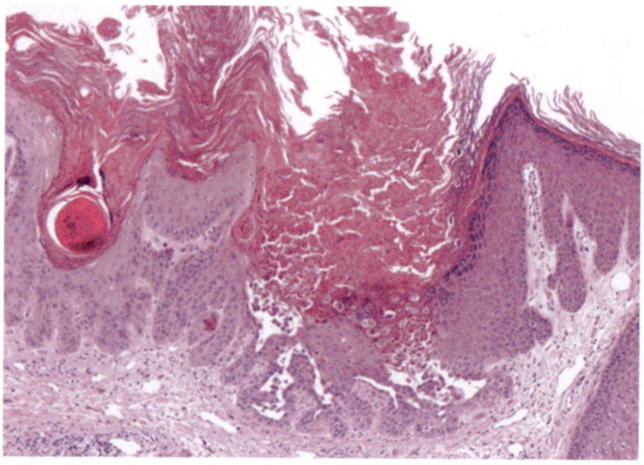

Fig. 7.3 Suprabasal split with acantholysis and dyskeratosis

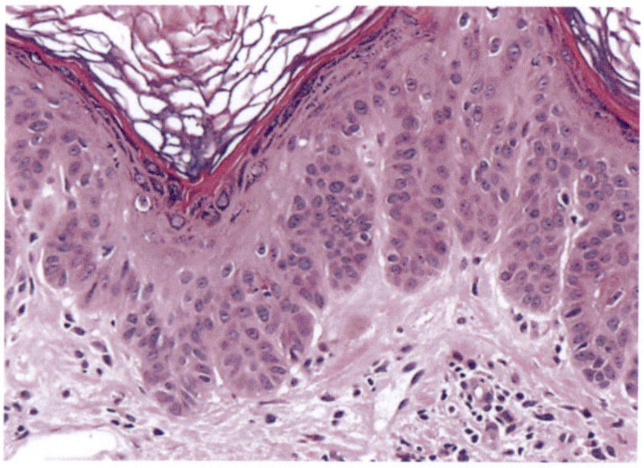

Fig. 7.4 "Finger-like" rete ridges with mildly increased pigment

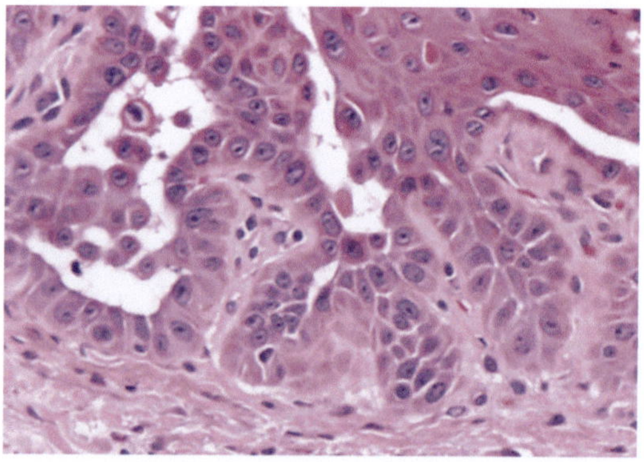

Fig. 7.5 Basal layer of the epidermis is preserved

Gauze

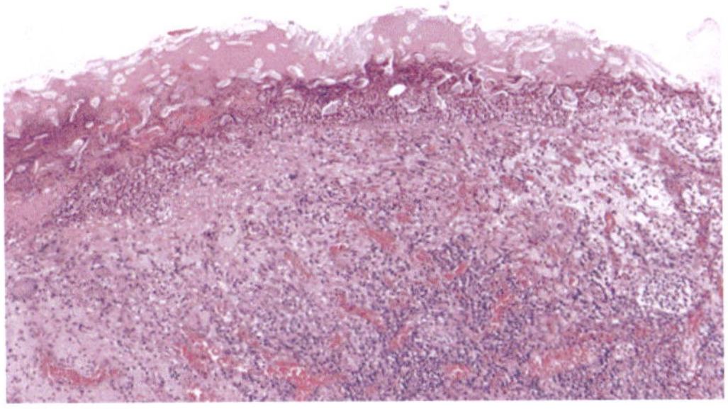

Fig. 7.6 Wound bed with granulation tissue

Histopathology (Figs. 7.6, 7.7, and 7.8)
- Foreign material found on the surface of the wound
- Gauze material is admixed with the serum crust
- Gauze material has oval shape with characteristic peripheral baby pink color and central dark pink slit
- Surrounding granulation tissue

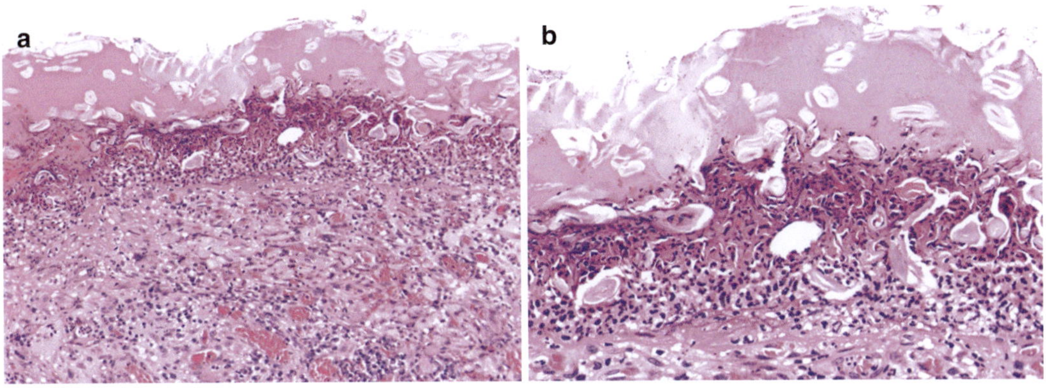

Fig. 7.7 (**a**, **b**) Granulation tissue with foreign body material in the superficial crust

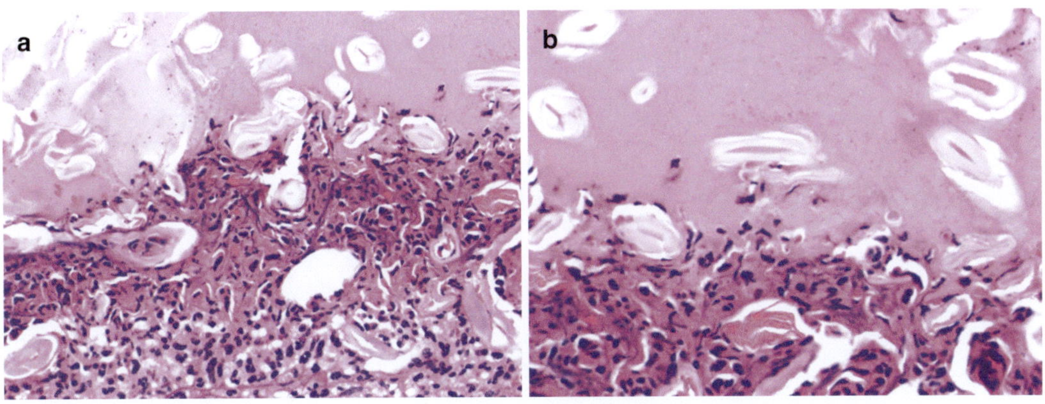

Fig. 7.8 (**a**, **b**) Irregular light pink oval fragments with central dark pink slit

Gelfoam

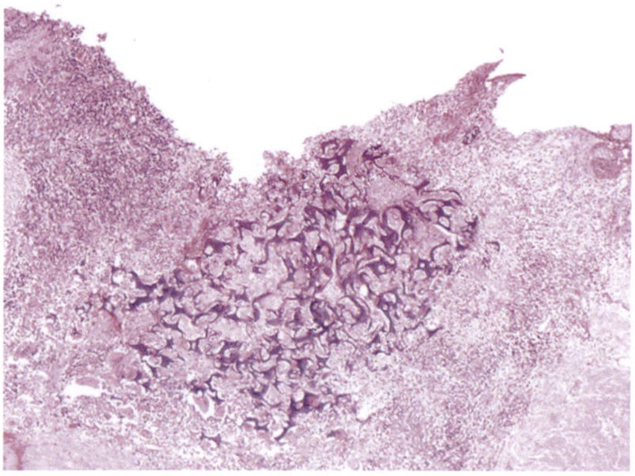

Fig. 7.9 Wound bed with foreign body material

Histopathology (Figs. 7.9, 7.10, 7.11, 7.12, and 7.13)

- Usually found in wound bed
- Distinctive branching architecture
- Foreign material with purple color and no birefringence
- Surrounding scar and granulation tissue

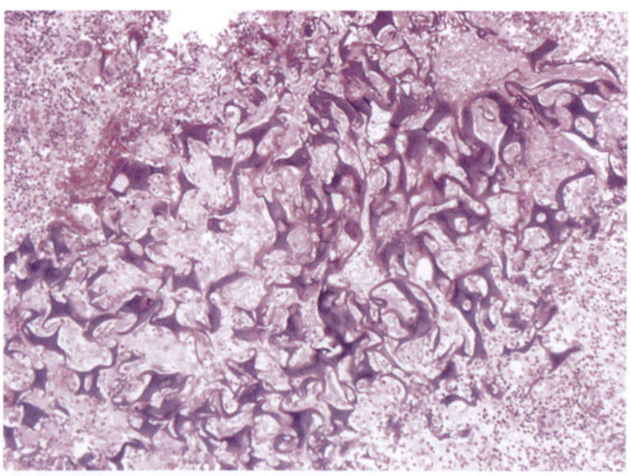

Fig. 7.10 Granulation tissue surrounds gelfoam

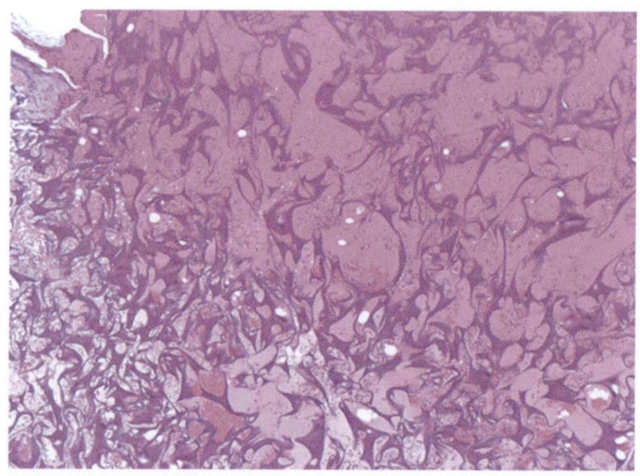

Fig. 7.11 Characteristic branching architecture

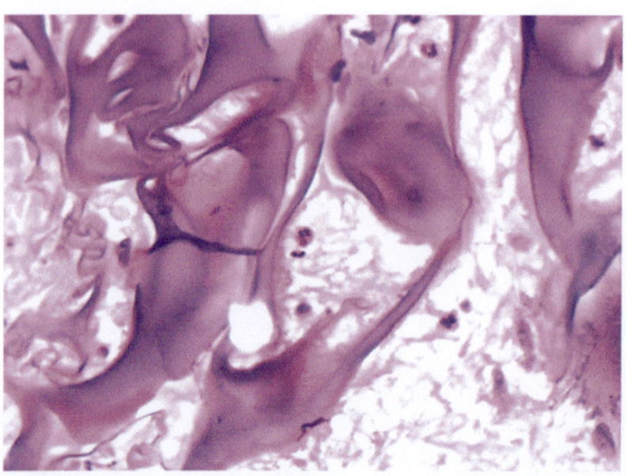

Fig. 7.12 Scattered neutrophils in between gelfoam

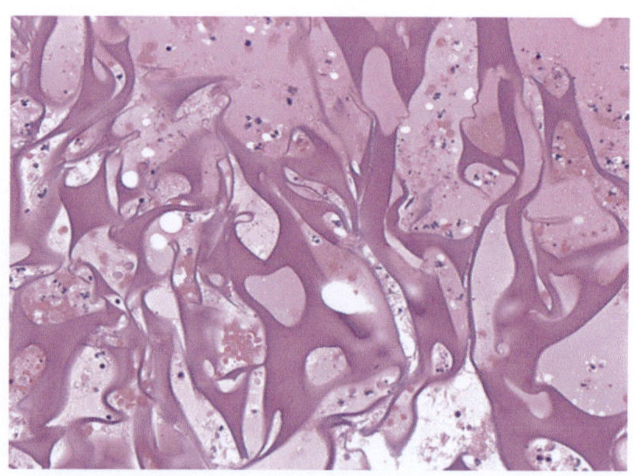

Fig. 7.13 Dark purple fragments of gelfoam

Generalized Eruptive Histiocytosis

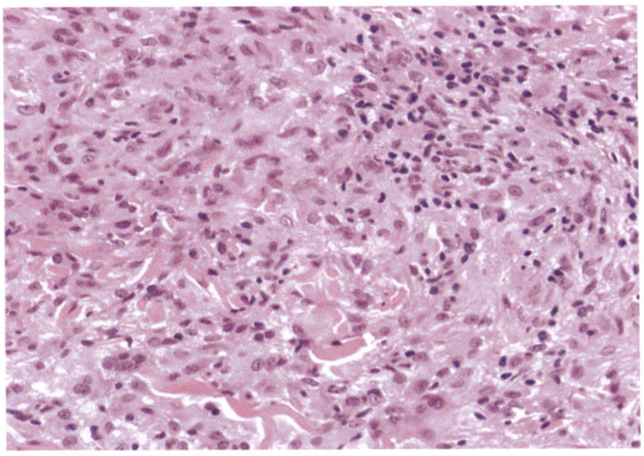

Fig. 7.14 Dermal pale histiocytic infiltrate

Histopathology (Figs. 7.14, 7.15, 7.16, 7.17, and 7.18)

- Dermal histiocytic infiltrate (CD68+, MAC387+)
- Histiocytes have pale cytoplasm and oval nuclei
- Absence of giant cells and xanthoma cells
- No lipid or PAS+ material present
- Variable number of lymphocytes and fibroblasts

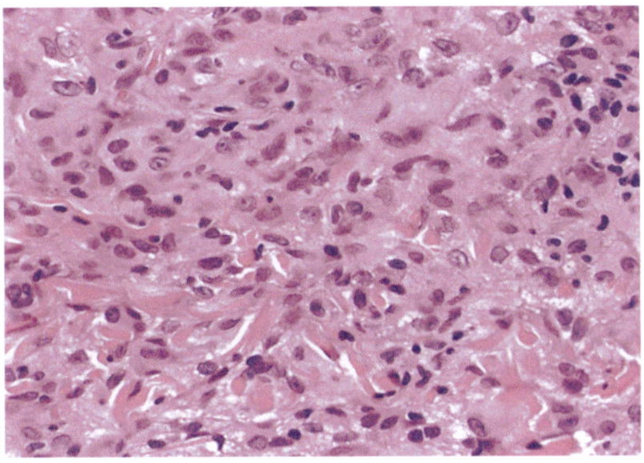

Fig. 7.15 Histiocytes have pale cytoplasm and oval pale nuclei

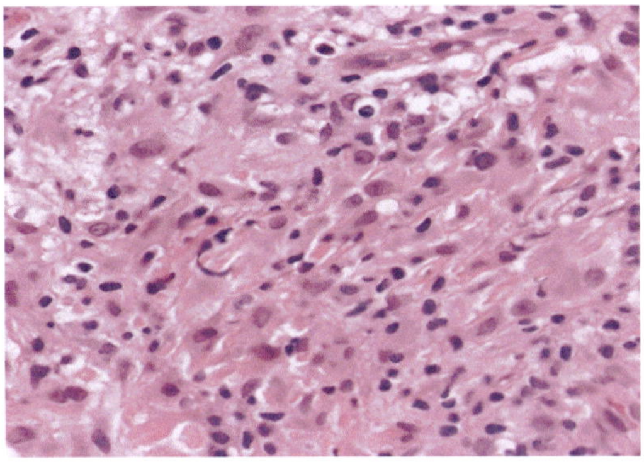

Fig. 7.16 Some histiocytes have bubbly cytoplasm but there is absence of lipid

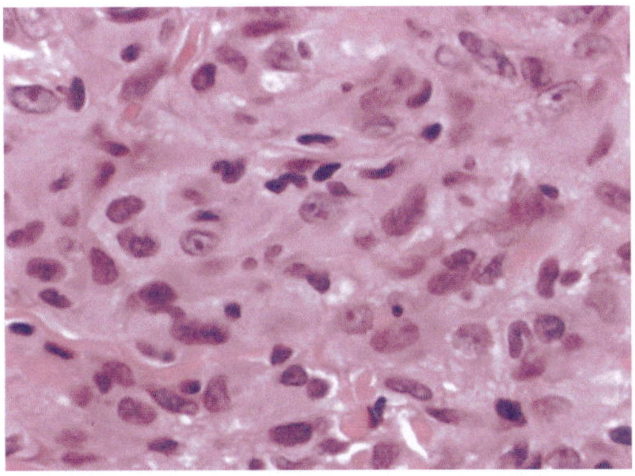

Fig. 7.17 Scattered lymphocytes and fibroblasts

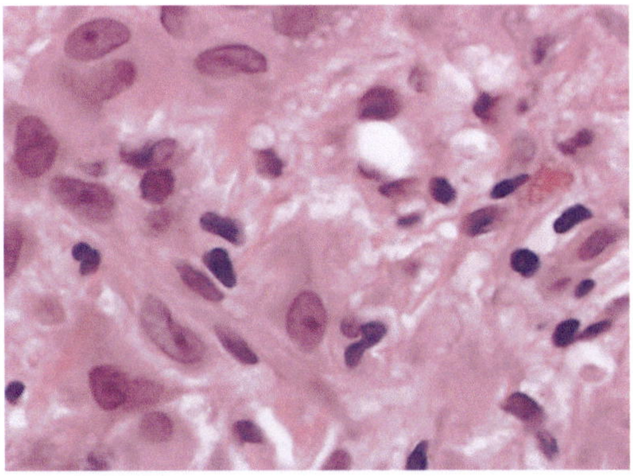

Fig. 7.18 Giant cells and genuine xanthoma cells are absent

Giant Cell Tumor of Tendon Sheath

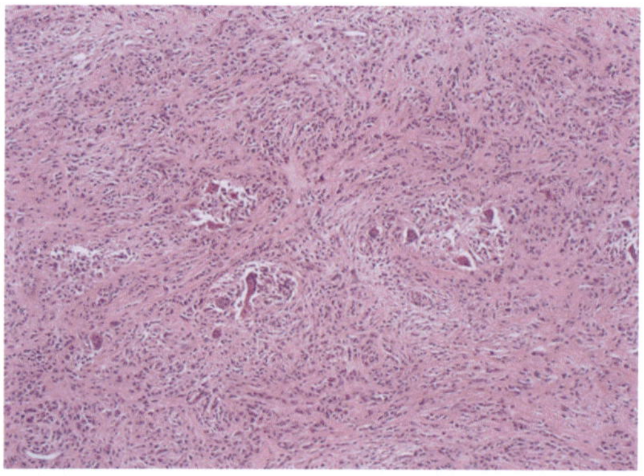

Fig. 7.19 Deep subcutaneous tumor nodule

Histopathology (Figs. 7.19, 7.20, 7.21, and 7.22)

- Nodular tumor attached to the tendon
- Mixture of histiocytes, numerous giant cells, and lymphocytes in fibrous stroma
- Giant cells have numerous nuclei
- Hemosiderin is usually present
- Variable number of mitoses
- Mononuclear and giant cells are CD68+

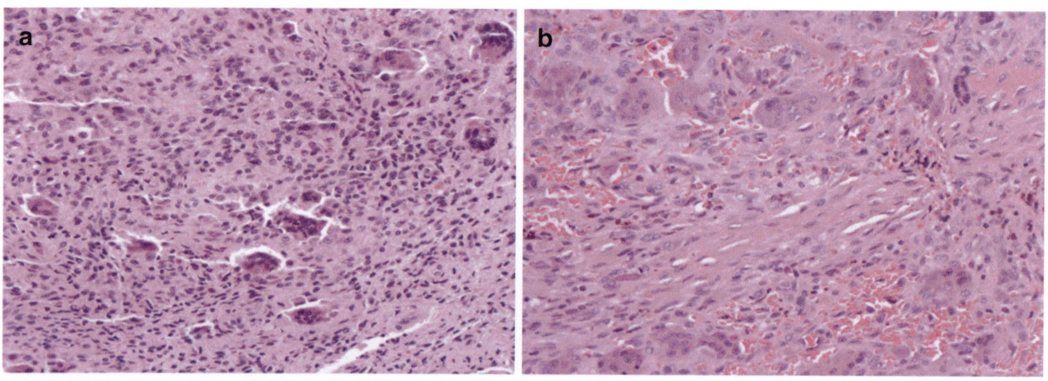

Fig. 7.20 (**a**, **b**) Tumor consists of histiocytes, numerous giant cells, and lymphocytes in dense stroma

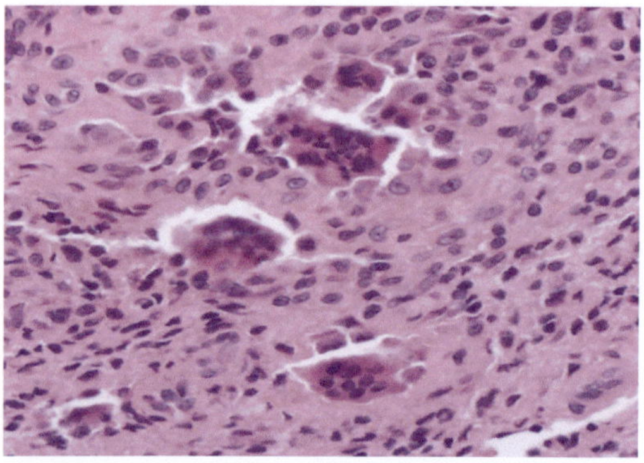

Fig. 7.21 Giant cells have numerous nuclei

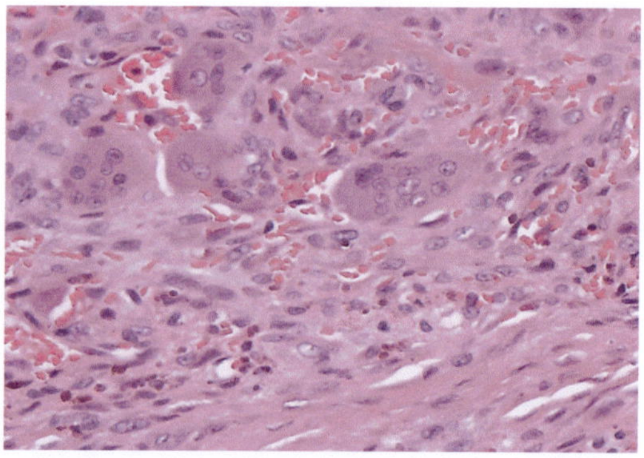

Fig. 7.22 Red blood cell extravasation and hemosiderin is present

Glomeruloid Hemangioma

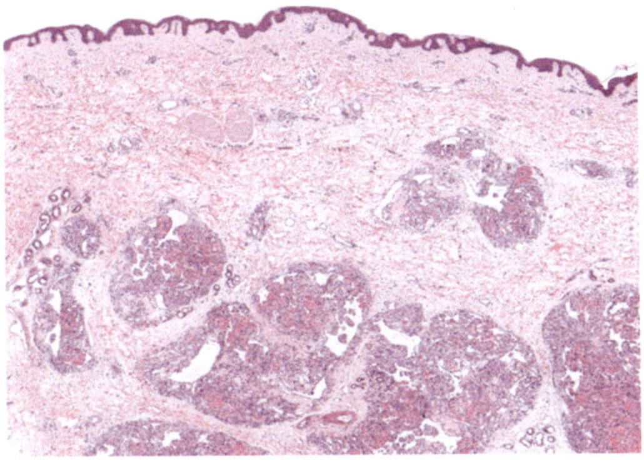

Fig. 7.23 Dermal vascular spaces

Histopathology (Figs. 7.23, 7.24, and 7.25)

- Dilated dermal vascular spaces
- Spaces are filled with vascular channels reminiscent of renal glomeruli
- Endothelial cells are plump but not atypical
- Endothelial cells contain eosinophilic globules

P.S. associated with Castleman and POEMS syndrome

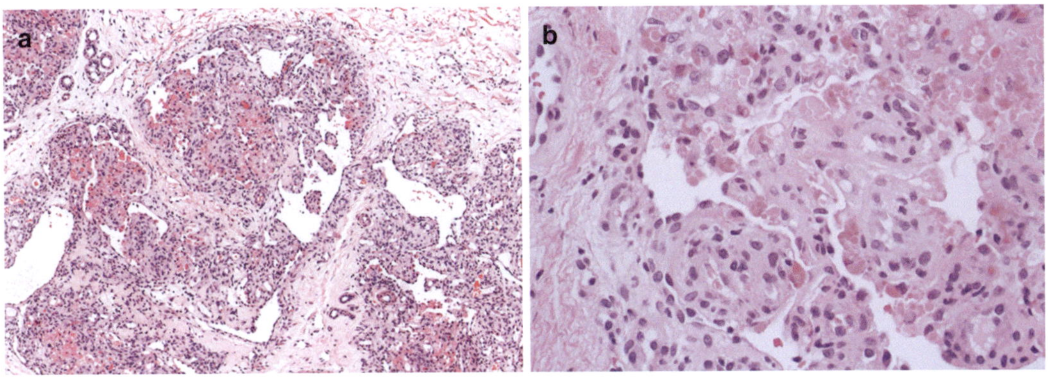

Fig. 7.24 (**a**, **b**) Dilated dermal vascular spaces filled with "grape-like" aggregates of small capillaries resembling glomeruli

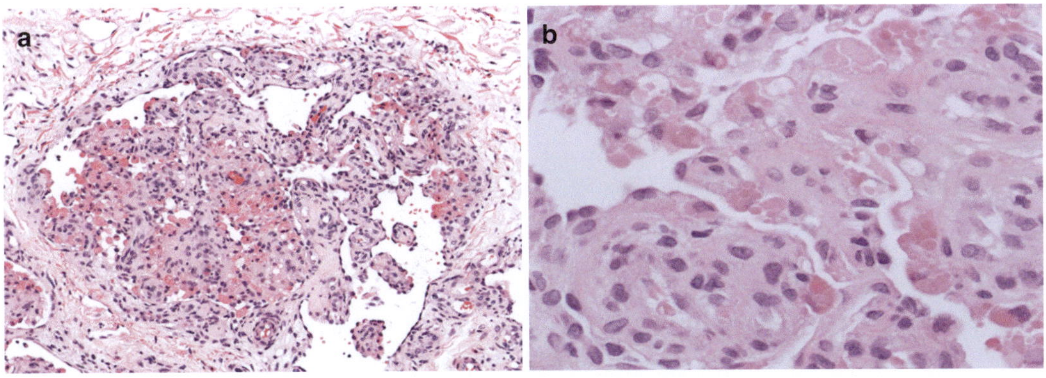

Fig. 7.25 (**a**, **b**) Endothelial cells are plump and contain eosinophilic globules

Glomangioma

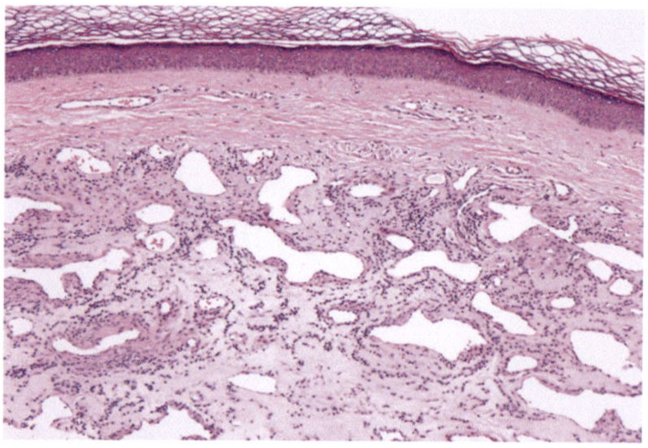

Fig. 7.26 Poorly circumscribed dermal tumor

Histopathology (Figs. 7.26, 7.27, 7.28, and 7.29)

- Poorly circumscribed not encapsulated dermal tumor
- Cavernous hemangioma-like vessels with various amount of red blood cells
- Vessels are surrounded by a few layers of uniform glomus cells
- Cells are SMA positive

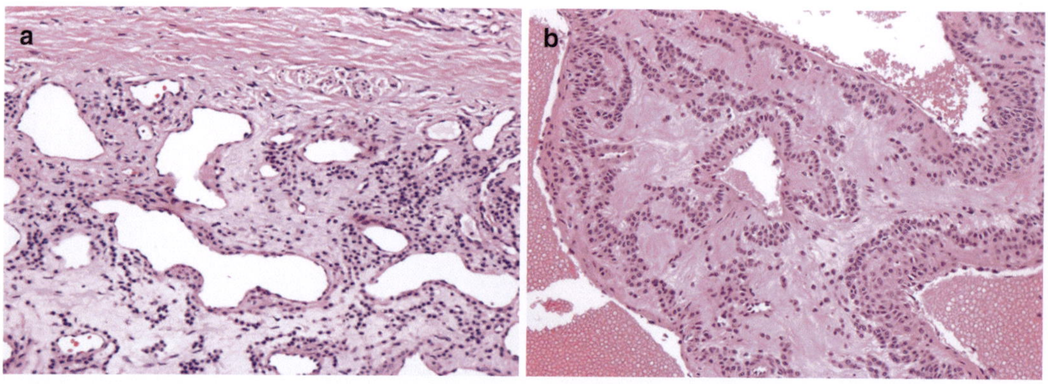

Fig. 7.27 (**a**, **b**) Dilated vascular channels surrounded by several layers of uniform cells

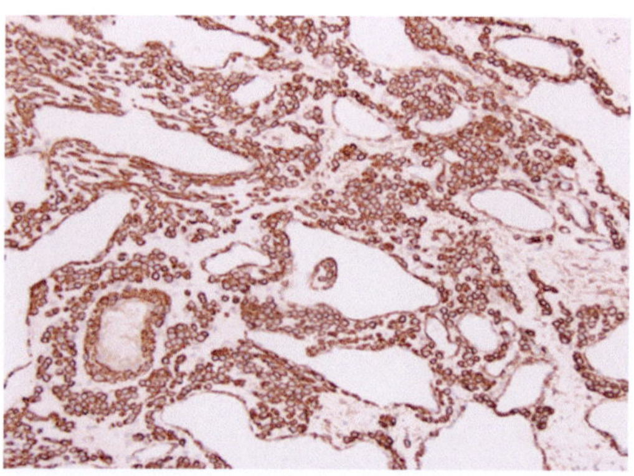

Fig. 7.28 Tumor cells are SMA positive

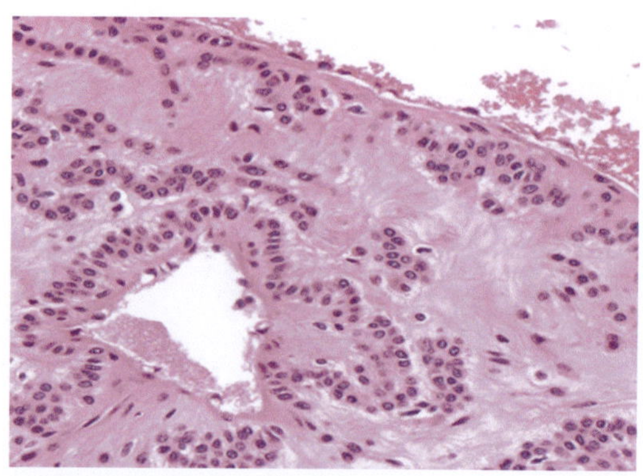

Fig. 7.29 Cells with uniform vesicular nuclei and eosinophilic cytoplasm

Glomus Tumor

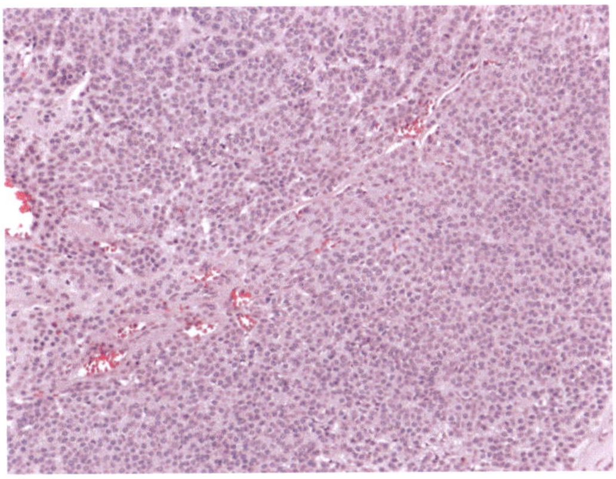

Fig. 7.30 Sheet of uniform cells

Histopathology (Figs. 7.30, 7.31, 7.32, and 7.33)

- Solid sheets or nests of glomoid cells
- Cells are uniform with eosinophilic cytoplasm and vesicular nuclei
- Cells surround inconspicuous vessels
- Lack of atypia or mitoses
- Cells are SMA positive

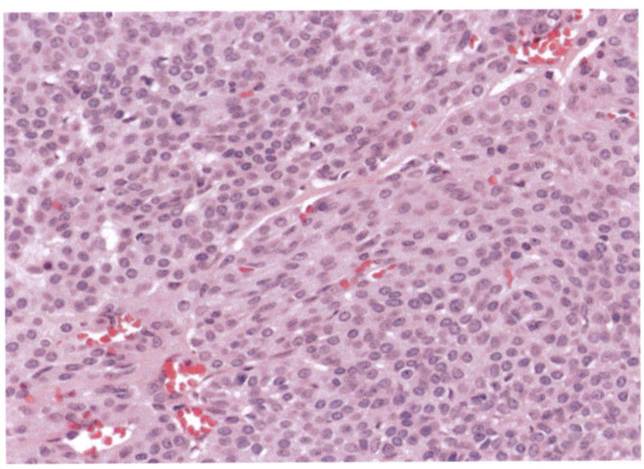

Fig. 7.31 Slit-like inconspicuous vessels compressed by tumor cells

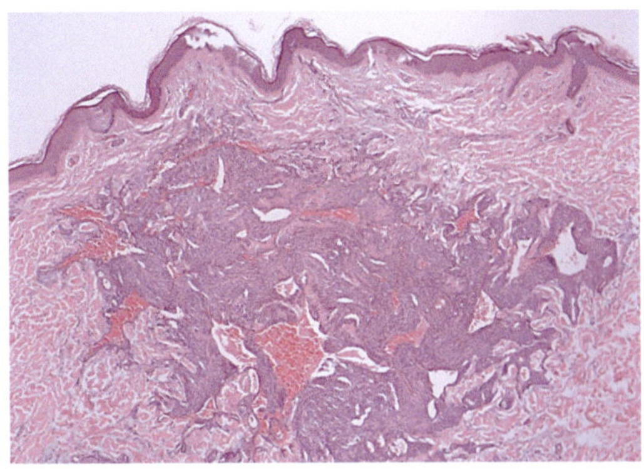

Fig. 7.32 Not encapsulated dermal tumor

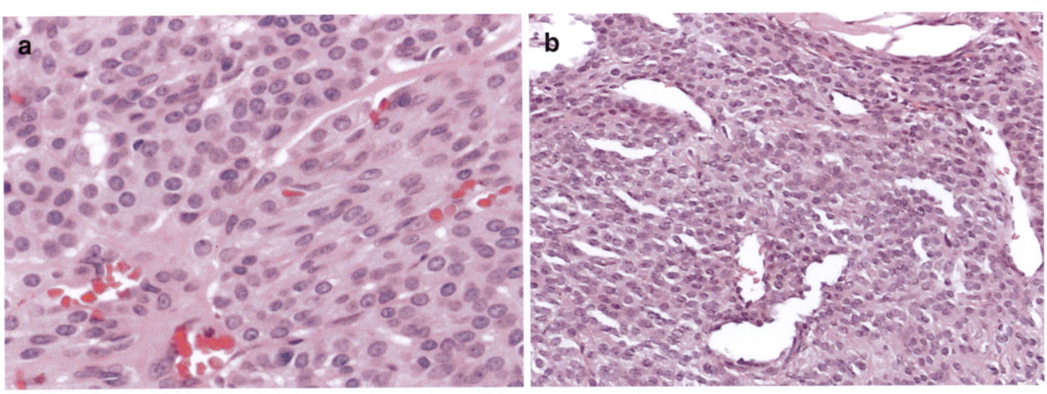

Fig. 7.33 (a, b) Cells with eosinophilic cytoplasm and vesicular nuclei with no atypia or mitoses

Gottron's Papule

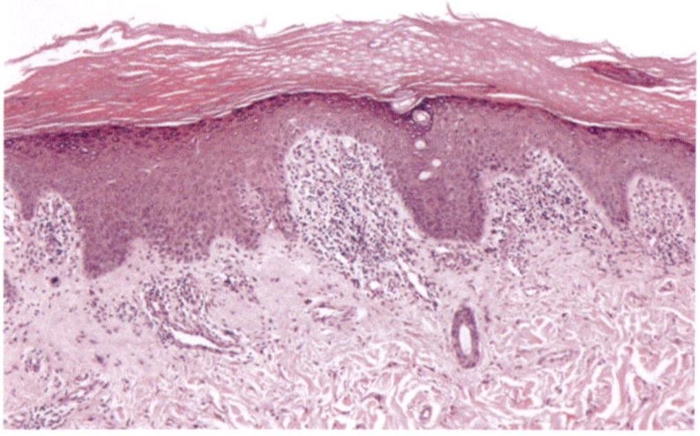

Fig. 7.34 Acanthotic, hyperkeratotic epidermis

Histopathology (Figs. 7.34, 7.35, 7.36, and 7.37)

- Acanthotic hyperkeratotic epidermis with irregular papillomatosis
- Epidermal hypergranulosis akin to one seen in lichen planus
- Interface vacuolar changes akin to one seen in dermatomyositis
- Dermal perivascular lymphocytic infiltrate
- Dermal mucin is increased

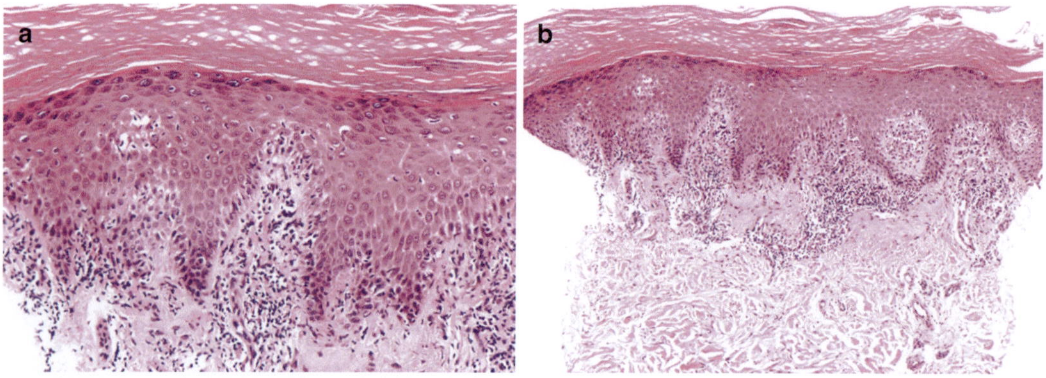

Fig. 7.35 (**a**, **b**) Epidermis appears like in lichen planus with hyperkeratotic, acanthotic epidermis and a pronounced granular layer

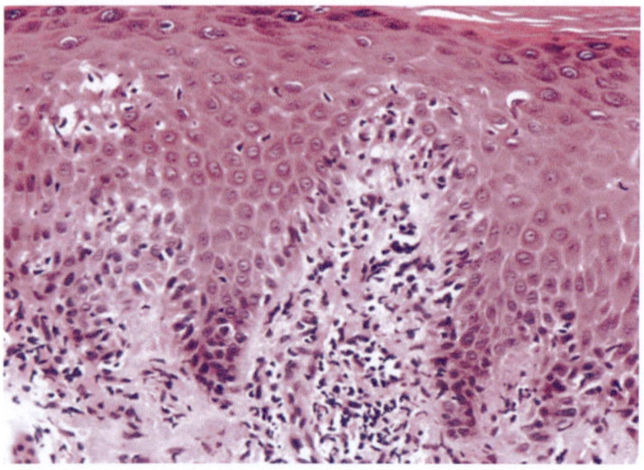

Fig. 7.36 Interface with vacuolar interface changes and occasional apoptotic keratinocytes

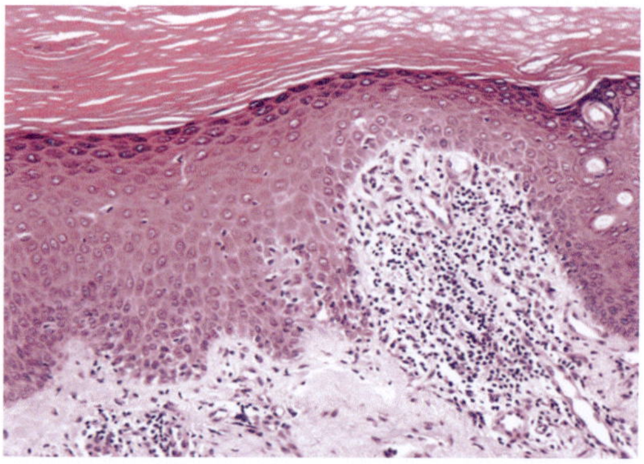

Fig. 7.37 Dermal perivascular lymphocytic infiltrate

Gout

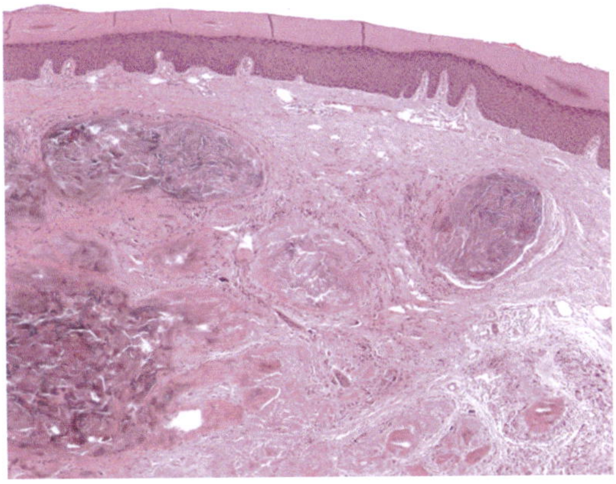

Fig. 7.38 Gouty deposits in alcohol fixed tissue

Histopathology (Figs. 7.38, 7.39, 7.40, 7.41, and 7.42)

- Deeply brown-gray amorphous dermal and subcutaneous deposits (if tissue is fixed in alcohol based fixative)
- Gray-pink deposits (if tissue is fixed in formalin)
- Deposits are surrounded by granulomatous reaction consisting of giant cells, lymphocytes, and histiocytes

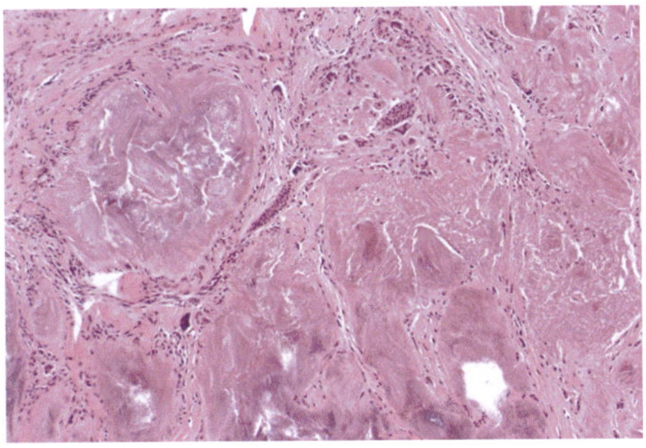

Fig. 7.39 Giant cells, histiocytes, and lymphocytes surround gouty deposits

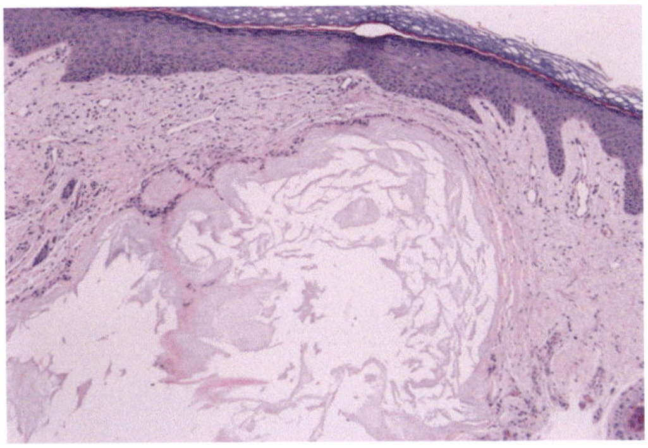

Fig. 7.40 Gouty deposits in formalin fixed tissue

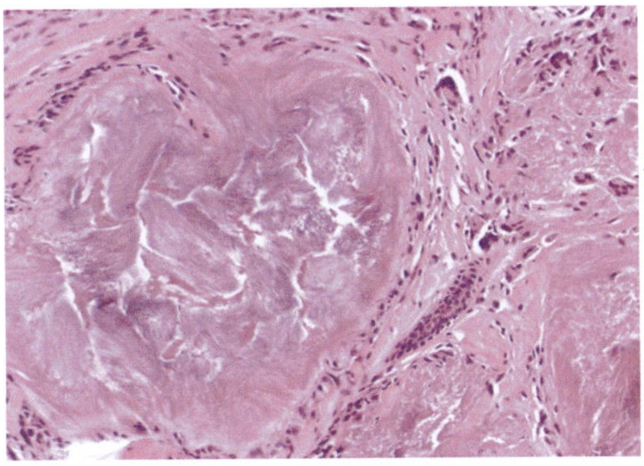

Fig. 7.41 Dirty appearing brown-gray deposits

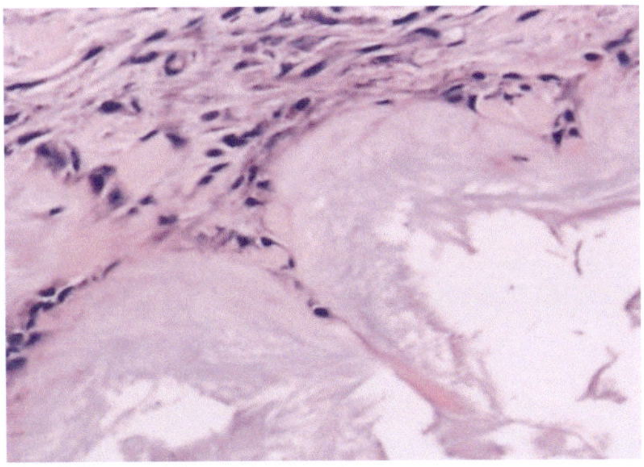

Fig. 7.42 Pink-gray deposits surrounded by giant cells

Graft-Versus-Host Disease

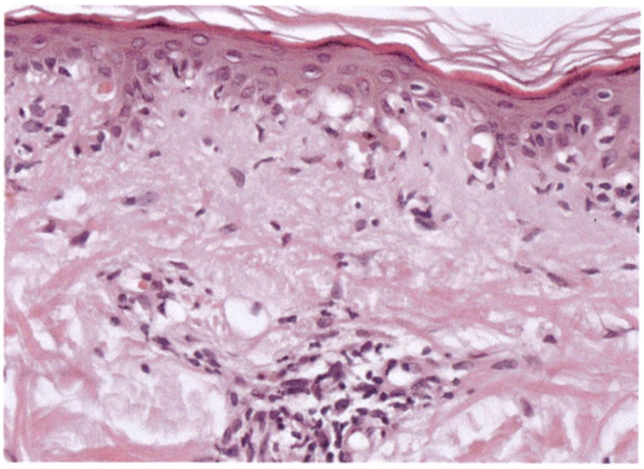

Fig. 7.43 **Acute grade 2 GvHD** with vacuolar changes, focal necrotic keratinocyte, and mild inflammation

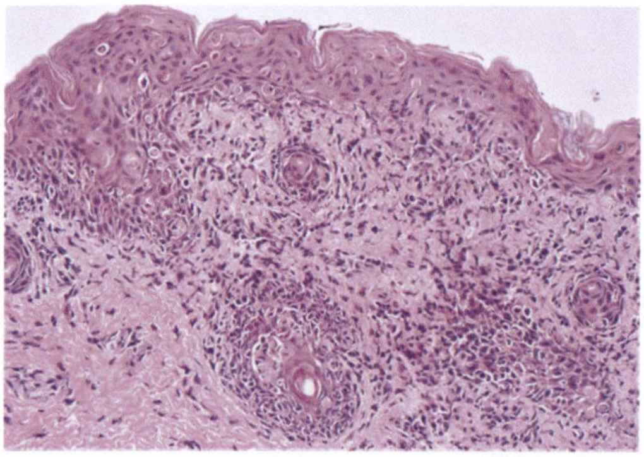

Fig. 7.44 **Acute grade 3 GvHD** with numerous necrotic keratinocytes and more pronounced inflammation

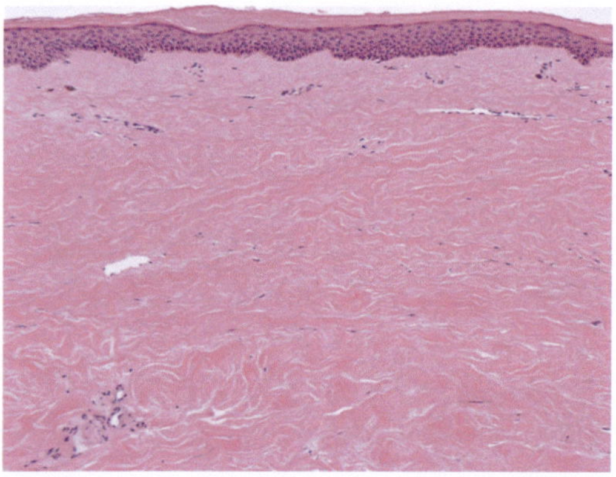

Fig. 7.46 **Chronic morphea type GvHD** with extensive sclerosis

Histopathology

Acute:

Grade 1—focal interface vacuolar changes

Grade 2—same as Grade 1 plus focal ecrotic keratinocytes, more pronounced interface vacuoles, and mild perivascular dermal inflammation (Fig. 7.43)

Grade 3—same as Grade 2 but with numerous necrotic keratinocytes and significant inflammation (Fig. 7.44)

Grade 4—same as Grade 3 plus separation of the epidermis from the dermis

Chronic:

- Lichenoid type (60 days or more after transplantation): appears like mild form of LP (Fig. 7.45)
- Morphea type (100 days or more after transplantation): appears like morphea (Fig. 7.46)

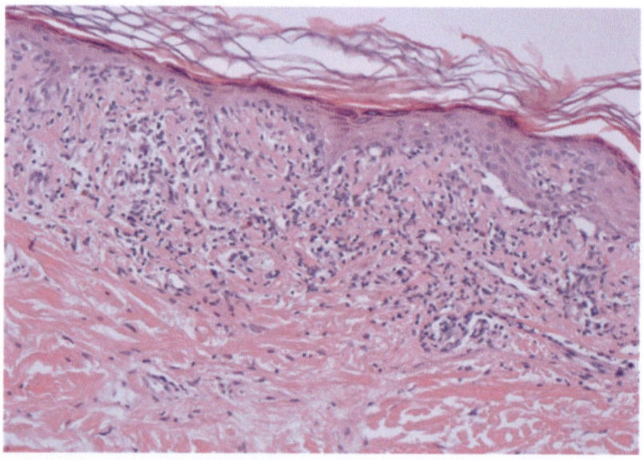

Fig. 7.45 **Chronic lichenoid GvHD** with band-like inflammation

Granular Cell Tumor

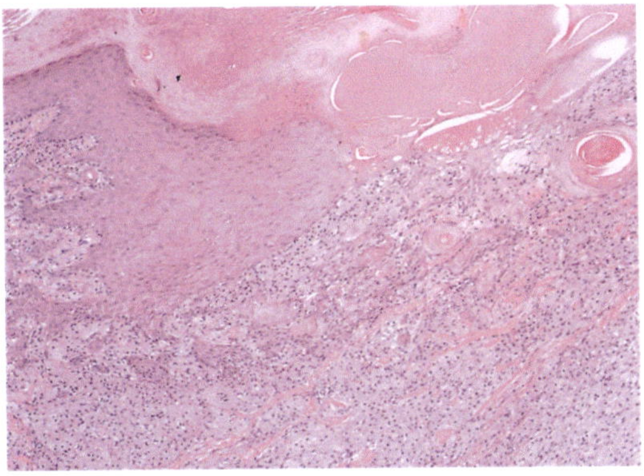

Fig. 7.47 Hyperkeratotic epidermis with pale dermis

Histopathology (Figs. 7.47, 7.48, and 7.49)
- Hyperkeratotic epidermis with pseudo-epitheliomatous hyperplasia
- Dermal/subcutaneous pale infiltrative tumor
- Round to oval pale cells (S-100+) with delicate eosinophilic cytoplasmic granules
- Minimal cellular pleomorphism and very rare mitosis

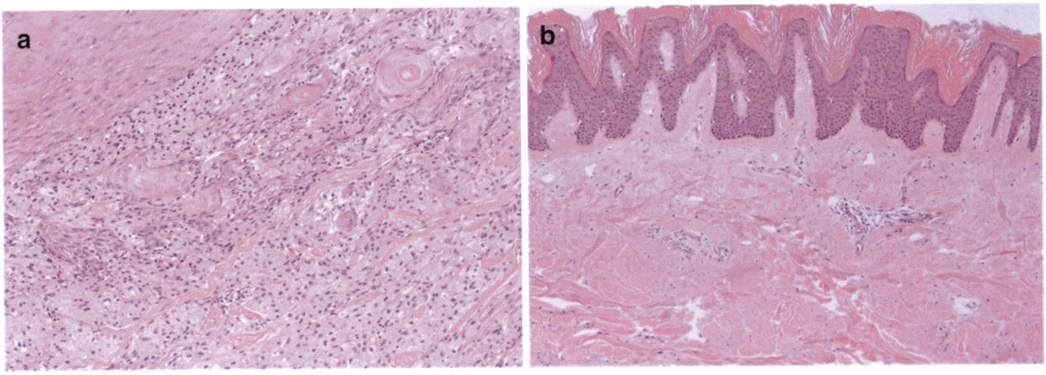

Fig. 7.48 (**a**, **b**) Pseudoepitheliomatous hyperplasia can overshadow dermal infiltrate (and be misdiagnosed as squamous cell carcinoma) which is particularly dangerous on the superficial shave biopsies

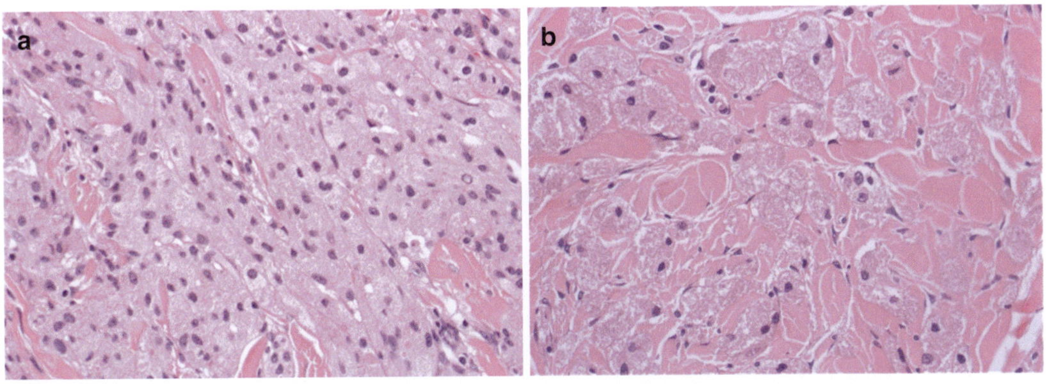

Fig. 7.49 (**a**, **b**) Uniform round to oval pale cells with fine granular cytoplasm

Granulation Tissue

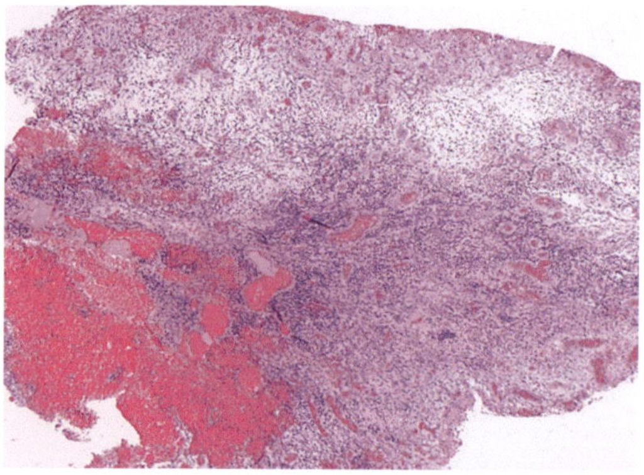

Fig. 7.50 Vascular, bloody biopsy with no epidermis

Synonym: Proud Flash

Histopathology (Figs. 7.50, 7.51, and 7.52)

- Proliferation of capillary network
- Admixed numerous lymphocytes, plasma cells, and some neutrophils
- Vessels are very congested
- As lesions age, vascular proliferation subsides and it is replaced by proliferating fibroblasts and eventual scar formation

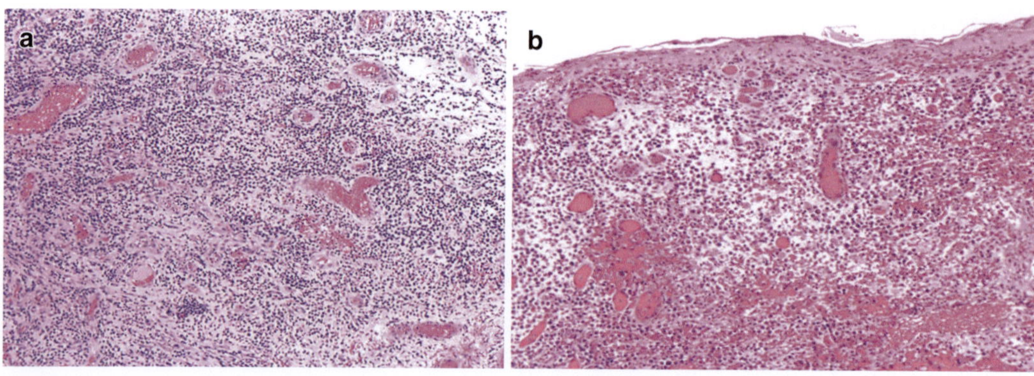

Fig. 7.51 (**a**, **b**) Random proliferation of congested capillaries and exuberant lymphoplasmocytic infiltrate

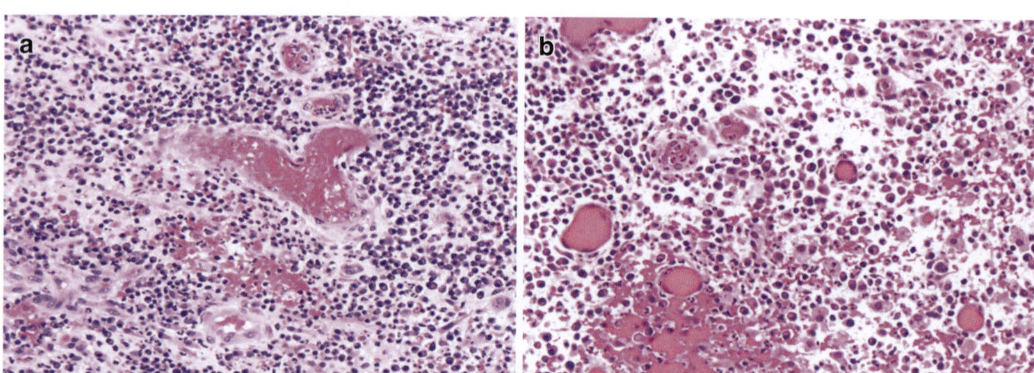

Fig. 7.52 (**a**, **b**) Capillaries have reactive endothelial cells but no real atypia

Granuloma Annulare

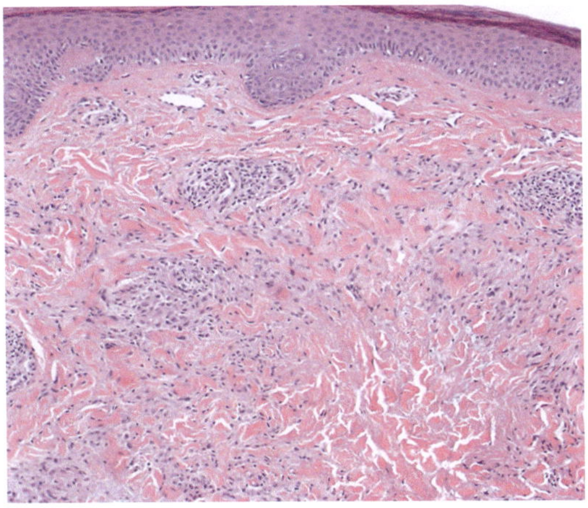

Fig. 7.53 **Granulomatous GA**

Histopathology

Granulomatous (palisaded) form: granulomatous dermatitis with central degenerated collagen (necrobiosis) with mucin and peripheral lymphohistiocytic infiltrate (Figs. 7.53 and 7.54)

Interstitial (diffuse) form: vaguely granulomatous appearance with lymphocytes and histiocytes arranged in between collagen (Figs. 7.55 and 7.56). Dermal mucin is present (Fig. 7.57).

Deep form: large area of granulomatous necrobiosis with mucin in the subcutis surrounded by exuberant lymphohistiocytic palisading

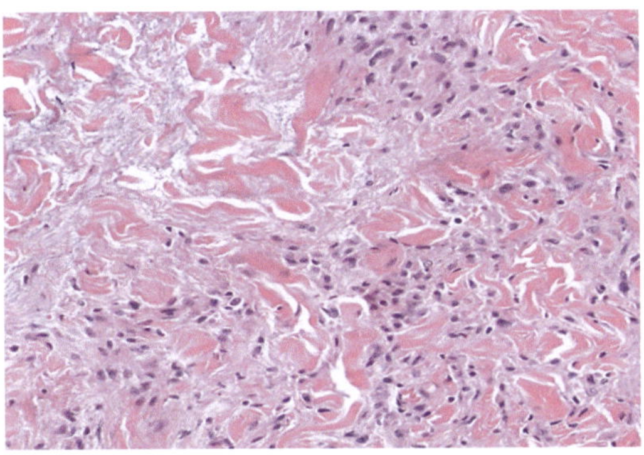

Fig. 7.54 Dermal granuloma with mucin and peripheral lymphocytes and histiocytes

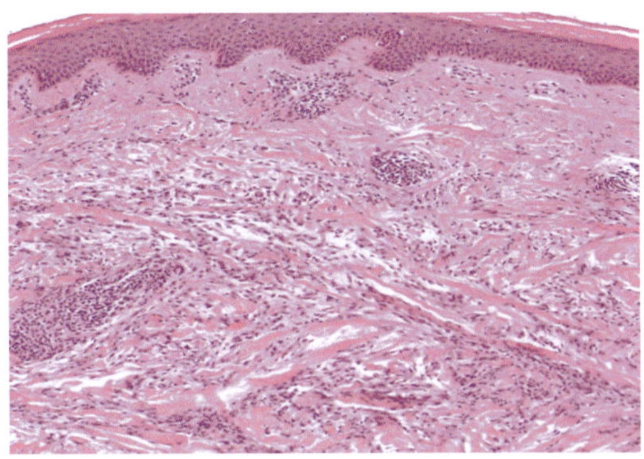

Fig. 7.55 **Interstitial GA**: Lymphocytes and histiocytes are interstitially distributed forming vague granulomas

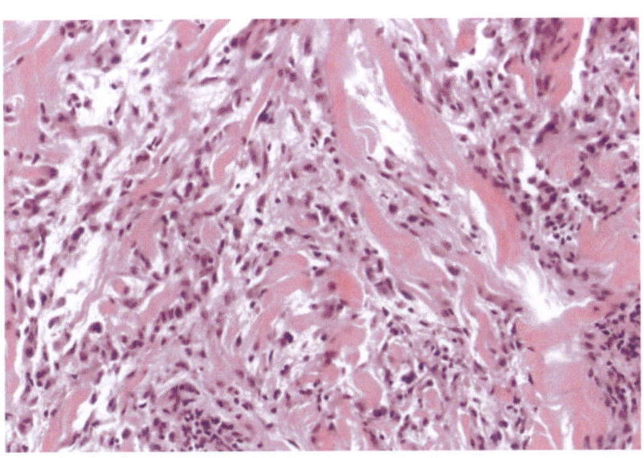

Fig. 7.56 Collagen fibers are thickened and eosinophilic with some mucin in between

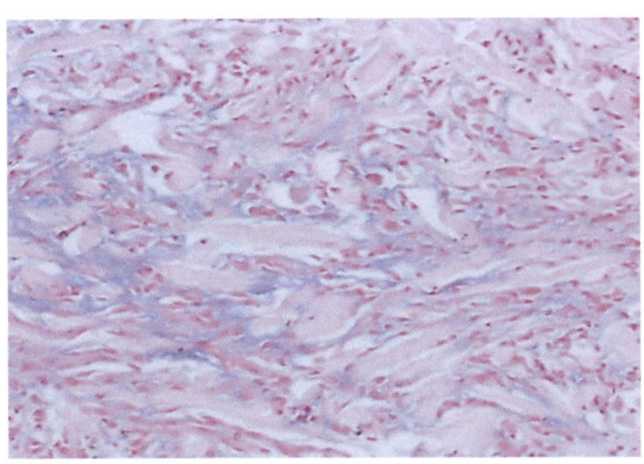

Fig. 7.57 Alcian Blue stain highlights mucin

Granuloma Faciale

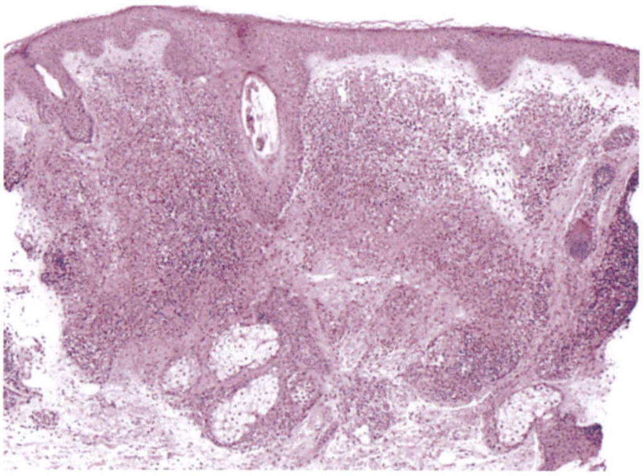

Fig. 7.58 Exuberant dermal mixed inflammation

Histopathology (Figs. 7.58, 7.59, 7.60, and 7.61)

- Dense dermal polymorphous infiltrate consisting of eosinophils, neutrophils, lymphocytes, histiocytes, and plasma cells
- Various degree of vascular damage with leukocytoclasia
- Separation of epidermis and dermal infiltrate by a narrow Grenz zone of normal collagen

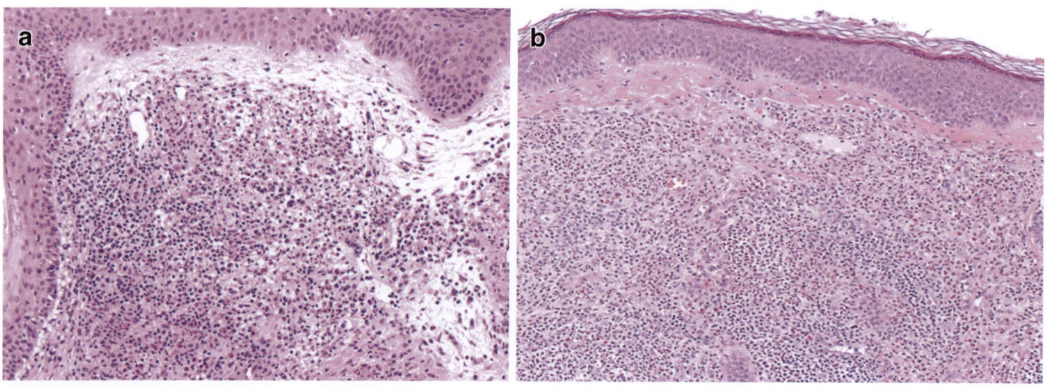

Fig. 7.59 (**a**, **b**) Grenz zone separates epidermis from dermal polymorphic inflammation

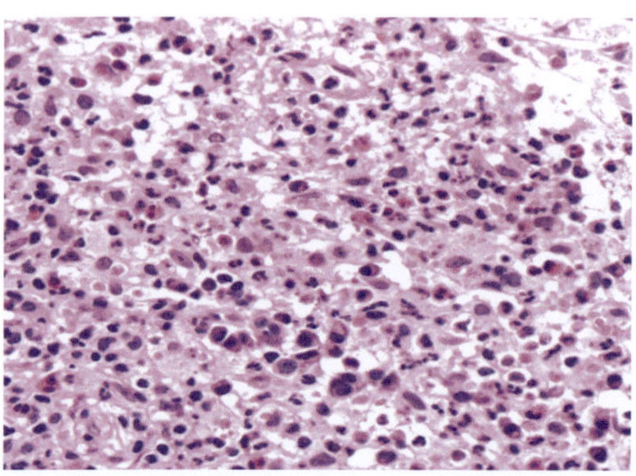

Fig. 7.60 Vascular damage with nuclear debris is present

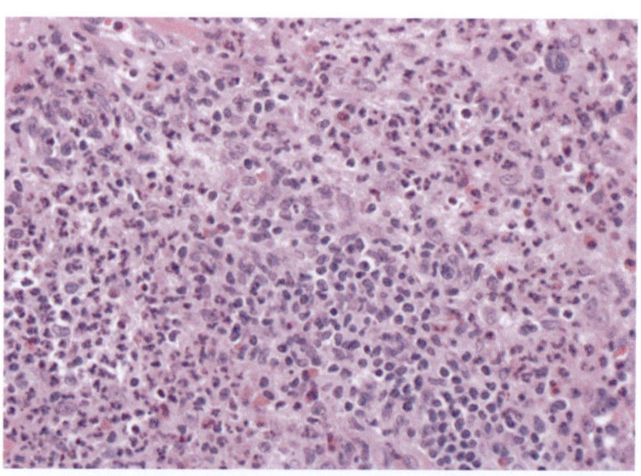

Fig. 7.61 Eosinophils, neutrophils, lymphocytes, histiocytes, and plasma cells compose the dermal infiltrate

Granuloma Inguinale

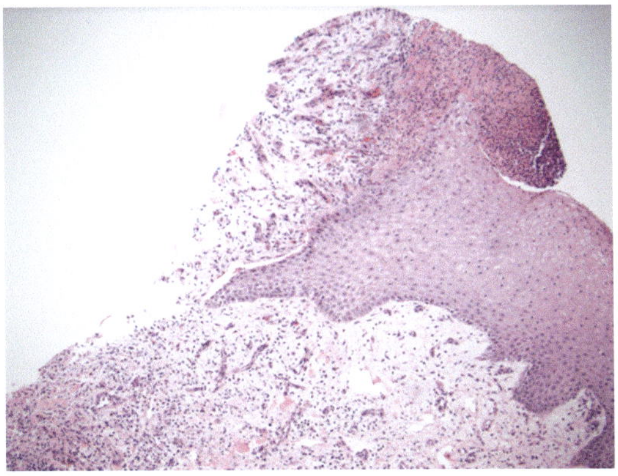

Fig. 7.62 Ulcerated skin with serum crust and adjacent pseudoepitheliomatous hyperplasia

Synonyms: Granuloma Venereum, Donovanosis

Histopathology (Figs. 7.62, 7.63, 7.64, and 7.65)

- Ulcerated skin with serum crust and granulation tissue with prominent vessels
- Margins of ulcer have pseudoepitheliomatous hyperplasia
- Inflammation consists of neutrophils, plasma cells, and histiocytes some of which are enlarged with organisms present in the cytoplasm
- Giemsa, Giemsa-Wright, and Warthin-Starry are the best special stains

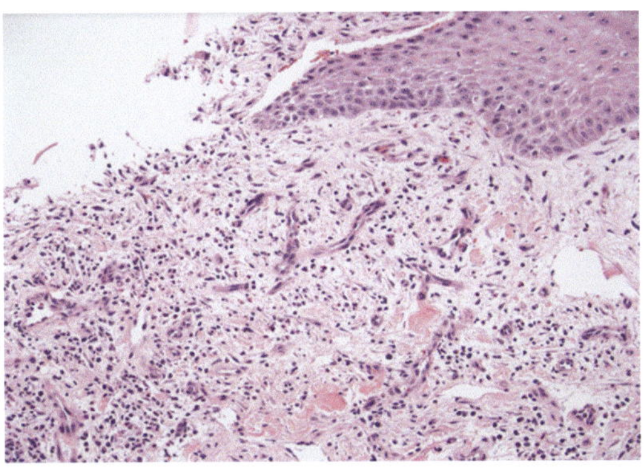

Fig. 7.63 Granulation tissue with prominent blood vessels

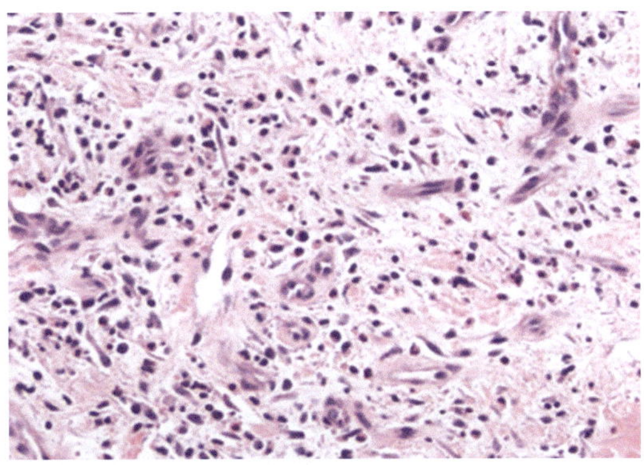

Fig. 7.64 Neutrophilic inflammation with few large histiocytes

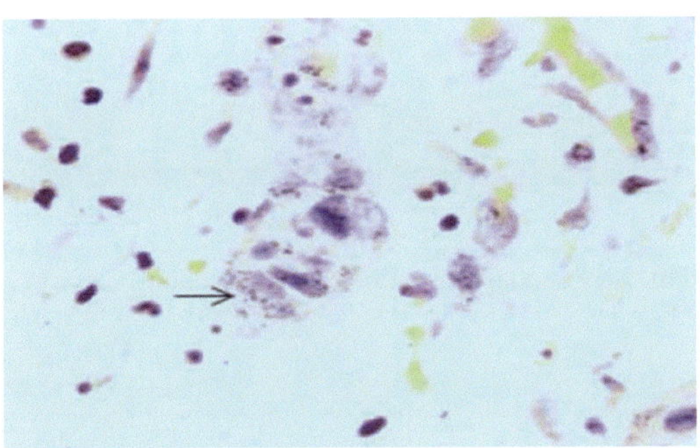

Fig. 7.65 Giemsa-Wright stain outlines purple organisms in the cytoplasm of the histiocytes

Grover's Disease

Synonym: Transient Acantholytic Dermatosis

Four different **histopathological** patterns of which more than one may be present:

Darier's pattern:

- Focal epidermal acantholysis with "corp ronds and corp grains" and suprabasal split (Fig. 7.66)

Hailey-Hailey pattern:

- Epidermal acantholysis with "dilapidated wall" appearance (Fig. 7.67)

Pemphigus Vulgaris pattern:

- Suprabasal epidermal acantholysis with "row of tombstones" (Fig. 7.68)

Spongiotic dermatitis pattern:

- Mild to moderate epidermal spongiosis with vesicle formation (Fig. 7.69)

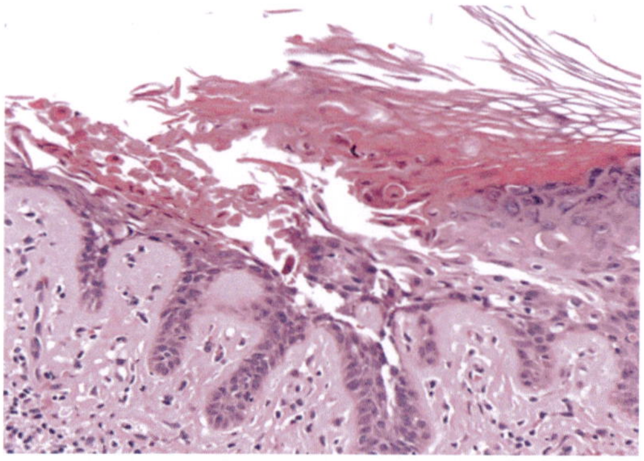

Fig. 7.66 "Corp ronds and corp grains"

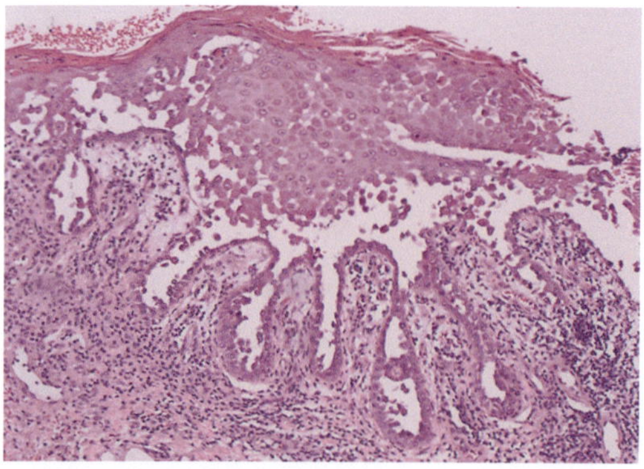

Fig. 7.67 "Dilapidated brick wall"

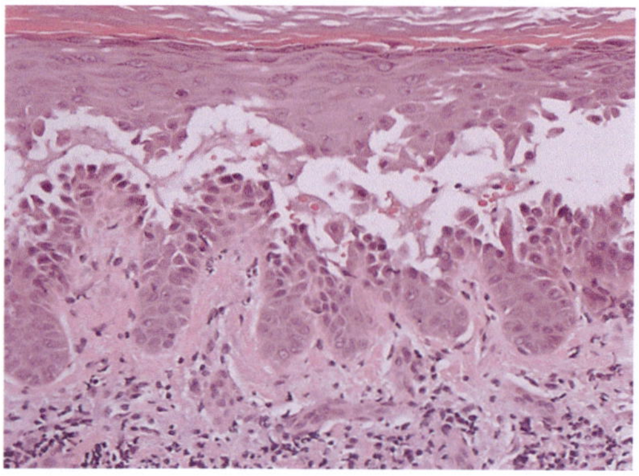

Fig. 7.68 "Row of tombstones"

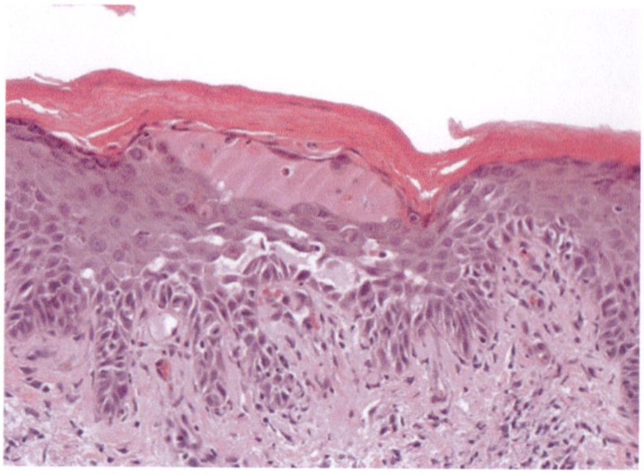

Fig. 7.69 Spongiosis with vesicle formation

Gynecomastia

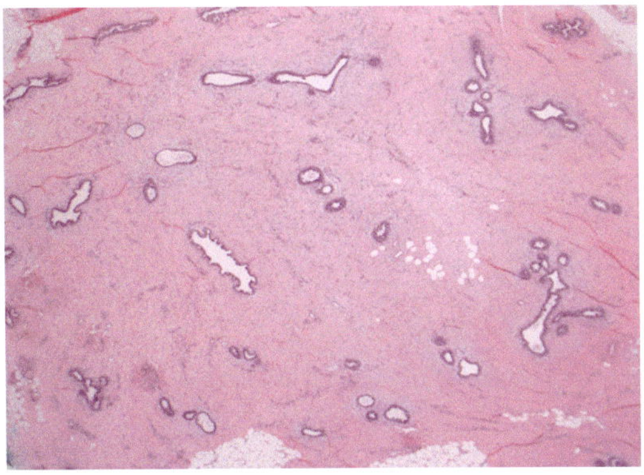

Fig. 7.70 Variably sized scattered ducts

Histopathology (Figs. 7.70, 7.71, 7.72, 7.73, and 7.74)

- Male breast with ductal hyperplasia with micropapillae
- In an early lesion there is periductal edema and in an older lesion there is periductal fibrosis
- Lobules are not present and there is no cytological atypia or mitoses

P.S. associated with Klinefelter's syndrome, use of anabolic steroids, digitalis, dilantin, isoniazid, antiretroviral medication

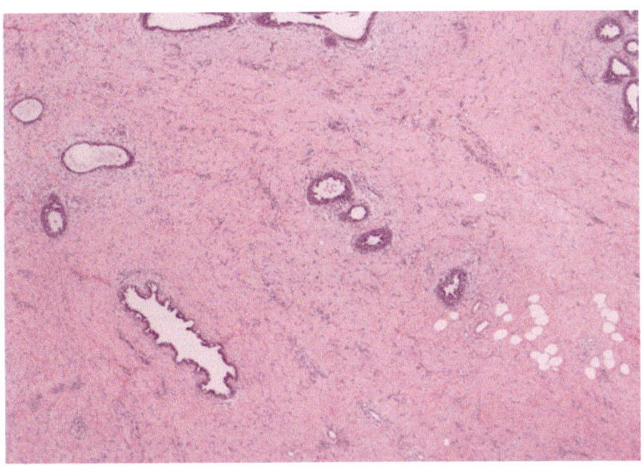

Fig. 7.71 Multiple dilated ducts but lobules not present

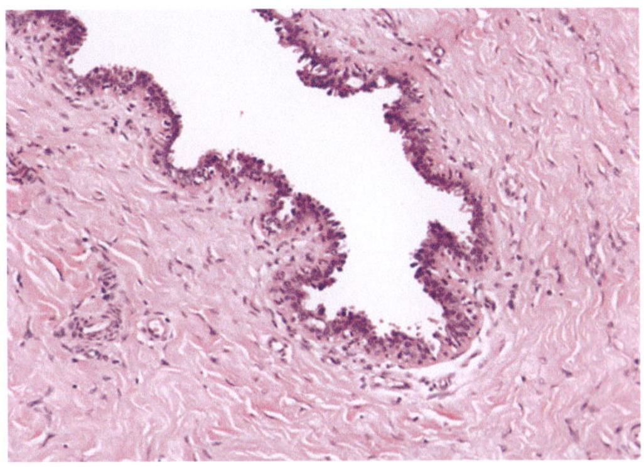

Fig. 7.72 Dilated duct with two cell layer

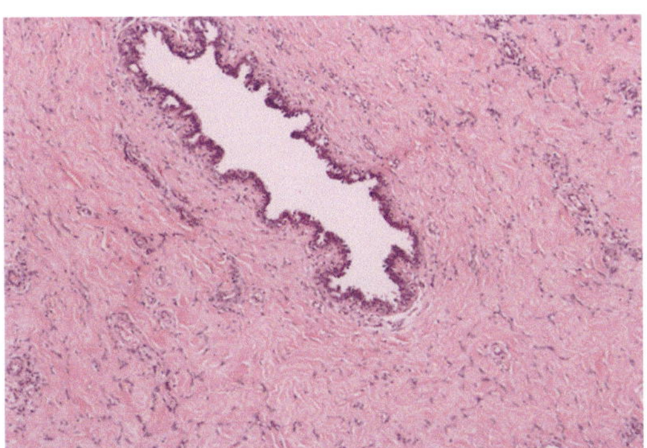

Fig. 7.73 Dilated ducts in fibrotic stroma

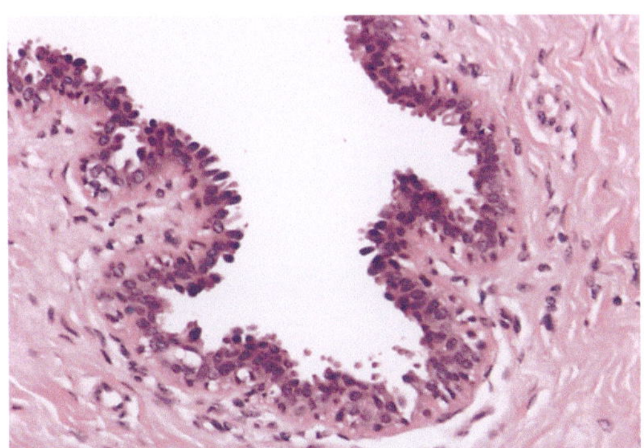

Fig. 7.74 Micropapillae are present

8 Dermatopathology H

V. Vincek, *Dermatopathology A–Z*, https://doi.org/10.1007/978-3-319-89486-7_8

Hailey-Hailey Disease

Synonym: Familial Benign Pemphigus

Histopathology (Figs. 8.1, 8.2, 8.3, and 8.4)

- Suprabasal clefting
- Epidermal acantholysis of stratum spinosum
- "Dilapidated brick wall" appearance
- Occasional dyskeratosis
- Mild dermal perivascular lymphocytic inflammation

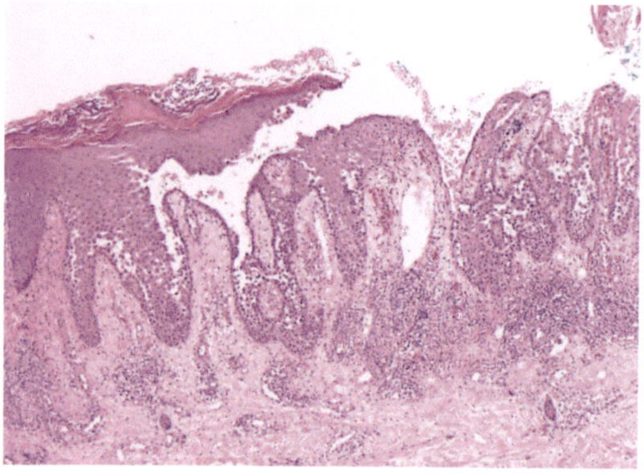

Fig. 8.1 Acanthotic epidermis that is disintegrating

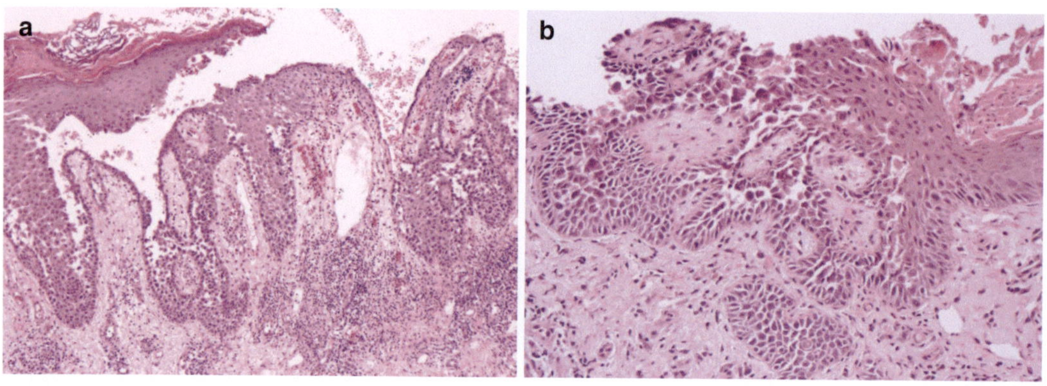

Fig. 8.2 (**a**, **b**) Acantholysis of stratum spinosum with dermal lymphocytic inflammation

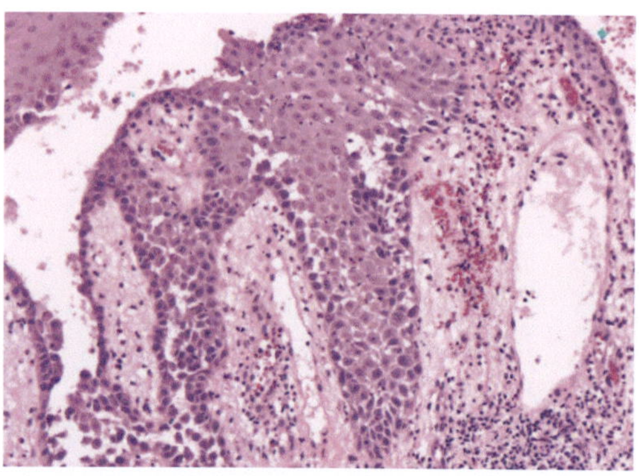

Fig. 8.3 Suprabasal clefting

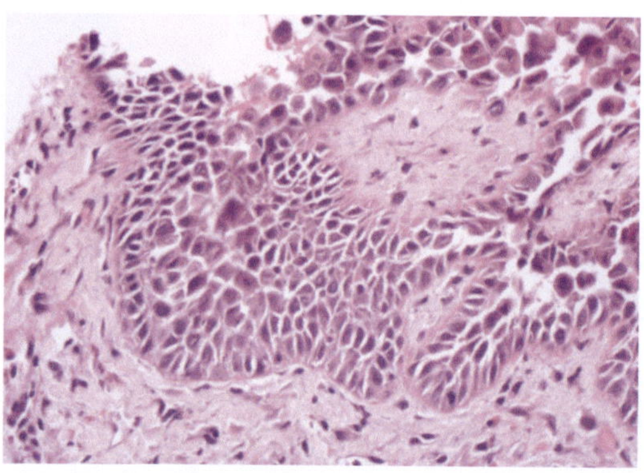

Fig. 8.4 "Dilapidated brick wall" appearance

Halo Nevus

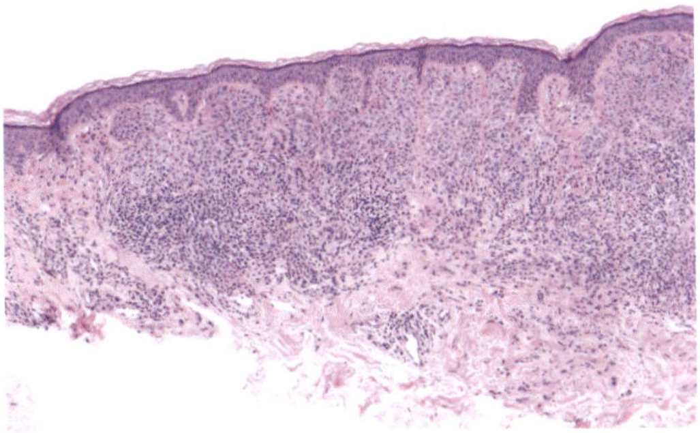

Fig. 8.5 Symmetrical compound nevus with lymphocytes

Synonym: Sutton's Nevus

Histopathology (Figs. 8.5, 8.6, and 8.7)

- Symmetrical junctional, compound, or dermal nevus
- Associated with well-circumscribed dense lymphocytic infiltrate
- Well defined interior margin
- Normal maturation of nevus cells with minimal cytological atypia

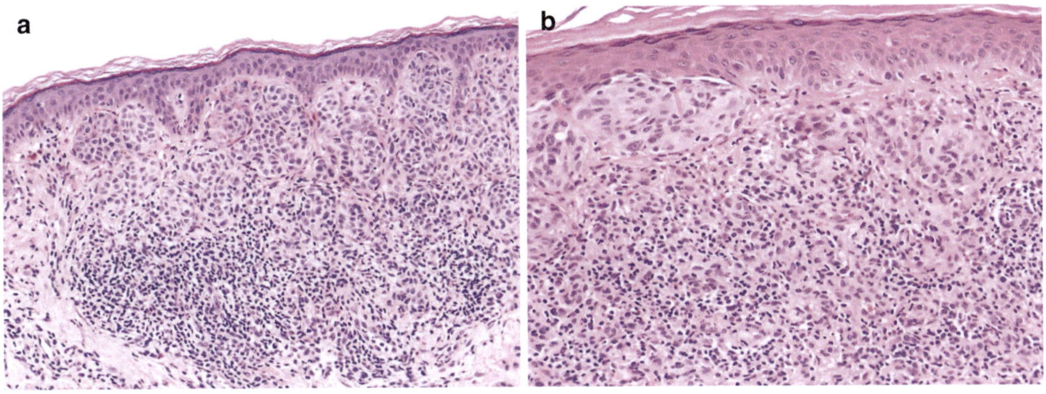

Fig. 8.6 (a, b) Numerous small lymphocytes surround nevus cells

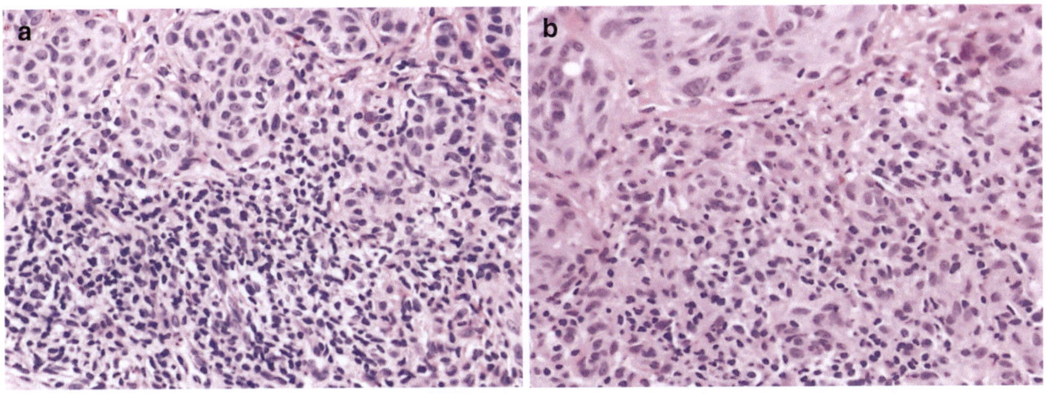

Fig. 8.7 (a, b) Dermal nevus cells among lymphocytes showing maturation with descent and no evidence of atypia

Halogenoderma

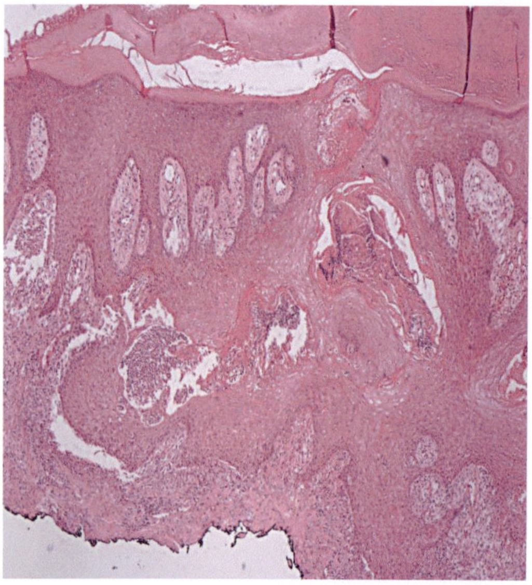

Fig. 8.8 Extensive irregular epidermal proliferation

Synonyms: Bromoderma, Fluoroderma, Iododerma

Histopathology (Figs. 8.8, 8.9, and 8.10)

- Extensive pseudoepitheliomatous hyperplasia
- Intraepidermal micropustules
- Dermal acute and chronic inflammation
- Occasional giant cells but not as many as in deep fungal infections

P.S. always exclude an infection. Clinical correlation is necessary.

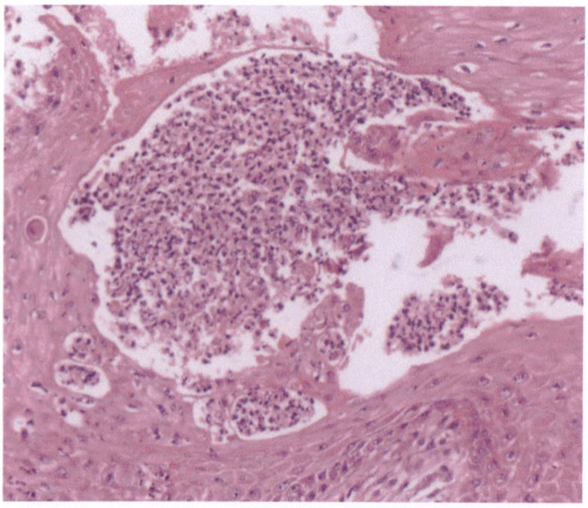

Fig. 8.9 Neutrophilic aggregates within the epidermis

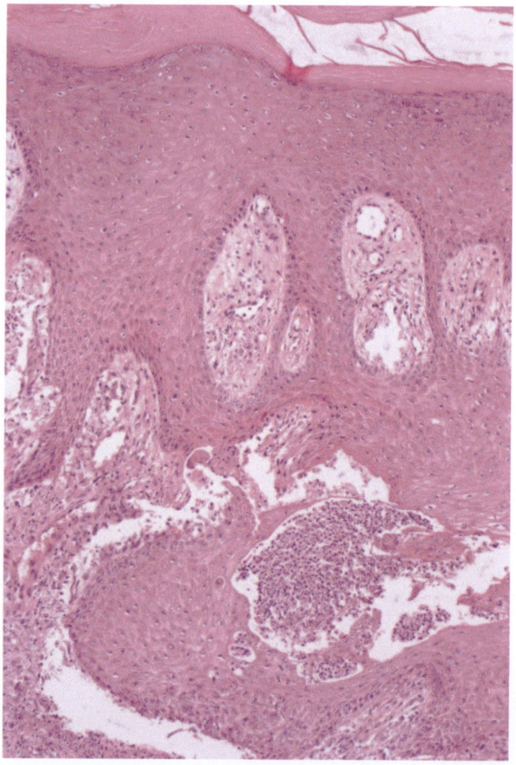

Fig. 8.10 No evidence of epidermal cytological atypia

Hand Foot and Mouth Disease

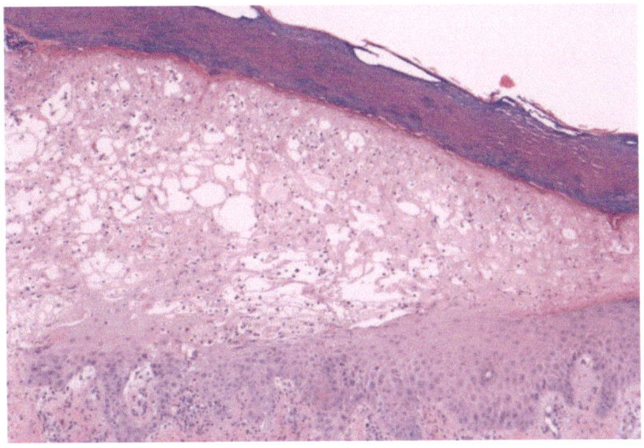

Fig. 8.11 Acral skin with epidermal necrosis

Histopathology (Figs. 8.11, 8.12, and 8.13)

- Acral skin with thick stratum corneum
- Epidermal necrosis with prominent reticular degeneration of keratinocytes
- Prominent ballooning of keratinocytes
- No inclusion bodies or giant cells
- Sparse scattered lymphocytes and neutrophils among degenerated keratinocytes

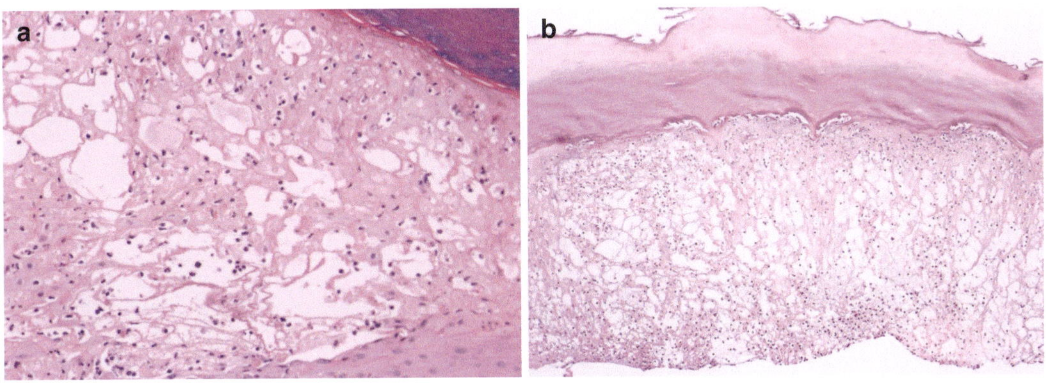

Fig. 8.12 (a, b) Characteristic full thickness reticular degeneration of keratinocytes

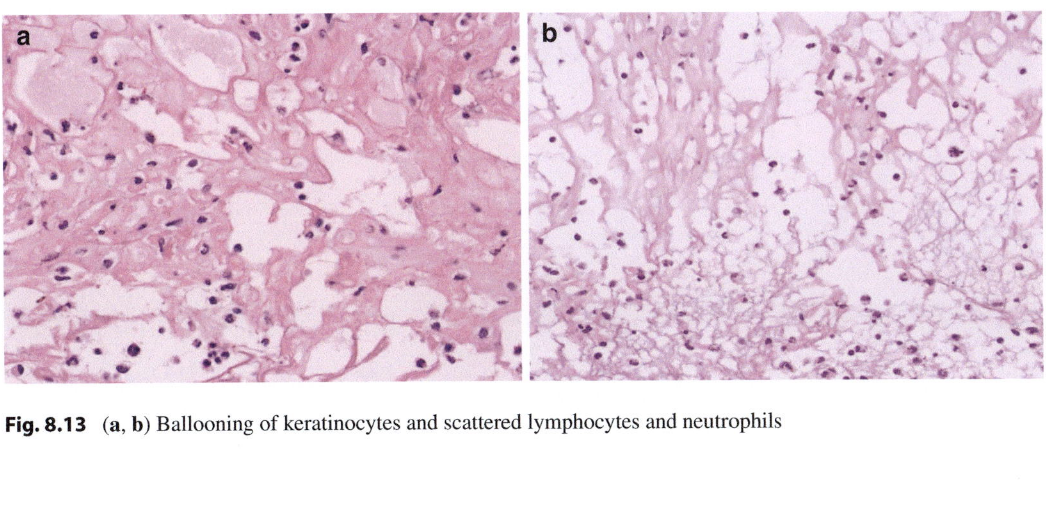

Fig. 8.13 (a, b) Ballooning of keratinocytes and scattered lymphocytes and neutrophils

Hemangioendothelioma

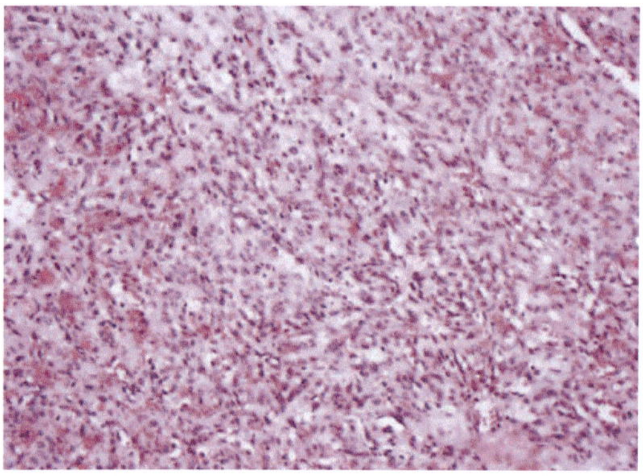

Fig. 8.14 Cellular vascular lesion with prominent RBCs

Histopathology (Figs. 8.14, 8.15, and 8.16)

- Infiltrating dermal/subcutaneous tumor
- Round/oval cells (CD31+, CD34+) with abundant eosinophilic cytoplasm and vesicular nuclei
- Intracytoplasmic lumina are characteristic
- Common red blood cell extravasation
- Cytological atypia and number of mitoses vary

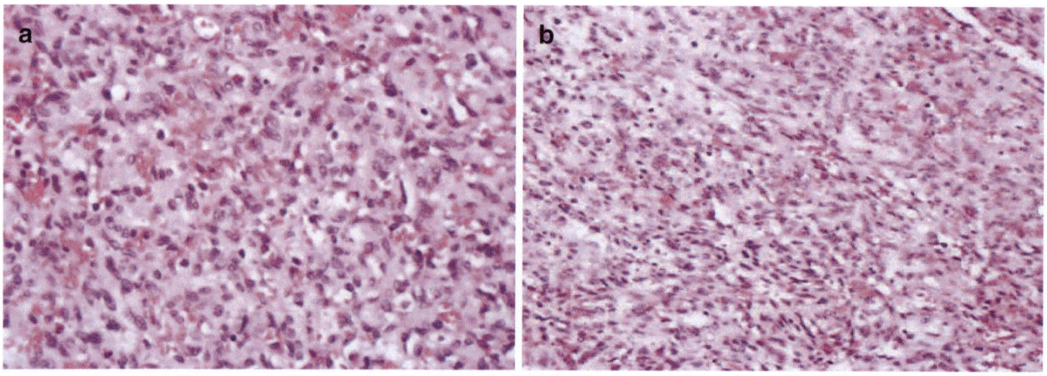

Fig. 8.15 (a, b) Cells with abundant cytoplasm and vesicular nuclei

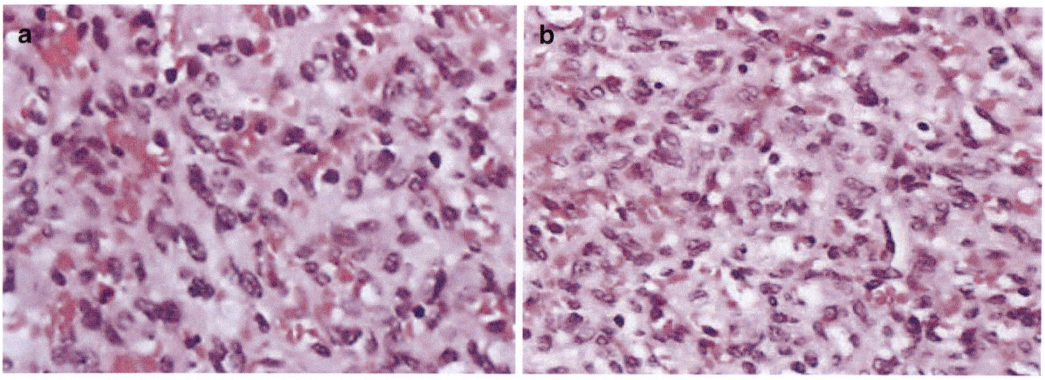

Fig. 8.16 (a, b) Intracytoplasmic lumina are present

Hemangioma

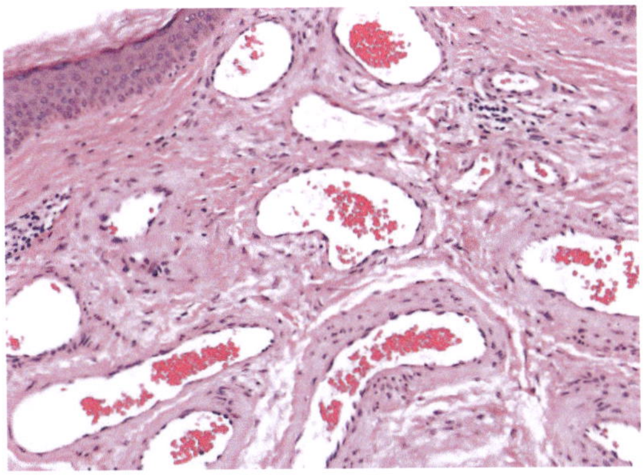

Fig. 8.17 **Arteriovenous hemangioma** with mixture of vessels with thick (arteries) and thin (veins) walls

Histopathology

- Proliferation of dermal and subcutaneous benign blood vessels
- Different subtypes based on the size and appearance of the vessels (Figs. 8.17, 8.18, 8.19, 8.20, 8.21, 8.22, 8.23, 8.24, and 8.25)

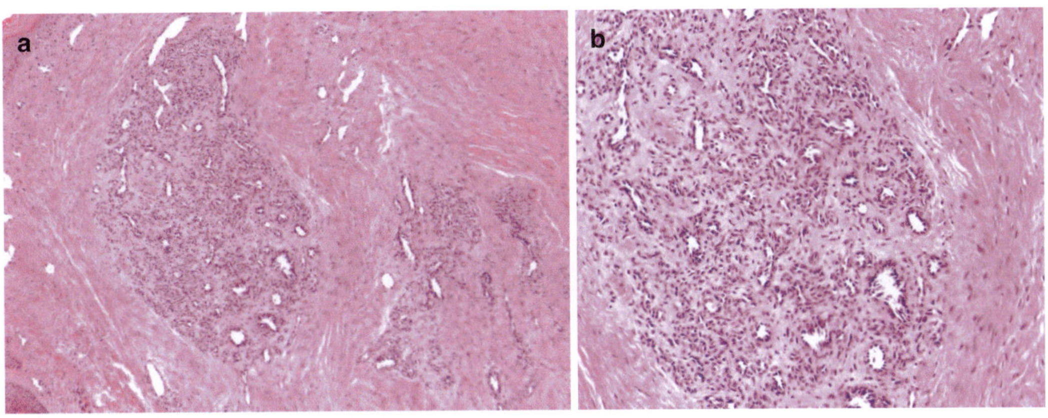

Fig. 8.18 (**a**, **b**) **Capillary hemangioma** with proliferation of small capillaries

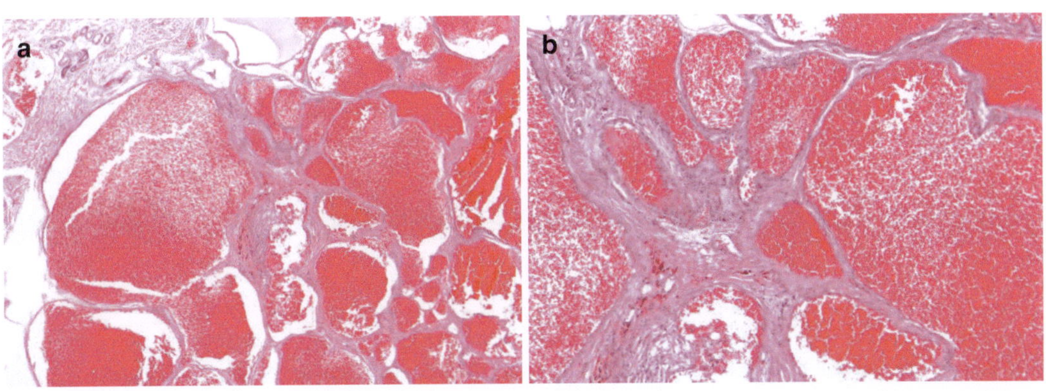

Fig. 8.19 (**a**, **b**) **Cavernous hemangioma** with proliferation of large cavernous vascular channels

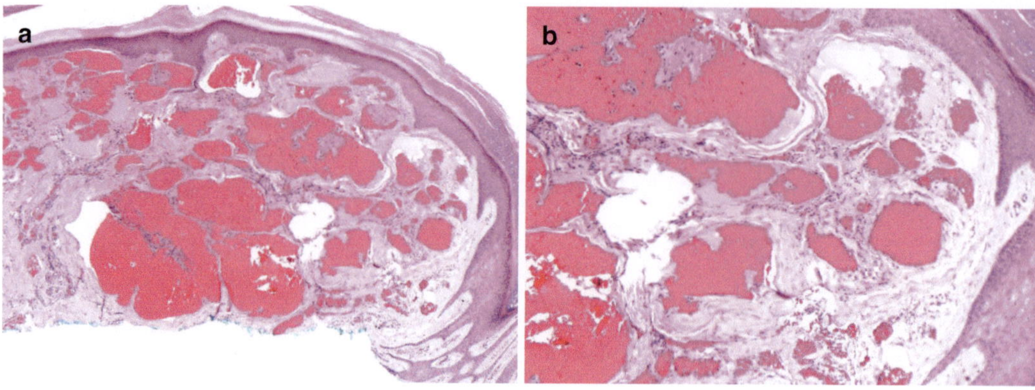

Fig. 8.20 (**a**, **b**) **Cherry angioma** with dermal proliferation of various size vessels with epidermal collarette

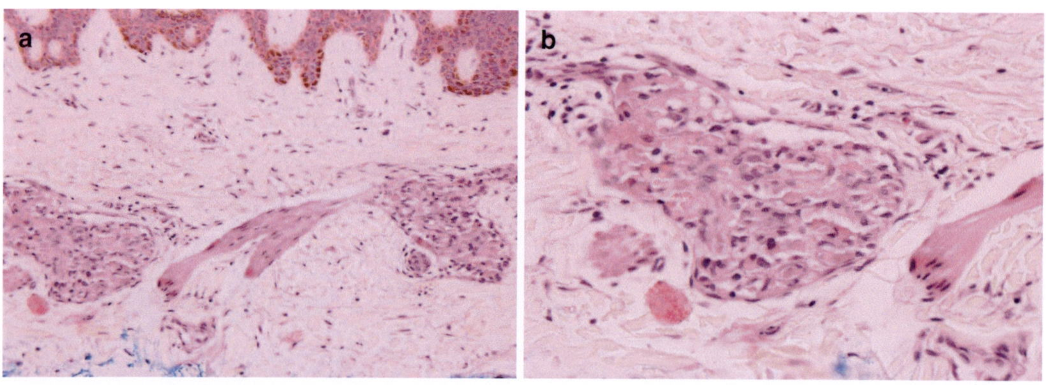

Fig. 8.21 (**a**, **b**) **Glomeruloid hemangioma** with "glomeruli-like" proliferation within dilated vessels

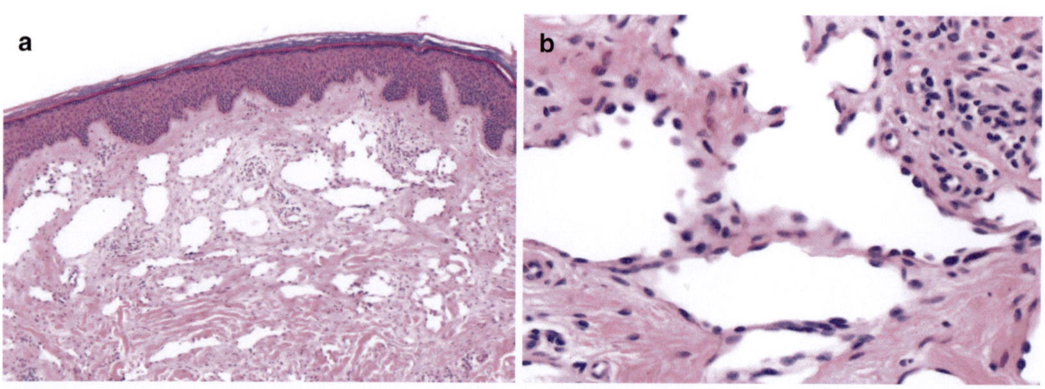

Fig. 8.22 (**a**, **b**) **Hobnail hemangioma** with endothelial cells showing characteristic "hobnail-like" nuclei

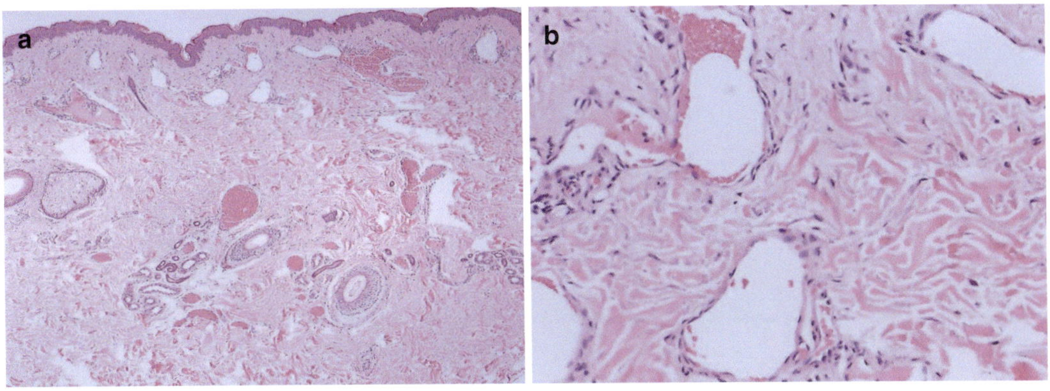

Fig. 8.23 (**a**, **b**) **Nevus flammeus** with dilated congested dermal vessels

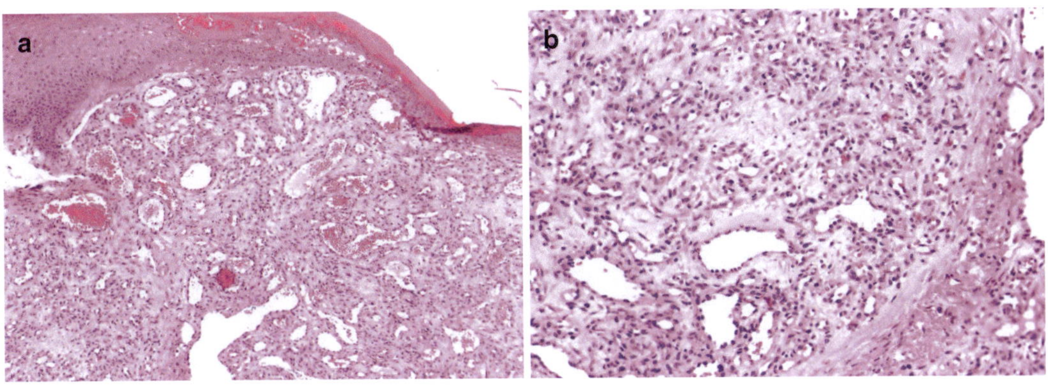

Fig. 8.24 (**a**, **b**) **Pyogenic granuloma** with excoriated epidermis and dermal lobular proliferation of capillaries

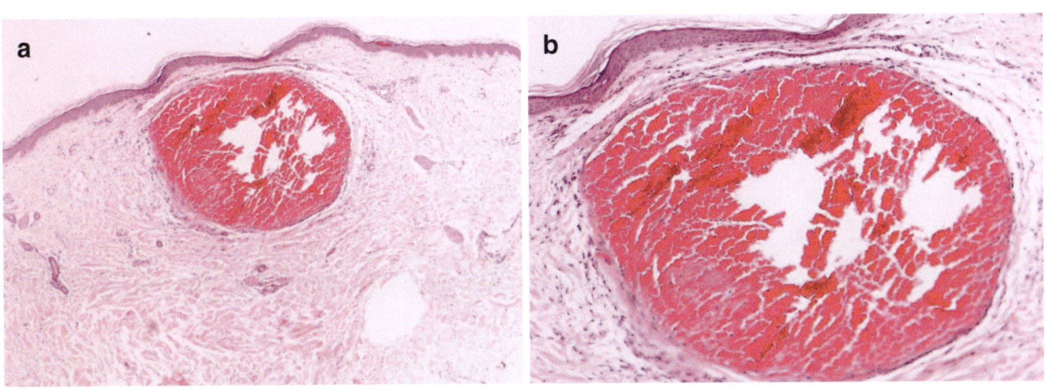

Fig. 8.25 (**a**, **b**) **Venous lake** with dilated vascular channel filled with red blood cells

Hemangiopericytoma

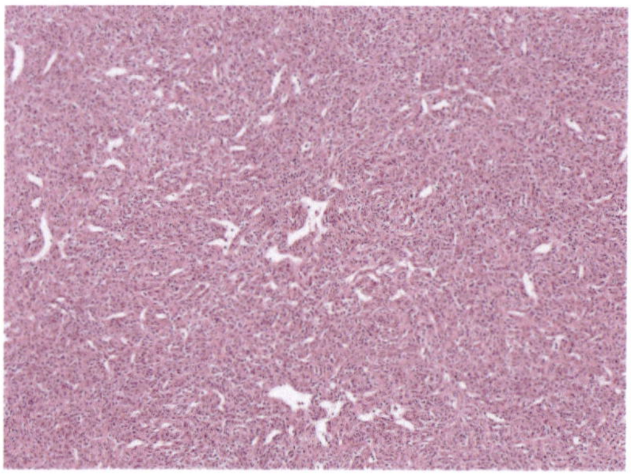

Fig. 8.26 Subcutaneous cellular tumor

Histopathology (Figs. 8.26, 8.27, 8.28, 8.29, and 8.30)
- Dermal and subcutaneous tumor
- Thin walled vessels of variable size with branching ("staghorn-like")
- Vessel covered by single layer of flattened endothelial cells
- Between vessels and encircling vessels are cells of round, oval or spindle shape (CD99+, CD34+)
- Cellularity varies from highly cellular to paucicellular with pronounced hyalinization

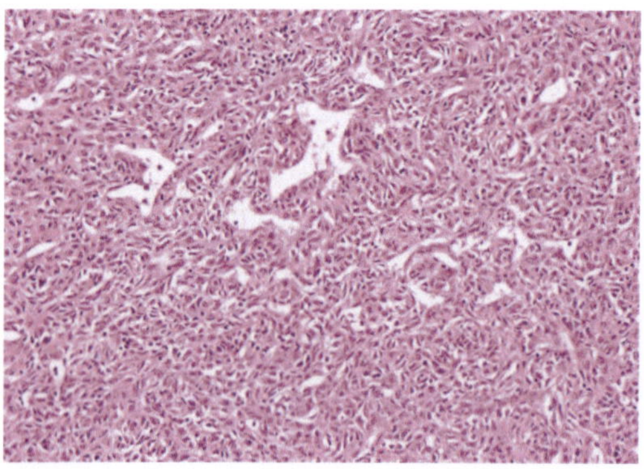

Fig. 8.27 "Staghorn-like" branching vessels

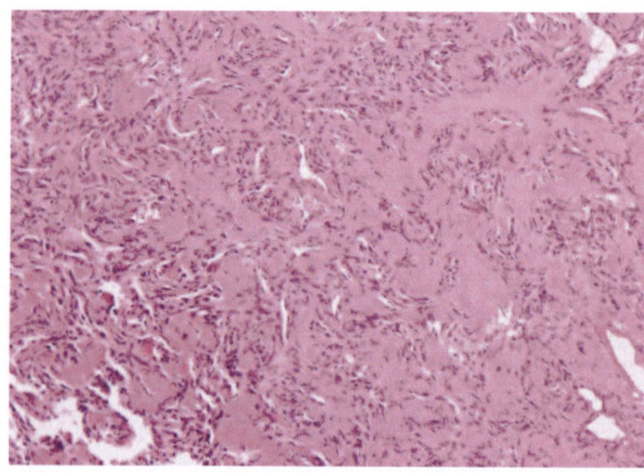

Fig. 8.28 Less cellular tumor with branching vessels

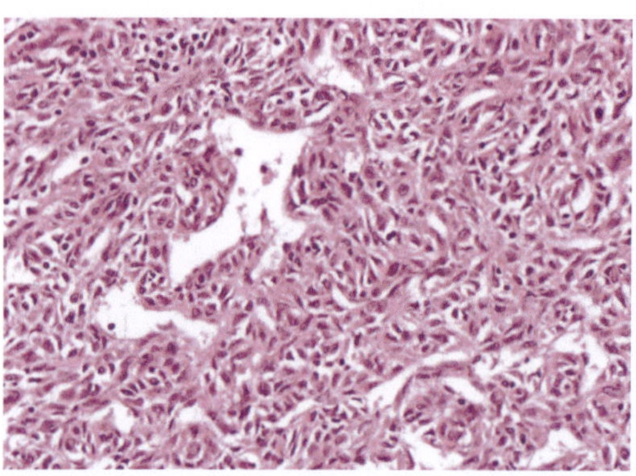

Fig. 8.29 Vessels surrounded by oval cells with vesicular nuclei and eosinophilic cytoplasm

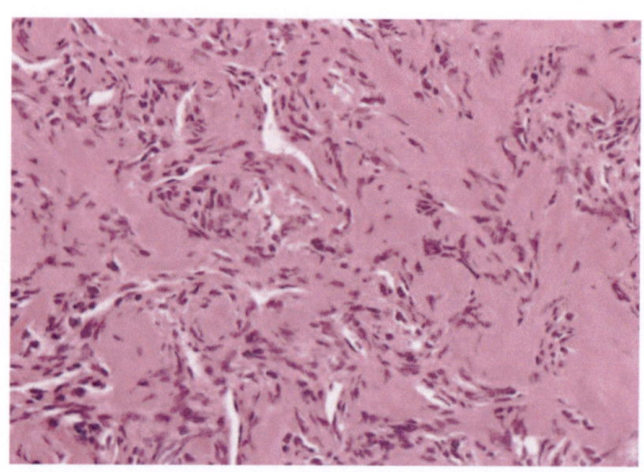

Fig. 8.30 Hyalinized stroma and elongated spindle cells

Henoch-Schönlein Purpura

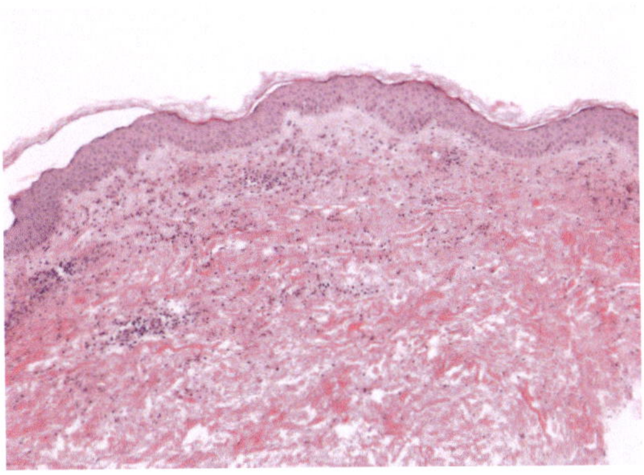

Fig. 8.31 Low power of dermis with numerous dark and red dots

Synonym: IgA Vasculitis

Histopathology is indistinguishable from other forms of leukocytoclastic vasculitis (Figs. 8.31, 8.32, and 8.33)

- Intra and perivascular neutrophilic infiltrate with neutrophilic degeneration (leukocytoclasia)
- Damaged capillaries with reactive endothelial cells, fibrin deposition and microthrombi
- Dermal red blood cell extravasation

P.S. DIF study demonstrates IgA depositions

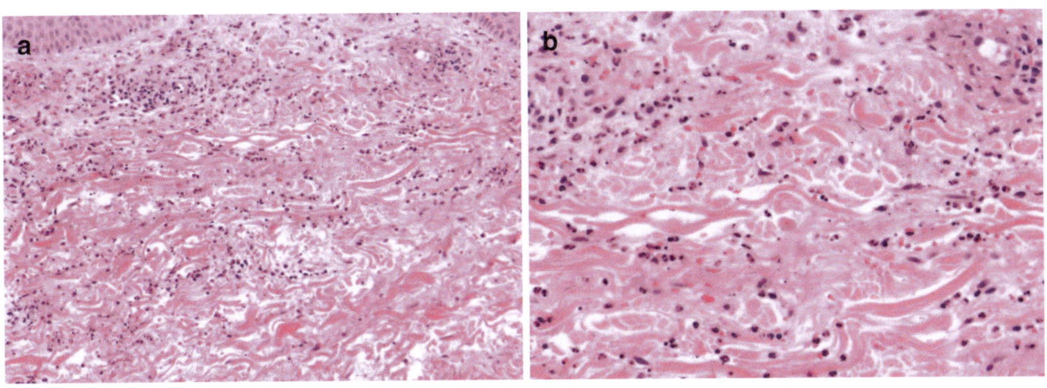

Fig. 8.32 (**a**, **b**) Perivascular and interstitial neutrophils with nuclear dust (leukocytoclasia)

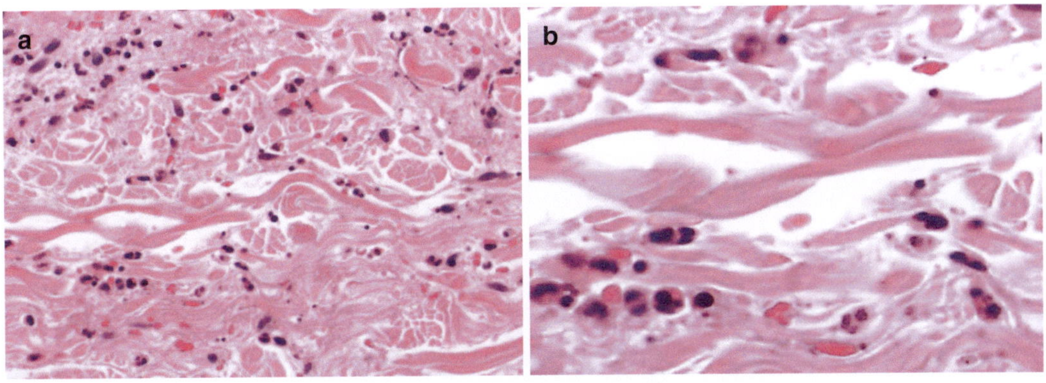

Fig. 8.33 (**a**, **b**) Neutrophils, nuclear debris, and red blood cell extravasation

Herpes Gestationis

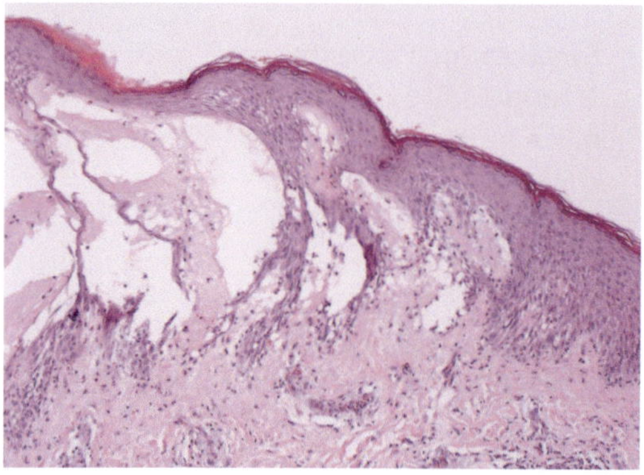

Fig. 8.34 Subepidermal blister

Synonym: Pemphigoid Gestationis

Histopathology (Figs. 8.34, 8.35, and 8.36)

- Subepidermal cleft with blister formation and focal necrosis of keratinocytes
- Blister contains eosinophils admixed with lymphocytes, histiocytes, and some neutrophils
- Similar infiltrate is present in the dermis
- DIF is required to confirm diagnosis

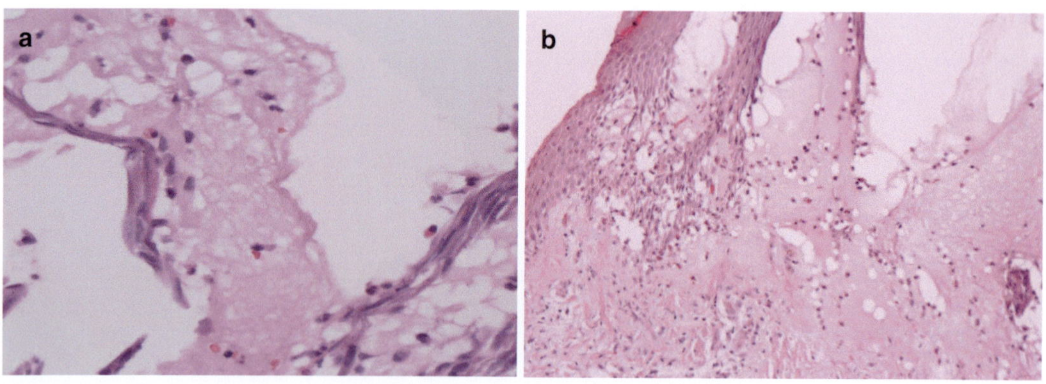

Fig. 8.35 (**a**, **b**) Blister with serous material admixed with eosinophils and lymphocytes

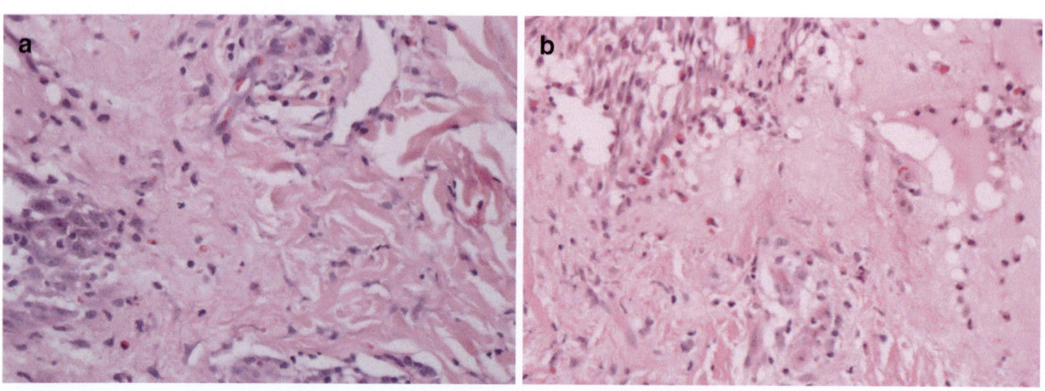

Fig. 8.36 (**a**, **b**) Dermal eosinophils with lymphocytes and occasional neutrophils

Herpes Virus

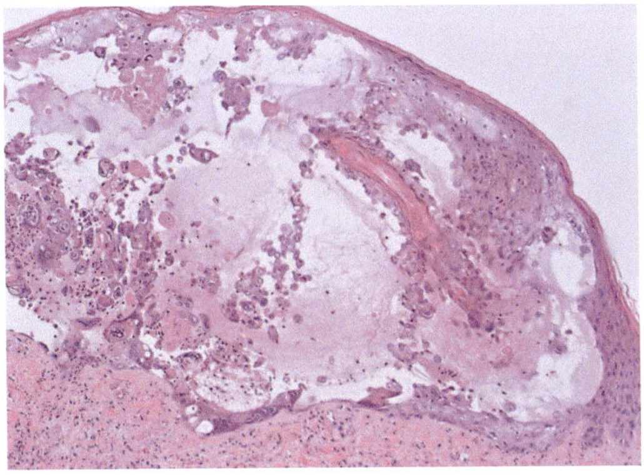

Fig. 8.37 Blister with acantholytic keratinocytes

Synonyms: **Herpes Simplex, Herpes Zoster, Chicken Pox, Varicella** (all these clinical entities demonstrate the same histopathology)

Histopathology (Figs. 8.37, 8.38, 8.39, 8.40, and 8.41)

- Blistered and/or ulcerated epidermis
- Acantholytic keratinocytes with "steel gray" nuclei
- Keratinocytes with intranuclear eosinophilic inclusion bodies
- Multinucleated giant cells with nuclear molding
- Dermal acute and chronic inflammation

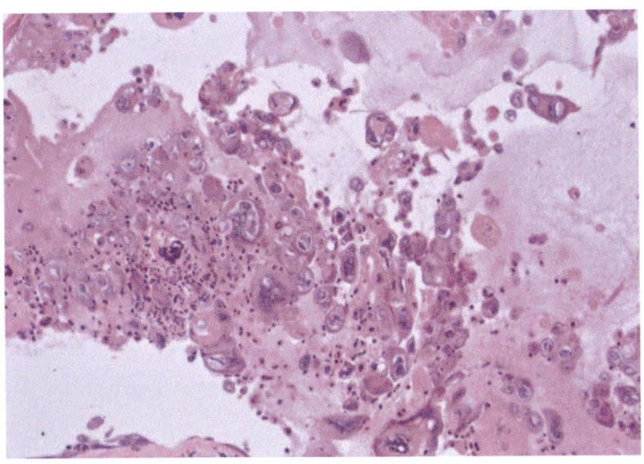

Fig. 8.38 Keratinocytes have "steel gray" nuclei

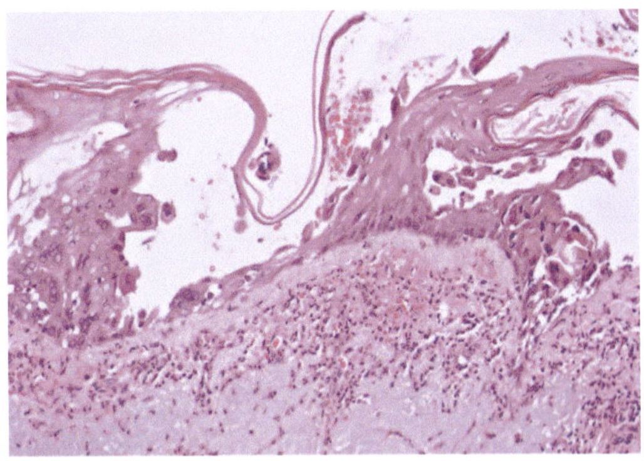

Fig. 8.39 Dermal mixed inflammation with numerous neutrophils

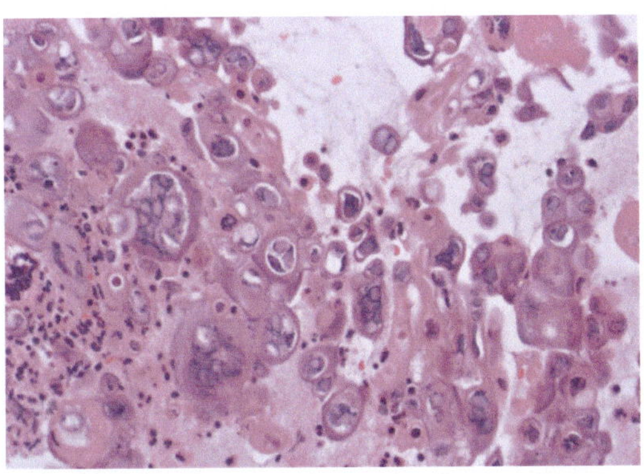

Fig. 8.40 Multinucleated cells with nuclear molding

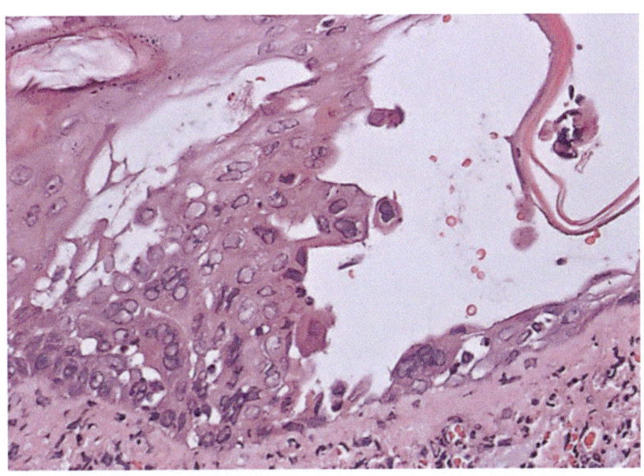

Fig. 8.41 Keratinocytes with intranuclear inclusions

Heterotopic Neural Tissue

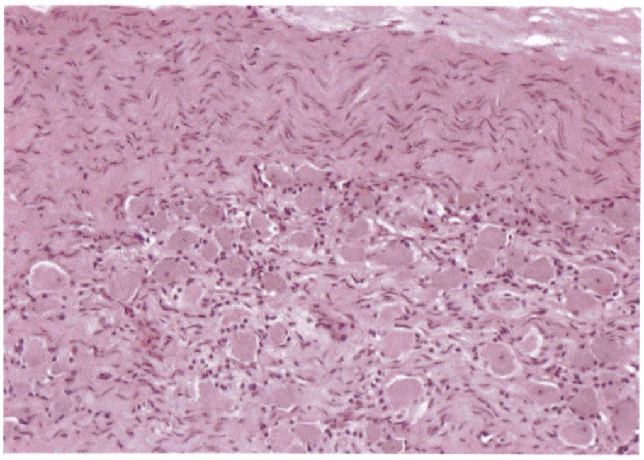

Fig. 8.42 Nodule made of normal appearing, disorganized neural tissue

Synonyms: Nasal Glioma, Neural Choristoma

Histopathology (Figs. 8.42, 8.43, 8.44, 8.45, and 8.46)

- Hamartoma formed of island of disorganized neural tissue in a neurofibrillary stroma
- Cells are GFAP+, S-100+

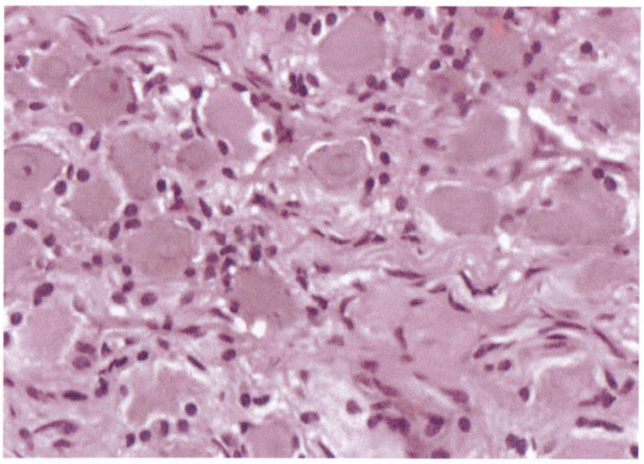

Fig. 8.43 Numerous neural ganglia

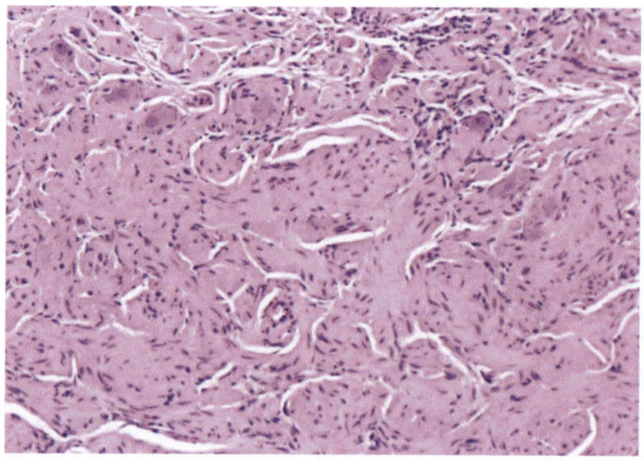

Fig. 8.44 Ganglions admixed with wavy neural fibers

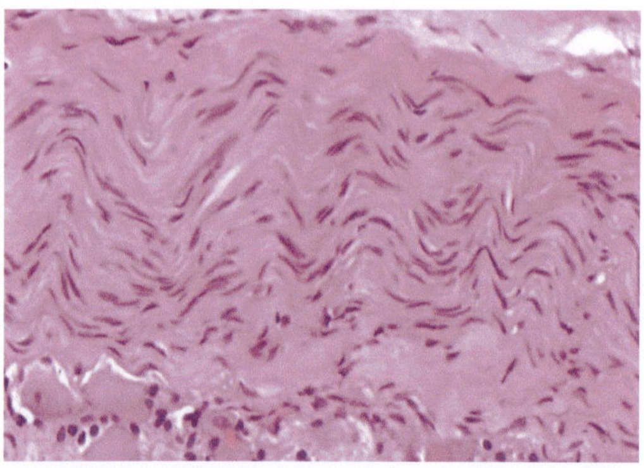

Fig. 8.45 Wavy neural tissue

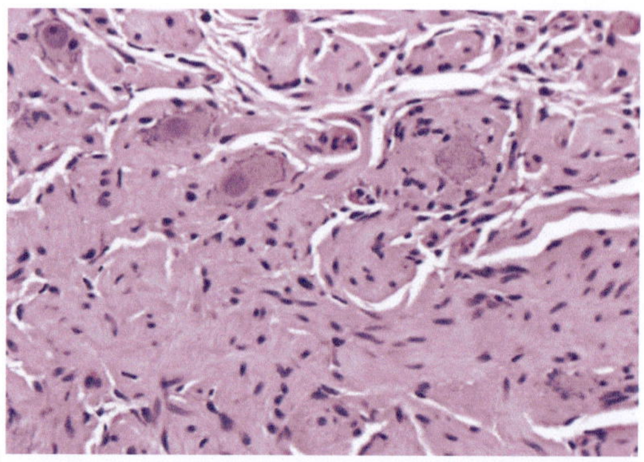

Fig. 8.46 Ganglions with prominent pink nuclei

Hibernoma

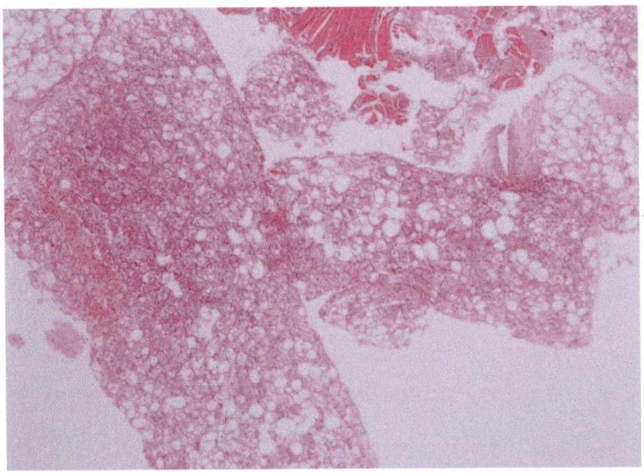

Fig. 8.47 Lobulated tumor of adipose tissue

Histopathology (Figs. 8.47, 8.48, and 8.49)

- Lobulated tumor of fetal brown adipose tissue
- Round or oval cells with granular, coarsely vacuolated eosinophilic cytoplasm admixed with some mature adipocytes
- Lipofuscin pigment commonly present
- Cells are S-100+, Oil Red O+, Sudan Black+

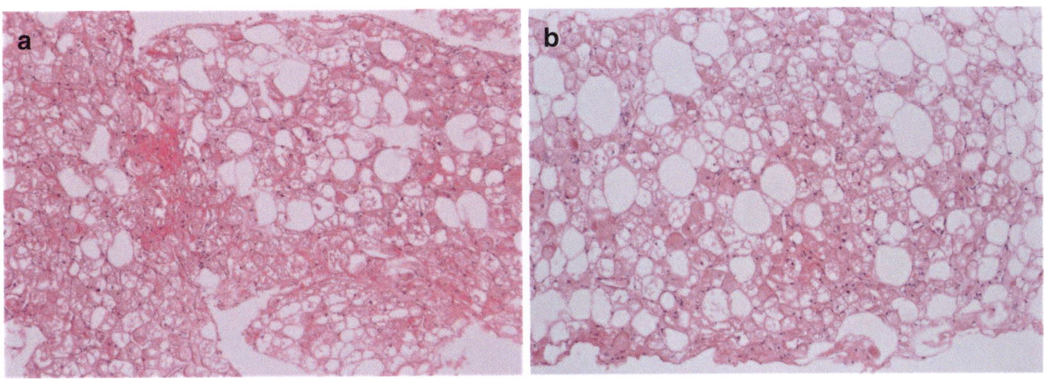

Fig. 8.48 (**a**, **b**) Admixture of mature univacuolated adipocytes and immature multivacuolated eosinophilic adipocytes

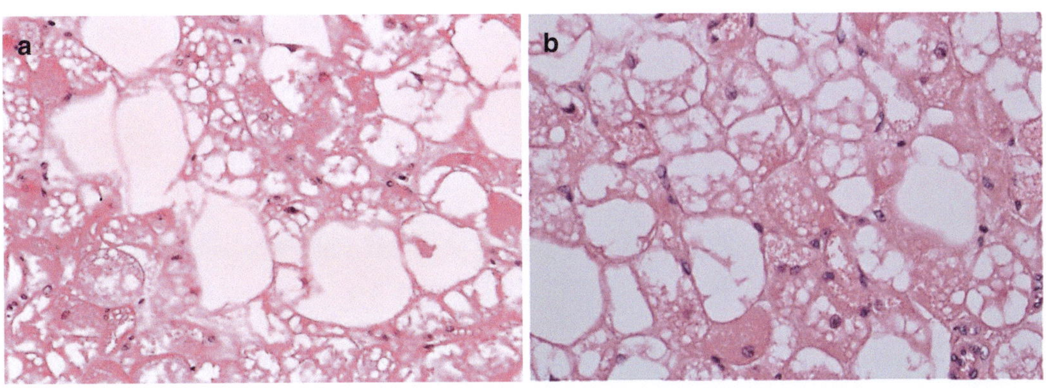

Fig. 8.49 (**a**, **b**) “Bubbly” immature adipocytes with eosinophilic granular cytoplasm with multiple small vacuoles

Hidradenoma Papilliferum

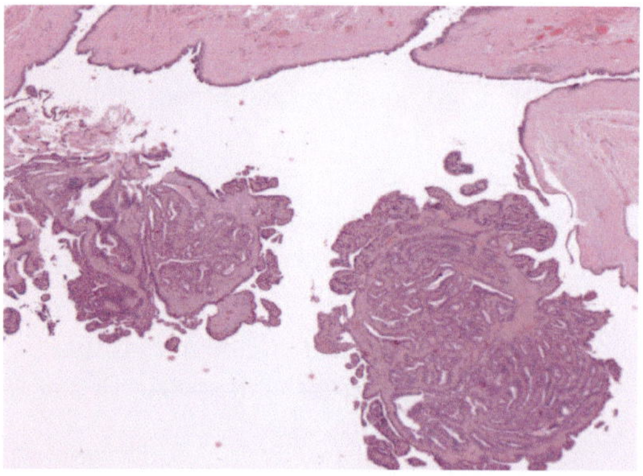

Fig. 8.50 Tumor nodules within cystic space

Histopathology (Figs. 8.50, 8.51, and 8.52)

- Well-circumscribed tumor nodule exclusively in women
- Complex glandular structures with no connection to the epidermis
- Two layer of cells; underlying myoepithelial cells and inner cuboidal/columnar epithelial cells (CK5/6+, ER+, androgen receptor+)
- Epithelial cells have apocrine snouts and papillary stroma is fibrotic with no plasma cells

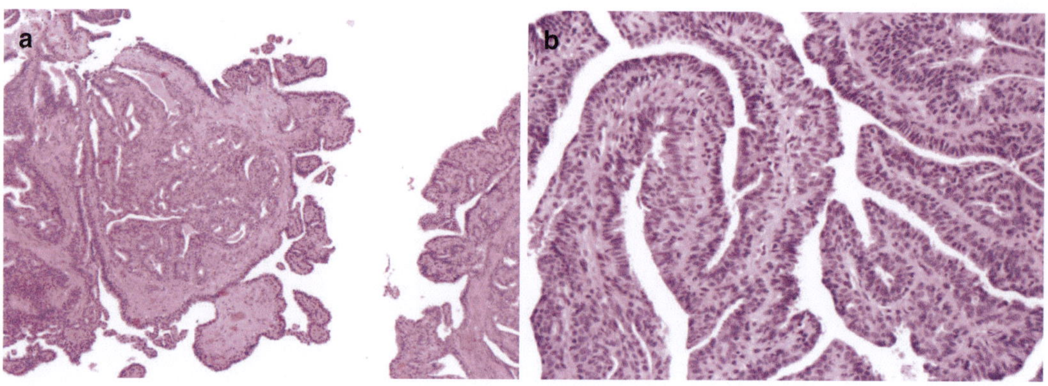

Fig. 8.51 (**a**, **b**) Complex papillary structures with fibrotic papillary stroma

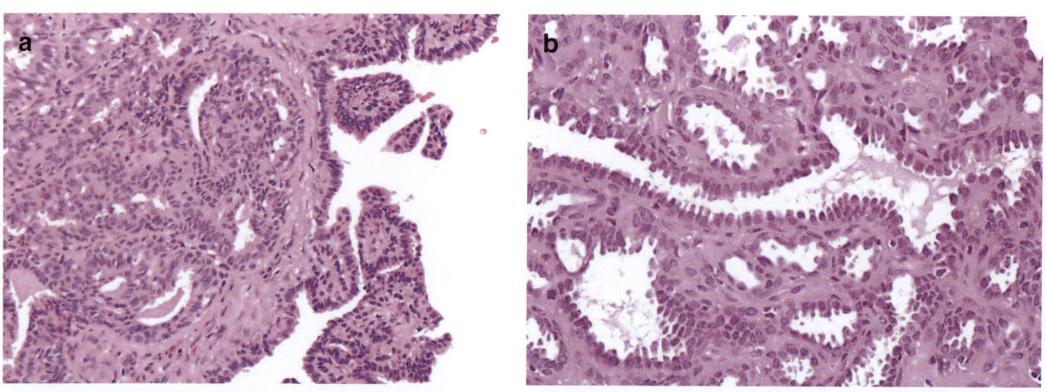

Fig. 8.52 (**a**, **b**) Outer flat myoepithelial cells and inner cuboidal cells with apocrine snouts ("nipple-like")

Hidroacanthoma Simplex

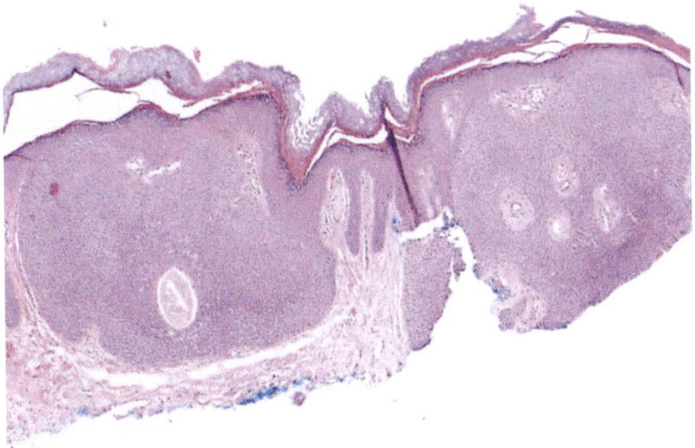

Fig. 8.53 Tumor nests limited to the epidermis and papillary dermis

Histopathology (Figs. 8.53, 8.54, 8.55, and 8.56)

- Intraepidermal well circumscribed nests that push into the papillary dermis
- Nests made of monotonous small basaloid cells
- There is no evidence of stromal retraction, peripheral palisading, or keratin filed cysts
- Duct-like structures (CEA highlighted) are present within the tumor

P.S. "poroma-like" tumor limited to epidermis and superficial dermis

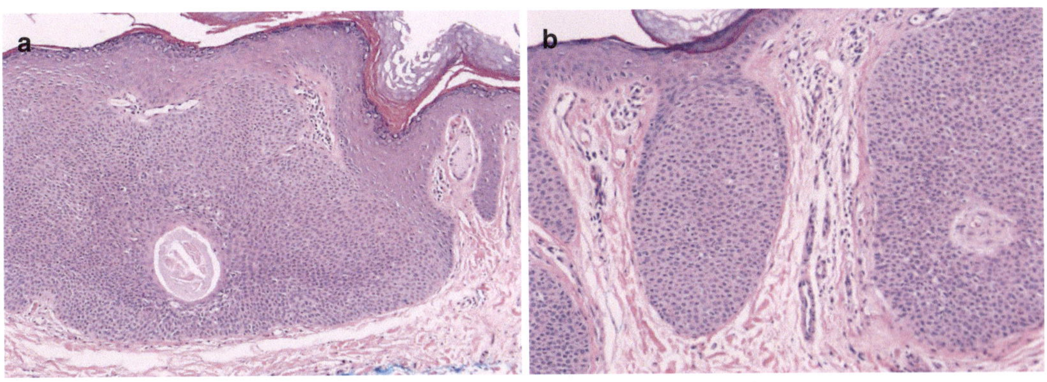

Fig. 8.54 (**a**, **b**) Tumor nests demonstrates pushing borders with no stromal retraction

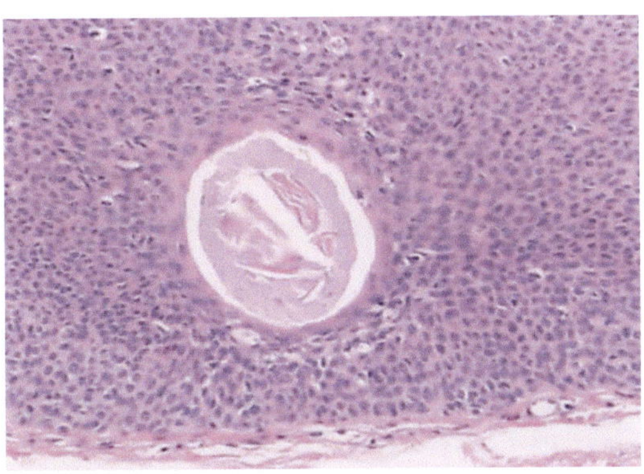

Fig. 8.55 Duct like structures are present

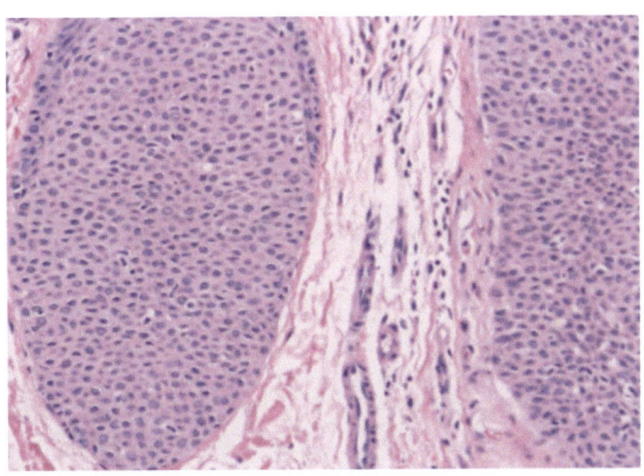

Fig. 8.56 Basaloid uniform cells with no atypia

Hidradenitis Suppurativa

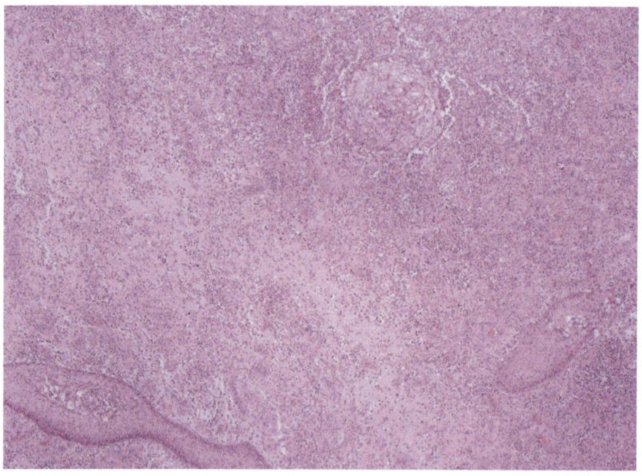

Fig. 8.57 Destruction of hair follicles and sweat glands

Synonyms: Acne Inversa, Apocrine Acne

Histopathology (Figs. 8.57, 8.58, 8.59, 8.60, and 8.61)

- Early lesions demonstrate acute folliculitis and apocrine/eccrine hidradenitis
- In established lesions hair follicles and sweat glands are destroyed and surrounded by exuberant acute inflammation
- There is abscess formation with scarring
- Keratin foreign body granulomas are present

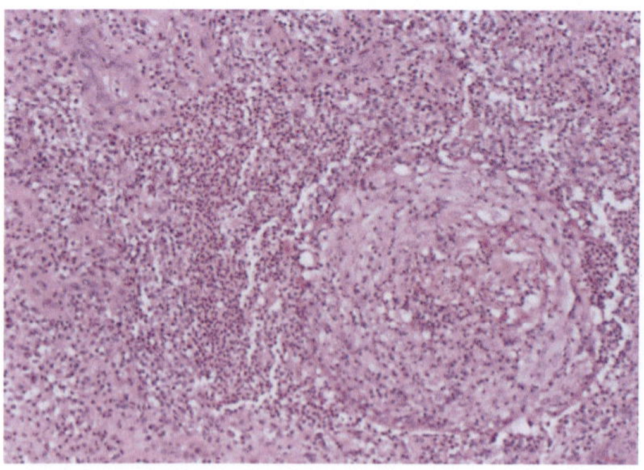

Fig. 8.58 Residual hair shaft with acute inflammation reaction

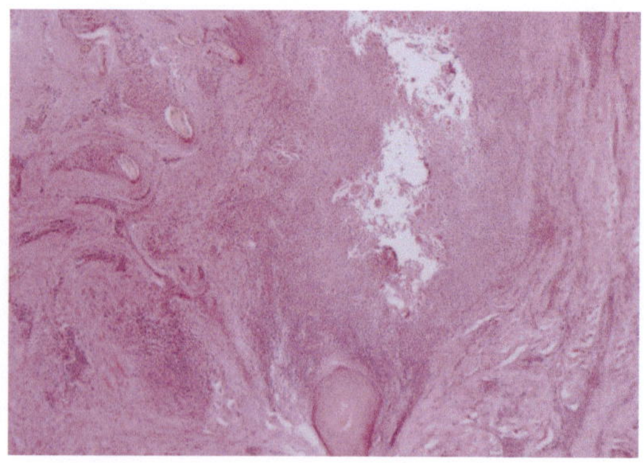

Fig. 8.59 Keratin giant cell reaction and scarring

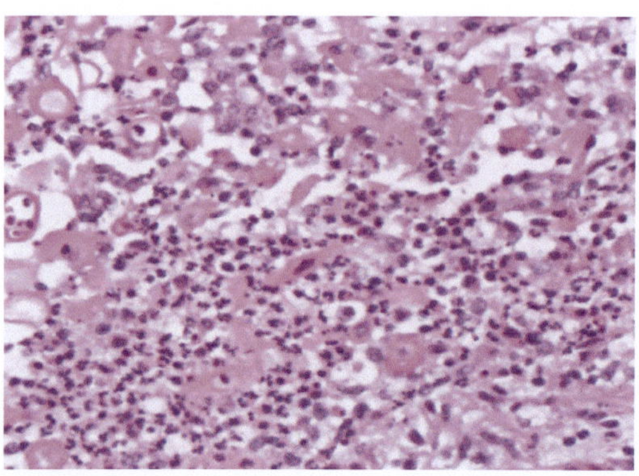

Fig. 8.60 Keratin flakes with acute inflammation and giant cells

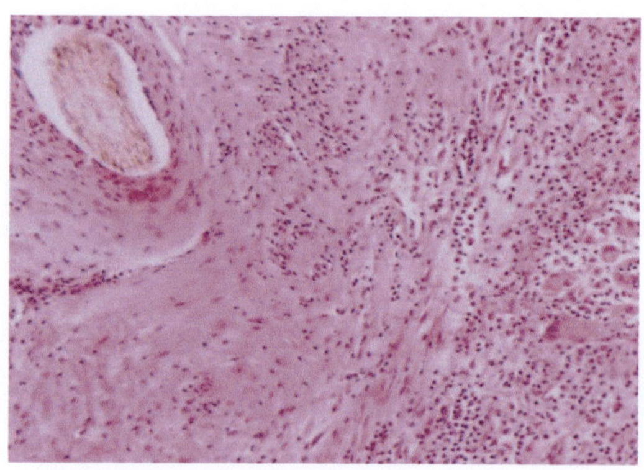

Fig. 8.61 Hair fragment with abscess

Hidrocystoma

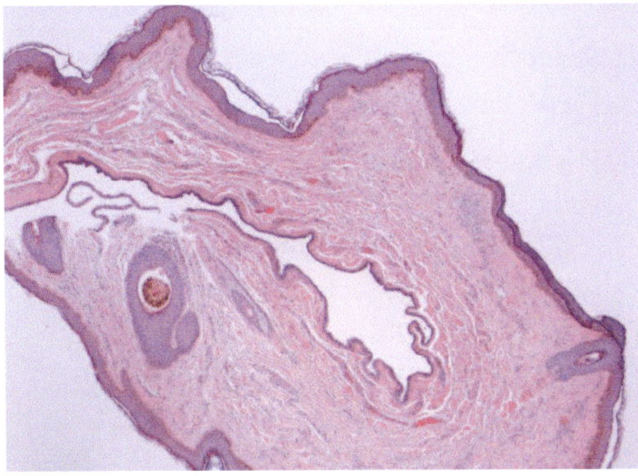

Fig. 8.62 Mildly corrugated cyst

Synonyms: Eccrine Hidrocystoma, Apocrine Hidrocystoma, Cystadenoma

Histopathology (Figs. 8.62, 8.63, 8.64, 8.65, and 8.66)

- Cyst with small papillary projections and the wall made of two layers of cells
- Outer layer of flat myoepithelial cells
- Inner layer of cells in eccrine type is made of cuboidal cells without snouts
- Inner layer of cells in apocrine type is made of cuboidal cells with cytoplasmic snouts

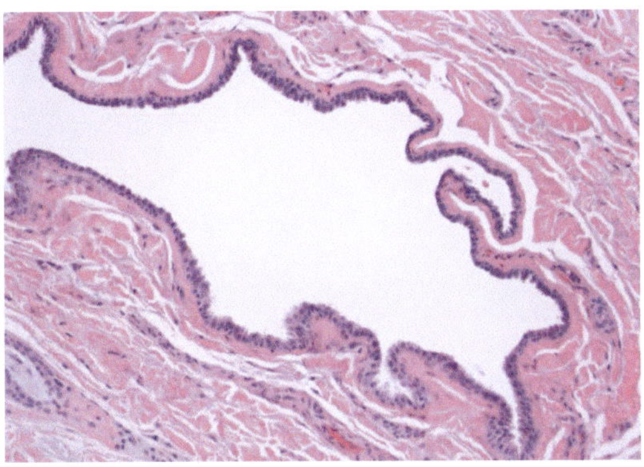

Fig. 8.63 Small papillae projecting into lumen

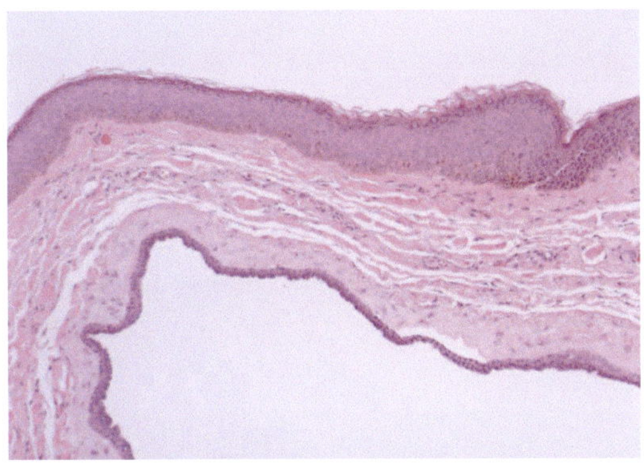

Fig. 8.64 Two cells layer lines dilated cyst

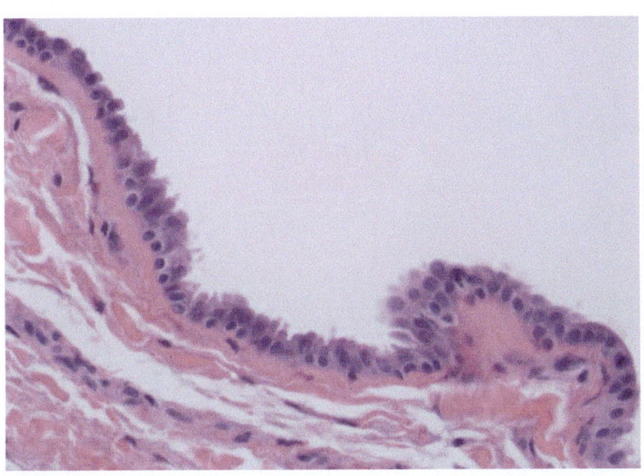

Fig. 8.65 Apocrine hidrocystoma with cuboidal cells with snouts

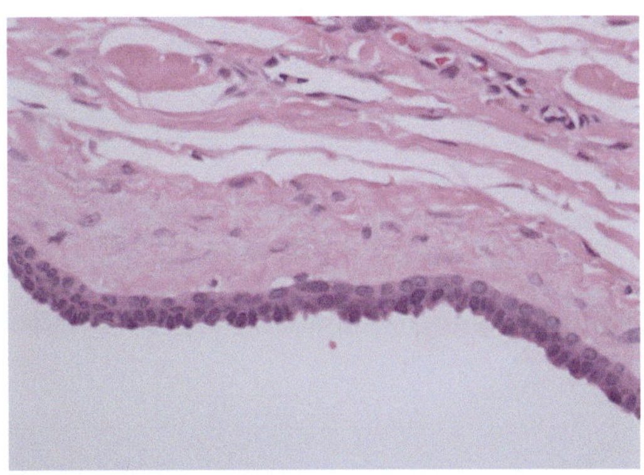

Fig. 8.66 Eccrine hidrocystoma with cuboidal cells without snouts

Histoplasmosis

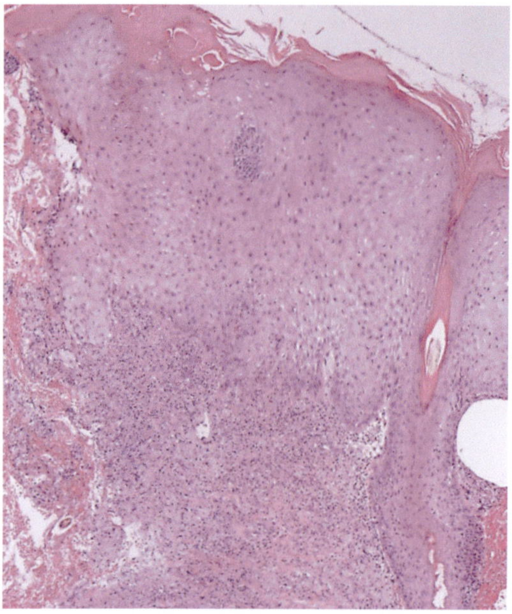

Fig. 8.67 Pseudoepitheliomatous hyperplasia

Synonyms: Darling's Disease, Cave Disease, Ohio Valley Disease

Histopathology (Figs. 8.67, 8.68, 8.69, and 8.70)

- Pseudoepitheliomatous hyperplasia
- Histiocytic/granulomatous infiltrate in the dermis and subcutis
- Yeast elements in histiocytes
- Yeast (2–4 µm in diameter) shows narrow-based budding and is often surrounded by clear halo

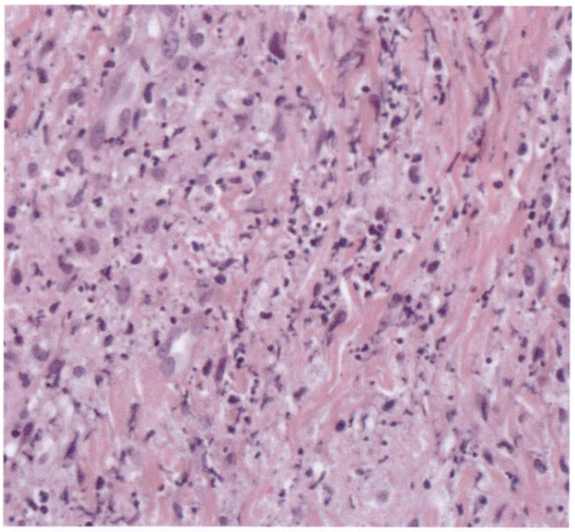

Fig. 8.68 Histiocytes, lymphocytes, and scattered neutrophils

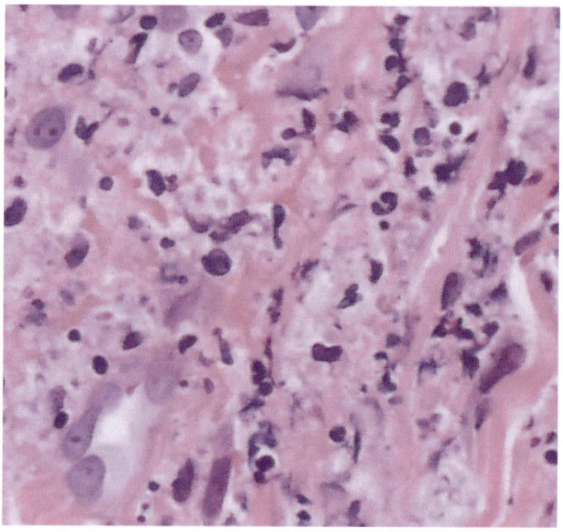

Fig. 8.69 Yeast elements seen as pink dots within the histiocytes

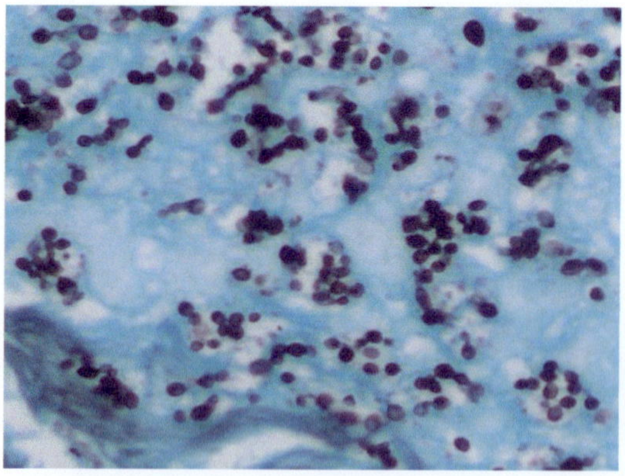

Fig. 8.70 Narrow based budding yeast (GMS)

Hobnail Hemangioma

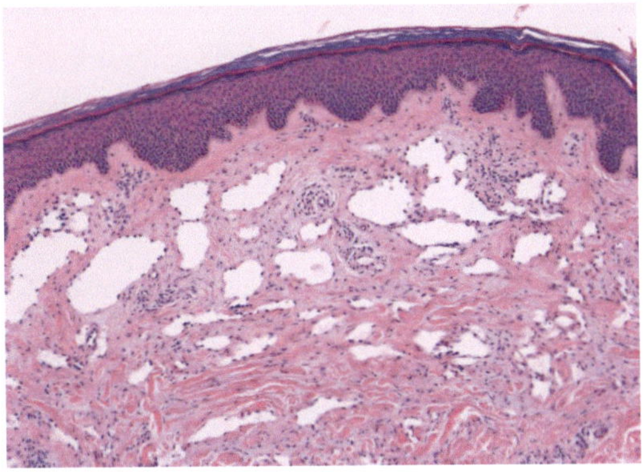

Fig. 8.71 Wedge shaped vascular lesion

Synonym: Targetoid Hemosiderotic Hemangioma

Histopathology (Figs. 8.71, 8.72, and 8.73)

- V shaped dermal vascular proliferation with wider side toward the epidermis
- Irregular vascular channels with focal papillary projections that are less apparent with descent
- Endothelial cell (CD31+, CD34+) are prominent and protrude into a lumen producing "hobnail" appearance
- Dermal hemosiderin can be prominent

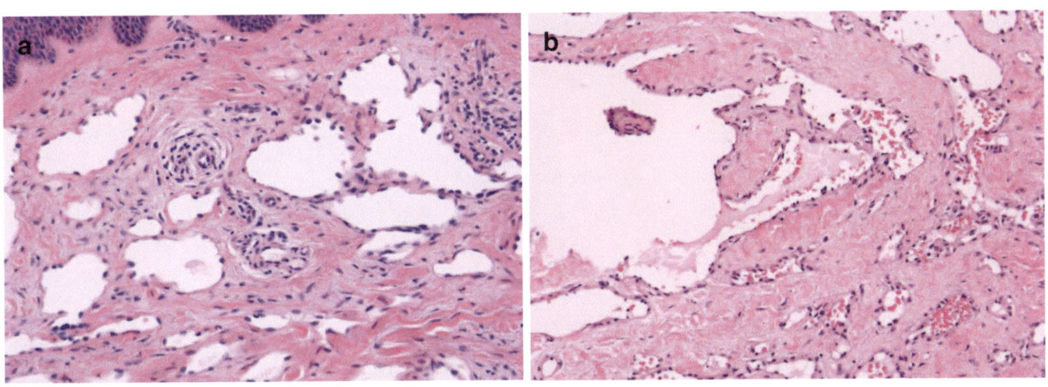

Fig. 8.72 (**a**, **b**) Vascular channels are dilated and irregular with focal papillary projections; with the descent the vascular channels become smaller

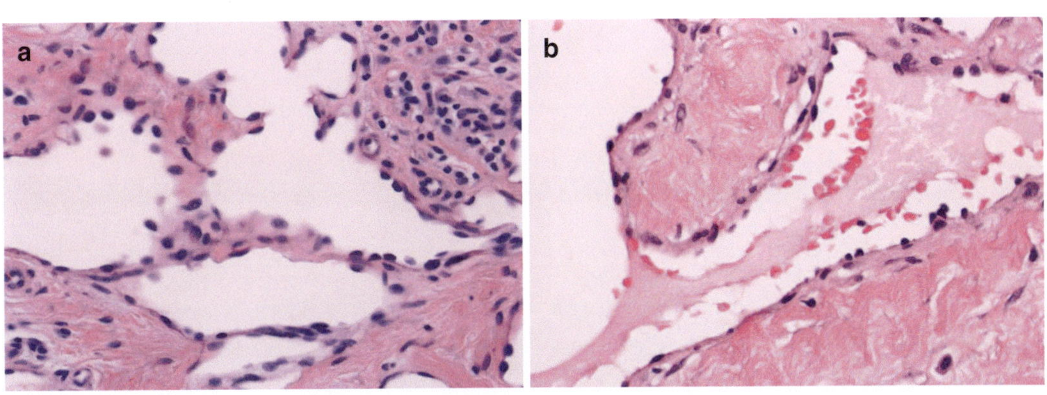

Fig. 8.73 (**a**, **b**) Nuclei of endothelial cell protrude in the lumen forming "hobnails"

Hodgkin's Disease

There are four types with different histopathology but nodular sclerosing type is the most common.

Histopathology (Figs. 8.74, 8.75, and 8.76)

- Nodular pattern with thick collagen separating nodules
- Reed-Sternberg and Hodgkin cells (CD15+, CD30+) in the background of lymphocytes, histiocytes, eosinophils, and plasma cells
- Reed-Sternberg cells have bilobal nucleus with prominent nuclei; Hodgkin cells have nucleus with prominent nucleolus

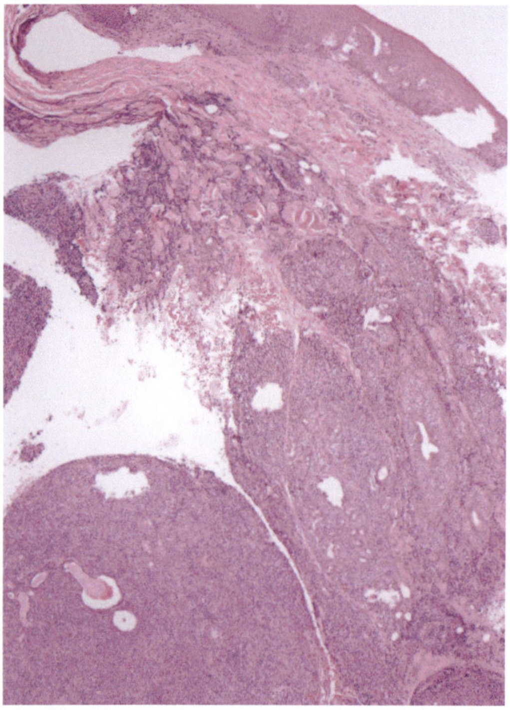

Fig. 8.74 Subcutaneous nodules separated by sclerotic stoma

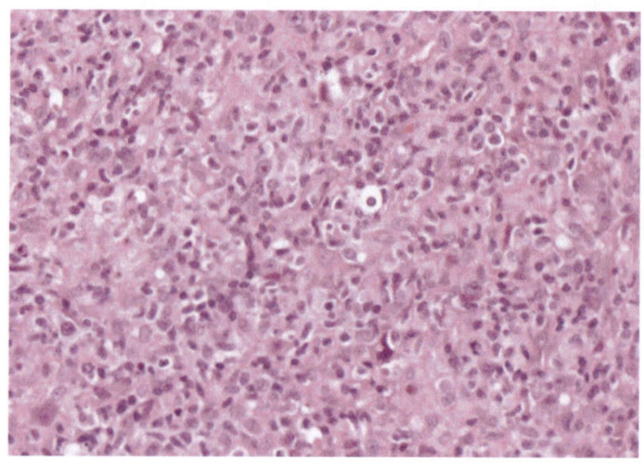

Fig. 8.75 Large pale tumor cells mixed with lymphocytes and histiocytes

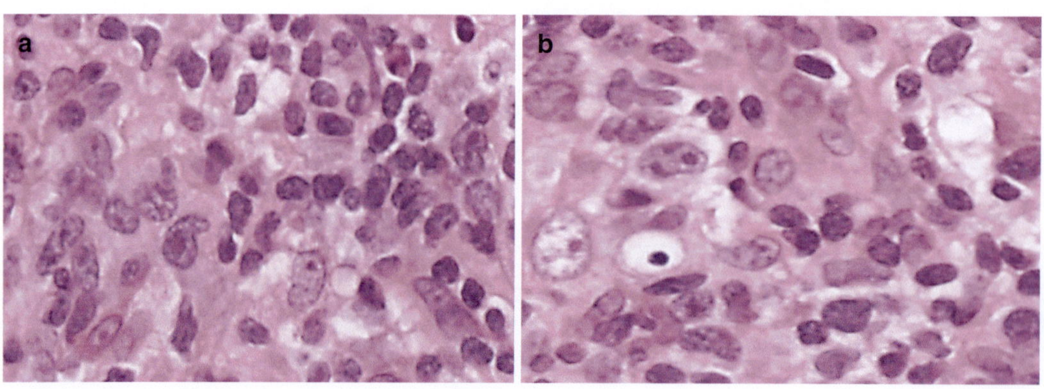

Fig. 8.76 (**a**, **b**) Hodgkin cells with prominent nucleoli ("owl eye")

Hyalinosis Cutis et Mucosae

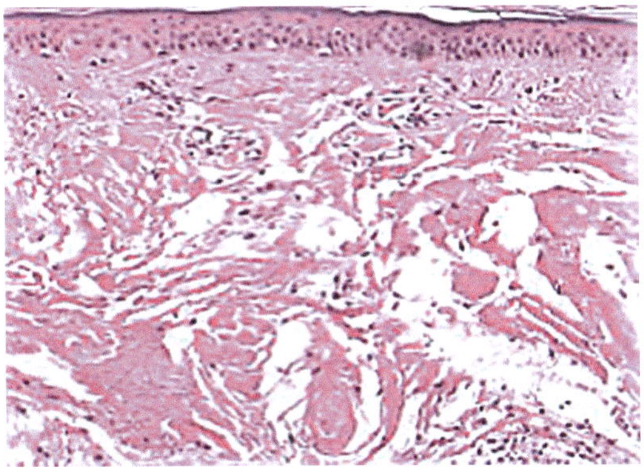

Fig. 8.77 Homogenous eosinophilic deposits in the dermis

Synonyms: Lipoid Proteinosis, Urbach-Wiethe Disease

Histopathology (Figs. 8.77, 8.78, 8.79, and 8.80)

- Homogenous eosinophilic material in the dermis
- Initially deposits are found around capillaries and sweat coils
- Later diffuse dermal deposits present
- Deposits stain with PAS (diastase-resistant) and only weekly with Congo red and thioflavine-T

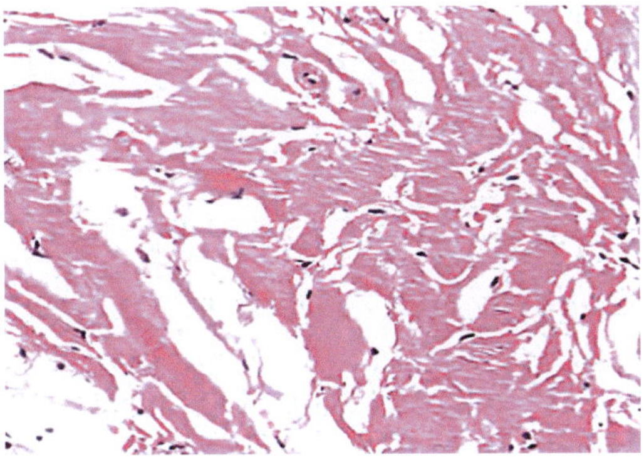

Fig. 8.78 Diffuse pink dermal deposit

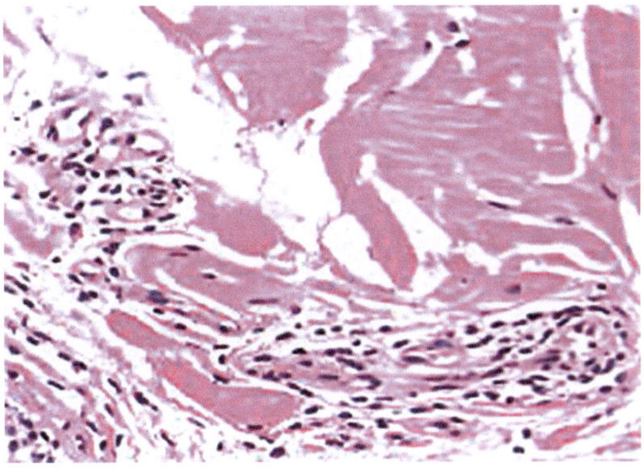

Fig. 8.79 Deposit around capillaries

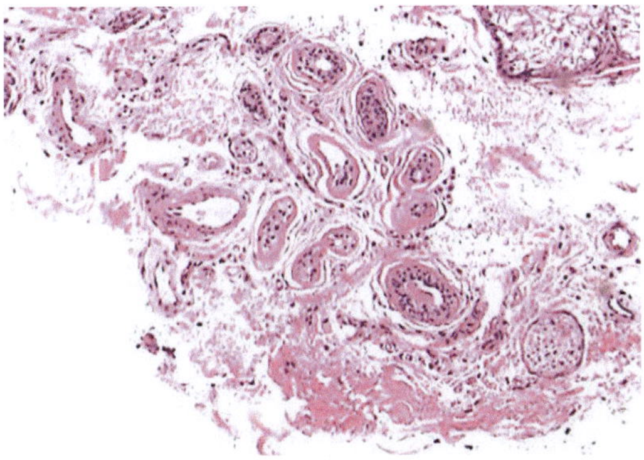

Fig. 8.80 Deposits around atrophic eccrine sweat glands

Hybrid Cyst

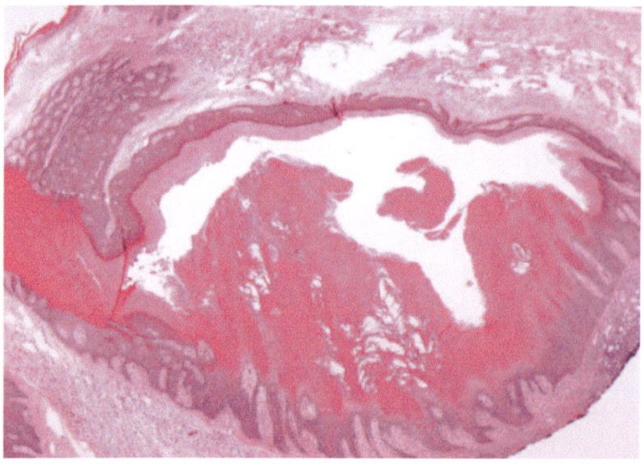

Fig. 8.81 Cyst with two different linings

Synonym: Follicular Hybrid Cyst

Histopathology (Figs. 8.81, 8.82, 8.83, 8.84, and 8.85)

- Cyst that is a hybrid between epidermal inclusion cyst and pilar cyst
- Usually upper part has lining of EIC and lower part has lining of pilar cyst
- There is sharp demarcation between two linings

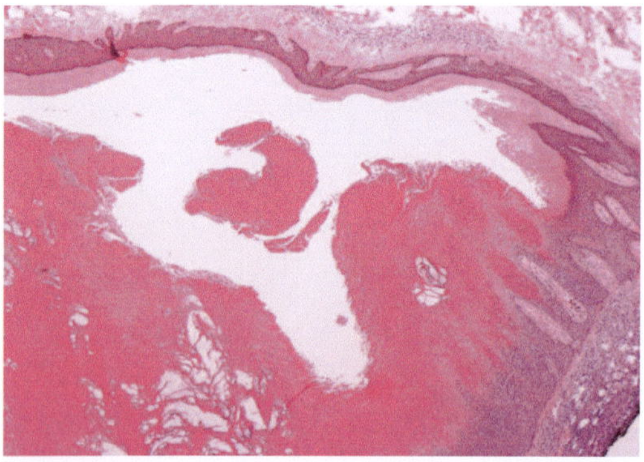

Fig. 8.82 Upper portion resembles EIC and the lower portion resembles pilar cyst

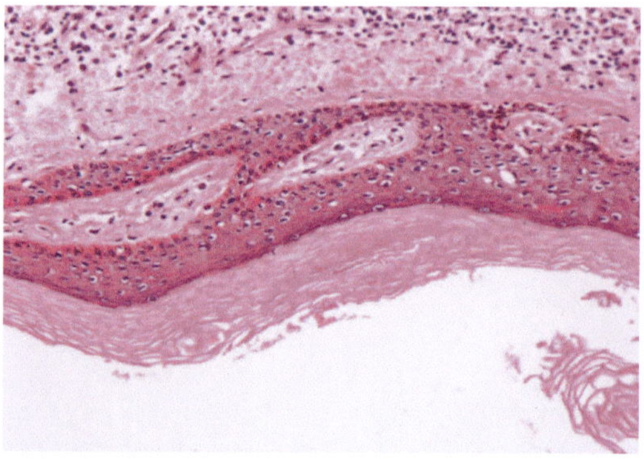

Fig. 8.83 Stratified squamous epithelium with granular layer

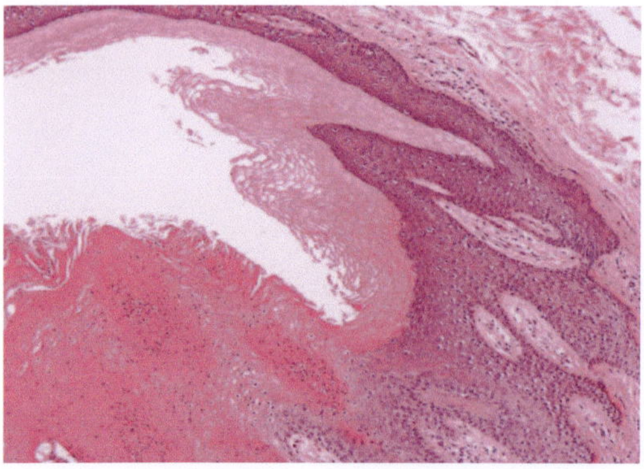

Fig. 8.84 Transition from epidermis with granular layer (above) to epidermis without granular layer (below)

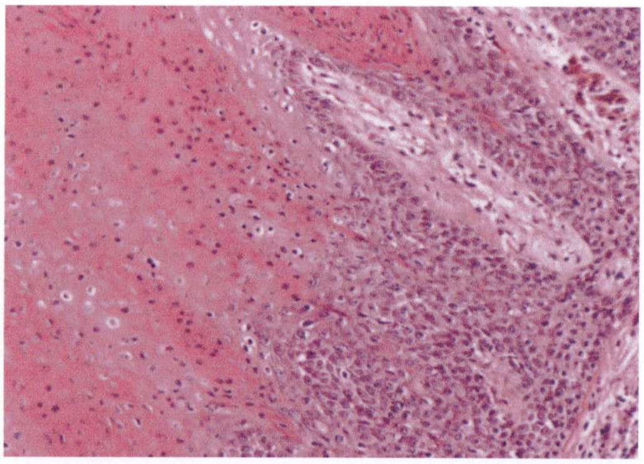

Fig. 8.85 Squamous epithelium with trichilemmal keratinization without granular layer

Hydroa Vacciniforme

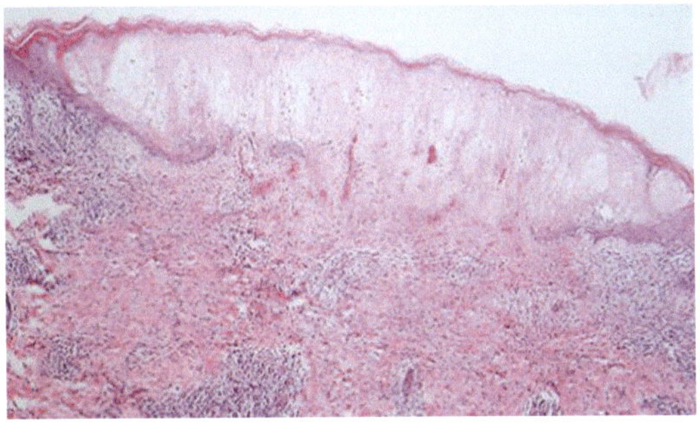

Fig. 8.86 Intraepidermal necrotic vesicle

Histopathology (Figs. 8.86, 8.87, and 8.88)
- Intraepidermal vesiculation
- Prominent reticular degeneration of keratinocytes
- Confluent necrosis above the vesicle
- Vesicle is filled with serum and inflammatory cells
- Dermal mixed inflammation is present

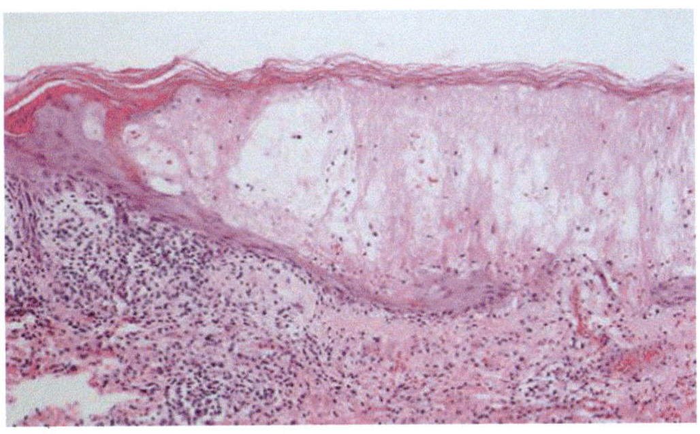

Fig. 8.87 Reticular degeneration and necrosis of keratinocytes

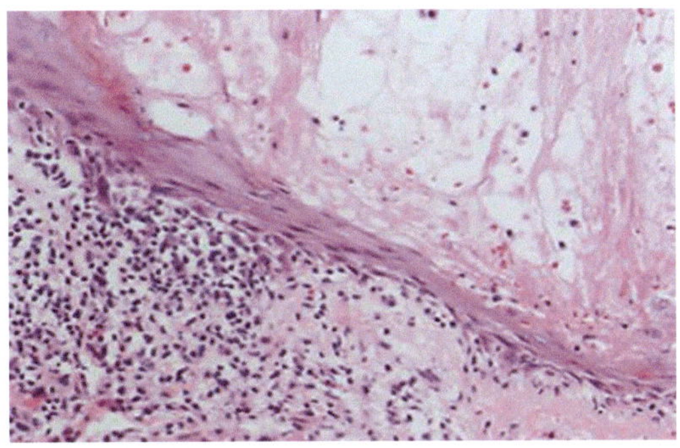

Fig. 8.88 Vesicle filled with serum and dermal lymphocytic inflammation

Hypertrophic Scar

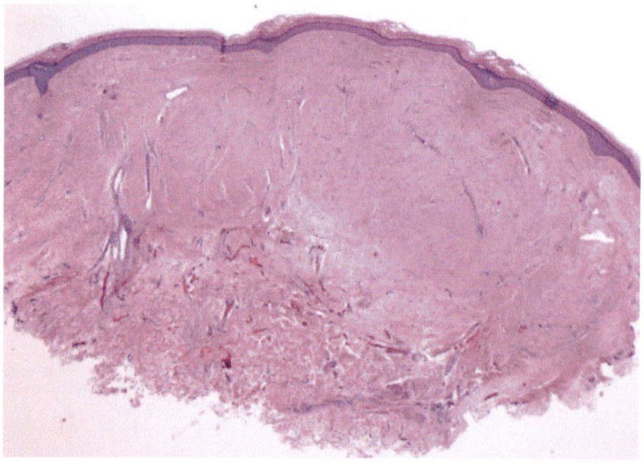

Fig. 8.89 Dermal fibrosis with absent adnexal structures

Histopathology (Figs. 8.89, 8.90, 8.91, 8.92, and 8.93)
- Atrophic epidermis
- Nodular scar replaces adnexal structures
- Thick hyalinized collagen bundles
- Compressed capillaries with tendency to be oriented perpendicular to the epidermis
- Mild chronic inflammation can be present

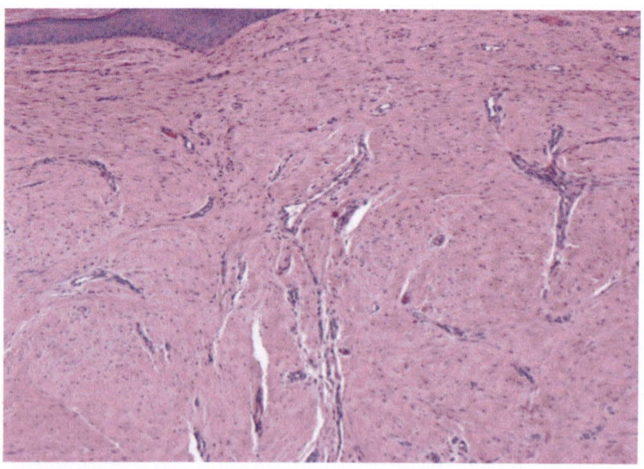

Fig. 8.90 Capillaries are compressed

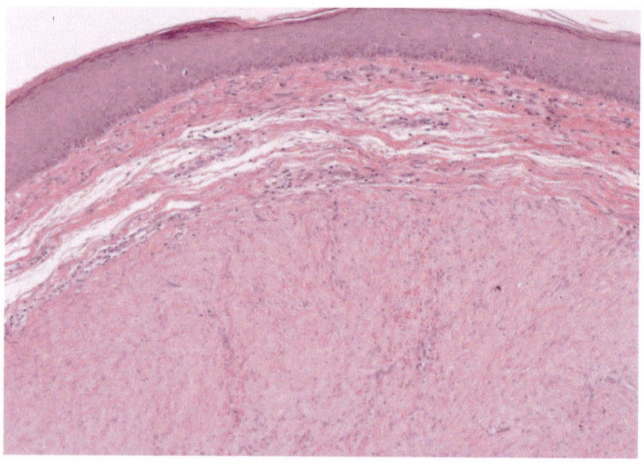

Fig. 8.91 Atrophic epidermis with nodular dermal scar

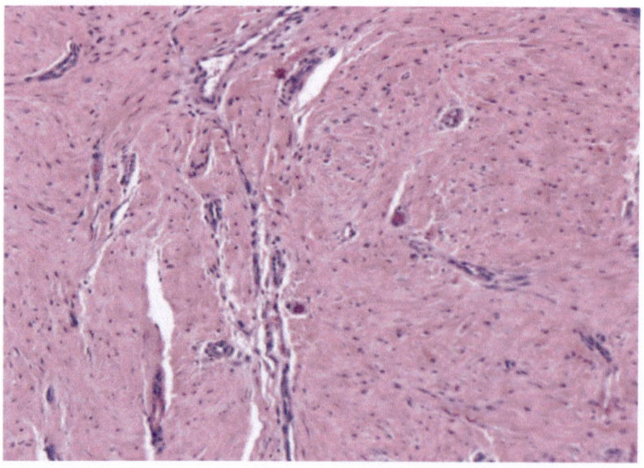

Fig. 8.92 Vessels are oriented perpendicularly to the epidermis

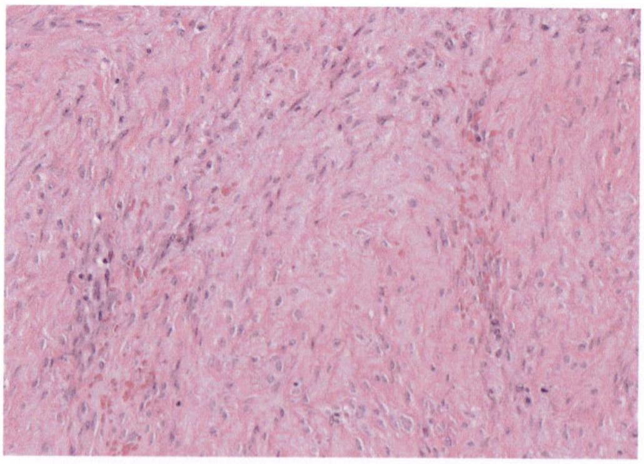

Fig. 8.93 Collagen bundles are thick and hyalinized

9 Dermatopathology I

V. Vincek, *Dermatopathology A–Z*, https://doi.org/10.1007/978-3-319-89486-7_9

Ichthyosis/Keratoderma

The term *Ichthyosis* encompasses large number of disorders of keratinization all of which have a prominent thickened stratum corneum (orthokeratosis). They can be divided into four groups.

Based on the presence or absence of a granular layer they can be divided into two groups.

Group 1: Orthokeratosis with **reduced stratum granulosum** (Fig. 9.1)

Prototypic disease is *Ichthyosis Vulgaris* but also includes following genodermatoses:

- *Tay Syndrome*
- *X-Linvked Dominant Ichthyosis*
- *Harlequin Ichthyosis*
- *Refsum Syndrome (can also be in group 2)*

Group 2: Orthokeratosis with **prominent stratum granulosum** (Figs. 9.2 and 9.3)

Prototypic disease is *X-linked Recessive Ichthyosis* but also includes following genodermatoses:

- *Erythrokeratoderma Variabilis*
- *IFAP inherited PRP*
- *KID syndrome*
- *Lamellar Ichthyosis*
- *Palmoplantar Keratoderma*
- *Sjögren Larsson Syndrome*

Based on the presence of parakeratosis and acantholysis they can be divided into two more groups.

Group 3: Variable granular layer with **prominent parakeratosis**

- *CHILD Syndrome* (granular layer is normal or thinned)
- *Comèl-Netherton Syndrome* (granular layer is usually thinned)

Group 4: Orthokeratosis with **prominent epidermolytic acantholysis** (Fig. 9.4)

Prototypic disease is *Epidermolytic Acanthoma* and can be seen in numerous disorders:

- *Bullous Ichthyosiform Erythroderma*
- *Epidermolytic Leukoplakia*
- *Ichthyosis Bullosa of Siemens*
- *Ichthyosis Hystrix*
- *Nevus Unis Lateralis*
- *Palmoplantar Keratoderma, Voerner type*

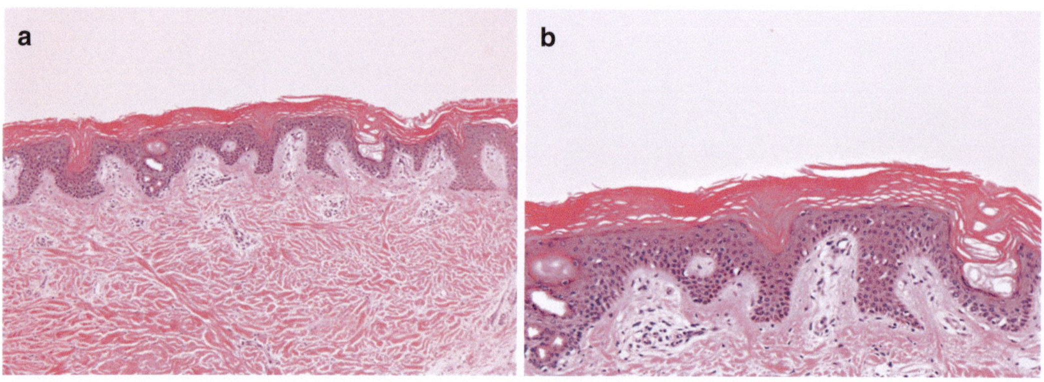

Fig. 9.1 (**a**, **b**) **Ichthyosis Vulgaris** with orthokeratosis and diminished granular layer

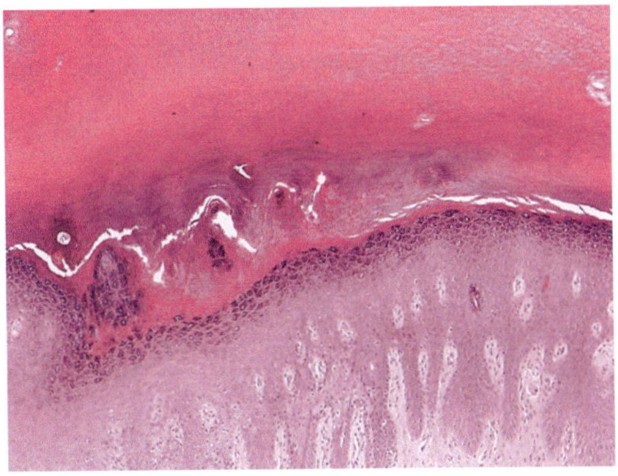

Fig. 9.2 **Palmoplantar keratoderma** with orthokeratosis and prominent granular layer

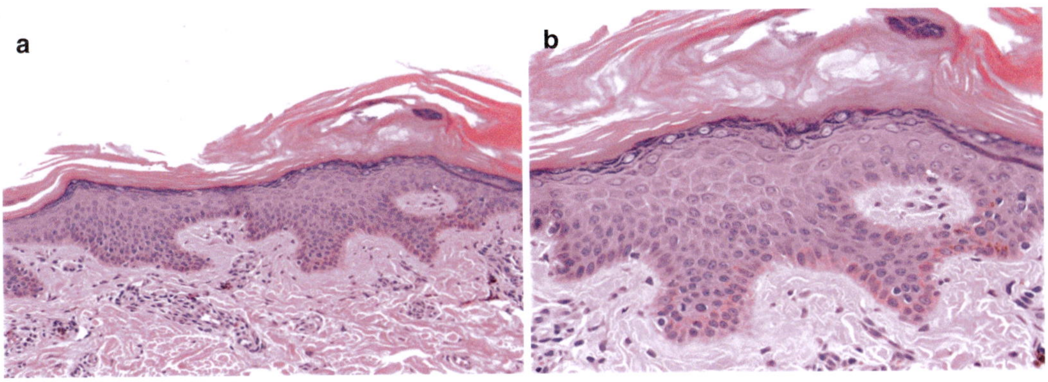

Fig. 9.3 (**a**, **b**) **X-linked Recessive Ichthyosis** with orthokeratosis and prominent granular layer

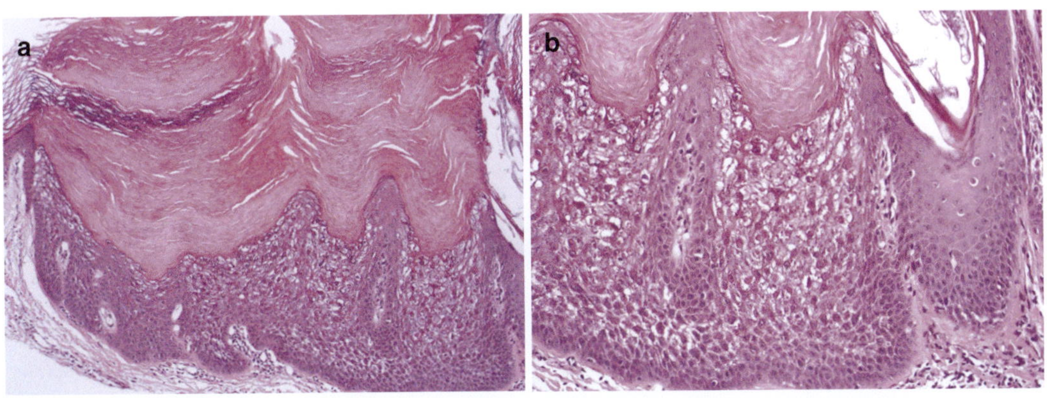

Fig. 9.4 (**a**, **b**) **Epidermolytic Acanthoma** with coarse eosinophilic granules present in the upper portion of stratum spinosum

Id Reaction

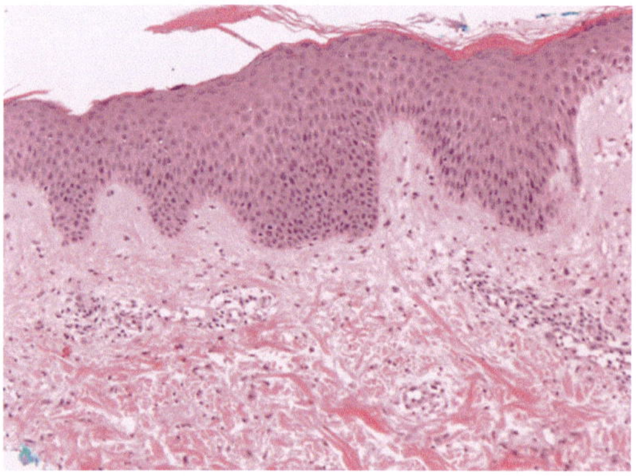

Fig. 9.5 Mildly spongiotic epidermis

Synonyms: Autoeczematization, Autosensitization

Histopathology (Figs. 9.5, 9.6, 9.7, 9.8, and 9.9)
- Findings are not specific and clinical correlation is required
- Variable epidermal spongiosis
- Mild perivascular lymphocytic inflammation
- Scattered eosinophils and mild dermal edema might be present

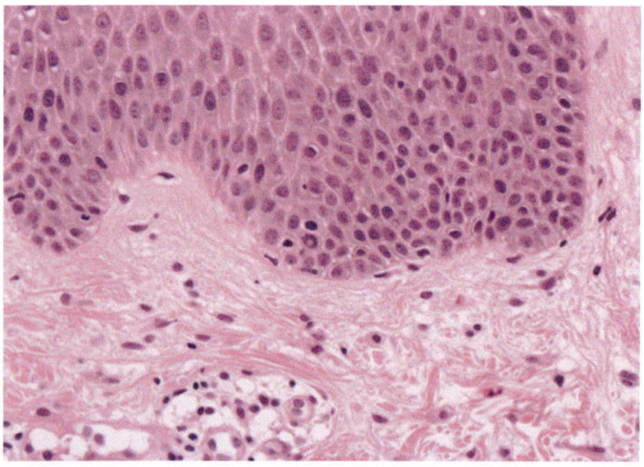

Fig. 9.6 Mild perivascular lymphocytic infiltrate

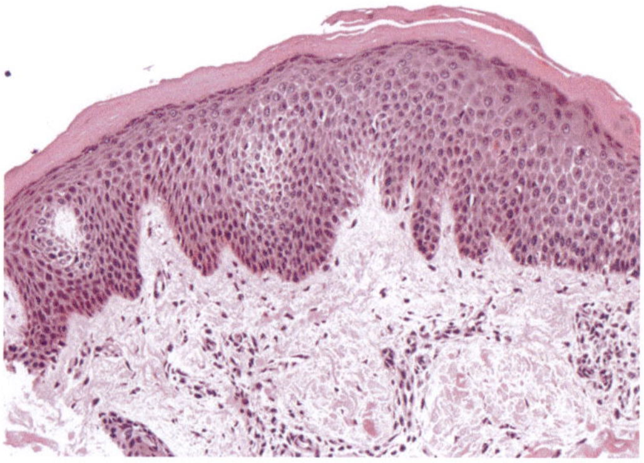

Fig. 9.7 Mild dermal edema

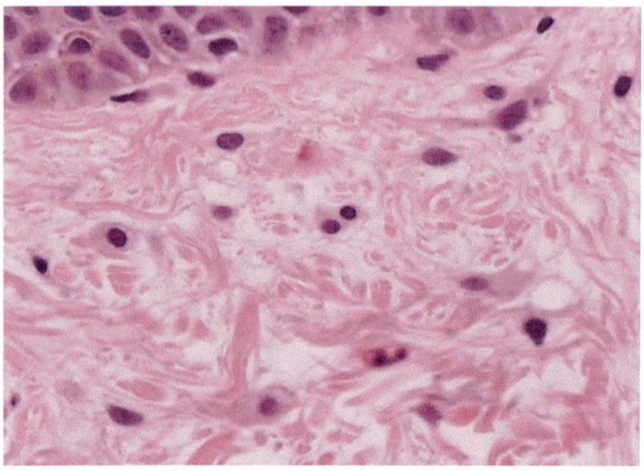

Fig. 9.8 Scattered dermal eosinophils

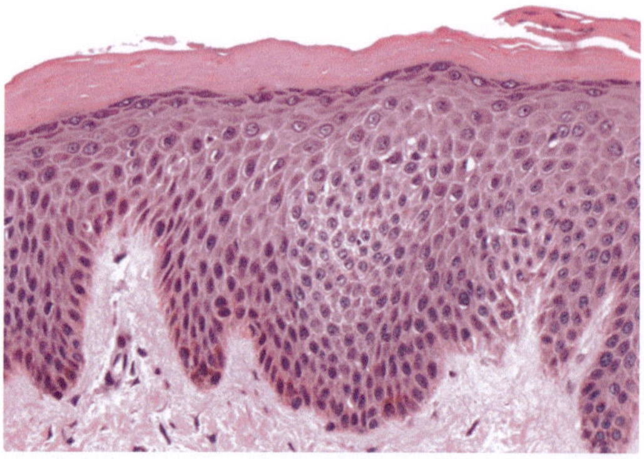

Fig. 9.9 Prominent desmosomes suggesting spongiosis

IgA Pemphigus

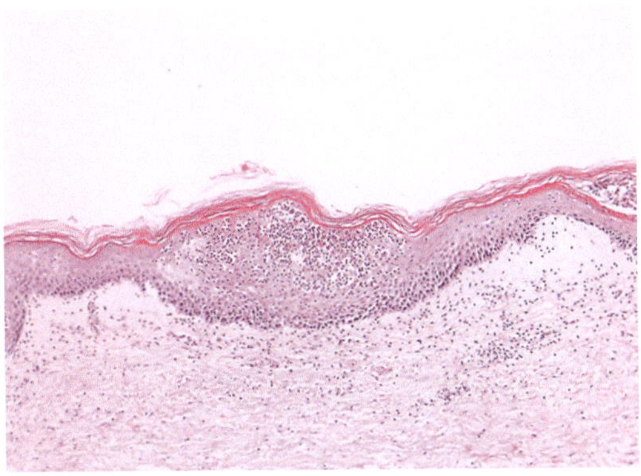

Fig. 9.10 Subcorneal pustule

Histopathology (Figs. 9.10, 9.11, and 9.12)
- Subcorneal and/or intraepidermal pustule
- Pustule is filled with neutrophils
- Mixed dermal inflammatory infiltrate
- Presence of IgA intercellular depositions on DIF

P.S. IgA pemphigus has almost identical histological features as *Sneddon Wilkinson disease*

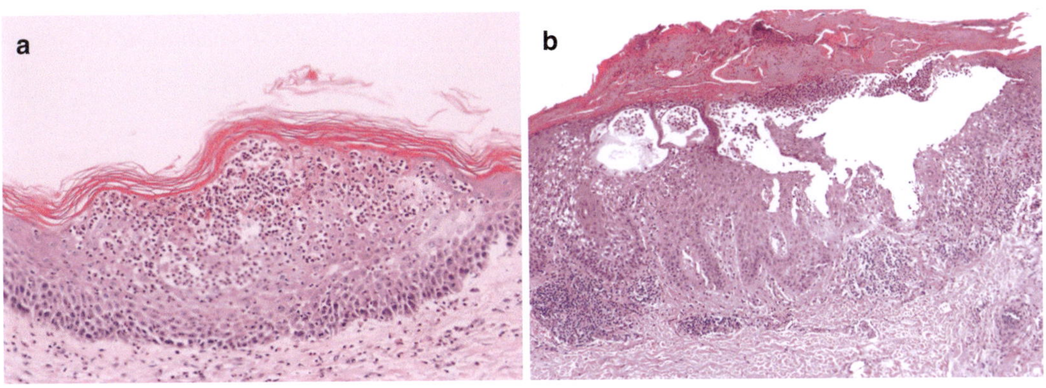

Fig. 9.11 (**a**, **b**) Subcorneal neutrophils filled pustule with mixed dermal inflammation

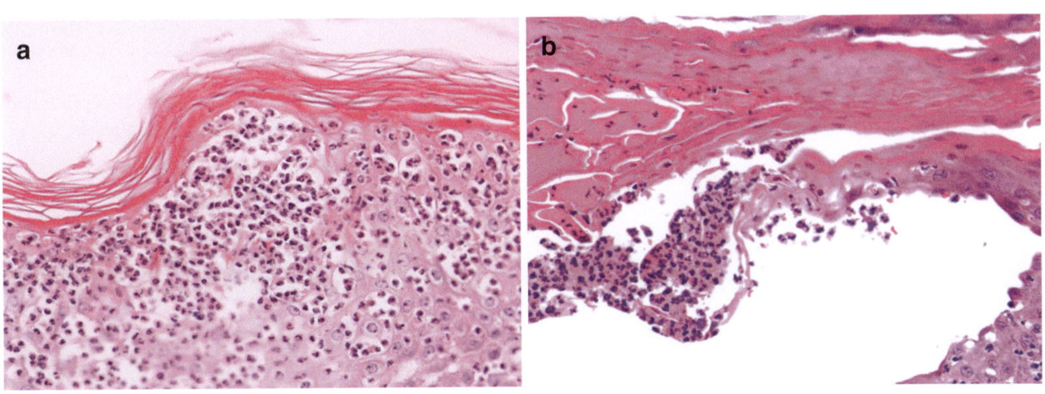

Fig. 9.12 (**a**, **b**) Neutrophilic pustule with minimal keratinocytic acantholysis

Incontinencia Pigmenti

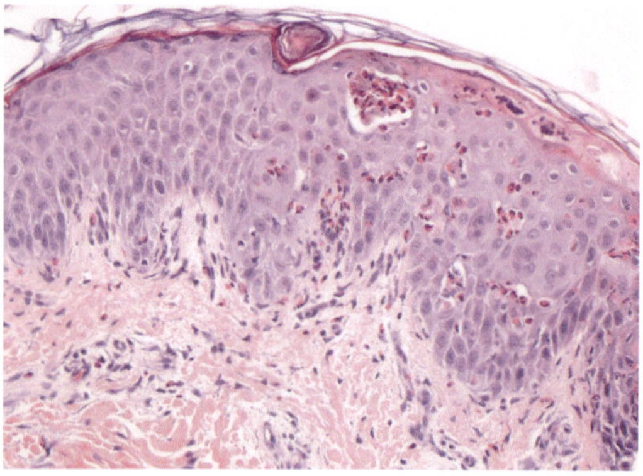

Fig. 9.13 The first stage with epidermal eosinophils and eosinophils filled vesicle

Synonym: Bloch-Sulzberger Disease

Histopathology is different in three disease stages:

The first stage: spongiosis with eosinophils that progress to intraepidermal vesicle with the eosinophil (Figs. 9.13 and 9.14)
The second stage: hyperkeratotic papillomatous epidermis with dyskeratotic cells and dermal eosinophils present in variable number (Figs. 9.15 and 9.16)
The third stage: significant dermal pigment incontinence (Fig. 9.17)

P.S. X-linked dominant disease with *IKBKG* mutation

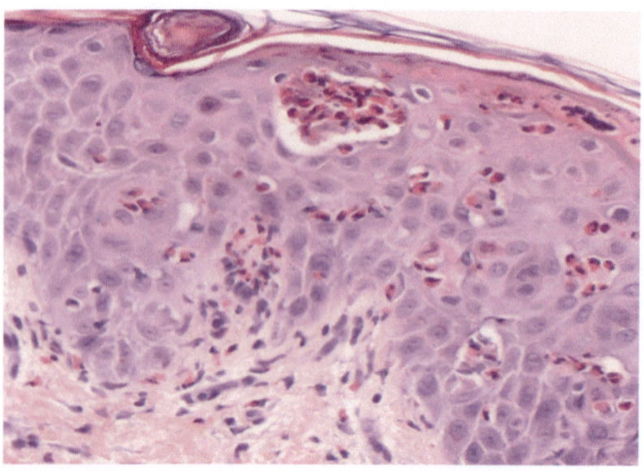

Fig. 9.14 Epidermal eosinophils are present

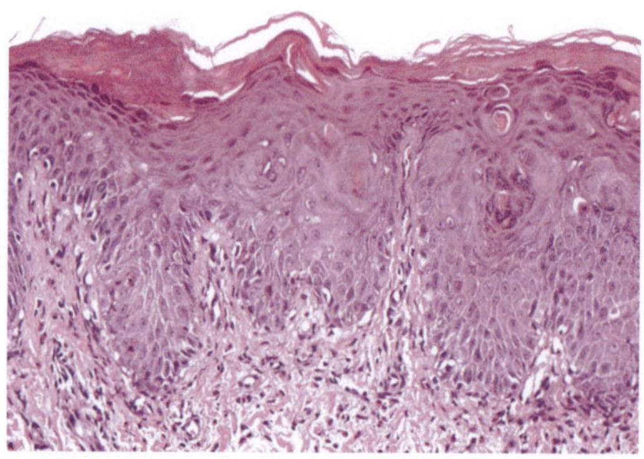

Fig. 9.15 The second stage with epidermal papillomatosis, hyperkeratosis and dyskeratotic keratinocytes

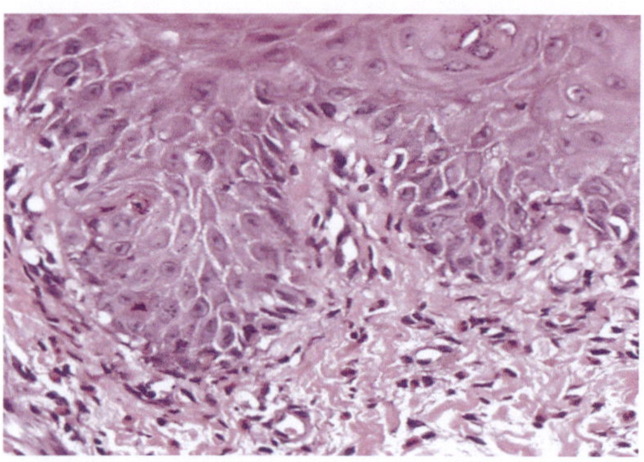

Fig. 9.16 Dermal eosinophils are present

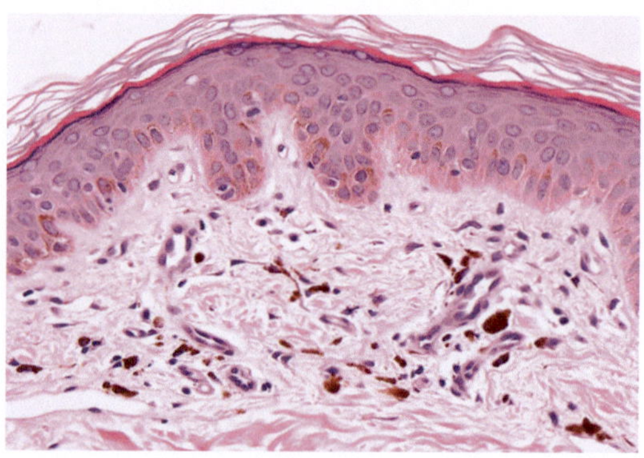

Fig. 9.17 The third stage with extensive dermal pigment incontinence

Infantile Acropustulosis

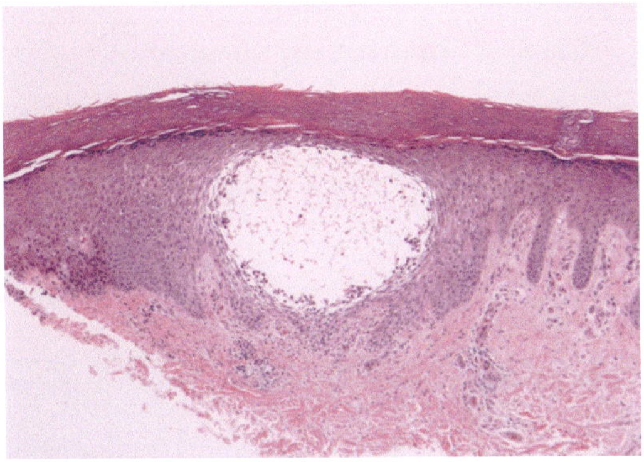

Fig. 9.18 Acral skin with intraepidermal vesicle

Histopathology

In early stages:

- Acral skin with epidermal spongiosis with neutrophils and some eosinophils

In later stages:

- Acral skin with intraepidermal pustule with neutrophils and varying number of eosinophils (Figs. 9.18, 9.19, and 9.20)

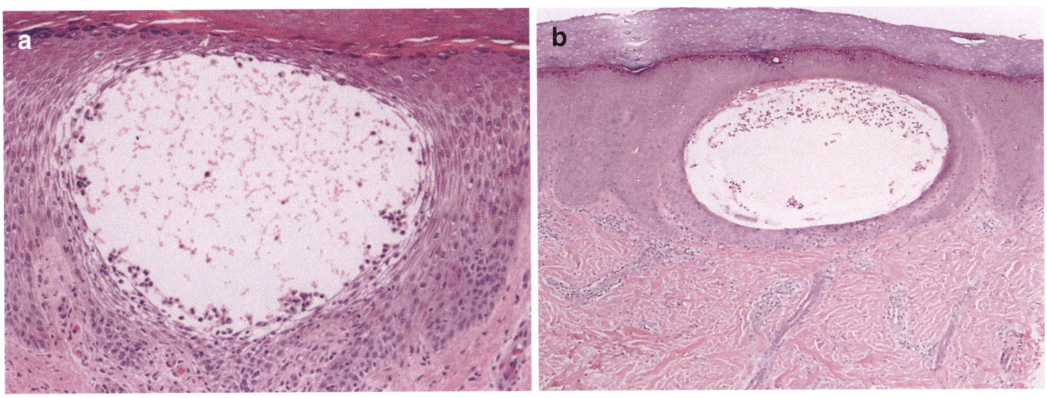

Fig. 9.19 (**a**, **b**) Vesicle is filled with neutrophils and some eosinophils

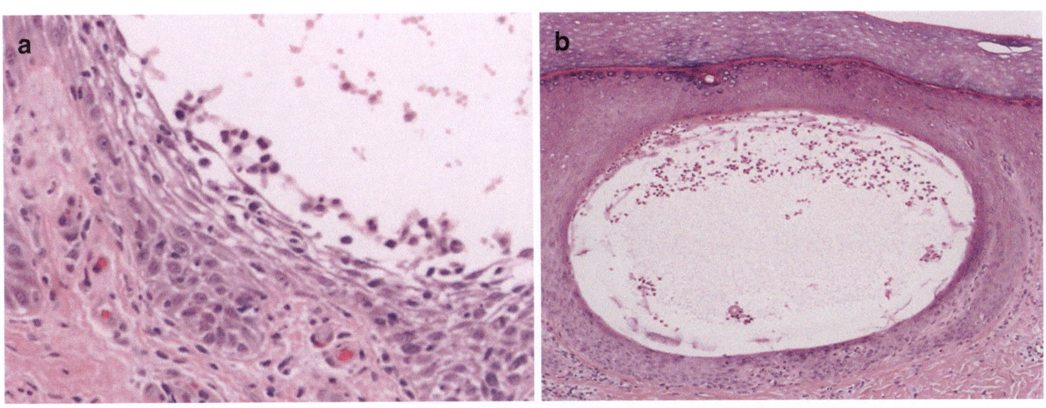

Fig. 9.20 (**a**, **b**) Intraepidermal vesicle with dermal neutrophilic inflammation and few eosinophils

Infantile Digital Fibromatosis

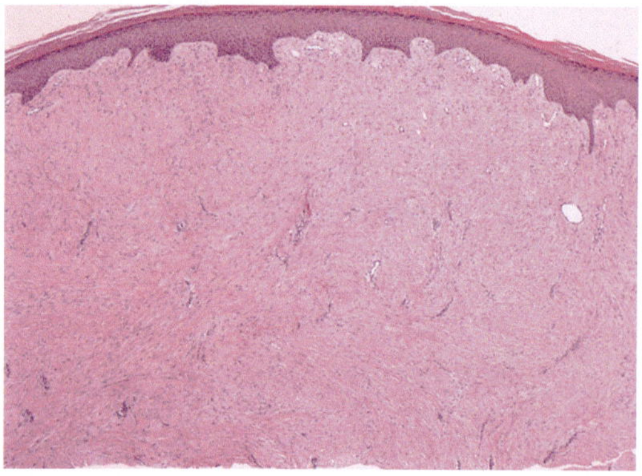

Fig. 9.21 Dermal and subcutaneous tumor nodule

Synonym: Inclusion Body Fibromatosis

Histopathology (Figs. 9.21, 9.22, 9.23, and 9.24)

- Dermal and subcutaneous uniform myofibroblastic proliferation
- Relatively uniform spindled myofibroblasts with no atypia embedded in fibrous stroma
- Characteristic eosinophilic intracytoplasmic inclusions
- Inclusions stain red with Trichrome stain
- Spindle cells are muscle actin+, calponin+, desmin+

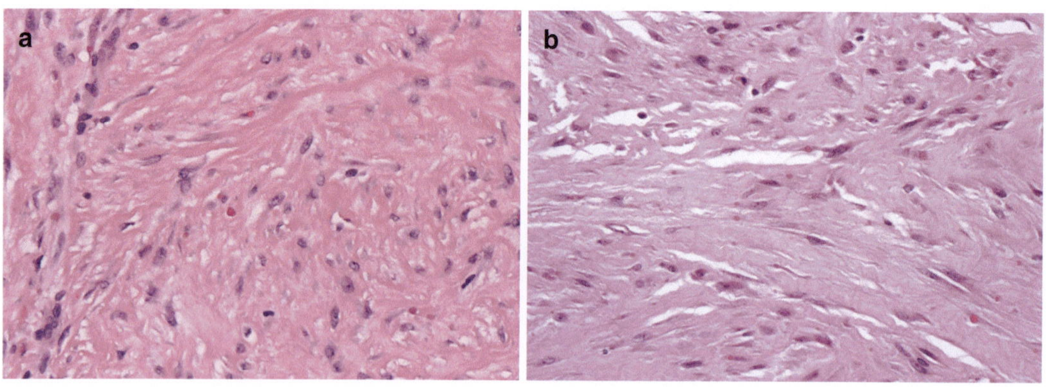

Fig. 9.22 (**a**, **b**) Elongated myofibroblasts with no cytological atypia embedded in thick fibrous stroma

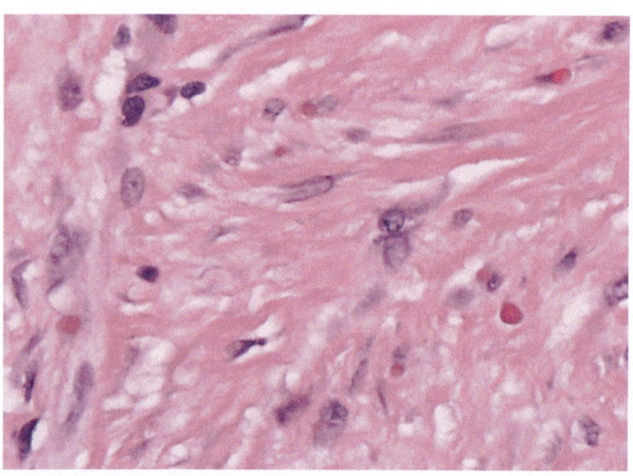

Fig. 9.23 Eosinophilic round intracytoplasmic inclusion are pathognomonic

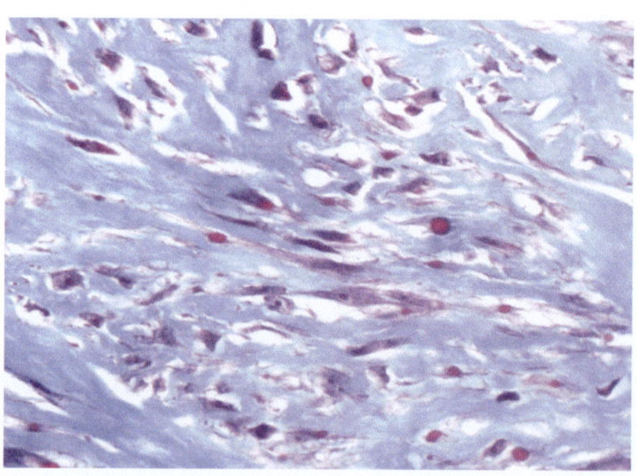

Fig. 9.24 Round inclusions stain red with Trichrome stain

Inflammatory Linear Verrucous Epidermal Nevus

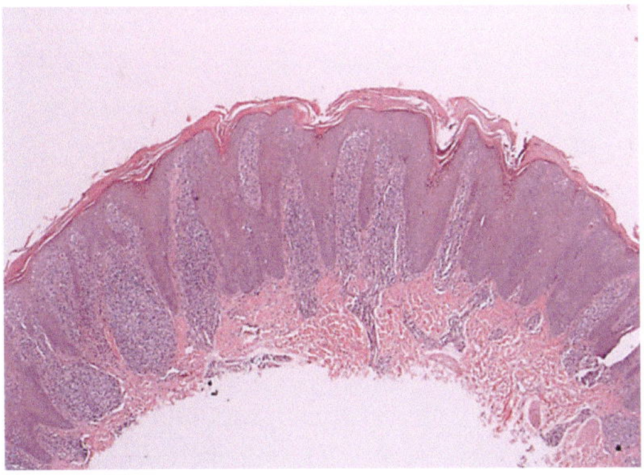

Fig. 9.25 Psoriasiform epidermal hyperplasia

Synonym: ILVEN

Histopathology (Figs. 9.25, 9.26, 9.27, and 9.28)

- Psoriasiform epidermal hyperplasia with hyperkeratosis
- Absence of granular layer
- Characteristic alternating parakeratosis and orthokeratosis
- Lymphocytic exocytosis is common
- Variable dermal lymphocytic inflammation

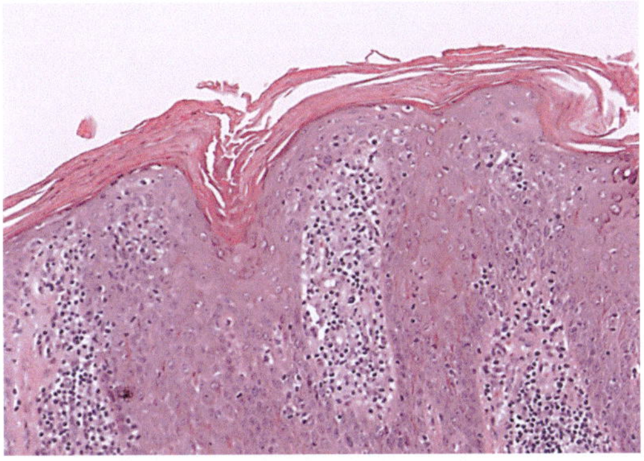

Fig. 9.26 Absence of granular layer underneath the parakeratosis

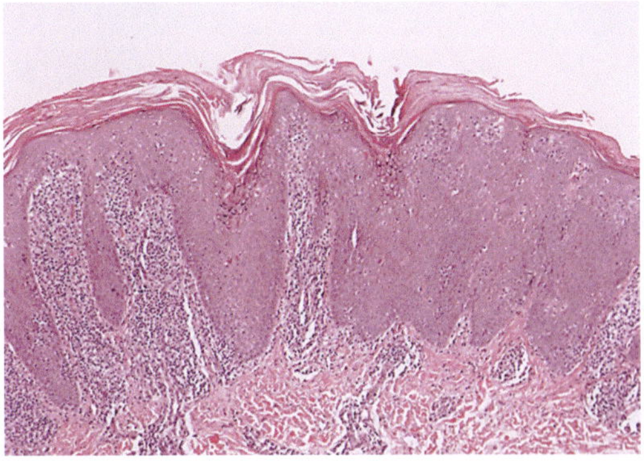

Fig. 9.27 Dermal lymphocytic inflammation

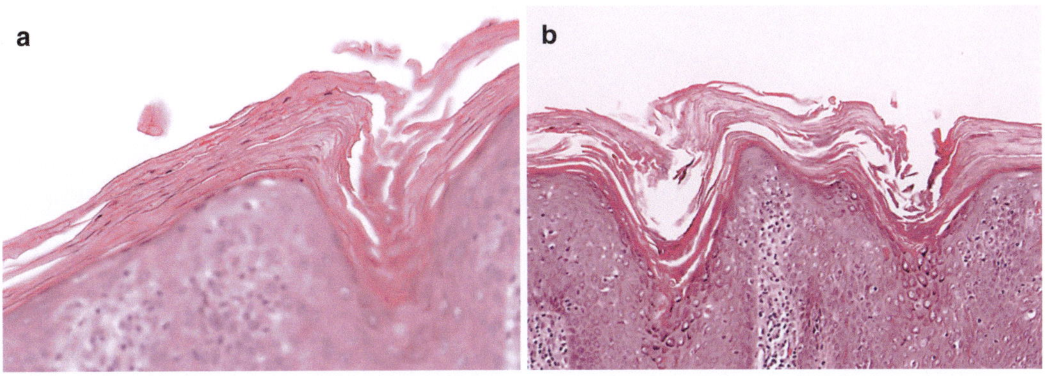

Fig. 9.28 (**a**, **b**) Alternating parakeratosis and orthokeratosis

Intravascular Large B-Cell Lymphoma

Rare type of extranodular large B cell lymphoma also referred as **angiotropic large-cell lymphoma**.

Histopathology (Figs. 9.29, 9.30, 9.31, 9.32, and 9.33)

- Characteristic growth of lymphoma cells within blood vessels
- Lymphoma cells are of large type
- Vessel wall mostly appears intact
- Tumor cells are CD20 positive

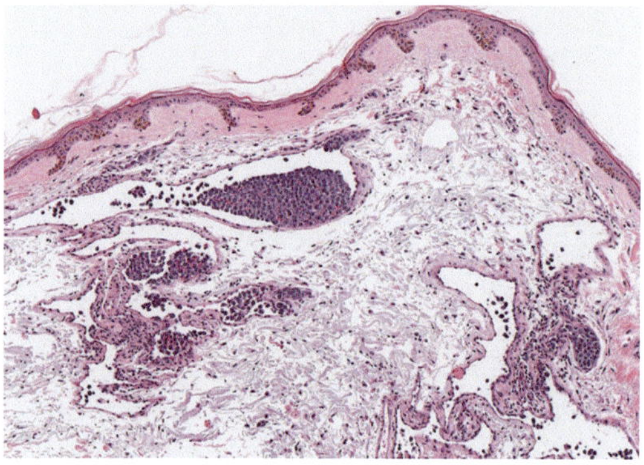

Fig. 9.29 Tumor within dilated vessels

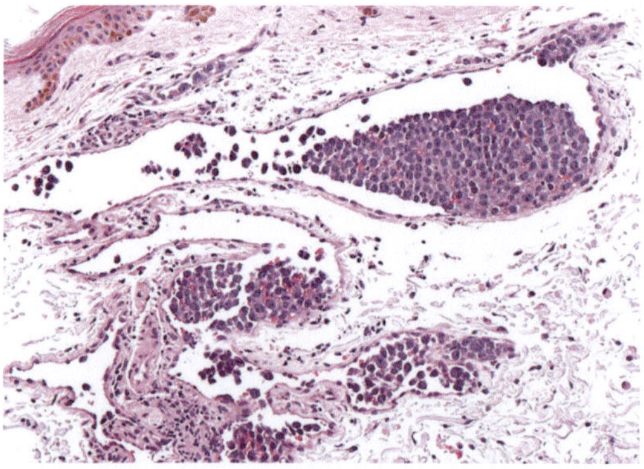

Fig. 9.30 Tumor filled vessels with no extravascular involvement

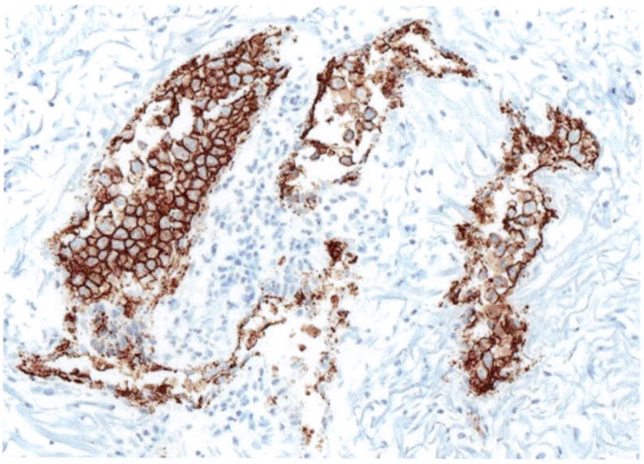

Fig. 9.31 Tumor cells are CD20 positive

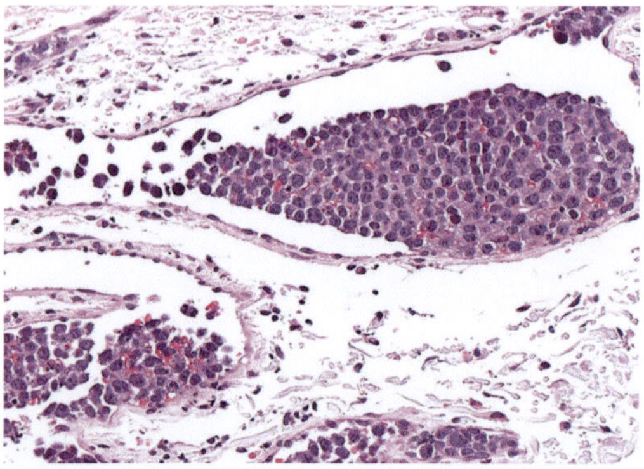

Fig. 9.32 Malignant lymphoma cells are of large type

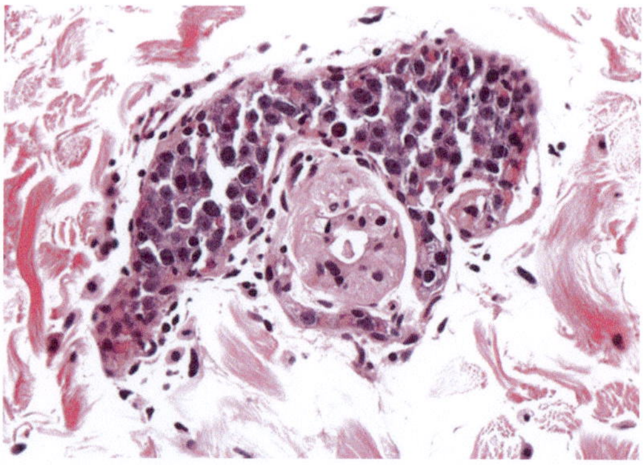

Fig. 9.33 Lymphoma filled vessel surrounds sweat duct

Intravascular Papillary Endothelial Hyperplasia

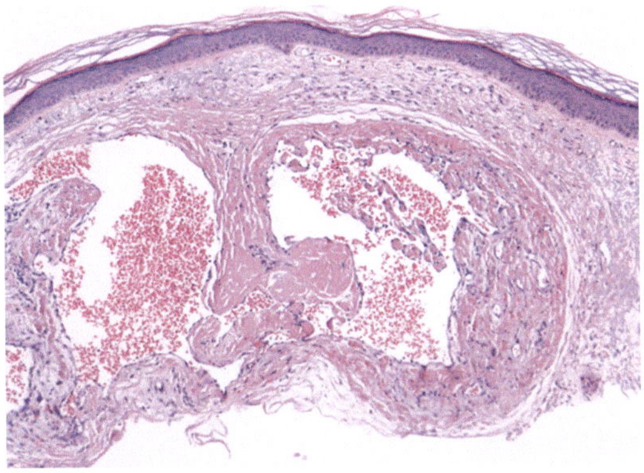

Fig. 9.34 Papillary proliferation within thrombosed vessel

Synonym: Masson's Tumor

Histopathology (Figs. 9.34, 9.35, and 9.36)

- Vascular tumor arising within thrombosed vessel or angioma
- Numerous papillary projections lined by plump endothelial cells
- Papillary stroma is hyalinized

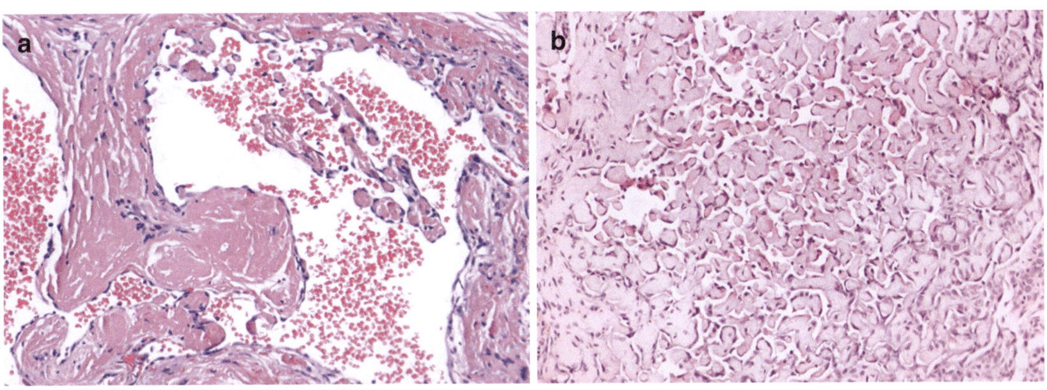

Fig. 9.35 (**a**, **b**) Anastomosing large and small papillae adjacent to organizing thrombus

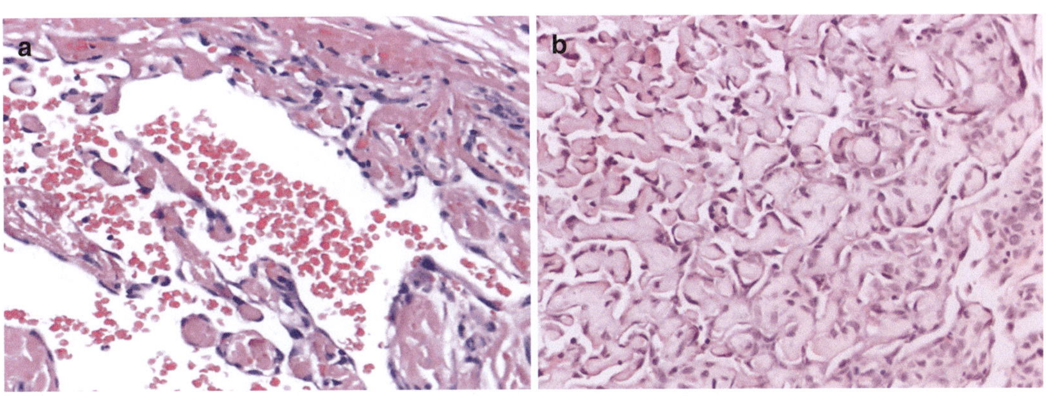

Fig. 9.36 (**a**, **b**) Papillae are made of hyalinized stroma and plump endothelial cells

Inverted Follicular Keratosis

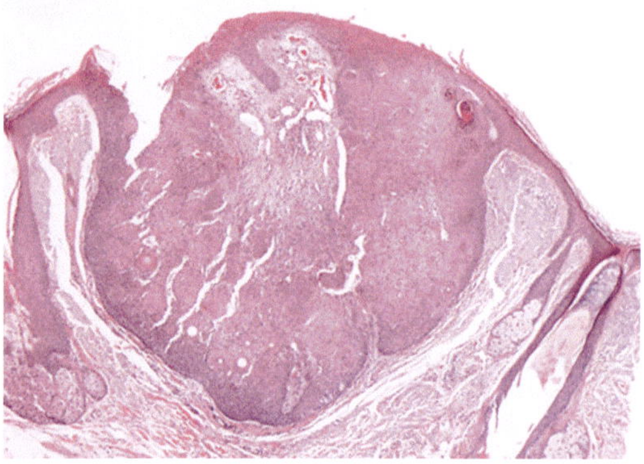

Fig. 9.37 Endophytic tumor invading dermis

A variant of seborrheic keratosis

Histopathology (Figs. 9.37, 9.38, and 9.39)
- Endophytic epithelial tumor
- Epithelial cells form lobules
- Basaloid cells at the periphery and squamoid cells toward the center
- Squamoid eddies are characteristic
- No major cellulvar atypia
- Occasional mitoses are present

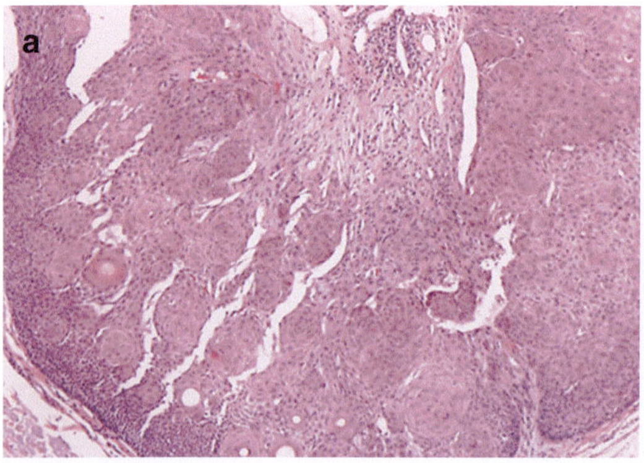

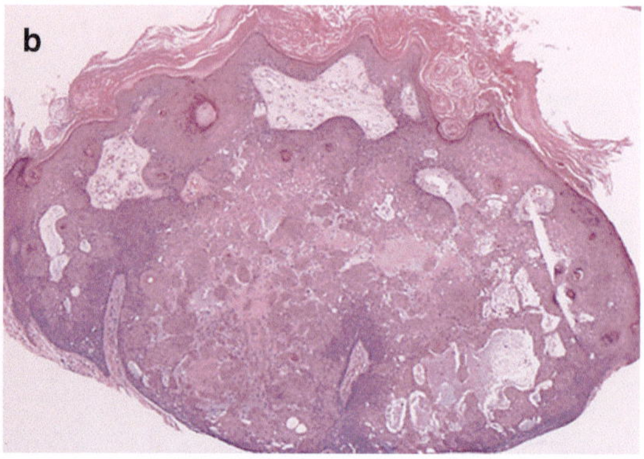

Fig. 9.38 (**a**, **b**) Peripheral cells are smaller and darker and central cells are paler and larger

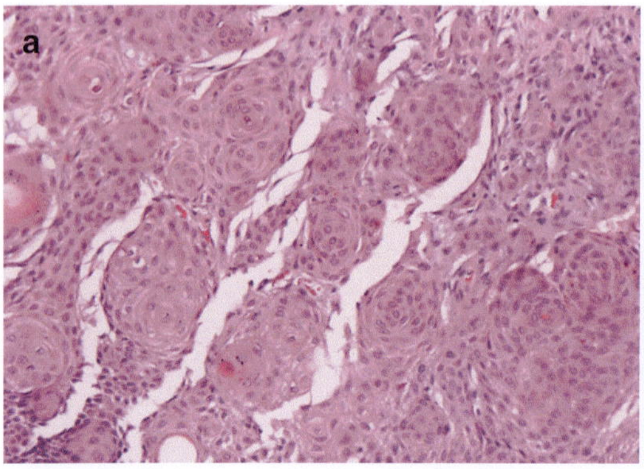

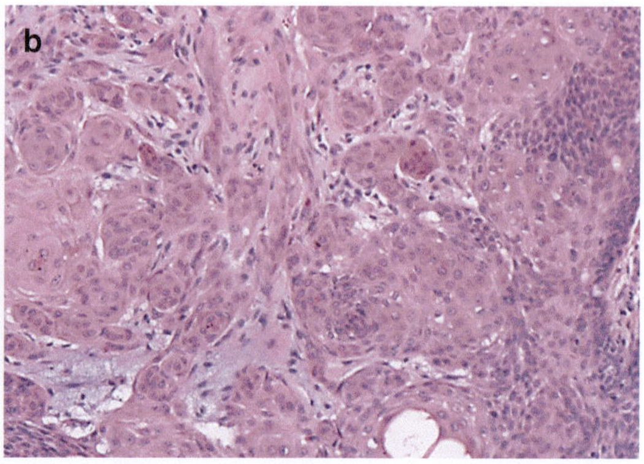

Fig. 9.39 (**a**, **b**) Cells are swirling forming characteristic squamous eddies with no evidence of cytological atypia

Impetigo

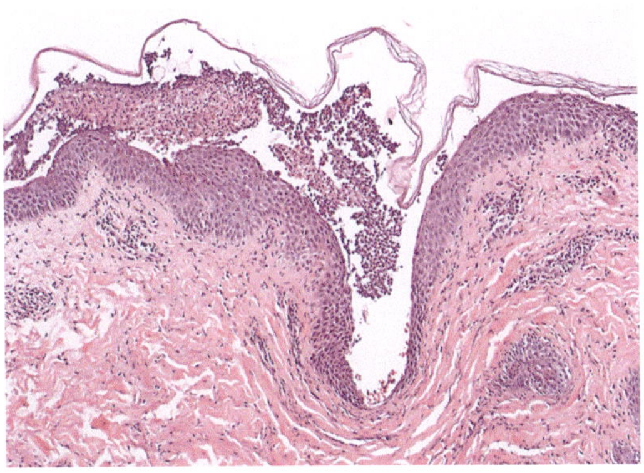

Fig. 9.40 Subcorneal pustule

Histopathology (Figs. 9.40, 9.41, 9.42, and 9.43)
- Split in the epidermis beneath the stratum granulosum
- Epidermal pustule filled with neutrophils
- Dermal neutrophilic and lymphocytic infiltrate
- Bacteria can be seen in the pustule

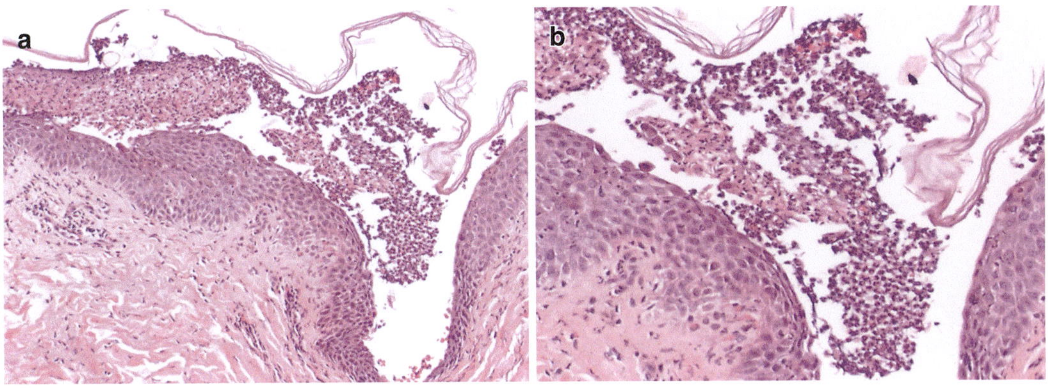

Fig. 9.41 (a, b) The split is below granular layer and acantholysis is minimal

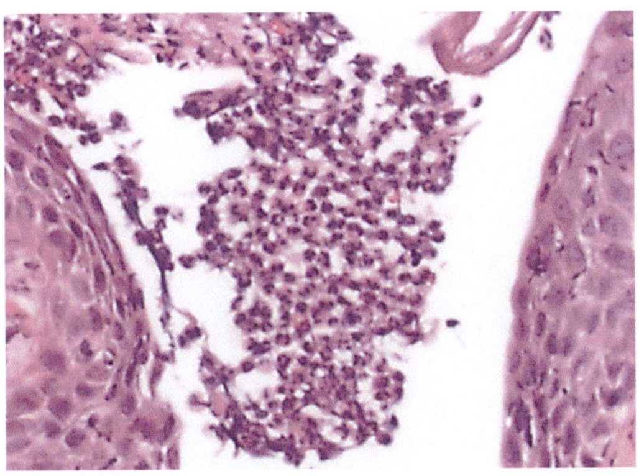

Fig. 9.42 Neutrophilic pustule

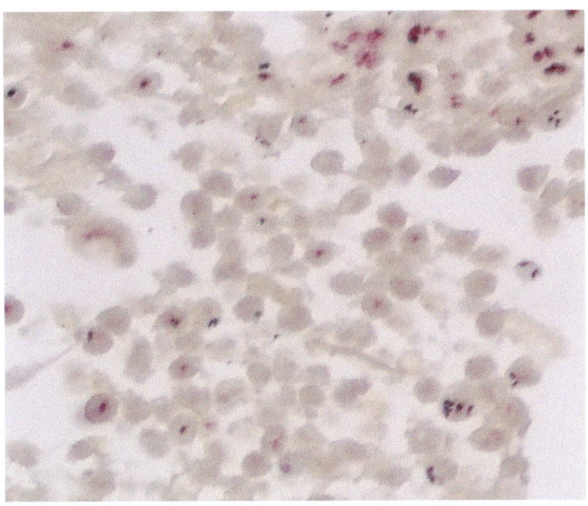

Fig. 9.43 Gram-positive cocci are highlighted with Gram stain

Irritant Contact Dermatitis

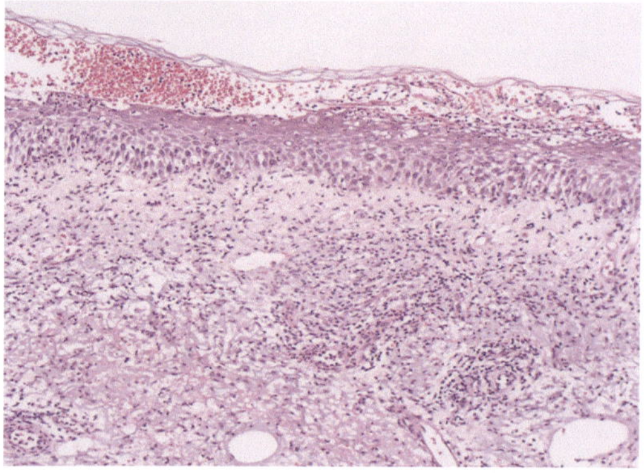

Fig. 9.44 **Acute** irritant contact dermatitis

Histopathology

Acute: epidermal spongiosis with intraepidermal vesicles containing lymphocytes and neutrophils; mild/moderate dermal inflammation with lymphocytes and neutrophils (Figs. 9.44, 9.45, and 9.46)

Subacute: psoriasiform epidermal hyperplasia with spongiosis and epidermal neutrophils; mild/moderate dermal inflammation with lymphocytes and neutrophils (Figs. 9.47 and 9.48)

Chronic: acanthotic, hyperkeratotic epidermis with minimal spongiosis; dermal fibrosis with occasional neutrophils

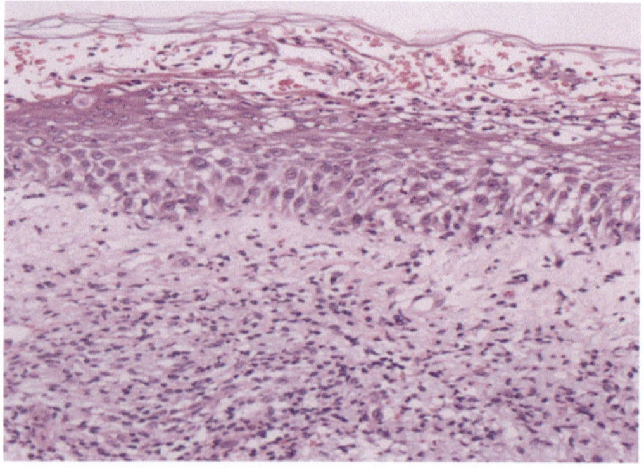

Fig. 9.45 Spongiotic epidermis with scattered neutrophils and neutrophils filled vesicle

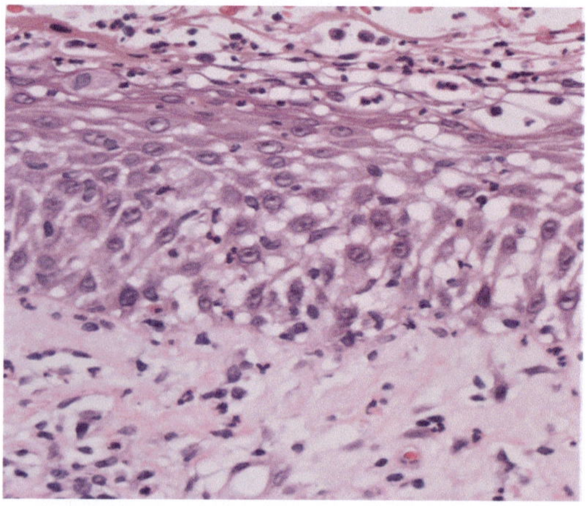

Fig. 9.46 Dermal neutrophils are present

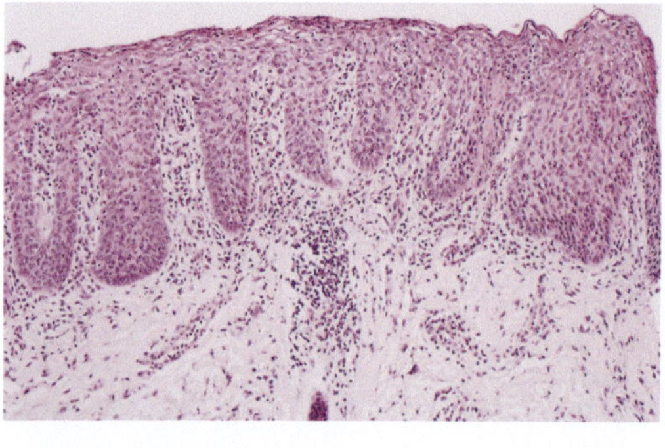

Fig. 9.47 **Subacute** irritant contact dermatitis with psoriasiform spongiotic epidermis

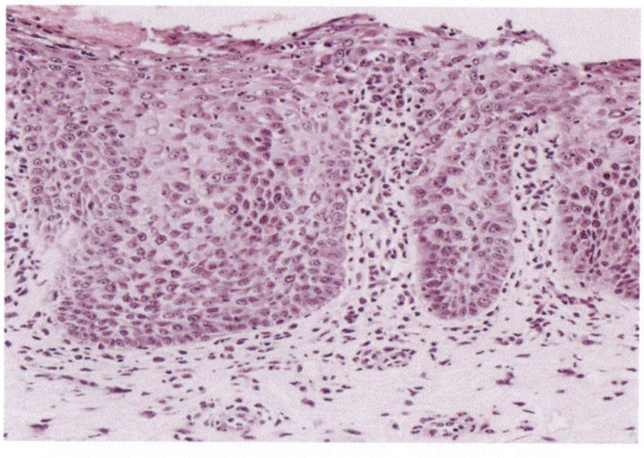

Fig. 9.48 Neutrophils are scattered in the epidermis

Ischemic Fasciitis

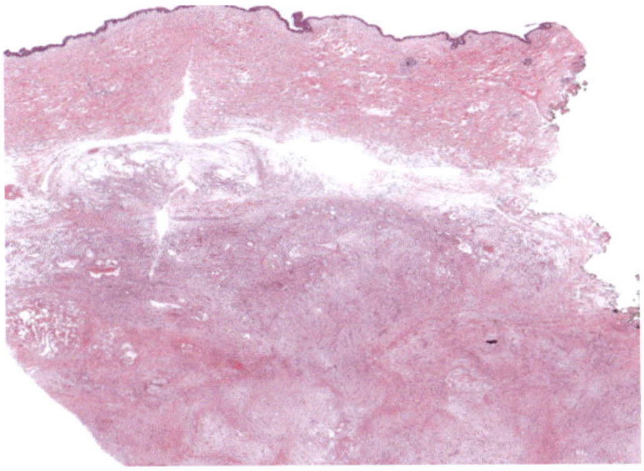

Fig. 9.49 Poorly defined subcutaneous lesion

Histopathology (Figs. 9.49, 9.50, and 9.51)

- Ill-defined lesion involving deep subcutis overlying bony prominence
- Zonal appearance with necrotic hypocellular area and viable cellular areas
- Cellular area consists of spindled and rounded fibroblasts
- Rounded cells can resemble ganglion cells seen in proliferating fasciitis

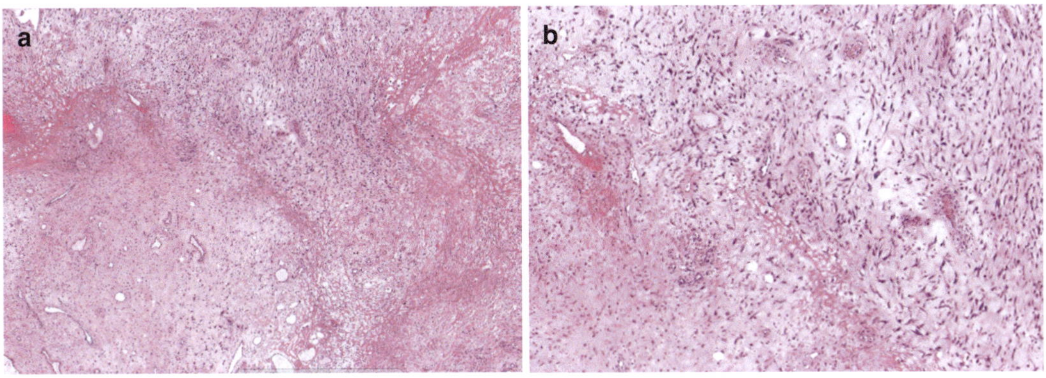

Fig. 9.50 (**a**, **b**) Necrotic area on the left with adjacent cellular area to the right

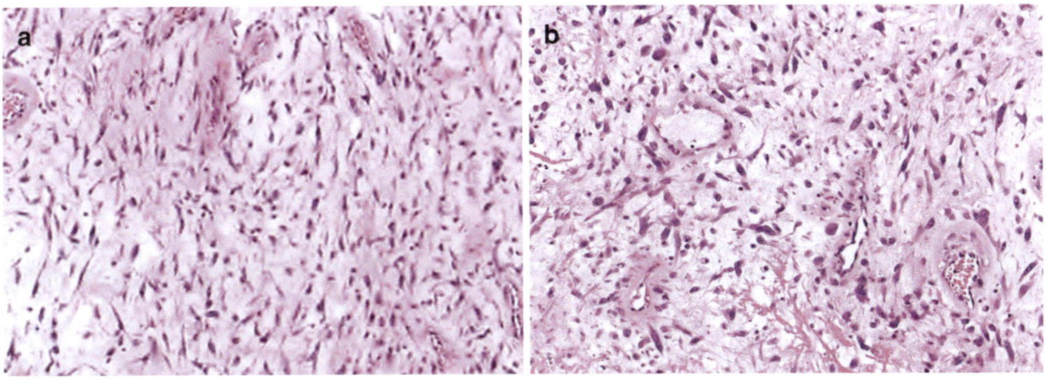

Fig. 9.51 (**a**, **b**) Spindled and rounded fibroblasts/myofibroblasts with cytological irregularity

10 Dermatopathology J

V. Vincek, *Dermatopathology A–Z*, https://doi.org/10.1007/978-3-319-89486-7_10

Jessner's Lymphocytic Infiltrate

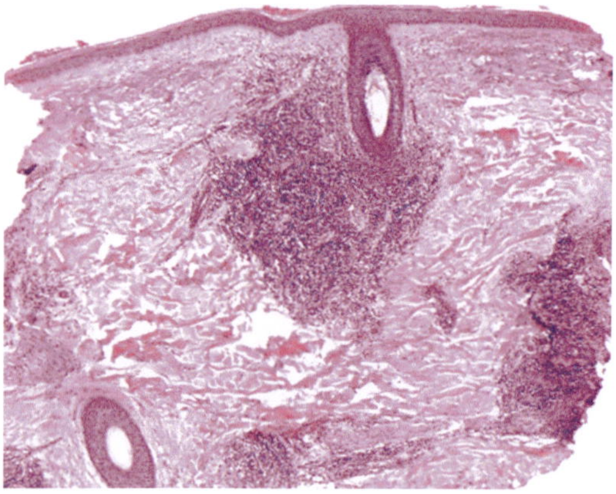

Fig. 10.1 Normal epidermis with perivascular and perifollicular inflammation

Synonym: T-Cell Pseudolymphoma

Histopathology (Figs. 10.1, 10.2, and 10.3)
- Normal epidermis
- Moderately dense perivascular and perifollicular lymphocytic infiltrate
- Infiltrate consists of CD4 positive small lymphocytes

P.S. *discoid lupus erythematous (DLE)* is in clinical and histological differential. However, in *DLE* the epidermis is affected unlike in *Jessner's*

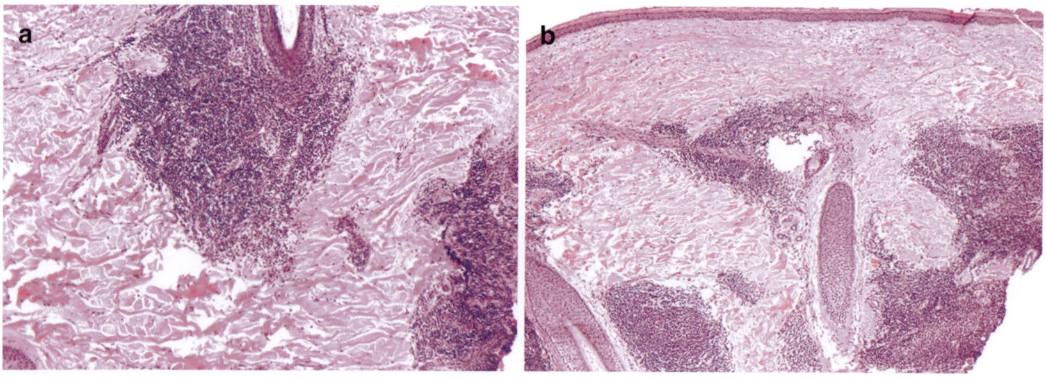

Fig. 10.2 (**a**, **b**) Densely grouped lymphocytic inflammation with minimal interstitial inflammation

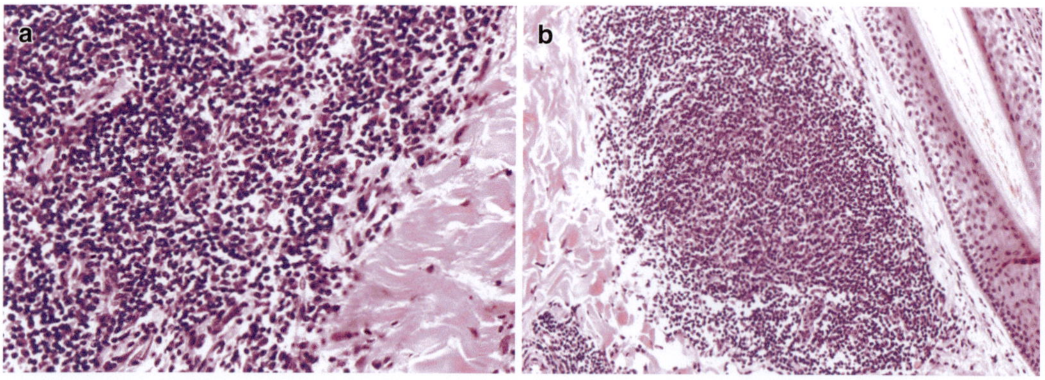

Fig. 10.3 (**a**, **b**) Infiltrate consists of small mature uniform lymphocytes

Junctional Nevus

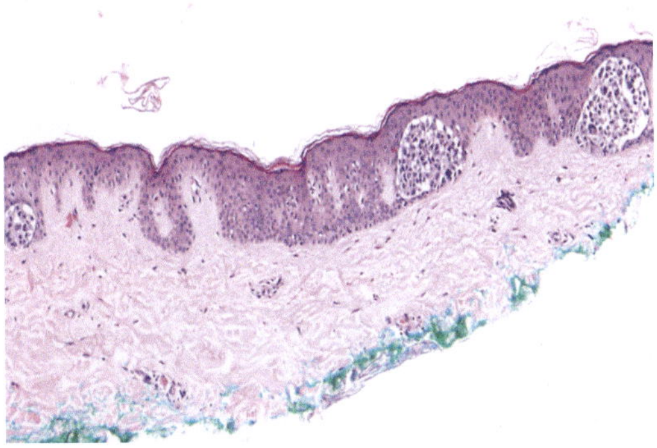

Fig. 10.4 Wavy epidermis with junctional nevus nests

Synonym: Junctional Melanocytic Nevus

Histopathology (Figs. 10.4, 10.5, 10.6, and 10.7)

- Nests of nevus cells on the tips of rete ridges
- Nests are cohesive and surrounded by a clear space
- Melanocytes do not show atypia or major variability within the nests
- Individual melanocytes can be present in the lower portion of the epidermis
- Minimal or no dermal inflammation

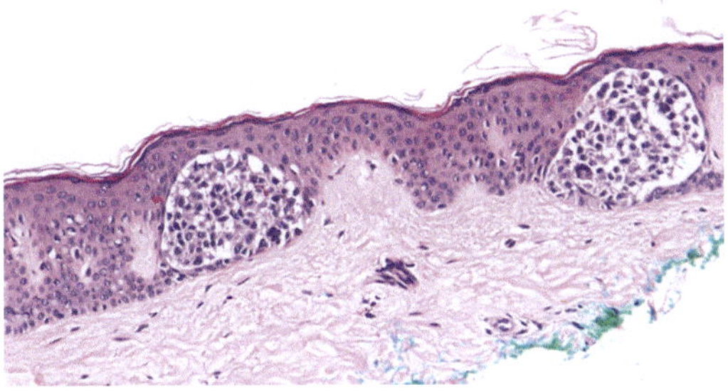

Fig. 10.5 Nests of nevus cells on the tips of the rete ridges

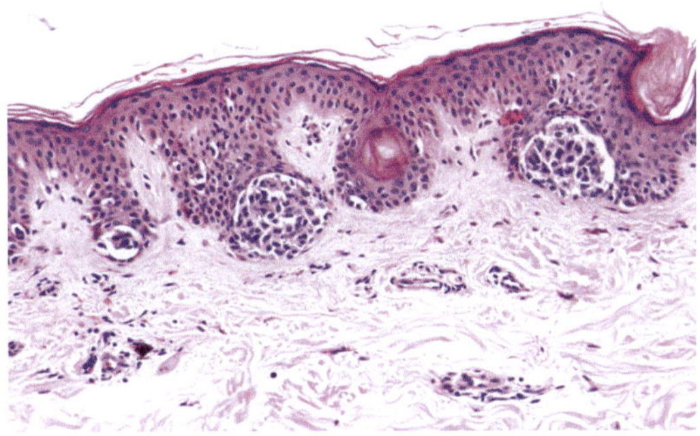

Fig. 10.6 Nests are slightly retracted from the epidermis

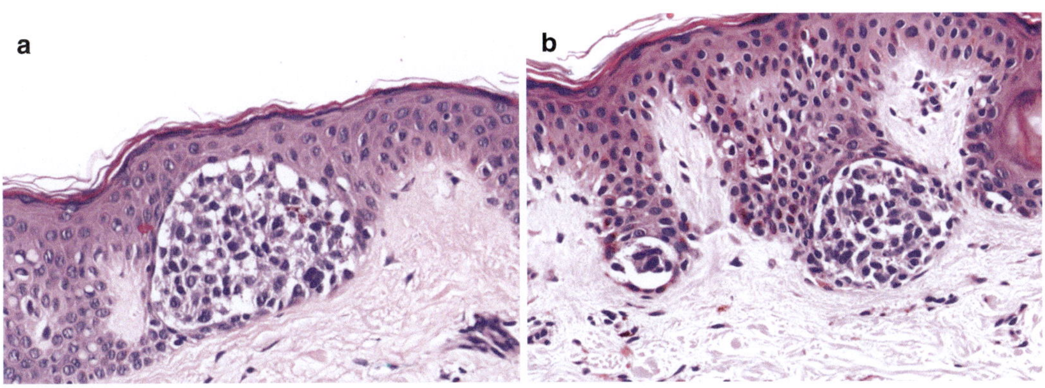

Fig. 10.7 (**a**, **b**) Melanocytes within the nests are uniform; some single melanocytes are present in the lower half of the epidermis

Juvenile Hyaline Fibromatosis

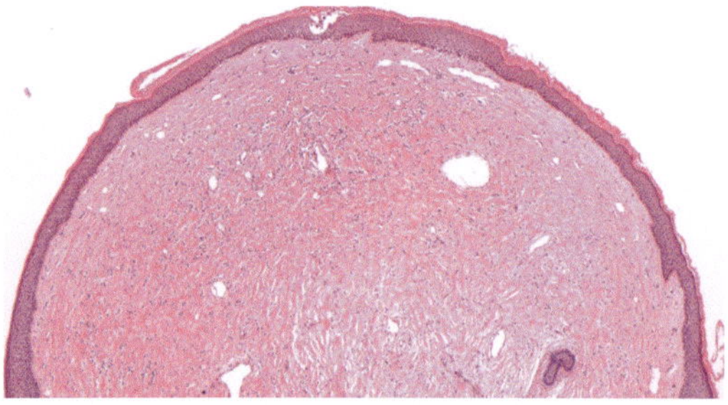

Fig. 10.8 Fibrotic tumor forming the nodule

Histopathology (Figs. 10.8, 10.9, and 10.10)

- Ill-defined dermal and subcutaneous lesion forming nodule
- Abundant amorphous hyalinized deeply eosinophilic stroma (PAS+)
- Scattered plumped fibroblasts focally vimentin and SMA+
- Autosomal recessive disease with *CMG2* mutation

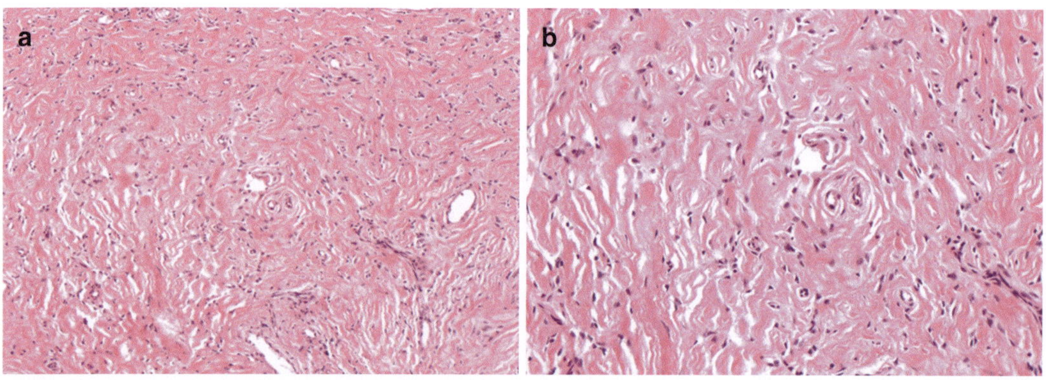

Fig. 10.9 (**a**, **b**) Hypocellular tumor with eosinophilic hyalinized stroma

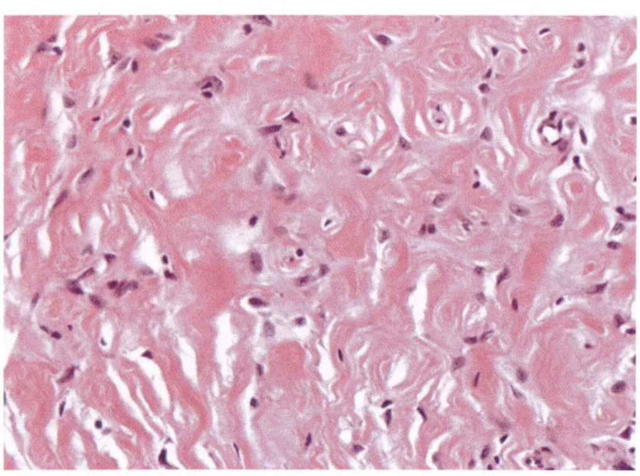

Fig. 10.10 Fibroblasts are plumped and scattered with no atypia or mitoses

Dermatopathology K 11

V. Vincek, *Dermatopathology A–Z*, https://doi.org/10.1007/978-3-319-89486-7_11

Kaposi's Sarcoma

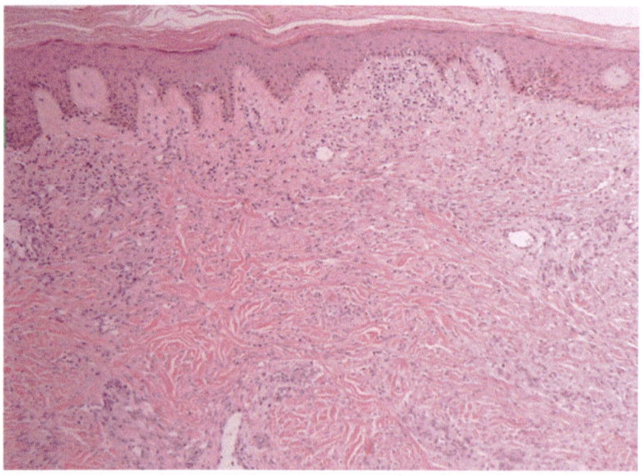

Fig. 11.1 **Patch stage KS**

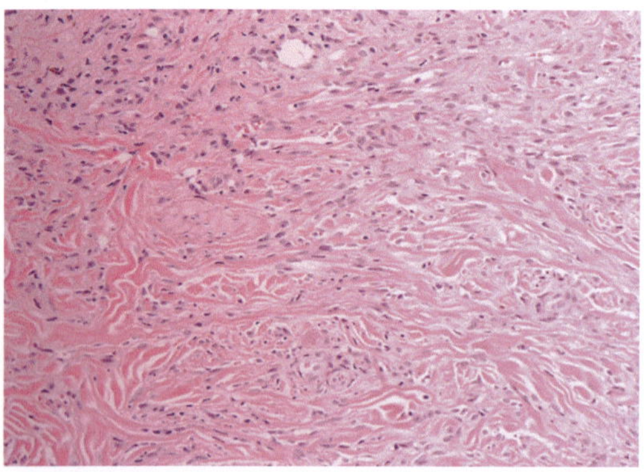

Fig. 11.2 Poorly defined dermal vascular proliferation

Histopathology

Patch stage (Figs. 11.1, 11.2, 11.3, and 11.4)

- Ill-defined dermal lesion
- Mild increase of elongated vessels with minimal endothelial atypia
- Perivascular lymphocytes and plasma cells
- Vessels dissect between collagen and surround larger vessels (the "promontory" sign)

Plaques stage (Figs. 11.5, 11.6, and 11.7)

- Easily detected dermal vascular proliferation
- Spindle cells with "slit-like" vascular spaces (HHV8+)
- Red blood cell extravasation with some hemosiderin

Nodular stage (Figs. 11.8, 11.9, and 11.10)

- Nodular proliferation of atypical spindle cells with delicate "slit-like" vascular spaces
- Red blood extravasation and hemosiderin can be seen

P.S.be careful HHV8 is also positive in Castleman's disease

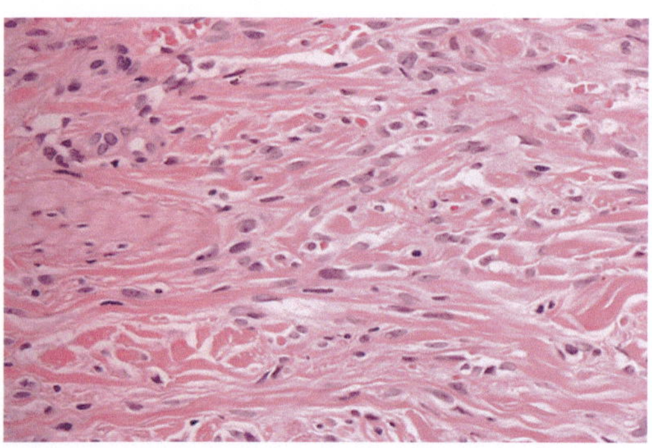

Fig. 11.3 Elongated vessels are dissecting collagen bundles; focal red blood cell extravasation present

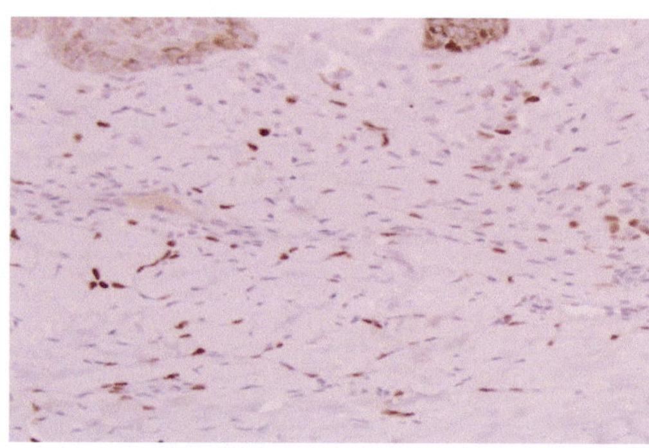

Fig. 11.4 Nuclear HHV8 staining (brown) is detected

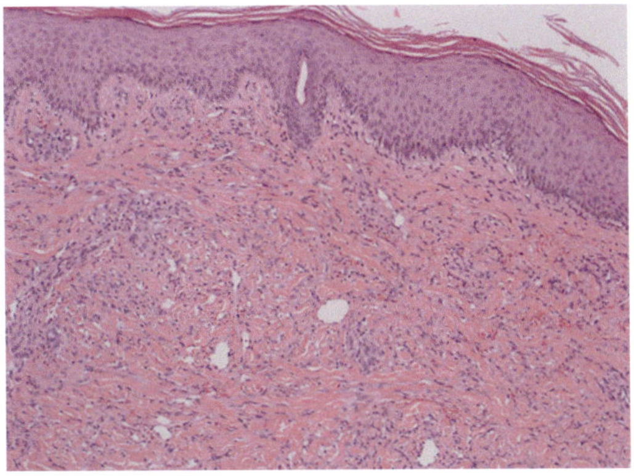

Fig. 11.5 Plaque stage KS

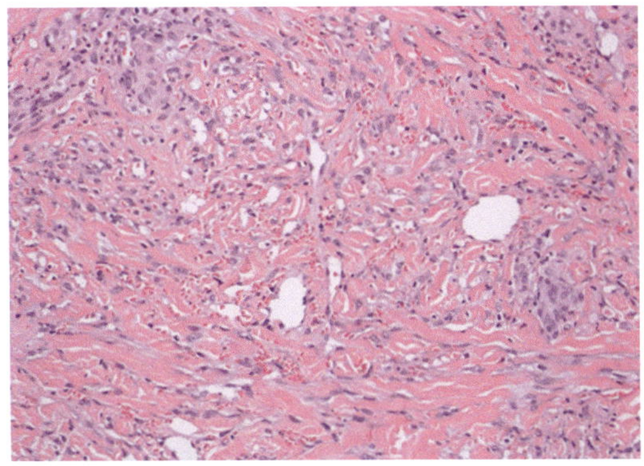

Fig. 11.6 Increased dermal vascular proliferation

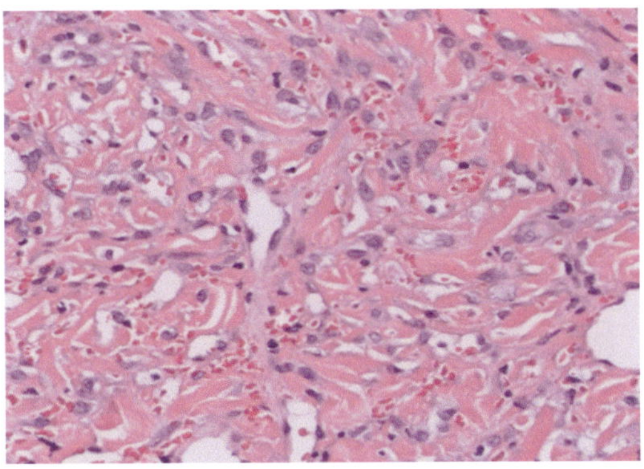

Fig. 11.7 "Slit-like" vascular channels surrounded by spindle cells and red blood cell extravasation

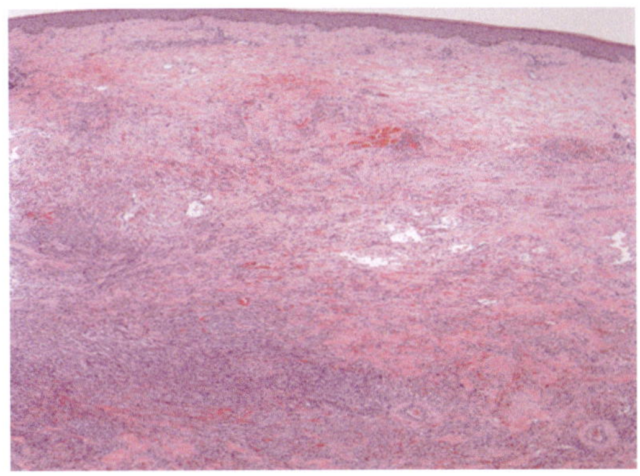

Fig. 11.8 Nodular stage KS

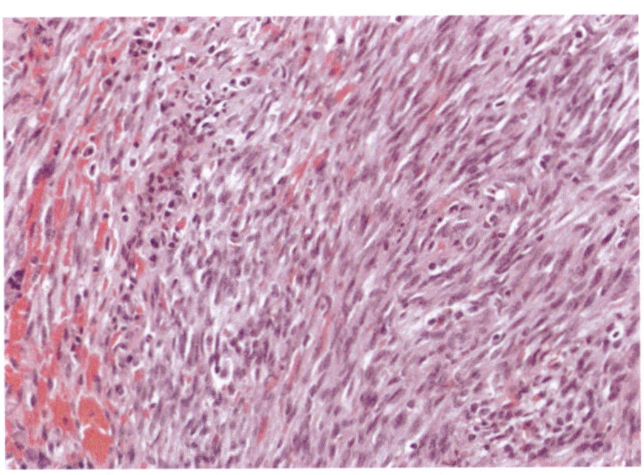

Fig. 11.9 Spindle cell proliferation consuming dermis and subcutis

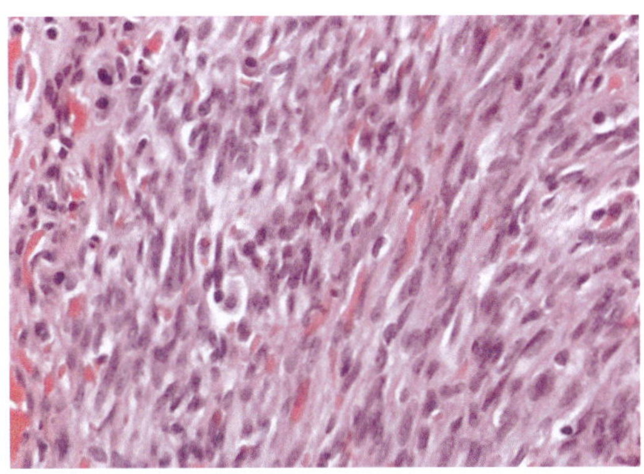

Fig. 11.10 Spindle cells forming fascicles with delicate "slit-like" spaces

Kaposiform Hemangioendothelioma

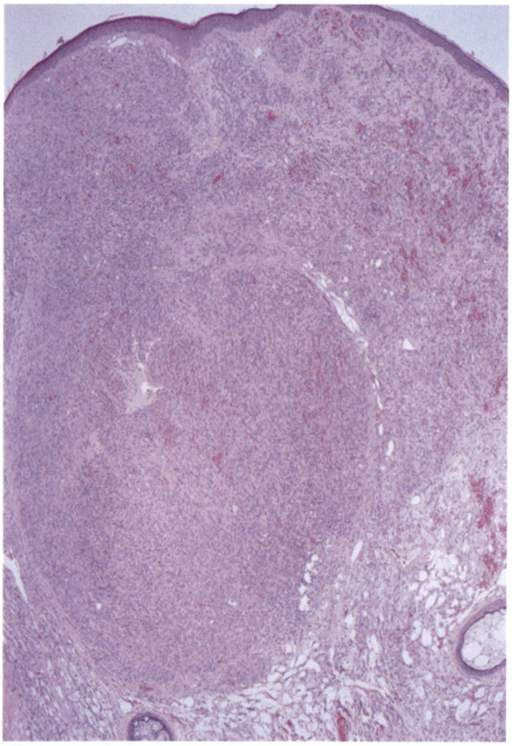

Fig. 11.11 Dermal and subcutaneous multinodular tumor with dense center and pale periphery

Histopathology (Figs. 11.11, 11.12, 11.13, and 11.14)

- Multinodular appearance
- Nodules made of spindle endothelial cells with "slit-like" spaces and red blood extravasation similar to *Kaposi's sarcoma*
- Periphery of the tumor has areas resembling capillary hemangioma
- Cells are CD31+, CD34+, FLI1+, HHV8−, GLUT−

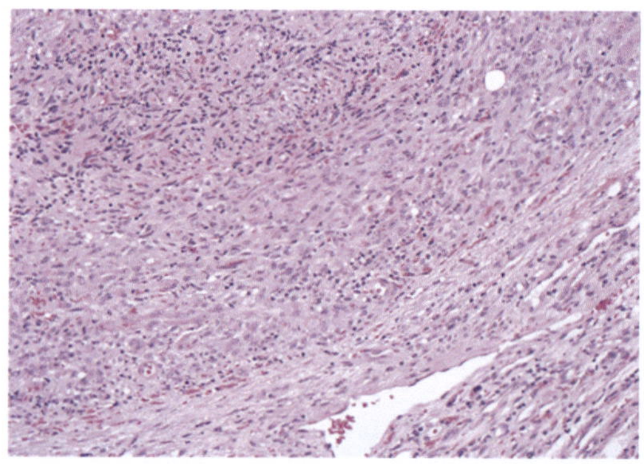

Fig. 11.12 Center of the tumor is made of spindle cells with small empty slits and RBCs extravasation

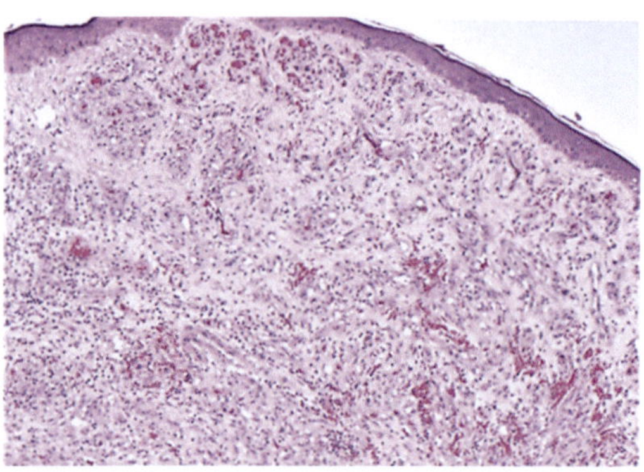

Fig. 11.13 Peripheral area resembles capillary hemangioma

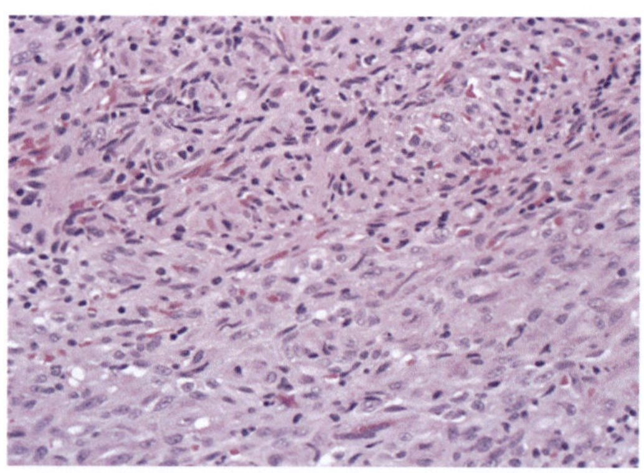

Fig. 11.14 Central area resembles Kaposi's sarcoma

Keloid

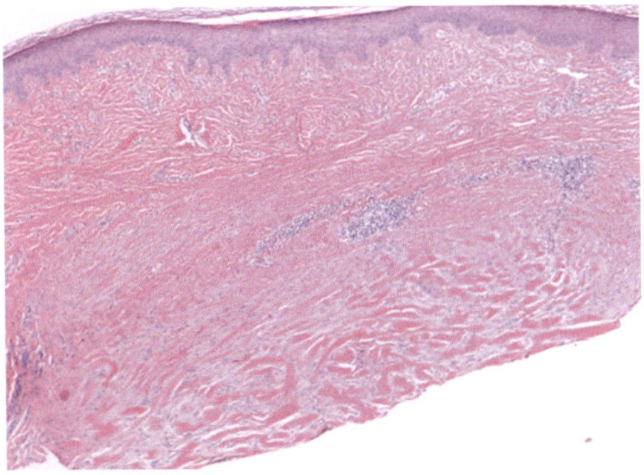

Fig. 11.15 Sclerotic dermis and subcutis with absent adnexal structures

Histopathology (Figs. 11.15, 11.16, 11.17, 11.18, and 11.19)

- Thick dermal collagen with broad hyalinized bundles
- Epidermis is usually normal or thin
- In early lesions chronic lymphocytic inflammation is usually present at the periphery
- Early lesions have bluish collagen in addition to typical thick pink collagen
- In late lesions, lymphocytes and bluish collagen are absent

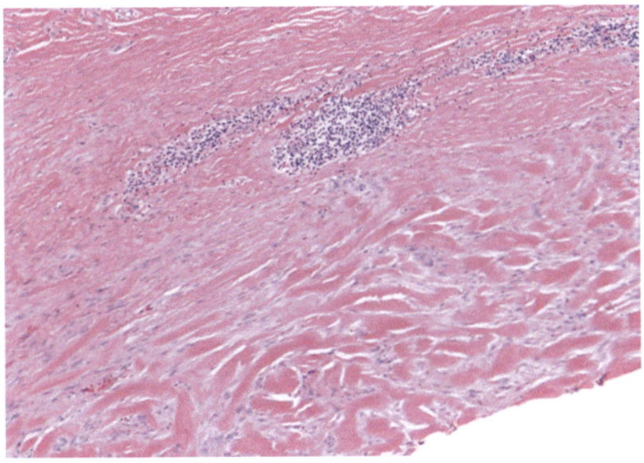

Fig. 11.16 Early, more cellular lesion with bluish and pink collagen

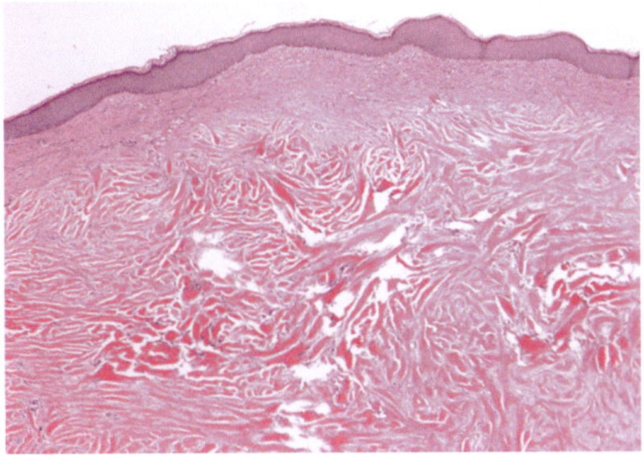

Fig. 11.17 Well established lesion is hypocellular

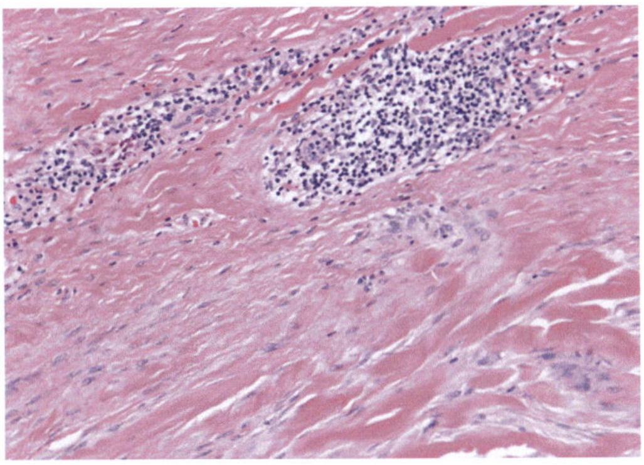

Fig. 11.18 Lymphocytic aggregates are common in early lesions

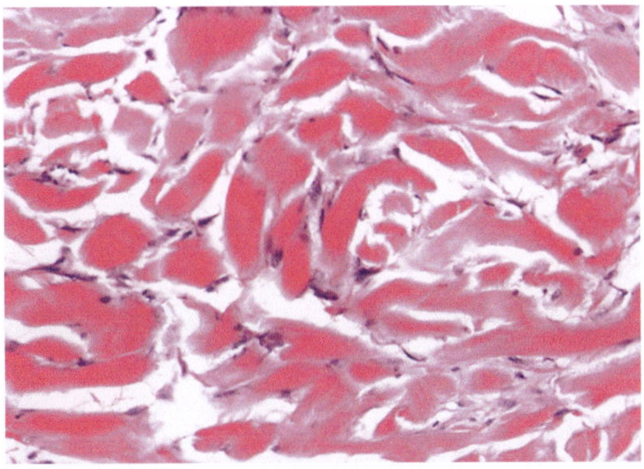

Fig. 11.19 Thick, darkly pink hyalinized collagen

Keratin Granuloma

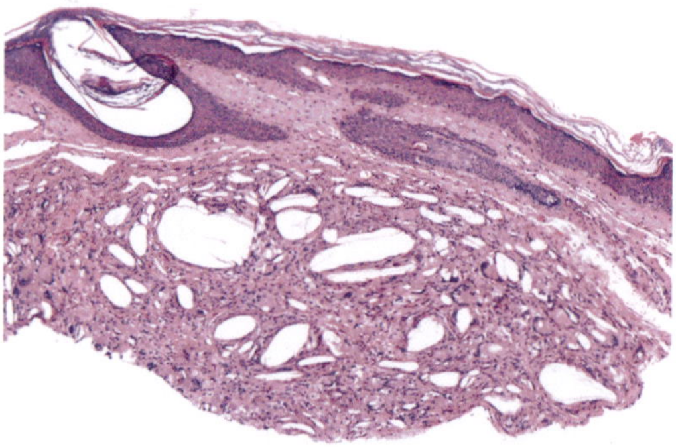

Fig. 11.20 Distorted hair follicle with underlying granuloma

Histopathology (Figs. 11.20, 11.21, 11.22, and 11.23)

- Keratin granuloma usually arises around ruptured follicle or cyst
- Multiple keratin fragments, many of them within multinucleated giant cells
- Numerous histiocytes and lymphocytes

P.S. be careful as keratin granuloma can also be seen in necrotic tumors

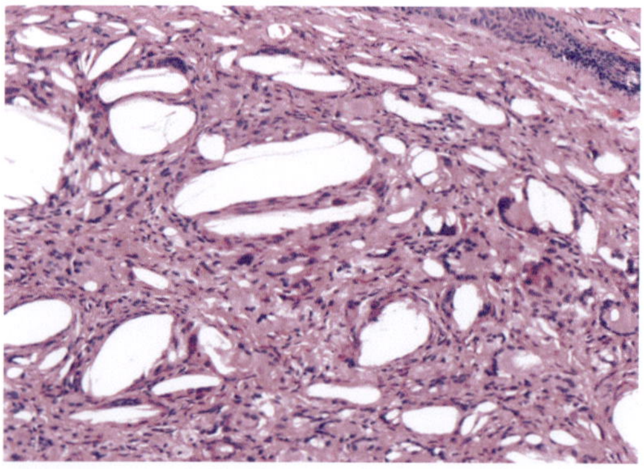

Fig. 11.21 Keratin flakes with surrounding giant cells and histiocytes

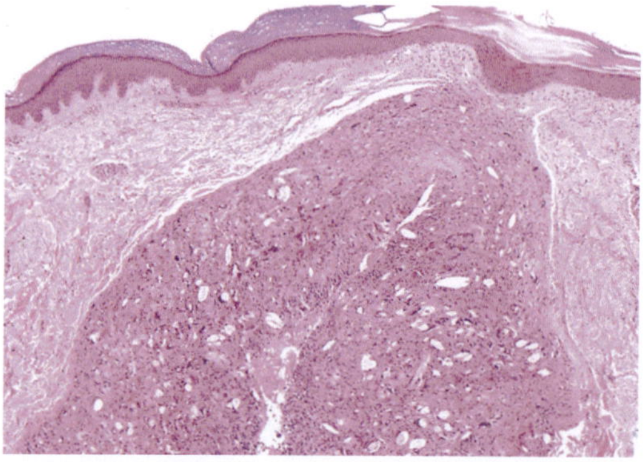

Fig. 11.22 Keratin granuloma surrounds ruptured hair follicle

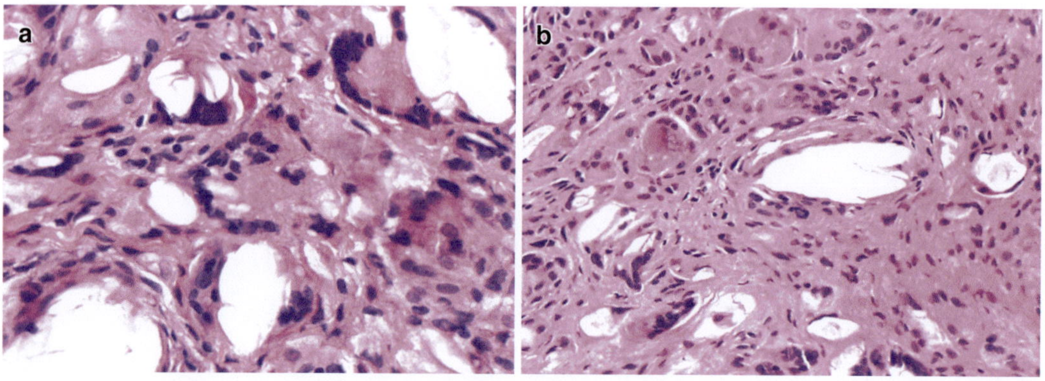

Fig. 11.23 (a, b) Many keratin fragments within multinucleated giant cells

Keratoacanthoma

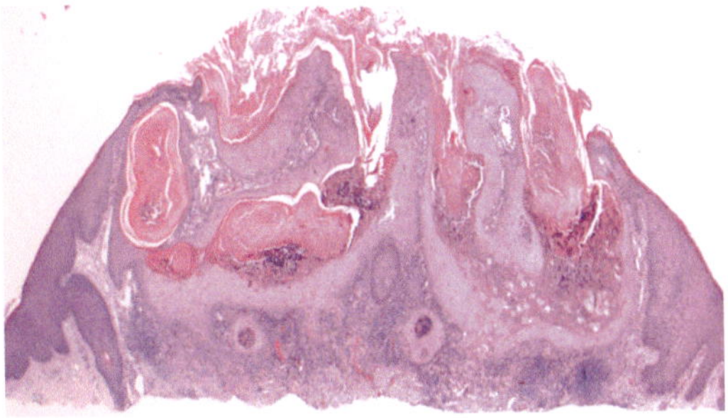

Fig. 11.24 "Crater-like" symmetrical epidermal lesion with epidermal collarette

Histopathology (Figs. 11.24, 11.25, 11.26, 11.27, and 11.28)

- Pear shaped symmetrical lesion with keratin filled center and epidermal collarette
- Invaginated squamous epithelium ranges from well differentiated to dysplastic
- Keratinocytes commonly have ground glass appearance and squamous pearls are common
- Intraepidermal neutrophilic microabscesses and dermal mixed inflammation present

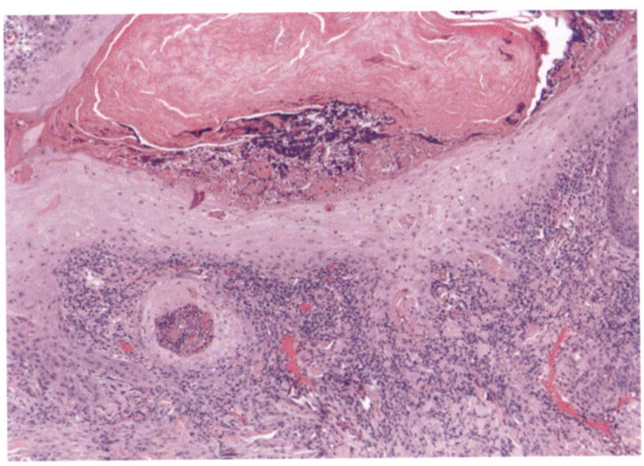

Fig. 11.25 Crater is filled with thick collagen. Epidermis is well differentiated with pushing borders

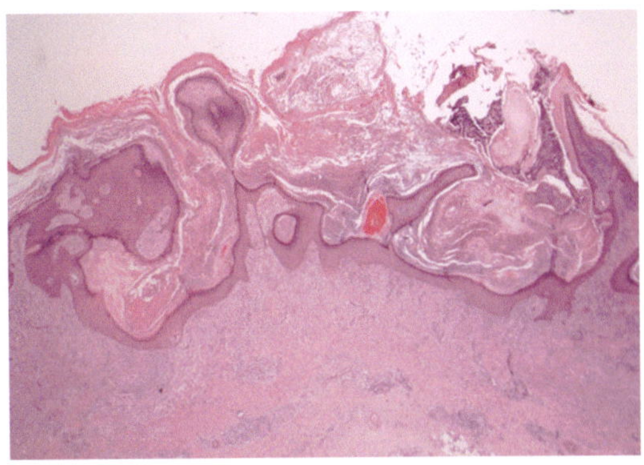

Fig. 11.26 Regressing keratoacanthoma filled with keratin

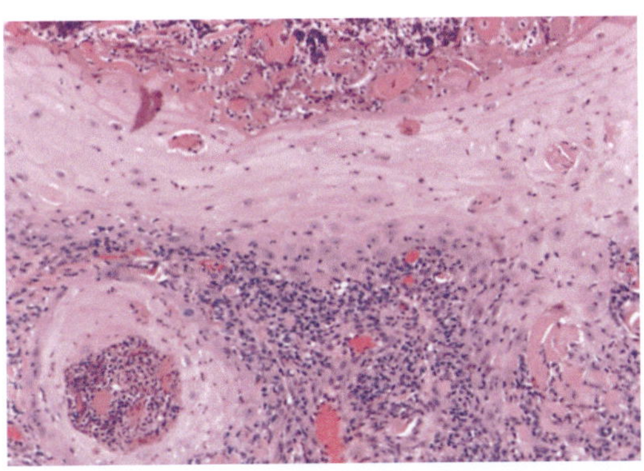

Fig. 11.27 Glassy keratinocytes and intraepidermal microabscess. Dermal mixed inflammation is present

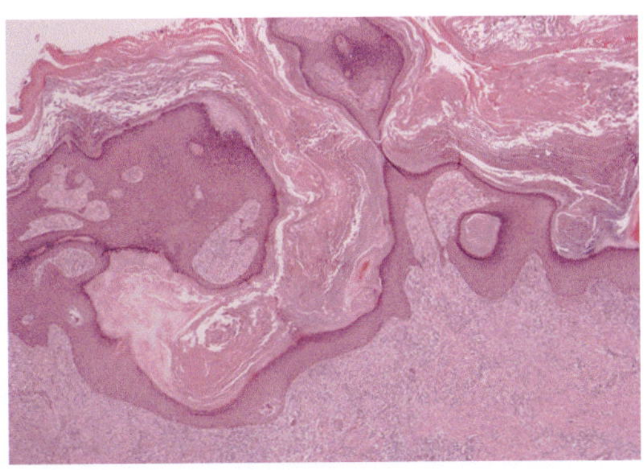

Fig. 11.28 The squamous epithelium is becoming atrophic with flattened bottom

Keratosis Pilaris

Synonyms: Lichen Spinulosus, Follicular Hyperkeratosis, Phrynoderma

Histopathology (Figs. 11.29, 11.30, and 11.31)

- Dilated infundibulum of the hair follicle filled with keratin
- Infundibular epithelium is atrophic
- No evidence of inflammation

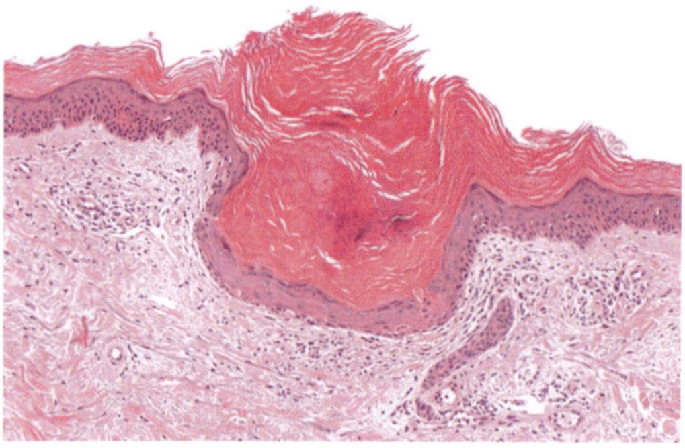

Fig. 11.29 Keratin filled dilated infundibulum

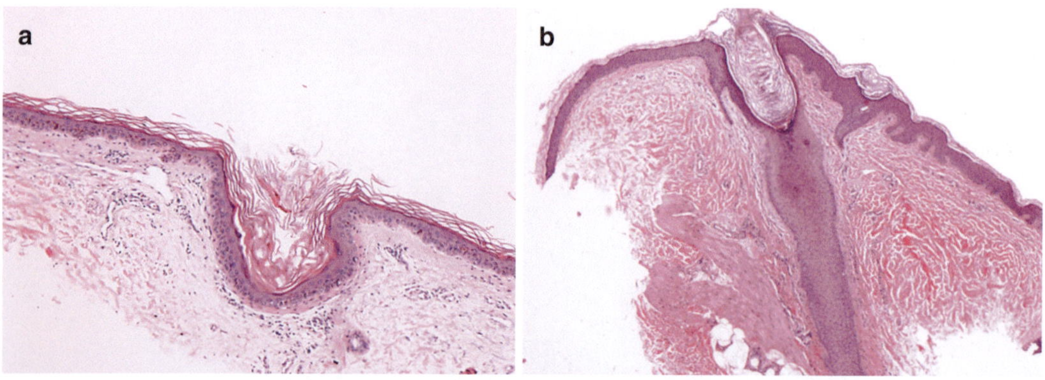

Fig. 11.30 (**a**, **b**) Dilated infundibulum filled with laminated keratin

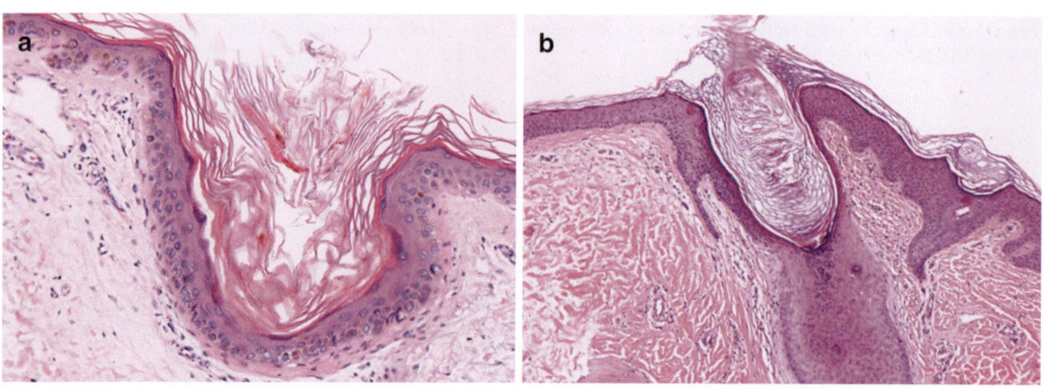

Fig. 11.31 (**a**, **b**) Epithelium is atrophic and there is no evidence of inflammation

Kimura's Disease

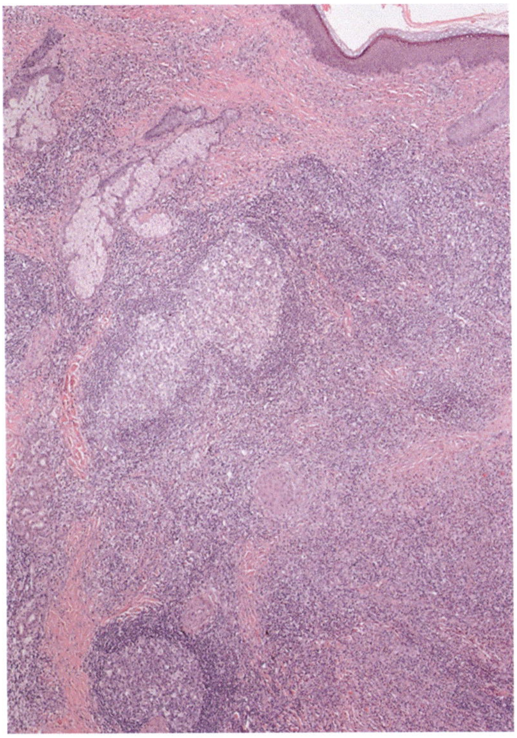

Fig. 11.32 Exuberant inflammation with scattered lymphoid follicle

Histopathology (Figs. 11.32, 11.33, 11.34, and 11.35)

- Dermal and subcutaneous inflammatory cell infiltrate with lymphoid follicles
- Germinal centers in addition to histiocytes can have some eosinophils
- Follicles are surrounded by smaller lymphocytes, histiocytes, and numerous eosinophils
- Vessels with plump endothelial cells are present

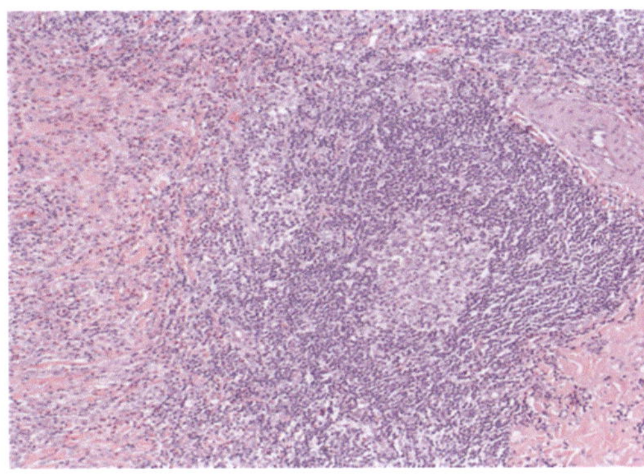

Fig. 11.33 Lymphoid follicle surrounded by smaller lymphocytes

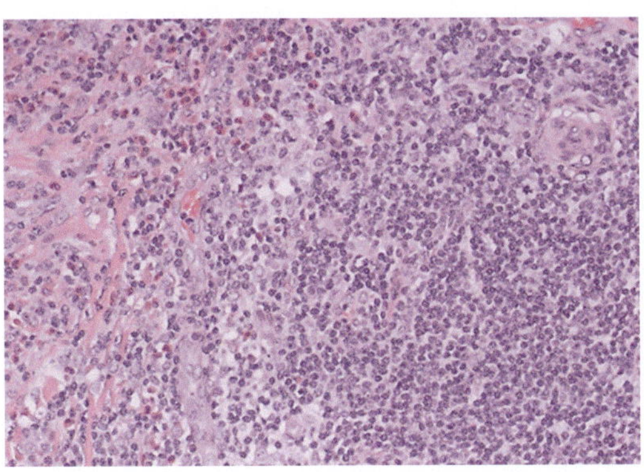

Fig. 11.34 Infiltrate consisting of lymphocytes, histiocytes, and eosinophils

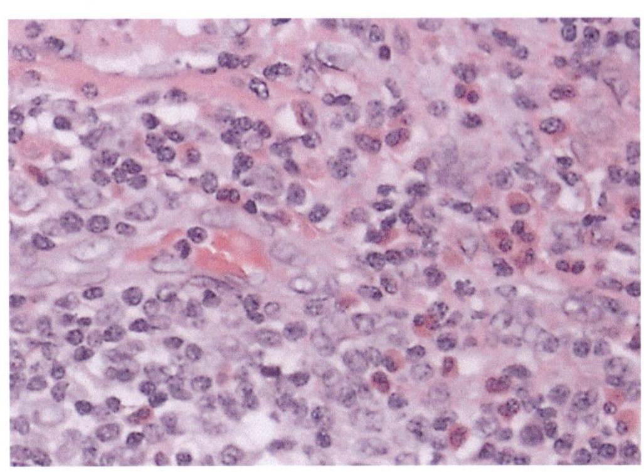

Fig. 11.35 Small vessels with plump endothelial cells surrounded by eosinophils

Knuckle Pad

Histopathology (Figs. 11.36, 11.37, and 11.38)
- Wavy epidermal papillomatosis
- Epidermal acanthosis and extensive hyperkeratosis
- Mild dermal fibrosis and inflammation

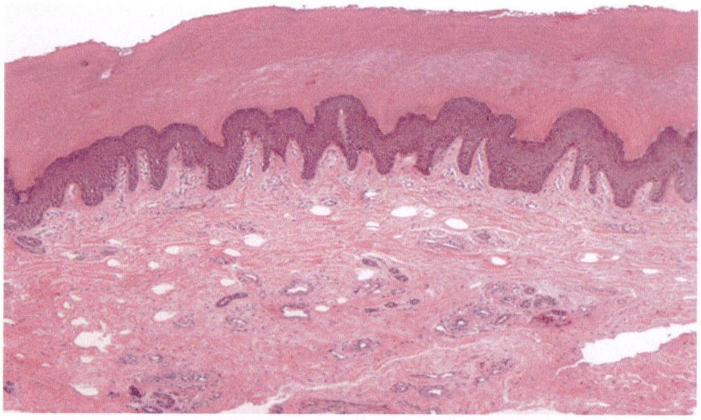

Fig. 11.36 Wavy epidermal papillomatosis

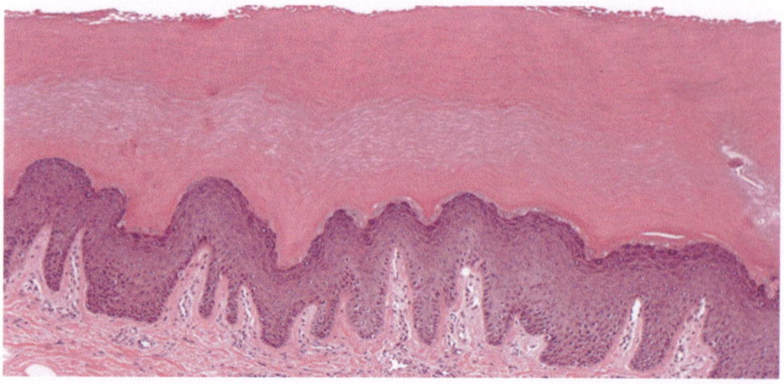

Fig. 11.37 Extensive epidermal hyperkeratosis

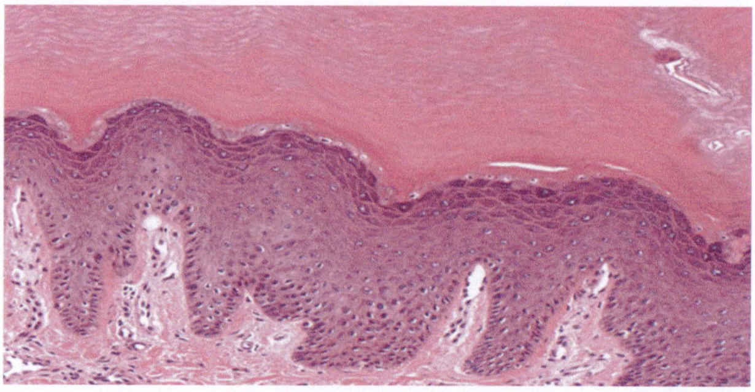

Fig. 11.38 Mild dermal fibrosis and minimal inflammation

Kyrle's Disease

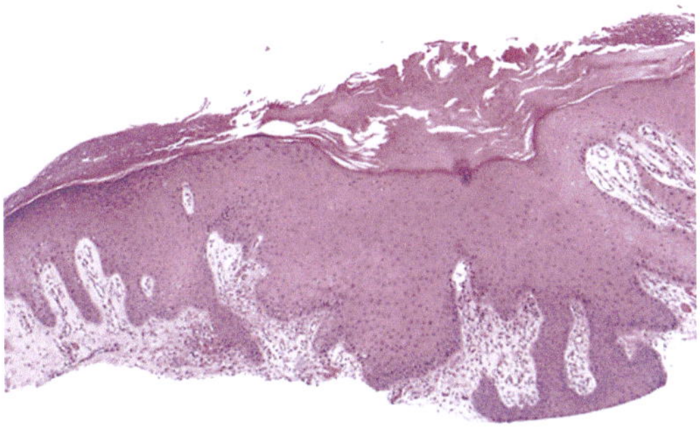

Fig. 11.39 Wide epidermal invagination filled with thick keratin

Synonym: Hyperkeratosis Follicularis et Parafollicularis in Cutem Penetrans

Histopathology (Figs. 11.39, 11.40, 11.41, 11.42, and 11.43)

- Epidermal invagination with wide plug filled with laminated keratin
- Parakeratosis in the deep part of the plug
- Plug can contain cellular debris and neutrophils but collagen and elastic fiber stains are negative in the crater

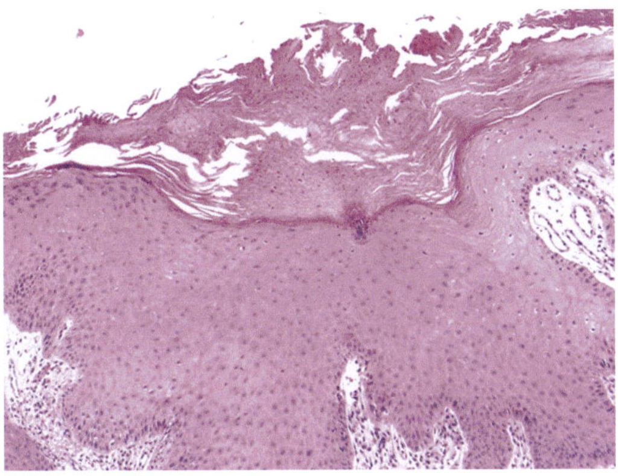

Fig. 11.40 Laminated keratin fill wide, shallow invagination

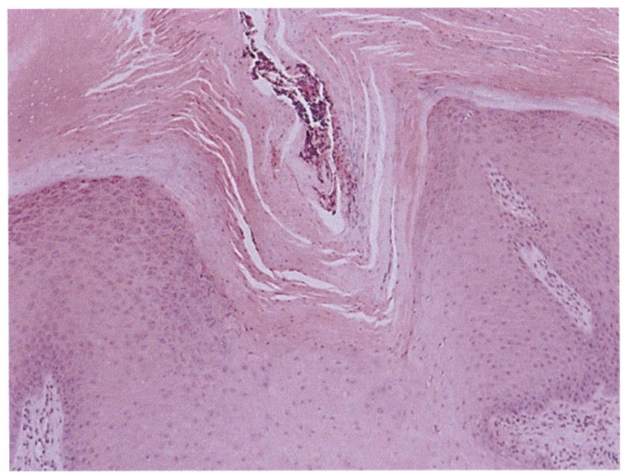

Fig. 11.41 No evidence of collagen or elastic fibers within the plug

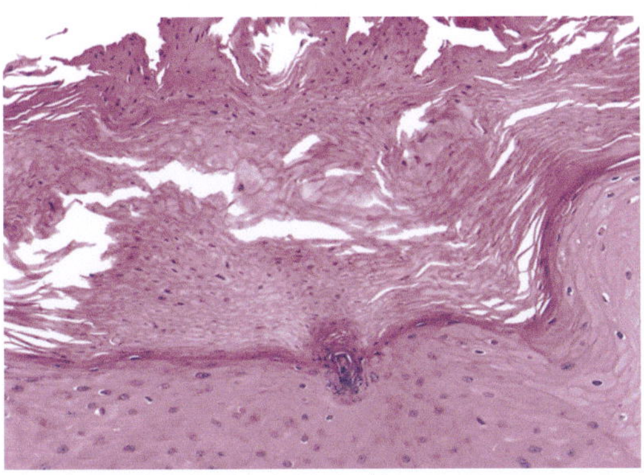

Fig. 11.42 Parakeratosis is present in the lower portion of the plug

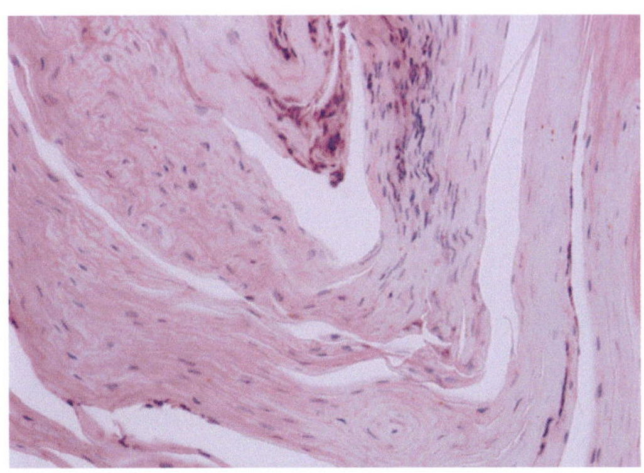

Fig. 11.43 Neutrophils and debris is present in the plug

12 Dermatopathology L

V. Vincek, *Dermatopathology A–Z*, https://doi.org/10.1007/978-3-319-89486-7_12

Langerhans Cell Histiocytosis

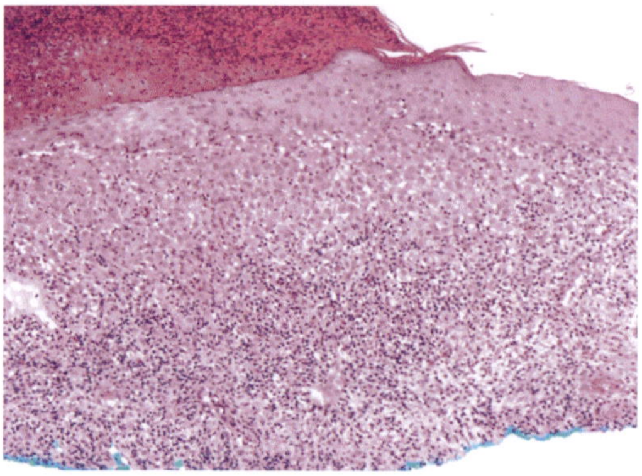

Fig. 12.1 Extensive dermal inflammation

Histopathology (Figs. 12.1, 12.2, 12.3, and 12.4)

- Dermal infiltrate of large histiocytic cells, with eosinophilic cytoplasm, demonstrating common epidermal invasion
- Some histiocytes have grooved nuclei and mitoses can be seen
- Lymphocytes and occasional eosinophils are admixed
- Giant cells can be present
- Tumor cells are S100+, CD1a+, CD207+

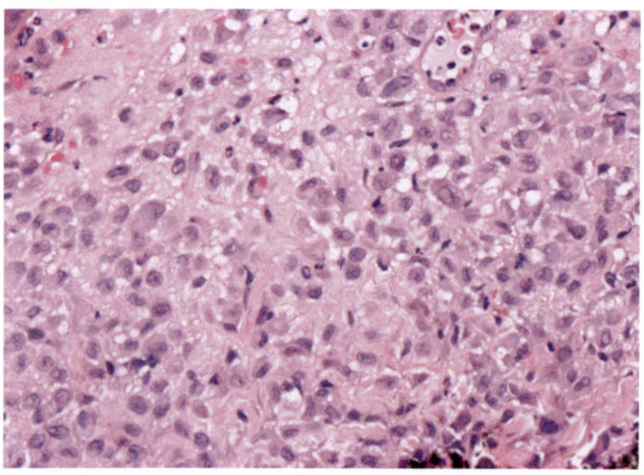

Fig. 12.2 Large histiocytes admixed with inflammatory cells

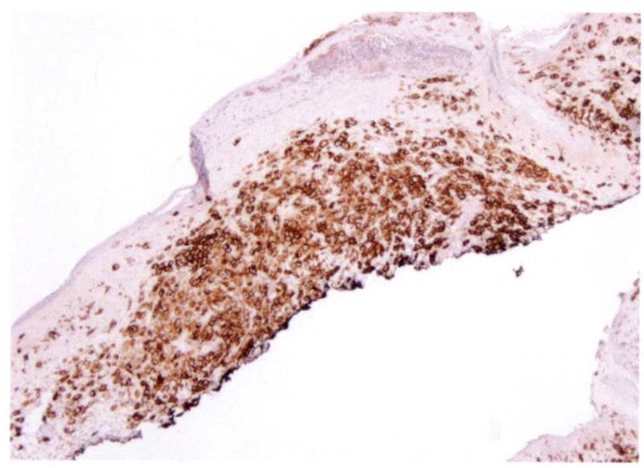

Fig. 12.3 Tumor cells are CD1a positive (brown)

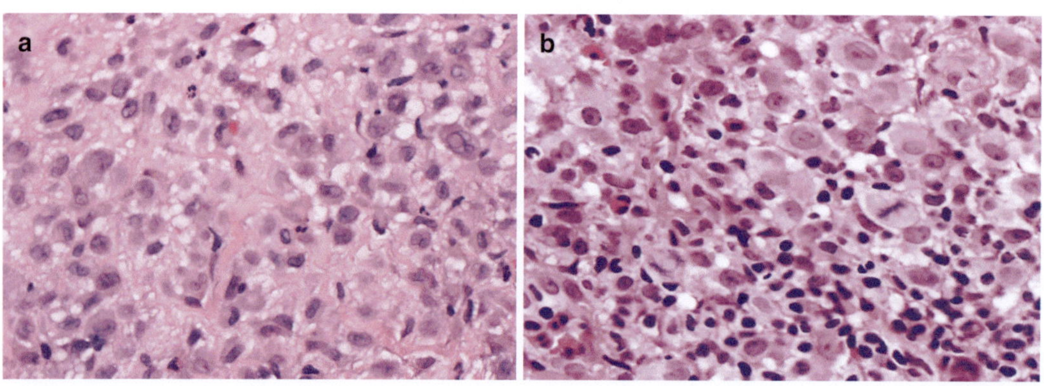

Fig. 12.4 (**a**, **b**) Large pale histiocytes, some with bean shaped nuclei, admixed with lymphocytes and eosinophils; mitosis can be seen

Large Cell Acanthoma

Histopathology (Figs. 12.5, 12.6, 12.7, 12.8, and 12.9)

- Epidermal hyperkeratosis
- Keratinocytes are enlarged with prominent nucleoli but not atypical
- The lesion is sharply demarcated from normal epidermis
- There is mild basal layer hyperpigmentation
- Epidermis can be flat or show bulbous rete

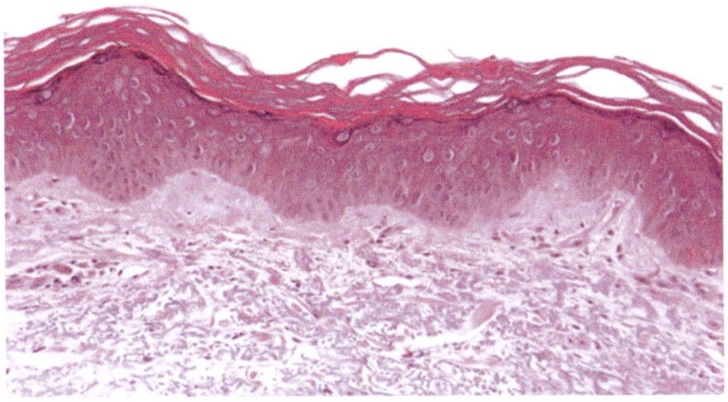

Fig. 12.5 Hypertrophic epidermis with prominent keratinocytes

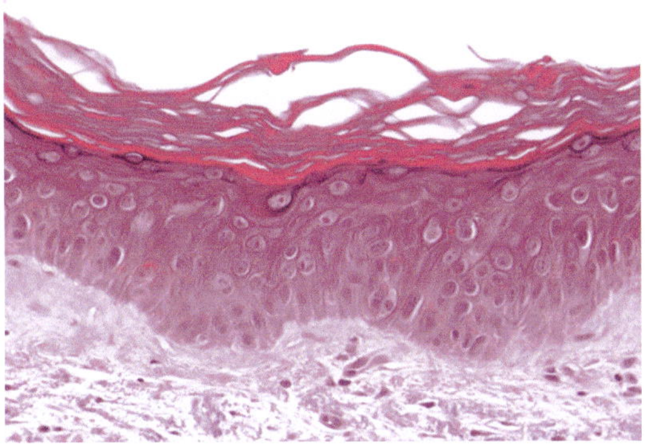

Fig. 12.6 Hyperkeratotic flat epidermis with granular layer

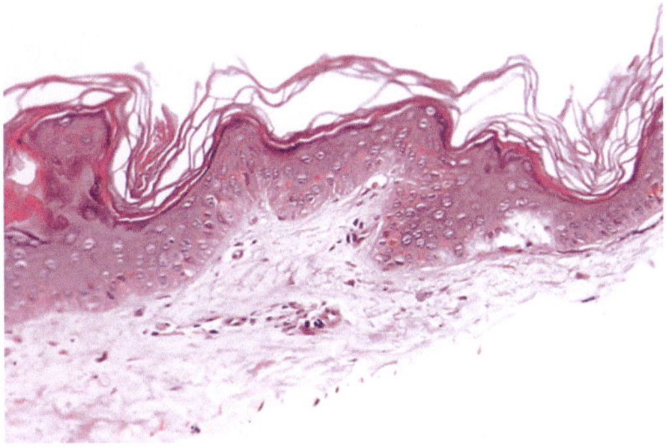

Fig. 12.7 Hyperkeratotic epidermis with bulbous rete ridges

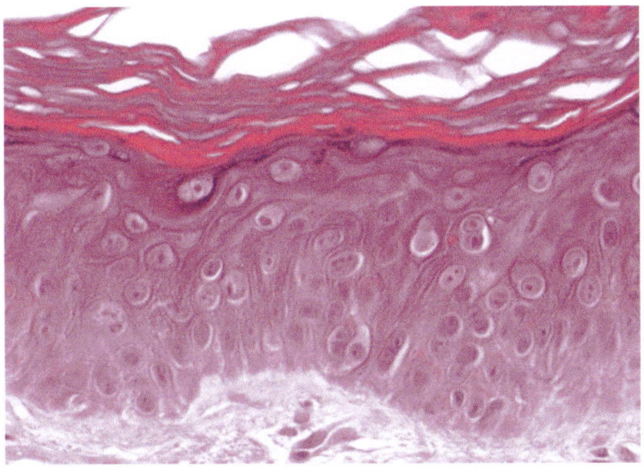

Fig. 12.8 Enlarged keratinocytes with prominent nucleoli

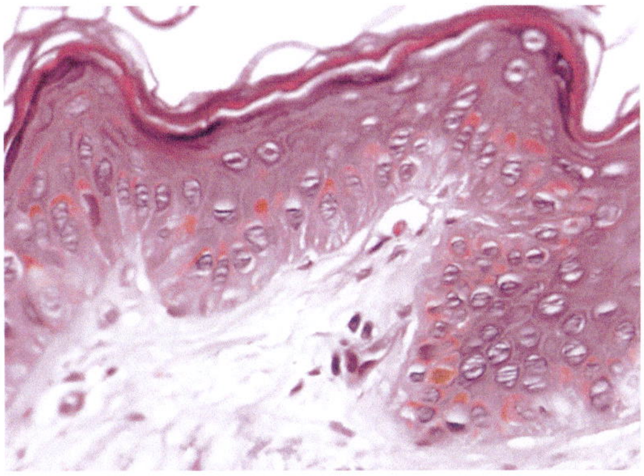

Fig. 12.9 Keratinocytes are enlarged and hyperpigmented

Larva Migrans

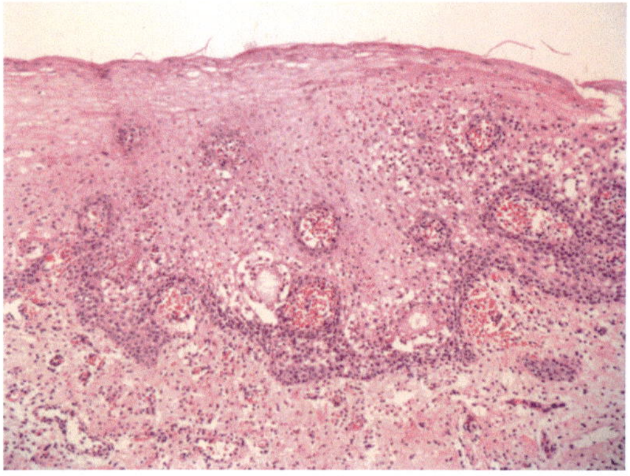

Fig. 12.10 A case of larva migrans affecting oral mucosa

Synonym: Creeping Eruption

Histopathology (Figs. 12.10, 12.11, and 12.12)

- *Ancylostoma braziliense* is the most common cause
- Larvae forms tunnel usually at the epidermo-dermal junction but can also be higher in the epidermis
- Epidermis around the tunnel is spongiotic
- Epidermal and dermal inflammation made of neutrophils and eosinophils

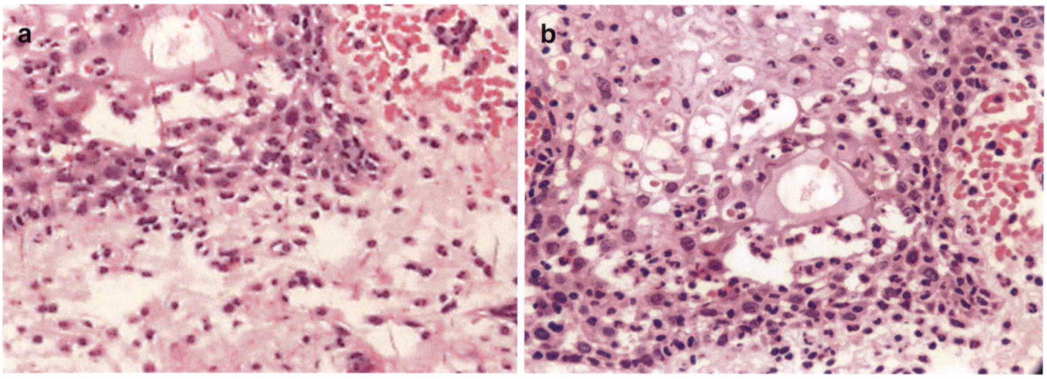

Fig. 12.11 (**a**, **b**) Epidermal spongiosis with epidermal and submucosal neutrophils and eosinophils

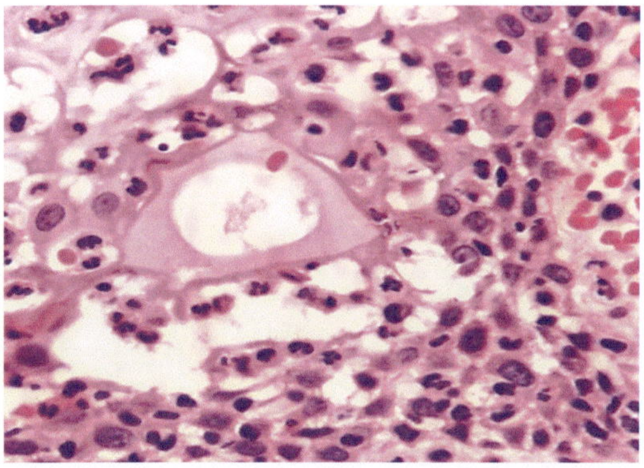

Fig. 12.12 Intraepidermal larva with eosinophilic cuticle

Leiomyoma

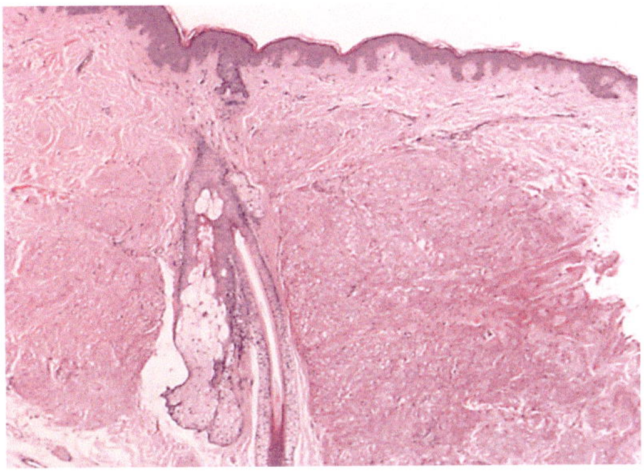

Fig. 12.13 Ill-defined tumor surrounds the hair follicle

Synonym: Pilar Leiomyoma

Histopathology (Figs. 12.13, 12.14, 12.15, and 12.16)

- Ill-defined lesion consisting of interlacing fascicles
- Tumor arises from pilar muscle and therefore tends to surround hair follicle
- Made of well differentiated smooth muscle spindle cells (SMA+, caldesmon+) with no mitoses
- Cells have eosinophilic cytoplasm and oval blunt-ended nuclei ("Cuban cigar" shaped)

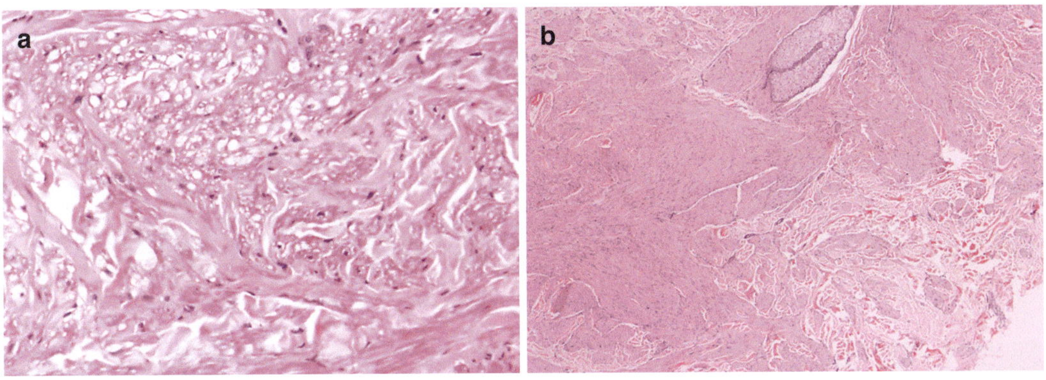

Fig. 12.14 (**a**, **b**) Fascicles of eosinophilic spindle cells

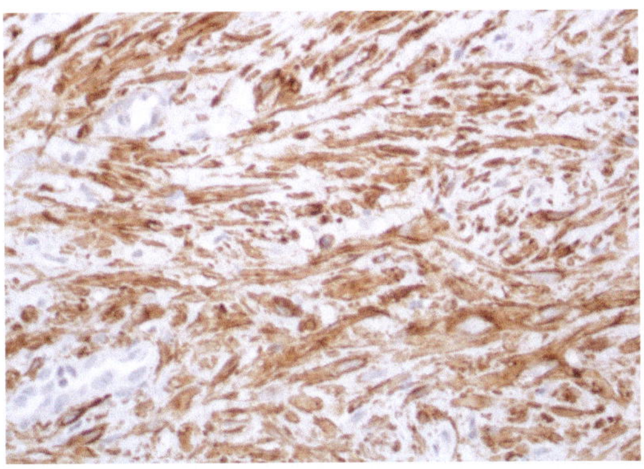

Fig. 12.15 Caldesmon stain confirms muscle origin

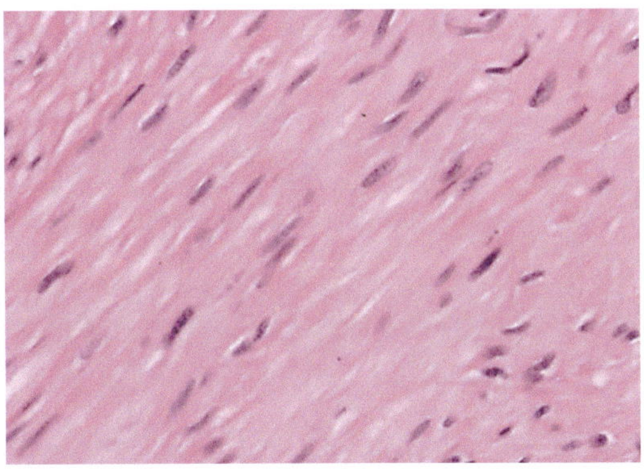

Fig. 12.16 Cells have elongated blunt-ended nuclei

Leiomyosarcoma

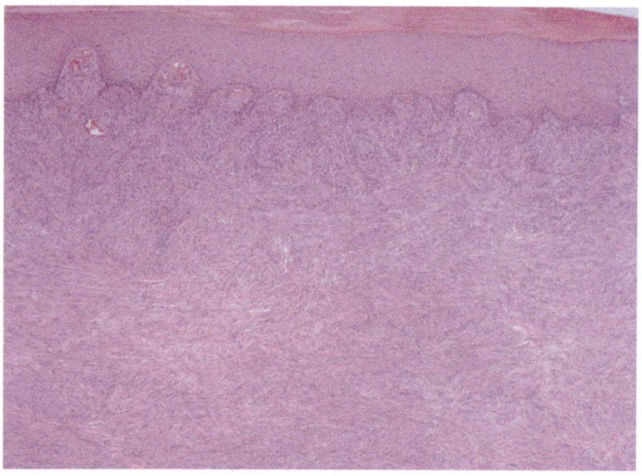

Fig. 12.17 Ill-defined spindle cell tumor

Histopathology (Figs. 12.17, 12.18, 12.19, 12.20, and 12.21)

- Ill-defined spindle cell lesion
- Spindle cells with eosinophilic cytoplasm and oval, "cigar-shaped" nuclei (SMA+, desmin+, caldesmon+)
- Cells form interlacing fascicles
- Nuclear polymorphism is seen
- Mitoses are present (2 or more per 10 hpf)
- Necrosis variably present

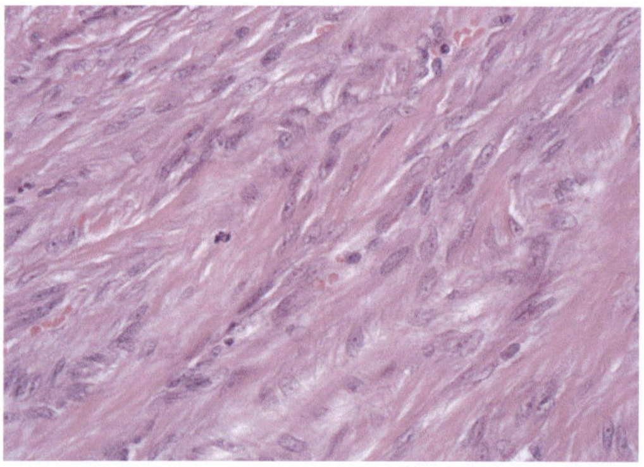

Fig. 12.18 Spindle cells with eosinophilic cytoplasm and atypia

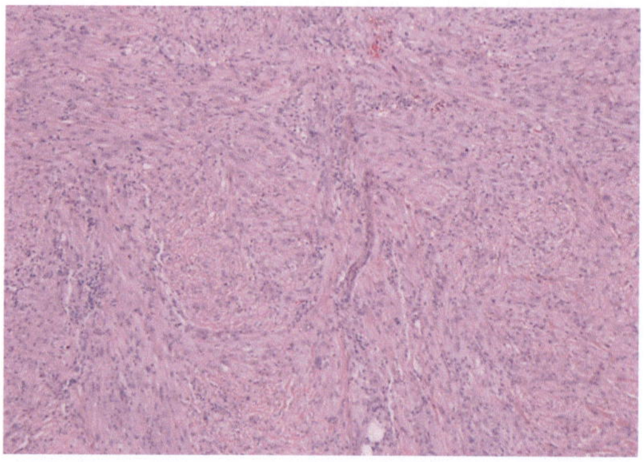

Fig. 12.19 Cells form interlacing poorly defined fascicles

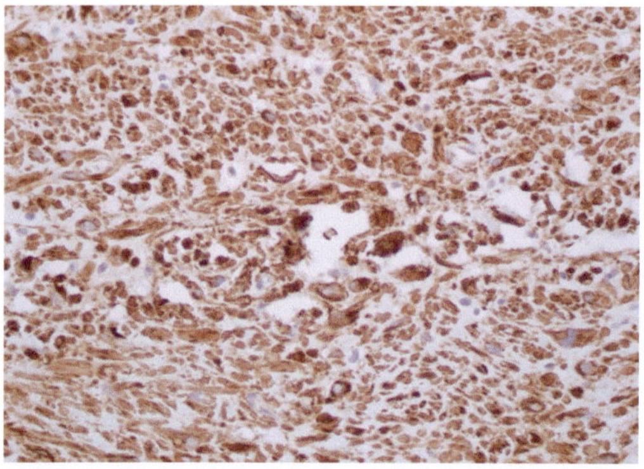

Fig. 12.20 Caldesmon stain confirms smooth muscle origin

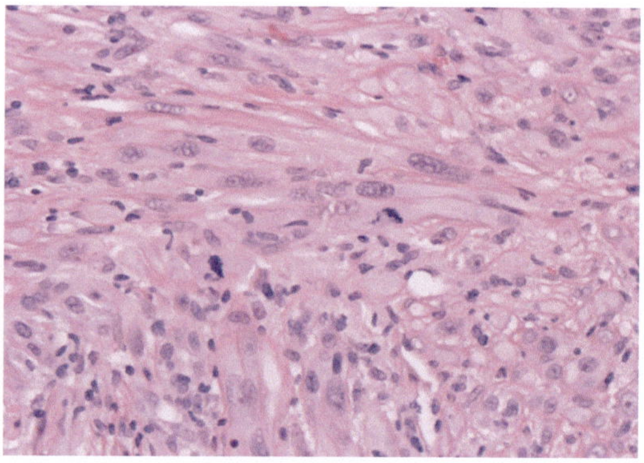

Fig. 12.21 Multiple mitoses are present

Leishmaniasis

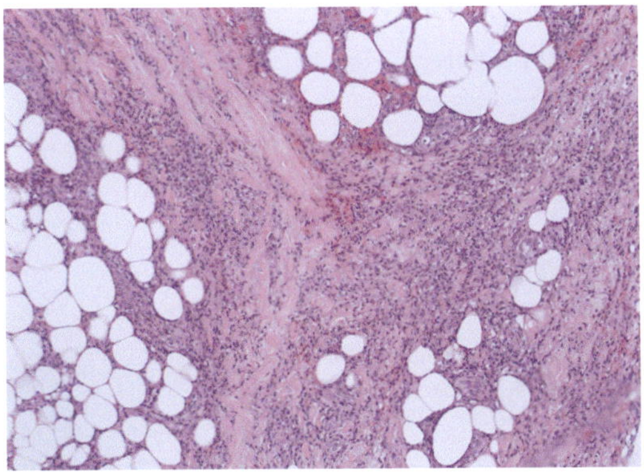

Fig. 12.22 Diffuse subcutaneous inflammation

Histopathology (Figs. 12.22, 12.23, 12.24, 12.25, and 12.26)

- Epidermis is frequently ulcerated
- Dermal and subcutaneous lymphohistiocytic infiltrate
- Some neutrophils, eosinophils, and plasma cells can be present
- Round to oval amastigotes are present in the histiocytes
- Giemsa stain is preferred special stain

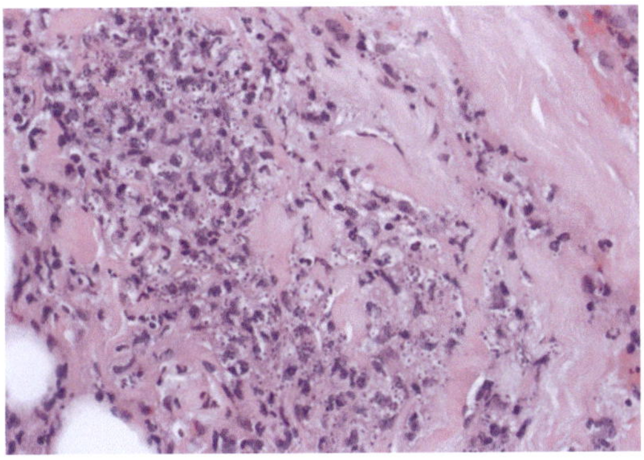

Fig. 12.23 Lymphohistiocytic infiltrate with RBCs extravasation

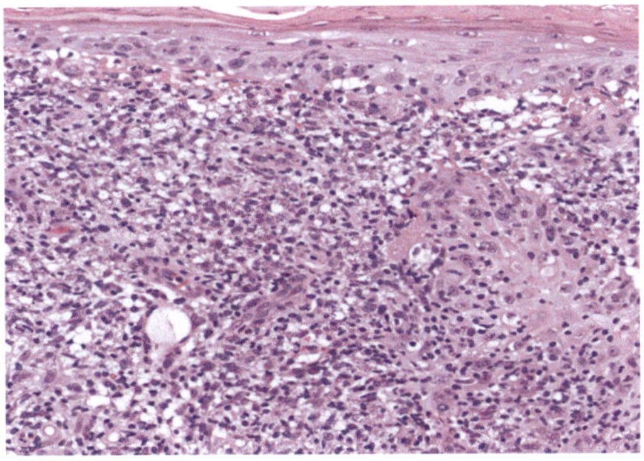

Fig. 12.24 Diffuse dermal infiltrate of histiocytes

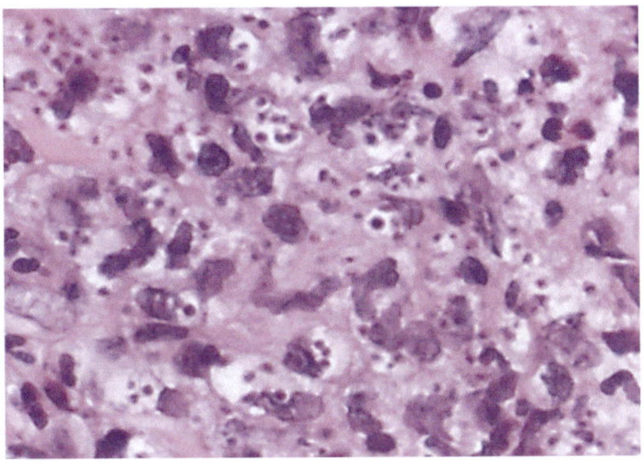

Fig. 12.25 Round to oval amastigotes within the histiocytes

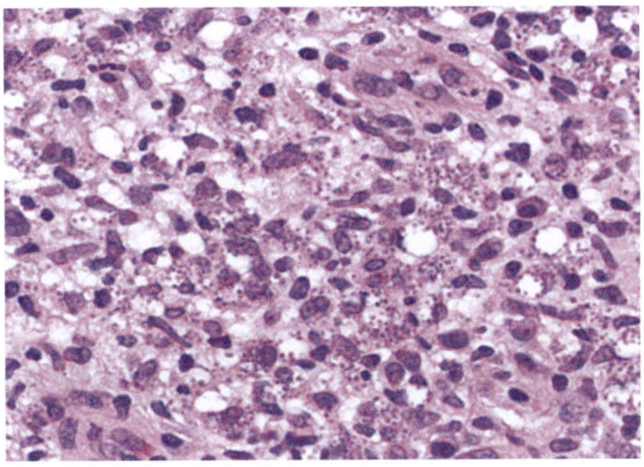

Fig. 12.26 Histiocytes with amastigotes in granular dust-like cytoplasm

Lentigo Simplex

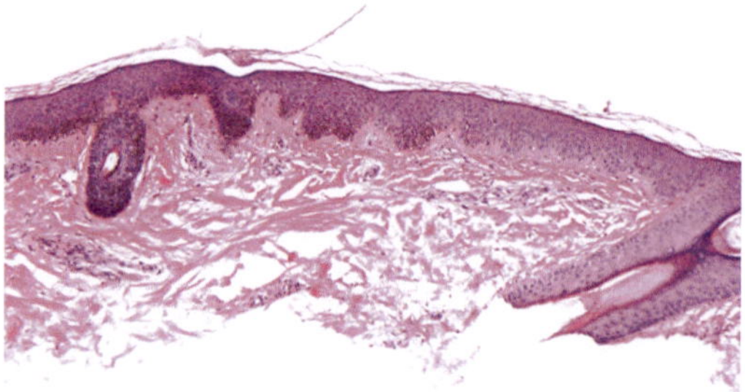

Fig. 12.27 Epidermal acanthosis with prominent pigmented rete ridges

Histopathology (Figs. 12.27, 12.28, 12.29, and 12.30)

- Epidermal acanthosis with elongation of rete ridges
- Increased pigmentation of the tips of epidermal retes
- Number of melanocytes is increased
- Dermal pigment incontinence but no significant solar elastosis

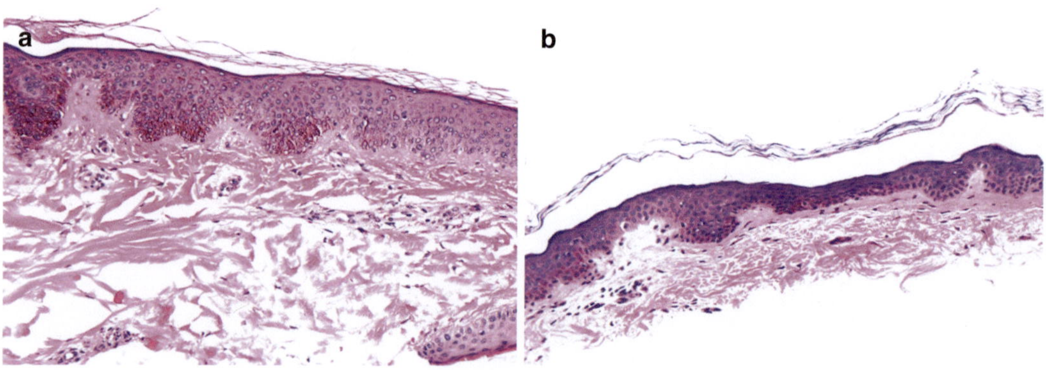

Fig. 12.28 (**a**, **b**) Elongation of pigmented rete ridges and no significant dermal solar elastosis

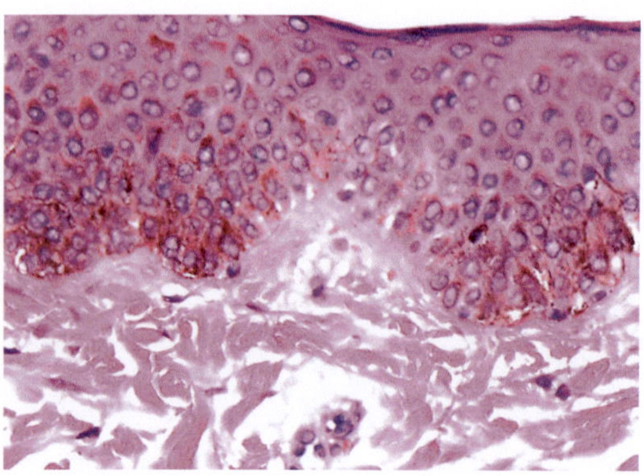

Fig. 12.29 Number of pigmented melanocytes is mildly increased

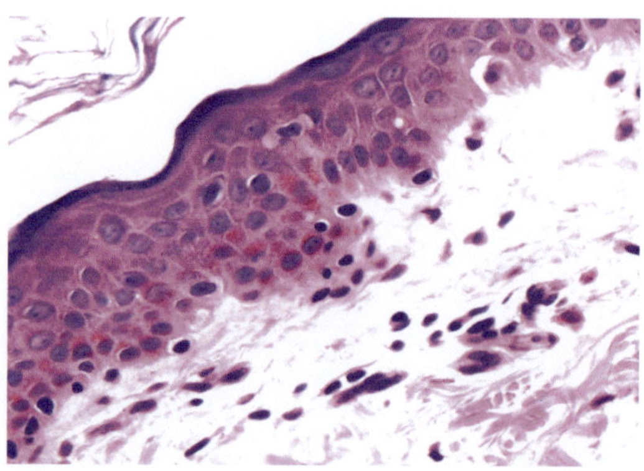

Fig. 12.30 Mild dermal inflammation

Leukemia Cutis

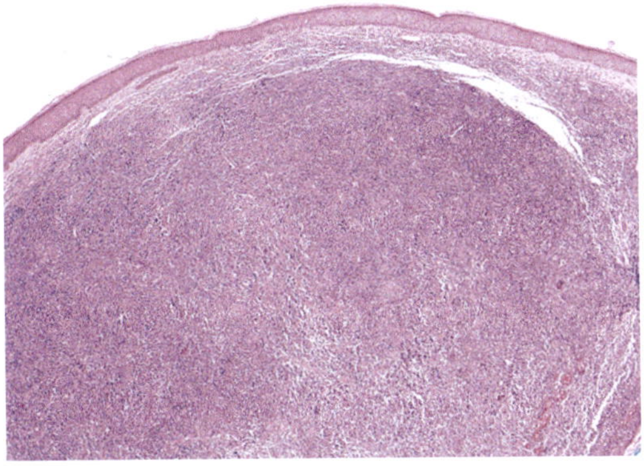

Fig. 12.31 Diffuse infiltrate with complete absence of adnexal structures

Synonym: Chloroma

Histopathology (Figs. 12.31, 12.32, 12.33, and 12.34)

- Diffuse skin infiltration by leukemic cells
- Most commonly acute myelomonocytic leukemia (AML-M4) and acute monocytic leukemia (AML-M5)
- Immunophenotype of cells depends on the type of leukemia
- Myeloperoxidase stain is usually positive

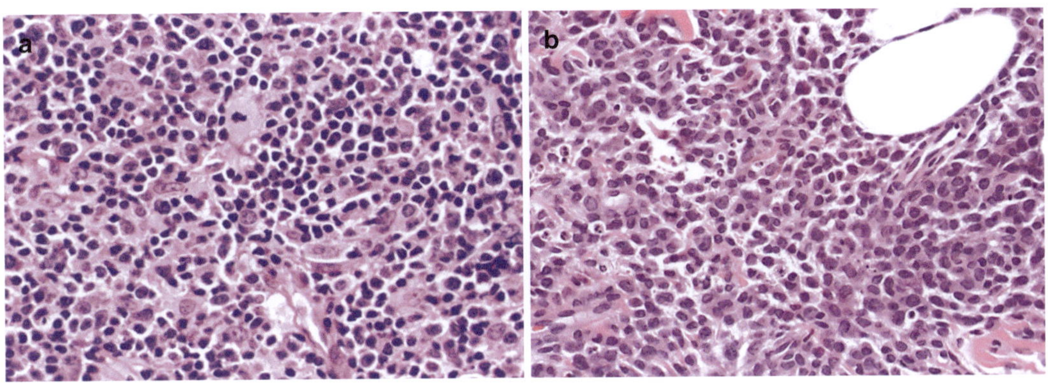

Fig. 12.32 (**a**, **b**) Sheet of atypical cells

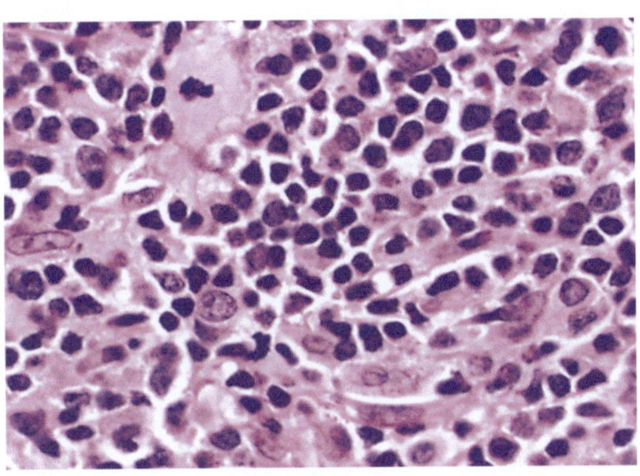

Fig. 12.33 Cells with irregular nuclei and scattered, very large, atypical cells

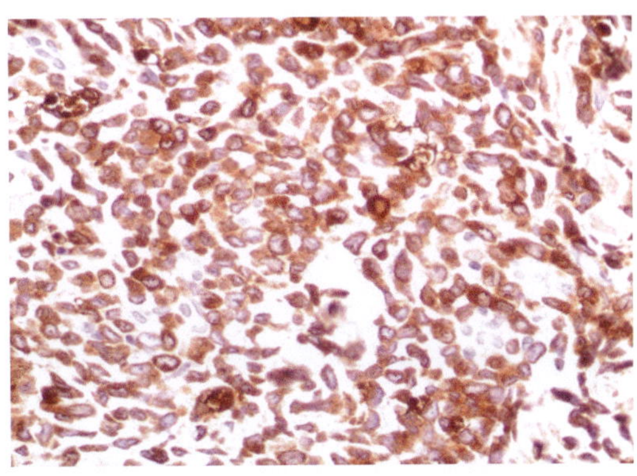

Fig. 12.34 Myeloperoxidase stain is positive

Leukocytoclastic Vasculitis

Histopathology (Figs. 12.35 and 12.36)
- Intra and perivascular neutrophilic infiltrate with neutrophilic degeneration (leukocytoclasia)
- Damaged capillaries with reactive endothelial cells, fibrin deposition, and microthrombi
- Dermal red blood cell extravasation

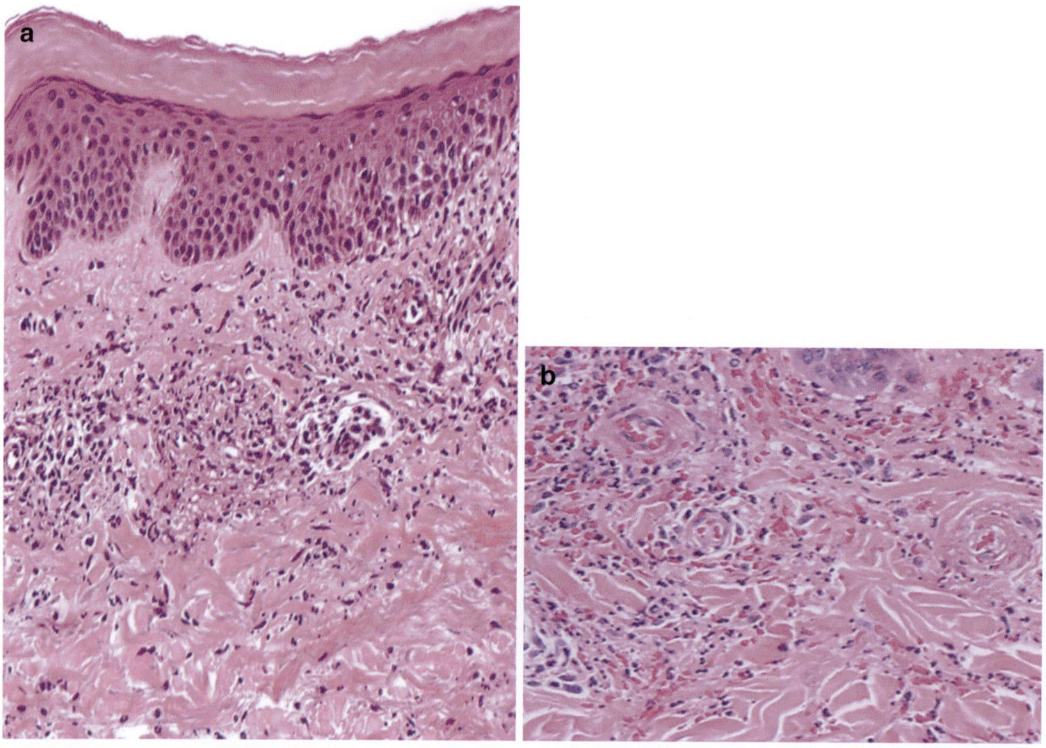

Fig. 12.35 (**a**, **b**) Dermis with red blood cell extravasation and nuclear dust

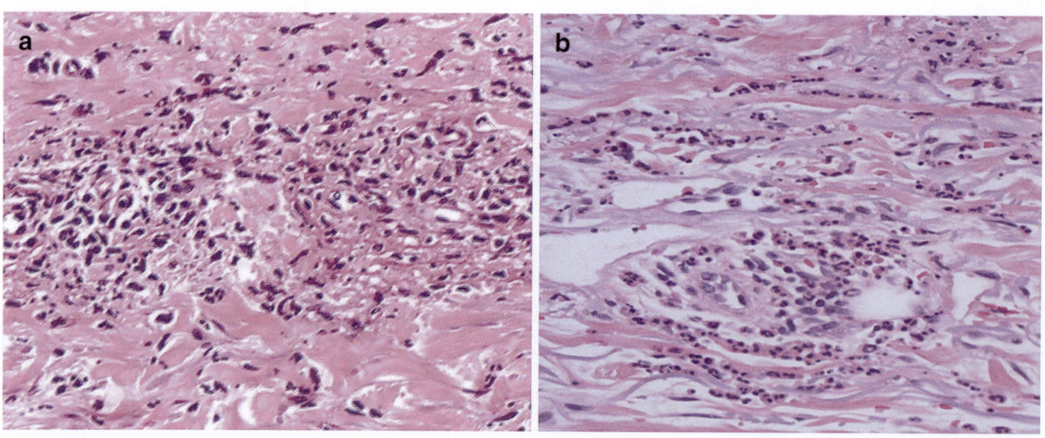

Fig. 12.36 (**a**, **b**) Fragmented intra and perivascular neutrophils with nuclear dust and red blood cell extravasation. Reactive endothelial cells and microthrombi

Leukoedema

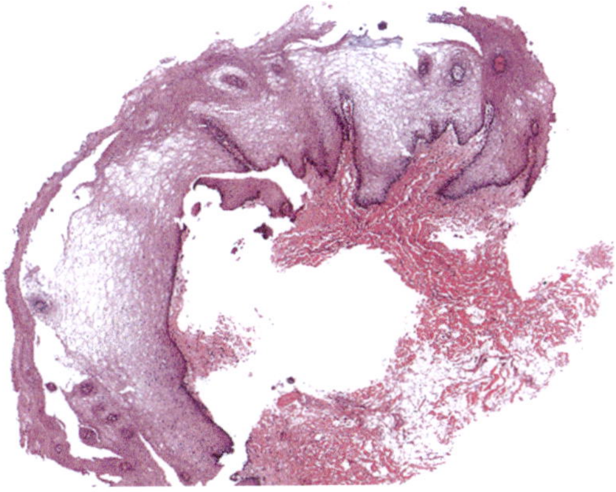

Fig. 12.37 Pale acanthotic squamous mucosa

Histopathology (Figs. 12.37, 12.38, and 12.39)

- Acanthotic squamous mucosa
- No evidence of parakeratosis
- Pale cells in the mid and superficial epidermis
- Characteristic "jigsaw-like" pattern of cell membranes

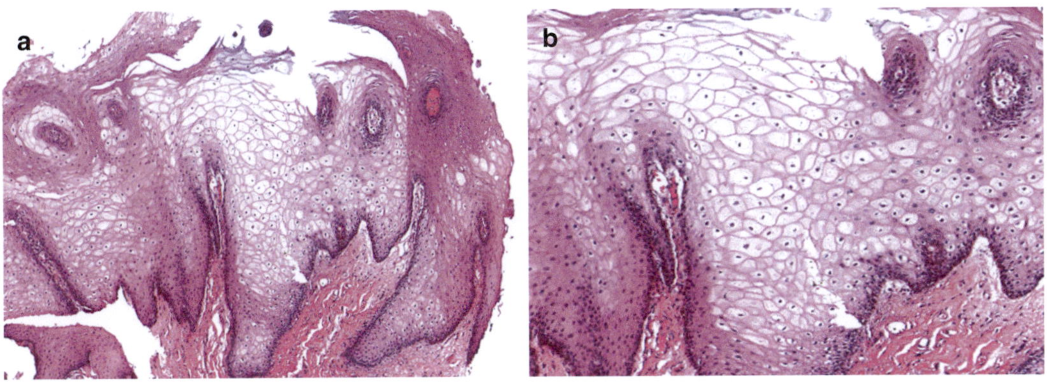

Fig. 12.38 (**a**, **b**) Ballooned cells in the middle and upper portion of the epidermis with no evidence of parakeratosis

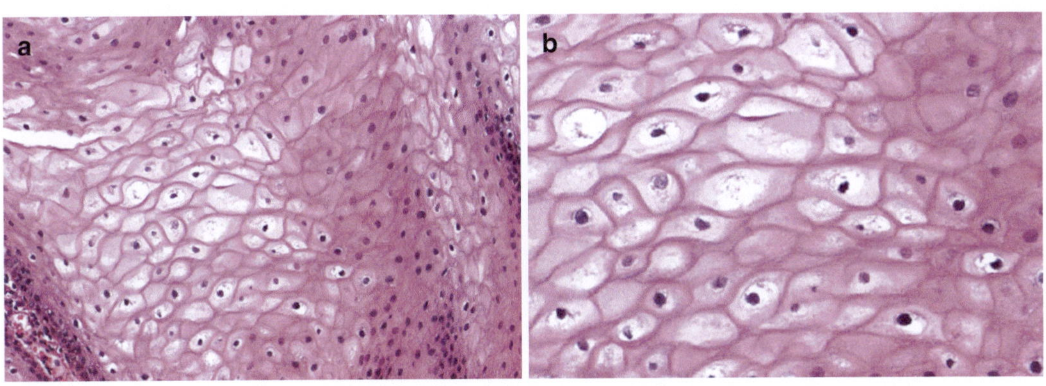

Fig. 12.39 (**a**, **b**) Cells with pale cytoplasm and "jigsaw-like" pattern of cellular membranes

Leukoplakia

Leukoplakia is clinical and not a histological designation.

Histopathology is not specific (Figs. 12.40, 12.41, and 12.42)
- Acanthotic squamous mucosa with mild parakeratosis and papillomatosis
- No cytological atypia

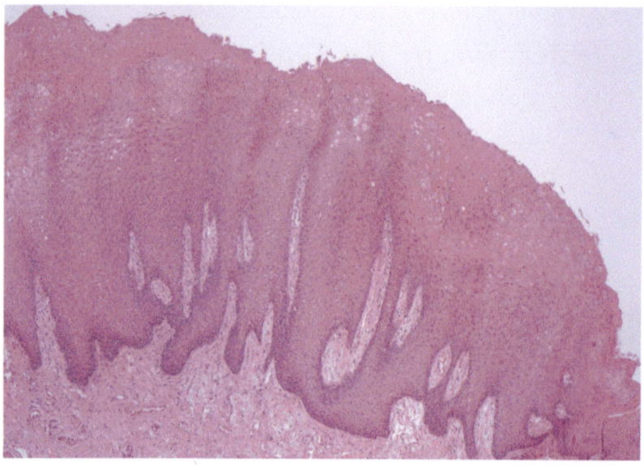

Fig. 12.40 Thickened irregular mucosal epithelium

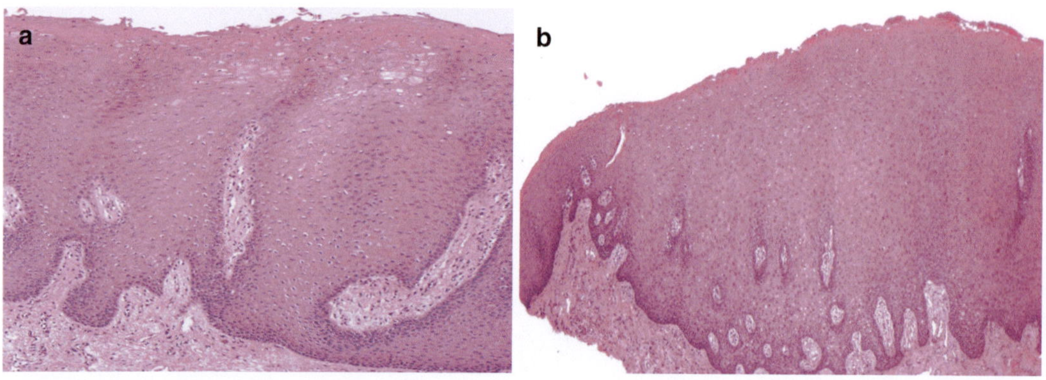

Fig. 12.41 (**a**, **b**) Irregular epidermal papillomatosis

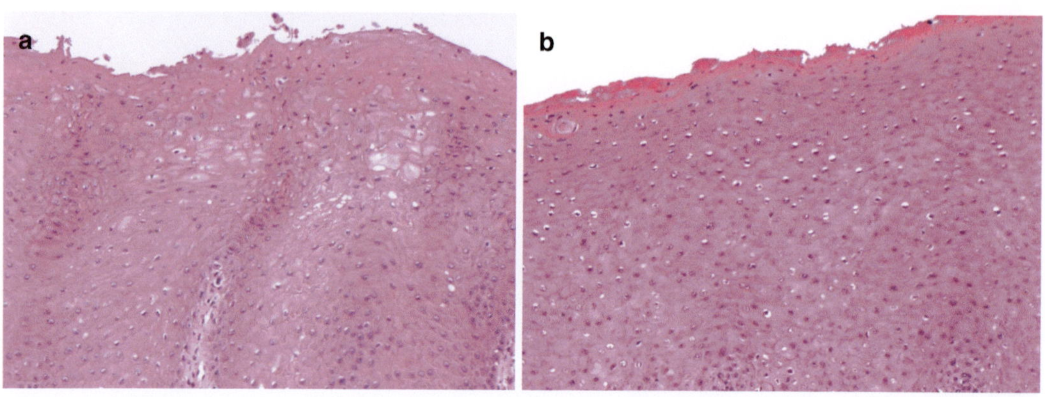

Fig. 12.42 (**a**, **b**) Mild parakeratosis and no cytological atypia

Leprosy-Lepromatous

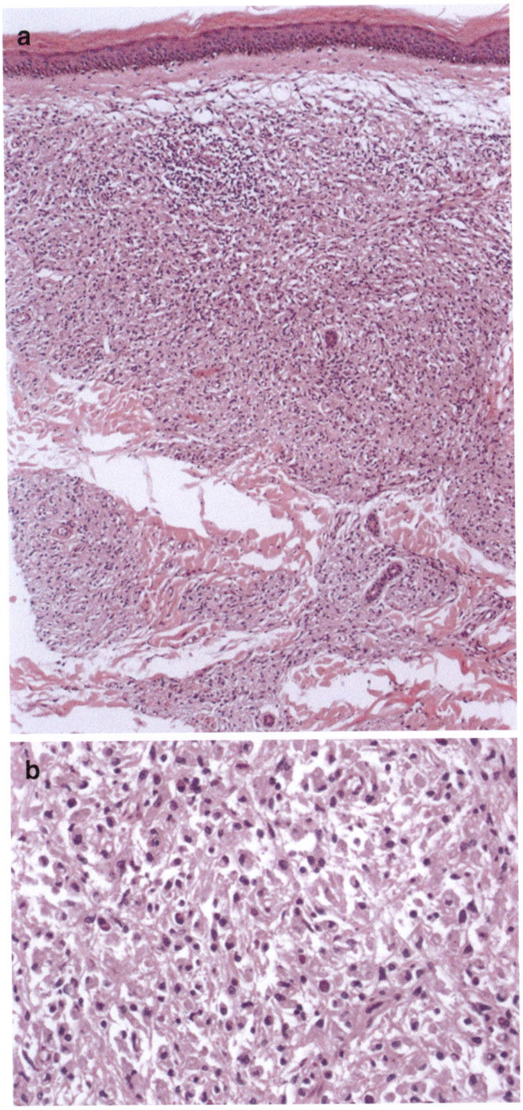

Fig. 12.43 (a, b) Sheath of foamy histiocytes consume the dermis and subcutis with giant cells absent

Synonym: Hansen's Disease

Histopathology

- Diffuse dermal infiltrate of foamy macrophages (Figs. 12.43 and 12.44)
- Adnexal structures are absent
- Numerous mycobacteria detected by Fite Faraco stain (Figs. 12.45)

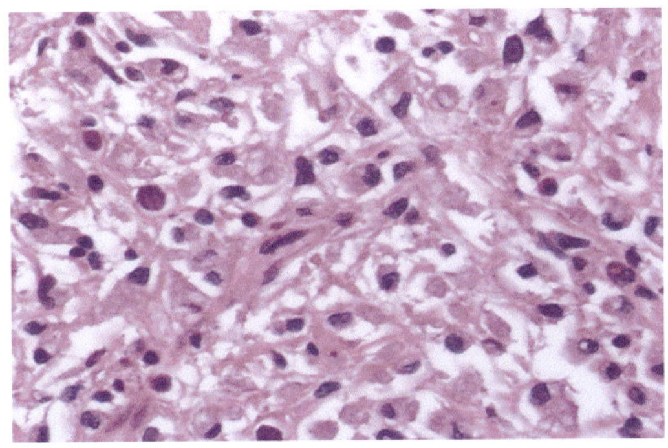

Fig. 12.44 Histiocytes with pink dusty cytoplasm

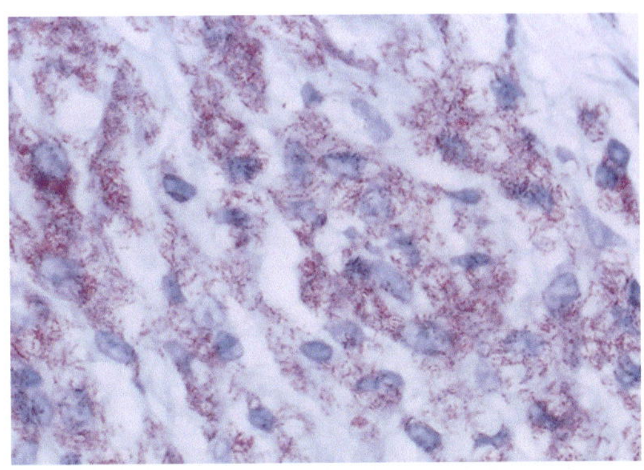

Fig. 12.45 Numerous mycobacteria stained with Fite Faraco stain

Leprosy-Tuberculoid

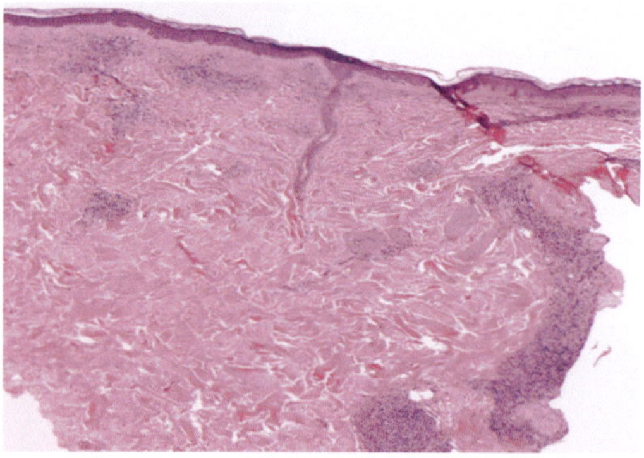

Fig. 12.46 Dermal perivascular and periadnexal inflammation

Histopathology (Figs. 12.46, 12.47, 12.48, and 12.49)

- Dermal perivascular and periadnexal histiocytic and lymphocytic aggregates
- Vague non-caseating granulomas with giant cells adjacent to vessels and nerves
- Fite Faraco stain is negative in most of the cases; positive cases demonstrate few mycobacteria unlike in the cases of lepromatous leprosy

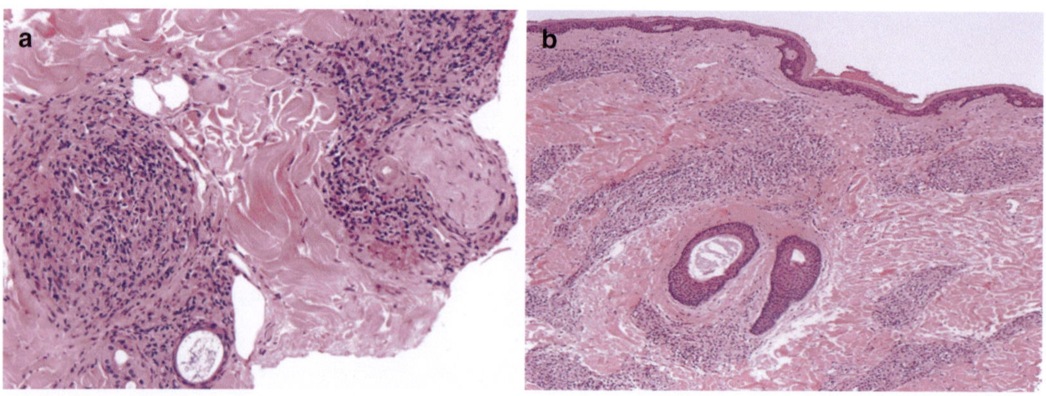

Fig. 12.47 (**a**, **b**) Dermal perivascular and periadnexal lymphocytic and histiocytic aggregates

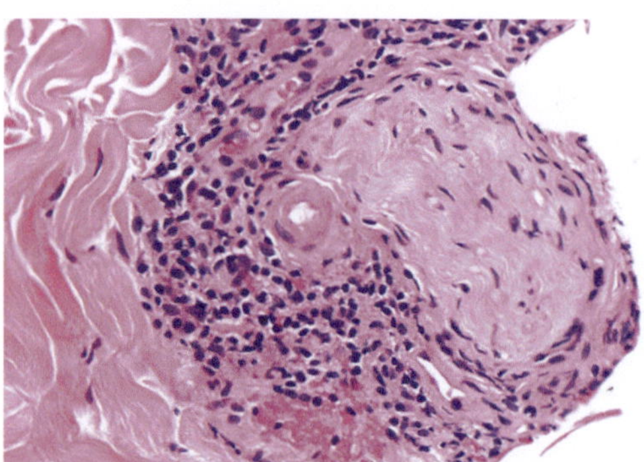

Fig. 12.48 Perineural lymphocytes and histiocytes

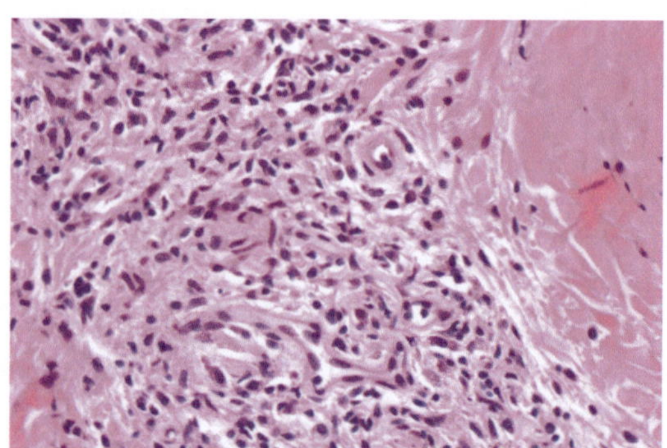

Fig. 12.49 Vague non-caseating granuloma with giant cell

Lichen Aureus

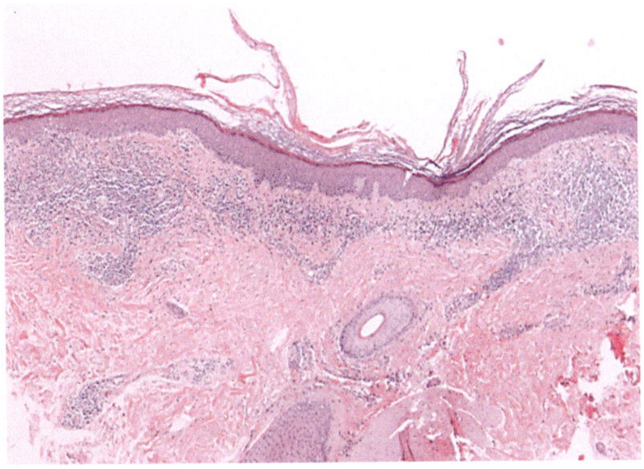

Fig. 12.50 Lichenoid dermal infiltrate

Synonym: Lichen Purpuricus

Histopathology (Figs. 12.50, 12.51, and 12.52)

- Lichenoid band-like lymphocytic infiltrate
- Grenz zone is present and epidermis is normal
- Dermal red blood cell extravasation
- Increased number of dermal capillaries
- Dermal hemosiderin is present

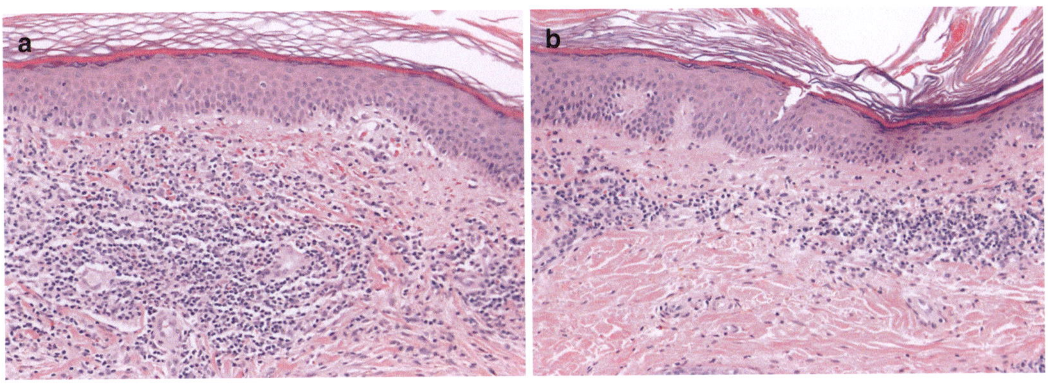

Fig. 12.51 (a, b) Band-like dermal lymphocytic infiltrate with Grenz zone and unremarkable epidermis

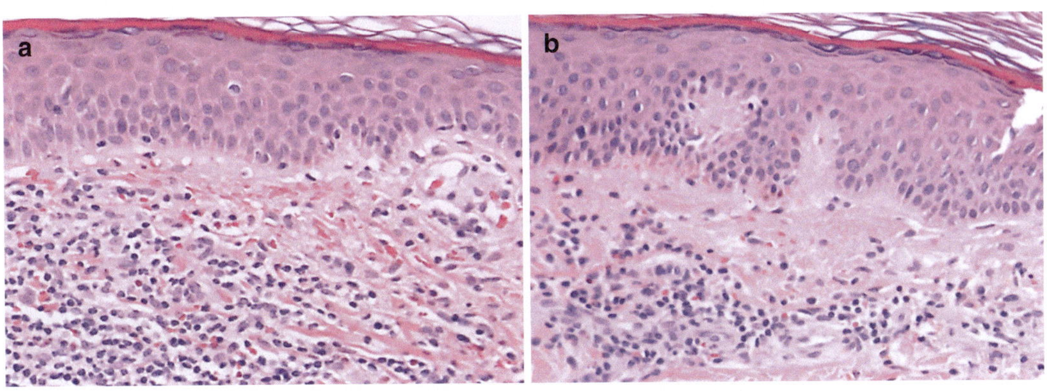

Fig. 12.52 (a, b) Dermal red blood cell extravasation and more prominent dermal capillaries

Lichen Myxedematosus

Disease has localized and generalized form.

Generalized form is known as **scleromyxedema**.

Histopathology (Figs. 12.53 and 12.54)

Early lesion—disorganized collagen with increased number of fibroblasts and easily found mucin separating collagen

Established lesion—increased number of fibroblasts with significant fibrosis

- Mucin is less evident or even absent
- Perivascular lymphocytic inflammation is present

Localized form has several variants including **discrete papular mucinosis, acral persistent papular mucinosis, papular mucinosis of infancy, self-healing papular mucinosis,** and **nodular mucinosis** with similar **histopathology** (Figs. 12.55 and 12.56)

- Papillary shaped lesion
- Resembles focal dermal mucinosis
- Slight proliferation of fibroblasts with mild thickening of collagen
- Amount of mucin is variable

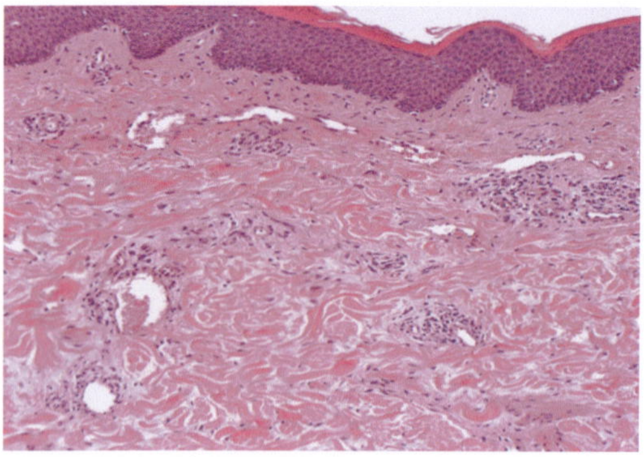

Fig. 12.53 **Scleromyxedema** with fibrosis and suggestion of bluish dermal mucin

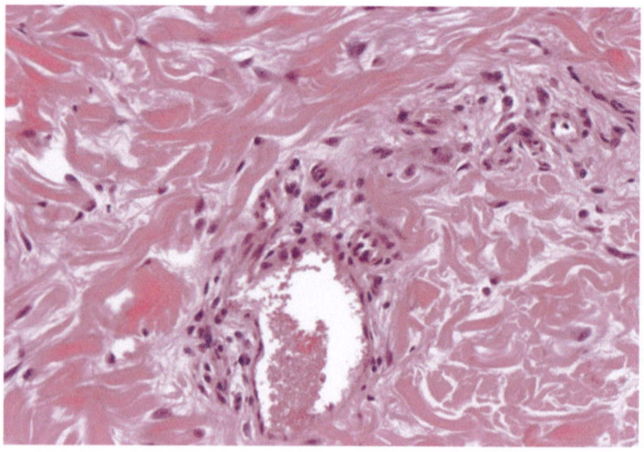

Fig. 12.54 Increased number of fibroblasts with dermal fibrosis and dermal mucin

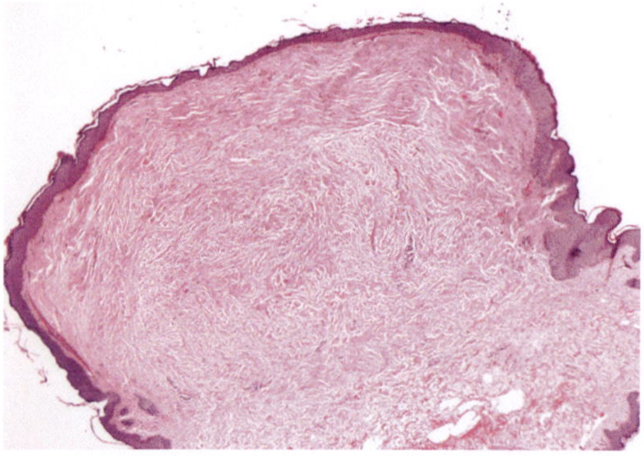

Fig. 12.55 Papillary lesion of **papular mucinosis** with pale dermal stroma

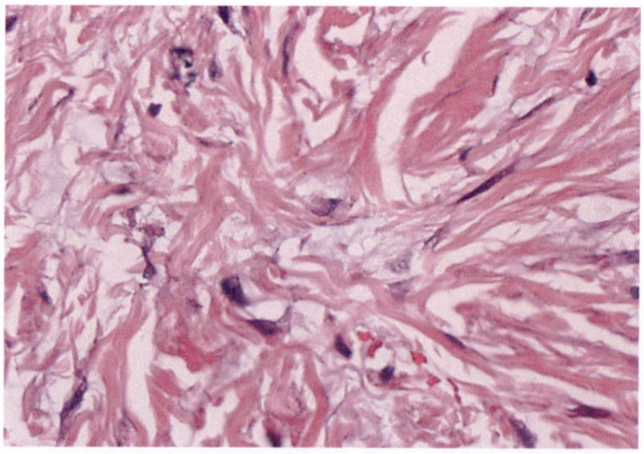

Fig. 12.56 Mild proliferation of fibroblasts among thickened collagen and dermal mucin

Lichen Nitidus

Histopathology (Figs. 12.57, 12.58, and 12.59)

- Thin epidermis with parakeratosis
- Subepidermal well circumscribed infiltrate of lymphocytes and histiocytes
- Epidermal collarettes extend around the lesion
- Giant cell may be present

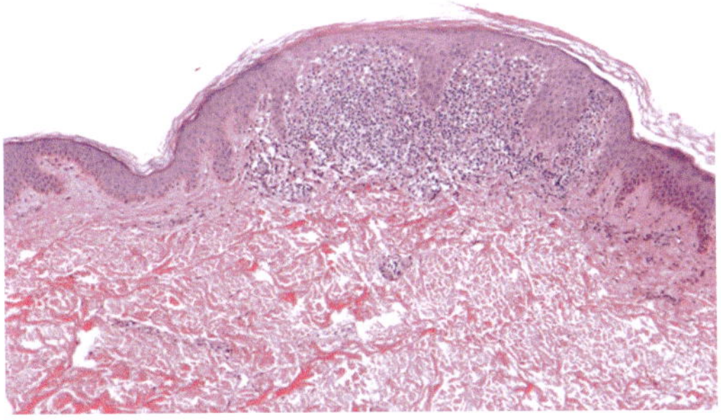

Fig. 12.57 Epidermal collarettes surround the infiltrate

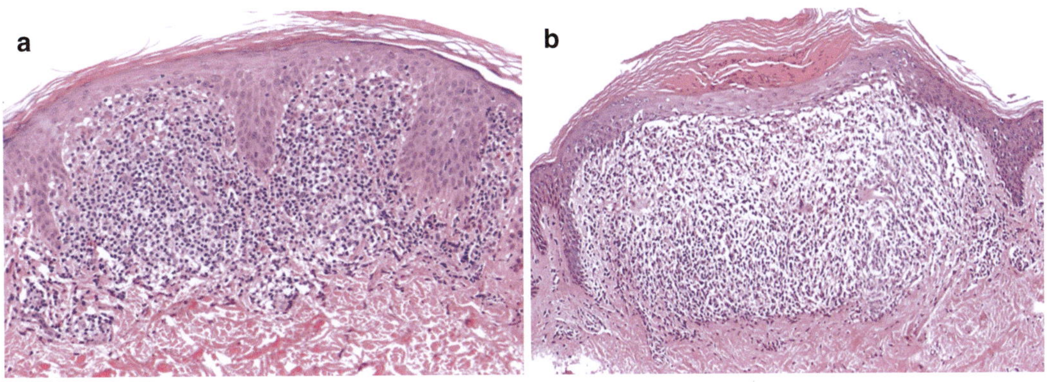

Fig. 12.58 (**a**, **b**) Epidermis is atrophic with parakeratosis

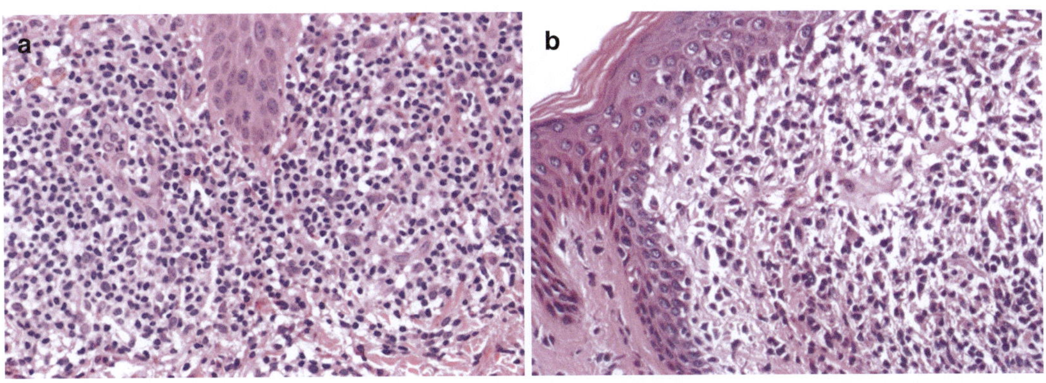

Fig. 12.59 (**a**, **b**) Dermal infiltrate consists of lymphocytes, histiocytes, and occasional giant cells

Lichen Planopilaris

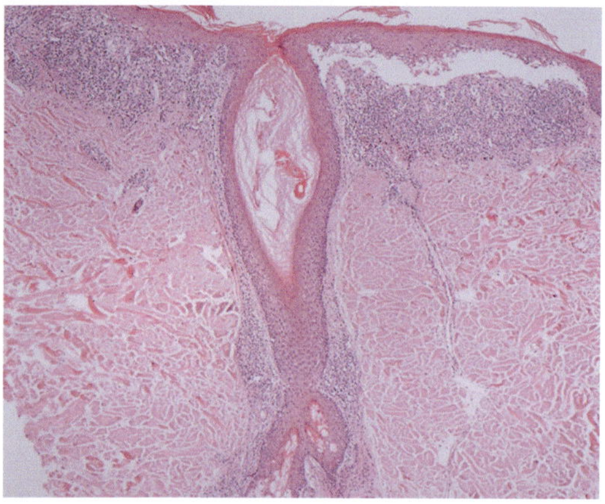

Fig. 12.60 Perifollicular and subepidermal lichenoid infiltrate

Histopathology (Figs. 12.60, 12.61, and 12.62)

- Perifollicular lichenoid lymphocytic infiltrate surrounding upper part of the follicle
- Infiltrate obscure epidermo-dermal junction
- There is no significant perivascular inflammation
- Epidermis between the follicles is involved in one third of cases with features of lichen planus
- If not treated, scarring alopecia develop with perifollicular fibrosis and loss of hair follicle

P.S. **frontal fibrosing alopecia** shows the same features but the epidermis is not involved

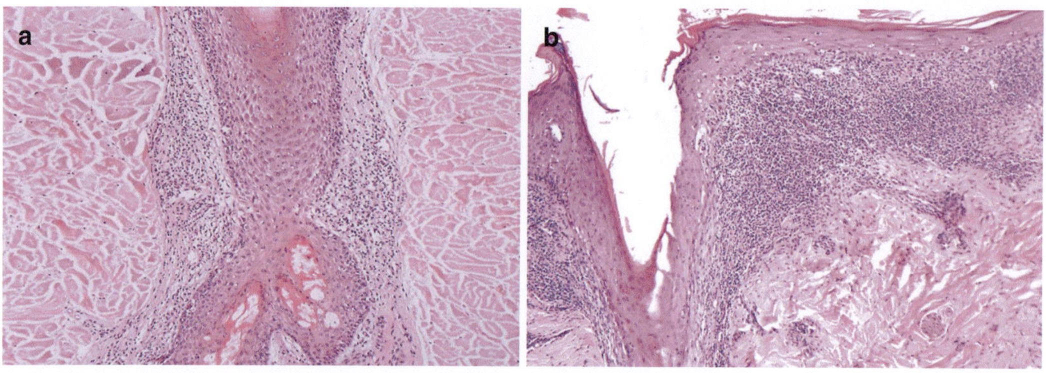

Fig. 12.61 (**a**, **b**) Lymphocytic infiltrate surrounds upper half of the hair follicle

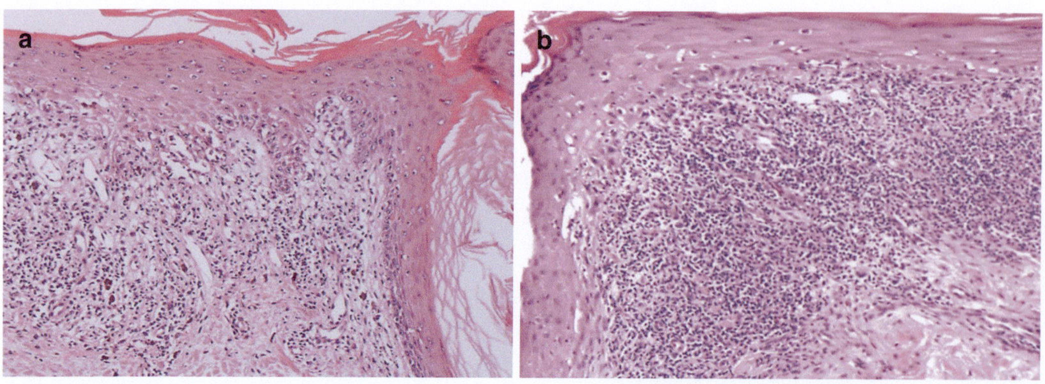

Fig. 12.62 (**a**, **b**) In one third of cases, the interfollicular epidermis shows features of lichen planus

Lichen Planus

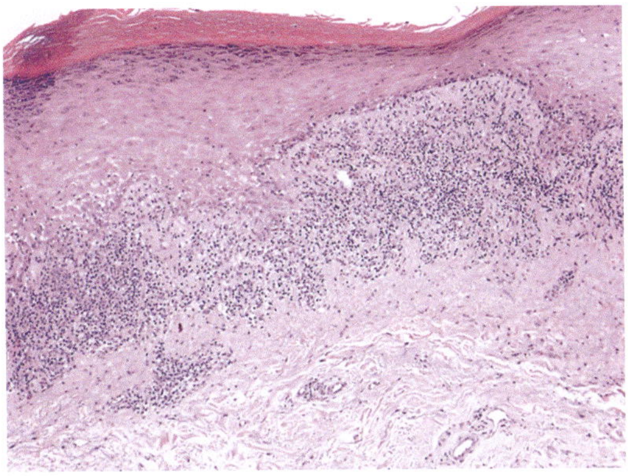

Fig. 12.63 Hypertrophic epidermis with lichenoid dermal infiltrate

Histopathology (Figs. 12.63, 12.64, and 12.65)

- Band-like dermal infiltrate abutting the epidermis with dermal pigment incontinence
- V shaped hypergranulosis with "saw-toothed" epidermal appearance
- Vacuolization of basal layer keratinocytes with some necrotic keratinocytes

Actinic type: same with atrophic epidermis

Hypertrophic type: same with acanthotic epidermis

Bullous type: same with subepidermal blister

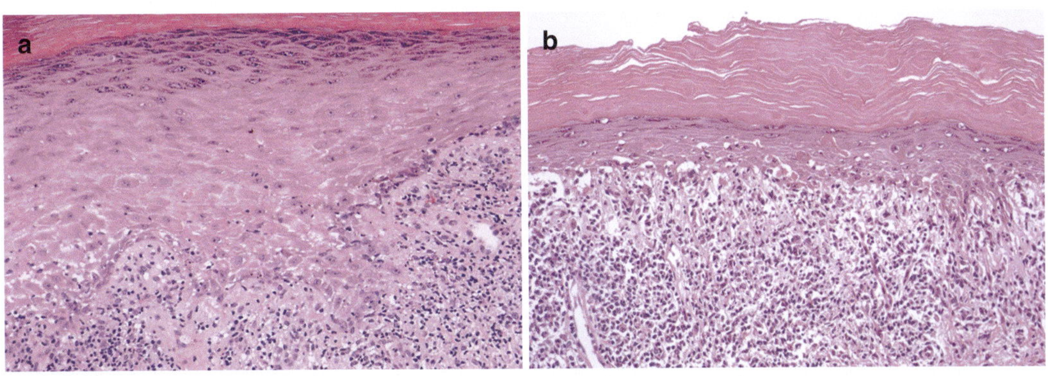

Fig. 12.64 (**a**, **b**) V shaped hypergranulosis with epidermal "saw-toothed" appearance and minimal or no parakeratosis

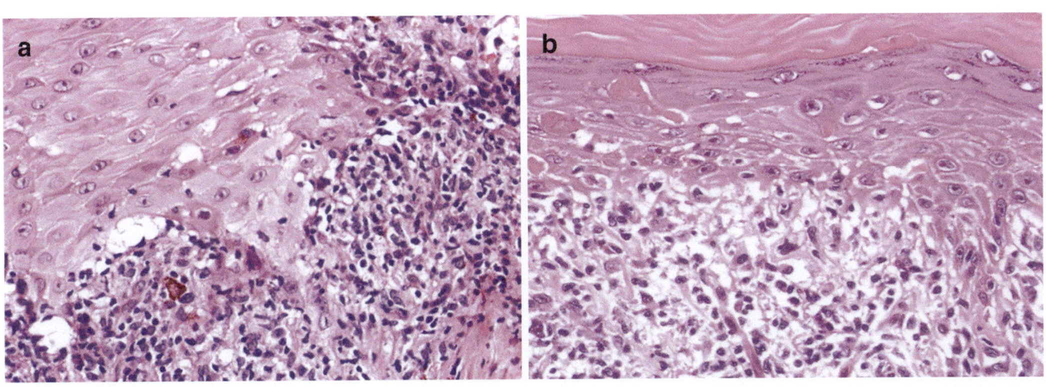

Fig. 12.65 (**a**, **b**) Degeneration of the basal layer with vacuolization and scattered necrosis with dermal pigment incontinence

Lichen Planus-Like Keratosis

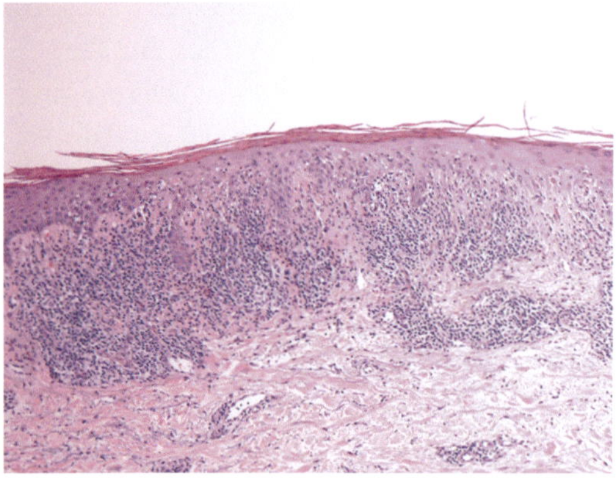

Fig. 12.66 Band like dermal lymphocytic infiltrate

Synonym: Benign Lichenoid Keratosis

Histopathology (Figs. 12.66, 12.67, and 12.68)

- Band-like dermal infiltrate abutting the epidermis with dermal pigment incontinence and adjacent solar lentigo
- Epidermal hypergranulosis and focal parakeratosis
- Vacuolization of basal layer keratinocytes with scattered necrotic keratinocytes

P.S. features are the same as in lichen planus with an additional focal epidermal parakeratosis and adjacent solar lentigo in LPLK

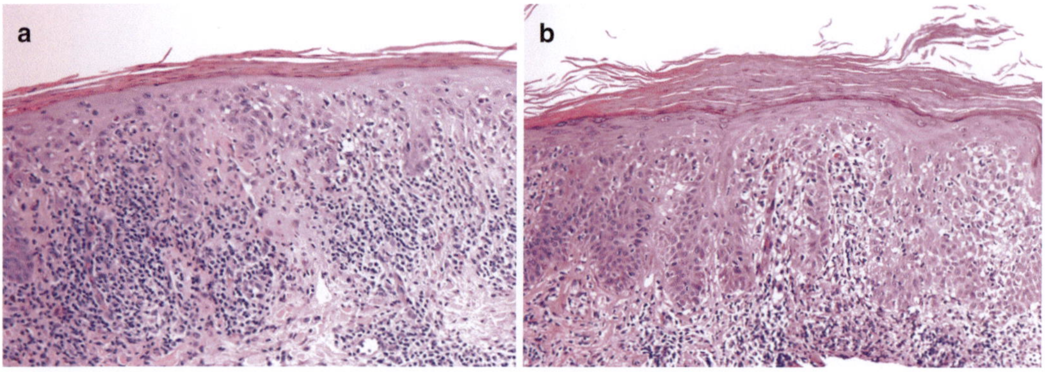

Fig. 12.67 (**a**, **b**) Epidermal hypergranulosis and focal parakeratosis with dermal lichenoid infiltrate

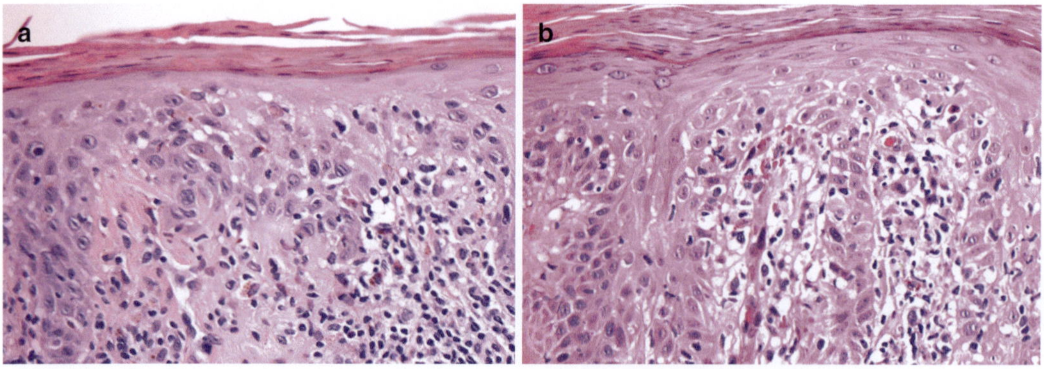

Fig. 12.68 (**a**, **b**) Interface vacuoles with focal necrotic keratinocyte and dermal pigment incontinence

Lichen Sclerosus et Atrophicus

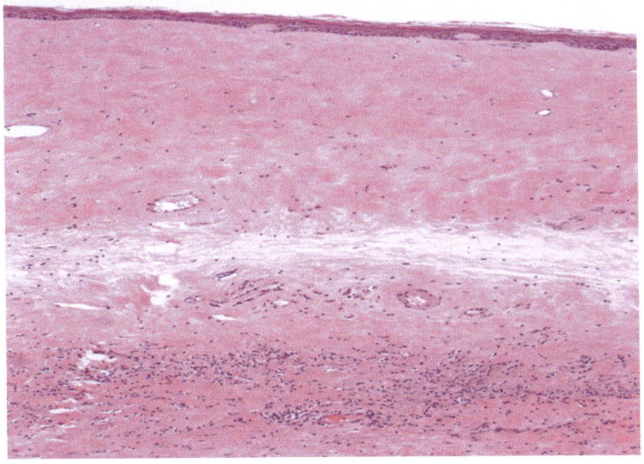

Fig. 12.69 Skin with appearance of **three colors**: purple epidermis, pink sclerosis, blue lichenoid infiltrate usually called red, white, blue

Synonyms: Kraurosis Vulvae (in females), Balanitis Xerotica Obliterans (in males)

Histopathology (Figs. 12.69, 12.70, and 12.71)

- Hyperkeratosis with epidermal atrophy
- Subepidermal dermal sclerosis
- Dilated capillaries in the sclerotic dermis
- Lichenoid infiltrate underneath the dermal sclerosis

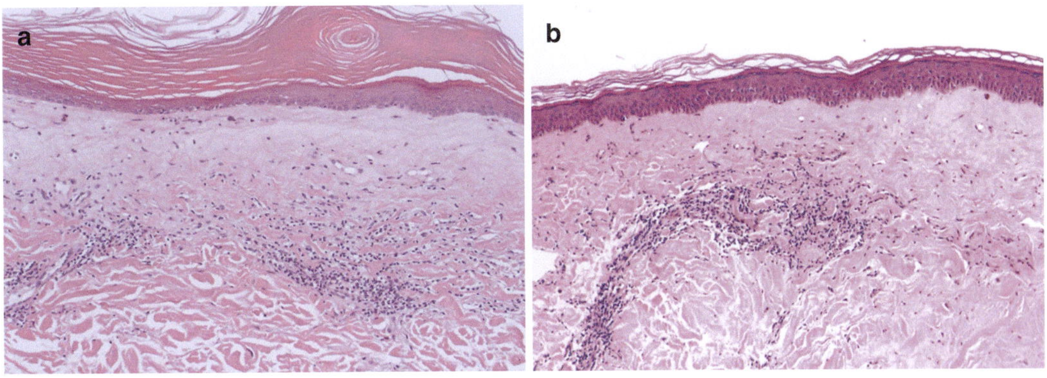

Fig. 12.70 (**a**, **b**) Hyperkeratotic atrophic epidermis with sclerosis of the upper dermis

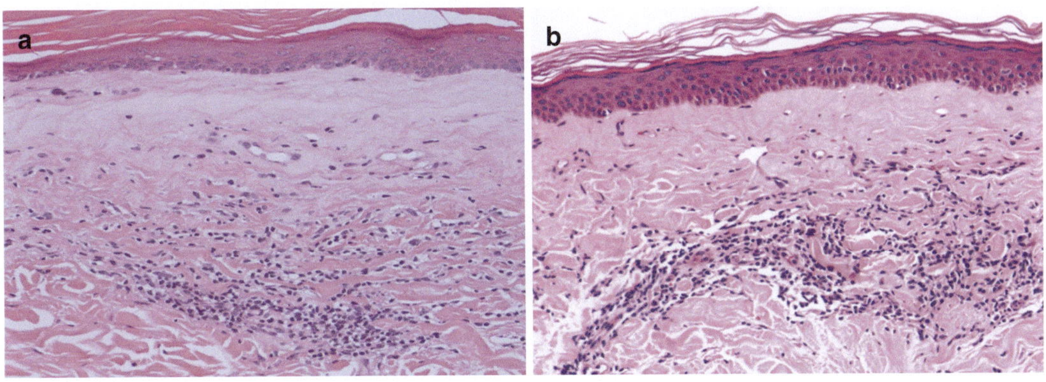

Fig. 12.71 (**a**, **b**) Dermal telangiectasias in the sclerotic dermis with underlying band-like lymphocytic infiltrate

Lichen Simplex Chronicus

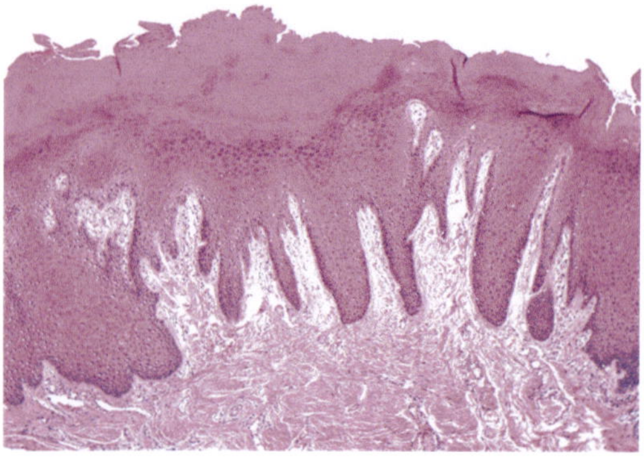

Fig. 12.72 Irregular psoriasiform hyperplasia

Synonym: Circumscribed Neurodermatitis

Histopathology (Figs. 12.72, 12.73, and 12.74)

- Irregular psoriasiform epidermis with elongated rete ridges
- Epidermal hyperkeratosis, acanthosis, and hypergranulosis
- Fibrosis of the papillary dermis
- Mild perivascular lymphocytic infiltrate

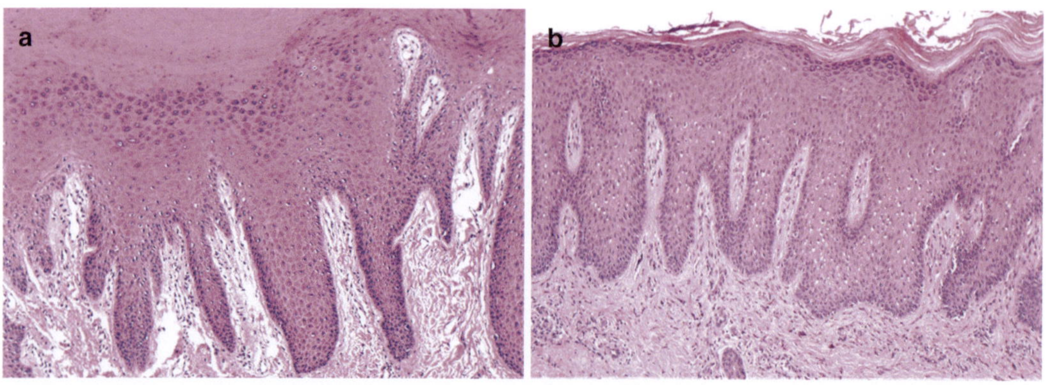

Fig. 12.73 (**a**, **b**) Orthokeratosis and hypergranulosis with elongated rete ridges

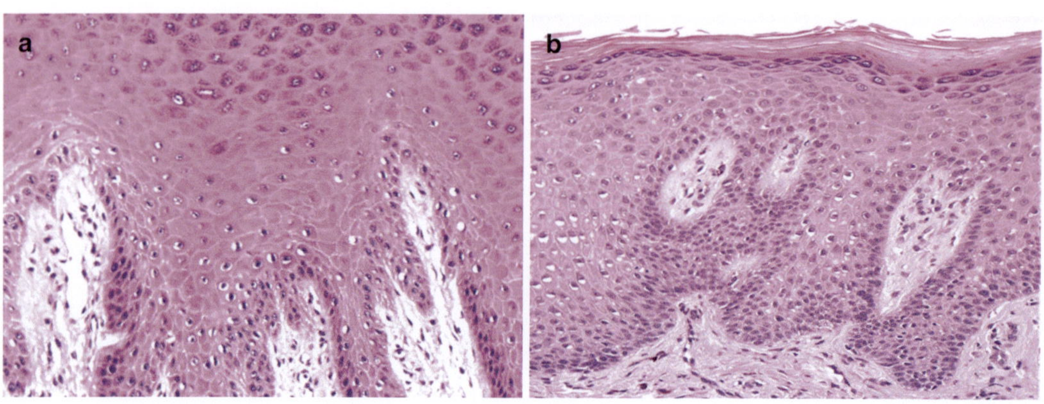

Fig. 12.74 (**a**, **b**) Papillary dermal fibrosis and mild dermal inflammation

Lichen Striatus

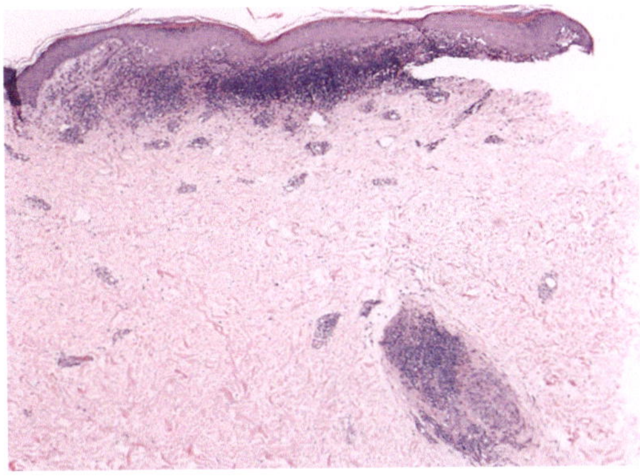

Fig. 12.75 Lichenoid dermatitis with deep dermal inflammation

Histopathology (Figs. 12.75, 12.76, 12.77, and 12.78)

- Lichenoid dermal infiltrate
- Exuberant periеccrine lymphocytic infiltrate
- Mild perivascular lymphocytic infiltrate

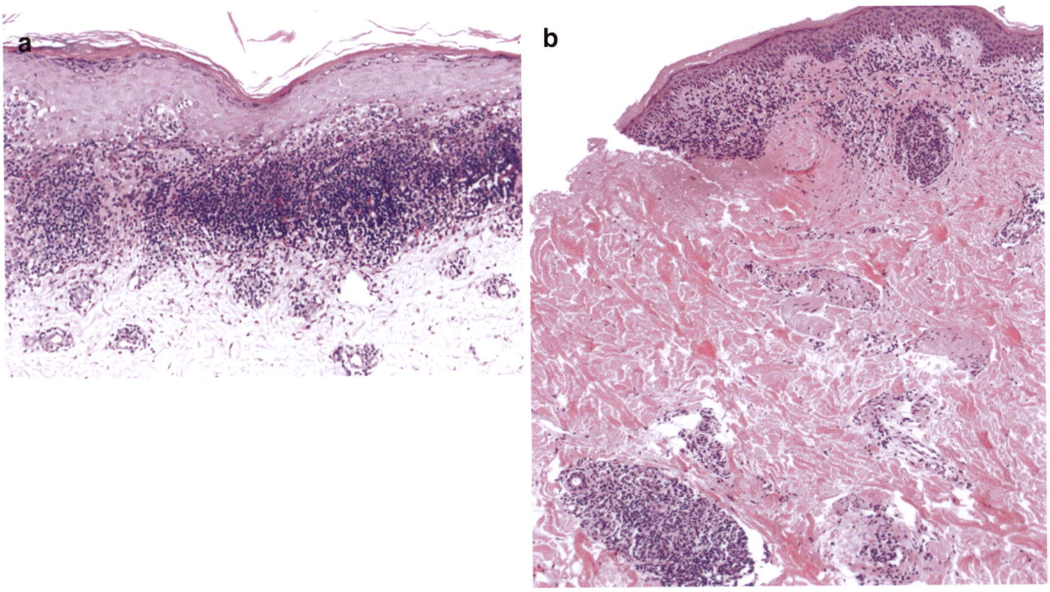

Fig. 12.76 (**a**, **b**) Superficial band-like inflammation and epidermal changes are indistinguishable from lichen planus

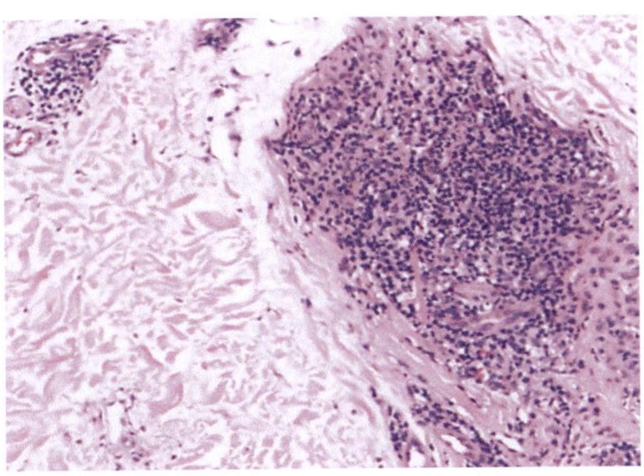

Fig. 12.77 Perivascular inflammation is present

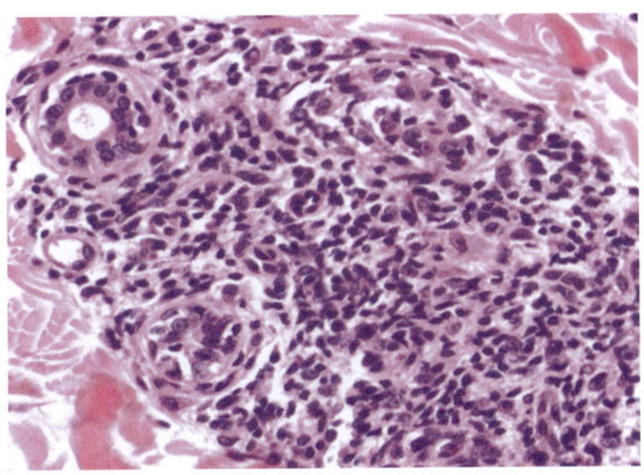

Fig. 12.78 Perieccrine lymphocytic inflammation is characteristic

Light Reaction

Acute reaction

Sunburn (Fig. 12.79)
- Individual necrotic keratinocytes ("sunburn cells")
- Mild dermal edema and inflammation

Photoallergic dermatitis (Fig. 12.80)
- Epidermal spongiosis with variable necrosis of keratinocytes particularly in the upper epidermis
- Dermal lymphocytic and eosinophilic inflammation

Phototoxic dermatitis (Fig. 12.81)
- Epidermal spongiosis with variable necrosis of keratinocytes particularly in the upper epidermis
- Dermal lymphocytic and neutrophilic inflammation

Polymorphous light eruption (Fig. 12.82)
- Mild epidermal spongiosis
- Dermal edema with superficial and deep perivascular lymphocytic inflammation
- Eosinophils and neutrophils can be present

Chronic reaction

Actinic prurigo (Fig. 12.83)
- Acute stage resembles polymorphous light eruption with dermal edema and perivascular lymphocytic infiltrate
- Chronic stage histologically is not specific and resembles prurigo nodularis; if the biopsy is taken from a lip lesion, dermal lymphoid follicles are present (follicular cheilitis)

Actinic reticuloid (Fig. 12.84)
- Epidermis with psoriasiform hyperplasia and fibrotic papillary dermis resembling lichen simplex chronicus
- Prominent dermal lymphocytic infiltrate
- Epidermal lymphocytic exocytosis resembling mycosis fungoides

Hydroa vacciniforme (Fig. 12.85)
- Epidermal necrosis
- Focal dermal necrosis with hemorrhage and perivascular and interstitial lymphocytic infiltrate

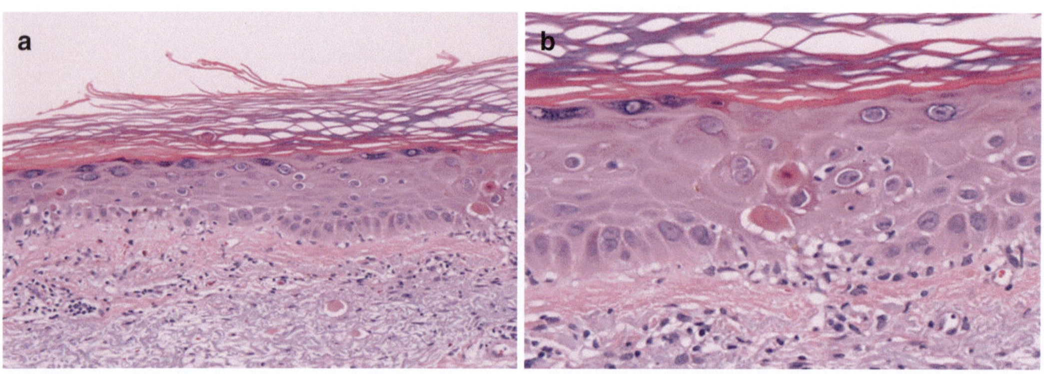

Fig. 12.79 (**a**, **b**) **Sunburn** with scattered necrotic keratinocytes and mild dermal inflammation

Light Reaction: Acute

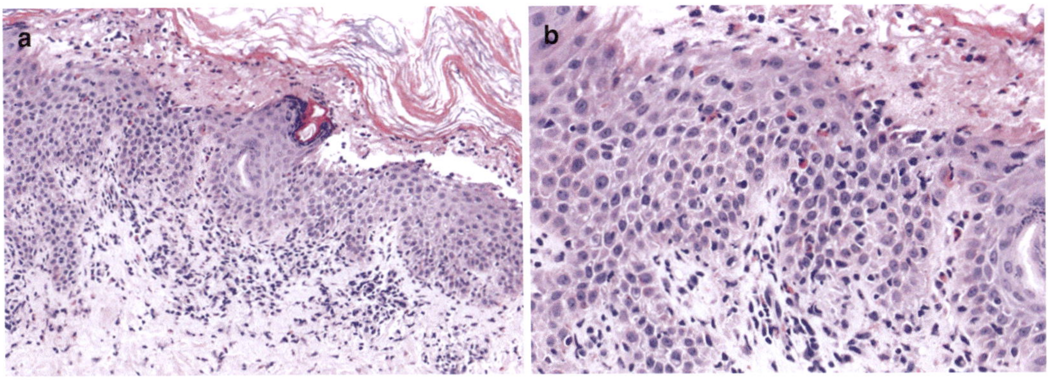

Fig. 12.80 (**a**, **b**) **Photoallergic** dermatitis with necrosis of the superficial epidermis and numerous epidermal and dermal eosinophils

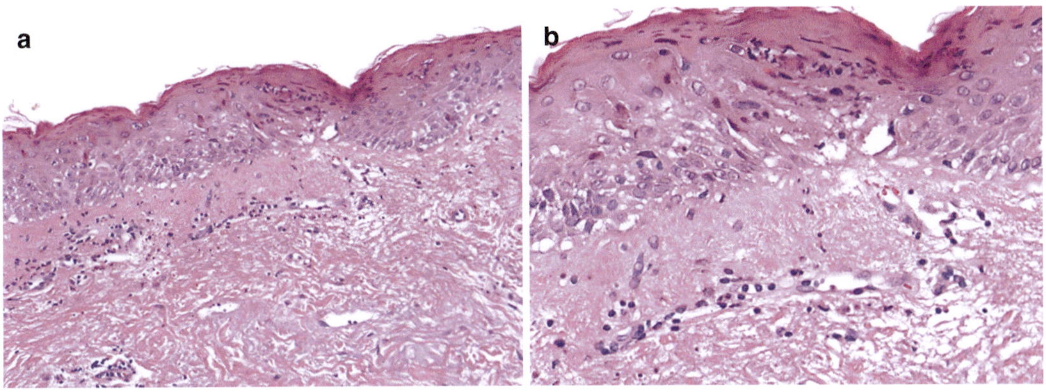

Fig. 12.81 (**a**, **b**) **Phototoxic** dermatitis with necrosis of the superficial epidermis and numerous epidermal and dermal neutrophils

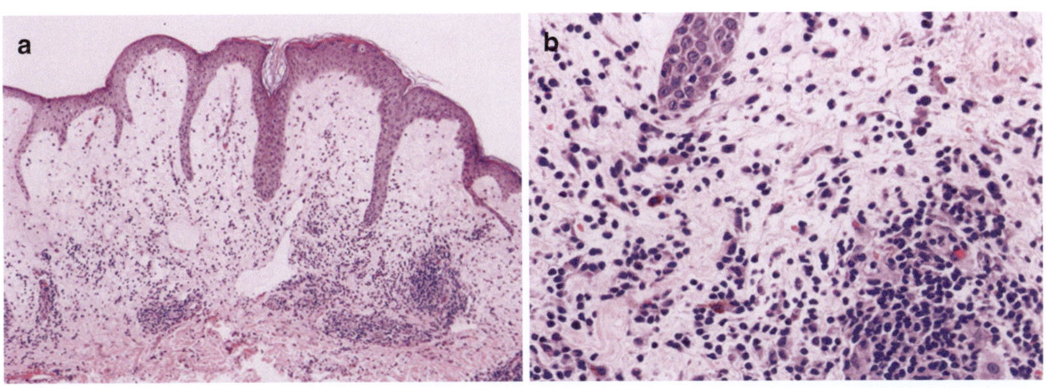

Fig. 12.82 (**a**, **b**) **Polymorphous light eruption** with wavy epidermis, extensive dermal edema, and dermal lymphocytes

Light Reaction: Chronic

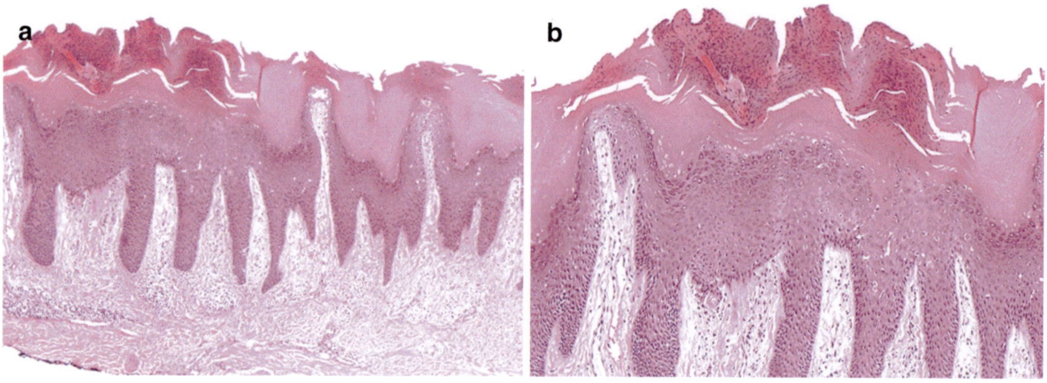

Fig. 12.83 (**a**, **b**) **Actinic prurigo** with epidermal acanthosis, hyperkeratosis, hypergranulosis, and dermal lymphocytic inflammation

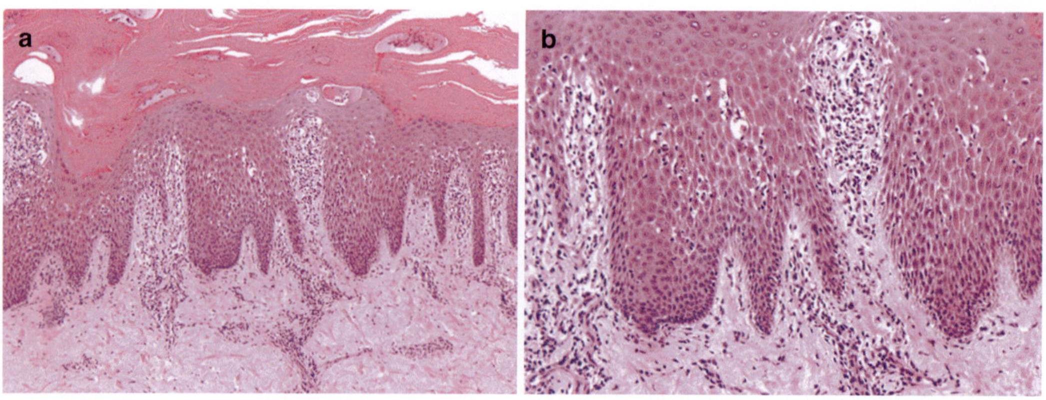

Fig. 12.84 (**a**, **b**) **Actinic reticuloid** with psoriasiform epidermis and epidermal lymphocytic exocytosis resembling mycosis fungoides

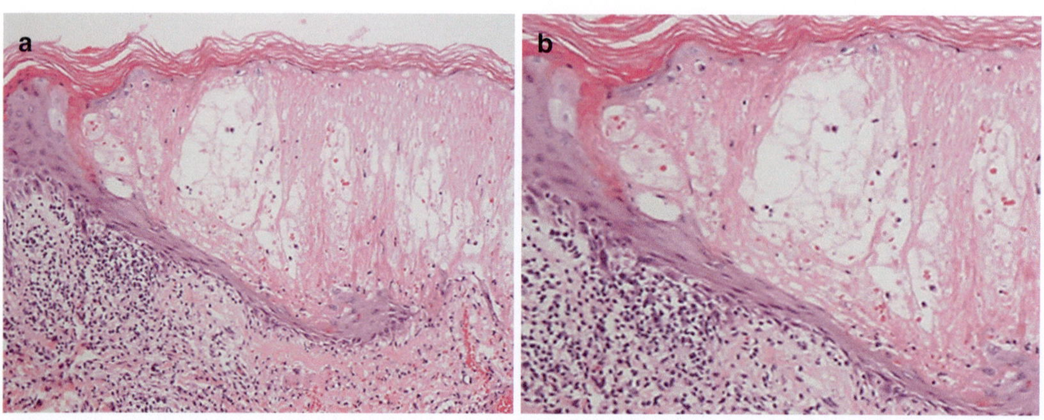

Fig. 12.85 (**a**, **b**) **Hydroa vacciniforme** with epidermal necrosis, vesicle formation, hemorrhage and dermal mixed inflammation

Linear IgA Bullous Dermatosis

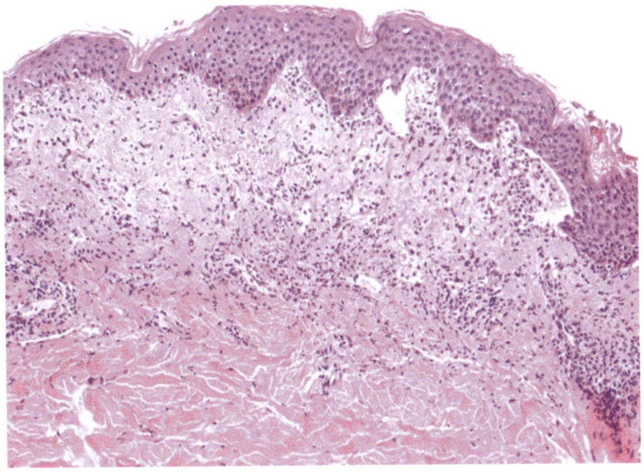

Fig. 12.86 Linear dermal neutrophilic infiltrate with small subepidermal blister

Histopathology (Figs. 12.86, 12.87, 12.88, and 12.89)

- Subepidermal split with blister formation
- Linear neutrophilic infiltrate in the blister and at the base of the blister
- Scattered neutrophils and lymphocytes in the dermis that is not split from the epidermis
- Linear IgA deposits at epidermal-dermal junction by DIF

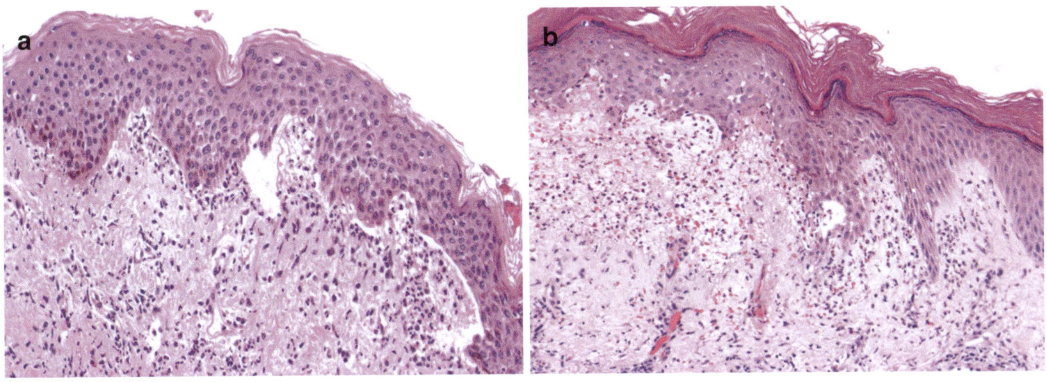

Fig. 12.87 (a, b) Neutrophils line up at the dermal-epidermal junction

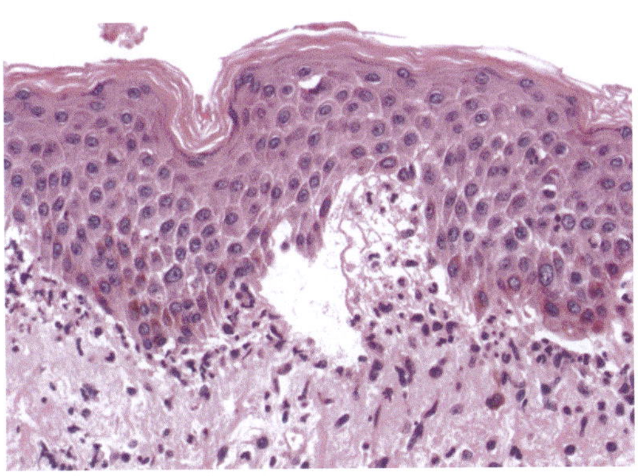

Fig. 12.88 Subepidermal blister with neutrophils

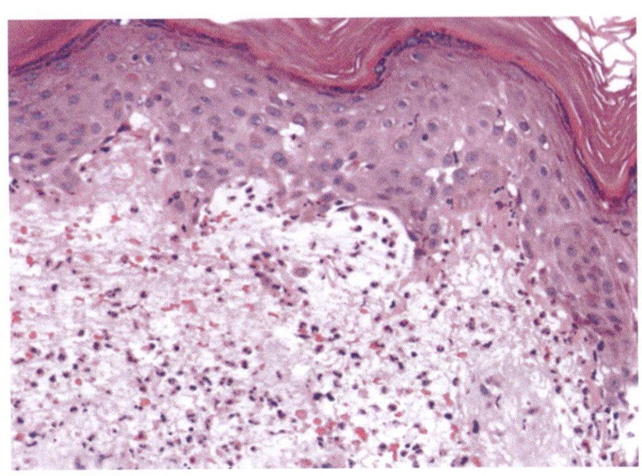

Fig. 12.89 Mild RBCs extravasation is present

Lipodermatosclerosis

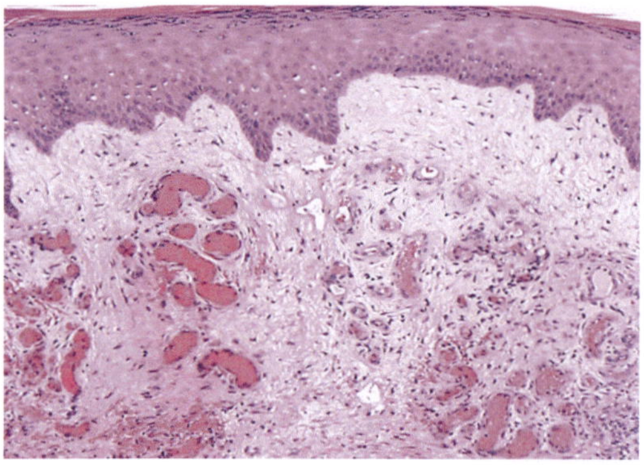

Fig. 12.90 Dermal proliferation of benign capillaries

Histopathology (Figs. 12.90, 12.91, 12.92, 12.93, and 12.94)
- Dermal fibrosis and proliferation of small capillaries in lobular pattern consistent with dermal stasis
- Subcutaneous septal fibrosis and sclerosis that spills over to the lobules
- Fat necrosis with variably sized adipocytes and "feathery" change (lipomembranous change)
- Pseudocysts can form from damaged adipocytes

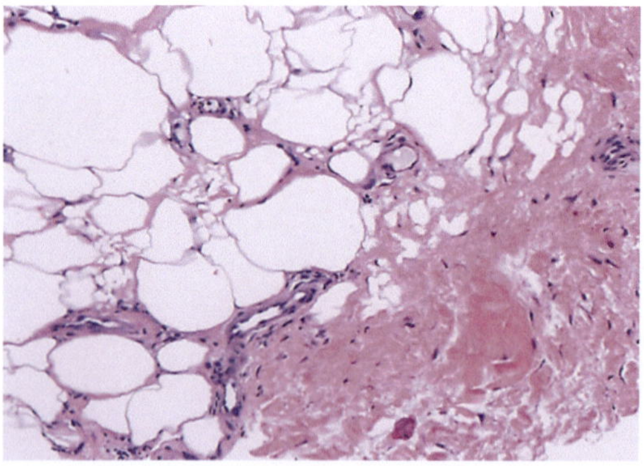

Fig. 12.91 Damaged adipocytes varying in size

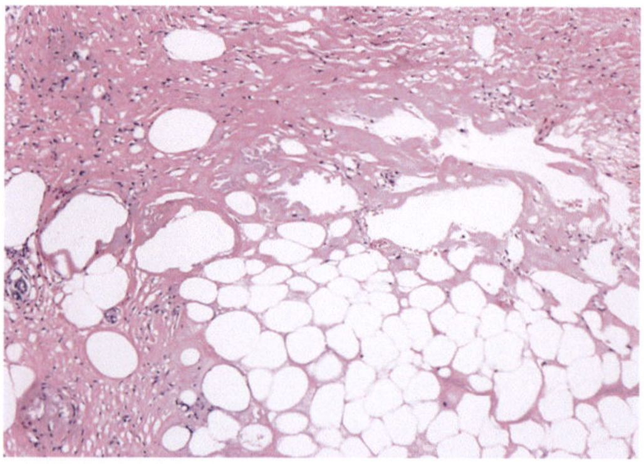

Fig. 12.92 Septal sclerosis that is spilling over to the lobules

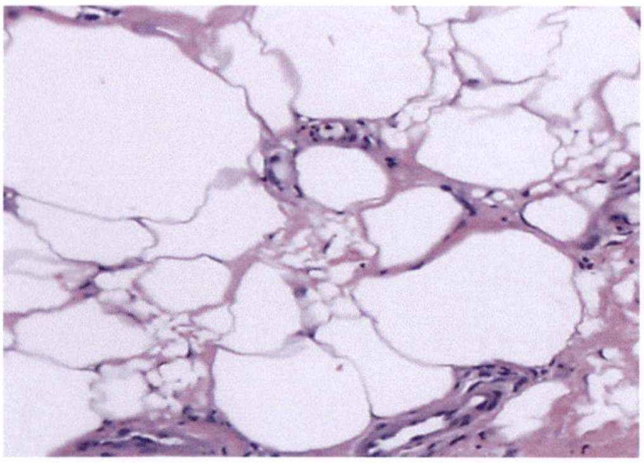

Fig. 12.93 Broken adipocytes form larger pseudocystic spaces

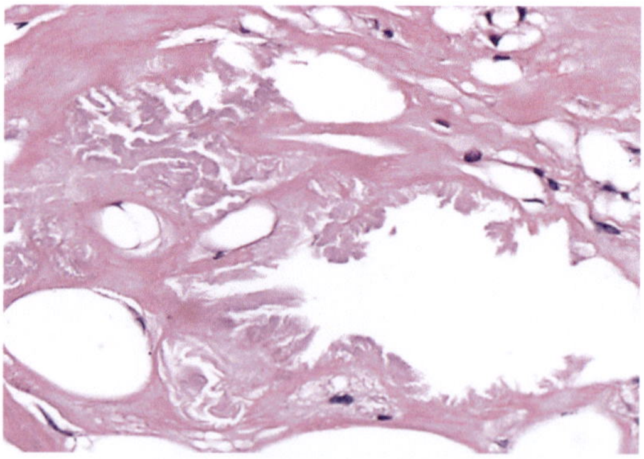

Fig. 12.94 Lipomembranous "feathery" changes

Lipoma

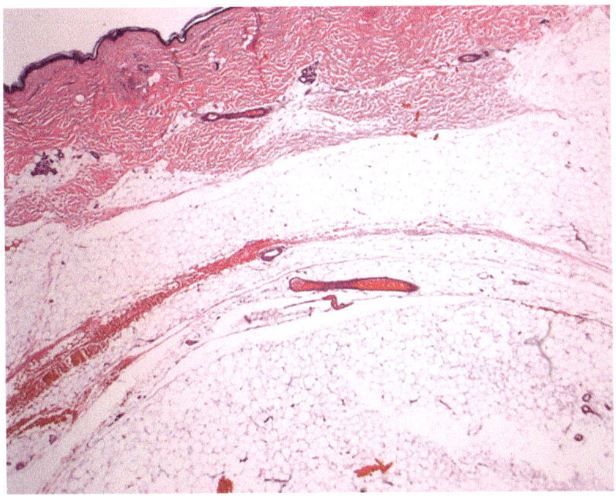

Fig. 12.95 Tumor nodule made of mature adipocytes with no fibrous septae

Histopathology

- Non encapsulated tumor made of mature adipocytes (S-100+) with thin or no fibrous septa (Figs. 12.95 and 12.96)

Angiolipoma:

- Increased number of small normal vascular channels (Fig. 12.97)

Pleomorphic lipoma:

- Multinucleated giant cells ("floret" cells) scattered among normal appearing adipocytes (Fig. 12.98)

Spindle cell lipoma:

- Uniform bland spindle cells in myxoid background among mature adipocytes (Fig. 12.99)

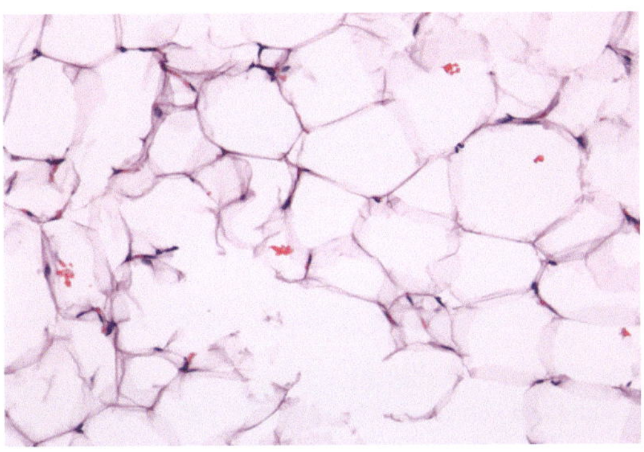

Fig. 12.96 **Lipoma** with normal adipocytes without atypia

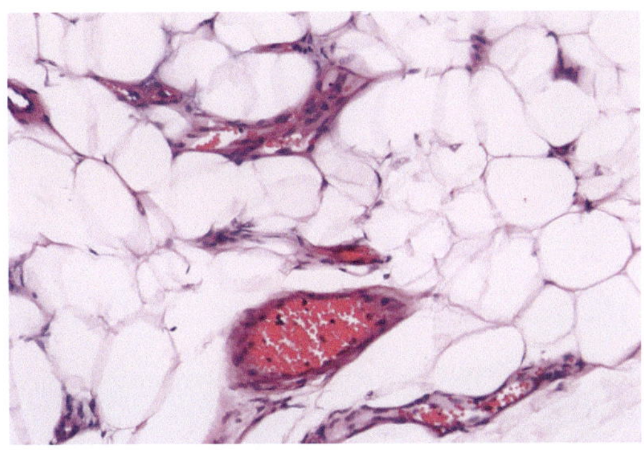

Fig. 12.97 **Angiolipoma** with increased number of capillaries

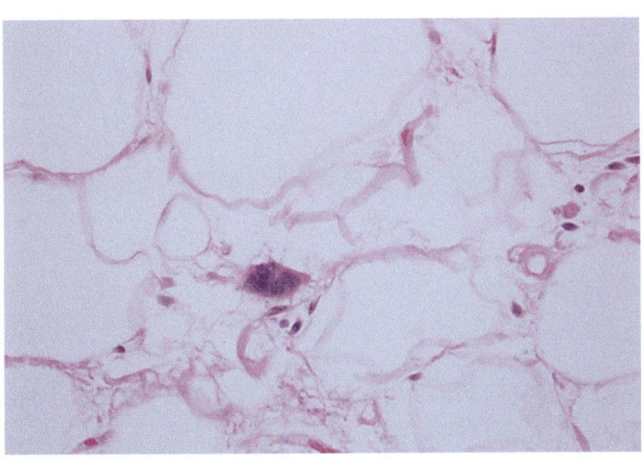

Fig. 12.98 **Pleomorphic lipoma** with "floret" cell

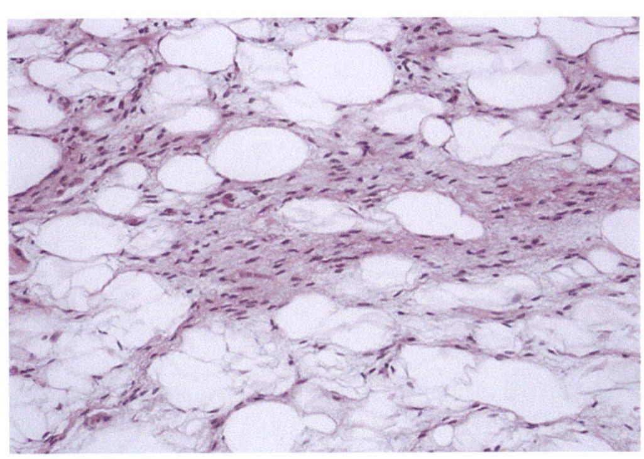

Fig. 12.99 **Spindle cell lipoma** with spindle cells in myxoid stroma

Liposarcoma

Histopathology

Well-differentiated liposarcoma/atypical lipoma (Fig. 12.100)
- Mature adipocytes with mildly atypical nuclei and rare lipoblasts

Myxoid and round cell liposarcoma (Figs. 12.101 and 12.102)
- Multilobular tumor with univacuolated and multivacuolated lipoblasts and round cells
- Diffuse myxoid background
- Capillary network in "chicken wire" pattern

Dedifferentiated liposarcoma:
- Atypical lipomatous tumor showing progression to sarcoma (usually non-lipogenic) of variable histological grade

Pleomorphic liposarcoma (Fig. 12.103)
- Bizarre lipoblasts
- Pleomorphic atypical cells
- Mitoses are frequent

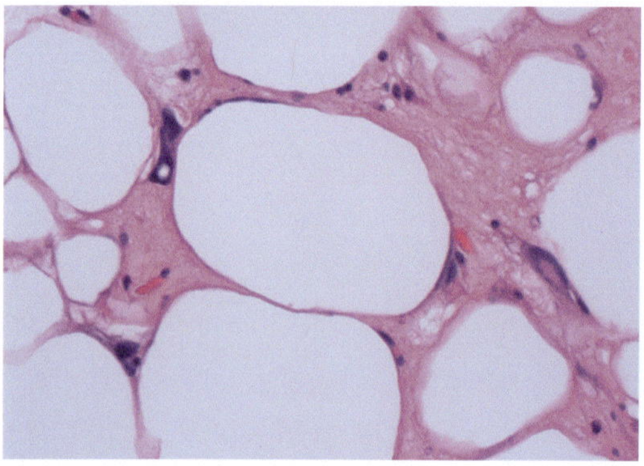

Fig. 12.100 **Well differentiated liposarcoma** with lipoblasts that have atypical nuclei

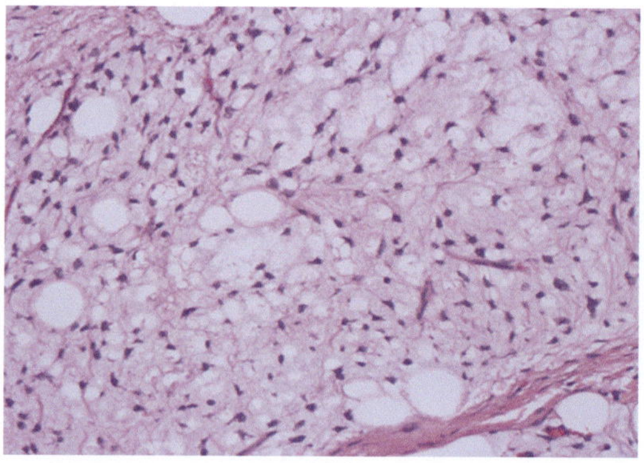

Fig. 12.101 **Myxoid liposarcoma** with myxoid background and vessels in "chicken wire" pattern

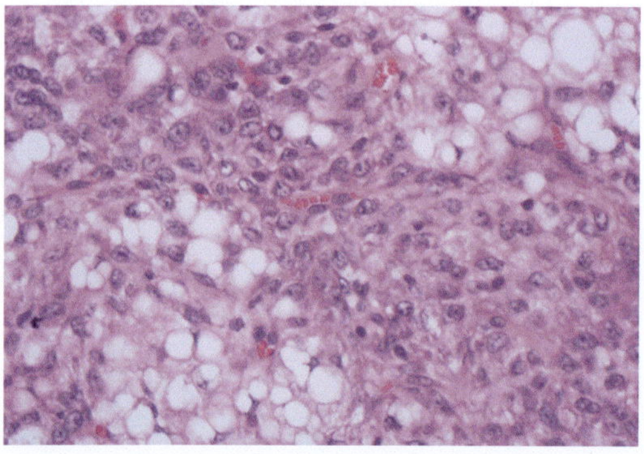

Fig. 12.102 **High grade myxoid liposarcoma** with atypical round cells admixed with mature looking adipocytes

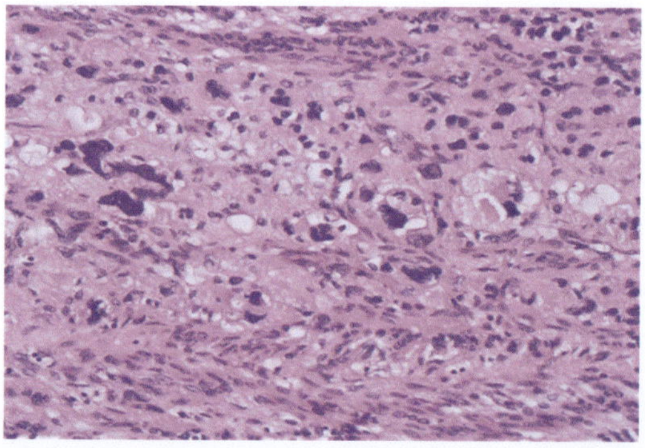

Fig. 12.103 **Pleomorphic liposarcoma** with pleomorphic cells that have bizarre nuclei

Livedo Reticularis

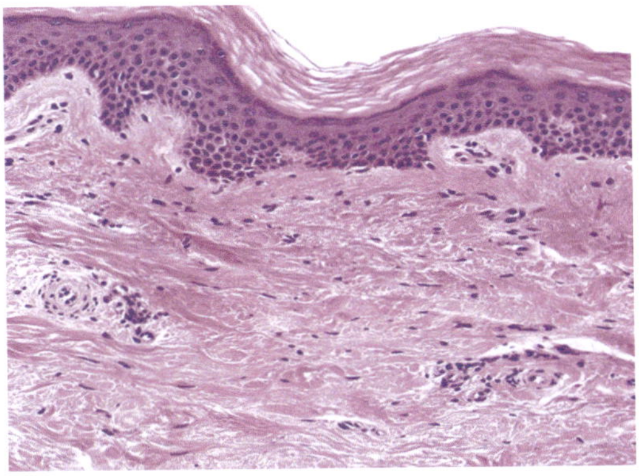

Fig. 12.104 Epidermal hyperkeratosis with subtle changes in dermal capillaries

It was always assumed that a biopsy from a clinically erythematous area is normal whereas a pale area shows pathological features. Recent reports contradict this, suggesting that both areas have similar subtle changes and therefore multiple biopsies are required to confirm diagnosis.

Histopathology (Figs. 12.104, 12.105, 12.106, 12.107, and 12.108)

- Epidermal hyperkeratosis
- Occasional capillaries with thickened wall and plump endothelial cells
- Occasional microthrombi in the deep capillaries

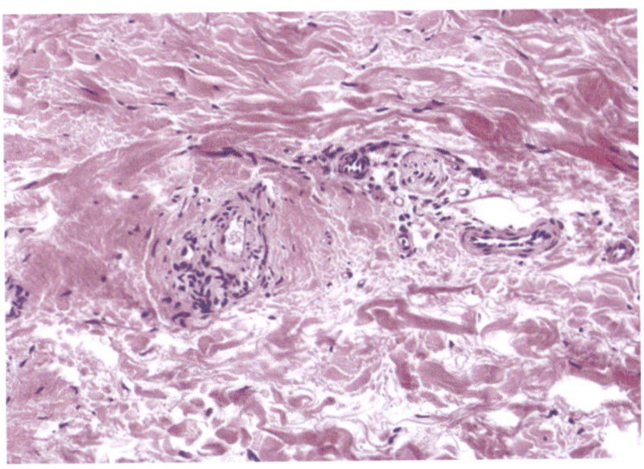

Fig. 12.105 Thickened wall of capillaries

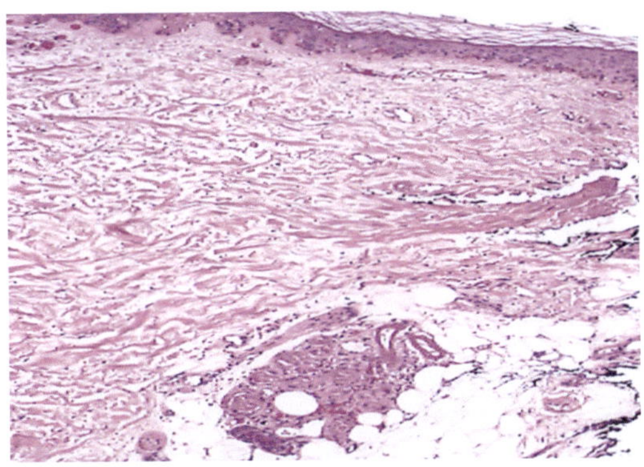

Fig. 12.106 Deep capillaries are affected

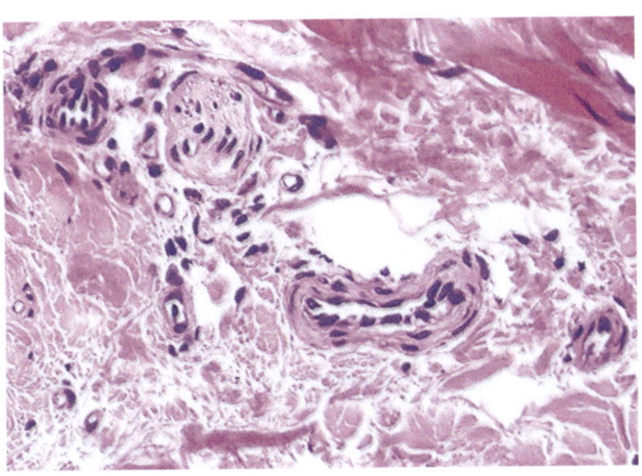

Fig. 12.107 Endothelial cells are prominent and plump

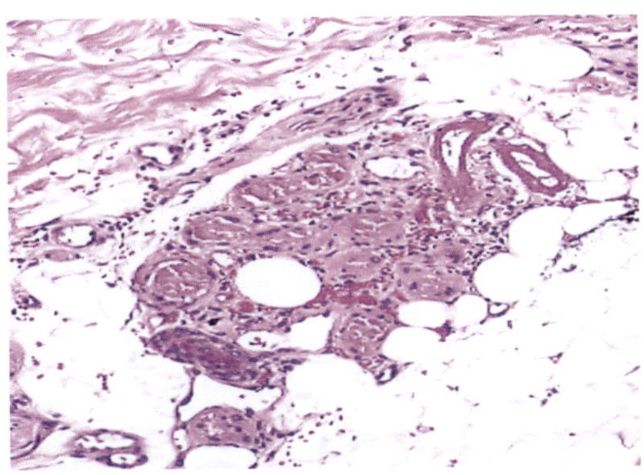

Fig. 12.108 Microthrombi in capillaries

Lobomycosis

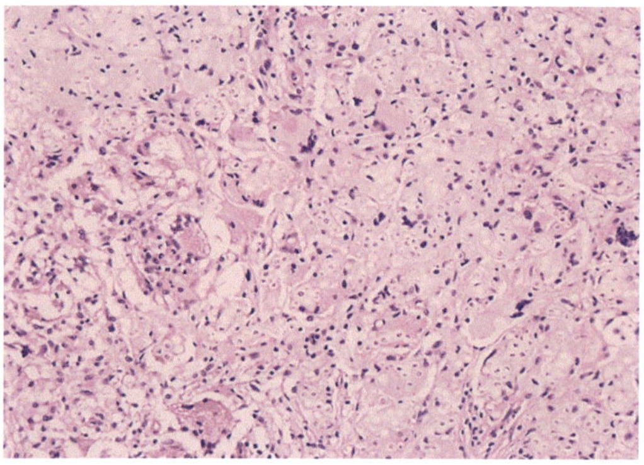

Fig. 12.109 Exuberant dermal infiltrate

Synonym: Keloidal Blastomycosis

Histopathology (Figs. 12.109, 12.110, 12.111, 12.112, and 12.113)

- Exuberant dermal infiltrate of histiocytes and some giant cells
- There are numerous fungal elements in histiocytes and giant cells
- Fungi are 6–12 μM in size and have thick wall
- Although clinically lesions have keloid appearance, fibroblasts appear in the lesion later

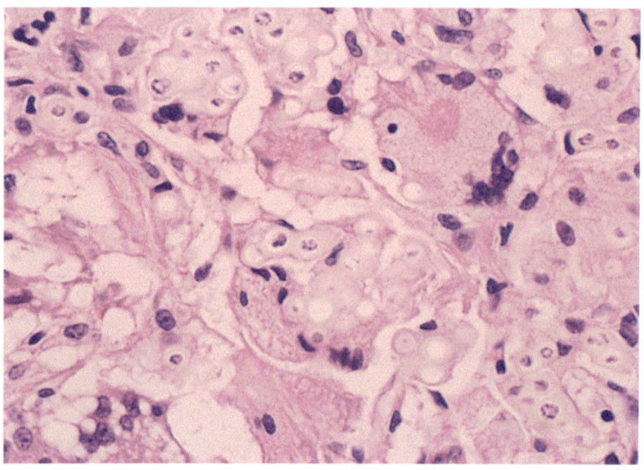

Fig. 12.110 Infiltrate consists of histiocytes and giant cells

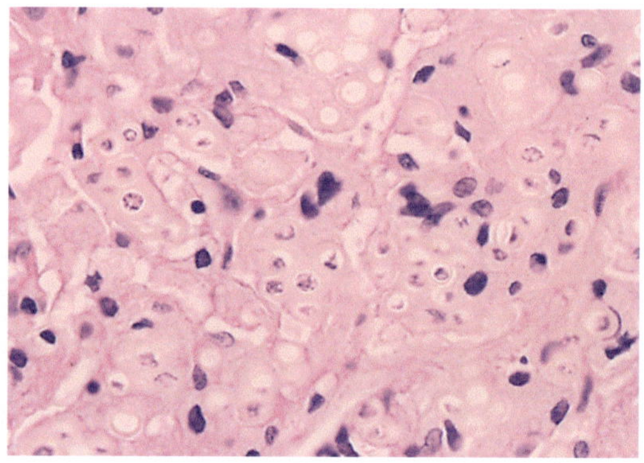

Fig. 12.111 Spores within histiocytes

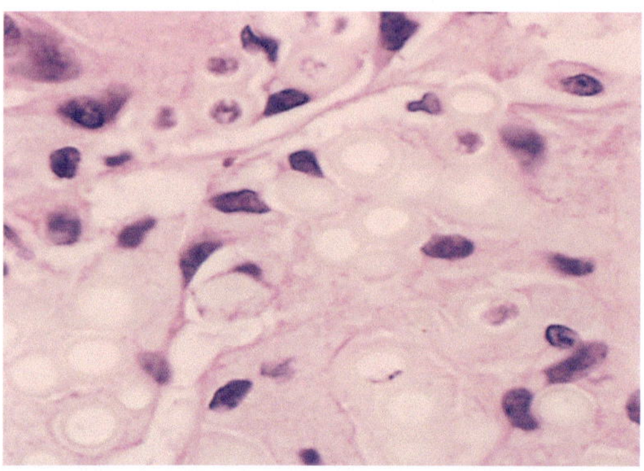

Fig. 12.112 Fungal elements are intra and extracellular

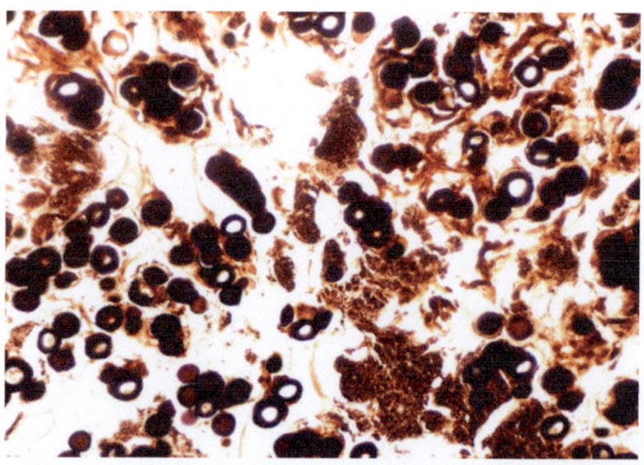

Fig. 12.113 Thick capsule better visualized using silver stain

Low Grade Fibromyxoid Sarcoma

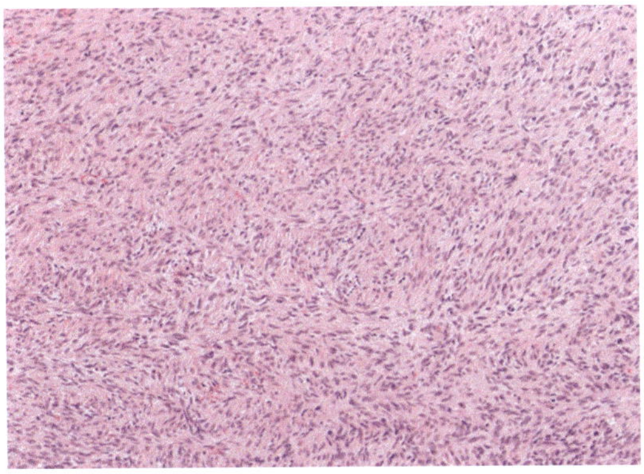

Fig. 12.114 Infiltrating moderately cellular tumor

Synonym: Evans tumor

Histopathology (Figs. 12.114, 12.115, 12.116, and 12.117)

- Infiltrating subcutaneous tumor with moderate cellularity
- Bland appearing spindle cells (CD99+, Bcl2+, EMA+) with minimal atypia and rare mitosis
- Swirling, whorled growth pattern
- Alternating fibrous and myxoid areas (MUC4+)
- Giant collagen rosettes in some cases

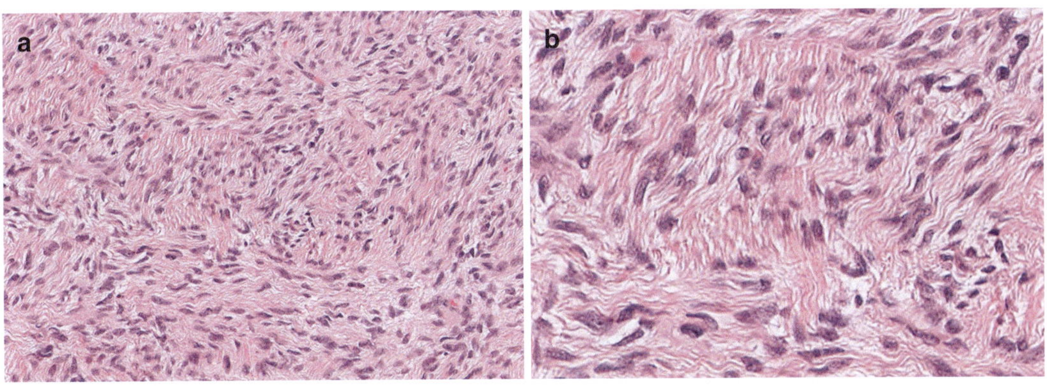

Fig. 12.115 (**a**, **b**) Swirling, whorled growth pattern

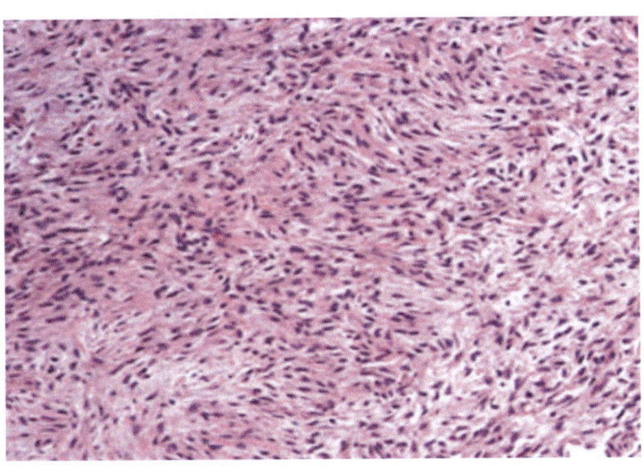

Fig. 12.116 Alternating fibrous and myxoid areas

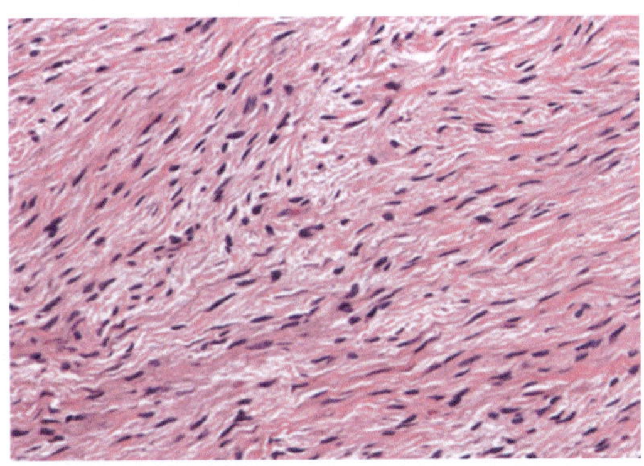

Fig. 12.117 Bland appearing spindle cells with no atypia or mitoses

Lupus Erythematosus

There are three major clinical forms and several variants.

Discoid lupus erythematosus (DLE) (Fig. 12.118)
- Atrophic epidermis with hyperkeratosis and follicular plugging
- Vacuolar degeneration of the basal layer keratinocytes with apoptotic keratinocytes
- Dermal mucin and thickening of the basement membrane in older lesions
- Perifollicular and perivascular lymphocytic infiltrate

Subacute cutaneous lupus erythematosus (SCLE) (Fig. 12.119)
- Flattened atrophic epidermis with hyperkeratosis
- Interface vacuolar changes with necrotic keratinocytes are present
- Lymphocytic infiltrate is confined to the superficial dermis and dermal mucin is detected

Systemic lupus erythematosus (SLE):
- Changes are identical to SCLE but everything is more subtle (Fig. 12.120)

Discoid lupus of tumid type (tumid lupus):
- Patchy superficial and deep perieccrine and perivascular lymphocytic infiltrate with significant amount of dermal mucin (Fig. 12.121)

Lupus panniculitis: half of the cases have epidermal changes of DLE in addition to patchy lobular lymphocytic aggregates and septal hyalinization (Fig. 12.122)

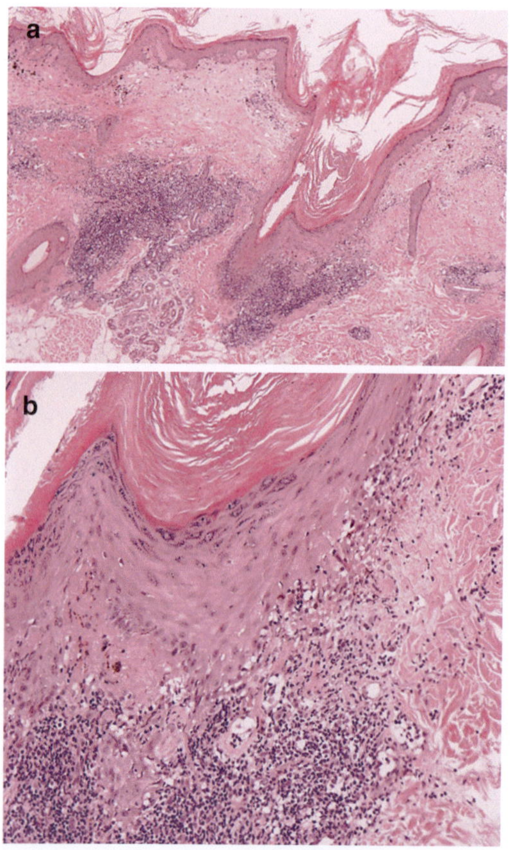

Fig. 12.118 (**a**, **b**) **DLE** with atrophic extremely hyperkeratotic epidermis and follicular plugging. Interface vacuolar changes with apoptotic keratinocytes and pigment incontinence. Perifollicular and perivascular lymphocytic inflammation

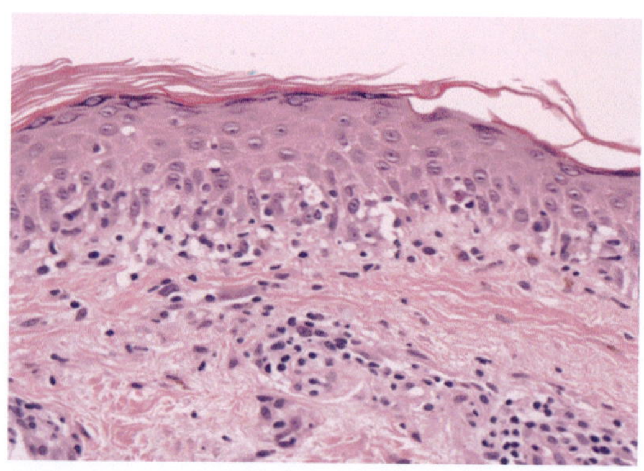

Fig. 12.119 **SCLE** with flattened atrophic epidermis. Interface vacuolar changes with apoptotic keratinocytes are present. Inflammation is restricted to the superficial dermis and is milder than in DLE

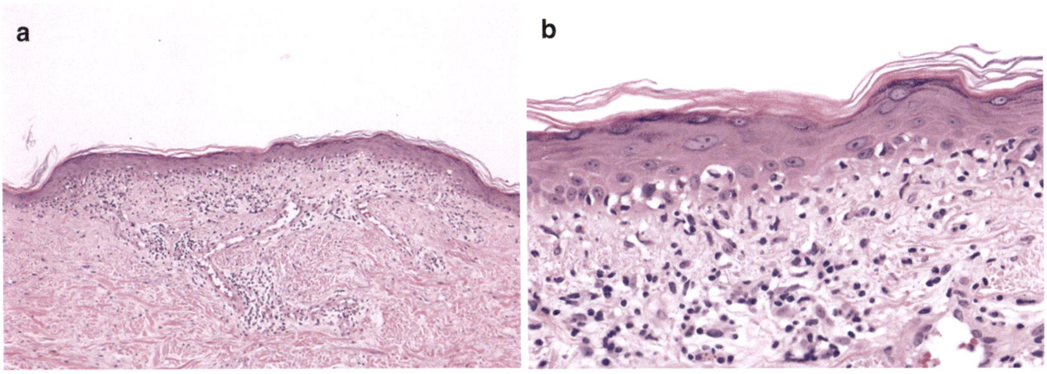

Fig. 12.120 (**a**, **b**) **SLE** with flattened atrophic epidermis with mild hyperkeratosis. Patchy interface vacuolar changes with apoptotic keratinocytes are present. Inflammation is restricted to the superficial dermis and is somewhat milder than in SCLE

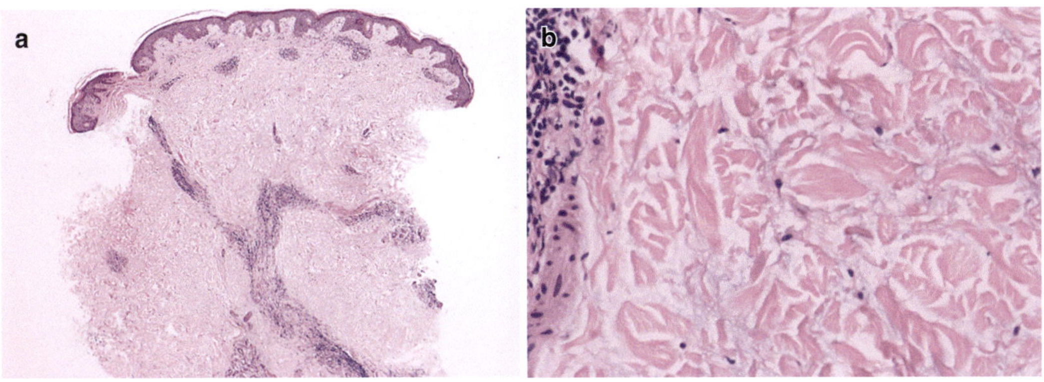

Fig. 12.121 (**a**, **b**) Only half of the cases of **tumid lupus** (variant of DLE) will have epidermal changes of DLE. The other half (like this one) have a normal epidermis. Superficial and deep perieccrine and perivascular lymphocytic infiltrate is seen. Collagen bundles are separated and extensive dermal mucin is present

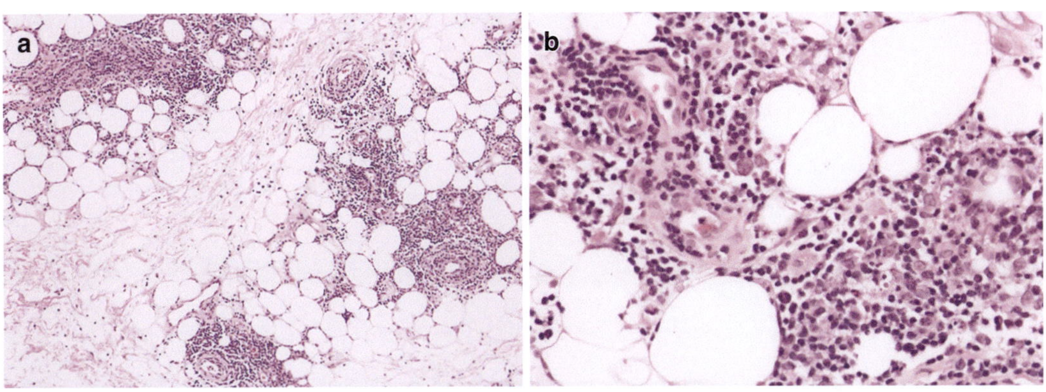

Fig. 12.122 (**a**, **b**) **Lupus panniculitis** with septal fibrosis and patches of paraseptal lymphocytes that extend into the lobules

Lupus Panniculitis

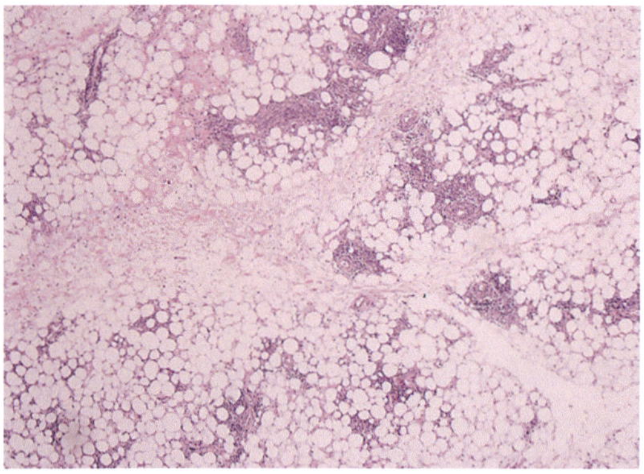

Fig. 12.123 Lobular panniculitis with septal fibrosis

Synonym: Lupus Profundus

Histopathology (Figs. 12.123, 12.124, and 12.125)

- Epidermis can be normal or have features of poikiloderma or DLE
- Dense lobular lymphocytic infiltrate in patchy distribution
- Plasma cells can be conspicuous
- The septa are thickened and there is focal hyalinization of the fat

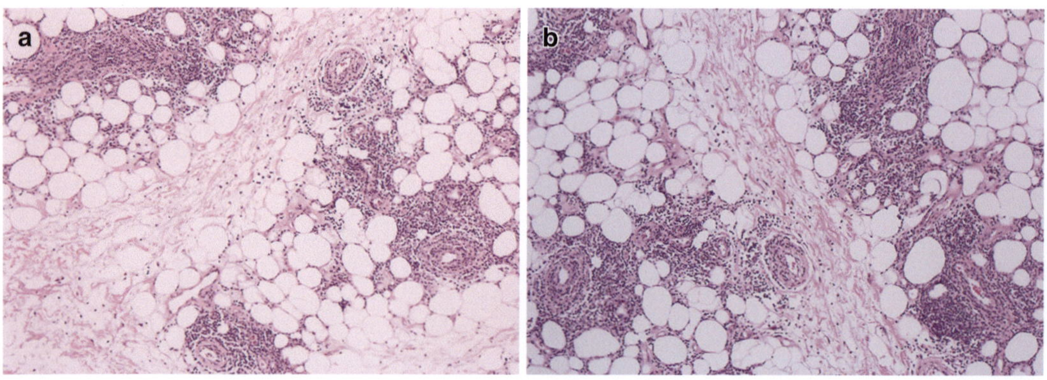

Fig. 12.124 (**a**, **b**) Septal fibrosis with focal hyalinized fat and periseptal lymphocytic infiltrate distributed in patchy pattern

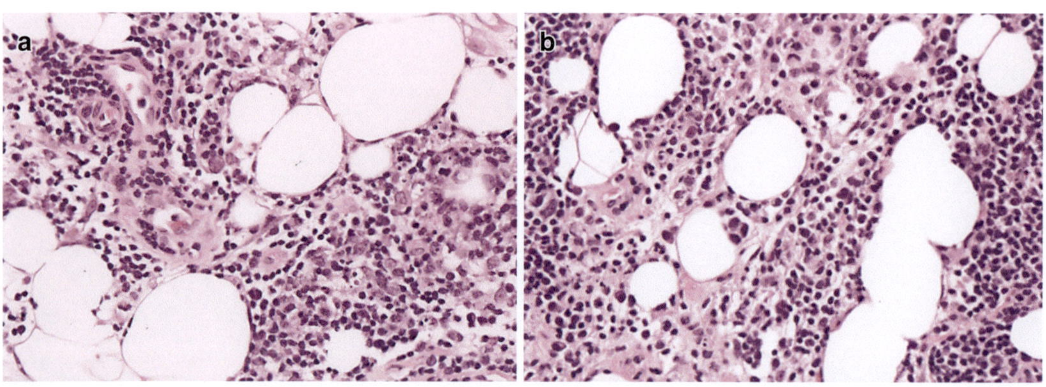

Fig. 12.125 (**a**, **b**) Lymphocytic infiltrate with significant number of plasma cells

Lupus Pernio

Like so many times in dermatology, the name is very misleading. *Lupus pernio* is the name for *sarcoidosis* on the cheeks, nose, ear, or forehead. It is granulomatous dermatitis with neither features of *lupus* nor *pernio.*

It is *different* from *chilblain (pernio) lupus erythematosus*, a *variant of lupus erythematosus*, that develops on the fingers, heels, and soles.

Histopathology (Figs. 12.126, 12.127, and 12.128)

- Lesion occurs on the facial skin
- Non necrotizing "naked" granulomas
- Granulomas are made of pale histiocytes with sparse lymphocytes around the granulomas
- No evidence of necrosis
- Giant cells can be seen but not too many

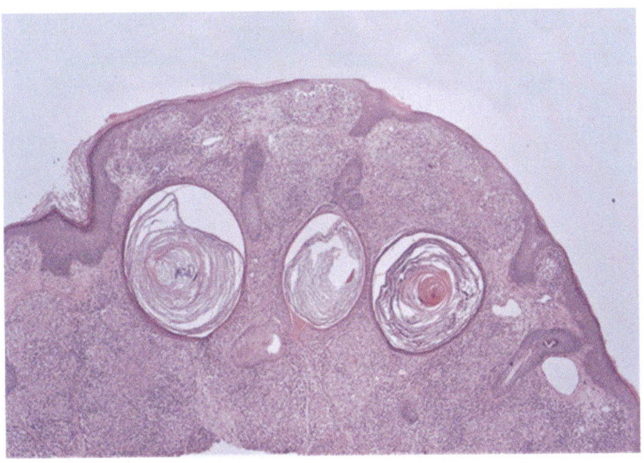

Fig. 12.126 Facial skin with granulomatous dermal infiltrate

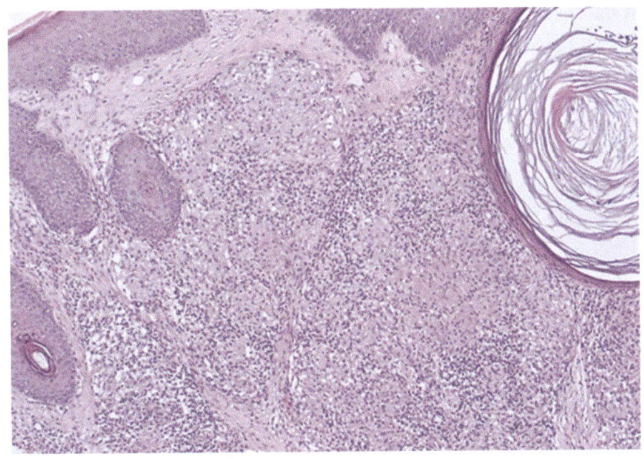

Fig. 12.127 Aggregates of pale histiocytes forming granuloma with sparse perigranulomatous lymphocytic inflammation

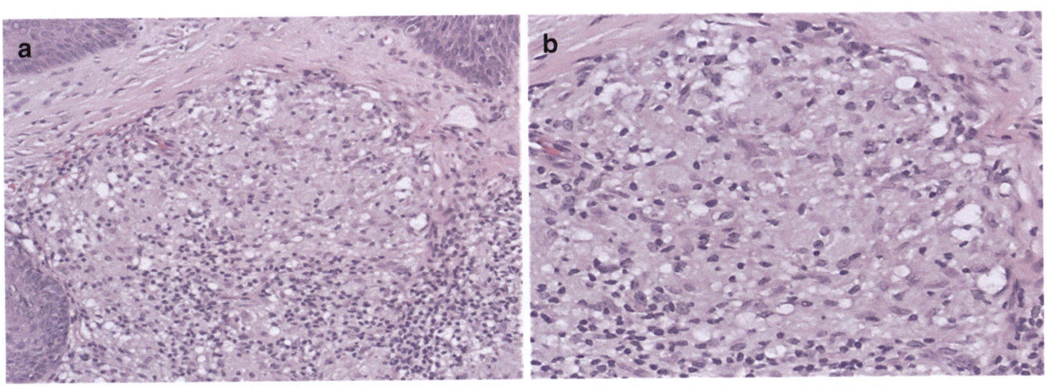

Fig. 12.128 (**a**, **b**) No evidence of necrosis within granuloma

Lyme Disease

Lyme disease can present in the skin as:
Erythema Migrans with subtle **histopathology** (Figs. 12.129 and 12.130)
- Superficial and deep perivascular and perieccrine inflammation consisting of lymphocytes and plasma cells
- Endothelial swelling and mild mucin can be detected

Acrodermatitis Chronica Atrophicans (Fig. 12.131)
- Acanthotic epidermis in early lesion and atrophic epidermis in older lesion
- Perivascular or lichenoid lymphoplasmocytic infiltrate in the early lesions and in the older lesions minimal inflammation with dermal sclerosis resembling *lichen sclerosus et atrophicus*

Lymphocytoma Cutis:
- Diffuse dermal lymphocytic infiltrate with admixed plasma cells and formation of germinal centers

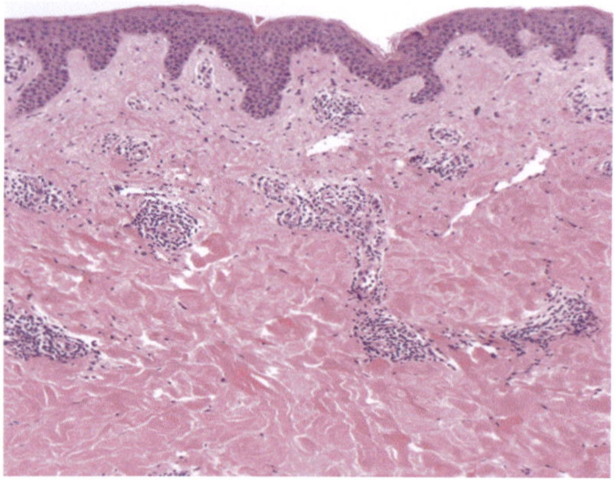

Fig. 12.129 **Erythema Migrans** with superficial and deep perivascular and perieccrine inflammation

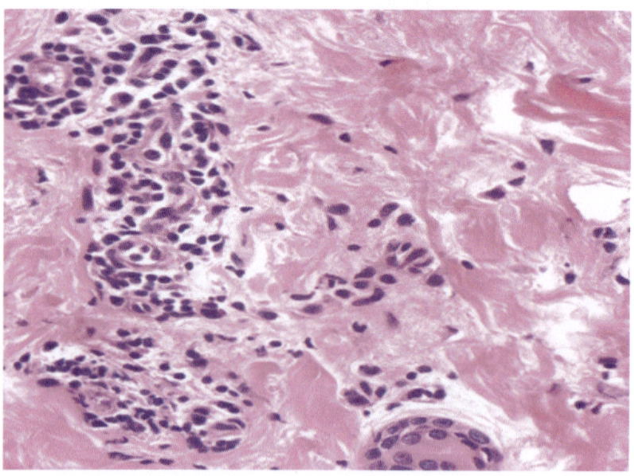

Fig. 12.130 Perieccrine lymphocytes and plasma cells

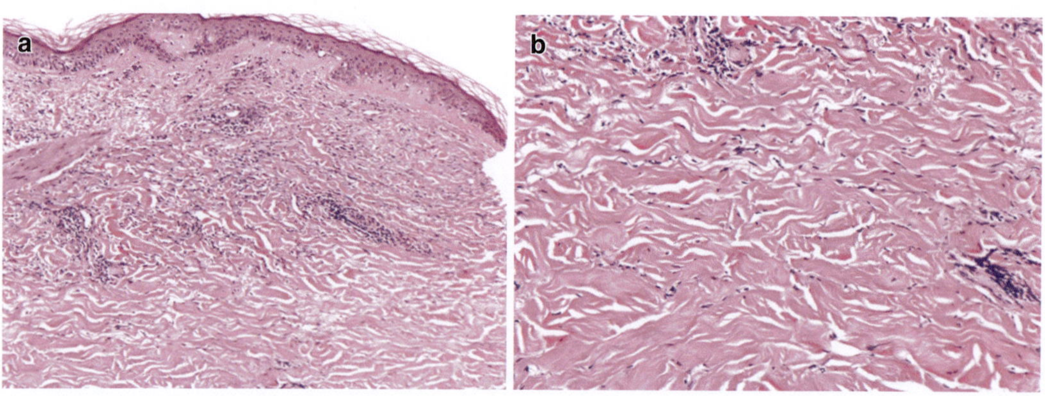

Fig. 12.131 (**a**, **b**) **Acrodermatitis Chronica Atrophicans** with flattened epidermis and dermal sclerosis

Lymphadenoma

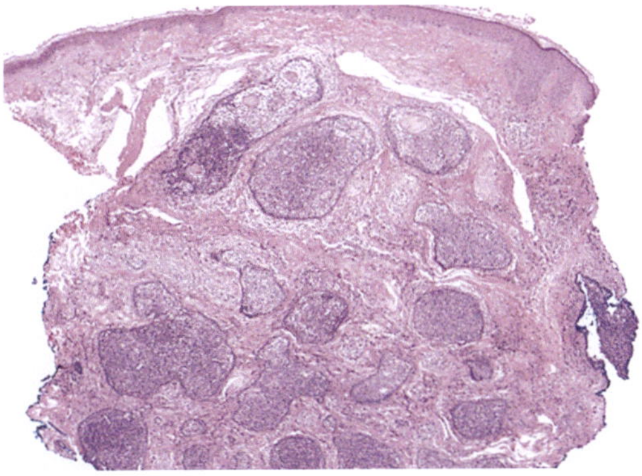

Fig. 12.132 Multiple lobules in the dermis and the subcutis

Synonyms: Cutaneous Lymphadenoma, Lymphoepithelial Tumor of Skin

Histopathology (Figs. 12.132, 12.133, 12.134, 12.135, and 12.136)

- Multilobular tumor of dermis and subcutis
- Round as well as irregularly shaped lobules with no stromal retraction
- Lobules are made of epithelioid pale cells in the center and basaloid dark cells rimming the lobules
- Lymphocytes infiltrate tumor lobules

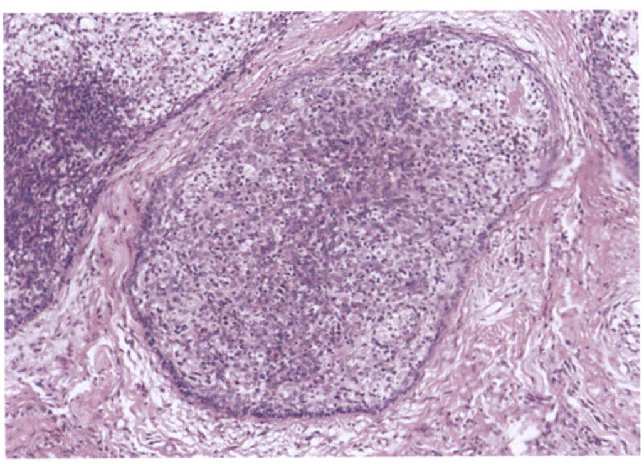

Fig. 12.133 Pale epitheliod cells form the tumor lobule and basaloid cells rim the lobule

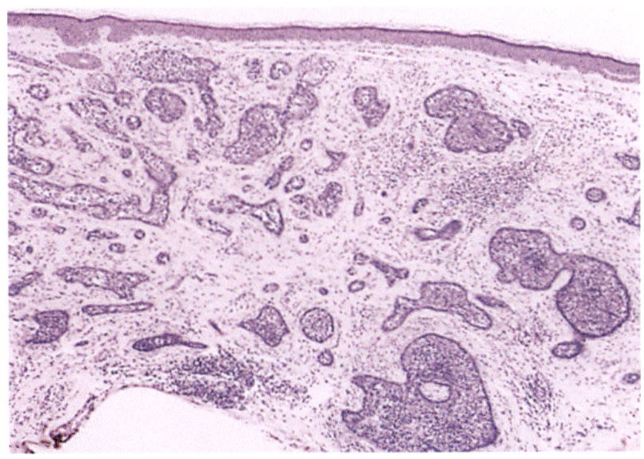

Fig. 12.134 Some lobules are rounded and some are irregular in shape

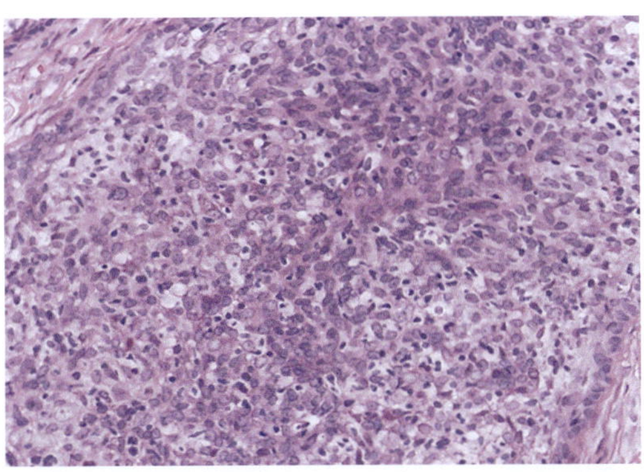

Fig. 12.135 Numerous small lymphocytes infiltrate tumor

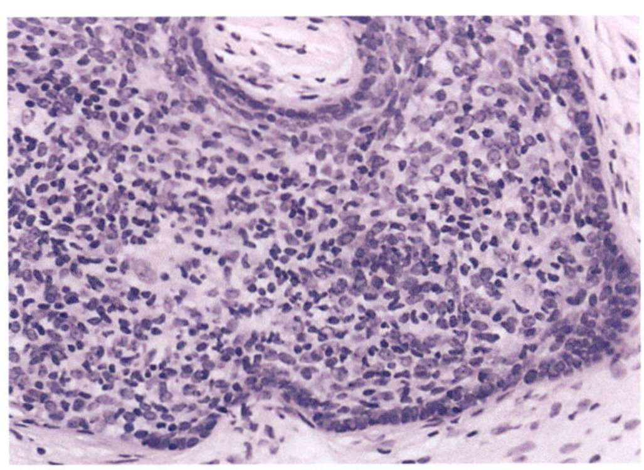

Fig. 12.136 Basaloid cells are palisading but there is no stromal retraction unlike in basal cell carcinoma

Lymphangioma

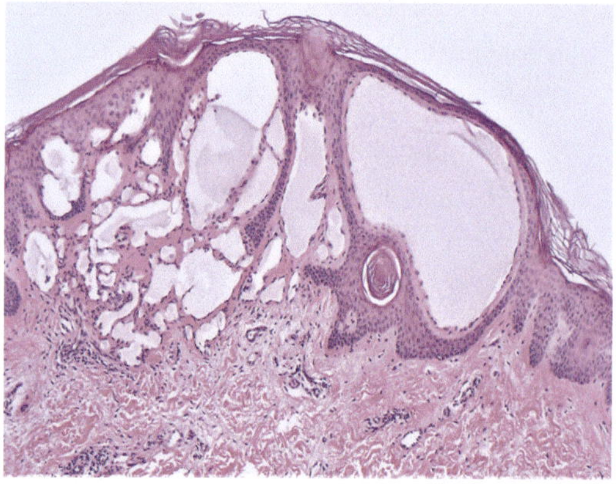

Fig. 12.137 Elevated atrophic epidermis covering dome shaped cystic tumor

Synonyms: Lymphangioma Circumscriptum, Cystic Hygroma

Histopathology (Figs. 12.137, 12.138, 12.139, 12.140, and 12.141)

- Ectatic lymphatic channels in the dermis (*lymphangioma circumscriptum and superficial lymphangioma*) or in the subcutaneous tissue (*cystic hygroma and cavernous lymphangioma*)
- Lymphatic channels with flaps are lined with flat, bland cells (D2-40+, CD31+, CD34+)
- Lumen is filled with delicate bluish acellular lymph and red blood cells can be present

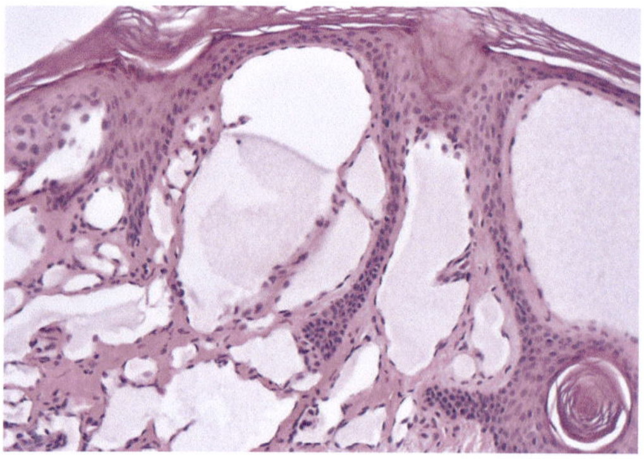

Fig. 12.138 Lymphatic channels lined with flat endothelial lining

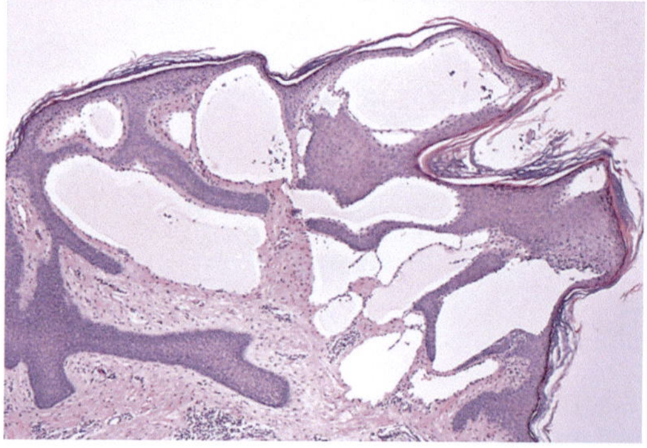

Fig. 12.139 Multiple irregular dilated lymphatic channels

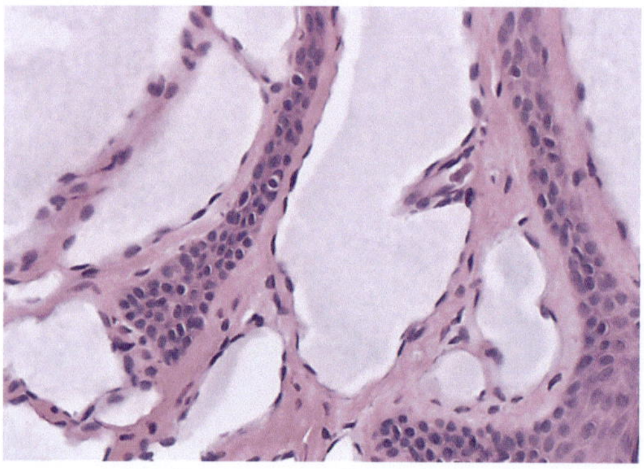

Fig. 12.140 Lymphatic flap projecting into the lumen

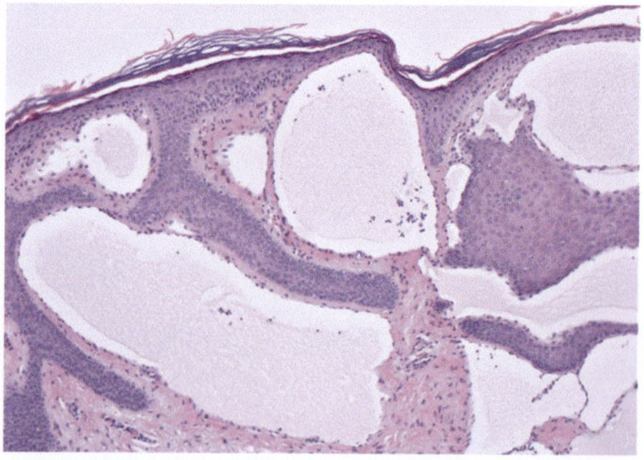

Fig. 12.141 The lumen is filled with delicate bluish lymph

Lymphedema

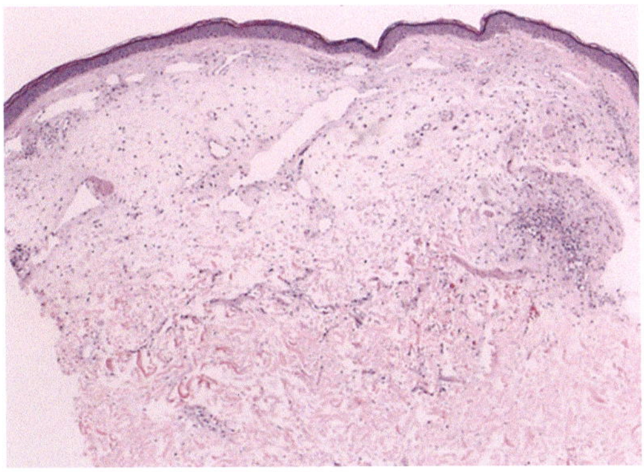

Fig. 12.142 Dermal and subcutaneous edema

Most commonly seen in cancer patients following a surgery to remove lymph nodes. Histopathology is different from one seen in massive localized lymphedema that is complication of morbid obesity.

Histopathology (Figs. 12.142, 12.143, and 12.144)
- Extensive dermal and subcutaneous edema
- Dilated lymphatic channels
- Fibroblasts appear "floating" in stroma

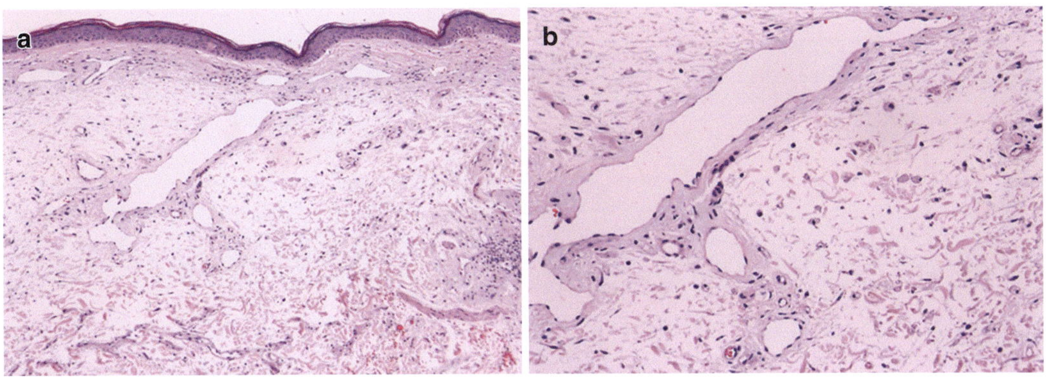

Fig. 12.143 (**a**, **b**) Dilated lymphatic channels with extensive edema

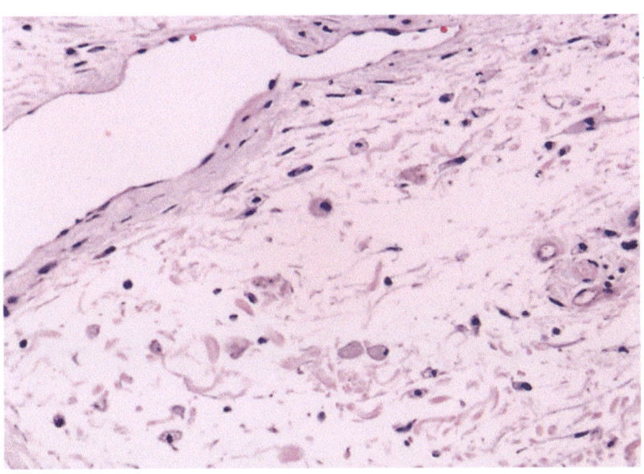

Fig. 12.144 Fibroblasts are "floating" in the loose pale stroma

Lymphoepithelioma-Like Carcinoma

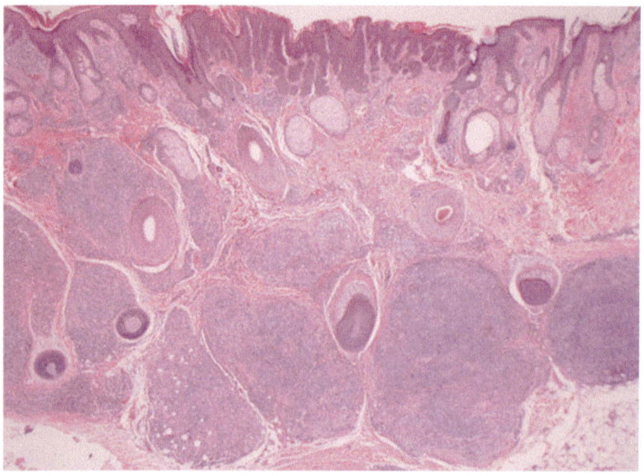

Fig. 12.145 Lobular tumor involving dermis and subcutaneous tissue

Histopathology (Figs. 12.145, 12.146, and 12.147)

- Lobulated tumor in dermis and subcutis
- Atypical cohesive epithelioid cells forming sheets (CK AE1/AE3+, p63+, EMA+)
- Mitoses are frequent
- Squamous differentiation is not a feature
- Adnexal differentiated can be seen
- Dense lymphocytic infiltrate (mixture of CD3 and CD20+ cells) obscures dermal epithelioid cells

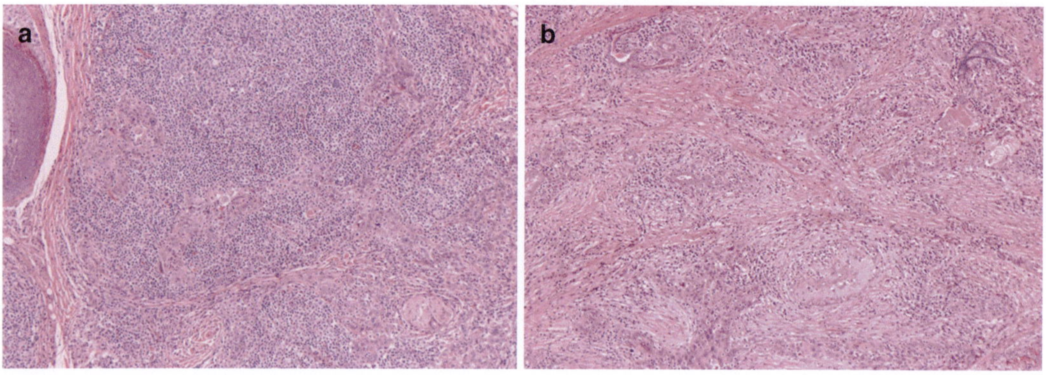

Fig. 12.146 (**a**, **b**) Epithelioid sheets obscured by lymphocytes

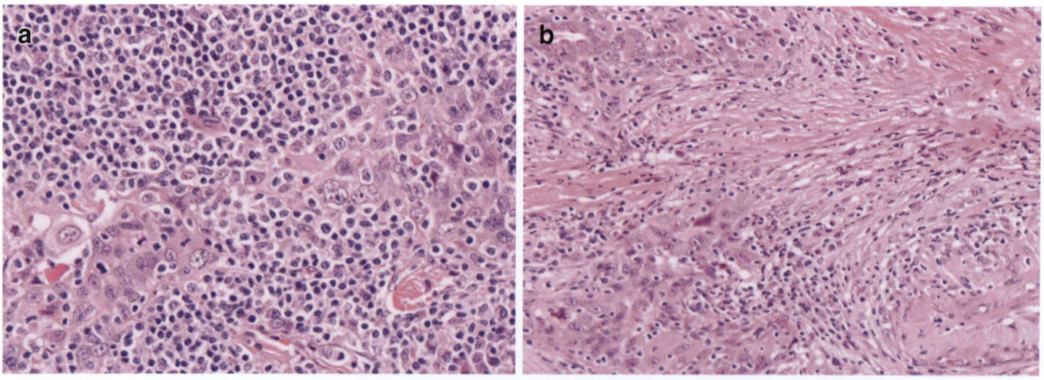

Fig. 12.147 (**a**, **b**) Epithelioid cells are cohesive and highly atypical with no clear squamous differentiation

Lymphogranuloma Venereum

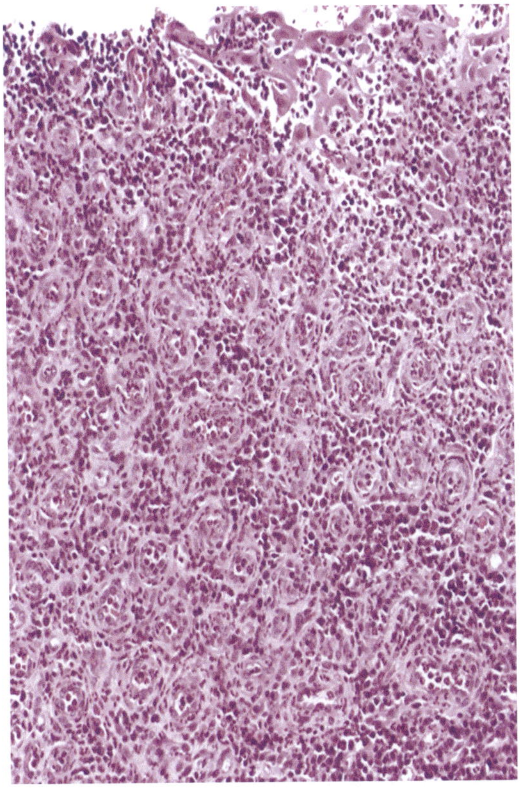

Fig. 12.148 Ulcer with exuberant granulation tissue

Histopathology

The 1st stage, consisting of ulcer is rarely biopsied:

- Ulceration with granulation tissue and numerous plasma cells (Figs. 12.148 and 12.149)

The 2nd stage consists of lymphadenopathy:

- Lymph node with multiple characteristic stellate necrotic microabscesses which may coalesce (Figs. 12.150 and 12.151)

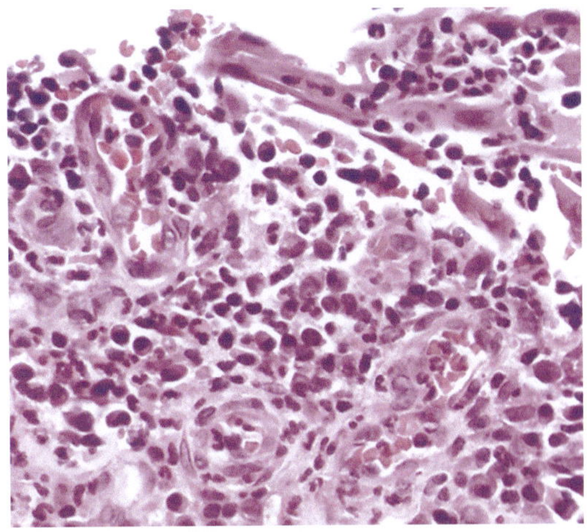

Fig. 12.149 Numerous plasma cells are present

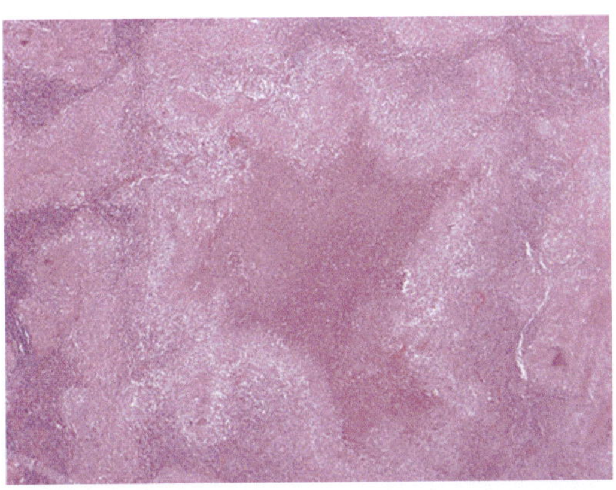

Fig. 12.150 Lymph node with stellate necrosis within an abscess

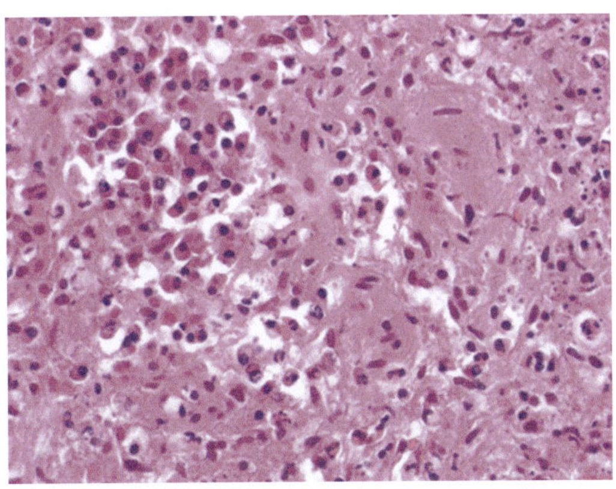

Fig. 12.151 Abscess with necrosis

Lymphomatoid Papulosis

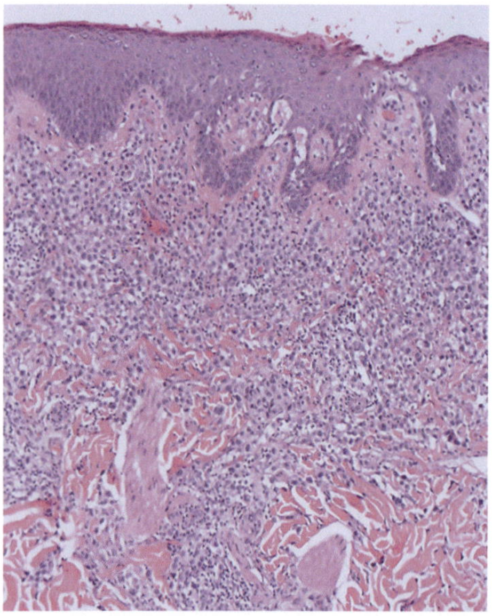

Fig. 12.152 **Type A** lymphomatoid papulosis with mixed cellular infiltrate

Four types (A, B, C, and D) characterized by CD30+ cells. Type A is the most frequent and **histopathology** is the most specific: (Figs. 12.152 and 12.153)

- Mixed population of superficial and deep lymphocytes (CD3 positive) admixed with larger pleomorphic atypical cells (CD30 positive, CD15 negative)
- Lymphocytic epidermotropism is focally present and eosinophils and red blood extravasation can be seen

Type B resembles plaque stage mycosis fungoides. (Figs. 12.154 and 12.155)

Type C resembles anaplastic large cell lymphoma.

Type D resembles CD8+ aggressive epidermotropic cytotoxic T-cell lymphoma

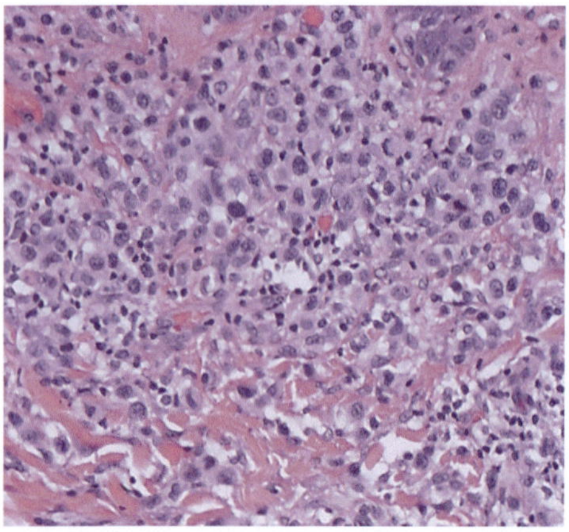

Fig. 12.153 Mixed cellular infiltrate made of smaller CD3 positive T cells and larger pleomorphic CD30 positive cells in **type A**

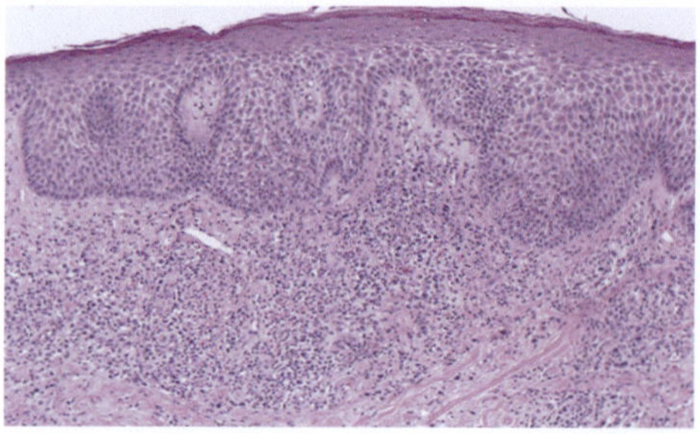

Fig. 12.154 **Type B** resembles MF with epidermotropism

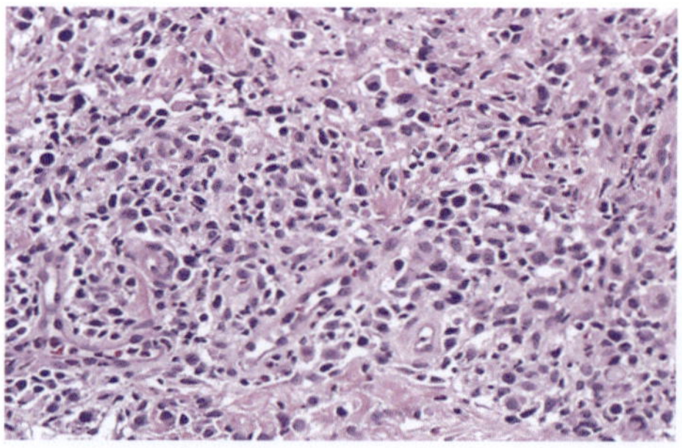

Fig. 12.155 Dermal small to medium size lymphocytes in **type B**

13 Dermatopathology M

V. Vincek, *Dermatopathology A–Z*, https://doi.org/10.1007/978-3-319-89486-7_13

Majocchi's Granuloma

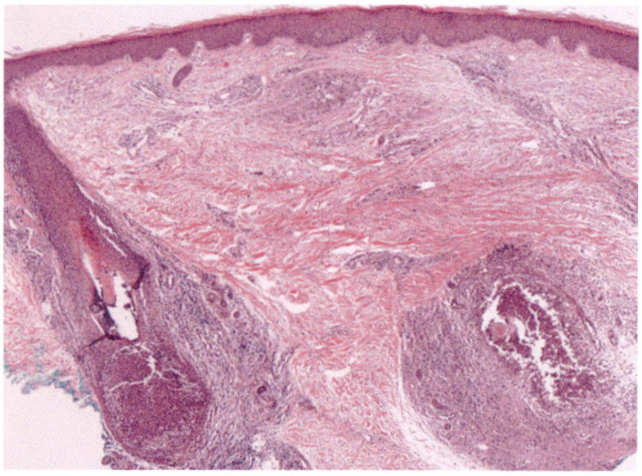

Fig. 13.1 Two ruptured acutely inflamed hair follicles

Synonym: Nodular Granulomatous Perifolliculitis

Histopathology (Figs. 13.1, 13.2, 13.3, and 13.4)

- Distorted, usually partially ruptured hair follicle
- Intense perifollicular acute neutrophilic inflammation
- Granuloma can be present
- Intrafollicular neutrophilic abscess
- Fungal spores and hyphae of dermatophytes are seen in and around hair shaft

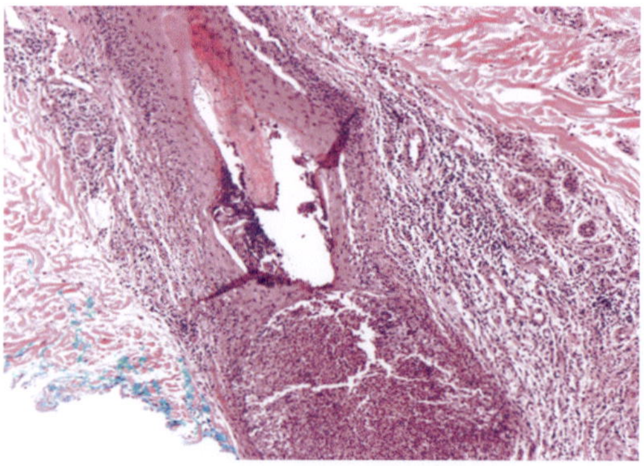

Fig. 13.2 Partially ruptured follicle with perifollicular and intrafollicular neutrophilic inflammation

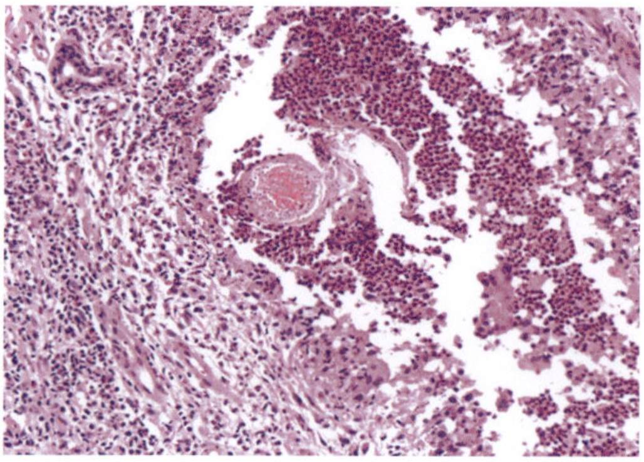

Fig. 13.3 Intrafollicular abscess around the hair shaft

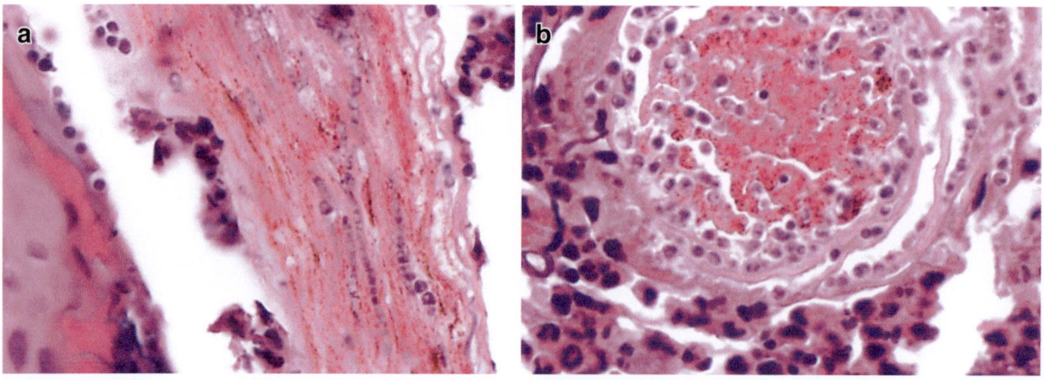

Fig. 13.4 (**a**, **b**) Dermatophyte spores and hyphae are present in the hair shaft

Malakoplakia

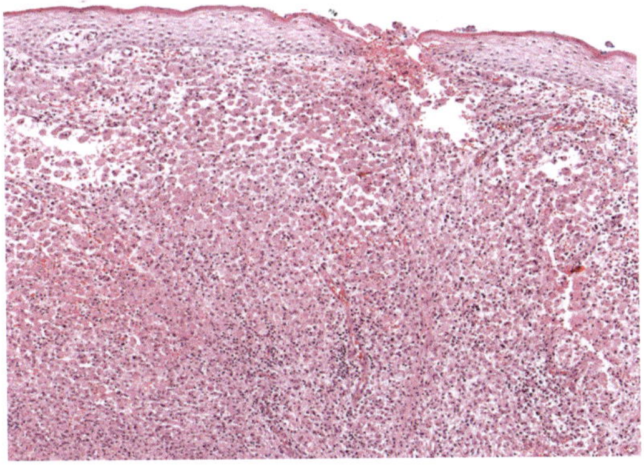

Fig. 13.5 Diffuse dermal and subcutaneous infiltrate

Histopathology (Figs. 13.5, 13.6, and 13.7)

- Diffuse dermal and subcutaneous histiocytic infiltrate (CD68+)
- Scattered lymphocytes and plasma cells
- Histiocytes have abundant granular eosinophilic cytoplasm (PAS+)
- Many histiocytes contain calcospherites inclusions (Michaelis-Gutmann bodies) that stain for iron and calcium and contain non-digested bacteria (usually *E. coli* or *Proteus*)

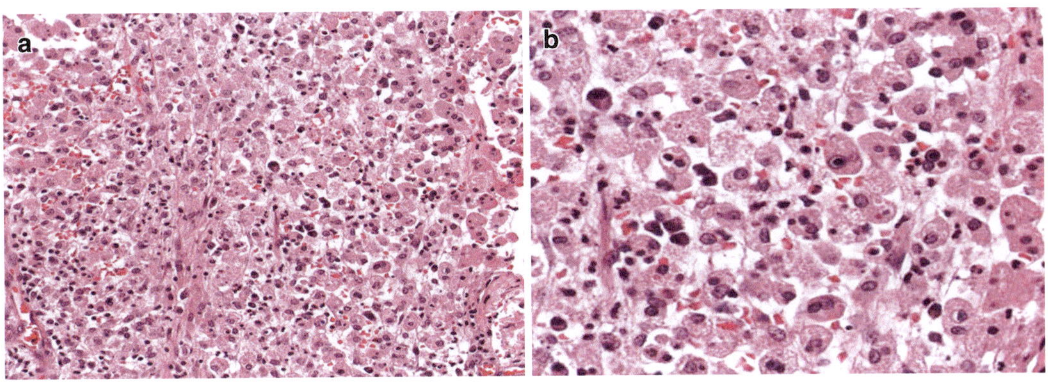

Fig. 13.6 (**a**, **b**) Histiocytes with abundant granular cytoplasm and inclusions admixed with lymphocytes

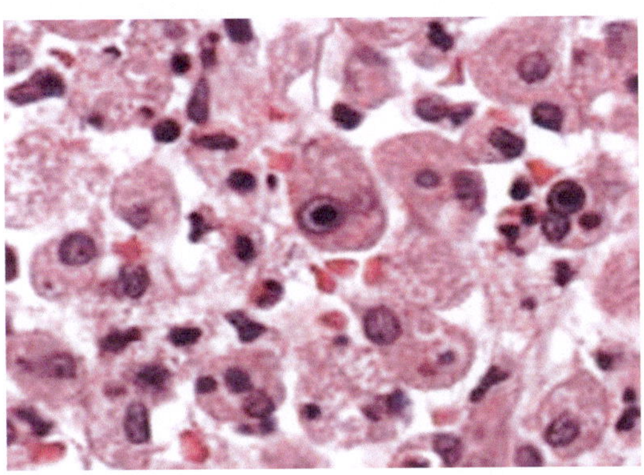

Fig. 13.7 Histiocytes with Michaelis-Gutmann bodies

Malignant Fibrous Histiocytoma

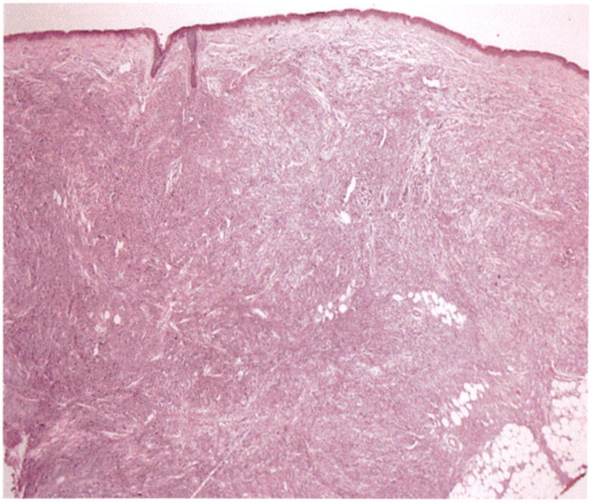

Fig. 13.8 Subcutaneous tumor extending to the dermis

Synonym: Undifferentiated Pleomorphic Sarcoma

Histopathological presentation with four types (Figs. 13.8, 13.9, 13.10, and 13.11)

Pleomorphic (the most common): subcutaneous tumor with storiform pattern formed by short fascicles made of bizarre pleomorphic cells and fibroblasts (CD68+, factor XIII+, CD10+)

Myxoid: same as pleomorphic but with at least 50% myxoid stroma

Giant cell: MFH with osteoclast-like giant cells

Inflammatory: pleomorphic MFH with extensive inflammation, xanthoma cells, and histiocytes

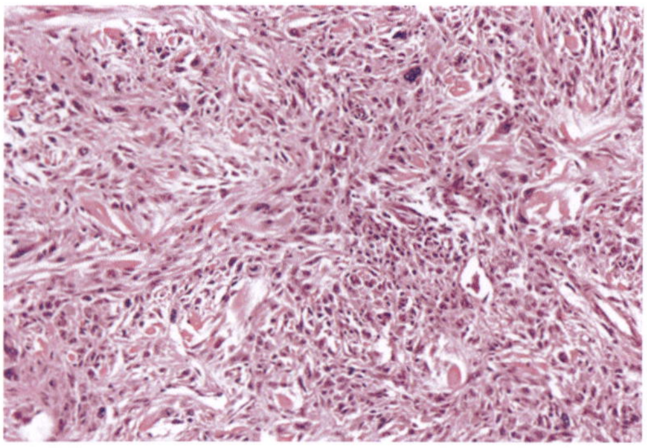

Fig. 13.9 Cellular tumor with bizarre cells and atypical fibroblasts

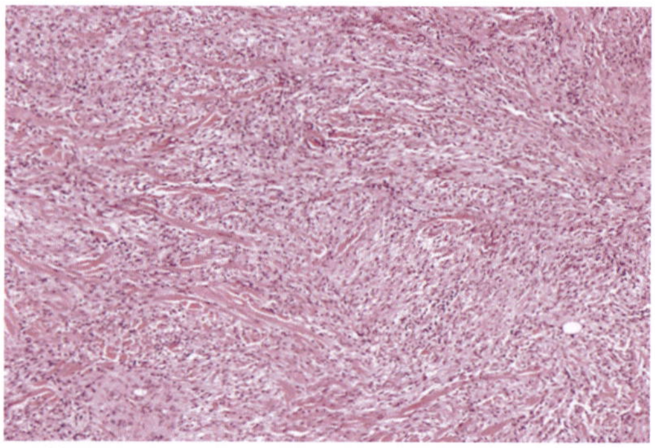

Fig. 13.10 Cells form fascicles organized in storiform pattern

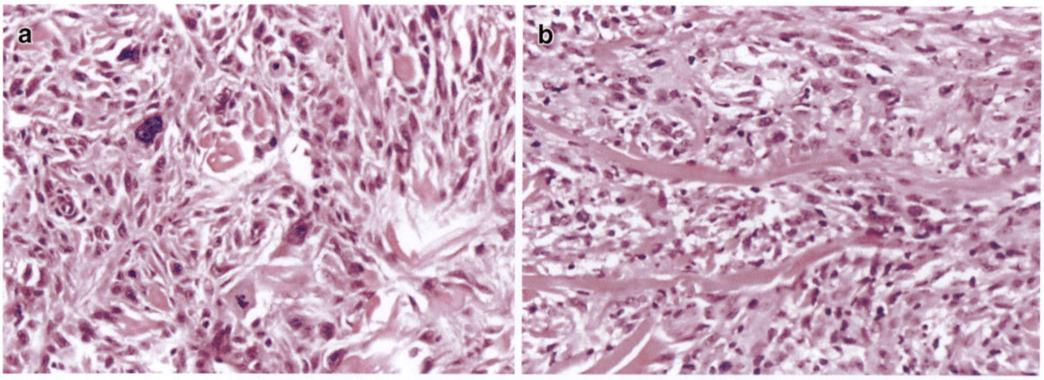

Fig. 13.11 (**a**, **b**) Tumor stroma is made of fibrotic collagen bundles

Malignant Peripheral Nerve Sheath Tumor

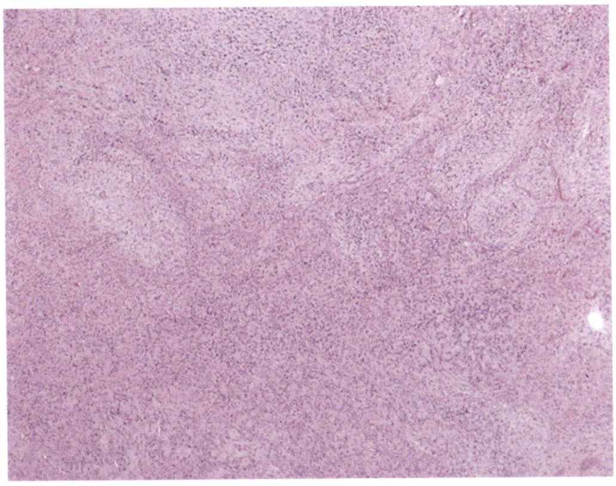

Fig. 13.12 Ill-defined spindle "marble-like" cell infiltrate

Synonym: Malignant Schwannoma

Histopathology (Figs. 13.12, 13.13, and 13.14)

- Fascicles made of elongated cells with wavy nuclei (CD99+, PGP9.5+, S-100 focally +)
- "Marble-like" hypercellular and myxoid hypocellular areas with vague nuclear palisading resembling Schwannoma and common mitoses and necrosis
- Heterologous elements such as bone and cartilage can be present; it is called **malignant Triton tumor** if rhabdomyosarcomatous bundles are present

P.S. 50% of cases are associated with NF

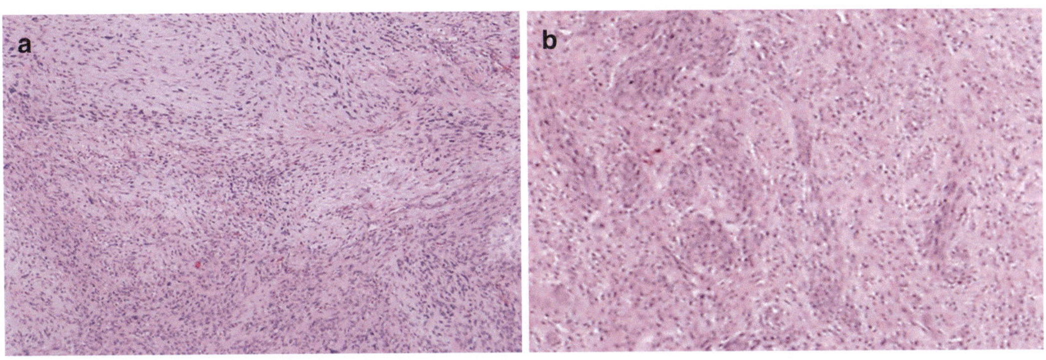

Fig. 13.13 (**a**, **b**) Dark hypercellular and pale myxoid hypocellular areas

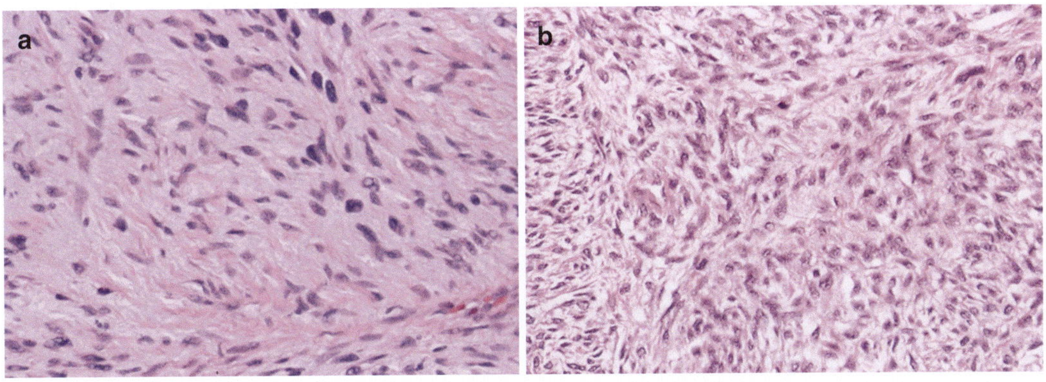

Fig. 13.14 (**a**, **b**) Pleomorphic spindle cells with vague nuclear palisading; scattered mitoses can be seen

Mastocytosis: Systemic

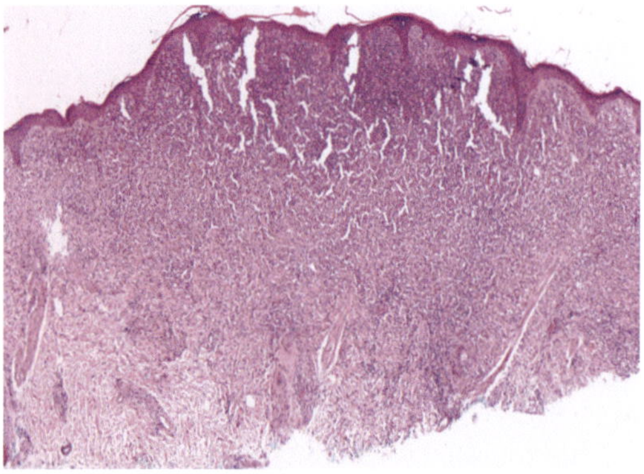

Fig. 13.15 Dermal infiltrate of uniform cells

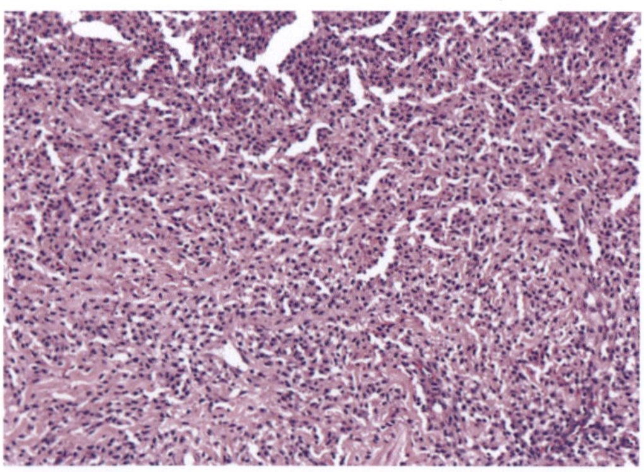

Fig. 13.16 Uniform mast cells with "fried egg" appearance

Systemic Mastocytoma, by definition, must have bone marrow involvement with more than 15 mast cells per aggregate.

Otherwise **histopathology** is identical to the one seen in *urticarial pigmentosa* with addition of solar elastosis (Figs. 13.15, 13.16, and 13.17)

- Diffuse dermal mast cells proliferation
- Mast cells are uniform with "fried egg" appearance (dark central nucleus and purple, finely granulated cytoplasm)
- Solar elastosis is present in surrounding normal dermis as lesion occurs mostly in adults
- Mast cells stain with Giemsa stain and toluidine blue stain special stains and mast cell tryptase and CD117 immunostains

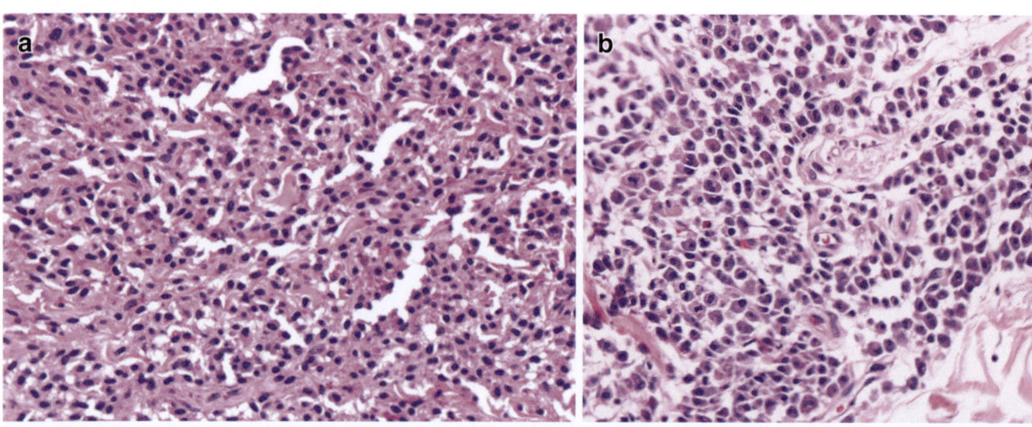

Fig. 13.17 (**a**, **b**) Mast cells have uniform dark nuclei and finely granular purple cytoplasm

Median Raphe Cyst

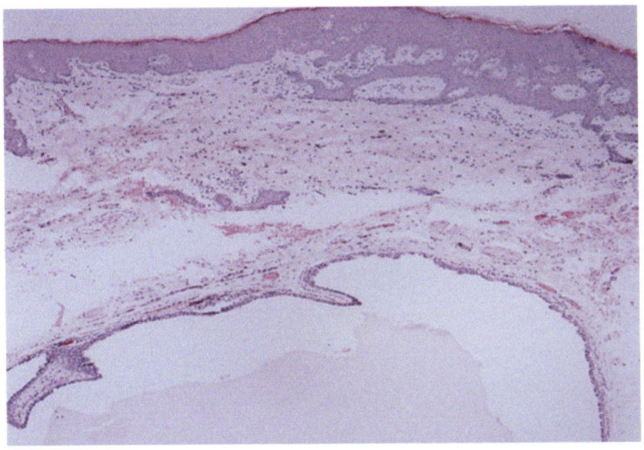

Fig. 13.18 Dilated cyst filled with eosinophilic, delicate, serous material

Histopathology (Figs. 13.18, 13.19, 13.20, and 13.21)

- Irregular cystic cavity that can be widely open or compressed
- Lining consists of a pseudostratified columnar epithelium
- Mucinous metaplasia can be seen
- Stroma vary from loose to dense

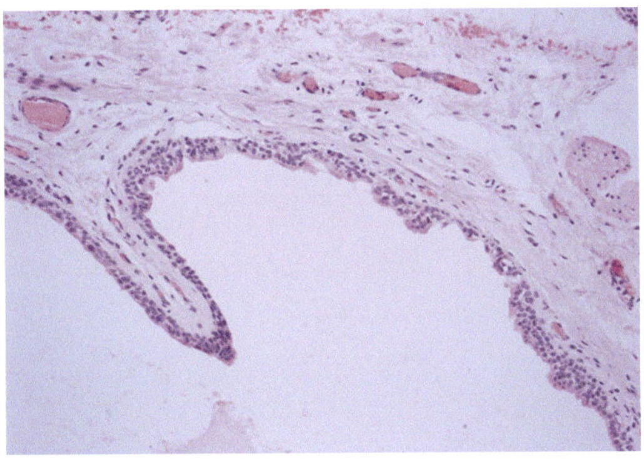

Fig. 13.19 Cyst wall surrounded by loose stroma

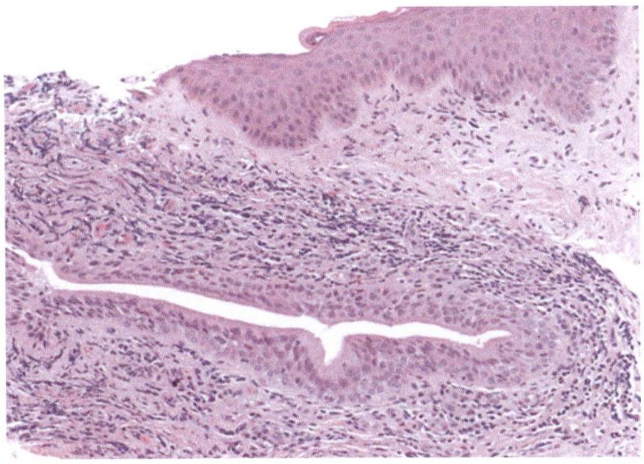

Fig. 13.20 Compressed cyst with dense stroma

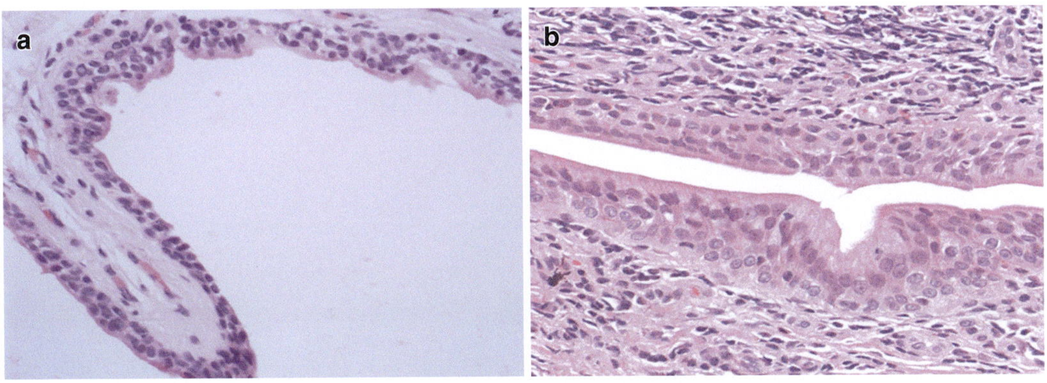

Fig. 13.21 (a, b) The cyst lining made of pseudostratified columnar epithelium

Melanoacanthoma

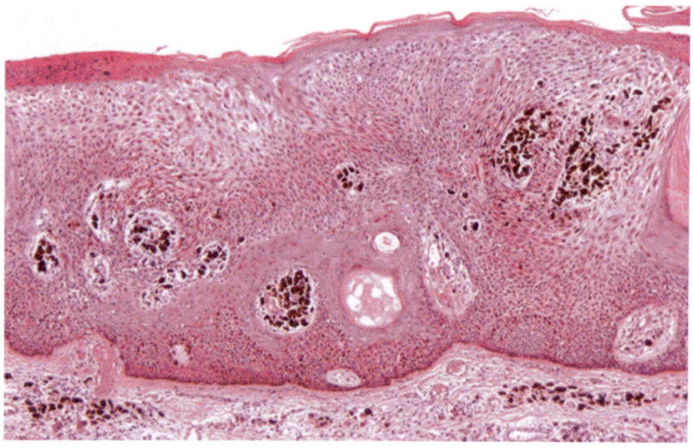

Fig. 13.22 **Melanoacanthoma of the skin** is pigmented seborrheic keratosis

Melanoacanthoma of the skin is pigmented seborrheic keratosis (Fig. 13.22).

Oral Melanoacanthoma is a different entity with unique **histopathology** (Figs. 13.23 and 13.24)

- Acanthotic oral mucosa with no granular layer
- Dendritic melanocytes in the epidermis with epidermal melanin globules
- Submucosal chronic inflammation with pigment incontinence

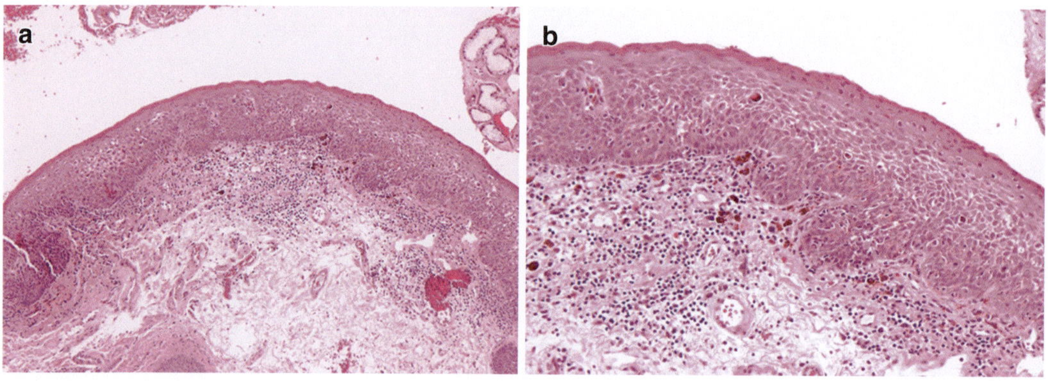

Fig. 13.23 (**a**, **b**) **Oral melanoacanthoma** with acanthotic oral mucosa that has prominent epidermal pigmentation. Submucosal chronic inflammation with pigment incontinence

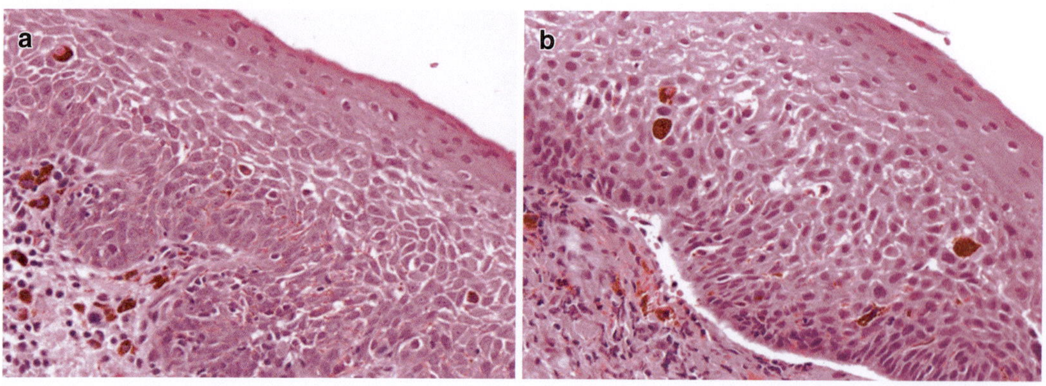

Fig. 13.24 (**a**, **b**) Oral mucosa with absent granular layer. Dendritic melanocytes with melanin globules are seen

Melanocytic Matricoma

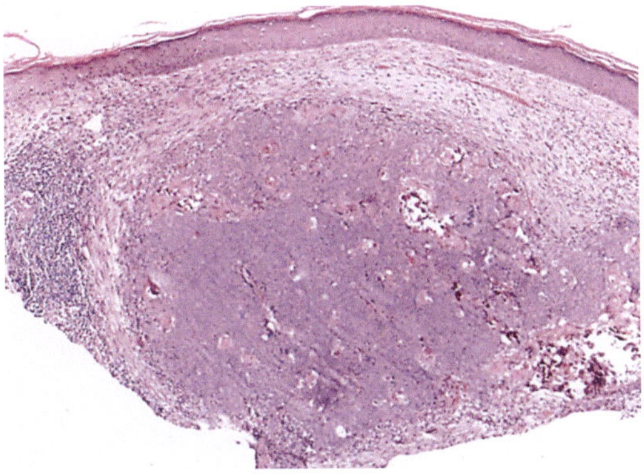

Fig. 13.25 Circumscribed dermal nodule

Synonym: Matricoma

Histopathology (Figs. 13.25, 13.26, 13.27, and 13.28)

- Well circumscribed dermal nodule with dual cell population
- Epithelial component of variable melanized matrical and supramatrical cells with shadow "ghost" cells admixed with dendritic pigmented melanocytic cells
- Cytological atypia and mitoses are present
- IHC demonstrates a mixture of cytokeratin positive cells and S-100/MelanA positive cells

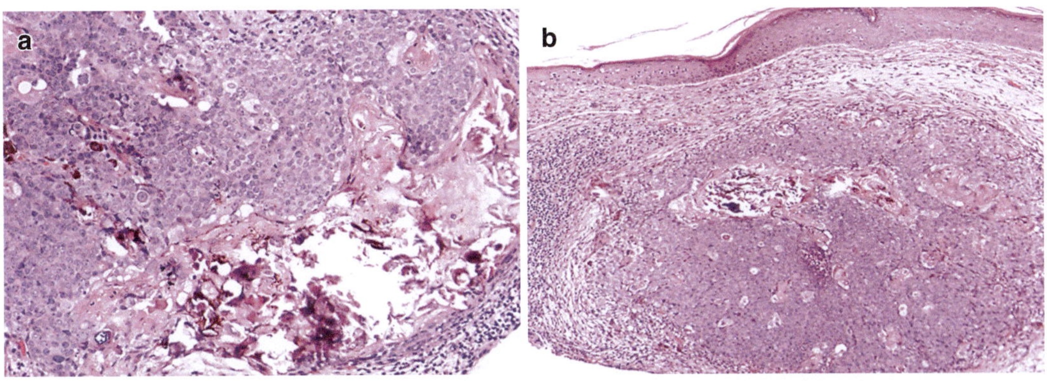

Fig. 13.26 (**a**, **b**) Basophilic cells admixed with eosinophilic "ghost" cells and scattered pigment

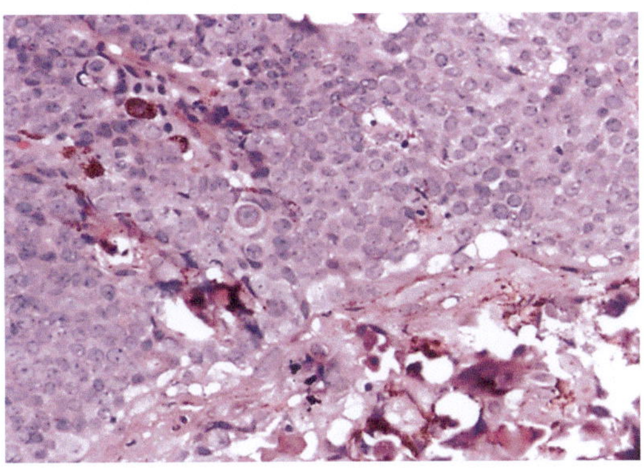

Fig. 13.27 Pigmented dendritic melanocytic cells are present

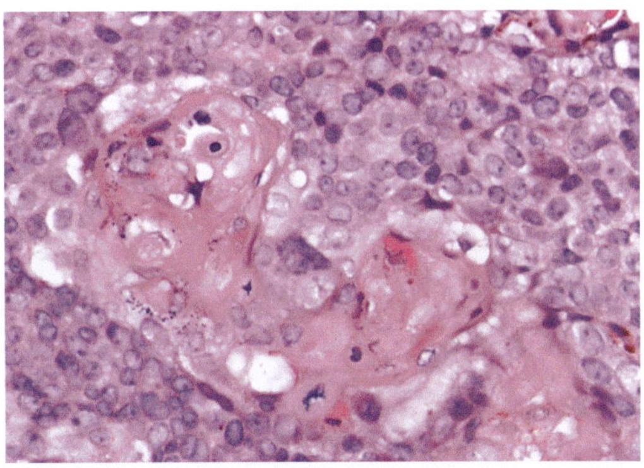

Fig. 13.28 Cytological atypia with scattered mitoses

Melanoma

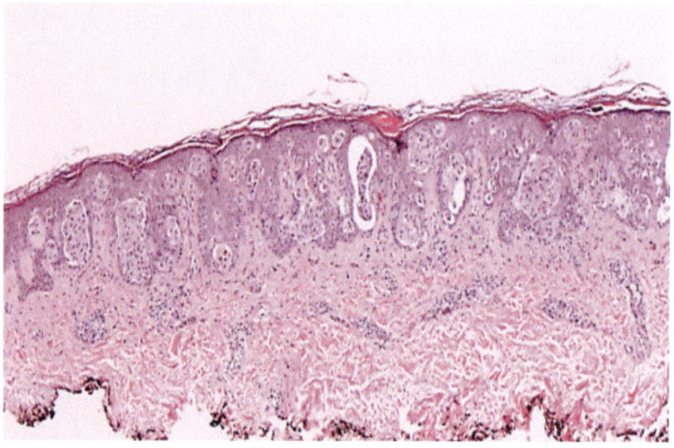

Fig. 13.29 In-situ melanoma

Histopathology varies depending on the type (see next four pages) but several features are in common:

- If present in the epidermis, malignant melanocytes cells try to consume epidermis either in a linear or pagetoid manner
- If present in the dermis, malignant melanocytes have similar histology at the top and the bottom of the lesion consistent with lack of maturation
- Cells demonstrate cytological atypia (Figs. 13.29, 13.30, 13.31, 13.32, 13.33, 13.34, 13.35, 13.36, 13.37, 13.38, 13.39, 13.40, 13.41, 13.42, 13.43, 13.44, 13.45, 13.46, 13.47, 13.48, 13.49, 13.50, 13.51, 13.52, 13.53, and 13.54)

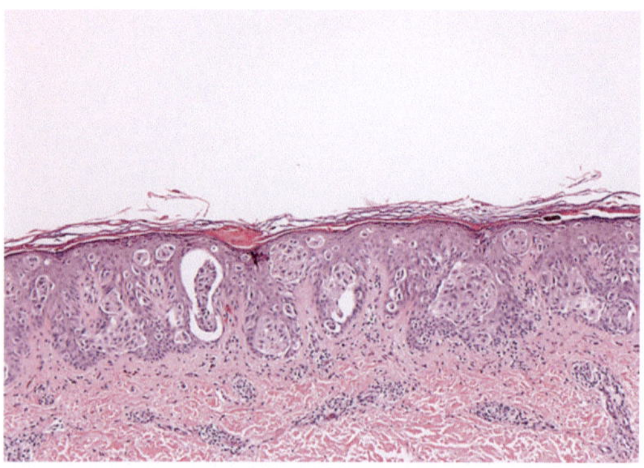

Fig. 13.30 Irregular junctional nests present in the tip of ridges but also in between. Numerous single cell melanocytes

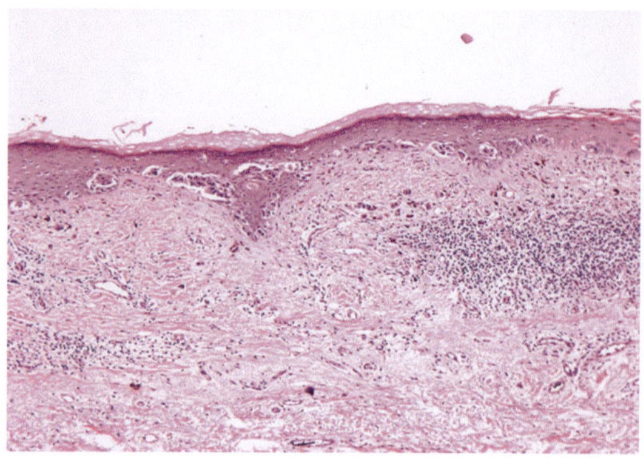

Fig. 13.31 Melanoma with signs of **regression**

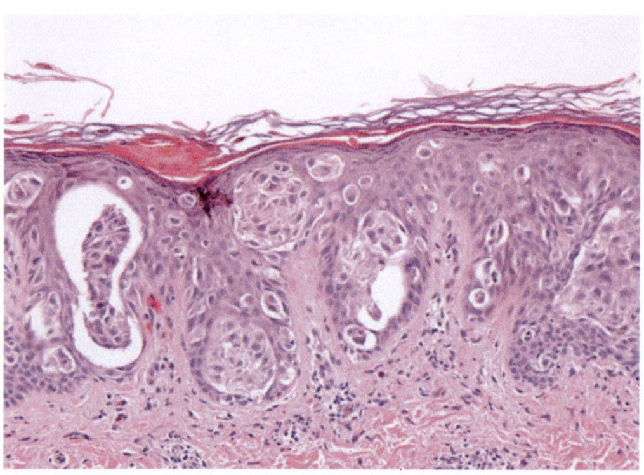

Fig. 13.32 Single melanocytes are scattered in pagetoid pattern. Individual cells are highly atypical

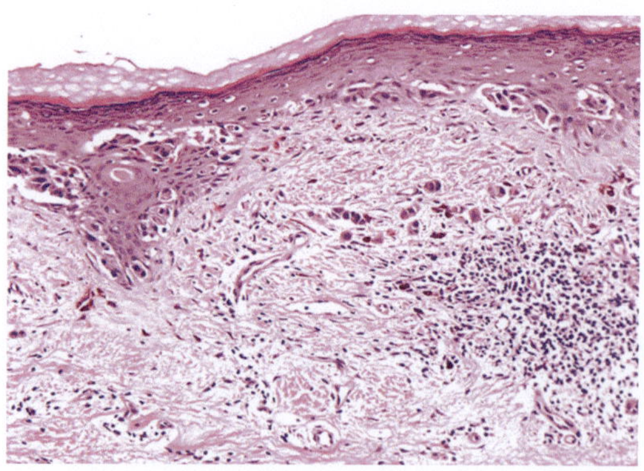

Fig. 13.33 **Superficial spreading melanoma** with dermal component. Junctional component is patchy. Dermal fibrosis and inflammation are present

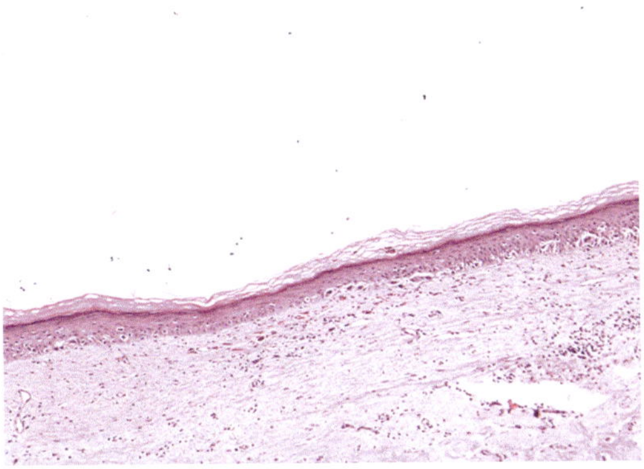

Fig. 13.34 Lentigo maligna melanoma

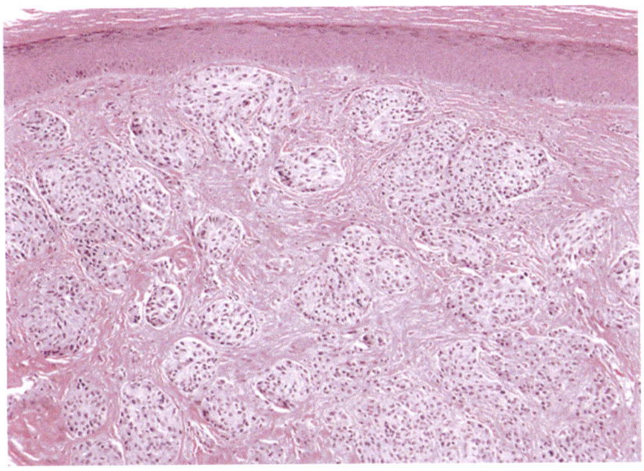

Fig. 13.35 Nevoid melanoma

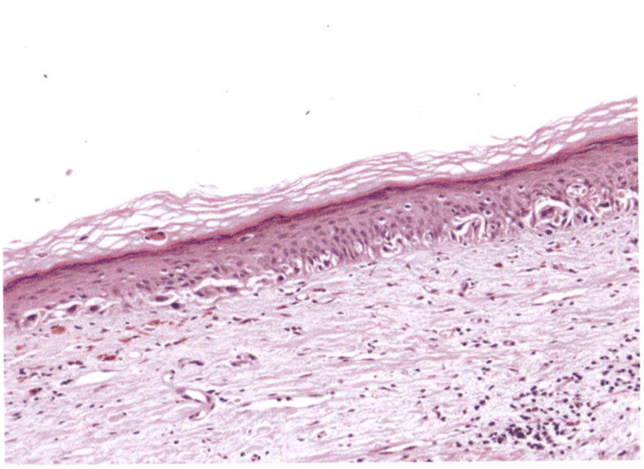

Fig. 13.36 Epidermis is atrophic and flattened

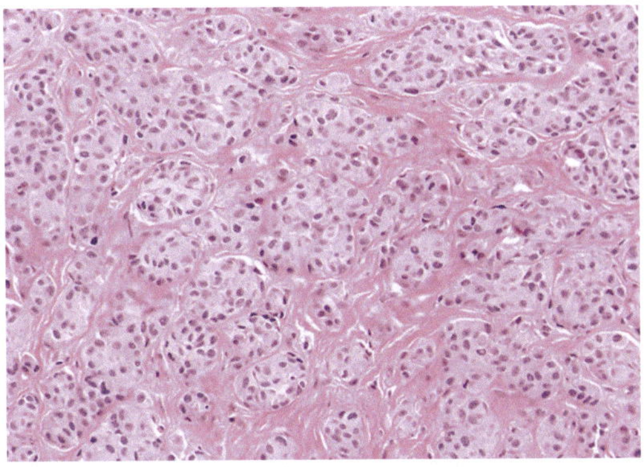

Fig. 13.37 Bland nevoid nests resembling dermal nevus. There is no evidence of dermal maturation

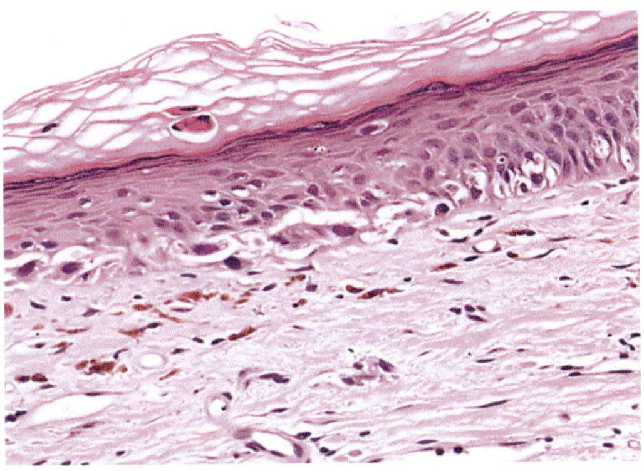

Fig. 13.38 Malignant melanocytes are predominantly along the epidermo-dermal junction

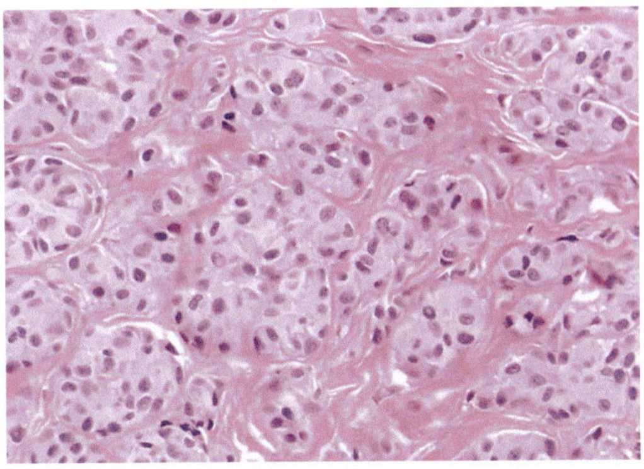

Fig. 13.39 Mitoses and apoptotic cells are present in the deep portion

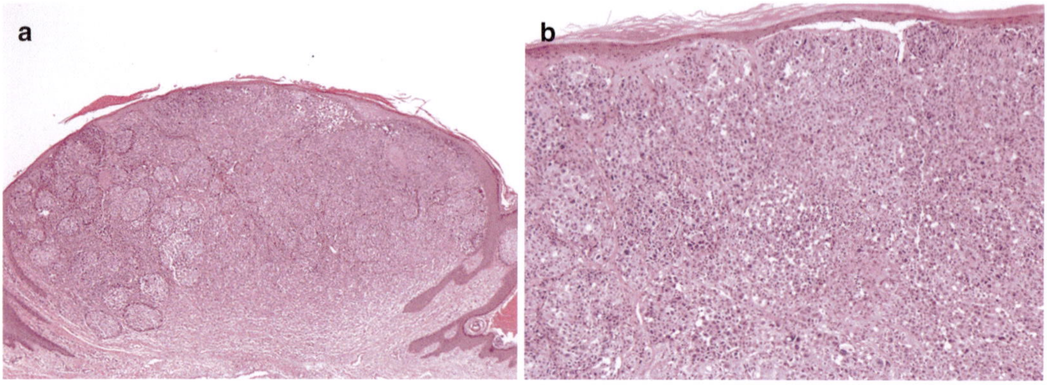

Fig. 13.40 (**a**, **b**) **Nodular melanoma** shows vertical growth so that epidermal involvement does not involve more than three epidermal rete ridges on either side of the nodule

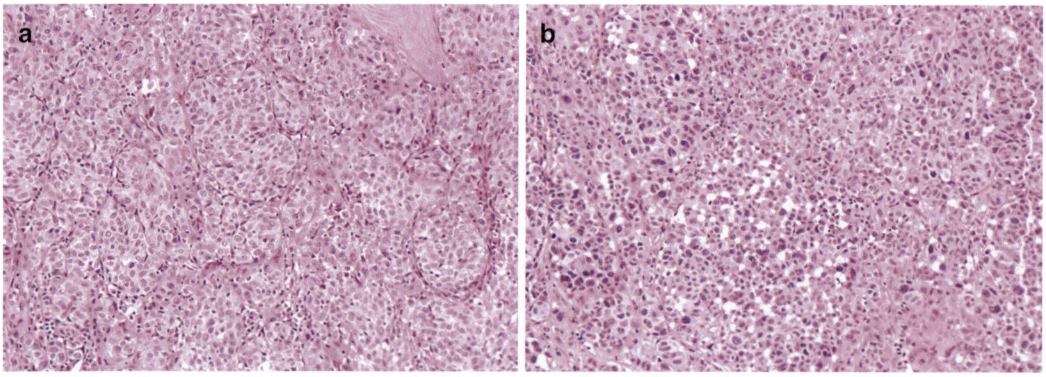

Fig. 13.41 (**a**, **b**) Tumor cells at the top and bottom of the nodule are of the same size indicating the absence of cell maturation

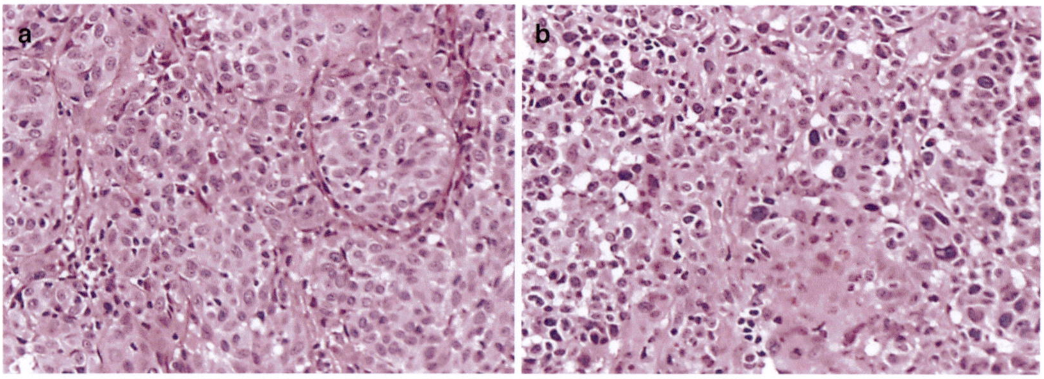

Fig. 13.42 (**a**, **b**) Cells have irregular nuclei with scattered apoptotic cells and mitoses

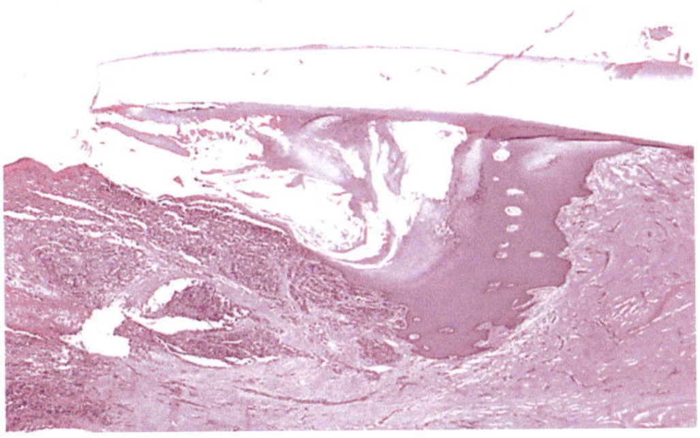

Fig. 13.43 Subungual acral melanoma

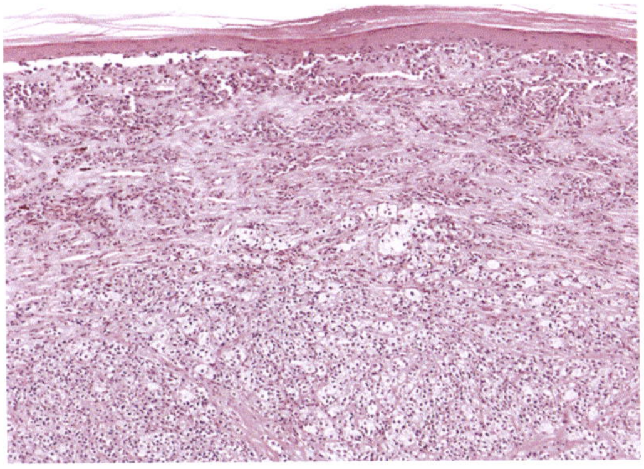

Fig. 13.44 Balloon cell melanoma in the dermis with regular superficial spreading melanoma in the epidermis

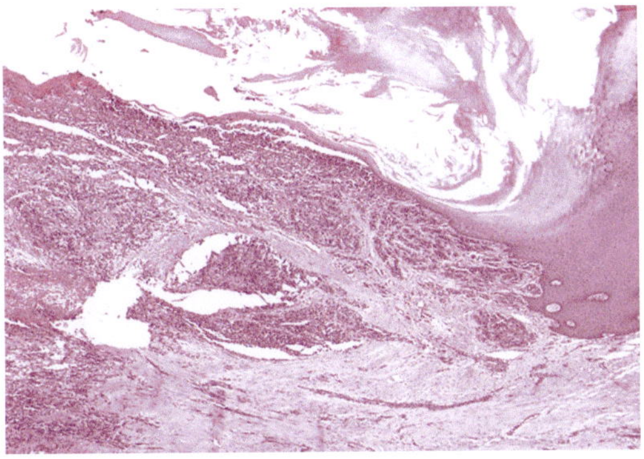

Fig. 13.45 Nail and nail bed with underlying melanoma invading dermis from the nail bed

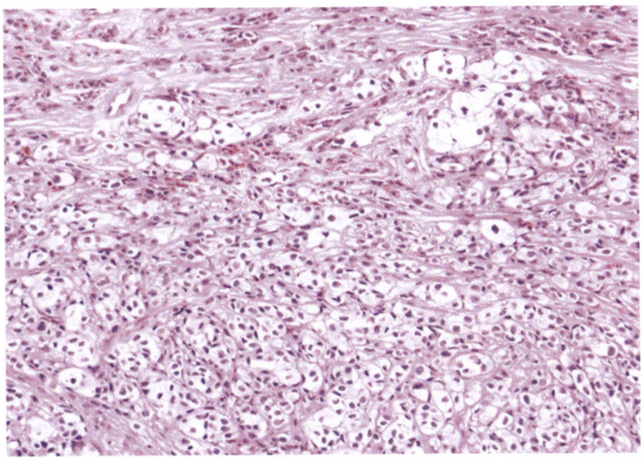

Fig. 13.46 Melanoma cells have abundant cytoplasm ("balloon-like")

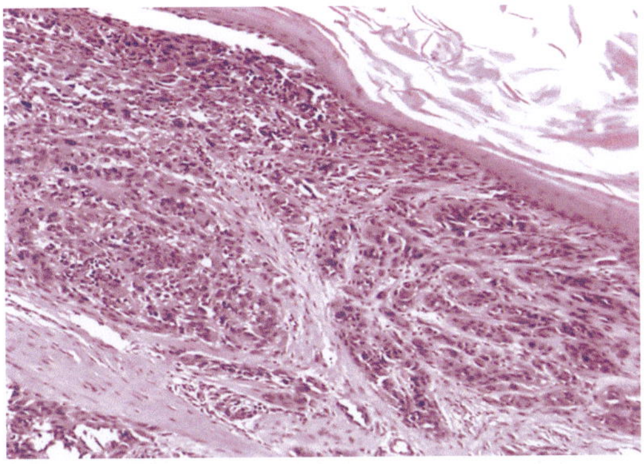

Fig. 13.47 Melanoma cells spread horizontally in nail bed. Pigment can be present in the nail itself

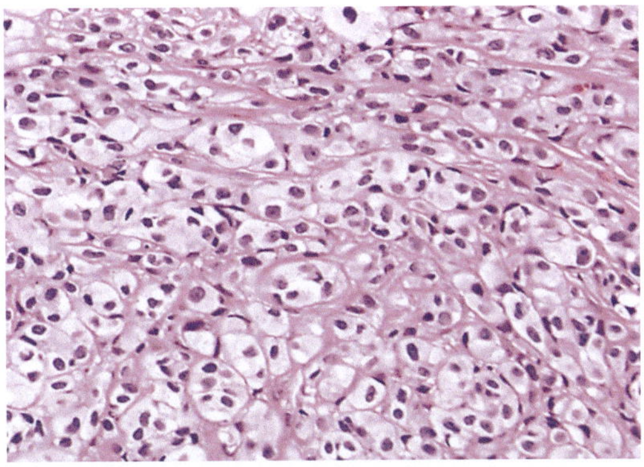

Fig. 13.48 "Balloon cells" have atypical nuclei and don't show signs of maturation

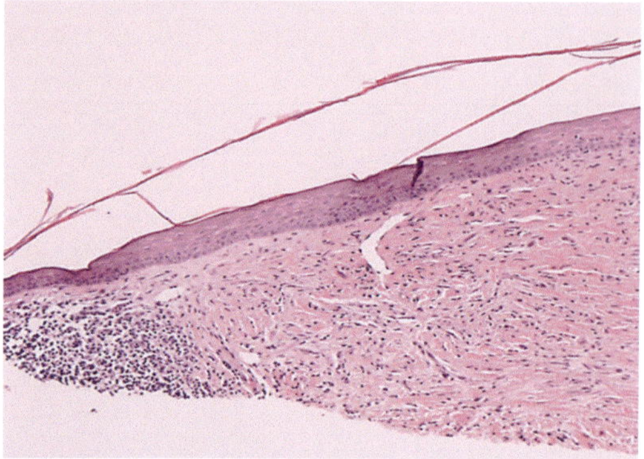

Fig. 13.49 **Desmoplastic melanoma** with scar-like appearance and characteristic adjacent lymphocytic aggregates

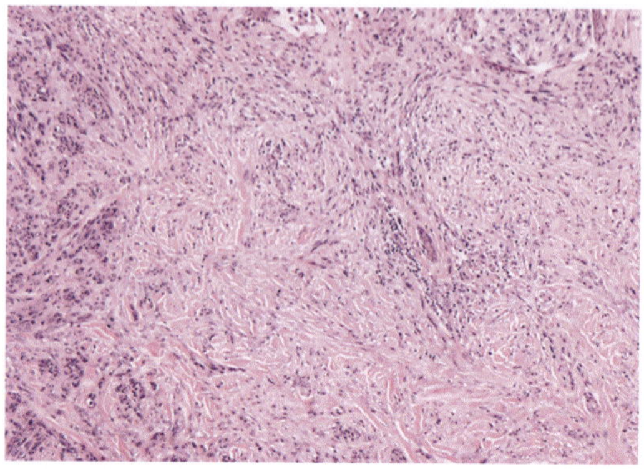

Fig. 13.50 **Spindle cell melanoma**

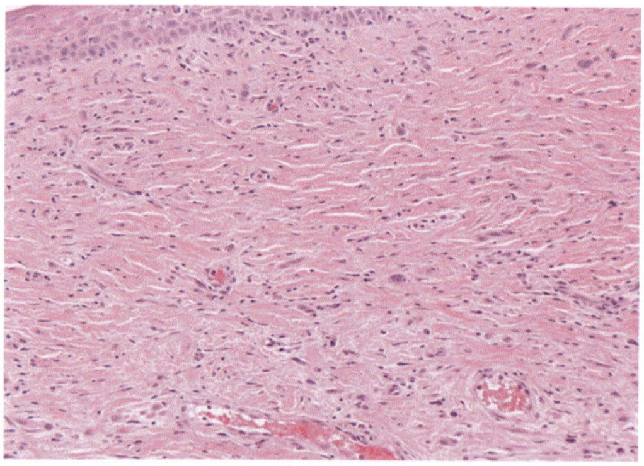

Fig. 13.51 The lesion appears hypocellular resembling dermal scar

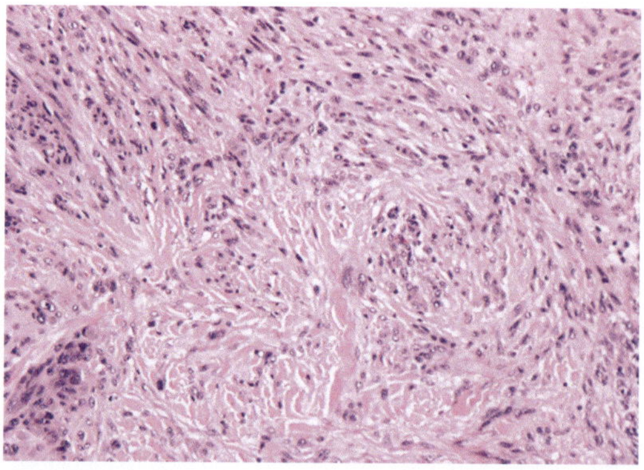

Fig. 13.52 Spindle cells forming irregular storiform pattern

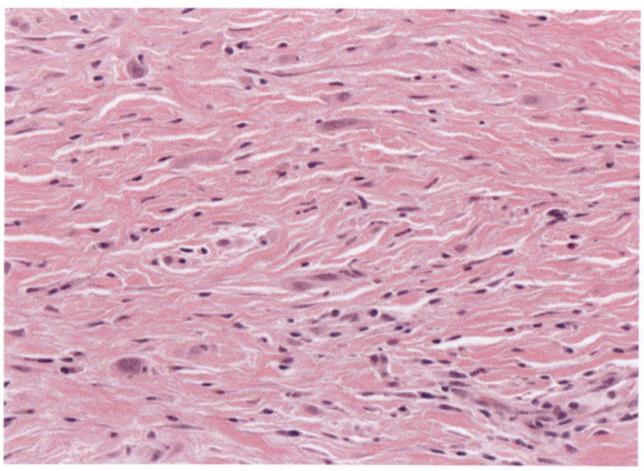

Fig. 13.53 Spindle cells with atypical nuclei that are S100+, SOX10+ but Melan A−, HMB45−

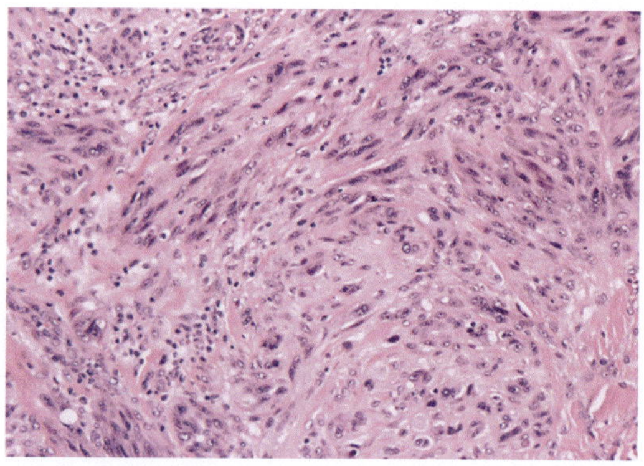

Fig. 13.54 Spindle cells have atypical irregular nuclei and scattered mitoses

Merkel Cell Carcinoma

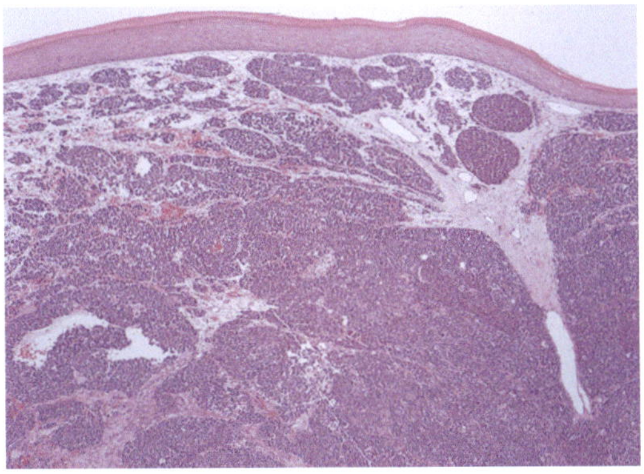

Fig. 13.55 Irregular nodules and sheets of basophilic tumor

Synonym: Neuroendocrine Carcinoma of Skin

Histopathology (Figs. 13.55, 13.56, and 13.57)

- Dermal infiltrate of small, round to oval uniform cells extending to the subcutis
- Tumor cells have scanty cytoplasm and dusky hazy purplish nuclei and form sheets and irregular nodules
- Mitoses and necrosis are common
- Tumor cells are cytokeratin 20, NSE, chromogranin, and synaptophysin positive

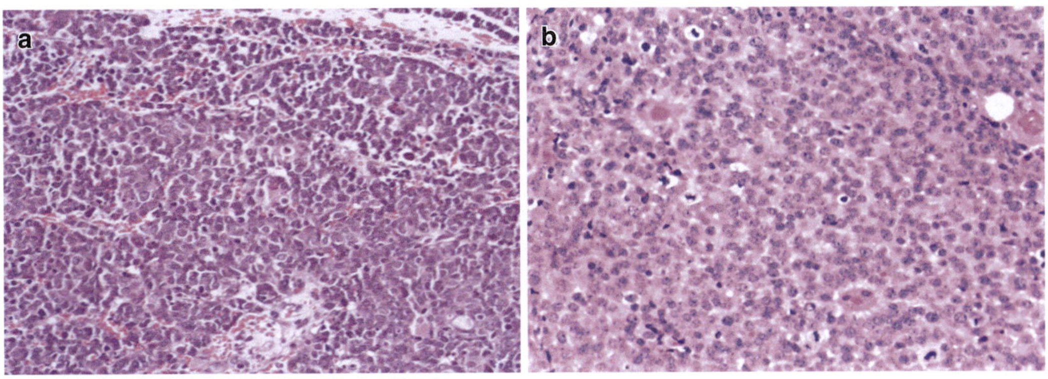

Fig. 13.56 (**a**, **b**) Cells with scanty cytoplasm and purplish hazy nuclei; nuclear molding of adjacent cells is present

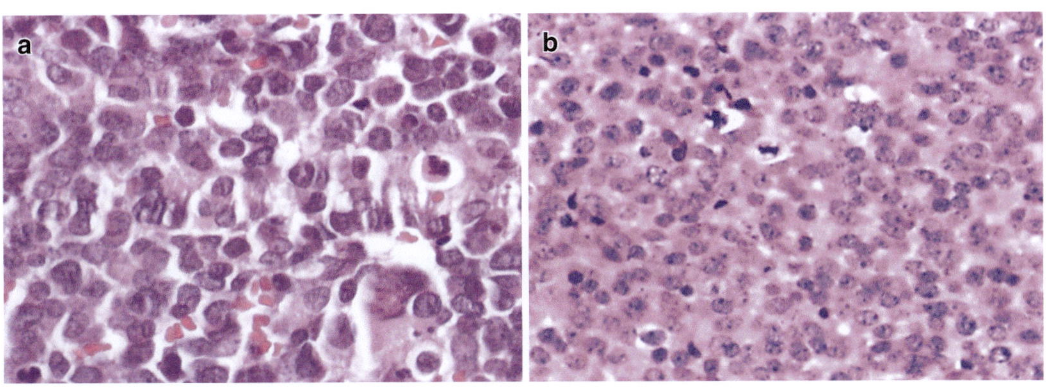

Fig. 13.57 (**a**, **b**) Numerous scattered mitoses can be seen

Meyerson's Nevus

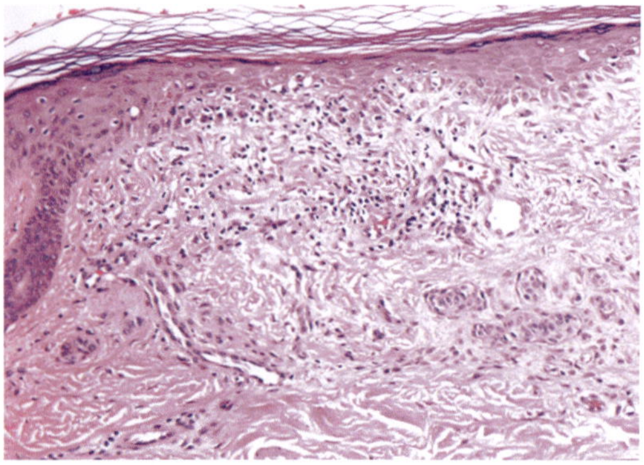

Fig. 13.58 Dermal nevus with spongiotic dermatitis

Histopathology (Figs. 13.58, 13.59, 13.60, and 13.61)

- Junctional, compound, or dermal nevus
- Epidermal spongiosis with hyperkeratosis and occasional parakeratosis
- Intraepidermal vesicle can form
- Dermal perivascular lymphocytic infiltrate
- Dermal eosinophils can be present

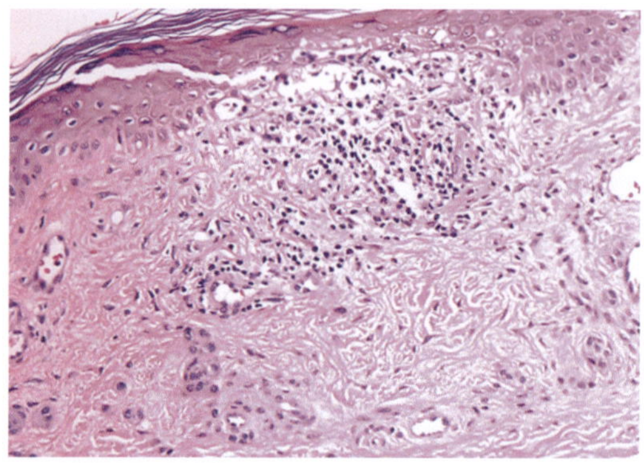

Fig. 13.59 Spongiotic dermatitis and nevus nests

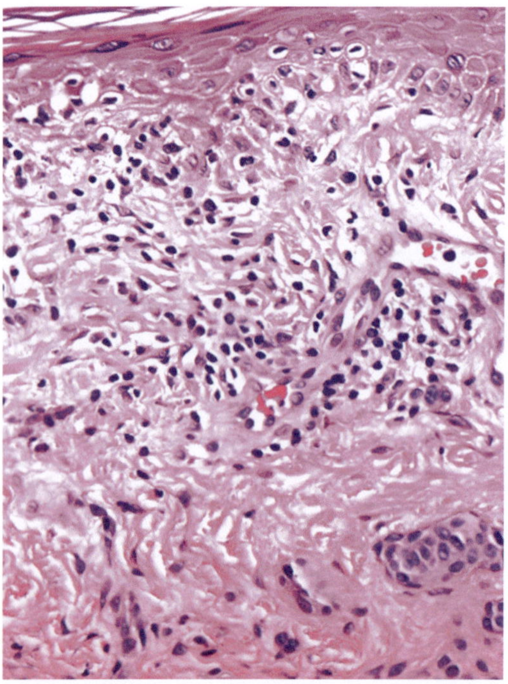

Fig. 13.60 Epidermal spongiosis and vacuolization. Dermal nevus and perivascular lymphocytic inflammation

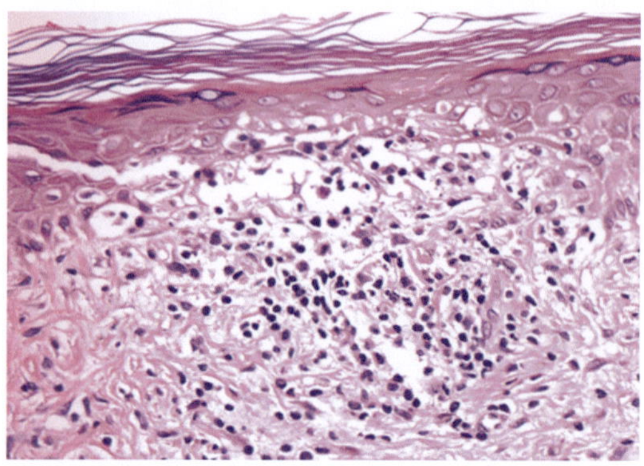

Fig. 13.61 Intraepidermal vesicles with dermal lymphocytes

Microcystic Adnexal Carcinoma (MAC)

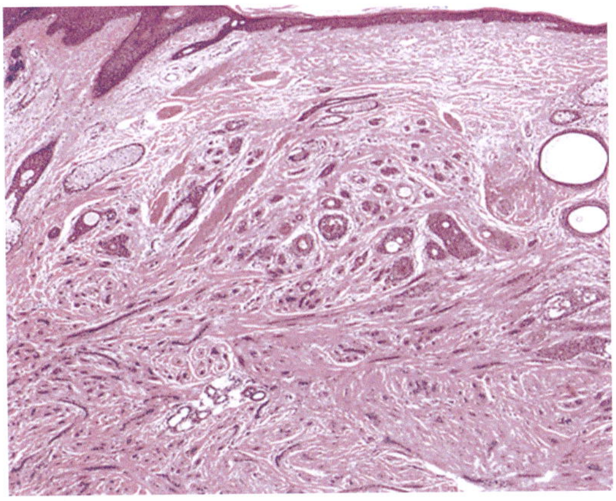

Fig. 13.62 Dermal tumor keratocysts and tumor ducts invading the subcutis

Histopathology (Figs. 13.62, 13.63, 13.64, 13.65, and 13.66)

- Tumor involves dermis and subcutis with small keratinous cyst and small ducts (EMA+, CEA+) more superficially
- Solid strands and cords of cells in sclerotic stroma infiltrate deeper subcutis
- Cytological atypia is minimal and mitoses are uncommon

P.S. *Syringoid Eccrine Carcinoma (SEC)* is probably a variant of *MAC* although some experts are separating them. In *SEC* some ducts have tadpole appearance with clear cell syringoid changes (Figs. 13.64 and 13.66)

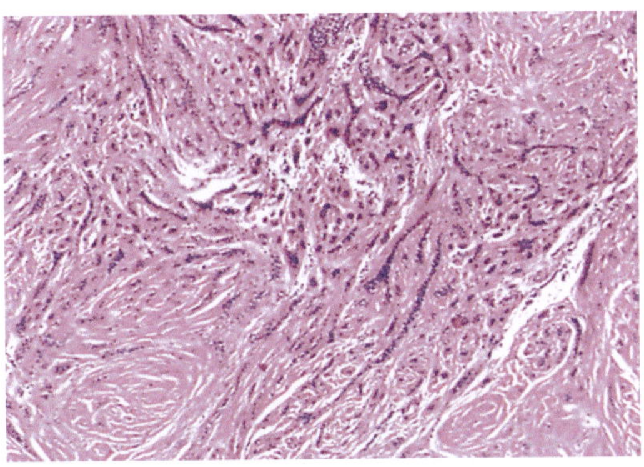

Fig. 13.63 Infiltrating tumor strands

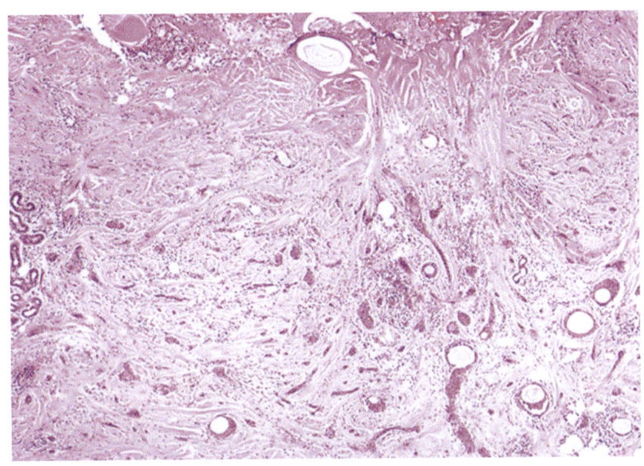

Fig. 13.64 Infiltrating SEC/MAC

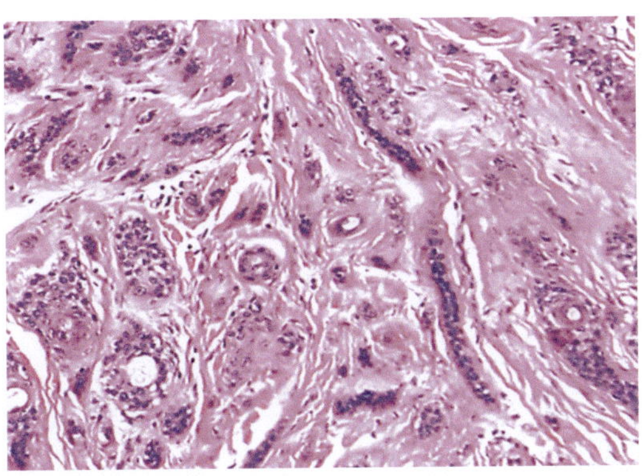

Fig. 13.65 Small ducts and narrow strands of relatively uniform cells in the sclerotic stroma

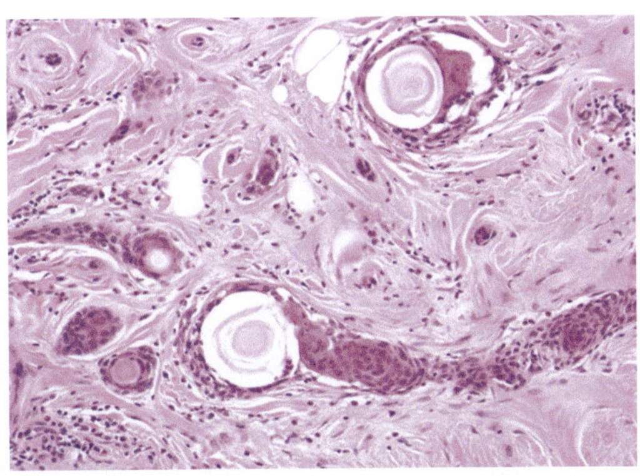

Fig. 13.66 Keratocysts and syringoid ducts with focal clear cell changes

Microscopic Polyangiitis

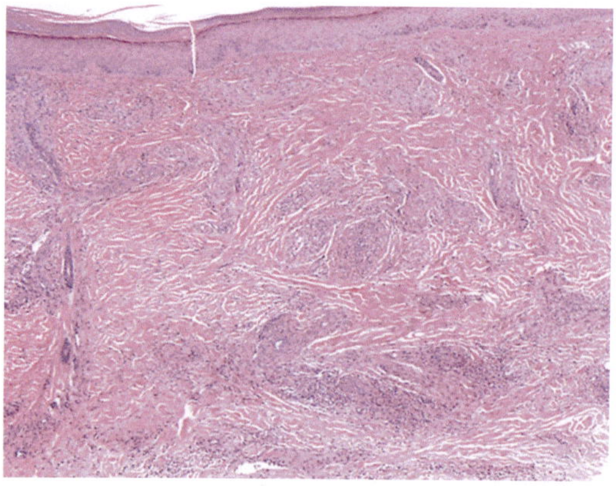

Fig. 13.67 Superficial and deep dermal perivascular inflammation

Synonym: Microscopic Polyartheritis

Histopathology (Figs. 13.67, 13.68, and 13.69)

- Present as small vessel cutaneous vasculitis with variable leukocytoclasia and associated glomerulonephritis and lung capillaritis
- Small arterioles, venules, and capillaries with neutrophilic inflammation and fibrinoid deposition
- Unlike LCV it also involves the deeper dermis and upper subcutis
- Medium size vessels are not affected unlike in Polyartheritis nodosa

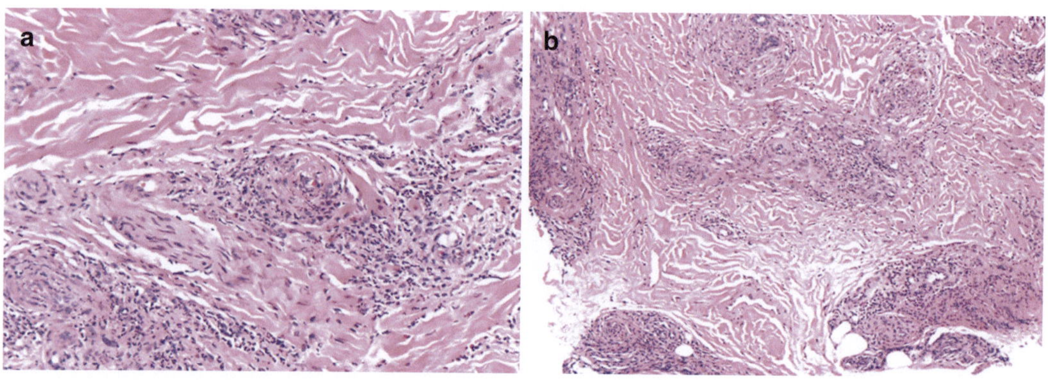

Fig. 13.68 (**a**, **b**) Neutrophilic inflammation affects capillaries but also small venules and arterioles

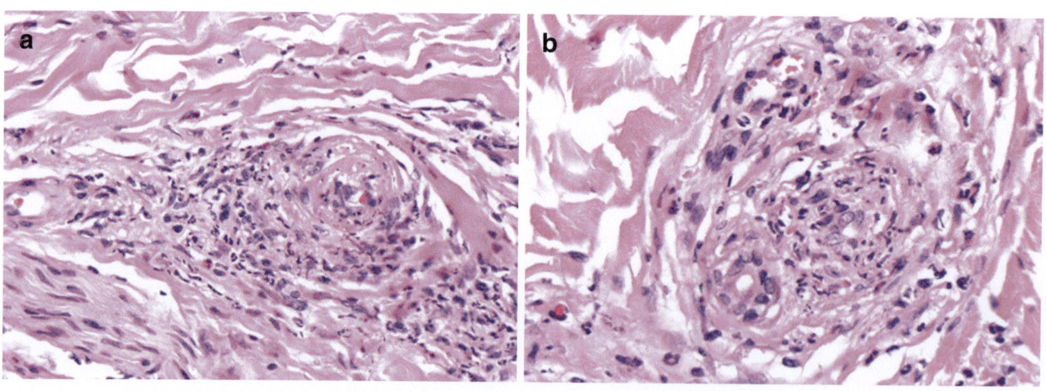

Fig. 13.69 (**a**, **b**) Perivascular neutrophils with fibrinoid necrosis and neutrophils within the vessel wall

Migratory Glossitis

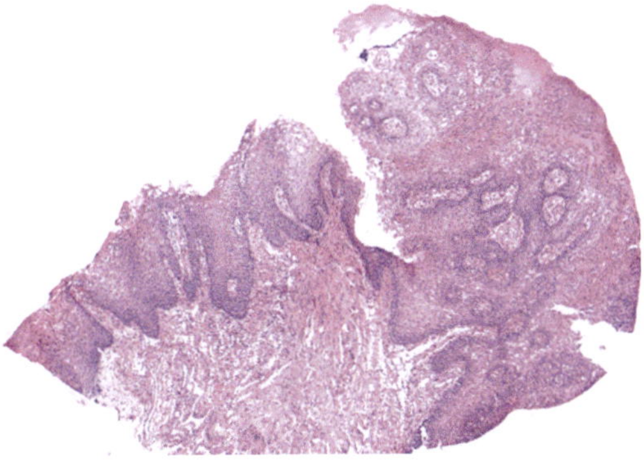

Fig. 13.70 Irregular acanthotic psoriasiform squamous mucosa

Synonym: Geographic Stomatitis

Histopathology (Figs. 13.70, 13.71, and 13.72)

- Mildly spongiotic irregular psoriasiform epithelial mucosa
- Neutrophilic aggregates forming pustules in the superficial epithelium
- Submucosal neutrophilic inflammation

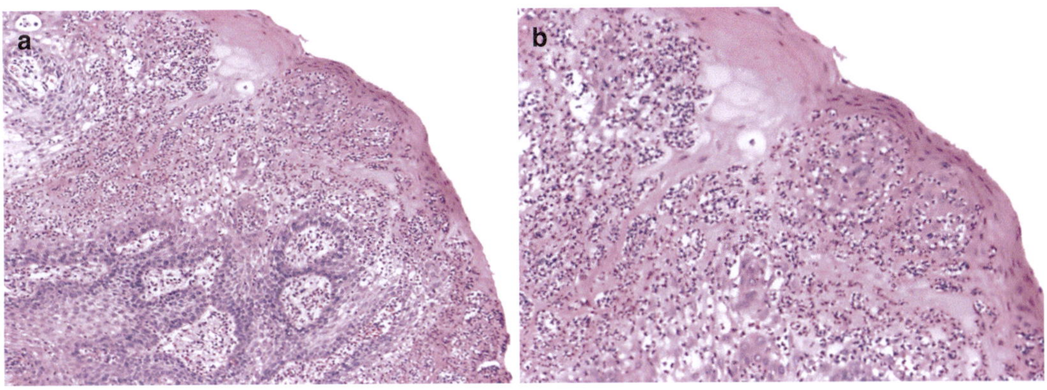

Fig. 13.71 (**a**, **b**) Neutrophils infiltrate the epithelium and form a pustule in the superficial portion

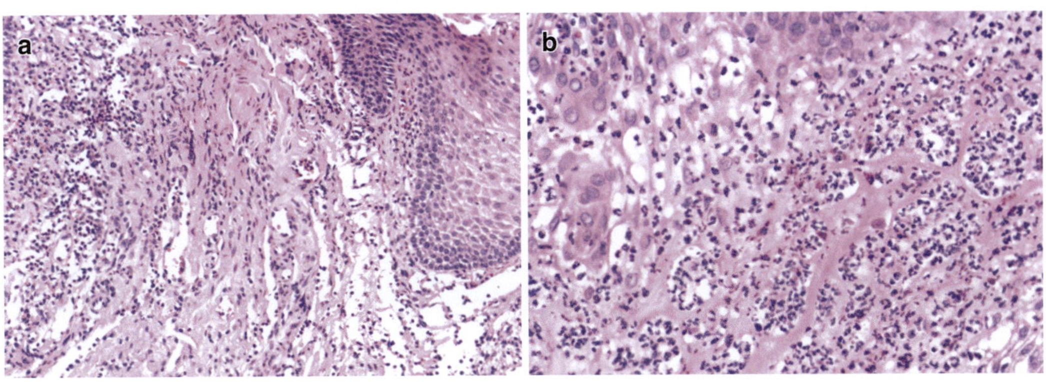

Fig. 13.72 (**a**, **b**) Neutrophils are present in the spongiotic epithelium and underlying submucosa

Miliaria

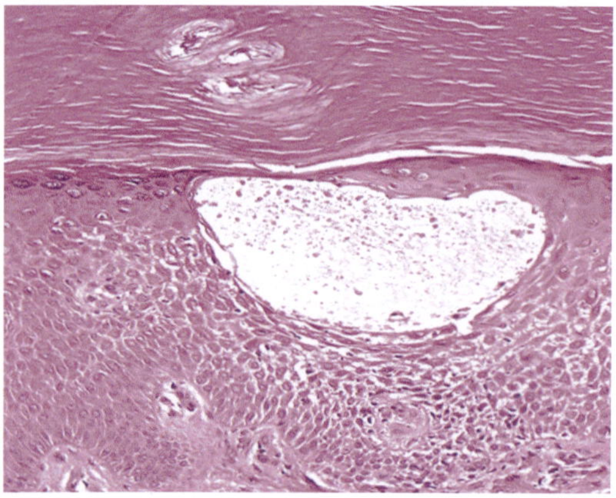

Fig. 13.73 Intraepidermal vesicle within the sweat duct

Histopathology

M. Crystalina: subcorneal "cell poor" vesicle associated with sweat duct in mildly spongiotic adjacent epidermis (Fig. 13.73)

M. Rubra: the same as *M. crystalina* but vesicle is within the stratum spinosum (Figs. 13.74 and 13.75)

M. Pustulosa: the same as *M. rubra* with neutrophils (Figs. 13.76 and 13.77)

M. Profunda: subepidermal vesicle associated with sweat duct

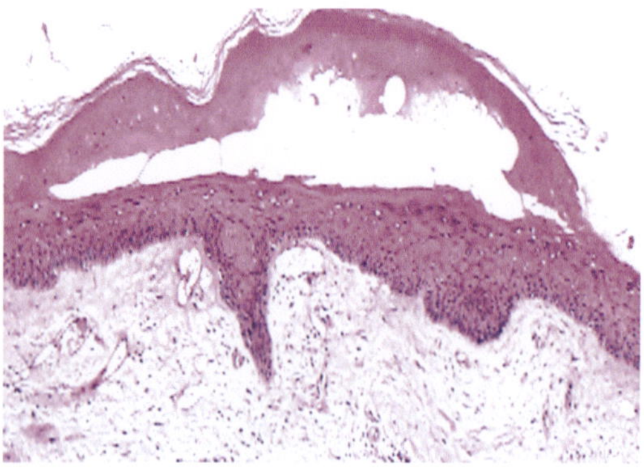

Fig. 13.74 M. crystalina/rubra

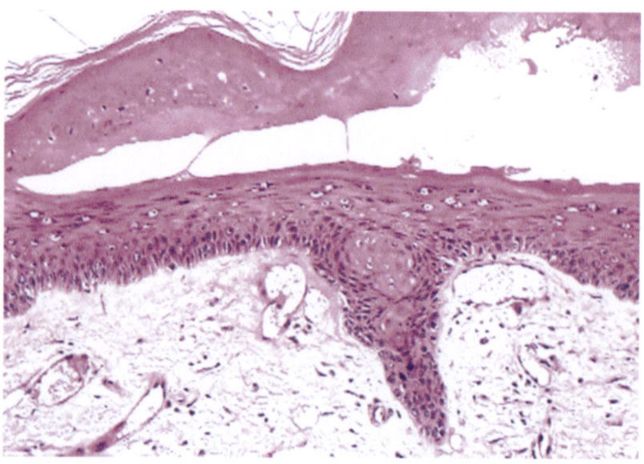

Fig. 13.75 Sweat duct associated intraepidermal vesicle without inflammation

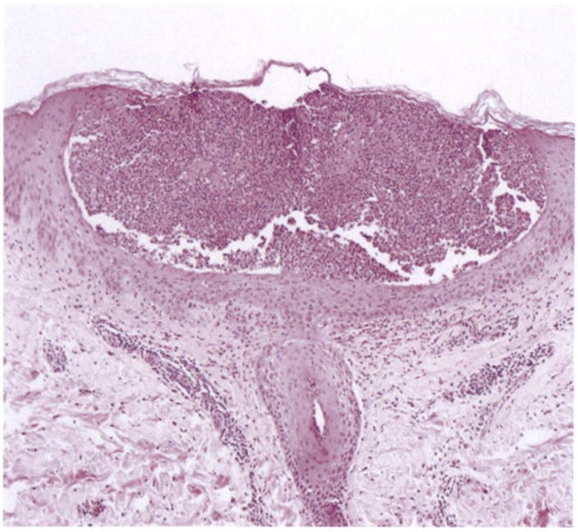

Fig. 13.76 Miliaria pustulosa

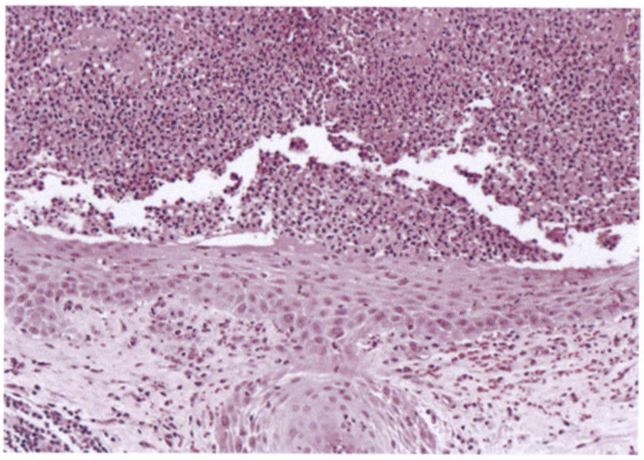

Fig. 13.77 Intraepidermal acrosyringium associated vesicle filled with neutrophils; dermal RBCs are present

Milia

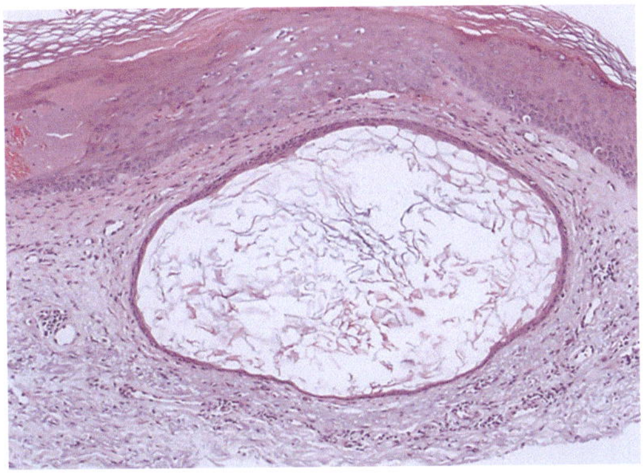

Fig. 13.78 Small dermal cyst

Histopathology (Figs. 13.78, 13.79, and 13.80)

- Small dermal cyst
- Lined with atrophic stratified squamous epithelium
- Filled with keratinous material
- Mild pericystic inflammation
- Appears like miniaturized epidermal inclusion cyst

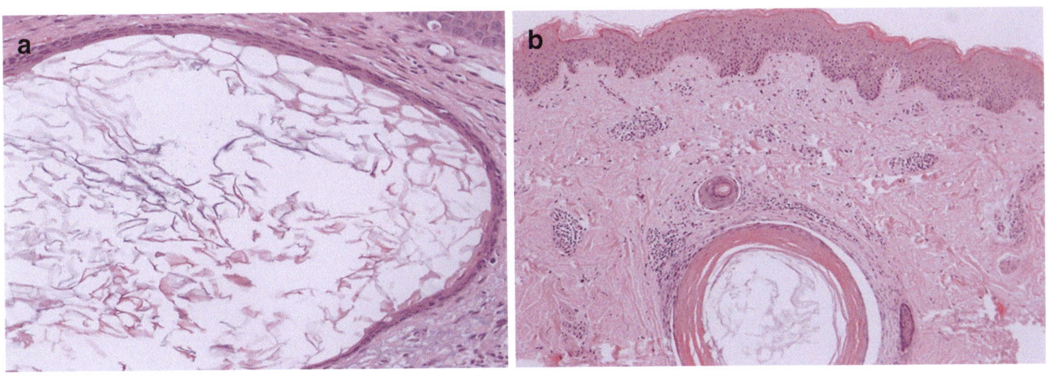

Fig. 13.79 (**a**, **b**) Laminated keratin is within the cyst

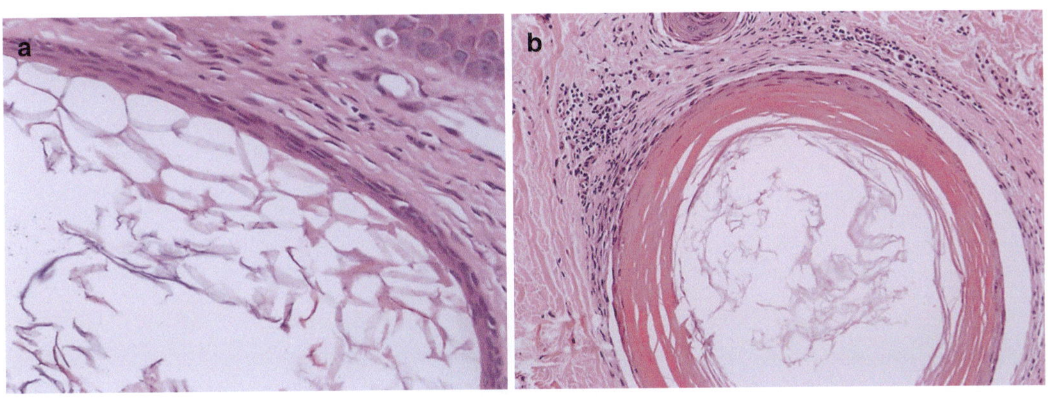

Fig. 13.80 (**a**, **b**) Atrophic squamous epithelium forms the wall of the cyst

Minocycline

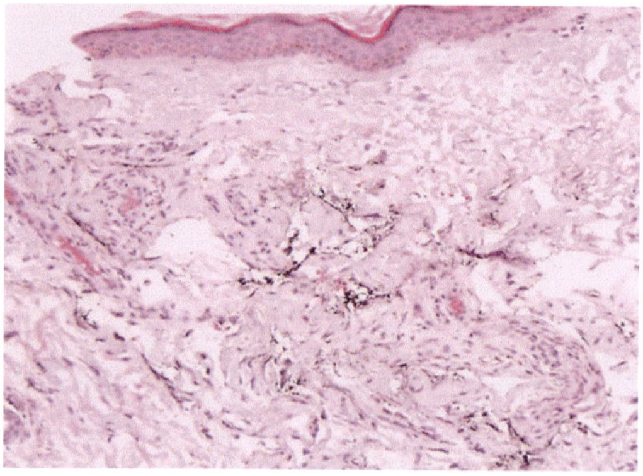

Fig. 13.81 Dark dermal pigment is present

Histopathology (Figs. 13.81, 13.82, 13.83, and 13.84)

- Dermal dark brown, black pigment
- Pigment is present in macrophages, dermal dendritic cells, and myoepithelial cells with perivascular tendency
- Pigment can also be extracellular deposited on elastic fibers
- Pigment is positive with iron (Perls' stain) and melanin stain (Fontana-Masson stain)

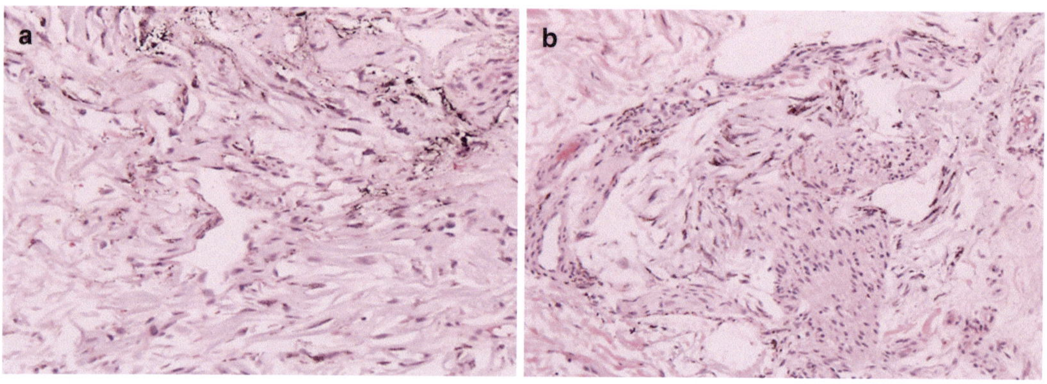

Fig. 13.82 (a, b) Dark pigment concentrated more around dermal vessels

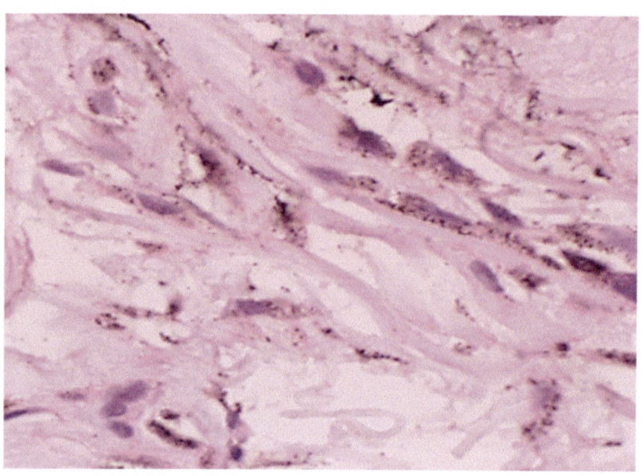

Fig. 13.83 Pigment is deposited on elastic fibers

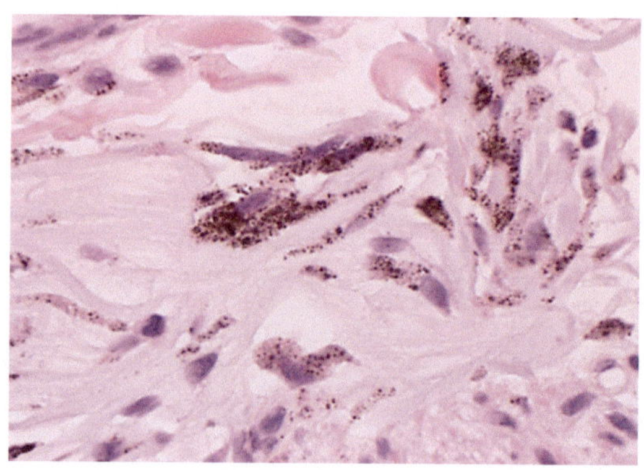

Fig. 13.84 Pigment is present within macrophages and dendrocytes

Molluscum Contagiosum

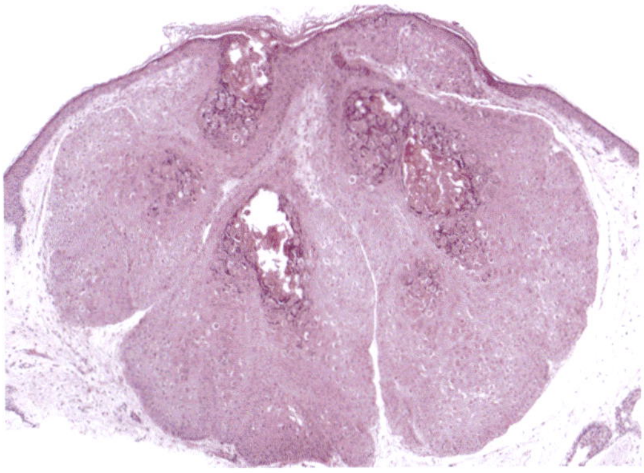

Fig. 13.85 Cup shaped inverted lesion

Histopathology (Figs. 13.85, 13.86, and 13.87)

- Cup shaped inverted acanthotic squamous epithelium
- Keratinocytes in the upper part of the epidermis contain large eosinophilic inclusion bodies (molluscum bodies)
- Molluscum body occupies almost the entire infected cell

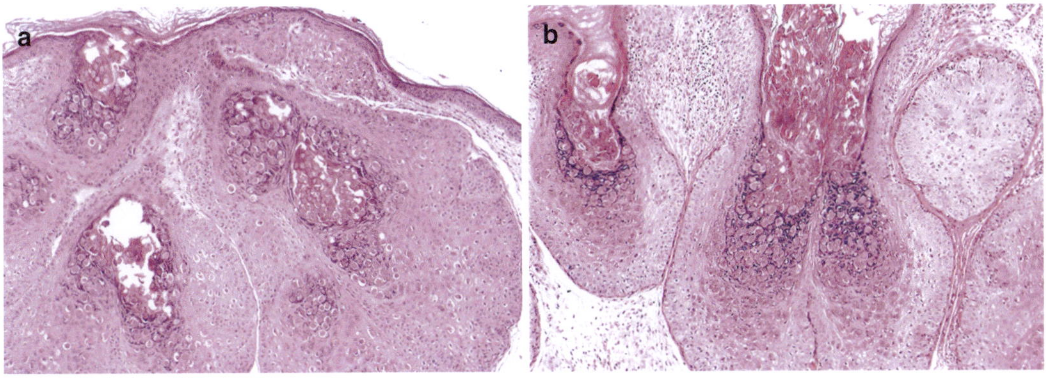

Fig. 13.86 (**a**, **b**) Numerous molluscum bodies present in the upper portion of the epidermis

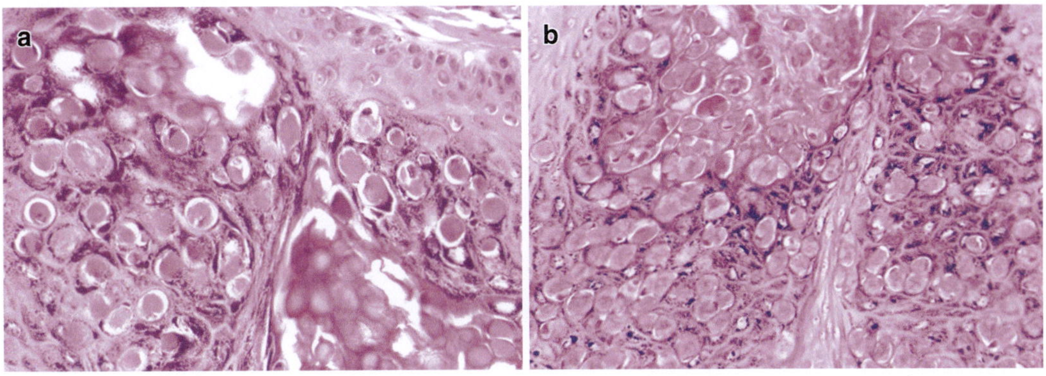

Fig. 13.87 (**a**, **b**) Eosinophilic molluscum bodies occupy the entire body of the keratinocytes

Mongolian Spot

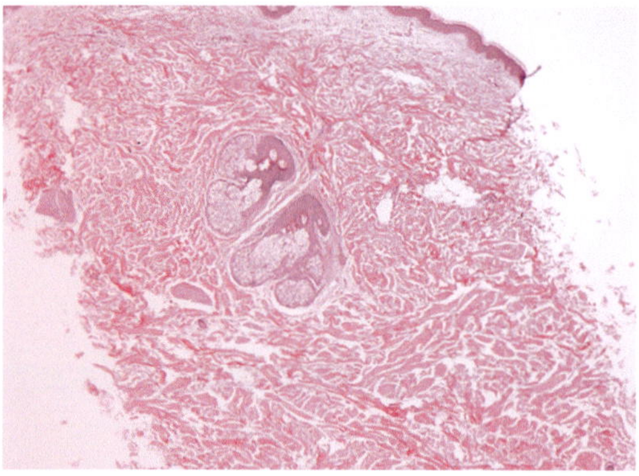

Fig. 13.88 On low power skin appears unremarkable

Histopathology (Figs. 13.88, 13.89, and 13.90)

- Heavily pigmented spindle dendritic melanocytes
- Pigmented cells are oriented parallel to collagen bundles
- Dendritic melanocytes are mostly in the deeper reticular dermis
- In *Nevus of Ota/Ito/Hori/Sun* dendritic melanocytes are located in the upper/ mid dermis

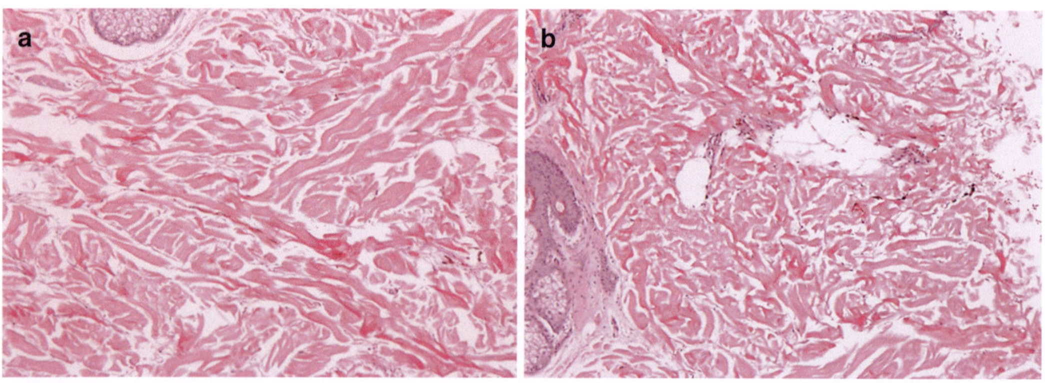

Fig. 13.89 (**a**, **b**) On medium magnification, trained eye can see pigmented dendritic melanocytes in the deeper dermis

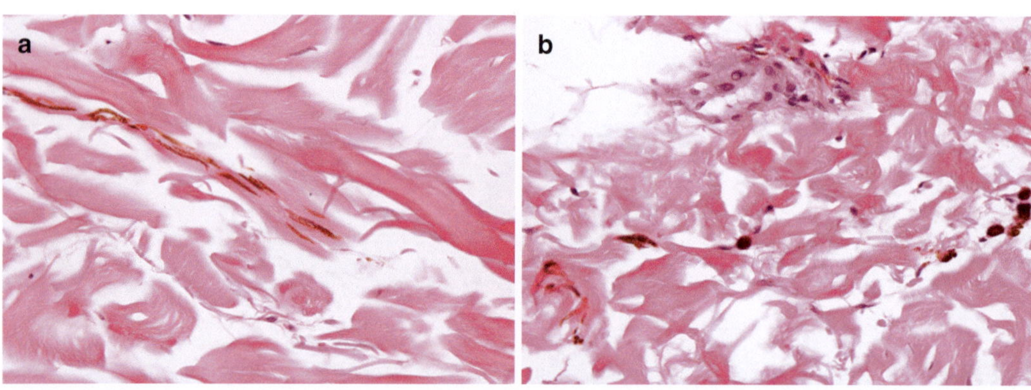

Fig. 13.90 (**a**, **b**) On high magnification, pigmented dendritic melanocytes are oriented parallel with the collagen

Monsel's Solution Reaction

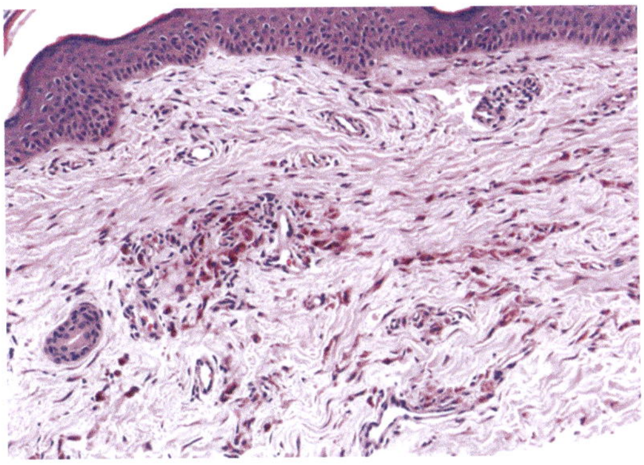

Fig. 13.91 Pigmented dermal scar

Monsel's solution is 20% ferric subsulfate used for homeostasis.

Histopathology (Figs. 13.91, 13.92, 13.93, and 13.94)

- Dermal scar with granules and clumps of dark brown pigment
- Pigment is present in dermis and in histiocytes (siderophages)
- Pigment stain strongly for iron (Perl's method)

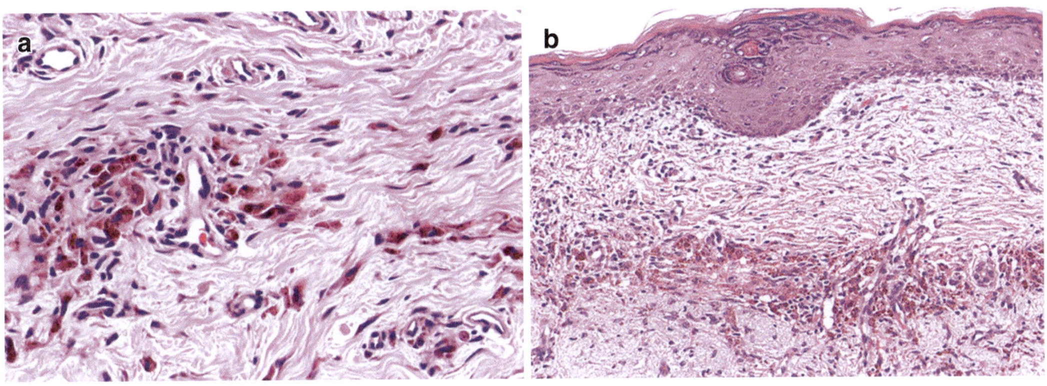

Fig. 13.92 (**a**, **b**) Dermal scar with lymphocytes, histiocytes, and dark brown pigment

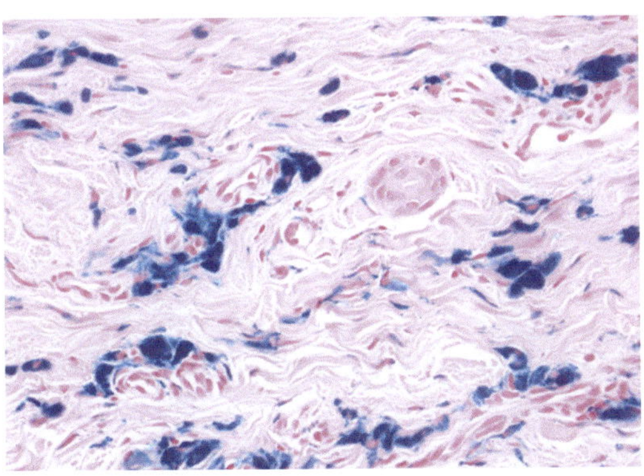

Fig. 13.93 Pigment stains blue (Perl's stain)

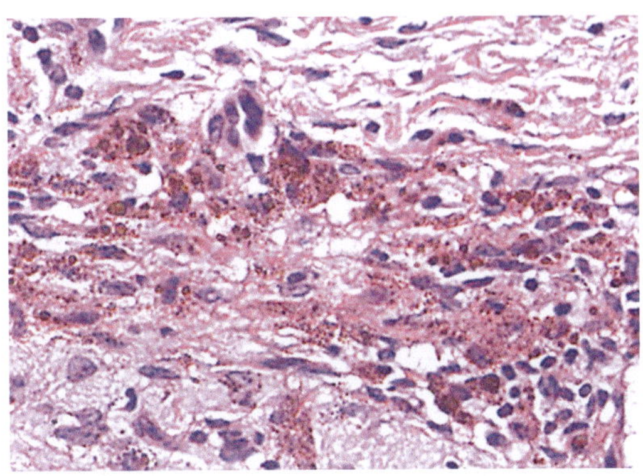

Fig. 13.94 Numerous siderophages with dark brown pigment

Montgomery's Tubercle

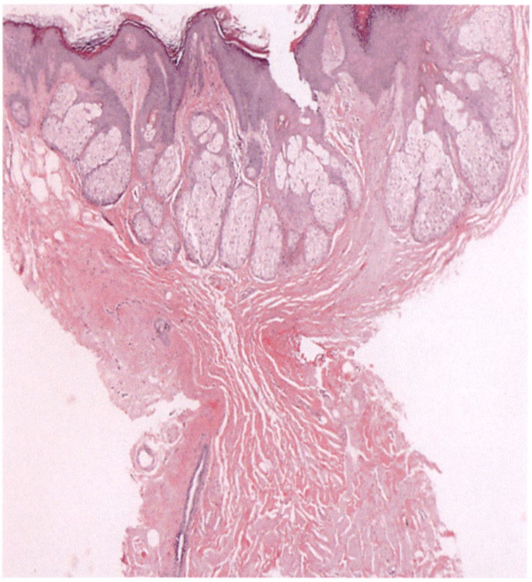

Fig. 13.95 Sebaceous hyperplasia with underlying lactiferous duct

Synonym: Sebaceous Hyperplasia of Nipple

Histopathology (Figs. 13.95, 13.96, 13.97, and 13.98)
- Sebaceous gland hyperplasia in nipple biopsy
- Four or more sebaceous glands attached to central infundibulum
- Normal ratio of basaloid and mature sebaceous cells
- Central infundibulum is usually dilated and filled with keratin
- Sebaceous hyperplasia is associated with vellus hair or lactiferous ducts

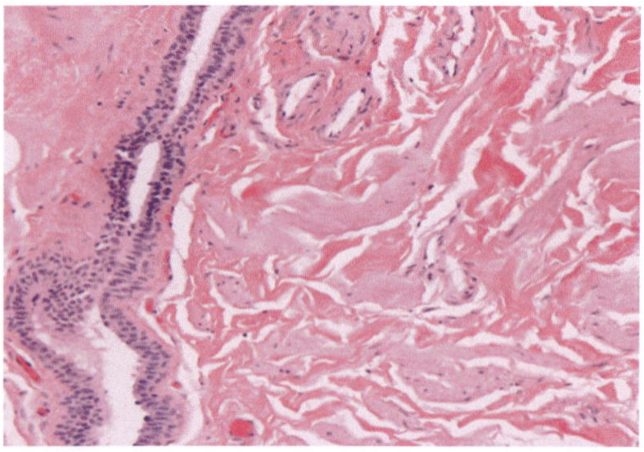

Fig. 13.96 Numerous pilar muscles consistent with the breast

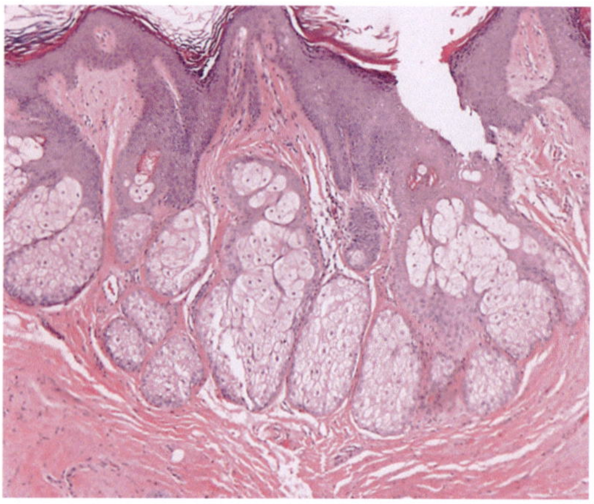

Fig. 13.97 Multiple benign appearing sebaceous glands are attached to the individual hair follicle

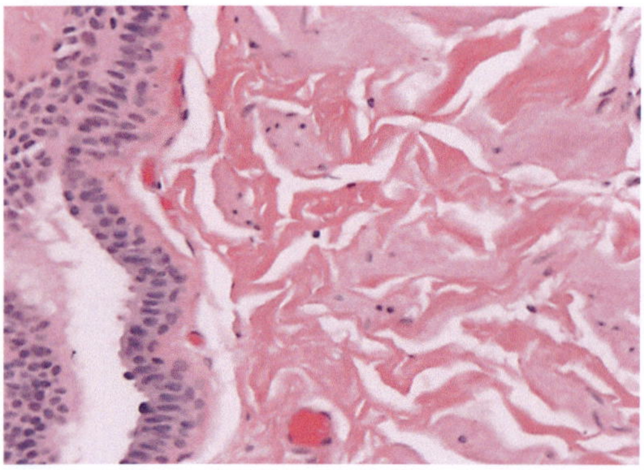

Fig. 13.98 Mammary duct lined with two cell layers

Morphea/Scleroderma

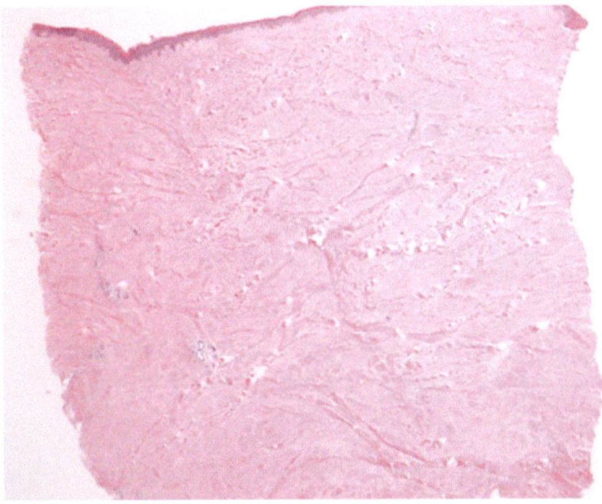

Fig. 13.99 Rectangular biopsy with sclerotic dermis and subcutis and completely absent adnexal structures

Histopathology (Figs. 13.99, 13.100, and 13.101)

- Dermal and subcutaneous thickening with sclerotic collagen making the biopsy rectangular in shape
- Atrophy or complete absence of adnexal structures
- Sclerosis also involves adipose tissue
- Superficial and deep perivascular inflammation is present particularly in newer lesion

P.S. in morphea and scleroderma histological findings are identical. Only difference, in my experience, is that inflammation is less marked in scleroderma

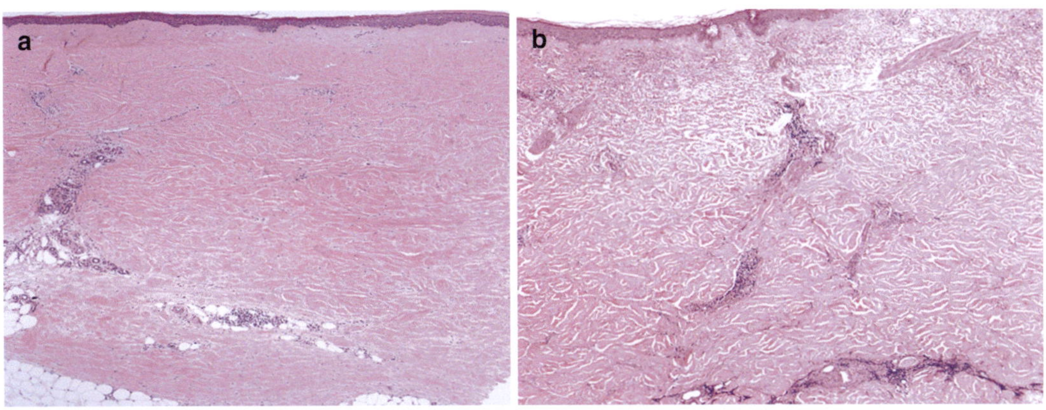

Fig. 13.100 (**a**, **b**) Dermal and subcutaneous sclerosis with superficial and deep perivascular inflammation

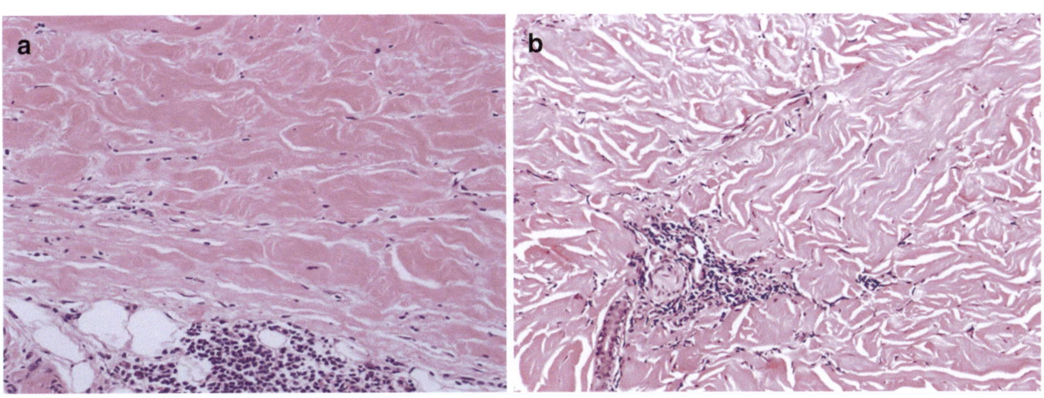

Fig. 13.101 (**a**, **b**) Eosinophilic thick collagen and perivascular lymphocytic inflammation

Mucinoses

There are several cutaneous disorders with an increased amount of cutaneous mucin. Here are the most common disorders:

Acral Papular Mucinosis: thin dorsal acral skin with well circumscribed deposition of dermal mucin separated from epidermis by Grenz zone (Fig. 13.102).

Digital Mucous Cyst: thick acral skin with dermal mucin deposit. There is no Grenz zone and epidermis forms collarette (Fig. 13.103).

Focal Dermal Mucinosis: slightly elevated nodule with atrophic epidermis and poorly circumscribed dermal mucin (Fig. 13.104).

Follicular Mucinosis: accumulation of mucin within the follicle. Intrafollicular and perifollicular lymphocytes with variable number of eosinophils (Fig. 13.105).

Mucocele: aggregate of submucosal mucin surrounded by lymphohistiocytic inflammation, granulation tissue, and muciphages (Fig. 13.106).

Papular Mucinosis (Lichen Myxedematosus): papillary shaped lesion with variable amount of dermal mucin. Slight proliferation of fibroblasts and mild collagen thickening (Fig. 13.107).

Pretibial Myxedema: prominent dermal and subcutaneous mucin with normal number of fibroblasts (Fig. 13.108).

Reticular Erythematous Mucinosis: perivascular lymphocytic infiltrate with mildly separated collagen and variable amount of dermal mucin (Fig. 13.109).

Scleredema: thick, sclerotic collagen separated by "empty" spaces. The "empty" spaces contain a minimal amount of mucin that decrease and disappear with maturation of the lesion (Fig. 13.110).

Scleromyxedema: in an early lesion there is disorganized collagen with an increased number of fibroblasts and easily found mucin separating collagen; in established lesions there is an increased number of fibroblasts with significant fibrosis and minimal mucin (Fig. 13.111).

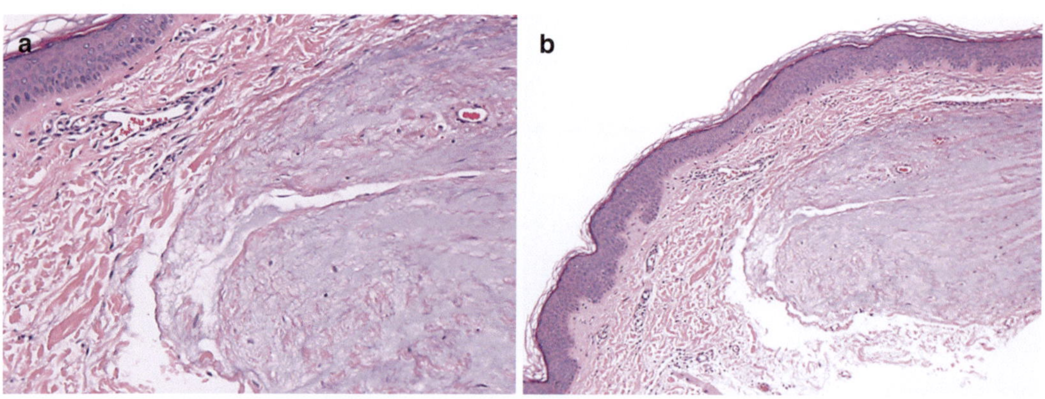

Fig. 13.102 (**a**, **b**) **Acral Papular Mucinosis** with well circumscribed deposition of dermal mucin separated from epidermis by Grenz zone

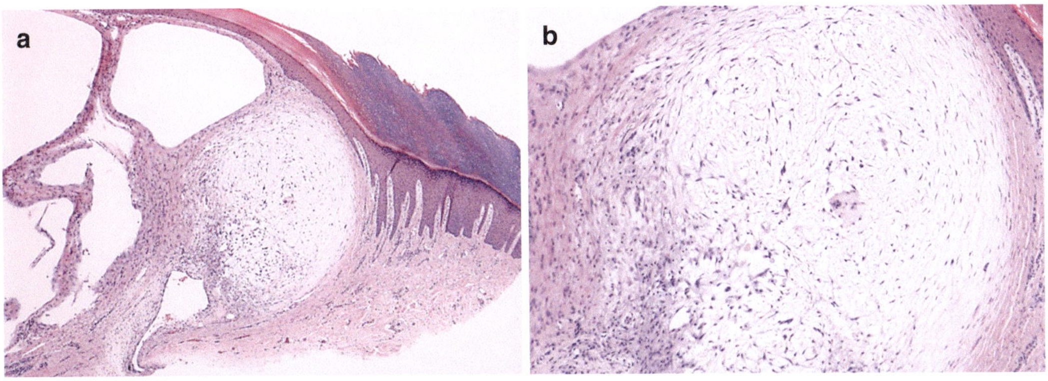

Fig. 13.103 (**a**, **b**) **Digital Mucous Cyst** arising underneath thick acral skin with collarette; mucin accumulation is well circumscribed and abuts the epidermis with no Grenz zone

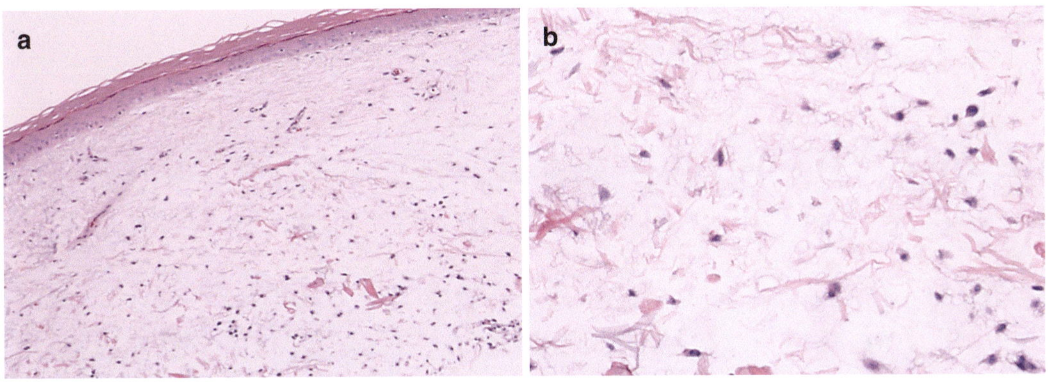

Fig. 13.104 (**a**, **b**) **Focal Dermal Mucinosis** with poorly circumscribed dermal mucin accumulating underneath the atrophic epidermis

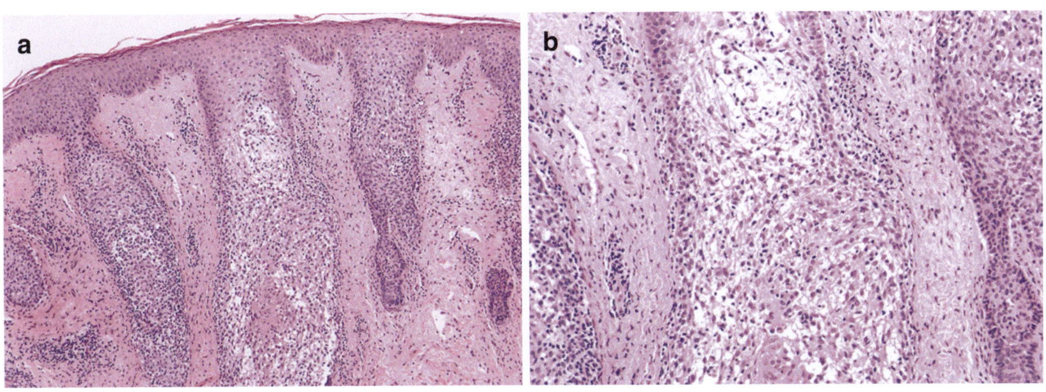

Fig. 13.105 (**a**, **b**) **Follicular Mucinosis** with accumulation of follicular mucin; intra and perifollicular lymphocytes are present

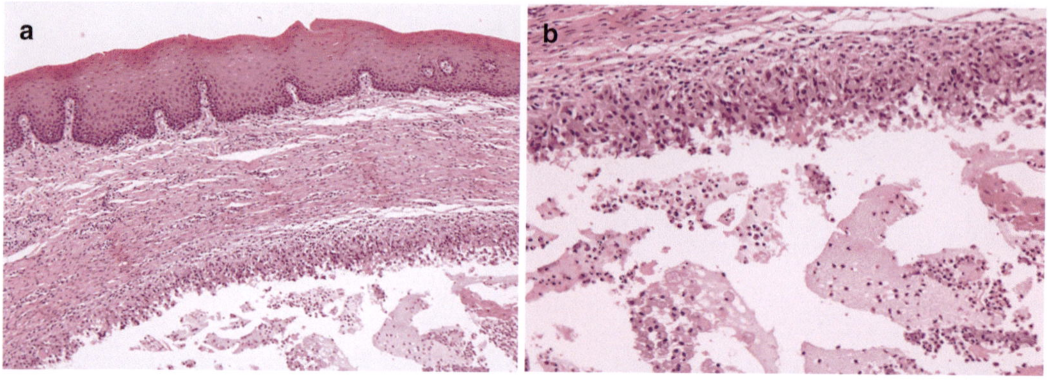

Fig. 13.106 (**a**, **b**) **Mucocele** with submucosal mucin surrounded by lymphocytes, histiocytes, and giant cells

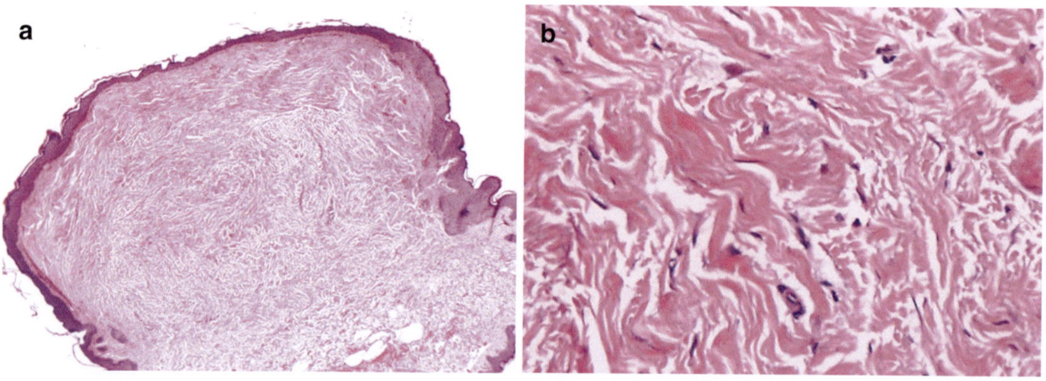

Fig. 13.107 (**a**, **b**) **Papular Mucinosis** with slight proliferation of fibroblasts and mild collagen thickening. Dermal mucin is present in between collagen

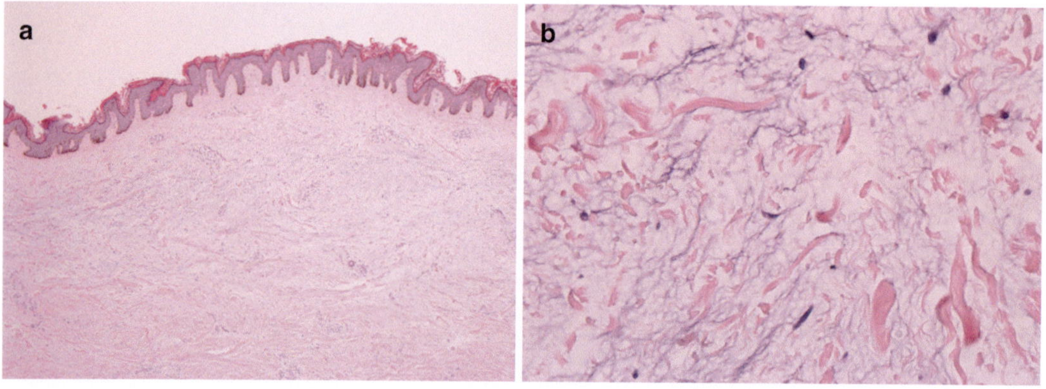

Fig. 13.108 (**a**, **b**) **Pretibial Myxedema** with extensive dermal and subcutaneous dermal deposition

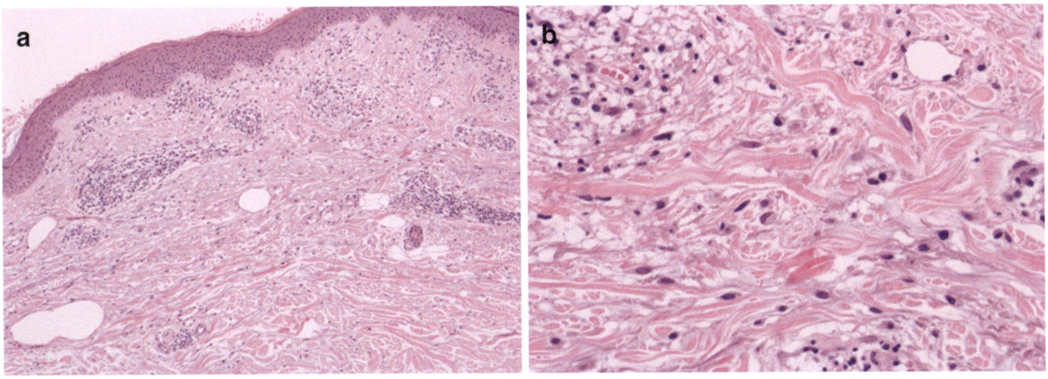

Fig. 13.109 (**a**, **b**) **Reticulated Erythematous Mucinosis** with perivascular lymphocytic infiltrate, mildly separated collagen, and variable amount of dermal mucin

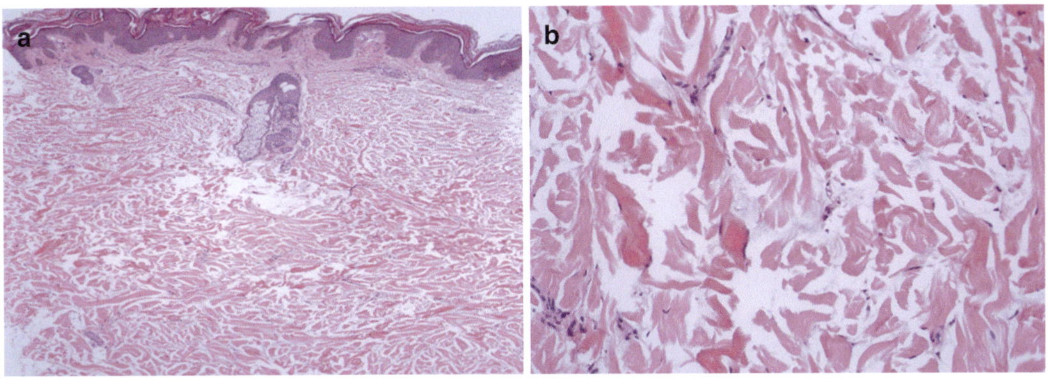

Fig. 13.110 (**a**, **b**) **Scleredema** with thick, sclerotic collagen separated by "empty" spaces that contain minimal amount of mucin

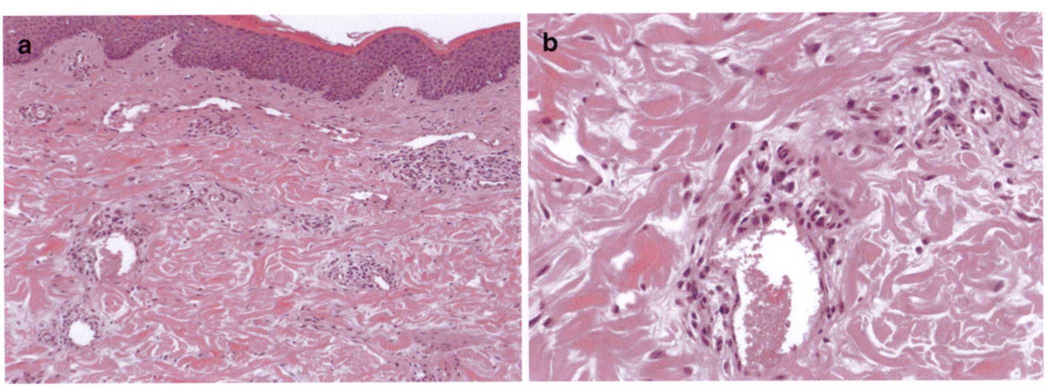

Fig. 13.111 (**a**, **b**) **Scleromyxedema** with disorganized collagen with increased number of fibroblasts and mucin separating collagen

Mucinous Carcinoma

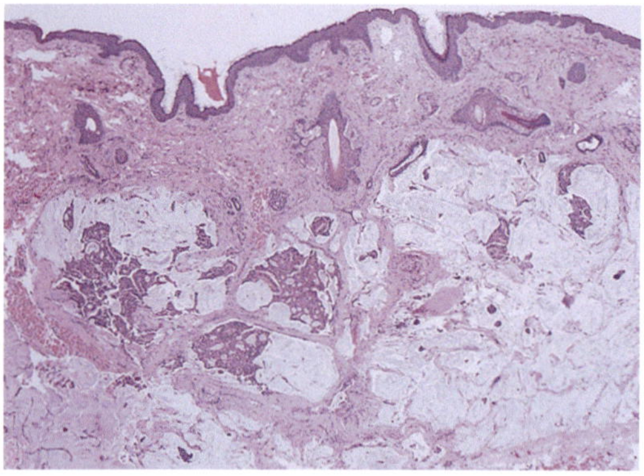

Fig. 13.112 Mucinous tumor infiltrates subcutis

Synonym: Colloid Carcinoma

Histopathology (Figs. 13.112, 13.113, 13.114, and 13.115)

- Dermal and subcutaneous tumor with large pools of mucin and pushing borders
- Malignant epithelial cells floating in mucin lakes
- Tumor cells can form trabeculae, glandular spaces with cribriform pattern, or focal solid area

P.S. primary tumor is rare. Breast and colon metastasis are more common

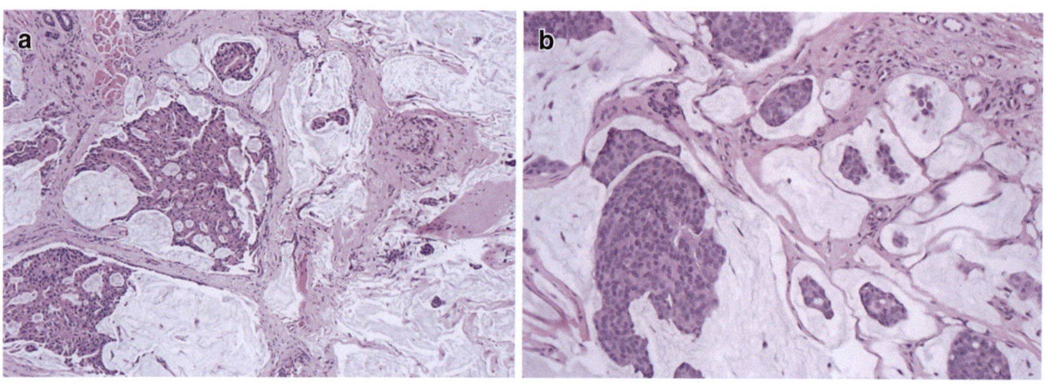

Fig. 13.113 (**a**, **b**) Tumor cells are present in large pools of dermal and subcutaneous mucin

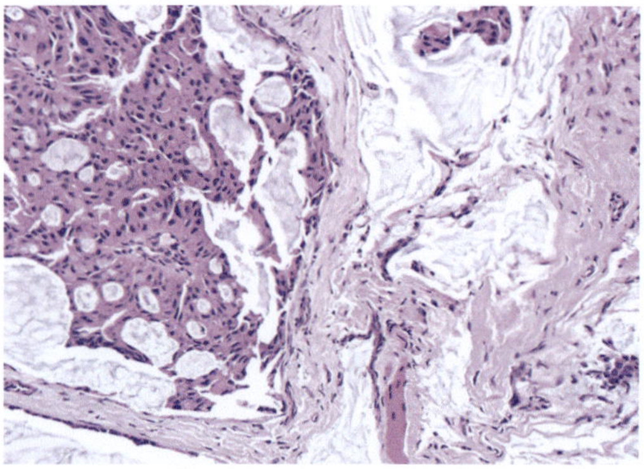

Fig. 13.114 Tumor cells in cribriform pattern

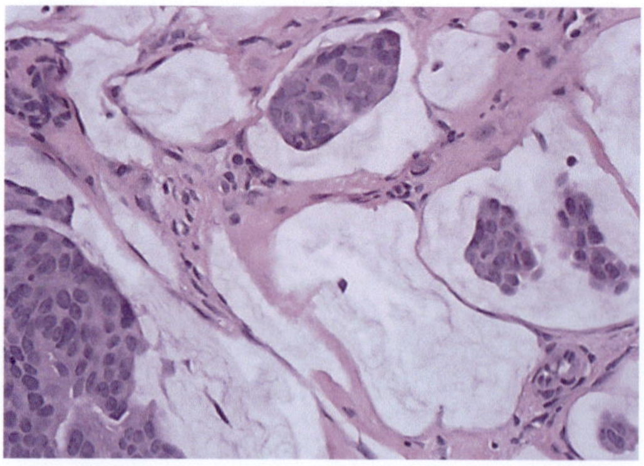

Fig. 13.115 Atypical tumor cells in small nests floating in the mucin

Mucocele

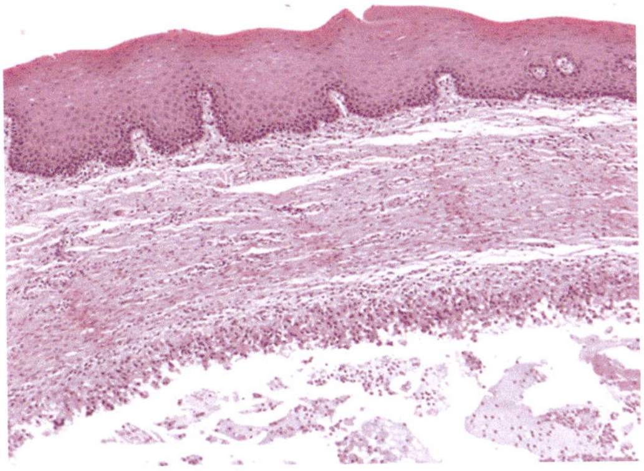

Fig. 13.116 Submucosal mucin filled pseudocyst

Synonym: Ranula

Histopathology (Figs. 13.116, 13.117, and 13.118)

- Aggregate of submucosal mucin
- Mucin is surrounded by lymphocytes, histiocytes, and granulation tissue with muciphages
- Salivary gland tissue is usually present in the vicinity

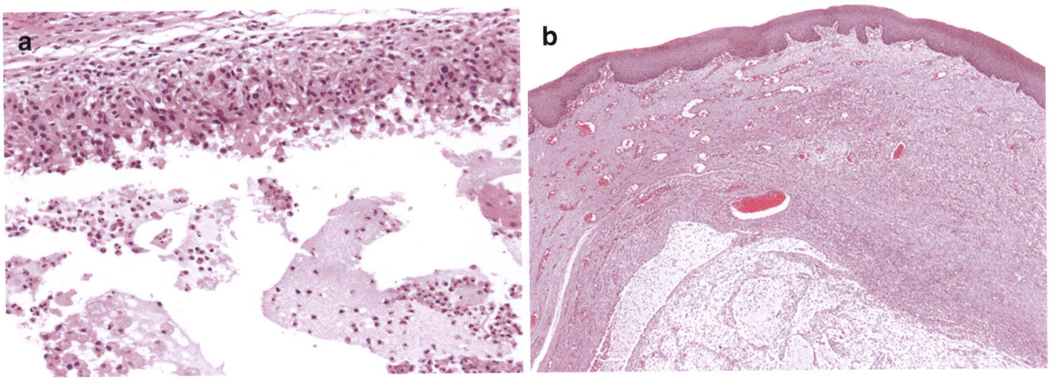

Fig. 13.117 (**a**, **b**) Mucin admixed with numerous neutrophils and surrounding granulation tissue and fibrosis

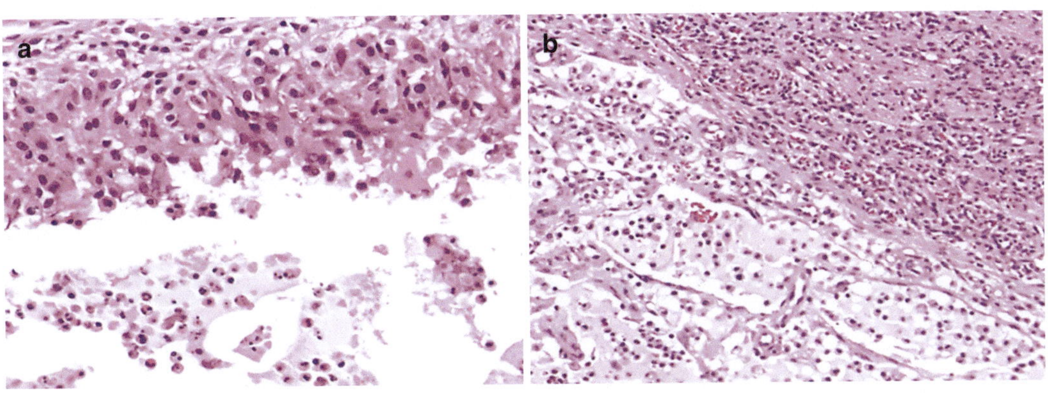

Fig. 13.118 (**a**, **b**) Central acutely inflamed mucinous material is surrounded by histiocytes, lymphocytes, and muciphages (macrophages with engulfed mucin)

Mucoepidermoid Carcinoma

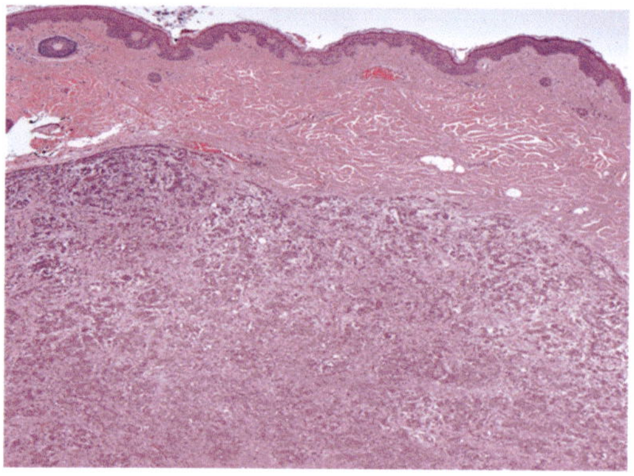

Fig. 13.119 Subcutaneous tumor nodule

Histopathology (Figs. 13.119, 13.120, 13.121, and 13.122)

- Mucous secreting ("goblet" cells) and epithelioid cells forming solid nests
- Tumor nests are in fibrous stroma admixed with extracellular mucin
- Epithelioid cells are large atypical cells with vesicular nuclei (CK7+, EMA+, CEA+, p63+)
- Extravasated mucin can excite foreign body reaction

P.S. *CRTC1* rearrangement is common

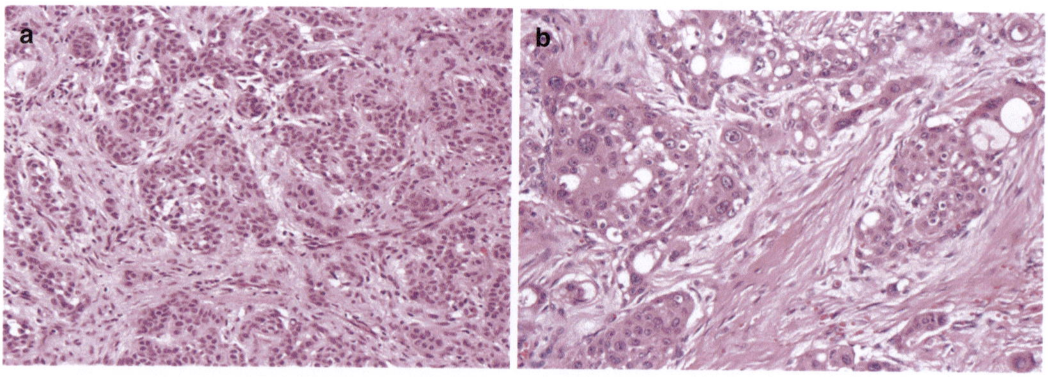

Fig. 13.120 (**a**, **b**) Atypical epithelioid cells and mucin producing cells form tumor islands embedded in fibrous stroma

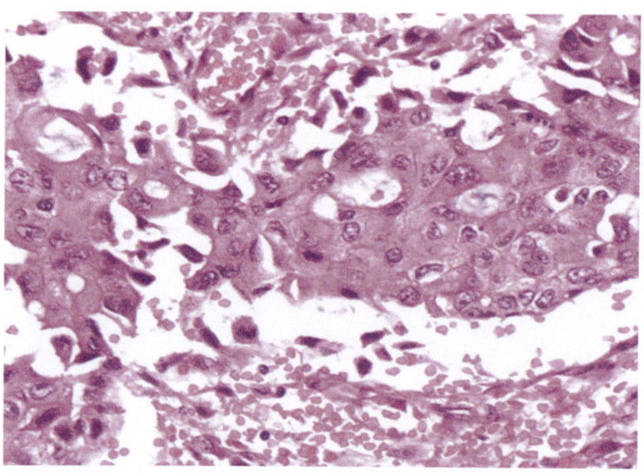

Fig. 13.121 Epithelioid cells are highly atypical

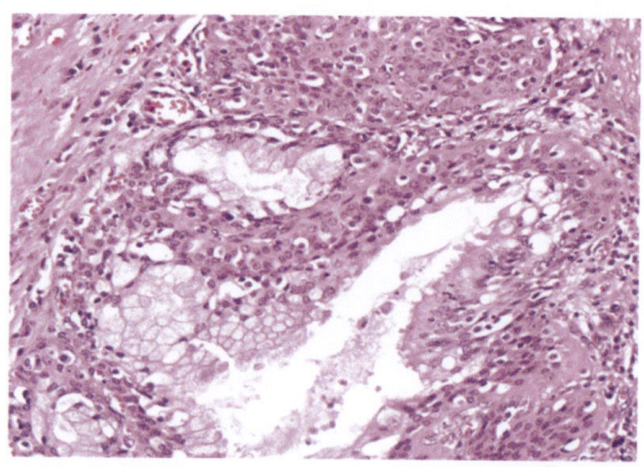

Fig. 13.122 Mucin is extracellular and within goblet cells

Mucormycosis

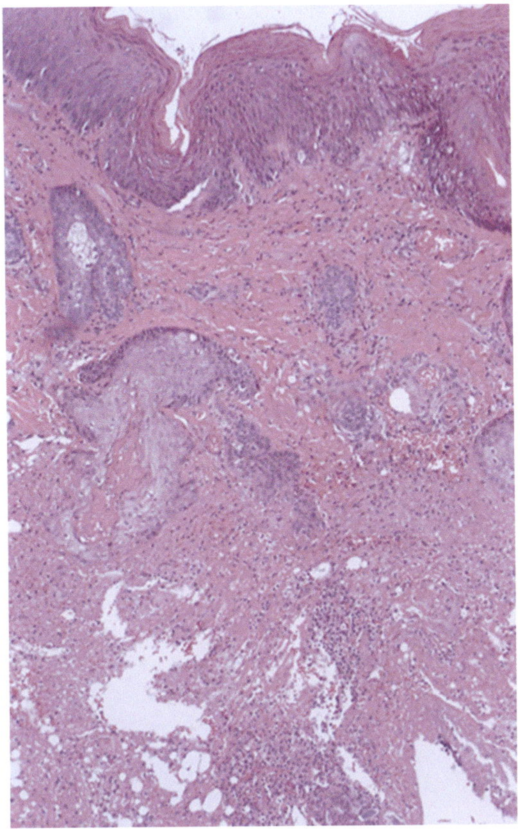

Fig. 13.123 Extensive dermal and subcutaneous necrosis

Synonym: Zygomycosis

Histopathology (Figs. 13.123, 13.124, 13.125, and 13.126)
- Dermal and subcutaneous acute and chronic inflammation
- Extensive necrosis is usually seen
- Broad, non-septated hyphae ("ribbon-like")
- Hyphae branch at 90° angles

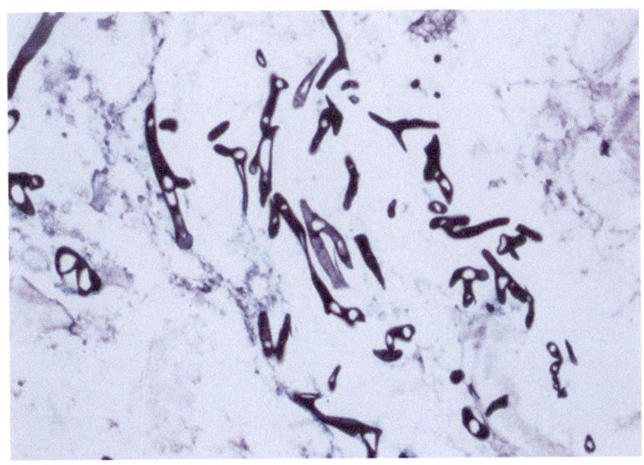

Fig. 13.124 "Ribbon-like" non-septated hyphae stained with GMS stain

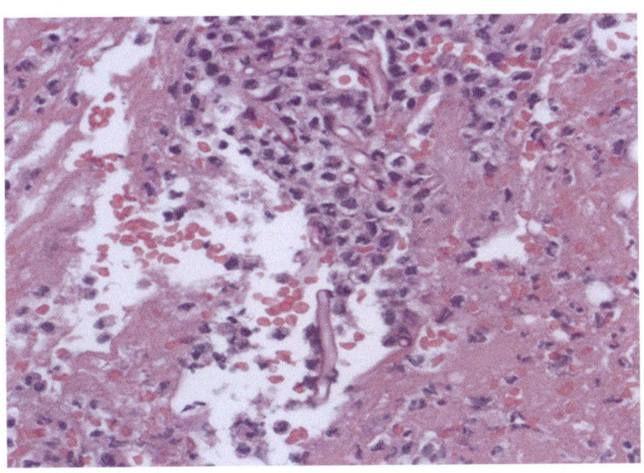

Fig. 13.125 Hyphae are seen in necrotic, acutely inflamed area

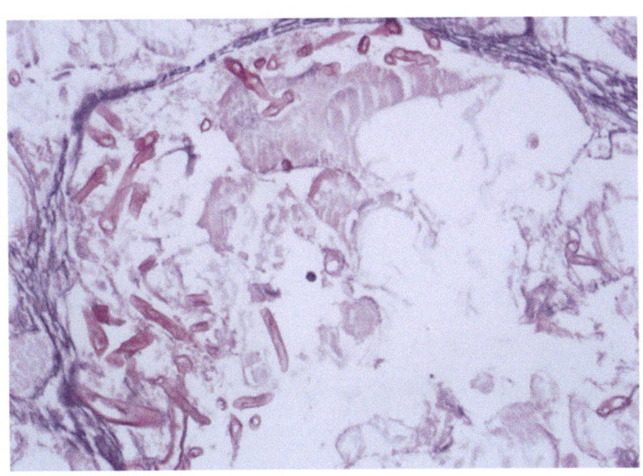

Fig. 13.126 PAS stain outlines hyphae branching at 90°

Mucosal Lentigo

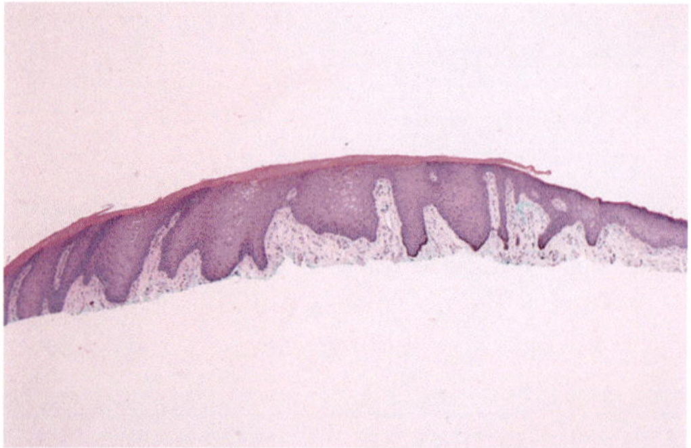

Fig. 13.127 Epithelium with broad, pigmented, and elongated rete ridges

Histopathology (Figs. 13.127, 13.128, and 13.129)
- Mucosal epithelium with no granular layer
- Elongation of broad rete ridges
- Hyperpigmentation of epidermal basal layer
- Mild increase in number of melanocytes

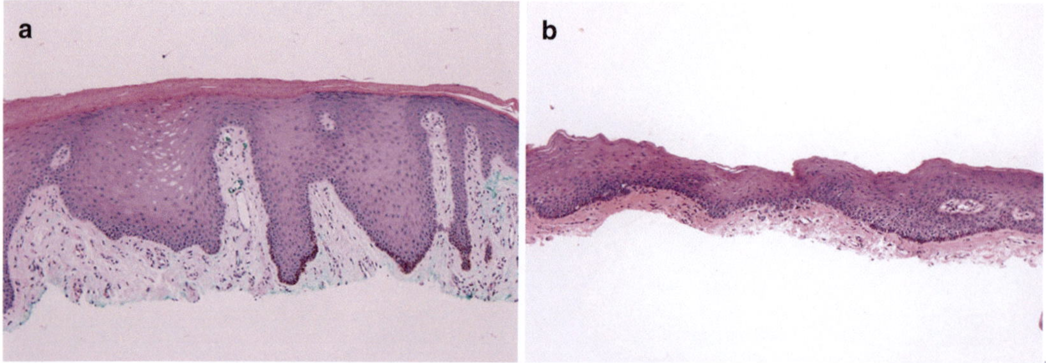

Fig. 13.128 (**a**, **b**) Mucosal epithelium with absent granular layer and broad elongated rete ridges

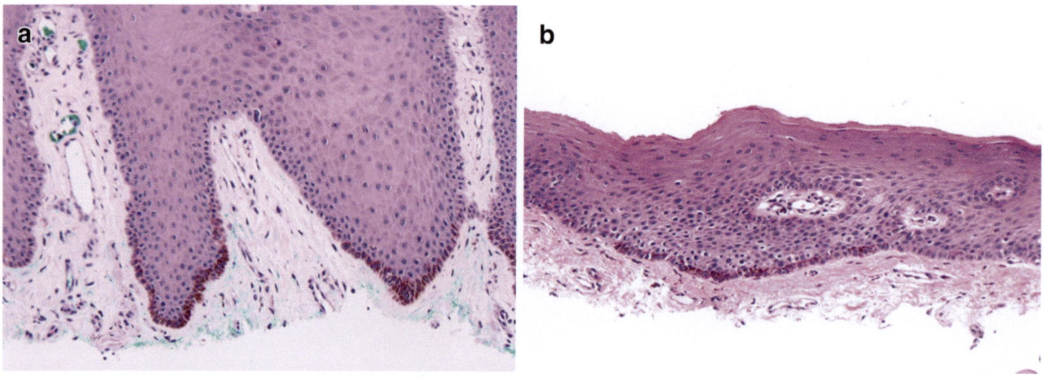

Fig. 13.129 (**a**, **b**) Hyperpigmentation of the basal layer keratinocytes

Multinucleated Cell Angiohistiocytoma

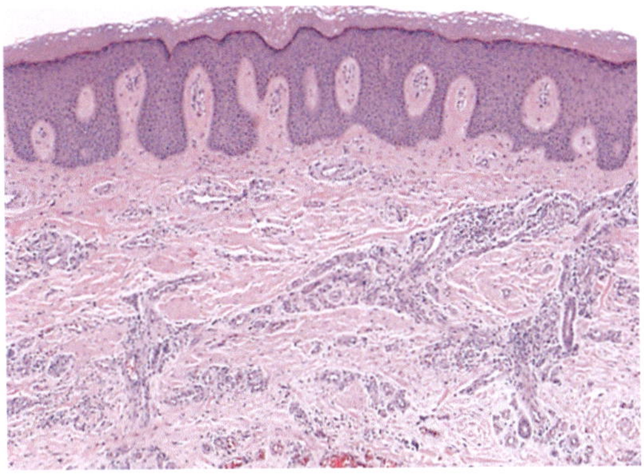

Fig. 13.130 Dermal vascular proliferation

Histopathology (Figs. 13.130, 13.131, and 13.132)
- Dermal proliferation of small blood vessels surrounded by fibrohistiocytic cells (factor XIII+)
- Scattered irregular multinucleated cells (CD68+) with scalloped borders
- Hyalinized stroma

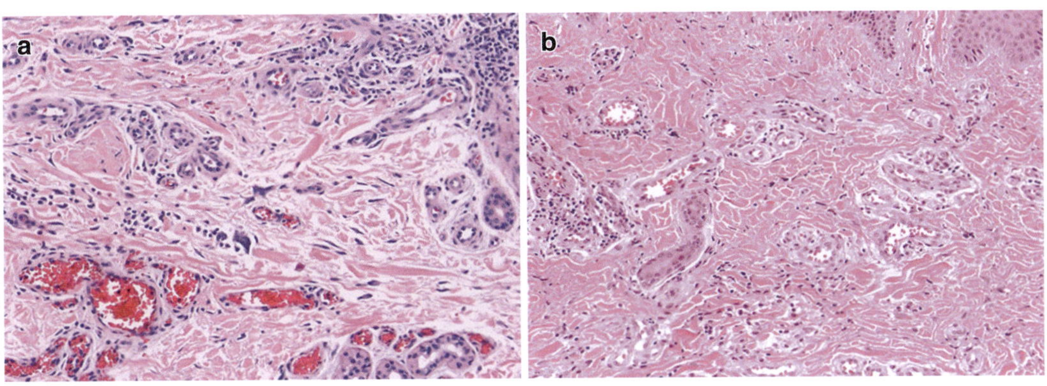

Fig. 13.131 (**a**, **b**) Haphazard proliferation of small vascular channels associated with fibrohistiocytic cells

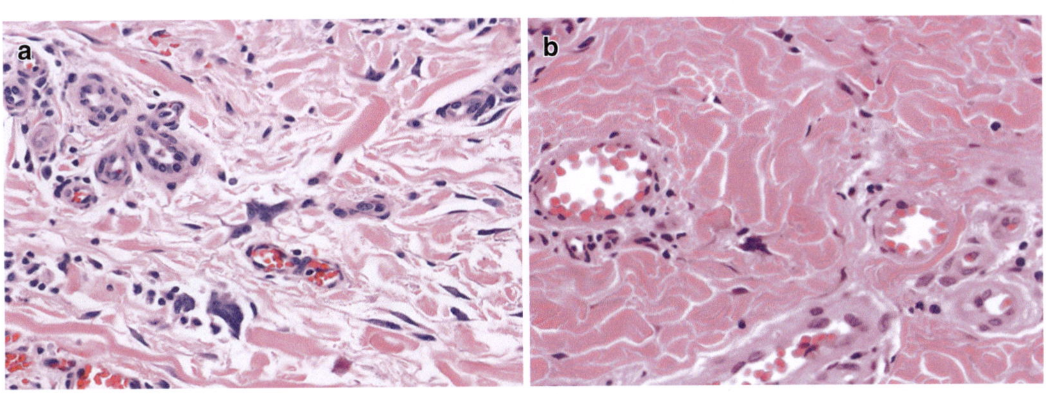

Fig. 13.132 (**a**, **b**) Conspicuous irregular scalloped, angulated multinucleated cells in the hyalinized stroma

Mycetoma

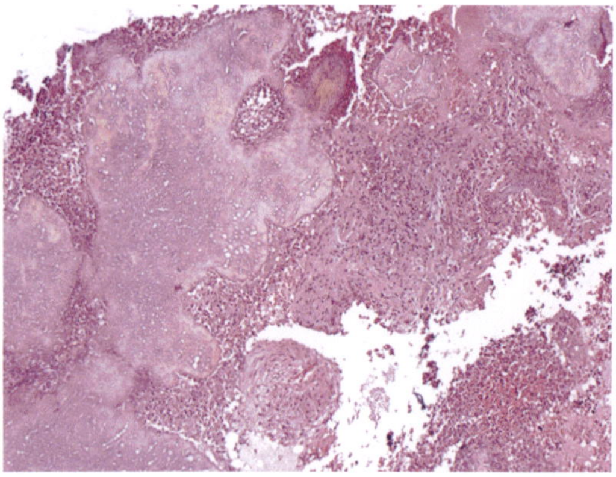

Fig. 13.133 Yellow-white granules within neutrophilic abscess

Synonym: Eumycetoma

Histopathology (Figs. 13.133, 13.134, 13.135, and 13.136)

- Characteristic granules within an exuberant neutrophilic inflammation
- Color of granules help in identifying organisms
- Black granules produced by *Madurella, Leptosphaeria, Pyrenochaeta,* and *Phialophora*
- Yellow-white granules produced by *Allescheria, Cephalosporium, Fusarium, Actinomadura,* and *Streptomyces*

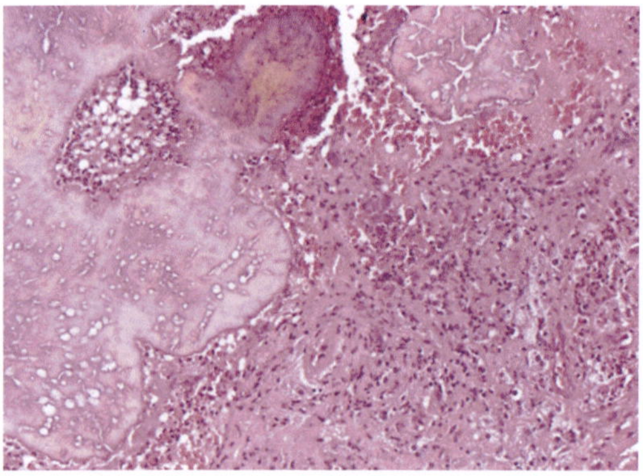

Fig. 13.134 Outlines of fungal hyphae can be seen even on H&E slide

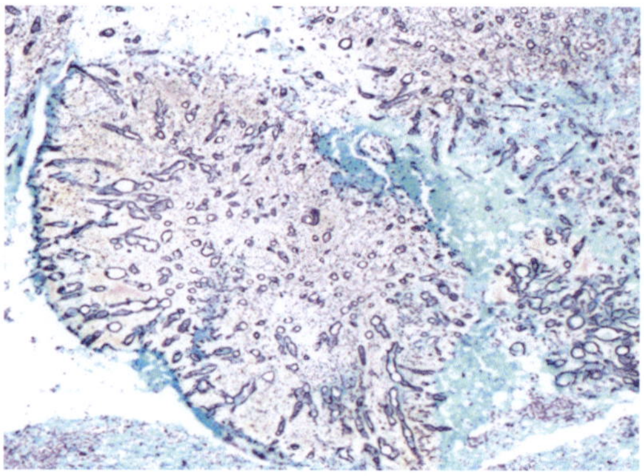

Fig. 13.135 GMS fungal stain highlights hyphae

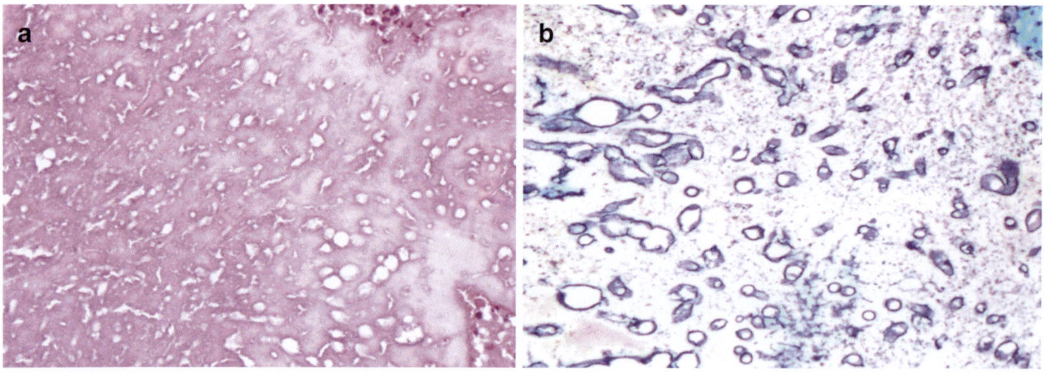

Fig. 13.136 (**a**, **b**) Irregularly shaped beaded hyphae

Mycosis Fungoides

Histopathology depends on the clinical stage.In all stages, epidermis can vary from spongiotic to psoriasiform to atrophic.

Patch stage (Figs. 13.137 and 13.138)
- Epidermotropic lymphocytes with nuclei larger than nuclei of dermal lymphocytes
- Lymphocytes like to form a line along the epidermal basal layer and have clear halo around the nuclei
- Focal intraepidermal lymphocytic collection (Pautrier's microabscesses)
- Dermal lymphocytes are mostly perivascular and are reactive and not part of the tumor

Plaque stage (Figs. 13.139 and 13.140)
- Epidermal lymphocytic presence is similar like in the patch stage but it is more pronounced
- Dermal lymphocytes start to form a band and are made of tumor lymphocytes with atypia similar to atypia of epidermal lymphocytes

Tumor stage (Figs. 13.141 and 13.142)
- Lymphocytic epidermotropism like in the patch stage but might be lost sometimes
- Dense dermal and subcutaneous infiltrate of atypical lymphocytes

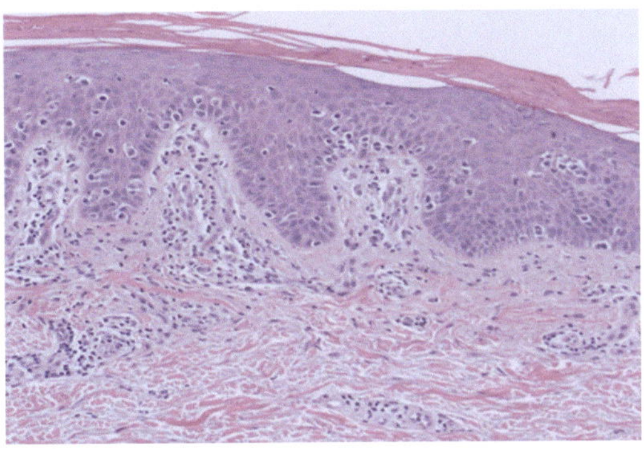

Fig. 13.137 **Patch stage MF** enlarged lymphocytes with clear halo present in the epidermis

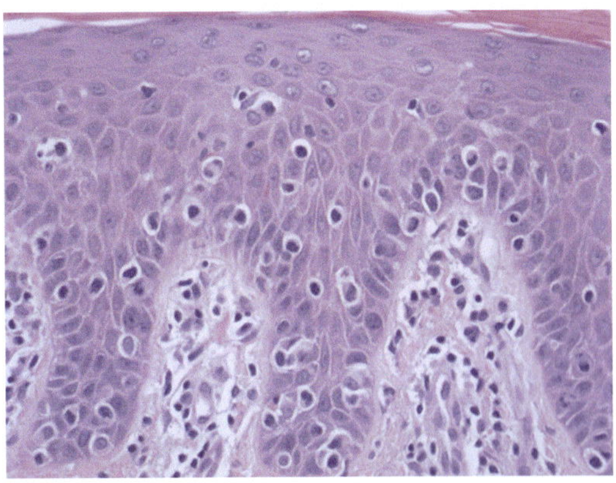

Fig. 13.138 Dermal perivascular lymphocytes are reactive, not malignant

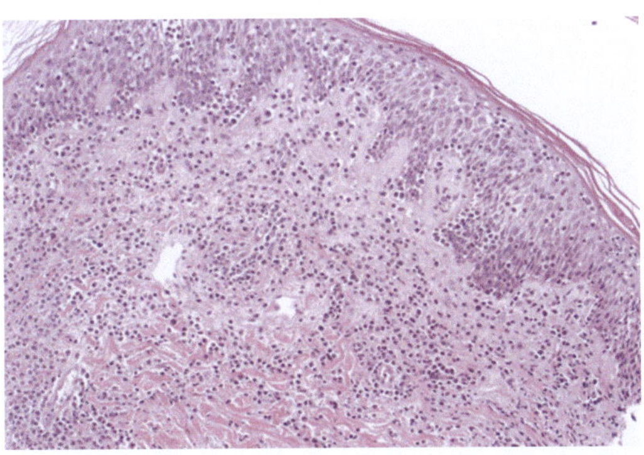

Fig. 13.139 **Plaque stage MF** with epidermal lymphocytes forming microabscesses and line at basal layer

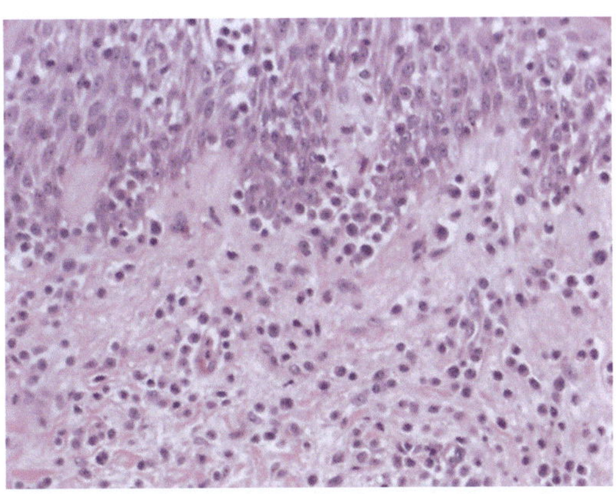

Fig. 13.140 Dermal lymphocytes are malignant, atypical and denser than in the patch stage

Multiple subtypes of *mycosis fungoides* exist.

In all of them lymphocytes are CD2+, CD3+, CD4+, CD8−, with the exception of hypopigmented MF, that is CD4− and CD8+.

Here are some of them:

- *Bullous MF*: with subepidermal blisters, dermal band-like lymphocytic infiltrate, and lymphocytic epidermotropism
- *Dyshidrotic MF*: with epidermal spongiosis and lymphocytes scattered in the epidermis and present within the vesicles
- *MF with follicular mucinosis:* follicular mucin with lymphocytes in the follicle
- *Granulomatous MF*: epidermal lymphocytes with dermal epithelioid granulomas (Figs. 13.143 and 13.144)
- *Hypopigmented MF*: with features of typical patch stage MF (CD4−, CD8+)
- *Pagetoid reticulosis*: hyperplastic epidermis with pagetoid lymphocytic epidermotropism
- *Pilotropic MF*: with dense perifollicular lymphocytic infiltrate without mucin
- *Poikilodermic MF*: epidermal atrophy with dermal telangiectasias and epidermal lymphocytes

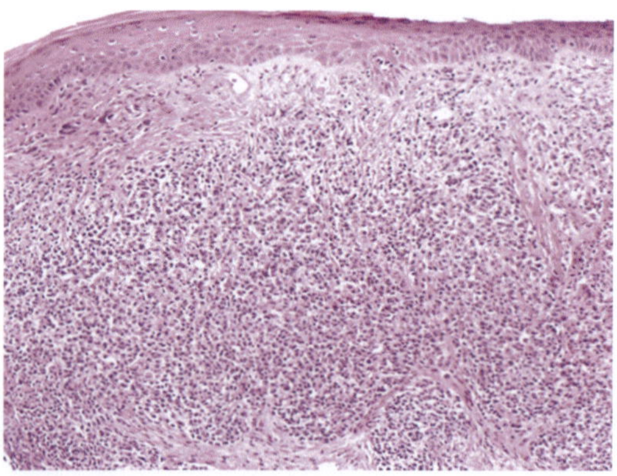

Fig. 13.141 Tumor stage MF

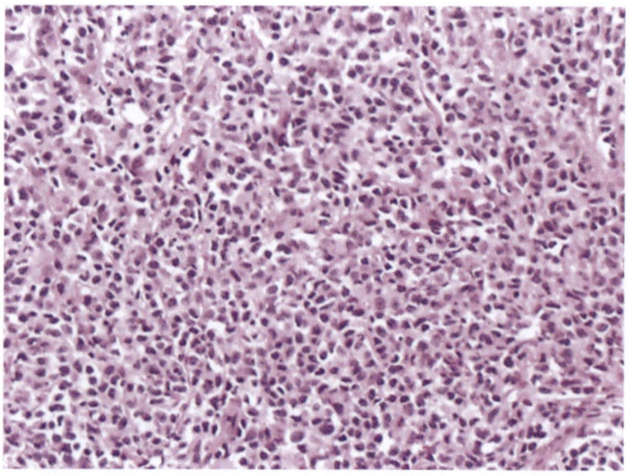

Fig. 13.142 Diffuse infiltrate of atypical lymphocytes

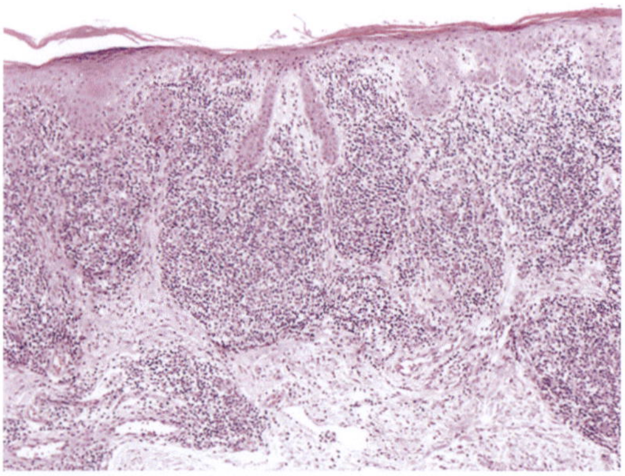

Fig. 13.143 Granulomatous MF

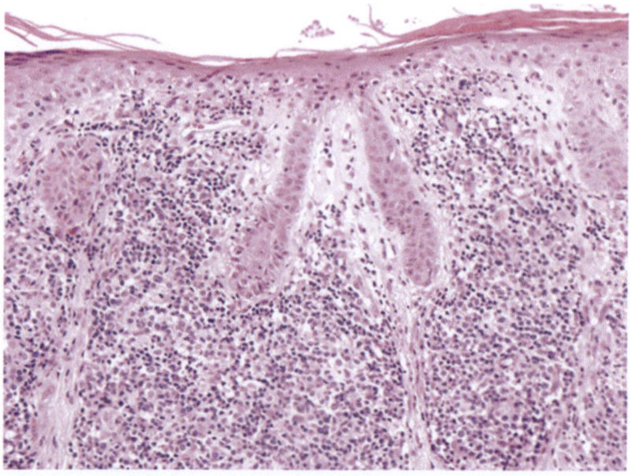

Fig. 13.144 Vague dermal epithelioid granulomas

Myiasis

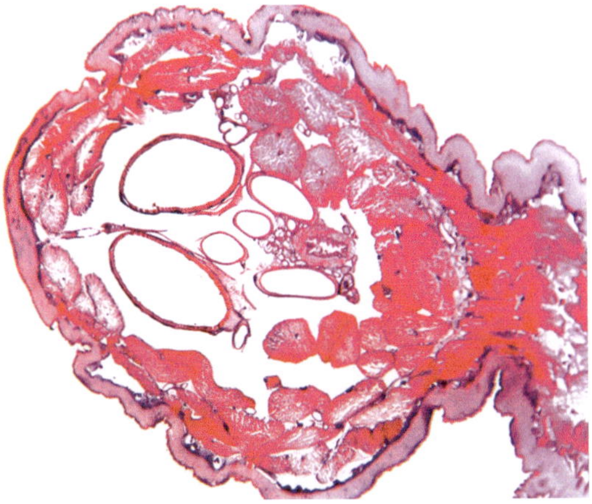

Fig. 13.145 Larva with chitinous cuticle with spines encapsulating the internal organs

Infestation by the larvae of *Diptera* flies.

Histopathology (Figs. 13.145 and 13.146)

- Cavity in the dermis containing larva
- Cavity is surrounded by reactive fibroblasts producing thick stroma
- Acute and chronic inflammation is present
- Larva (up to 20 mm in size) is present within the cavity
- Larva has a thick chitinous cuticle with spines

Muscle and internal organs can be seen

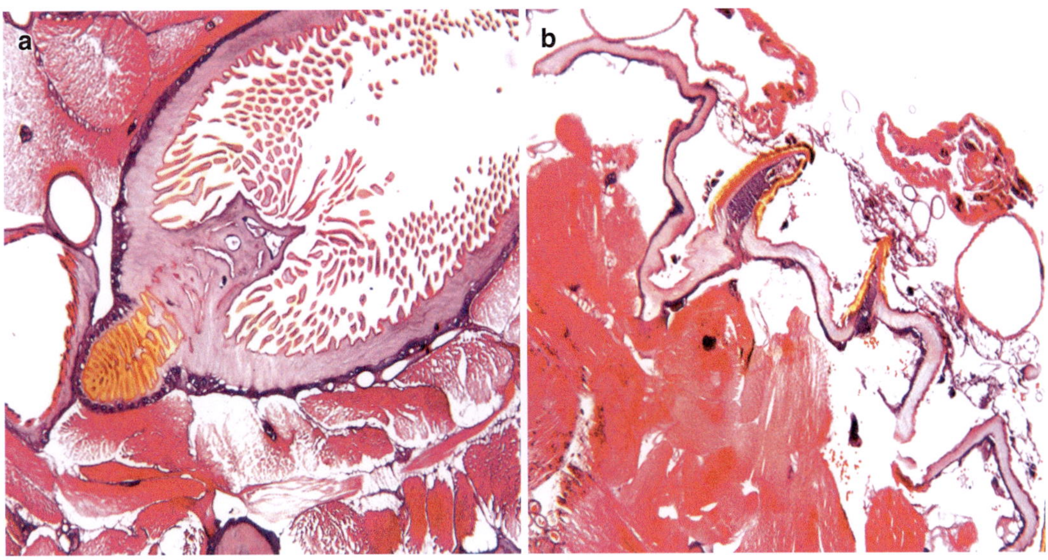

Fig. 13.146 (**a**, **b**) The mouth piece and skeletal muscle

Myoepithelioma

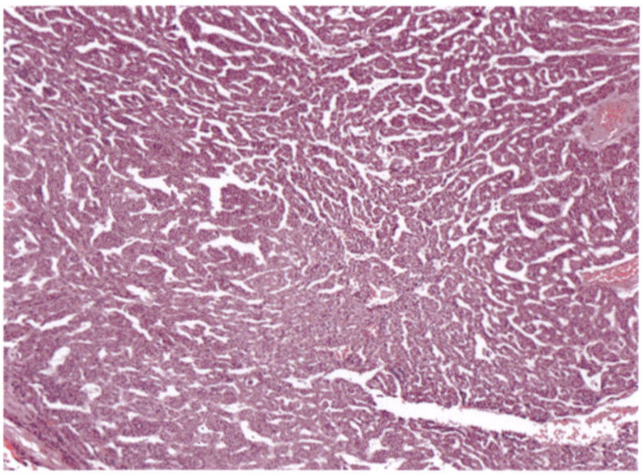

Fig. 13.147 Epithelioid tumor cells forming nodule

Histopathology (Figs. 13.147, 13.148, 13.149, 13.150, and 13.151)

- Dermal nodule made of uniform cells
- Cells are usually epithelioid but can also be spindle or plasmacytoid
- Cells form sheaths or have reticuloid/fascicular ("pericytoma-like") organization in myxoid stroma
- There is minimal cytological atypia but scanty mitoses can be seen
- Cells are S-100+, calponin+, EMA+, and keratin and SMA variable +

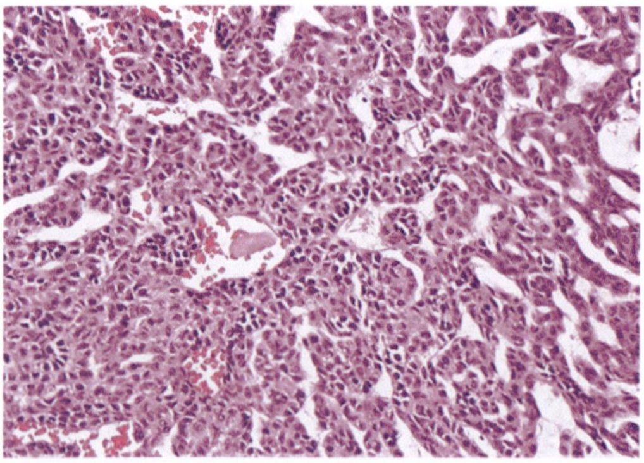

Fig. 13.148 Uniform epithelioid cells in reticuloid pattern

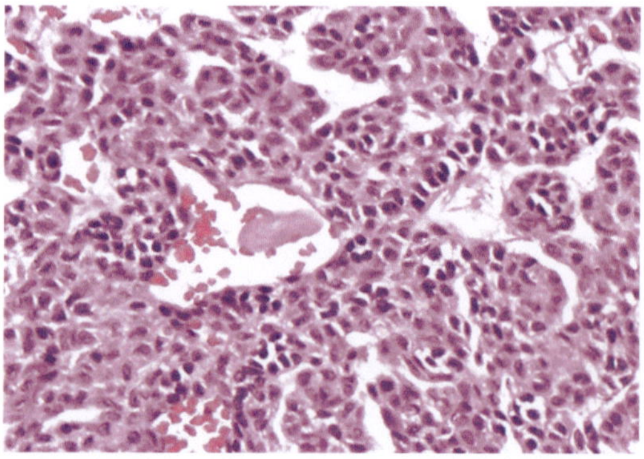

Fig. 13.149 Tumor cells are embedded in the myxoid stroma

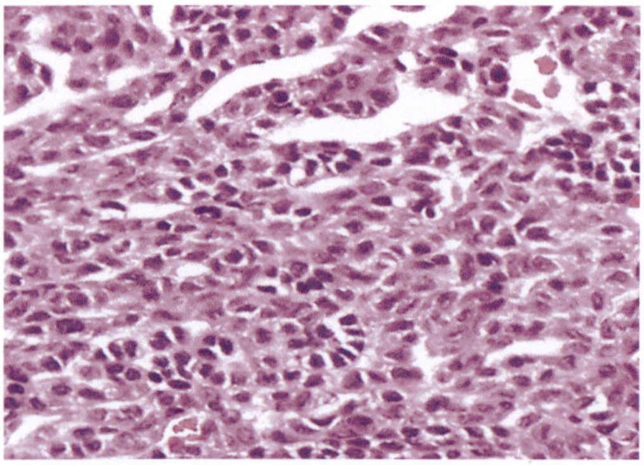

Fig. 13.150 Occasional mitoses can be present (left to the center)

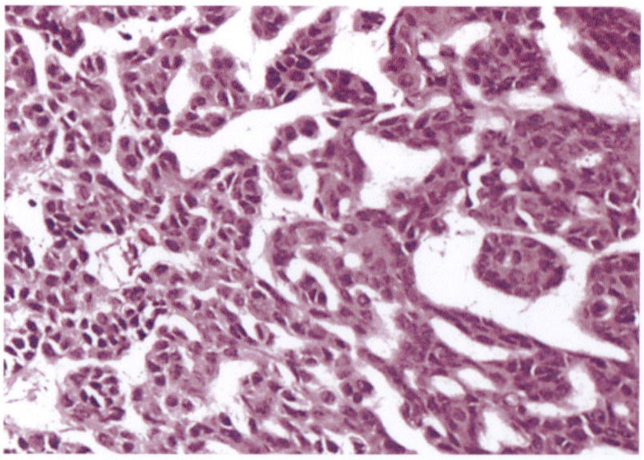

Fig. 13.151 Cells have eosinophilic cytoplasm and vesicular nuclei

Myofibroma

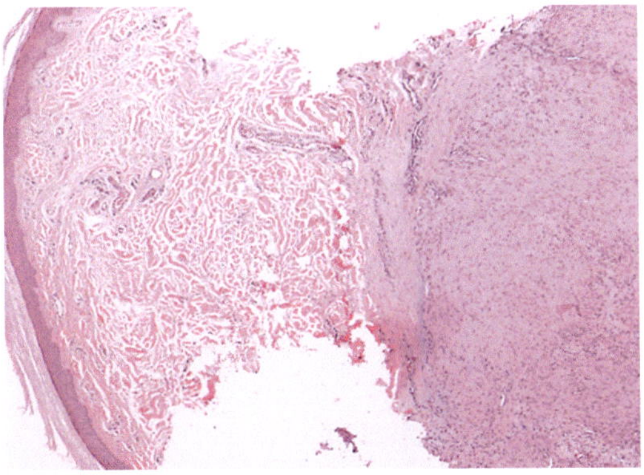

Fig. 13.152 Subcutaneous nodular tumor

Synonyms: Solitary Myofibroma (in adult) and Infantile Myofibromatosis (in young children)

Histopathology (Figs. 13.152, 13.153, 13.154, 13.155, and 13.156)

- Well circumscribed not encapsulated nodule made of plump to elongated SMA positive spindle cells forming short fascicles or whorls organized in two zones
- Central more cellular zone shows vascular network that is hemangiopericytoma-like
- Peripheral less cellular zone is leiomyoma-like

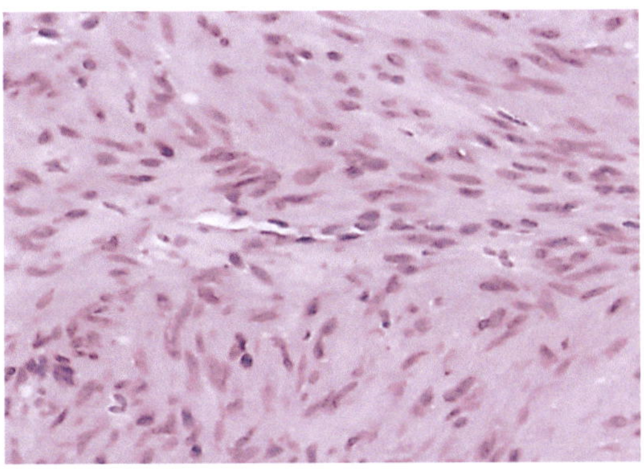

Fig. 13.153 Central area is more cellular with slit-like vessels

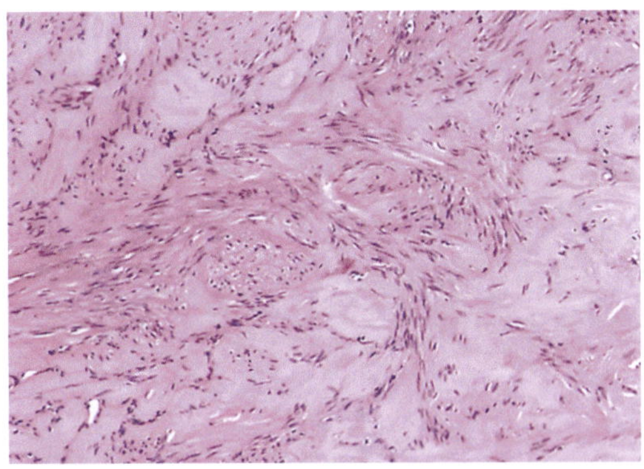

Fig. 13.154 Peripheral less cellular area that resemble muscle bundles

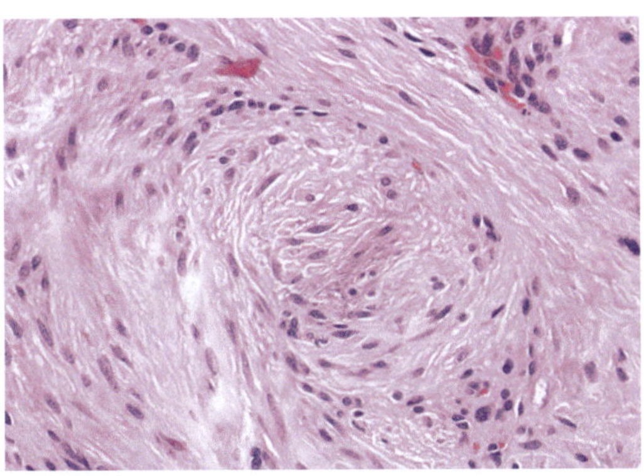

Fig. 13.155 Spindle cells forming whorls

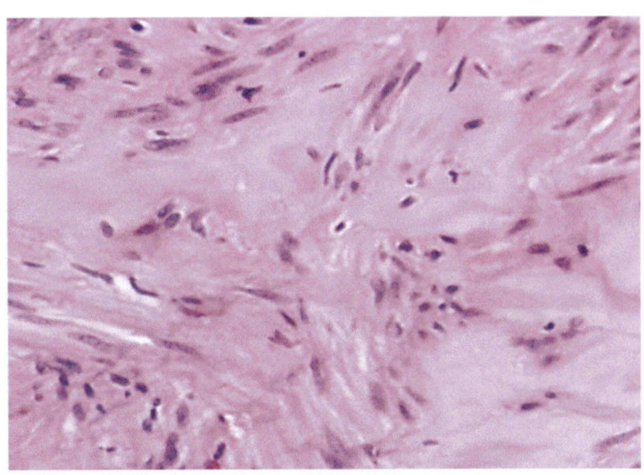

Fig. 13.156 Elongated cigar-shaped nuclei and prominent cytoplasm

Myxoma

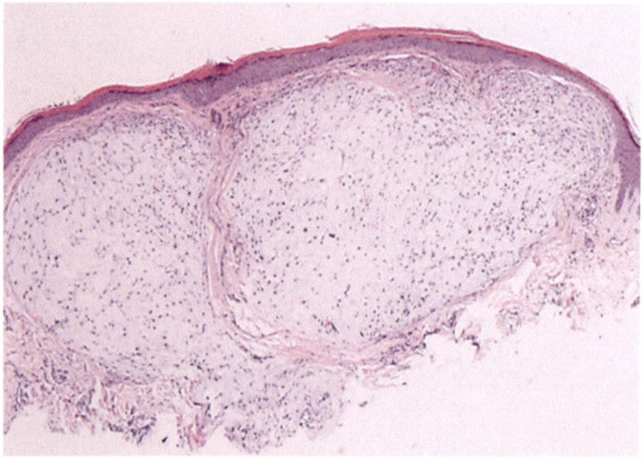

Fig. 13.157 Myxoid tumor with Grenz zone

Histopathology (Figs. 13.157, 13.158, 13.159, and 13.160)

- Sharply circumscribed not encapsulated dermal tumor with Grenz zone separating it from the epidermis
- Mucinous matrix with variably shaped fibroblasts

P.S. myxoma is sharply circumscribed comparing to focal mucinosis and contains more fibroblasts than focal mucinosis. Multiple myxomas are associated with Carney complex and Mazabraud syndrome

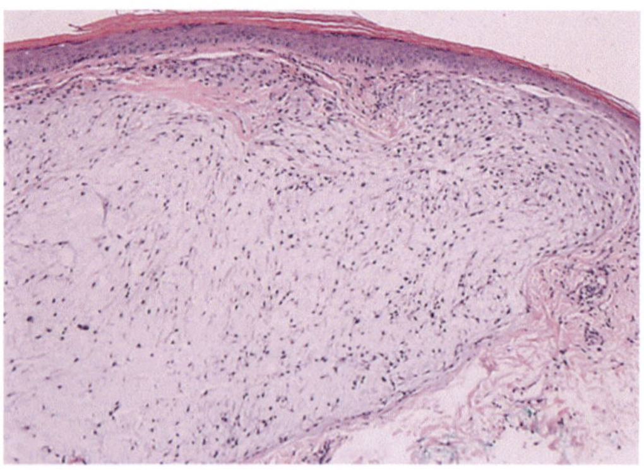

Fig. 13.158 Borders of the tumor are relatively well demarcated

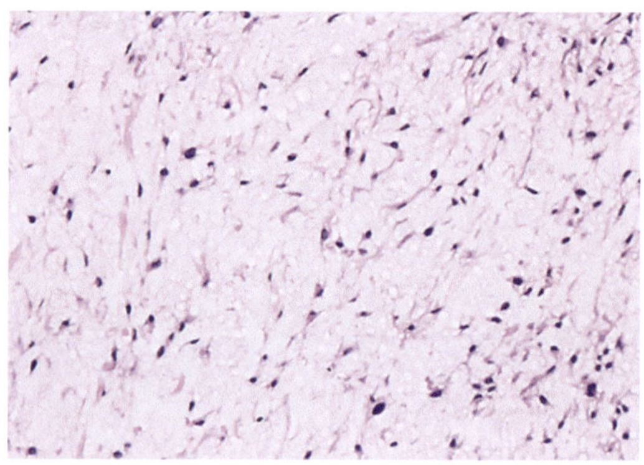

Fig. 13.159 Fibroblasts are more numerous than in the focal mucinosis

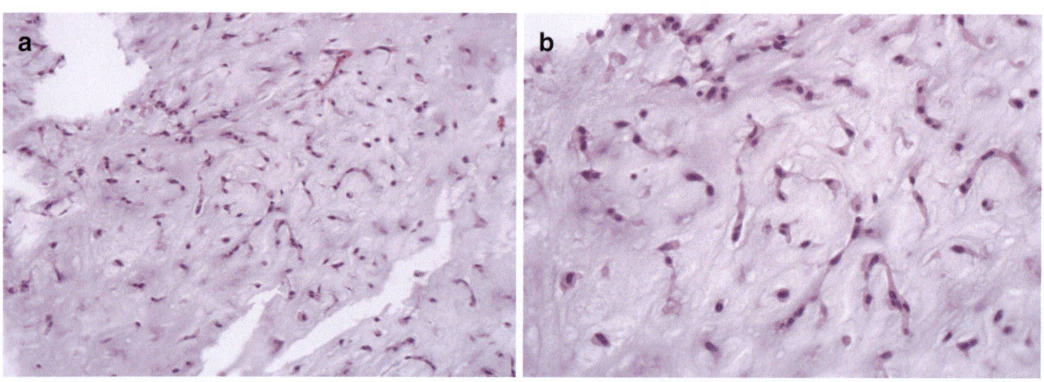

Fig. 13.160 (**a**, **b**) Numerous fibroblasts of various shapes are present in myxoid stroma

Dermatopathology N

14

V. Vincek, *Dermatopathology A–Z*, https://doi.org/10.1007/978-3-319-89486-7_14

Necrobiosis Lipoidica

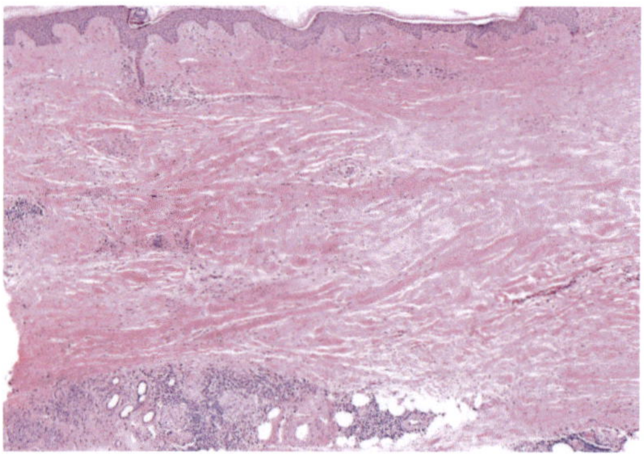

Fig. 14.1 Dermis and subcutis have layered light and dark appearance alternating collagen and inflammation

Histopathology (Figs. 14.1, 14.2, 14.3, 14.4, and 14.5)
- Normal to slightly atrophic epidermis
- Large zone of degenerated, hypocellular, and pale staining collagen
- Surrounding hypocellular area is a horizontally oriented palisade of histiocytes and lymphocytes
- Deep perivascular lymphocytic infiltrate with numerous plasma cells
- Dermal mucin is not present unlike in granuloma annulare

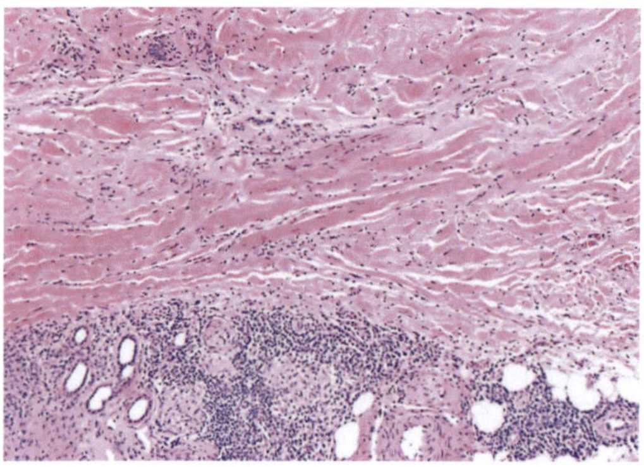

Fig. 14.2 Deep perivascular lymphocytic infiltrate

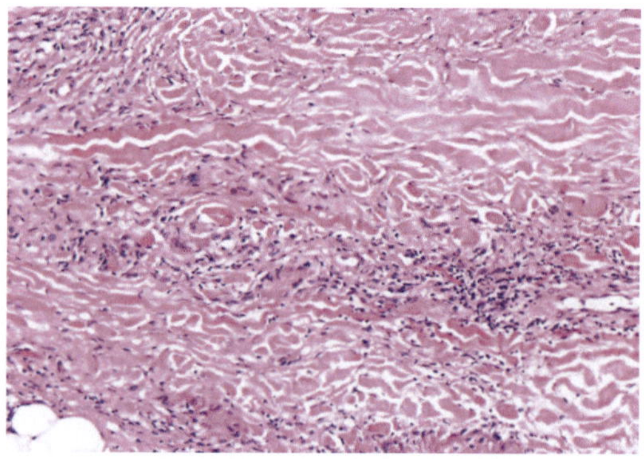

Fig. 14.3 Degenerated pale collagen

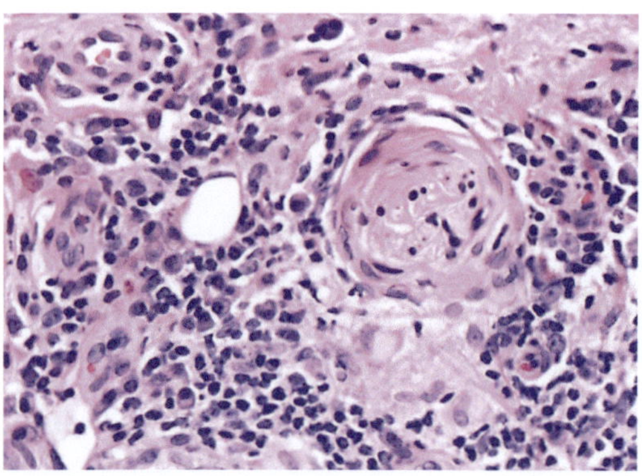

Fig. 14.4 Numerous plasma cells

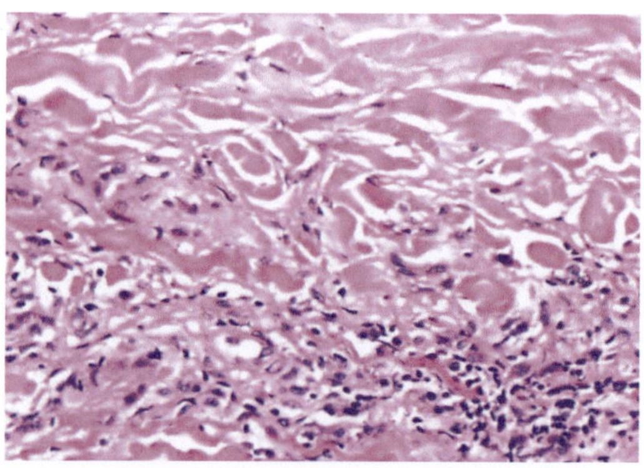

Fig. 14.5 Palisaded histiocytes and lymphocytes

Necrobiotic Xanthogranuloma

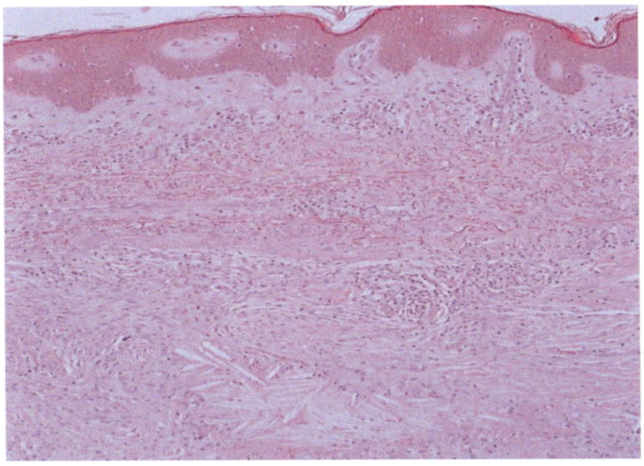

Fig. 14.6 Dermal and subcutaneous inflammatory process with areas of necrobiosis

Histopathology (Figs. 14.6, 14.7, 14.8, and 14.9)

- Infiltrate extends from the dermis into subcutis
- Central area of necrobiosis
- Numerous cholesterol clefts in necrobiotic area
- Peripheral lymphohistiocytic inflammation with giant cells
- Oil Red O stain may reveal focal lipid

P.S. associated with IgG paraproteinemia

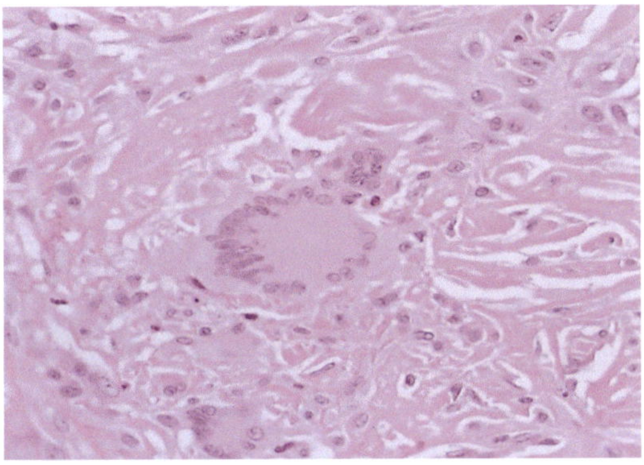

Fig. 14.7 Giants cells are scattered in the inflammatory infiltrate

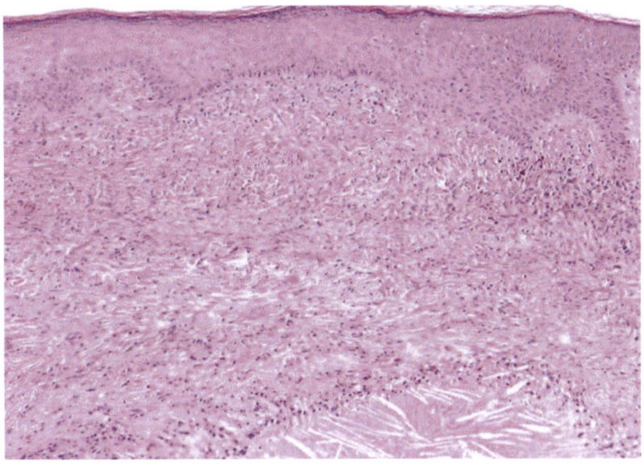

Fig. 14.8 Necrobiosis surrounded by lymphohistiocytic infiltrate

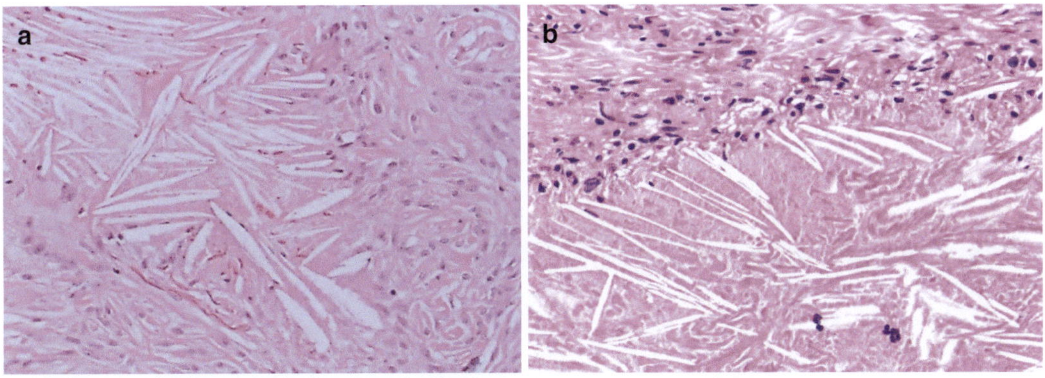

Fig. 14.9 (**a**, **b**) Cholesterol clefts are a characteristic feature

Necrolytic Migratory Erythema

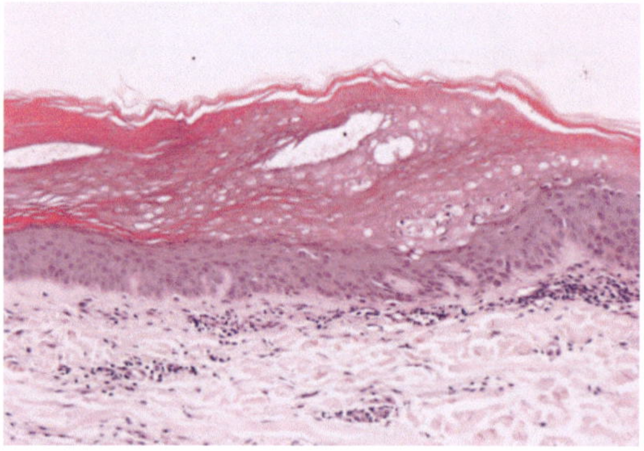

Fig. 14.10 **Early lesion** with mildly psoriasiform epidermis with pallor of the superficial portion of the epidermis

Histopathology (Figs. 14.10, 14.11, 14.12, 14.13, and 14.14)

- In early lesions, the granular layer is missing and there is pallor of keratinocytes in the upper layers of the epidermis
- In late lesions, there is confluent parakeratosis of psoriasiform epidermis and no evidence of granular layer or epidermal pallor. Scattered necrotic keratinocytes can be present in the upper portion of the epidermis.

P.S. **Glucagonoma Syndrome** and **Acrodermatitis Enteropathica** shows similar histopathology

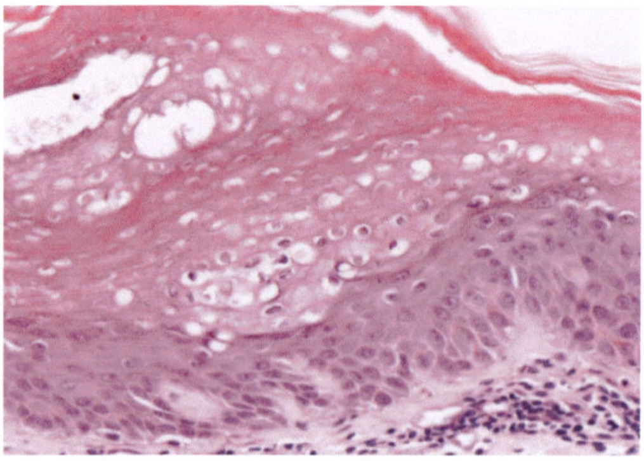

Fig. 14.11 Vacuolated "ghost-like" keratinocytes

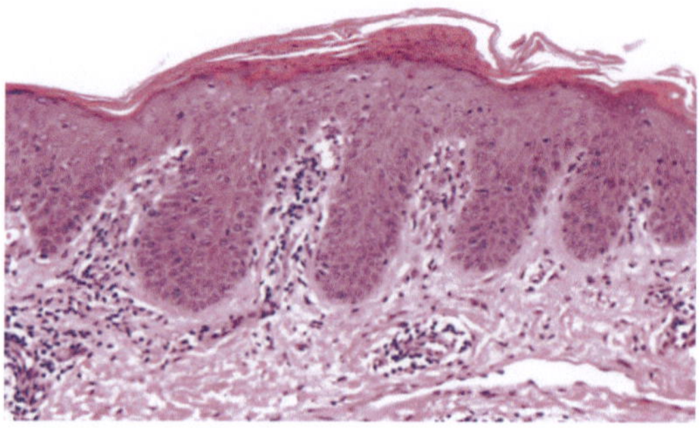

Fig. 14.12 **Late lesion** with psoriasiform epidermis with confluent parakeratosis

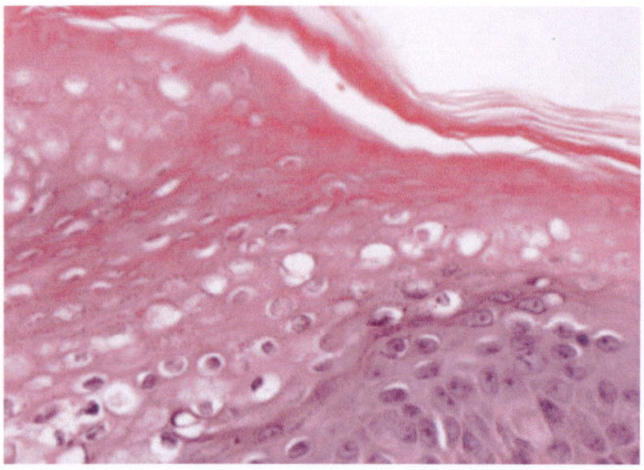

Fig. 14.13 Granular layer is missing above pale keratinocytes

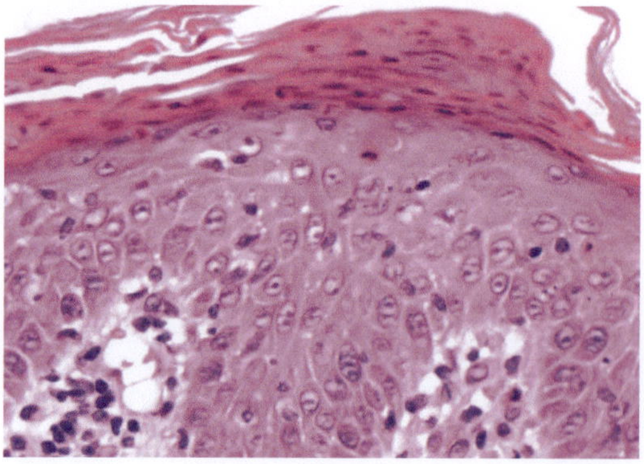

Fig. 14.14 Granular layer and epidermal pallor are absent. Focal necrotic keratinocytes are present

Necrotizing Fasciitis

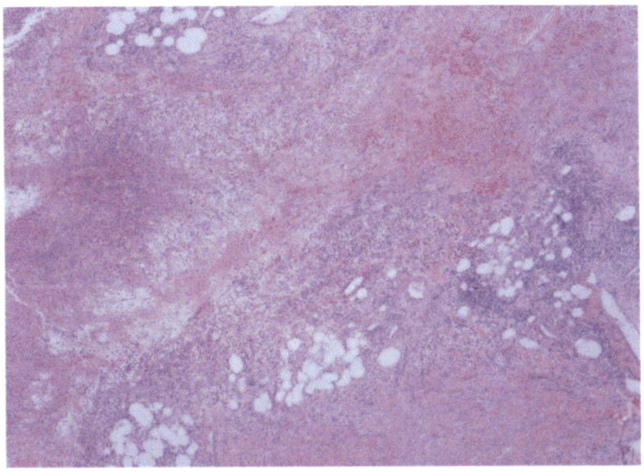

Fig. 14.15 Acute inflammation infiltrating deep tissue

Histopathology (Figs. 14.15, 14.16, 14.17, 14.18, and 14.19)

- Exuberant diffuse neutrophilic inflammation of subcutis, fascia, and muscle
- Large areas of necrosis and edema
- Hemorrhage and thrombosis is common
- Gram-positive cocci identified by special stain

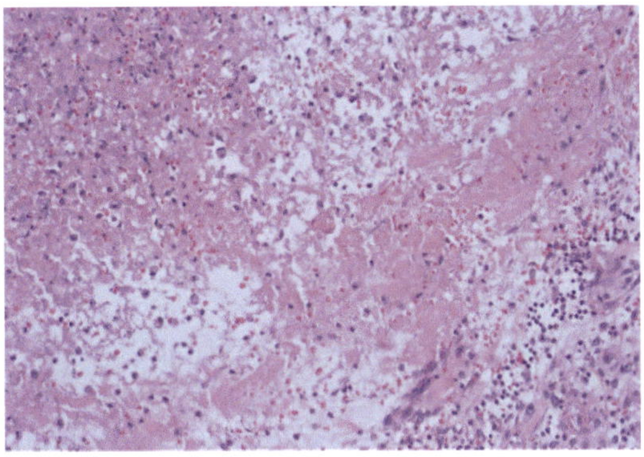

Fig. 14.16 Extensive necrosis with neutrophilic infiltrate and red blood cell extravasation

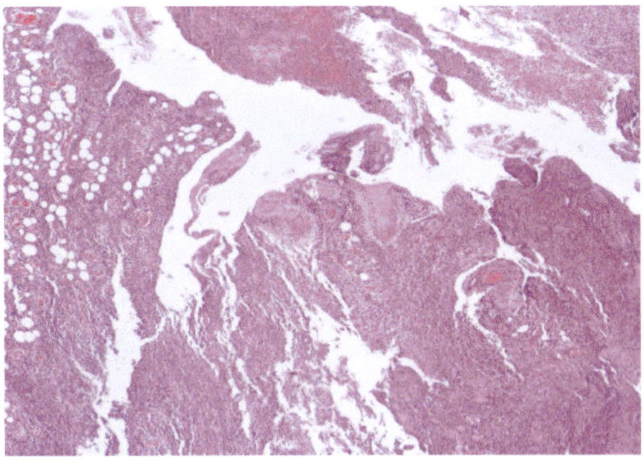

Fig. 14.17 Exuberant neutrophilic infiltrate consuming the subcutis and extending into the fascia

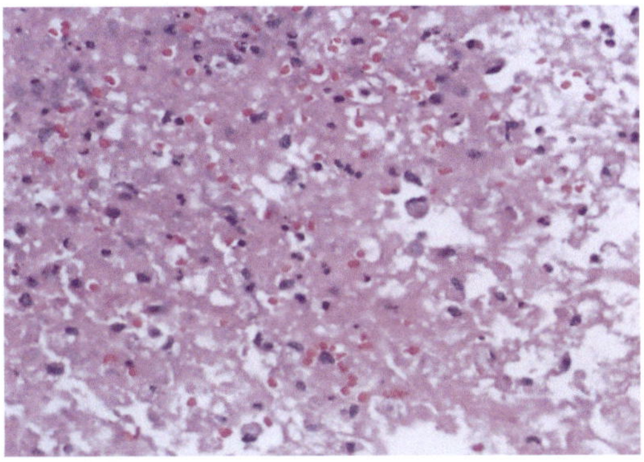

Fig. 14.18 Fragmented neutrophils in necrotic background

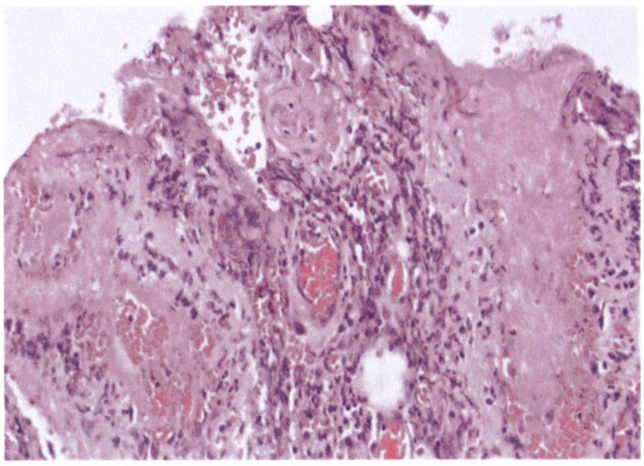

Fig. 14.19 Neutrophilic infiltrate with congested blood vessels and thrombi

Necrotizing Sialometaplasia

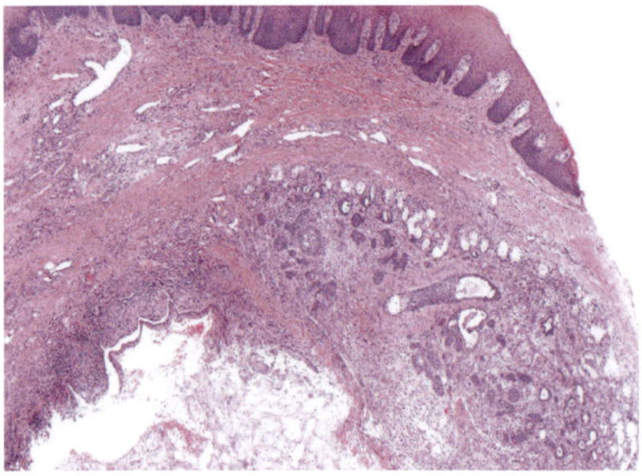

Fig. 14.20 Necrosis of salivary glands

Histopathology (Figs. 14.20, 14.21, 14.22, and 14.23)

- Necrosis of salivary glands with preservation of just their vague outlines
- Prominent squamous metaplasia of glands
- Metaplastic glands are not cytologically atypical
- Prominent acute and chronic inflammation

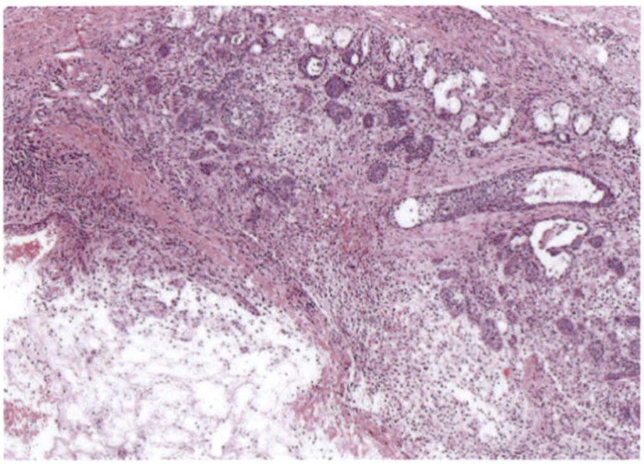

Fig. 14.21 Preservation of the lobular structure of salivary glands

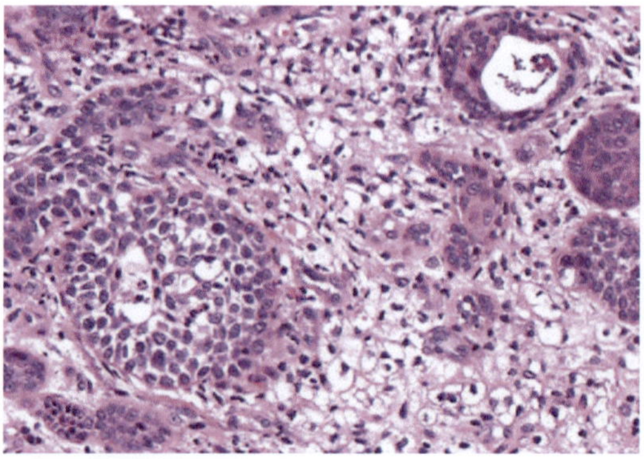

Fig. 14.22 Glands with squamous metaplasia surrounded by lymphocytes and neutrophils

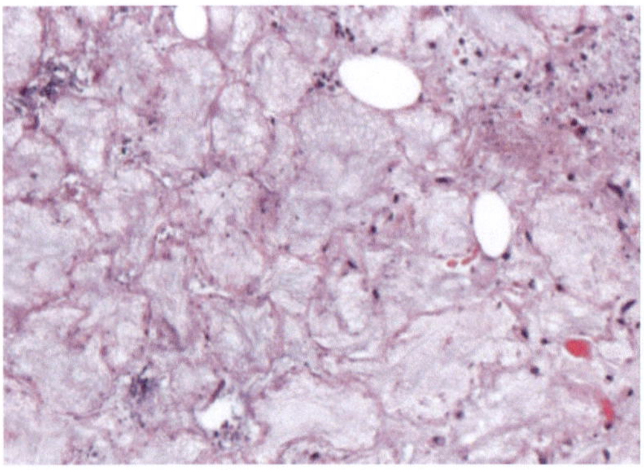

Fig. 14.23 Complete necrosis of salivary glands with preservation of vague lobular outlines

Nephrogenic Systemic Fibrosis

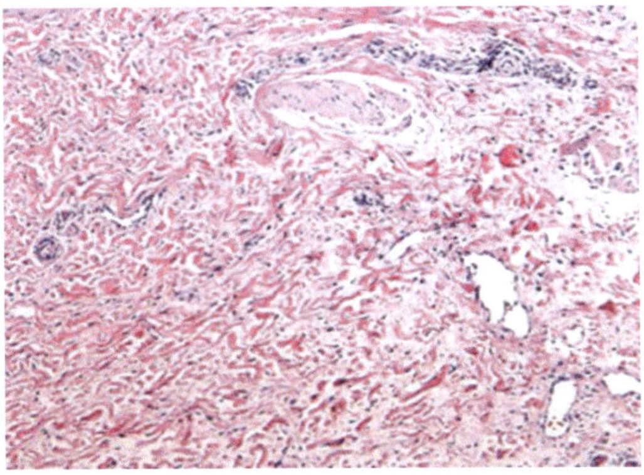

Fig. 14.24 Dermal and subcutaneous fibrosis

Histopathology is indistinguishable from scleromyxedema: (Figs. 14.24, 14.25, 14.26, 14.27, and 14.28)

- Fibrous thickening of dermis and subcutis
- Proliferation of dermal fibroblasts and thickened collagen bundles
- Mucin is focally present

P.S. caused by gadolinium exposure used in imaging of renal insufficiency patients

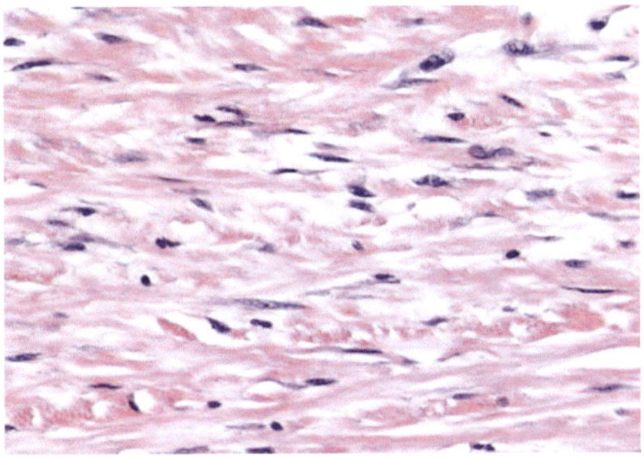

Fig. 14.25 Fibrotic collagen bundles with spaces filled with mucin

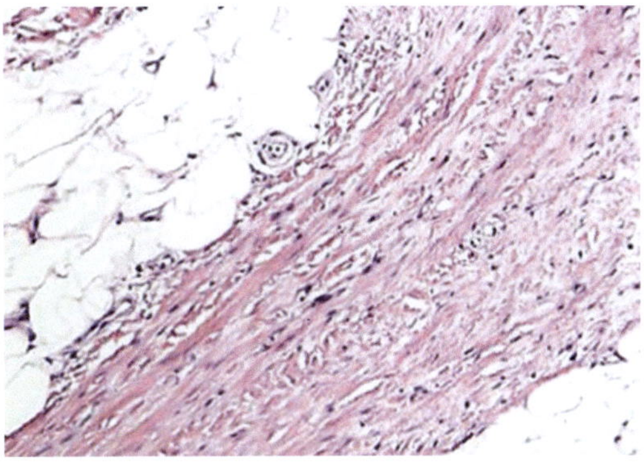

Fig. 14.26 Fibrosis extends into subcutis

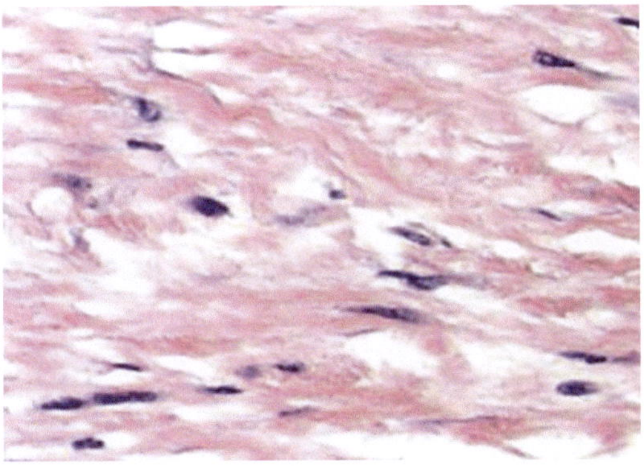

Fig. 14.27 Increased number of fibroblasts

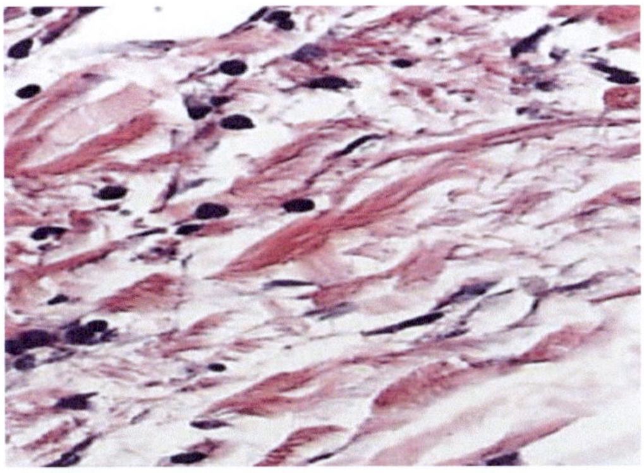

Fig. 14.28 Mucin is present among sclerotic collagen bundles

Neurofibroma

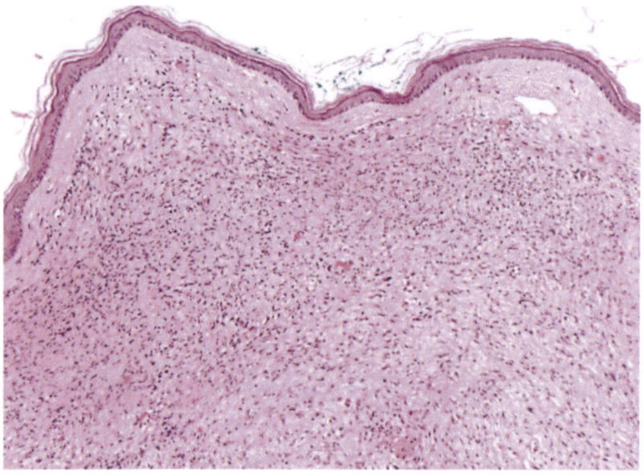

Fig. 14.29 Dermal tumor sparring papillary dermis (Grenz zone)

Histopathology (Figs. 14.29, 14.30, 14.31, 14.32, and 14.33)

- Ill-defined dermal/subcutaneous nodule
- Tumor demonstrates Grenz zone separating it from unremarkable epidermis
- Tumor is made of spindle cells with wavy serpentine nuclei (S-100+)
- Scattered mast cells are present
- Stroma is pale with delicate collagen
- Stroma can be myxoid

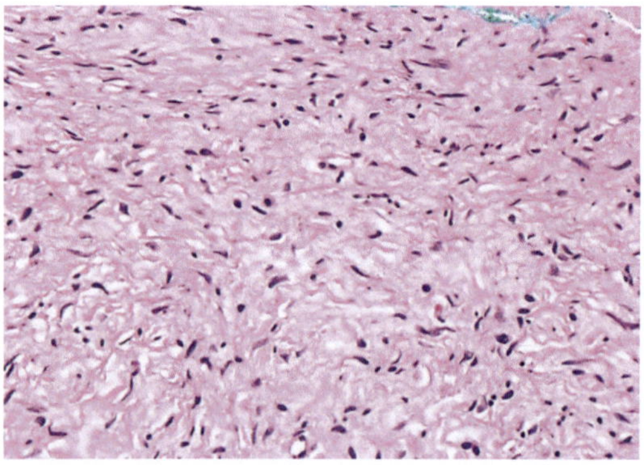

Fig. 14.30 Spindle uniform wavy cells in pale delicate stroma

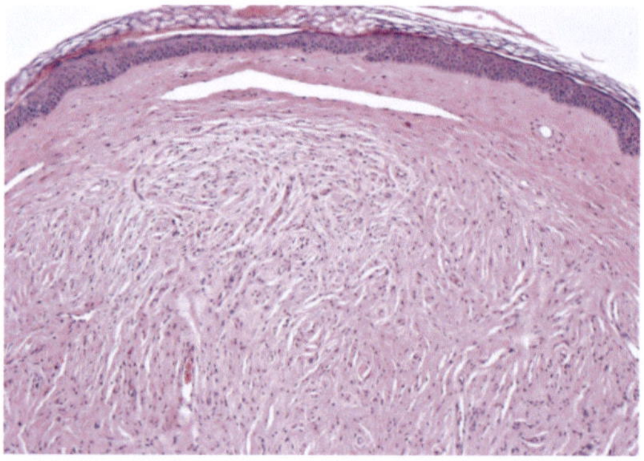

Fig. 14.31 Dermal tumor in bluish myxoid stroma

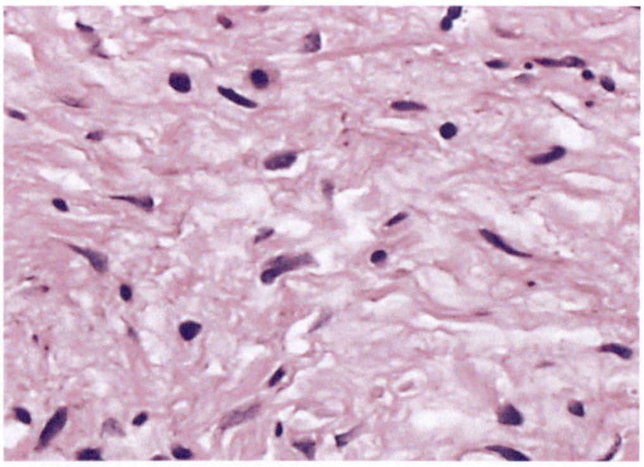

Fig. 14.32 Scattered mast cells with purple cytoplasm are present

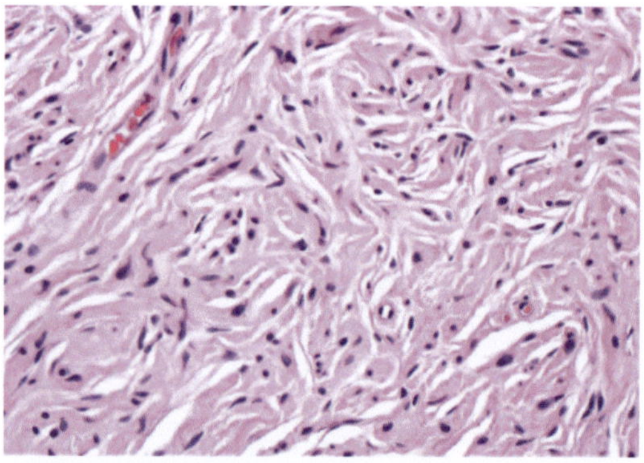

Fig. 14.33 No evidence of cytological atypia or mitoses

Neurofollicular Hamartoma

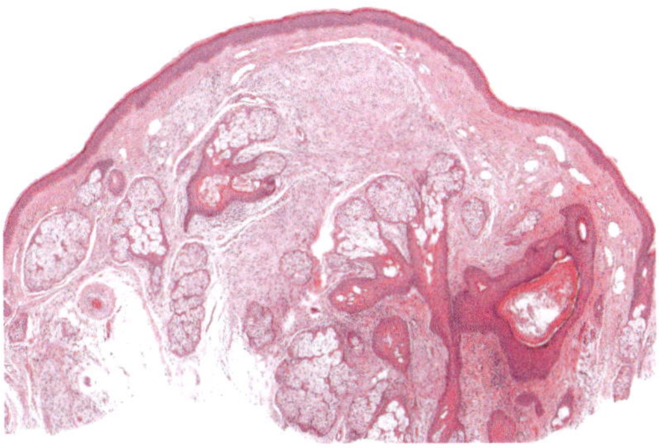

Fig. 14.34 Distorted pilosebaceous units

Histopathology (Figs. 14.34, 14.35, and 14.36)
- Distorted, hyperplastic pilosebaceous units
- Prominent sebaceous glands
- Surrounding myxoid stroma
- Stroma contains numerous spindle cells (NSE+, S-100+, CD34−) resembling neural tissue

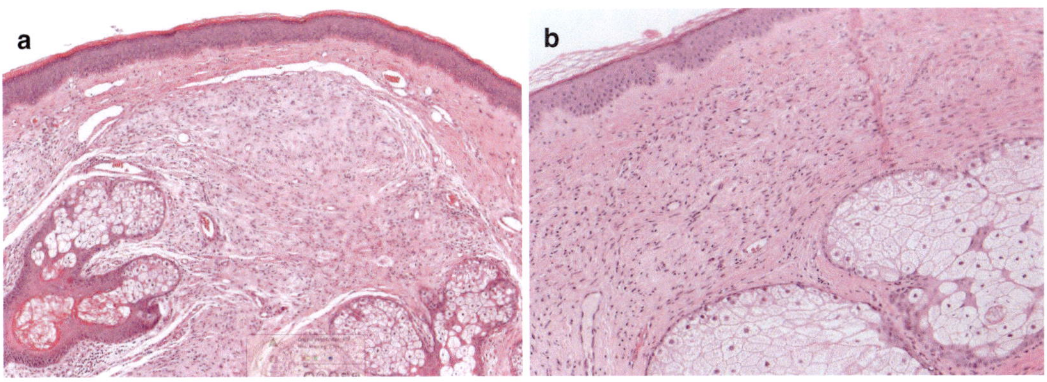

Fig. 14.35 (**a**, **b**) Prominent sebaceous glands surrounded by cellular myxoid stroma

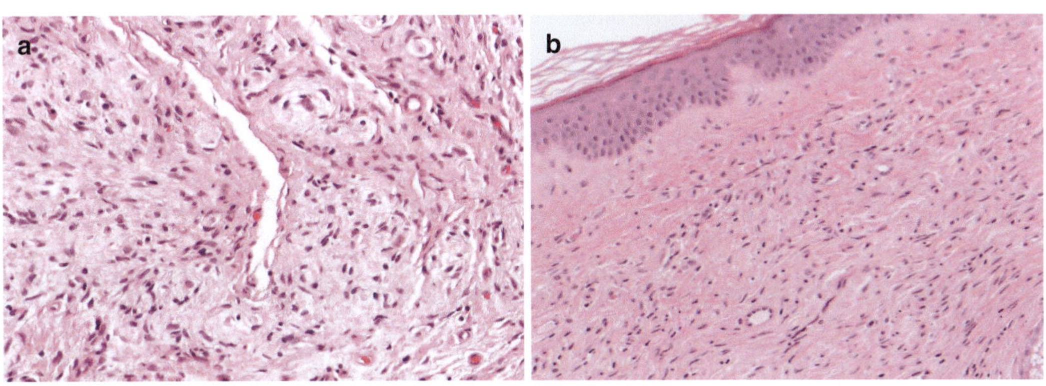

Fig. 14.36 (**a**, **b**) Stromal spindle cells resembling neurofibroma cells

Neurothekeoma

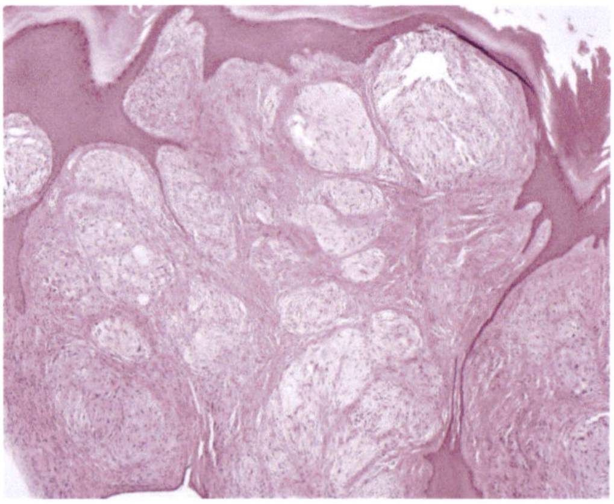

Fig. 14.37 Nodular myxoid tumor

Synonym: Nerve Sheath Myxoma

Histopathology: (Figs. 14.37, 14.38, and 14.39)

- Multilobular tumor made of uniform spindle cells with no atypia or mitoses
- Cells are arranged in a swirling pattern in myxoid stroma forming nests separated by fibrous stroma

Cellular neurothekeoma:

- Ill-defined cellular tumor with poorly defined nests made of mostly rounded and less spindle cells; cells are mildly atypical with pale cytoplasm, vesicular nuclei, and occasional mitoses (Figs. 14.40 and 14.41)

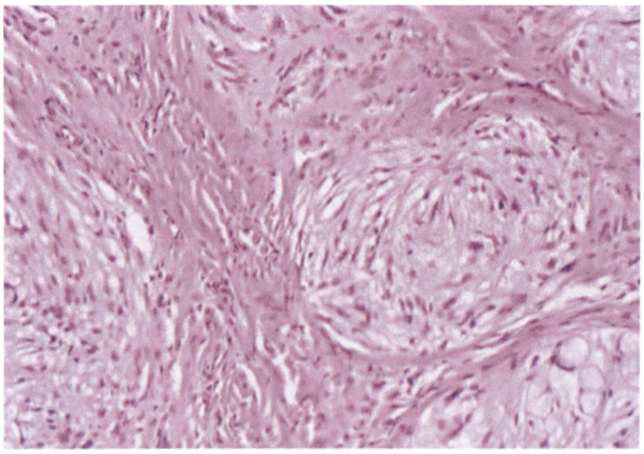

Fig. 14.38 Myxoid nests separated by fibrous stroma

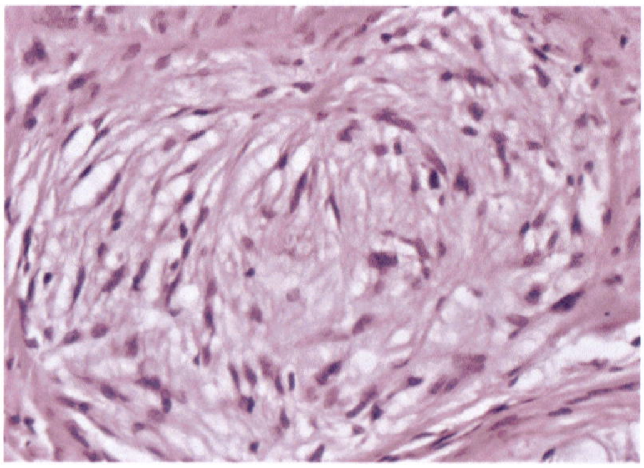

Fig. 14.39 Spindle cells arranged in a swirling pattern

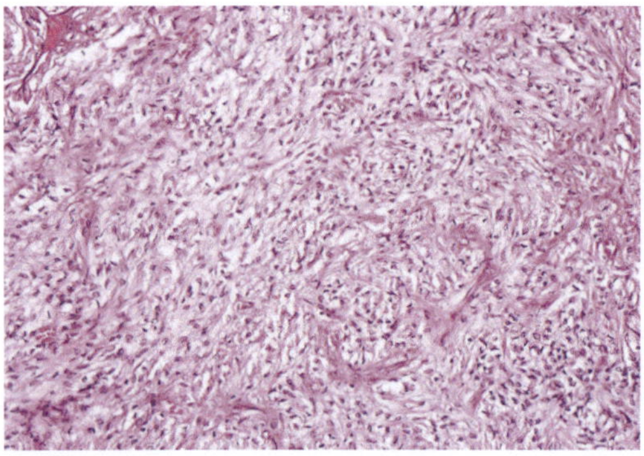

Fig. 14.40 Cellular neurothekeoma with poorly defined lobules

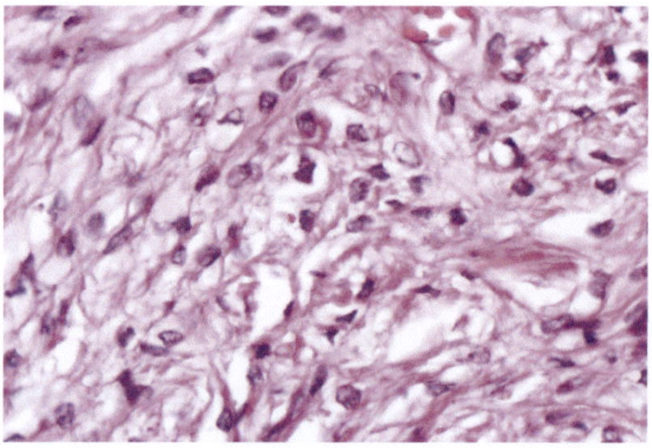

Fig. 14.41 Epithelioid cells with pale cytoplasm and vesicular nuclei

Neutrophilic Eccrine Hidradenitis

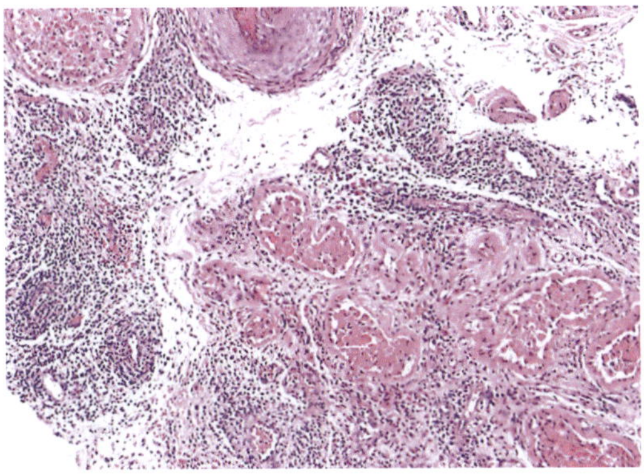

Fig. 14.42 Necrosis and inflammation involving the eccrine glands

Histopathology (Figs. 14.42, 14.43, 14.44, and 14.45)

- Neutrophilic infiltrate around eccrine glands
- Necrosis of eccrine gland
- Ducts of eccrine glands are usually spared
- Syringosquamous metaplasia can be present

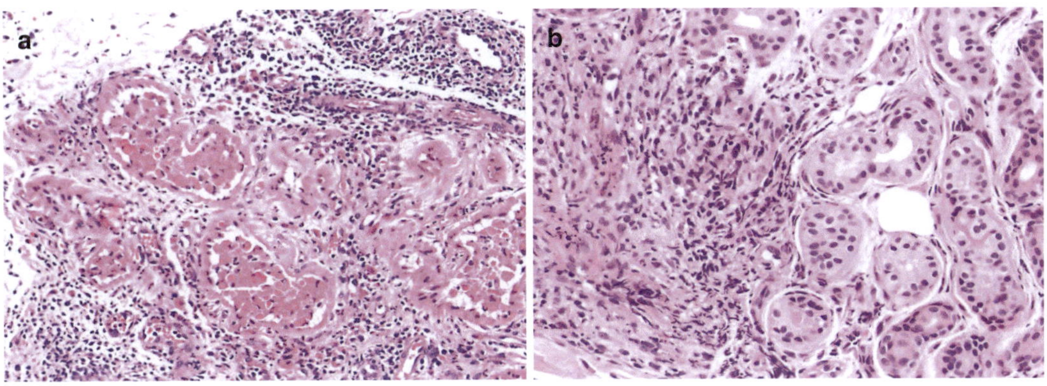

Fig. 14.43 (**a**, **b**) Neutrophils surround necrotic secretory part of eccrine glands some of which show squamous metaplasia

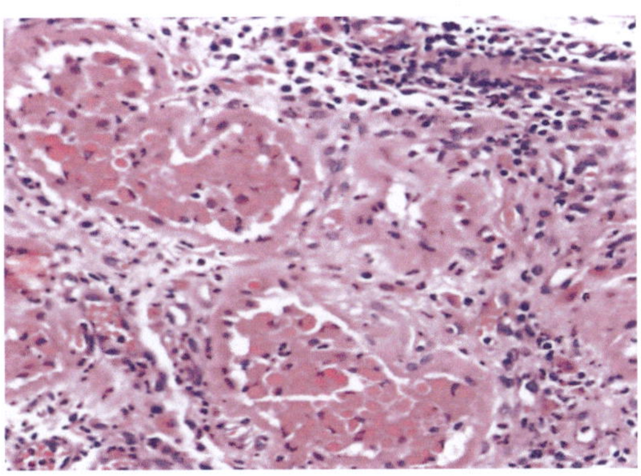

Fig. 14.44 Necrotic debris within eccrine glands

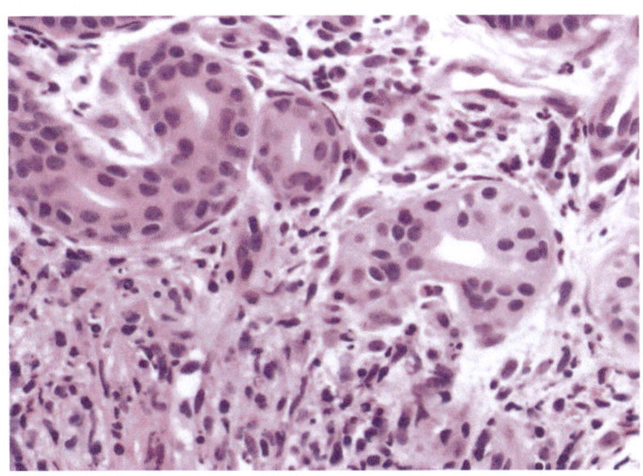

Fig. 14.45 Ducts of eccrine glands are spared of necrosis

Nevus Comedonicus

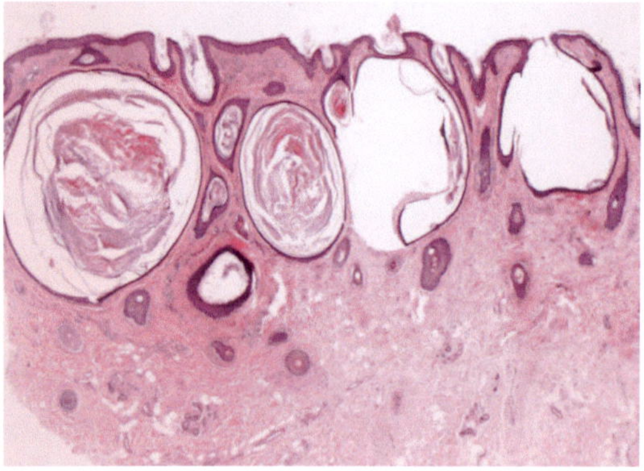

Fig. 14.46 Multiple open and closed comedones

Synonym: Comedo Nevus

Histopathology (Figs. 14.46, 14.47, and 14.48)

- Multiple open and closed comedones
- Comedone is cystically dilated hair follicle
- Lumen is filled with keratin debris
- Sebaceous glands are decreased in number or completely absent

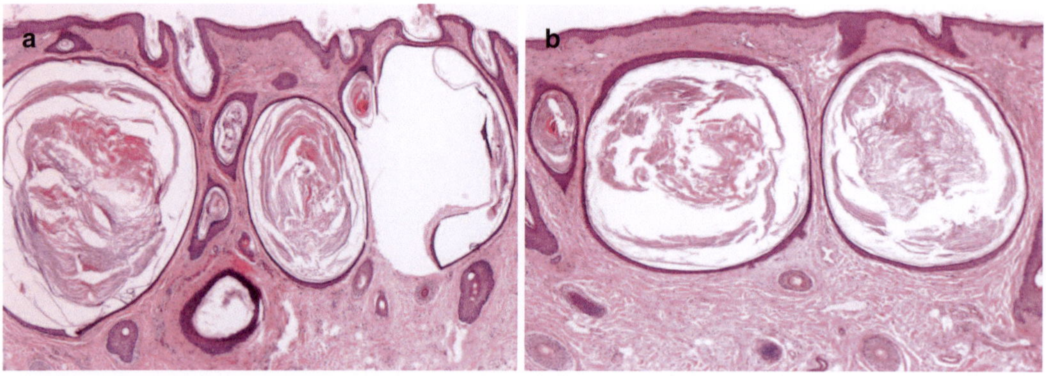

Fig. 14.47 (**a**, **b**) Sebaceous glands are missing

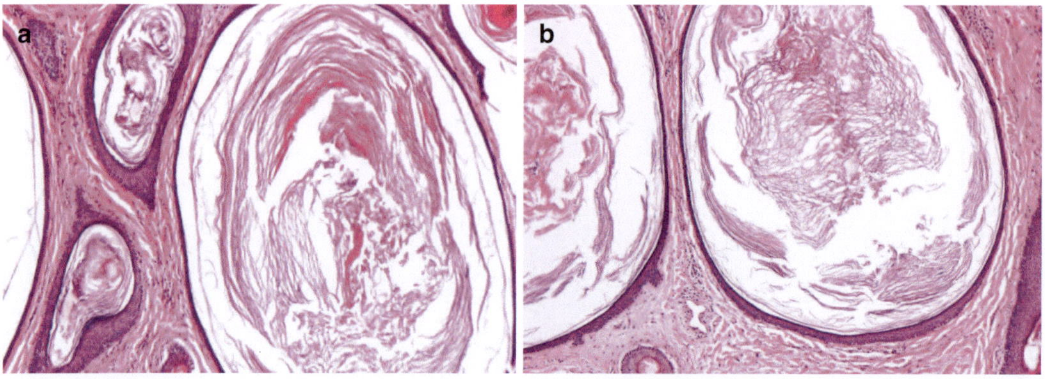

Fig. 14.48 (**a**, **b**) Comedones have atrophic wall and are filled with laminated keratin

Nevus Depigmentosus

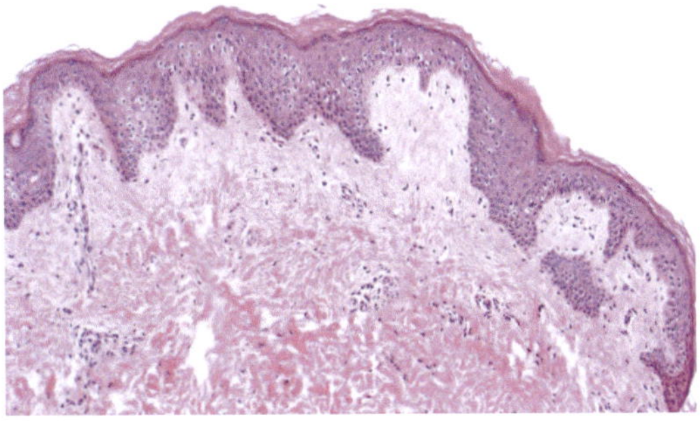

Fig. 14.49 Unremarkable skin

Synonym: Nevus Achromicus

Histopathology (Figs. 14.49, 14.50, and 14.51)

- Normal appearing epidermis on H&E slides
- Number of melanocytes is normal
- Amount of epidermal melanin is decreased

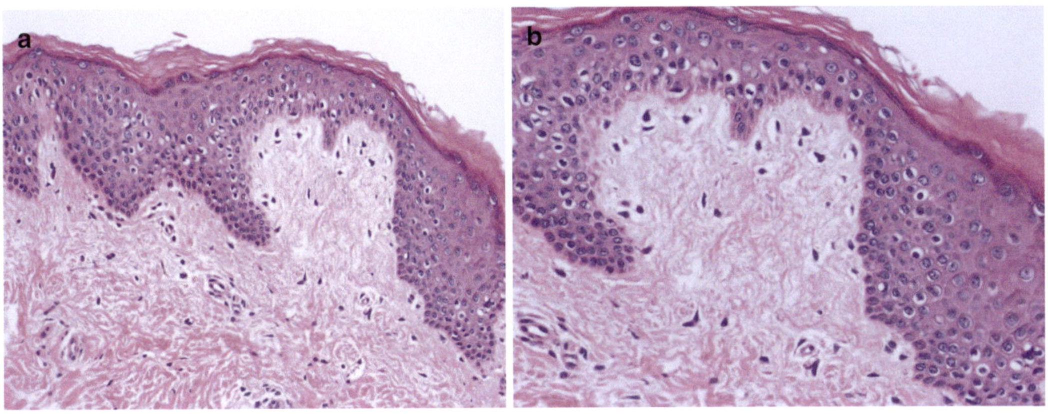

Fig. 14.50 (**a**, **b**) Normal appearing epidermis and dermis

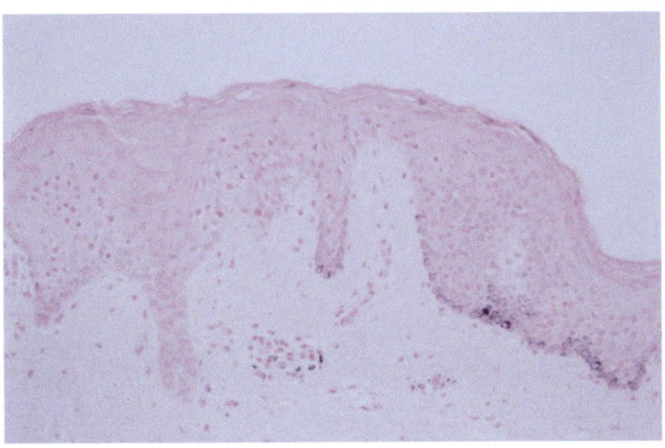

Fig. 14.51 Fontana Masson stain demonstrates that epidermal melanin (black) is decreased

Nevus Flammeus

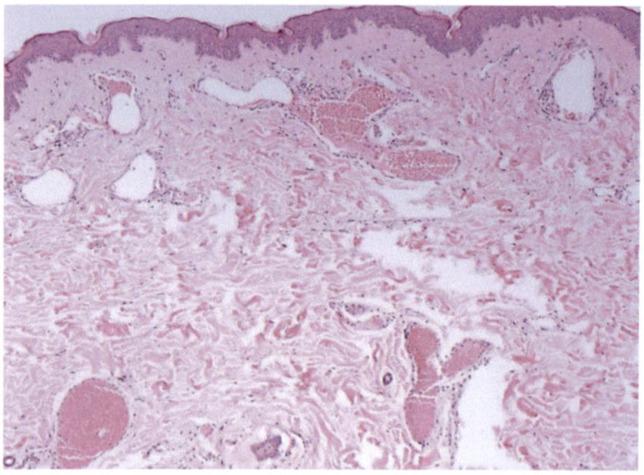

Fig. 14.52 Dermal capillaries of various sizes

Synonyms: Port Wine Stain, Salmon Patch

Histopathology (Figs. 14.52, 14.53, 14.54, and 14.55)

- Widely dilated thin walled capillaries in the dermis
- Congestion of capillaries is prominent

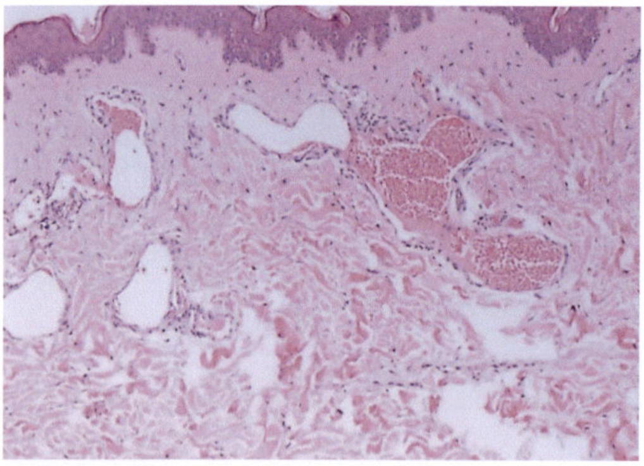

Fig. 14.53 Many capillaries are congested with red blood cells

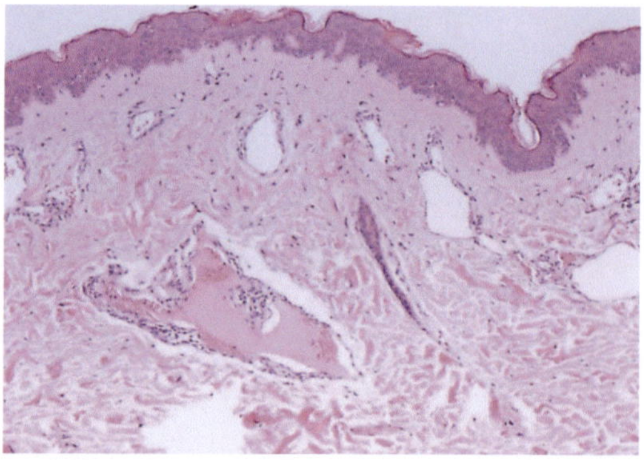

Fig. 14.54 Irregular dilated capillaries

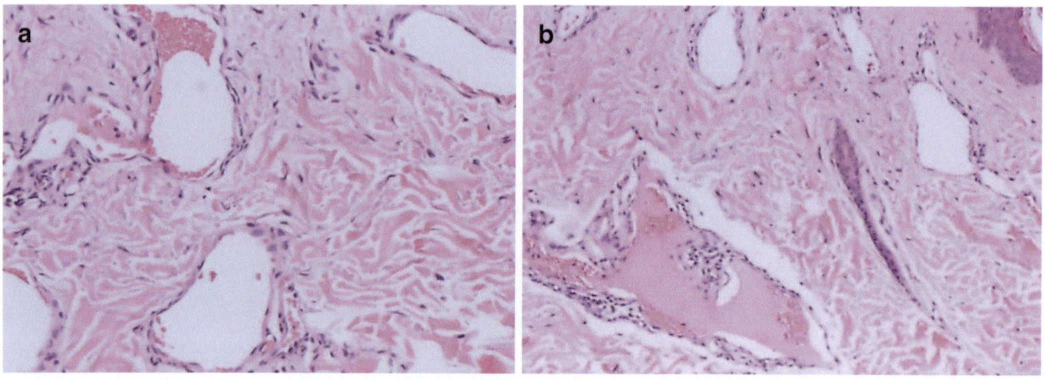

Fig. 14.55 (a, b) Flat endothelial cells with no atypia line the wall of capillaries

Nevus Lipomatosus

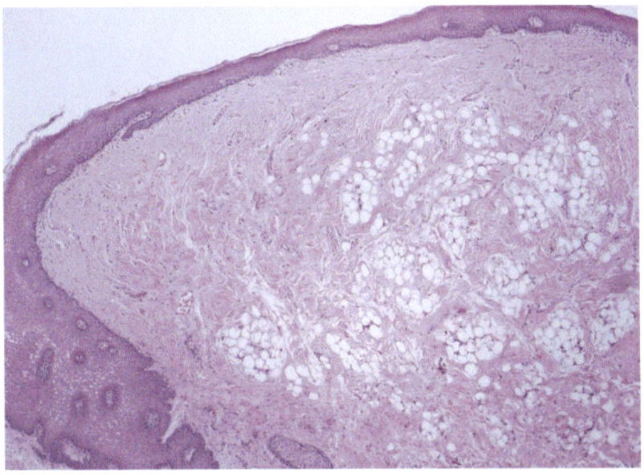

Fig. 14.56 Polypoid lesion with fibroadipose tissue

Synonym: Nevus Lipomatosus Superficialis of Hoffman and Zurhellen

Histopathology (Figs. 14.56, 14.57, and 14.58)

- Presence of mature adipose tissue within the superficial dermis
- Adnexal structures are absent

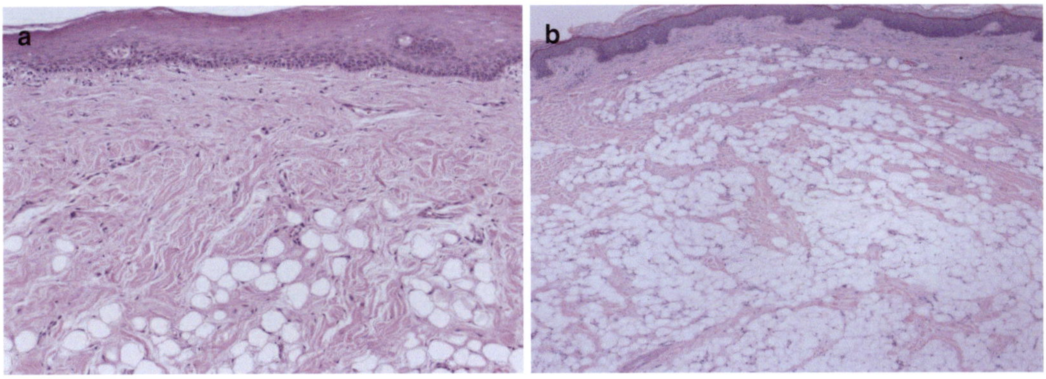

Fig. 14.57 (**a**, **b**) Mature adipose tissue infiltrates superficial dermis and adnexal structures are missing

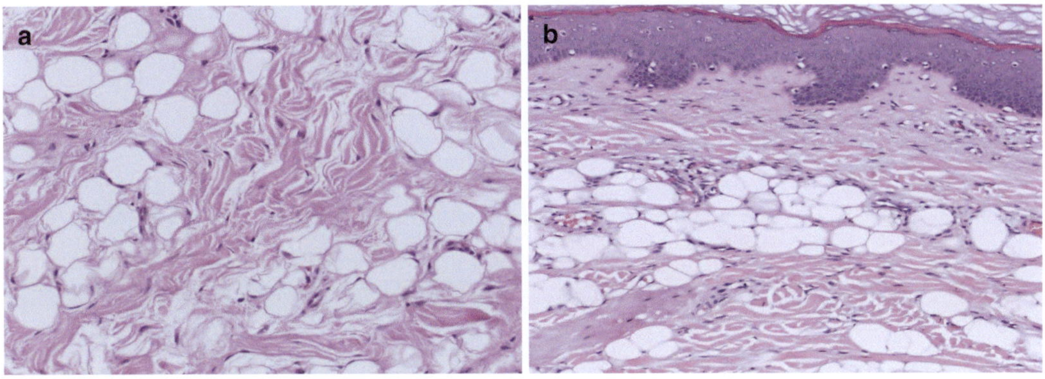

Fig. 14.58 (**a**, **b**) Mature adipocytes are separated by fibrous stroma

Nevus of Ito/Ota/Hori/Sun

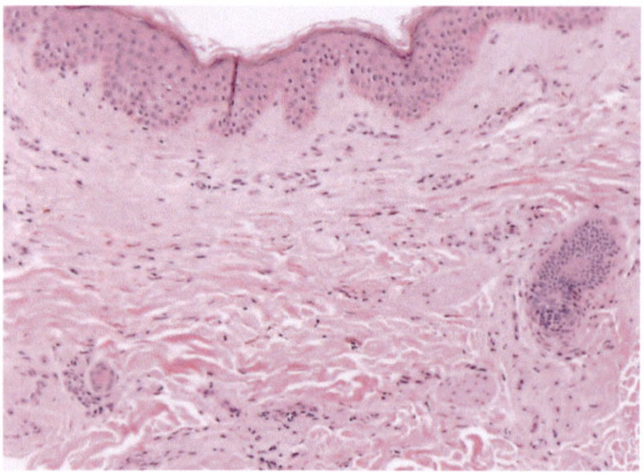

Fig. 14.59 Pigmented melanocytes oriented parallel to the epidermis

Synonym: Dermal Melanocytosis

Histopathology (Figs. 14.59, 14.60, and 14.61)

- Heavily pigmented spindle dendritic melanocytes
- Pigmented cells have tendency to be oriented parallel to the surface or circular around appendages
- In *Nevus of Ota/Ito/Hori/Sun* dendritic melanocytes are located in the upper and mid dermis but each has a different anatomic distribution

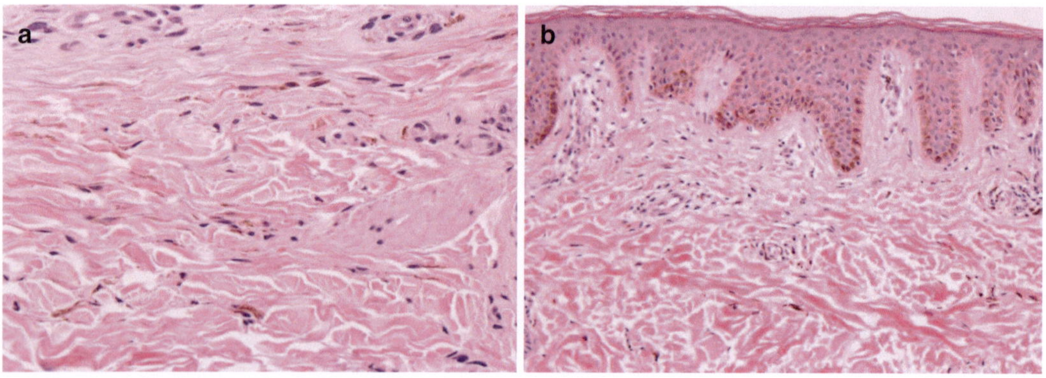

Fig. 14.60 (**a**, **b**) Upper and mid dermis contains scattered pigmented dendritic melanocytes

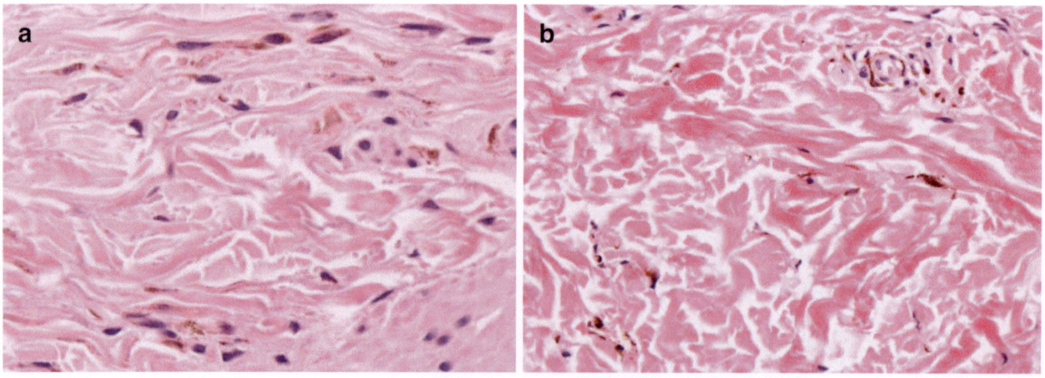

Fig. 14.61 (**a**, **b**) Wavy spindle pigmented melanocytes within fibrotic hypocellular stroma

Nevus Sebaceus of Jadassohn

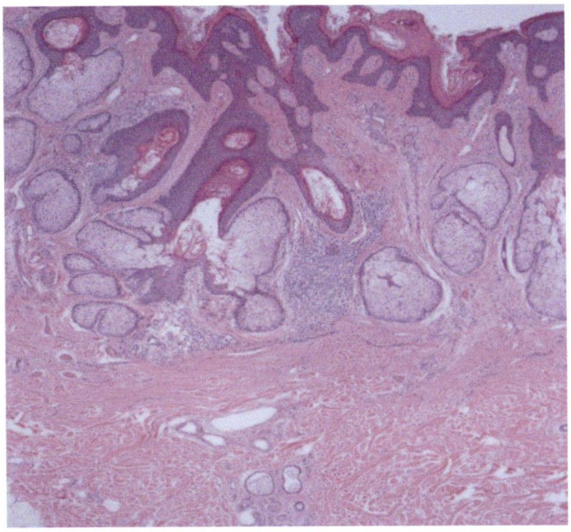

Fig. 14.62 **18 year old's** nevus sebaceous

Synonym: Organoid nevus

Histopathology (Figs. 14.62, 14.63, 14.64, 14.65, and 14.66)

- Epidermal papillomatosis and hyperkeratosis
- **In infants/young children** pilosebaceous units are immature whereas **at puberty** sebaceous glands become hyperplastic
- Mature hair follicles are absent or decreased in number
- Sebaceous glands commonly communicate directly with the epidermis and apocrine glands are present in the lower dermis
- **With increasing age,** sebaceous glands regress

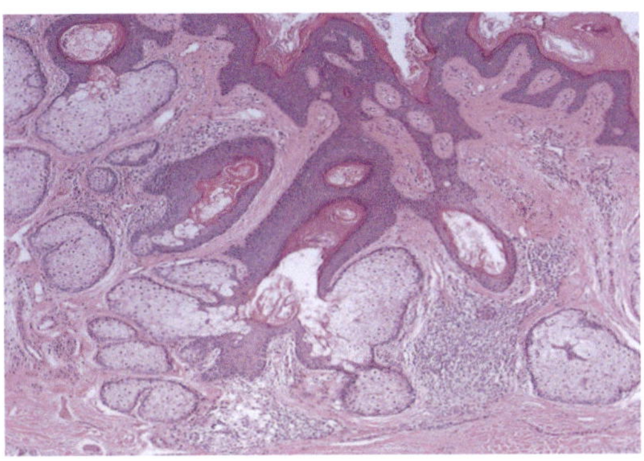

Fig. 14.63 Epidermal hyperplasia with sebaceous hyperplasia

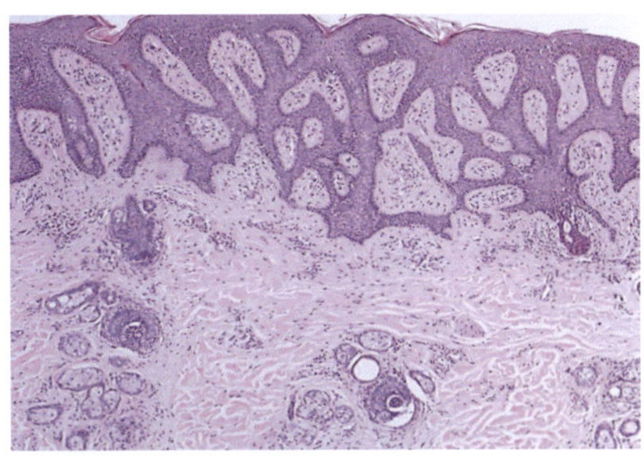

Fig. 14.64 Nevus sebaceous of **young child** with hypoplastic sebaceous glands

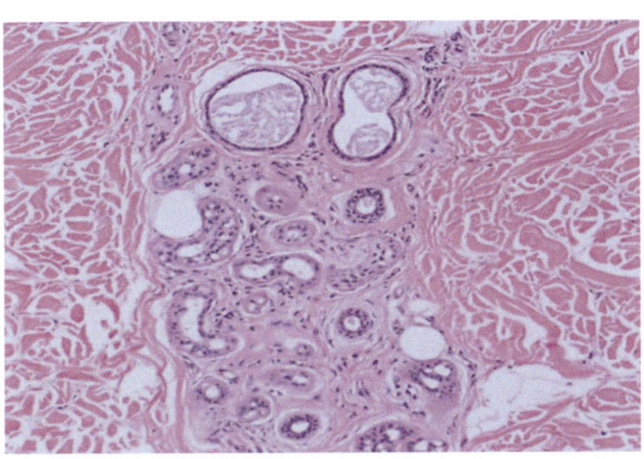

Fig. 14.65 Apocrine glands are present in the dermis

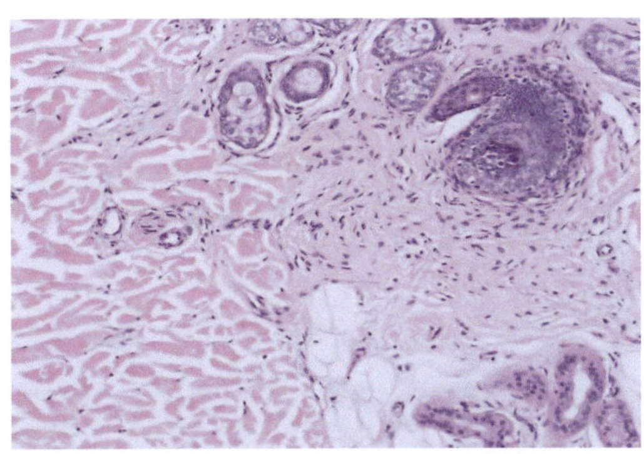

Fig. 14.66 Immature hair follicles and apocrine glands

Nevus Spilus

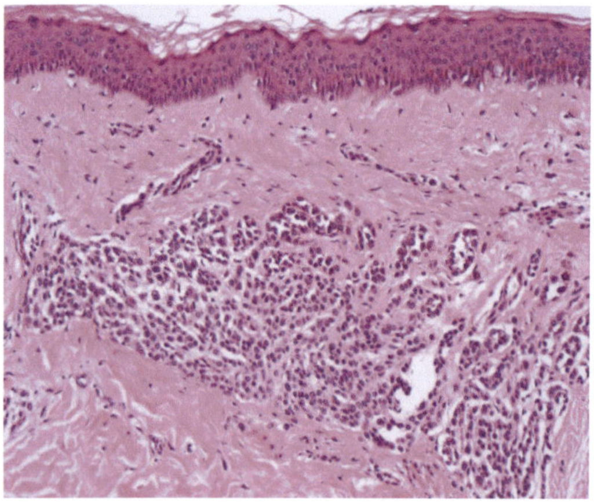

Fig. 14.67 Dermal nevus area

Synonym: Speckled Lentiginous Nevus

Histopathology:

- In the darkly pigmented speckled area junctional, dermal, or compound nevus is present (Figs. 14.67 and 14.68)
- In the lighter intervening skin there are features of lentigo simplex (Figs. 14.69 and 14.70)

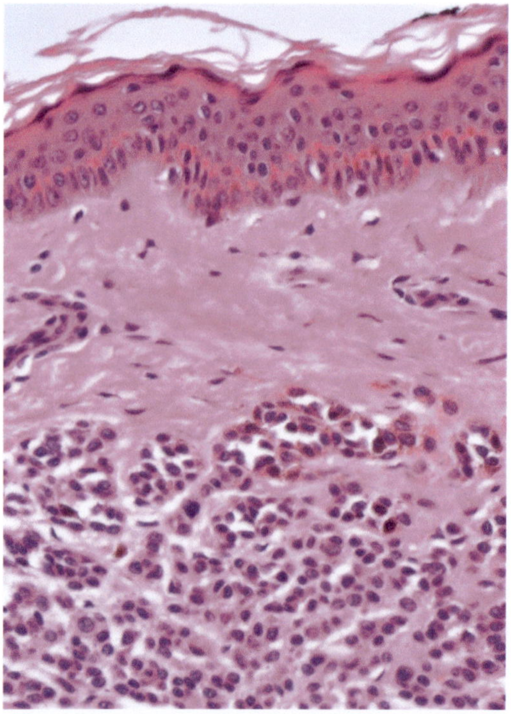

Fig. 14.68 Maturing dermal melanocytes

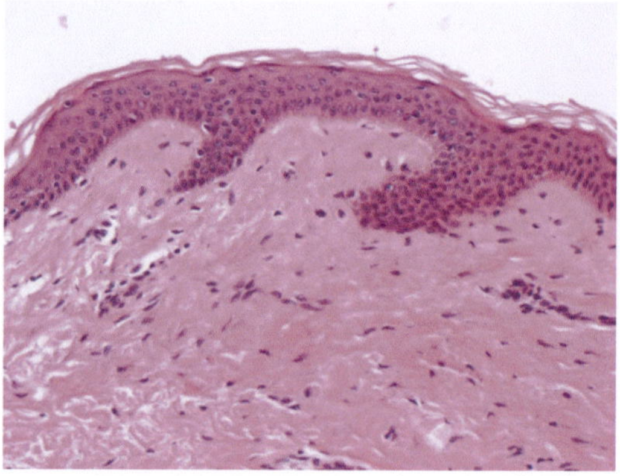

Fig. 14.69 Lentigo simplex area

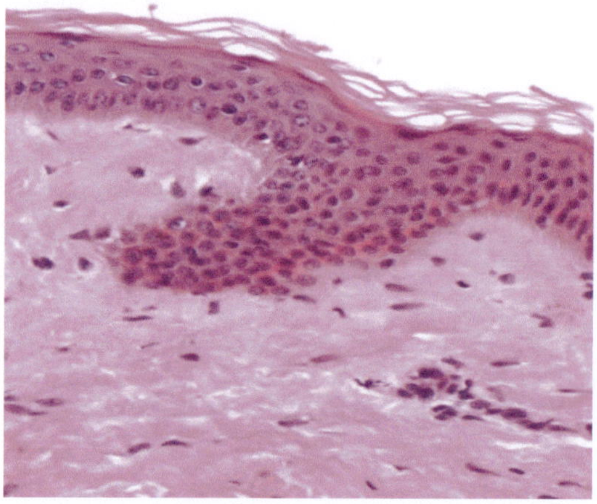

Fig. 14.70 Elongated pigmented epidermal rete ridges

Nipple Adenoma

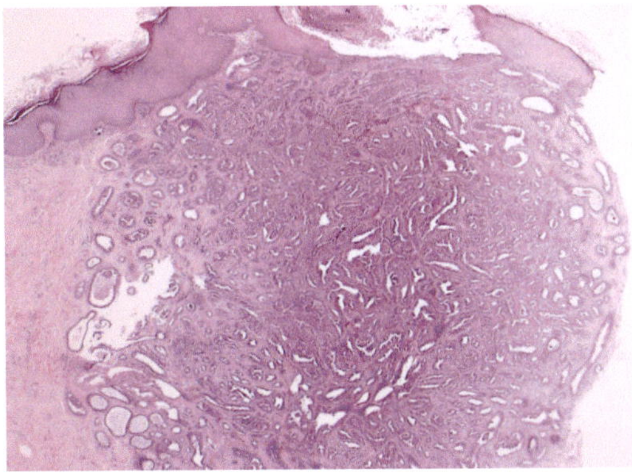

Fig. 14.71 Nodular tumor connected to the epidermis with no evidence of invasive infiltration

Synonyms: Erosive Adenomatosis of the Nipple, Florid Papillomatosis, Papillary Adenomatosis

Histopathology (Figs. 14.71, 14.72, 14.73, 14.74, and 14.75)

- Well circumscribed non encapsulated tumor made of variably sized ducts in fibrotic stroma
- Tumor connects to the surface epithelium
- Ducts are lined with inner cuboidal cells (CK7+) with apocrine secretion and outside myoepithelial cells (p63+, SMA+, calponin+)
- Some ducts have small papillary projections and can have cribriform appearance

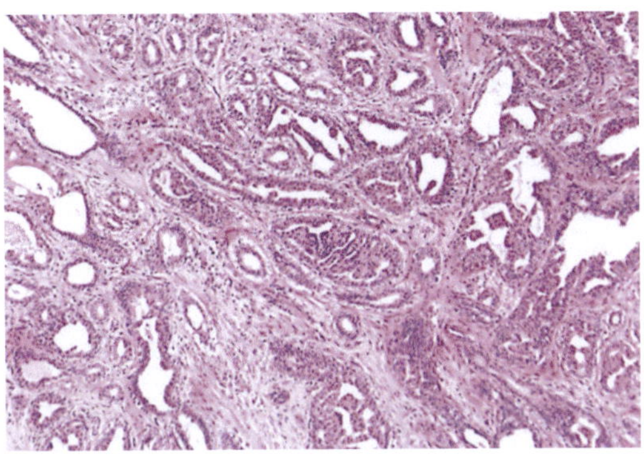

Fig. 14.72 Ducts of various sizes embedded in fibrous stroma

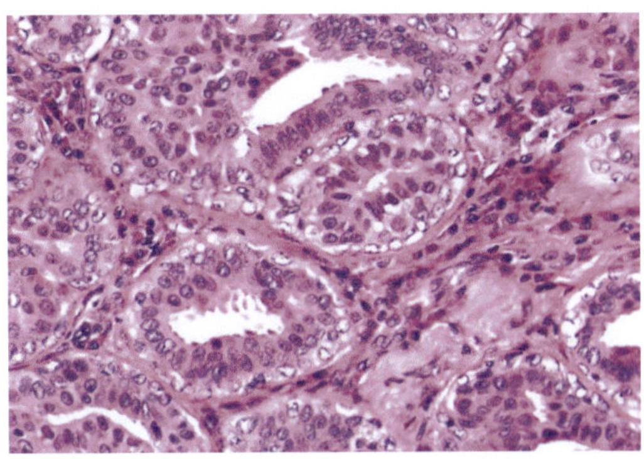

Fig. 14.73 Ducts lined with two cell layer showing apocrine secretion

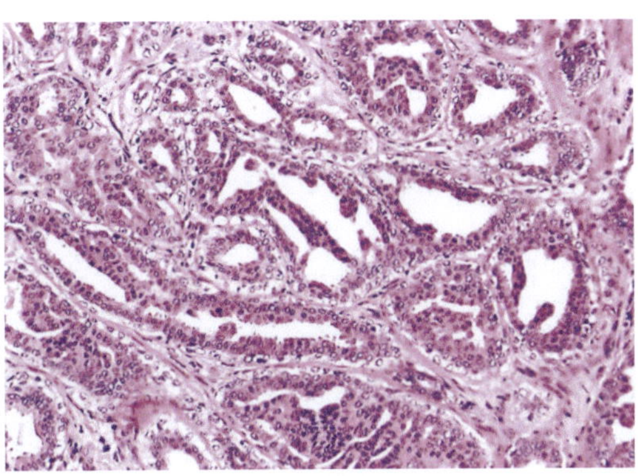

Fig. 14.74 Focal cribriform appearance

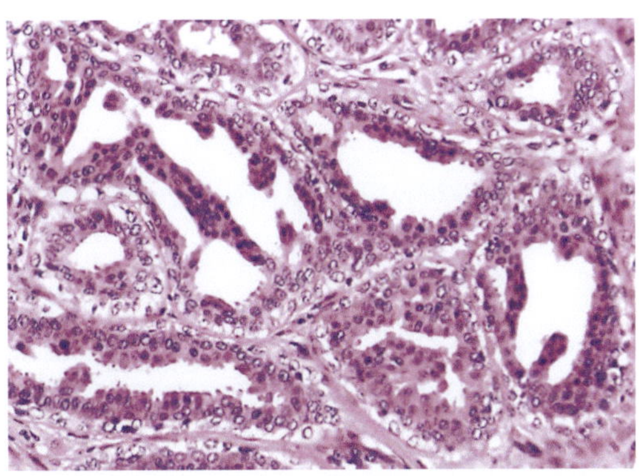

Fig. 14.75 Small papillae without central core are present

Nocardiosis

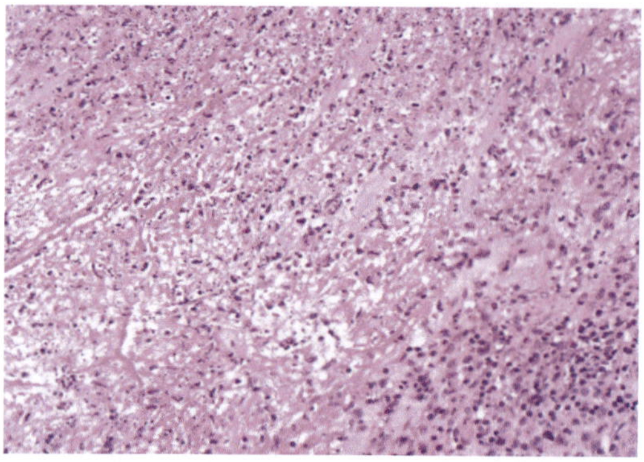

Fig. 14.76 Exuberant subcutaneous acute inflammation

Histopathology (Figs. 14.76, 14.77, and 14.78)

- Dense neutrophilic infiltrate in the dermis and/or subcutis
- Frequent abscess formation
- Necrosis and hemorrhage are common
- Fine filamentous bacteria can be seen using Fite-Faraco and Gram stains

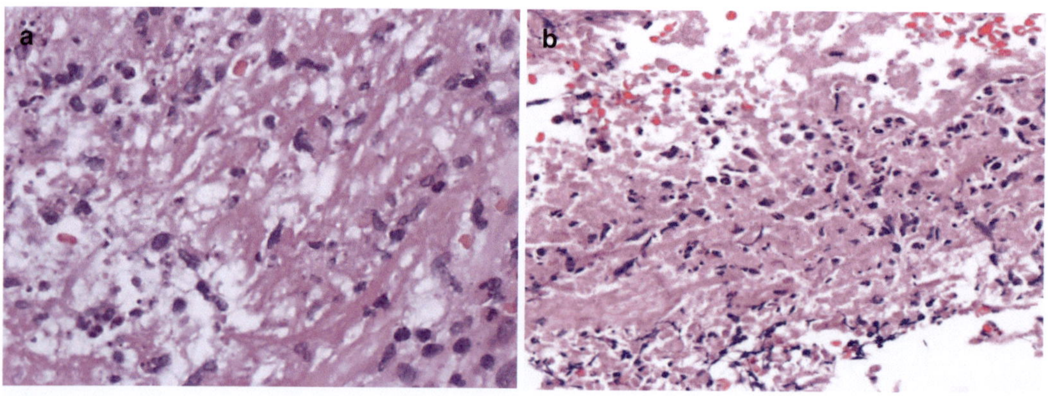

Fig. 14.77 (**a**, **b**) Neutrophilic infiltrate with extensive necrosis

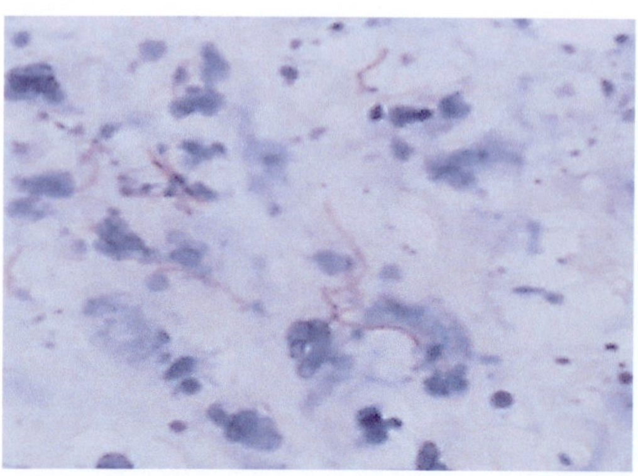

Fig. 14.78 Fite Faraco stain outlines pink filamentous bacteria

Nodular Fasciitis

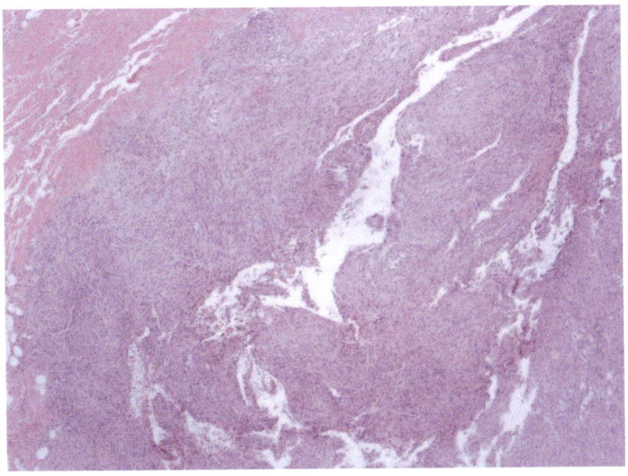

Fig. 14.79 Subcutaneous well circumscribed nodule

Histopathology (Figs. 14.79, 14.80, 14.81, 14.82, and 14.83)

- Relatively well circumscribed nodule in the deep subcutis
- Composed of plump spindle fibroblasts arranged in haphazard or focally storiform pattern ("tissue culture" appearance)
- Hypocellular areas have prominent myxoid stroma
- Mitoses are present but are not atypical and scattered lymphocytes are present
- Cells are SMA+, calponin+ with *MYH9-USP9* translocation

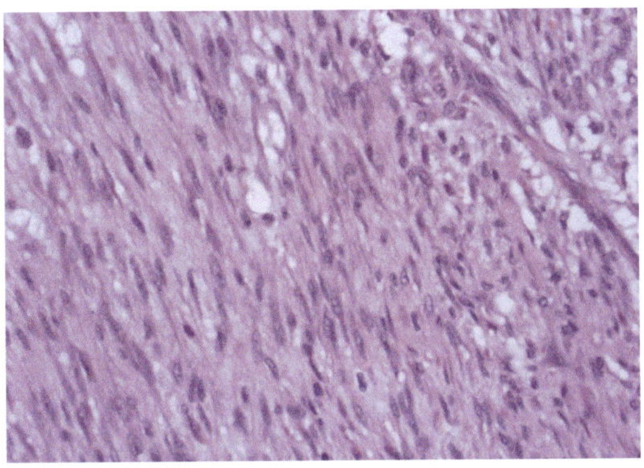

Fig. 14.80 Plump elongated fibroblasts

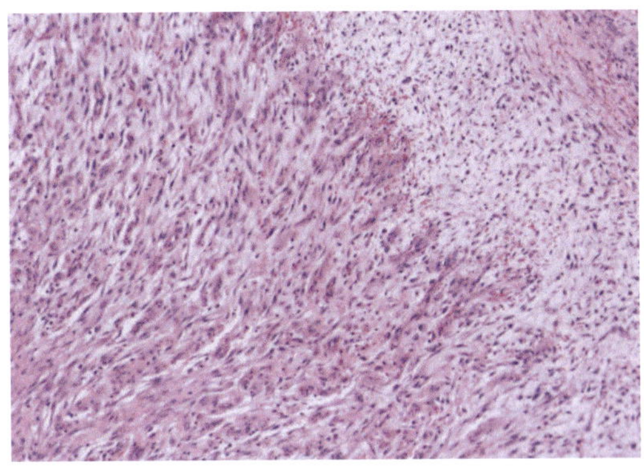

Fig. 14.81 Hyper and hypocellular areas

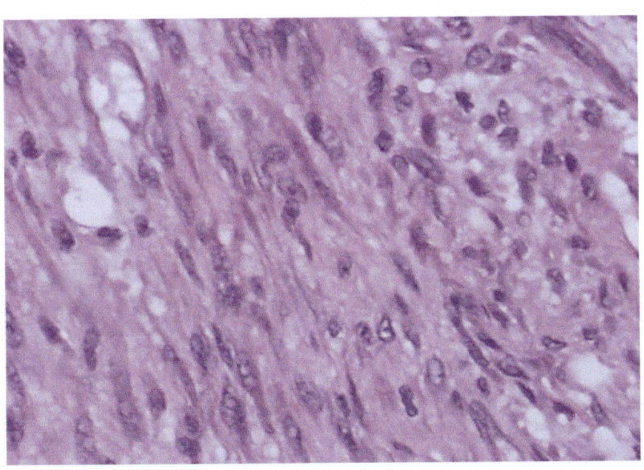

Fig. 14.82 Scattered mitoses are seen

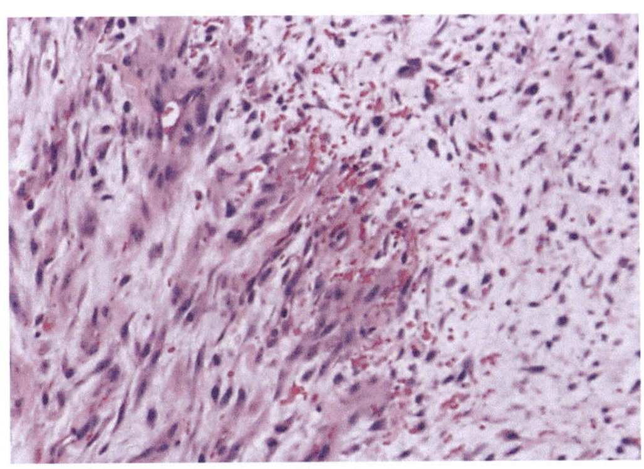

Fig. 14.83 Myxoid background with appearance of "tissue culture"

Non-Langerhans Cell Histiocytosis of Skin and Mucosa

Multiple clinically different disorders with similar **histomorphology**. They all belong to C group of histiocytosis.

1. Cutaneous Non-Langerhans Cell Histiocytosis
   (a) Xanthogranuloma (XG) family
   - *Juvenile xanthogranuloma (JXG)*
   - *Adult Xanthogranuloma (AXG)*
   - *Solitary Reticulohistiocytoma (SRH)*
   - *Benign Cephalic Histiocytosis (BCH)*
   - *Generalized Eruptive Histiocytosis (GEH)*
   - *Progressive Nodular Histiocytosis (PNH)*

   (b) Non Xanthogranuloma family
   - *Cutaneous Rosai-Dorfman Disease (RDD)*
   - *Necrobiotic Xanthogranuloma (NXG)*
2. Cutaneous Non-Langerhans Cell Histiocytosis with a major systemic component
   (a) *Xanthoma Disseminatum (XD)*
   (b) *Multicentric Reticulohistiocytoma (MRH)*

JXG, AXG, BCH, and XD **have similar histology:** (Fig. 14.84)

- Nodular dermal histiocytic proliferation that abut but does not excoriate the epidermis
- Many histiocytes have foamy, xanthomatous appearance
- There are scattered Touton giant cells
- Lymphocytes and eosinophils can be admixed

SRX and MRH **have identical histomorphology:** (Fig. 14.85)

- Circumscribed non encapsulated dermal nodule
- Made of histiocytes and giant cells with central glassy dark pink cytoplasm (PAS+)
- Small number of lymphocytes and neutrophils
- Xanthoma cells are not prominent

GEH has similar histomorphology to *JXG* group but giant cells are absent. Histiocytes are pale but devoid of intracytoplasmic lipids.

RDD is made of large histiocytes (CD68+, S100+, CD1a-) with abundant cytoplasm and admixed lymphocytes, plasma cells, and red blood cells. Histiocytes engulf other cells forming "bean bag" cells (Fig. 14.86).

NXG made of histiocytic infiltrate with central area of necrobiosis with cholesterol clefts. Scattered lymphocytes and giant cells are present (Fig. 14.87).

PNH resembles cellular dermatofibroma with scattered xanthoma cells (see P72, Figs. 16.238).

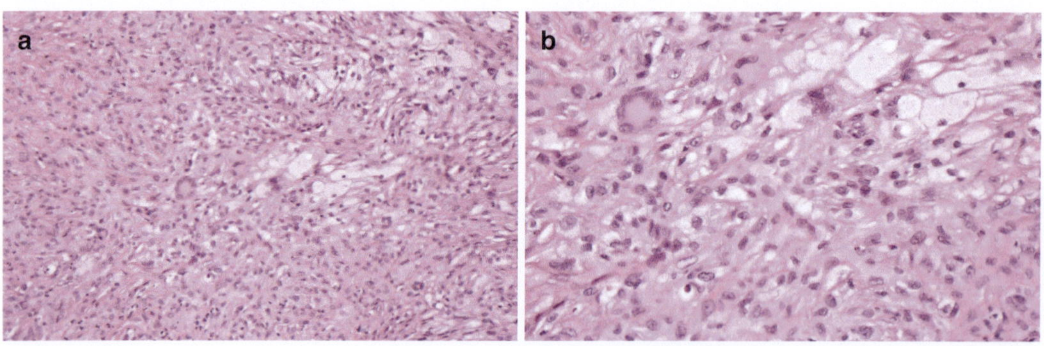

Fig. 14.84 (**a**, **b**) **Xanthogranuloma** made of sheet of histiocytes some with foamy cytoplasm, scattered giant cells, and lymphocytes

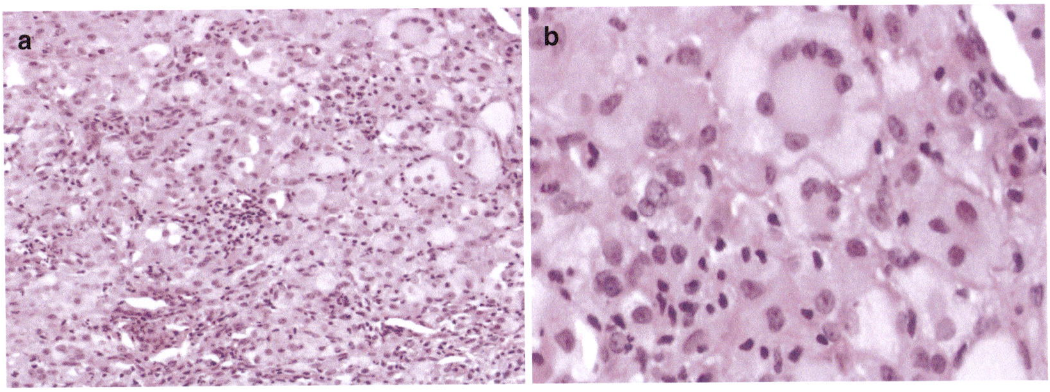

Fig. 14.85 (**a**, **b**) **Reticulohistiocytosis** with giant cells containing characteristic dark pink intracytoplasmic inclusion

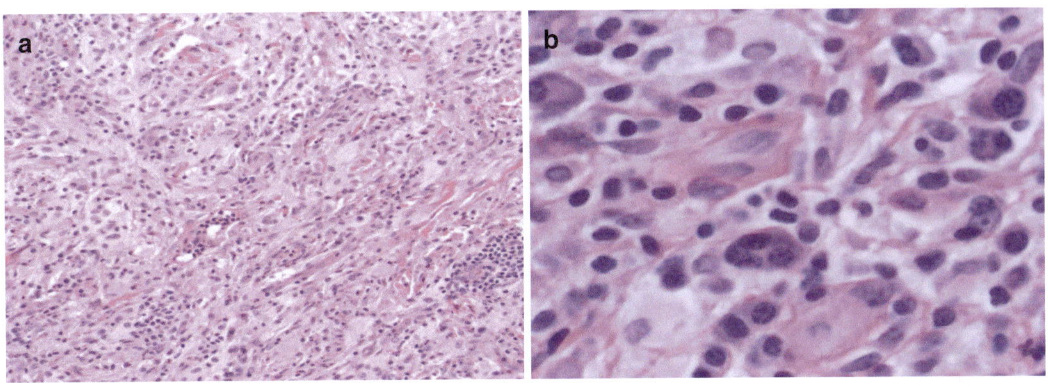

Fig. 14.86 (**a**, **b**) **Rosai Dorfman Disease** with characteristic "bean bag" cells

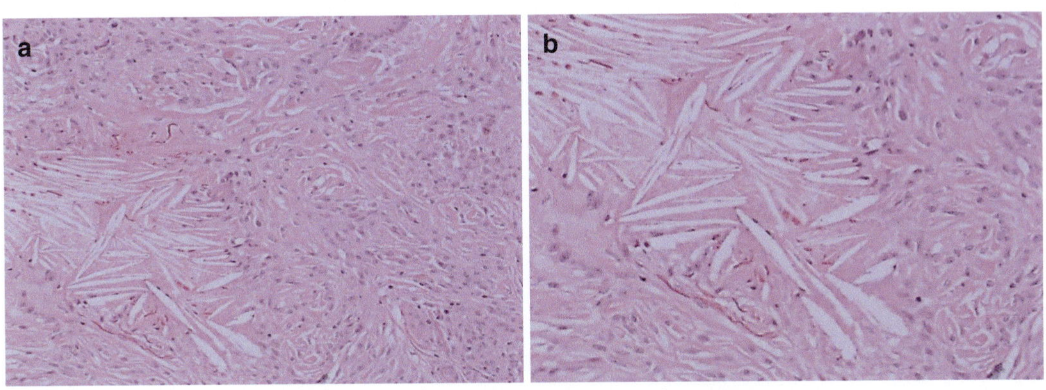

Fig. 14.87 (**a**, **b**) **Necrobiotic Xanthogranuloma** with characteristic cholesterol clefts

Nummular Dermatitis

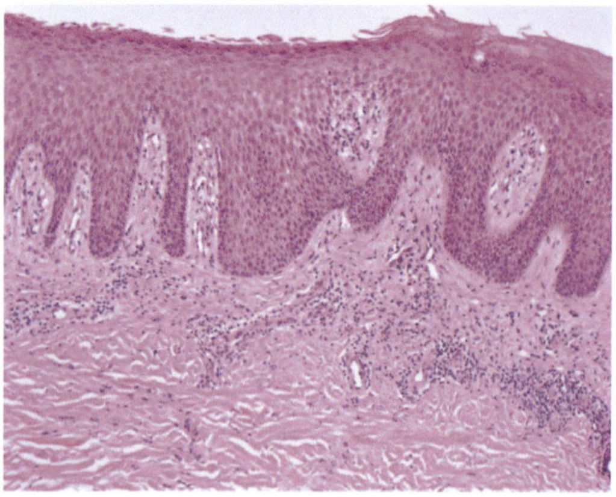

Fig. 14.88 Irregular epidermal psoriasiform acanthosis

Synonym: Discoid Dermatitis

Histopathological findings are not specific and clinical correlation is necessary (Figs. 14.88, 14.89, 14.90, and 14.91).

Early lesions (that are usually not biopsied):

- Acute spongiotic dermatitis

Older lesions:

- Epidermal subacute spongiosis, acanthosis, and psoriasiform hyperplasia
- Focal lymphocytic epidermal exocytosis
- Mild/moderate perivascular lymphocytic infiltrate

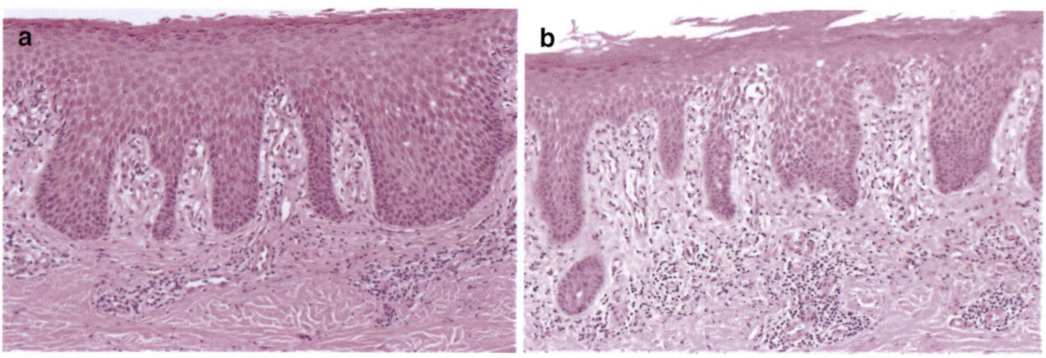

Fig. 14.89 (**a**, **b**) Mild epidermal spongiosis with dermal perivascular inflammation

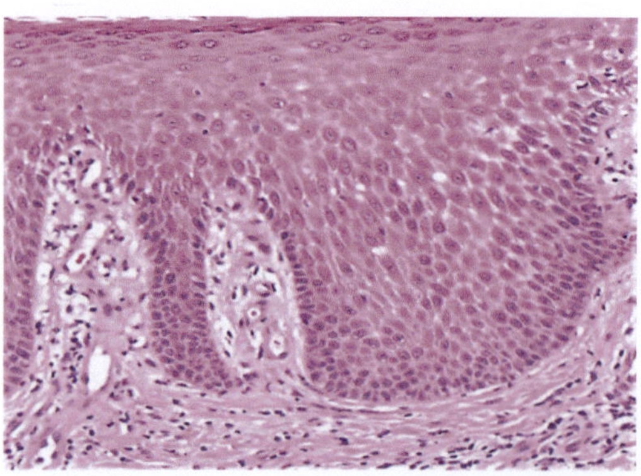

Fig. 14.90 Epidermal spongiosis and mild perivascular lymphocytic infiltrate

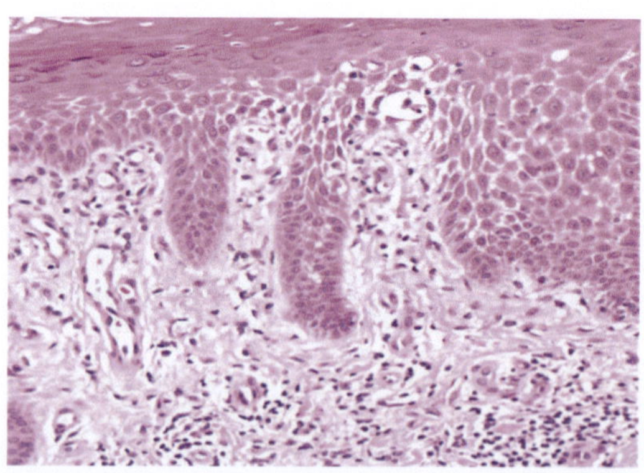

Fig. 14.91 Focal epidermal vesicle with some epidermal lymphocytes

15 Dermatopathology O

V. Vincek, *Dermatopathology A–Z*, https://doi.org/10.1007/978-3-319-89486-7_15

Ochronosis

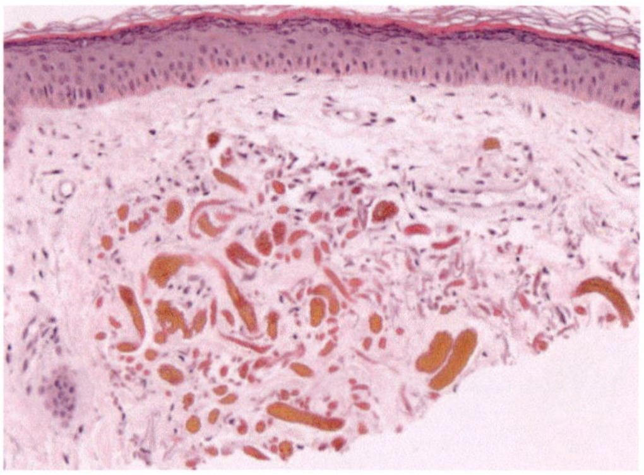

Fig. 15.1 Dermal pigmented deposits

Histopathology (Figs. 15.1, 15.2, and 15.3)
- Yellow brown "ochre" color dermal deposits
- Deposits have crescent or banana-shaped contour
- No inflammation
- Deposits are autofluorescent and stain black with Methylene Blue stain

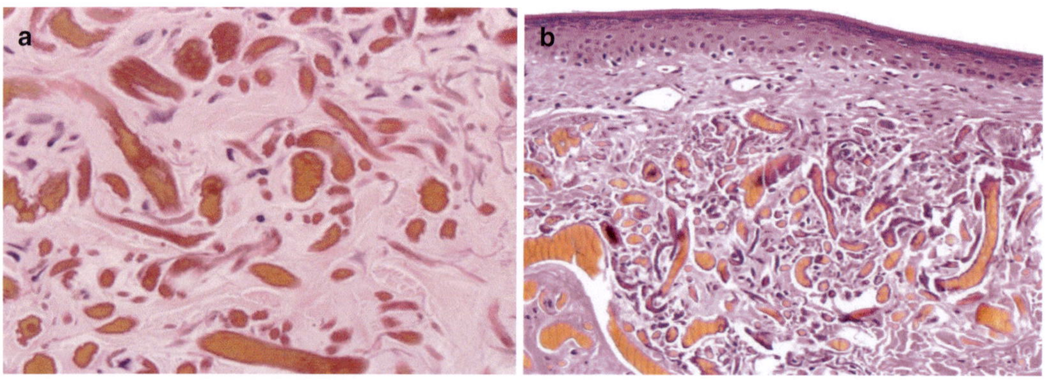

Fig. 15.2 (**a**, **b**) Golden brown/ochre colored dermal deposits with no dermal inflammation

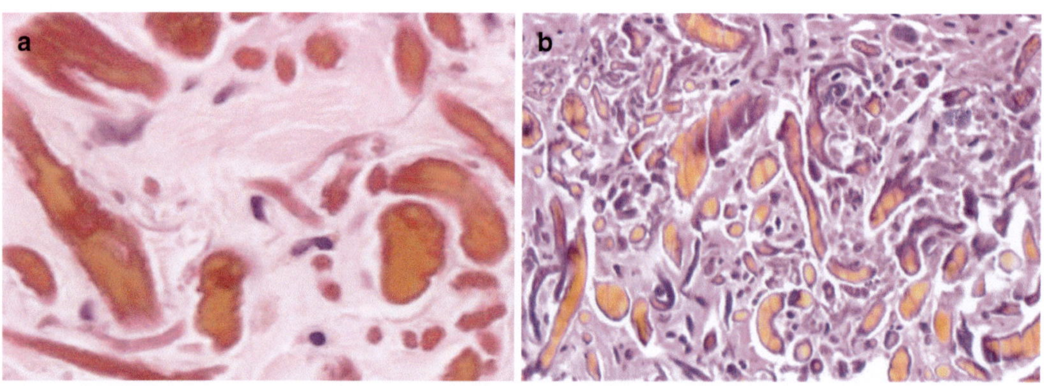

Fig. 15.3 (**a**, **b**) Irregular globules some of which have banana-like shape

Omphalomesenteric Duct Remnant

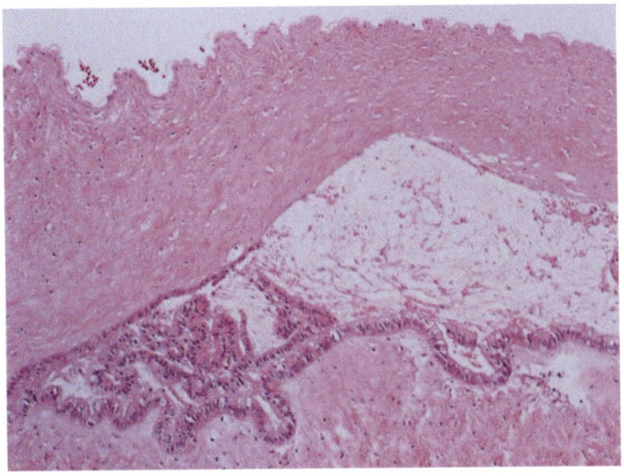

Fig. 15.4 Irregular cyst surrounded by fibroconnective tissue

Synonyms: Umbilical Granuloma, Vitello-intestinal Anomaly, Enteroteratoma, Raspberry Tumor

Histopathology (Figs. 15.4, 15.5, and 15.6)

- Cyst or fistula covered with columnar gastrointestinal epithelium that can resemble any part of gastrointestinal tract
- Lumen is filled with serous material
- Mild lymphocytic inflammation can be present

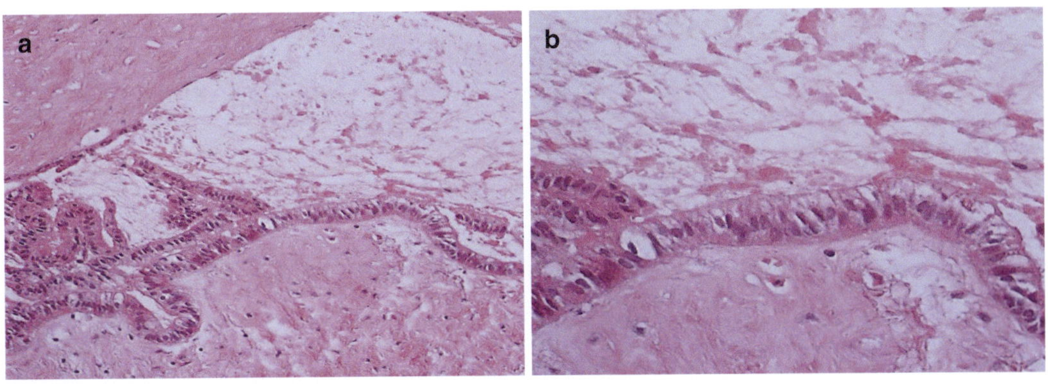

Fig. 15.5 (**a**, **b**) Cyst lined with columnar cells with admixed goblet cells. There is no evidence of cytological atypia

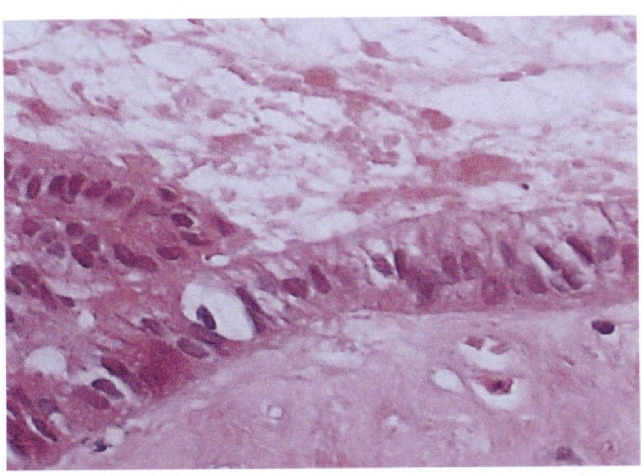

Fig. 15.6 The lumen is filled with pink serous secretion

Onchocerciasis

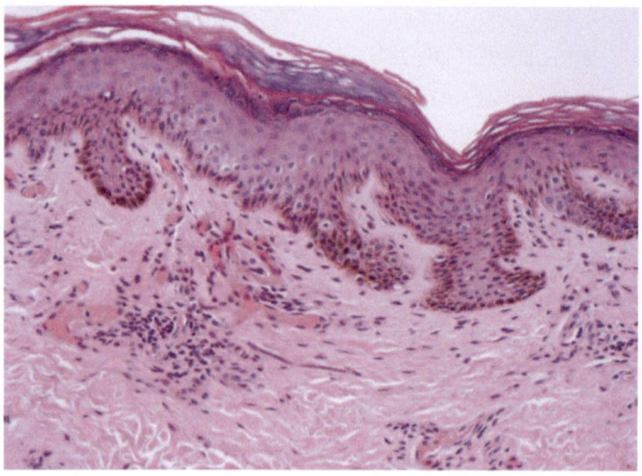

Fig. 15.7 Dermal mixed inflammation

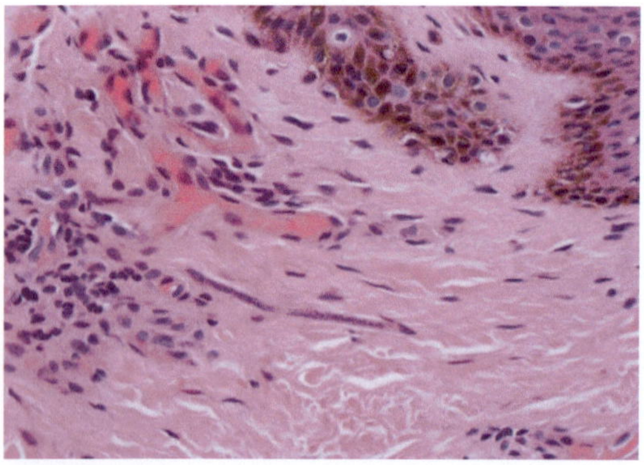

Fig. 15.8 Elongated microfilaris with pointed ends

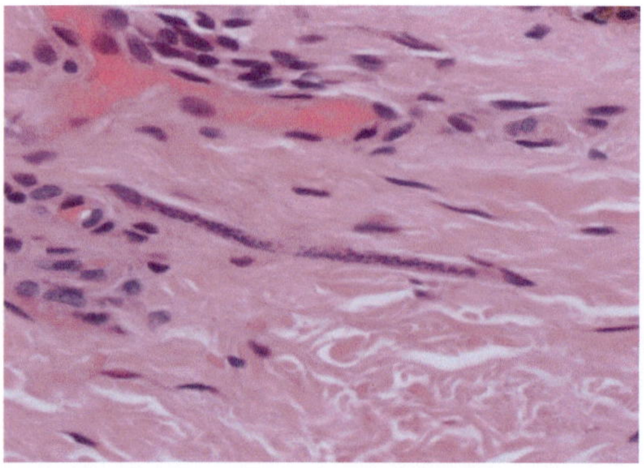

Fig. 15.9 Elongated body filled with speckles

Synonyms: Microfilariasis, River Blindness

Histopathology (Figs. 15.7, 15.8, 15.9, and 15.10)

- Microfilariae can be detected in the dermis and eye
- They are elongated and slender with pointed ends
- The body is filled with purple/blue granules
- Surrounding dermal mixed inflammation is present
- The larvae develop into worms in the subcutis
- Worms can entangle and form a nodule called "onchocercoma"
- "Onchocercoma" contain an adult worm with surrounding inflammation, necrosis and scarring

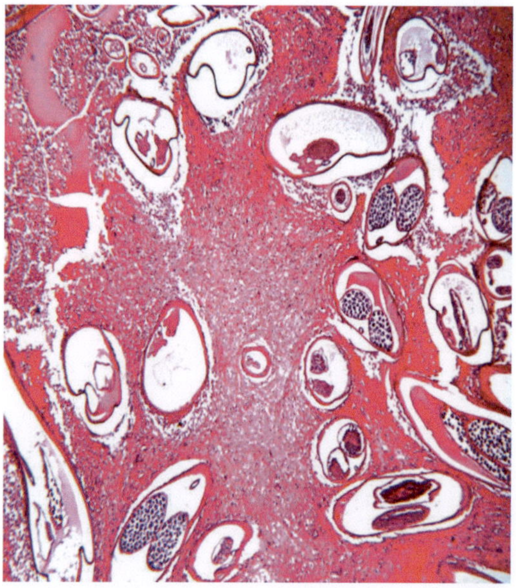

Fig. 15.10 Cross sections of onchocercoma with adult worm and extensive surrounding necrosis

Onychomycosis

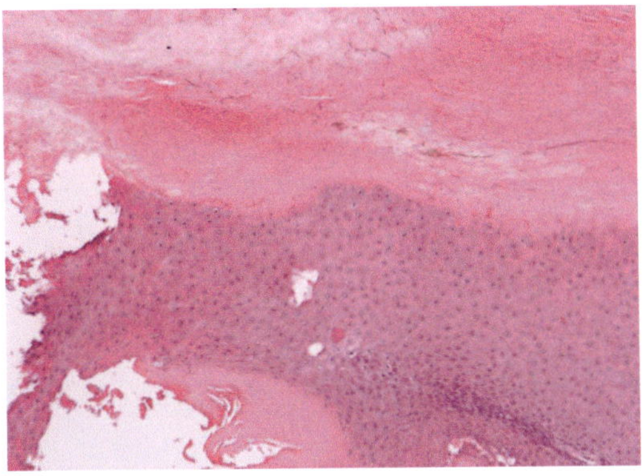

Fig. 15.11 Nail with nail matrix

Synonym: Tinea Unguium

Histopathology (Figs. 15.11, 15.12, 15.13, and 15.14)

- About 85% of cases are caused by dermatophytes among which *Trichophyton rubrum and Trichophyton mentagrophytes* are the most common. In those cases, straight septate hyphae are arranged parallel with nail keratin plates.
- About 15% are caused by yeast and *Candida Albicans* is the most common. In those cases, small round yeast forms and pseudohyphae are present between keratin plates.

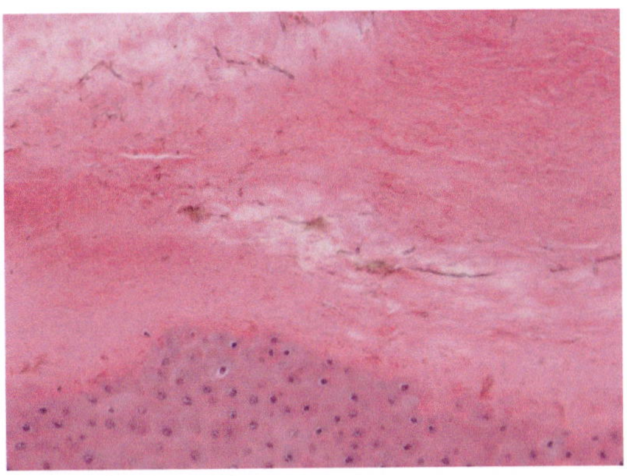

Fig. 15.12 Dermatophytes barely seen on H&E slides

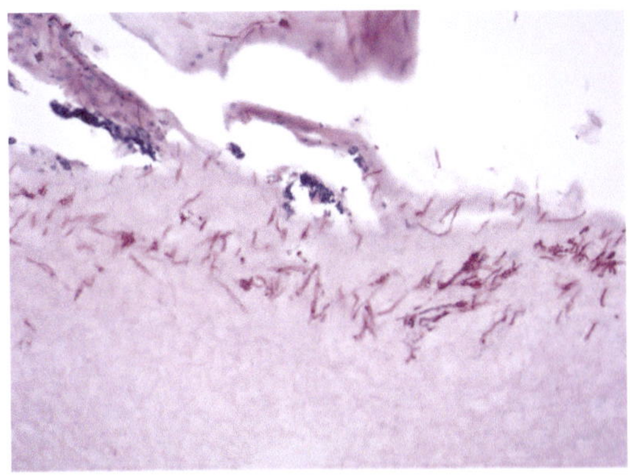

Fig. 15.13 Hyphae highlighted by PAS stain

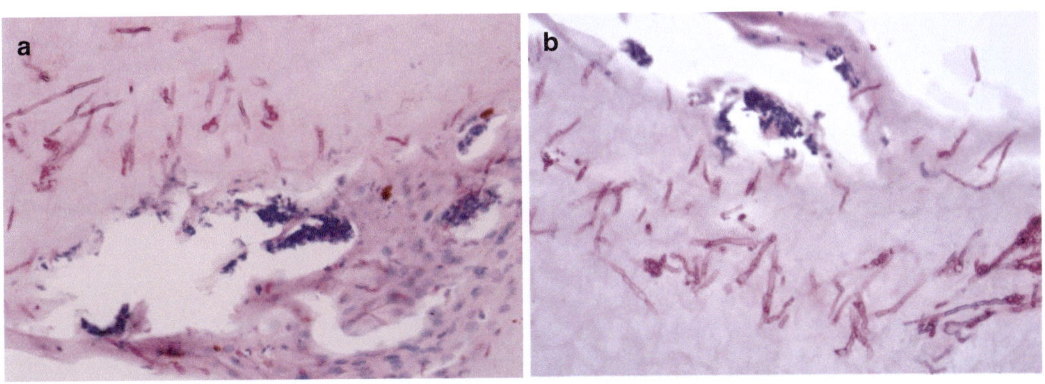

Fig. 15.14 (**a**, **b**) Relatively straight septate hyphae in between keratin lamellae (PAS)

Onychomatricoma

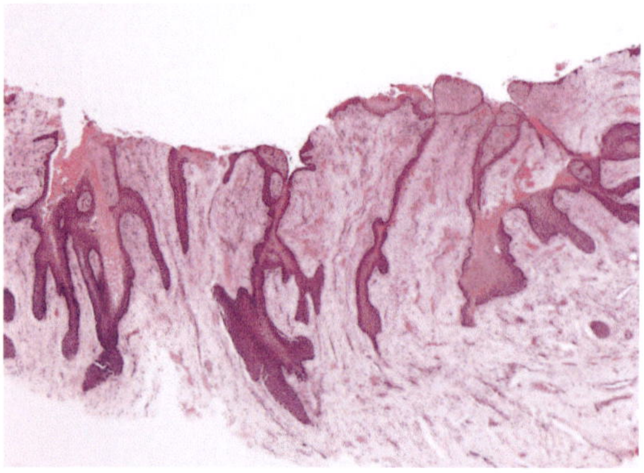

Fig. 15.15 "Finger-like" epithelial projections in nail bed

Histopathology (Figs. 15.15, 15.16, and 15.17)

- Nail bed with multiple "finger-like" projections covered with squamous epithelium with no granular layer
- The stroma shows increased cellularity with CD34 positive fibroblasts
- Pleomorphic large fibroblasts can occasionally be seen
- Increased number of mast cells can be present

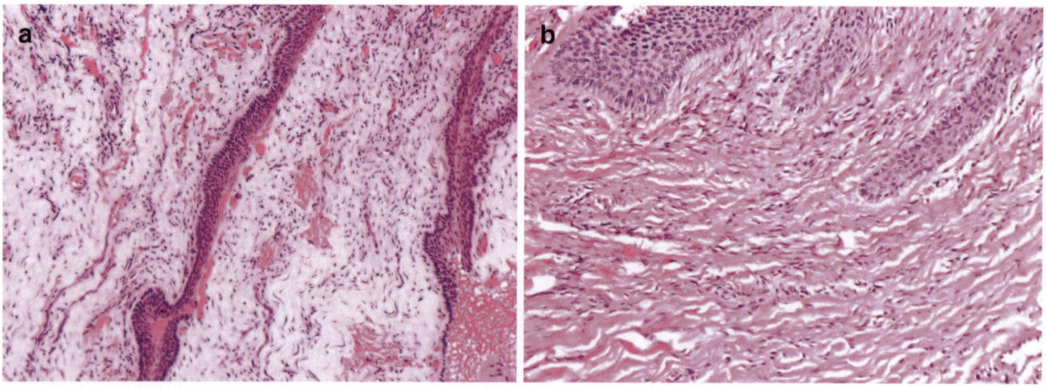

Fig. 15.16 (**a**, **b**) Epithelial projections with no granular layer are embedded in cellular stroma

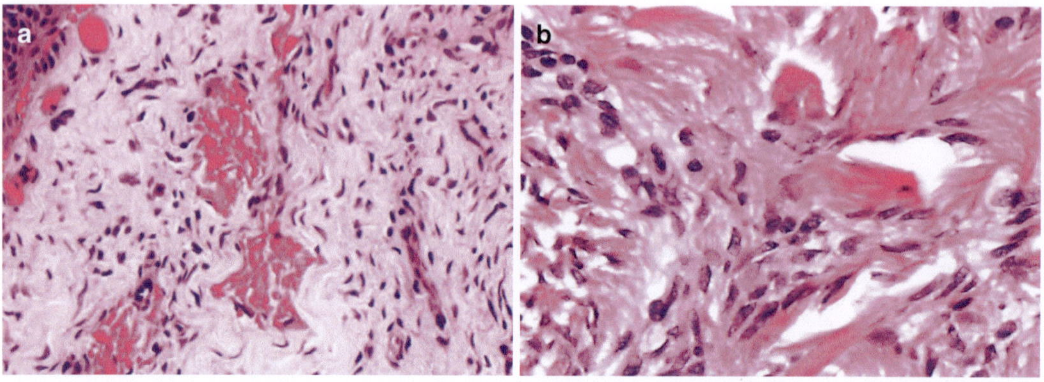

Fig. 15.17 (**a**, **b**) Some fibroblasts are pleomorphic; mast cells are present

Oral Fibroma

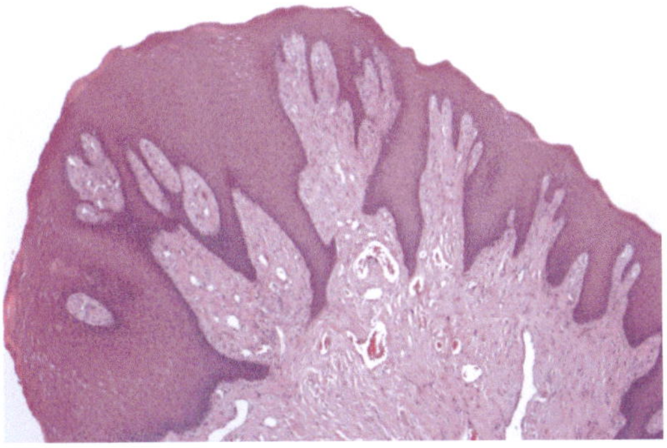

Fig. 15.18 Dome shaped lesion

Synonyms: Dental Fibroma, Irritation Fibroma, Bite Fibroma

Histopathology (Figs. 15.18, 15.19, and 15.20)

- Dome shaped lesion
- Acanthotic, papillomatous squamous mucosa with frequent hyperkeratosis
- Fibrotic, hypocellular stroma with scattered blood vessels
- Occasional reactive fibroblasts are present

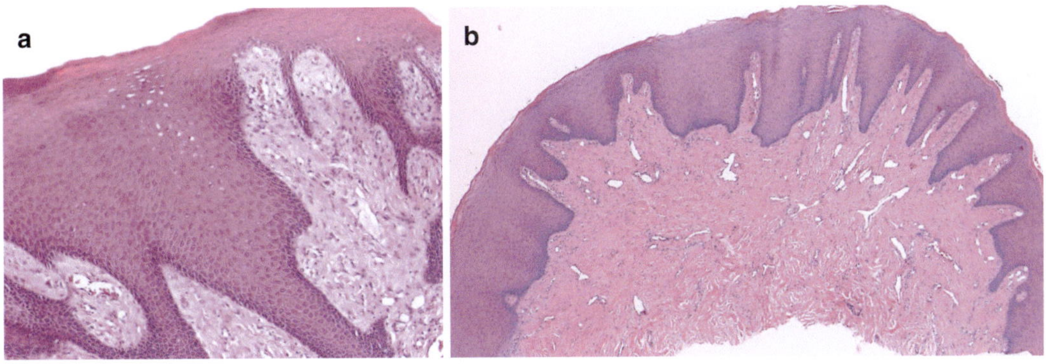

Fig. 15.19 (**a**, **b**) Thickened irregularly papillomatous epidermis without granular layer and with focal hyperkeratosis

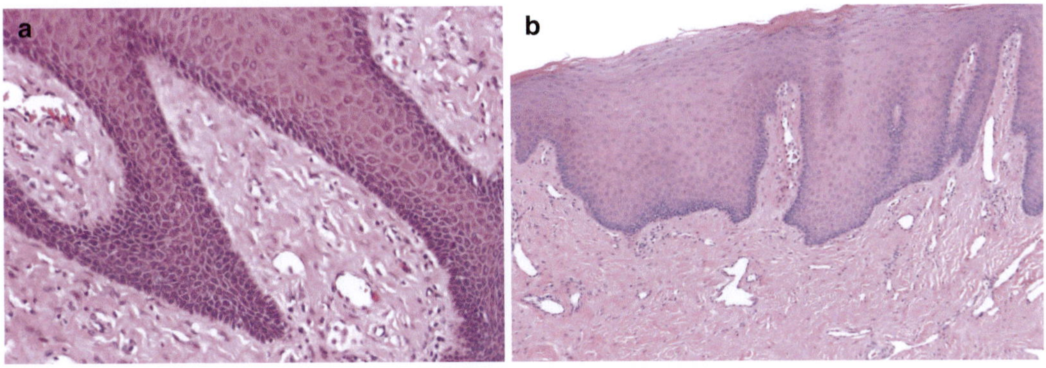

Fig. 15.20 (**a**, **b**) Fibrotic stroma with some reactive fibroblasts and dilated capillaries

Oral Hairy Leukoplakia

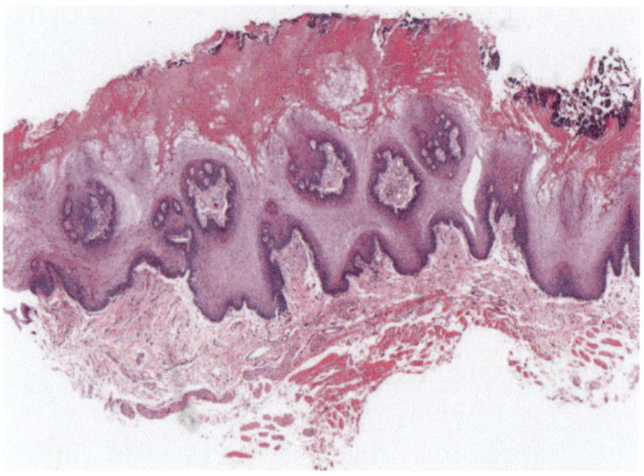

Fig. 15.21 Papillomatous epidermis with hyperkeratosis

Synonyms: Viral Leukoplakia, Hairy Leukoplakia

Histopathology (Figs. 15.21, 15.22, 15.23, and 15.24)

- Papillomatous epithelium with hyperkeratosis and hyperparakeratosis
- Beneath parakeratosis there are pale "balloon-like" cells
- Nuclear condensation with "beaded" appearance
- There is no evidence of cytological atypia
- Inflammation is absent

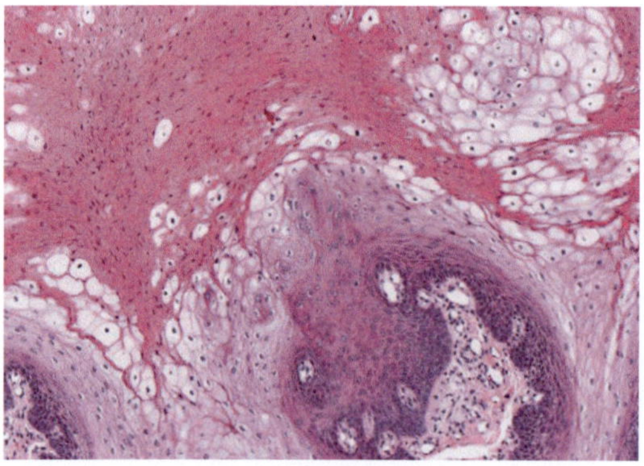

Fig. 15.22 Extensive epidermal parakeratosis

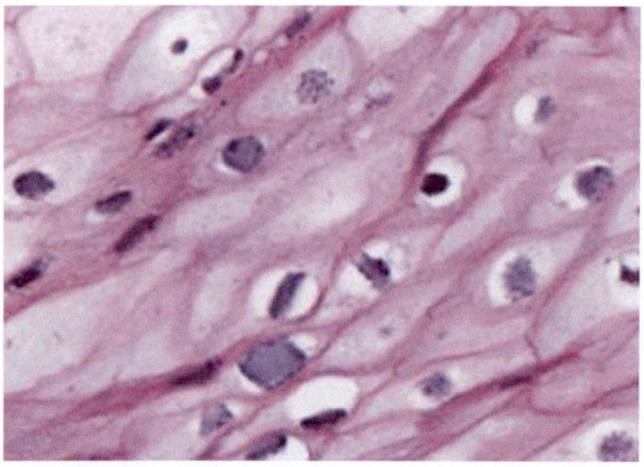

Fig. 15.23 Nuclear condensation with "beaded" appearance

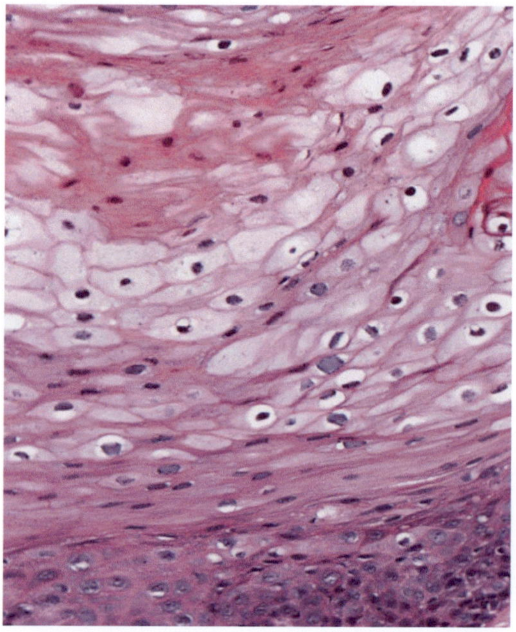

Fig. 15.24 Vacuolated "balloon-like" cells under the layer of parakeratotic keratinocytes

ORF

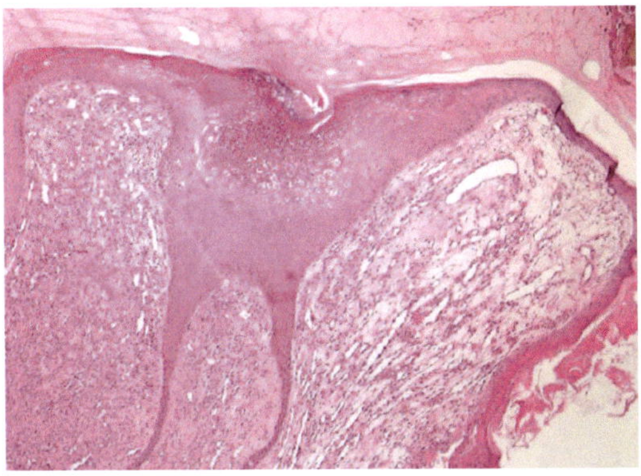

Fig. 15.25 Pedunculated lesion with acanthotic epidermis and vascular dermal proliferation

Synonym: Echtyma Contagiosum

Histopathology (Figs. 15.25, 15.26, 15.27, and 15.28)

- Nodule with epidermal acanthosis and pale keratinocytes in the upper epidermis
- Cytoplasmic inclusions are present
- Extensive dermal capillary proliferation
- Older lesions ulcerate and become necrotic with neutrophilic inflammation

P.S. inclusions are similar to molluscum inclusions but are smaller

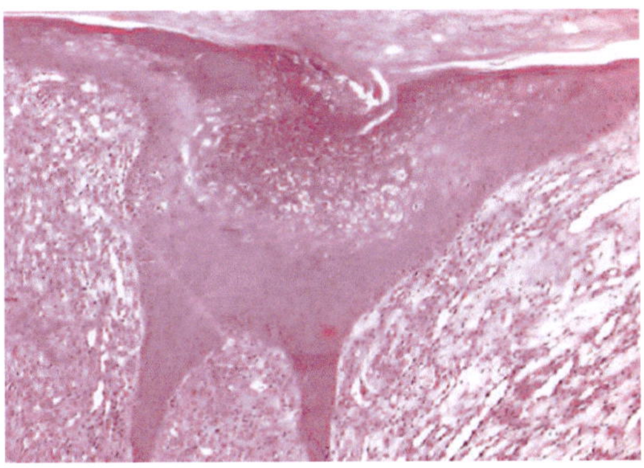

Fig. 15.26 Dermal capillary proliferation

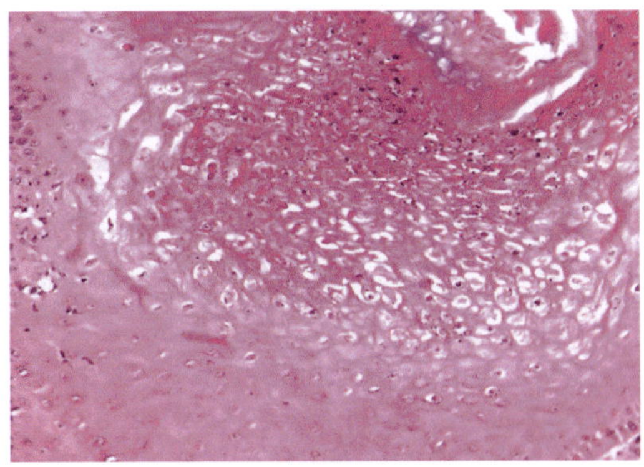

Fig. 15.27 Eosinophilic intracytoplasmic inclusions

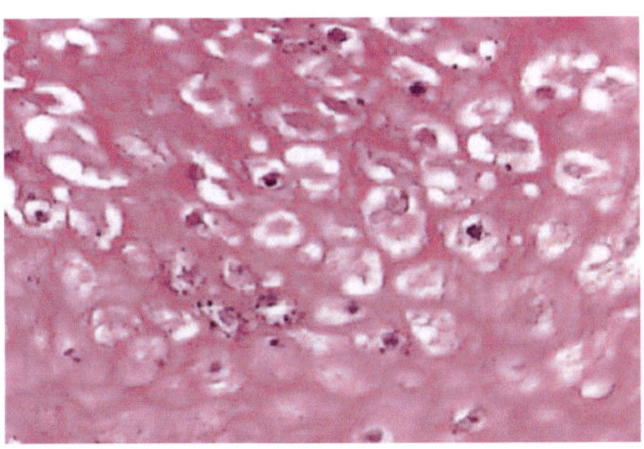

Fig. 15.28 Pale keratinocytes contain characteristic eosinophilic inclusions

Orofacial Granulomatosis

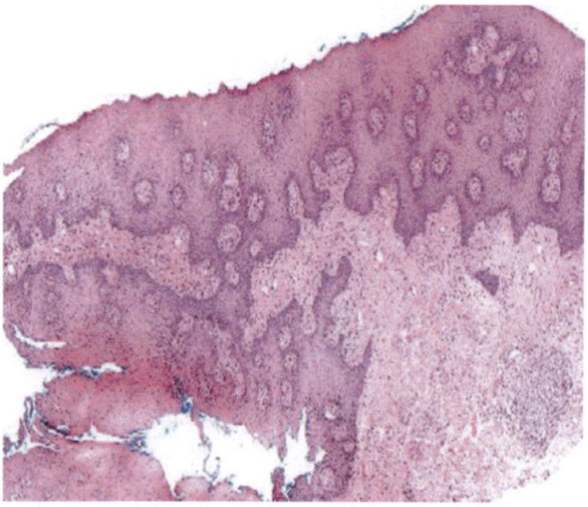

Fig. 15.29 Oral mucosa with one granuloma in lamina propria

Synonym: Cheilitis Granulomatosa

Histopathology (Figs. 15.29, 15.30, 15.31, and 15.32)

- Non-necrotizing granuloma in lamina propria
- Granuloma(s) are usually very subtle and frequently only one is present
- Granulomas are made of histiocytes and some lymphocytes
- Giant cells are variable in number
- There is minimal to mild surrounding inflammation

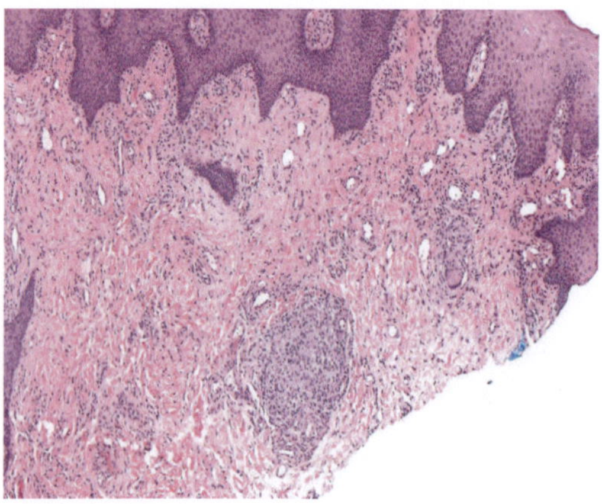

Fig. 15.30 Mild submucosal inflammation is present

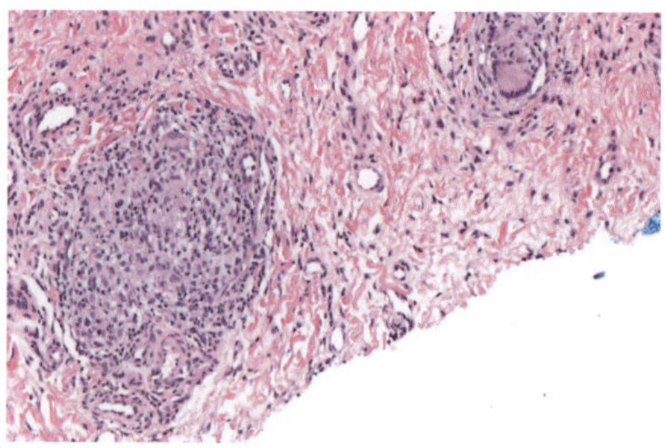

Fig. 15.31 Granuloma with adjacent giant cell (right)

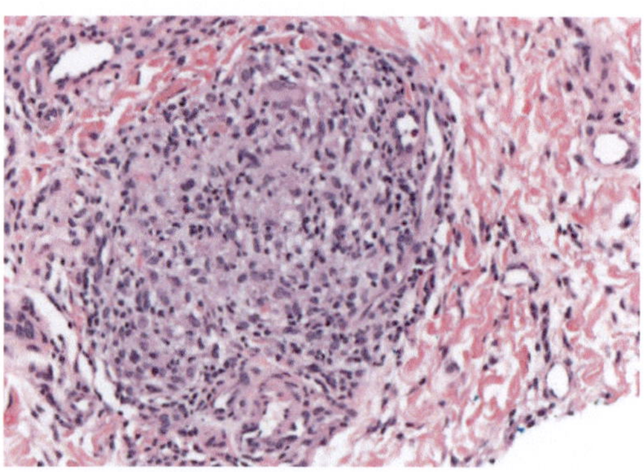

Fig. 15.32 Non-necrotizing granuloma with adjacent lymphocytes

Ossifying Fibromyxoid Tumor

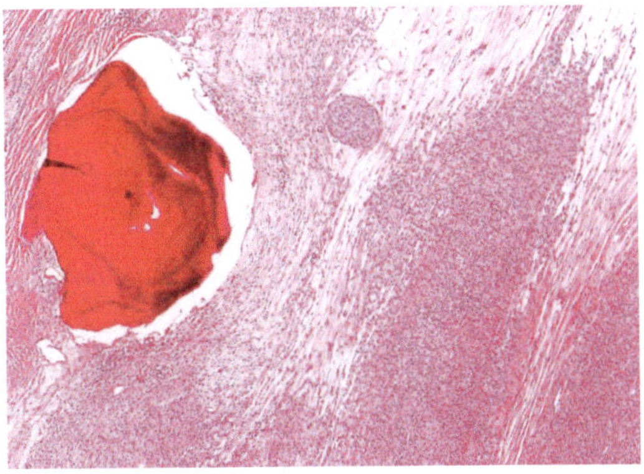

Fig. 15.33 Poorly defined tumor with peripheral bone

Histopathology (Figs. 15.33, 15.34, and 15.35)

- Poorly defined subcutaneous tumor nodules
- Presence of peripheral lamellar bone
- Small polygonal to spindle cells (S100+ in 75% cases) with vesicular nuclei and eosinophilic cytoplasm
- Cells are arranged in cords, trabeculae, or clusters
- No cytological atypia but rare malignant variant exists with increased mitoses
- Focal loose fibromyxoid stroma

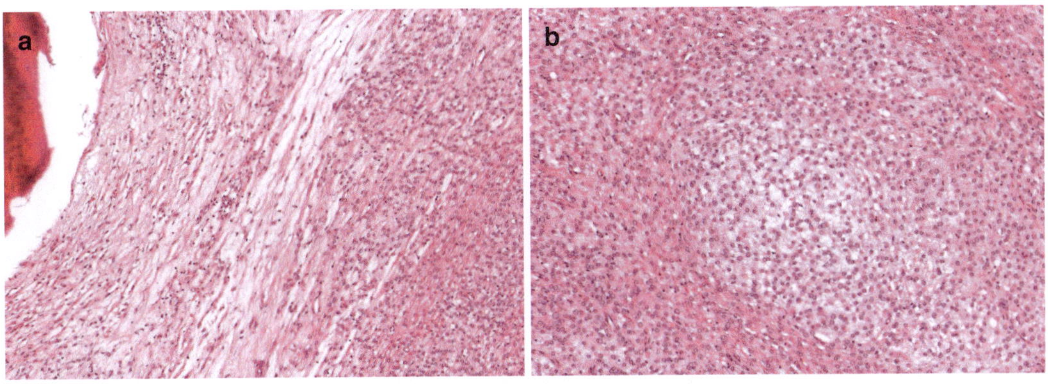

Fig. 15.34 (**a**, **b**) Cords and trabeculae of relatively uniform cells in focally myxoid stroma

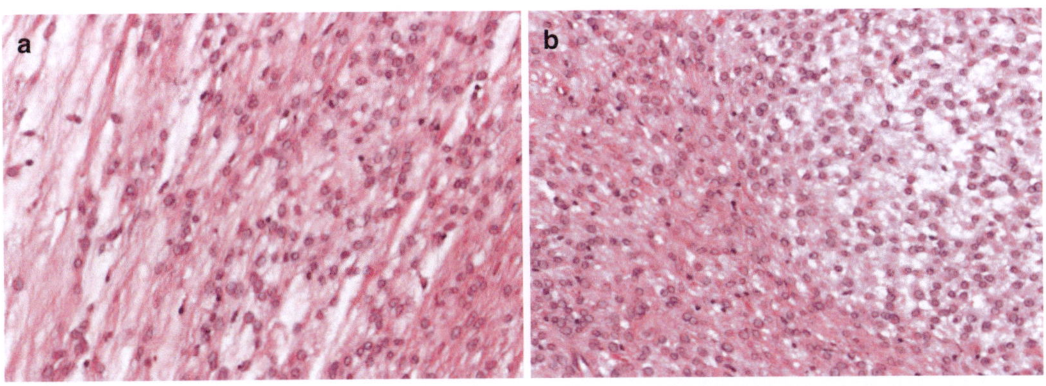

Fig. 15.35 (**a**, **b**) Small polygonal cells with vesicular nuclei and eosinophilic cytoplasm and no significant atypia or mitoses

Osteoma

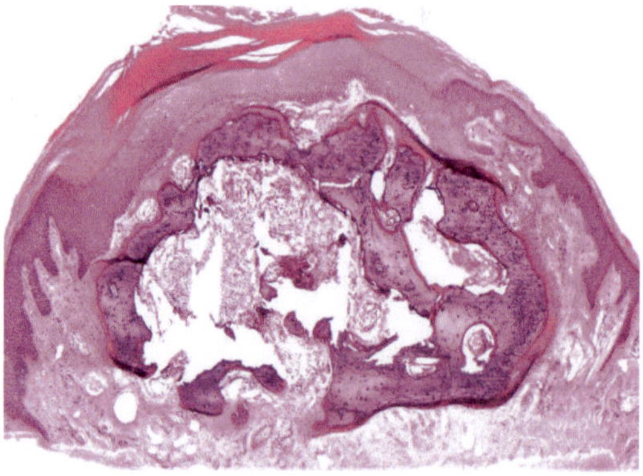

Fig. 15.36 Nodule of mature calcified lamellar bone

Histopathology (Figs. 15.36, 15.37, and 15.38)

- Well-circumscribed dermal/subcutaneous nodule
- Nodule is formed from fragments of matured lamellar bones
- Osteoblasts are present within the bone
- Multinucleated osteoclast cells are also seen
- Well-formed marrow can be present

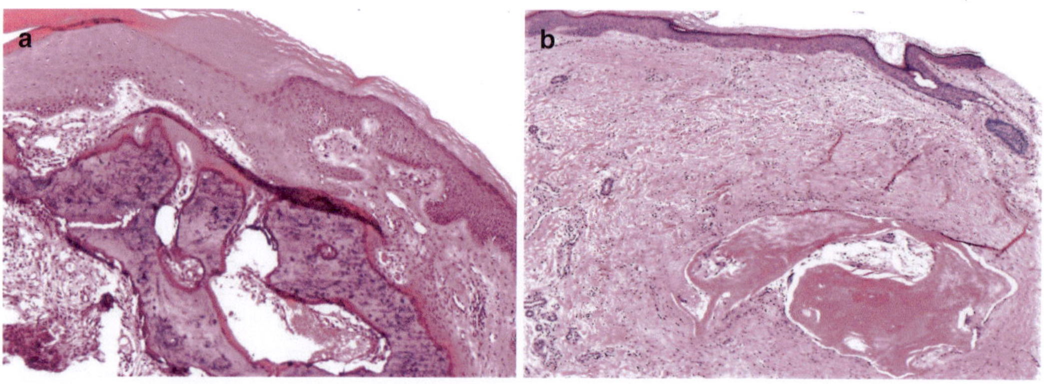

Fig. 15.37 (**a**, **b**) Fibrotic reactive connective tissue surrounds the nodules

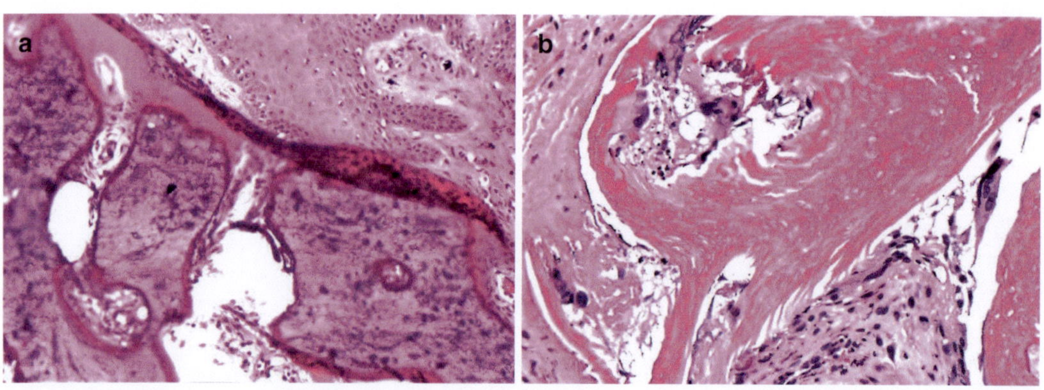

Fig. 15.38 (**a**, **b**) Osteoblasts and multinucleated osteoclasts are present

Osteo-Nevus of Nanta

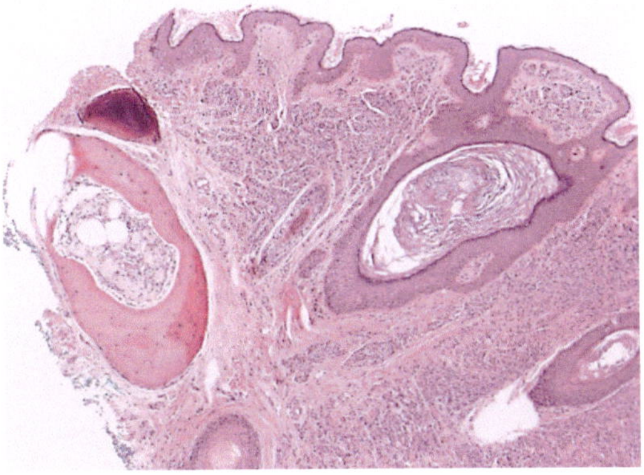

Fig. 15.39 Benign dermal nevus

Synonyms: Nevus of Nanta, Osseous Metaplasia in a Benign Intradermal Nevus

Histopathology (Figs. 15.39, 15.40, 15.41, and 15.42)

- Benign dermal nevus with regular maturation and no cytological atypia
- Presence of osteoma usually at the base of the melanocytic lesion
- Osteoma is made of lamellar bone with osteoblast

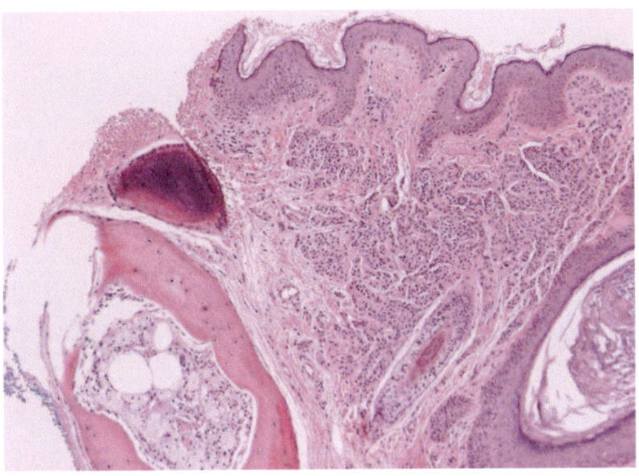

Fig. 15.40 Mature lamellar bone is present underneath the dermal nevus

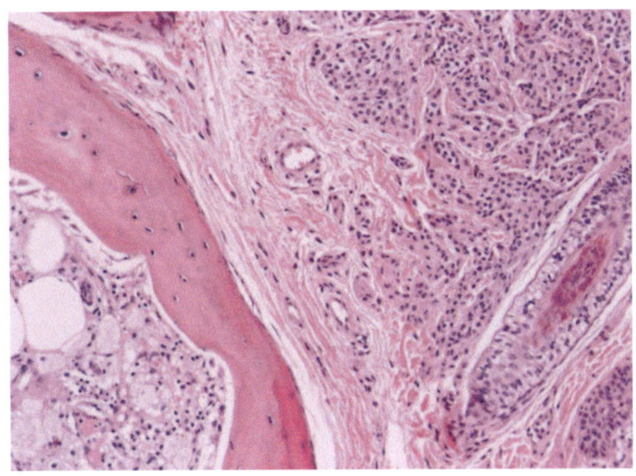

Fig. 15.41 Lamellar bone with osteoblasts and bone marrow

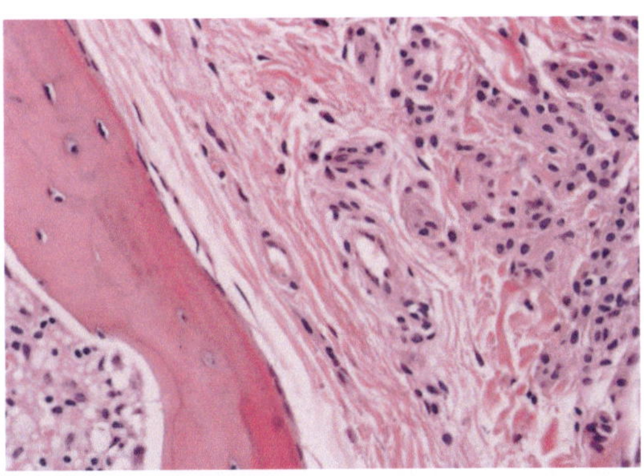

Fig. 15.42 Lamellar bone next to dermal nevus cells

Osteosarcoma

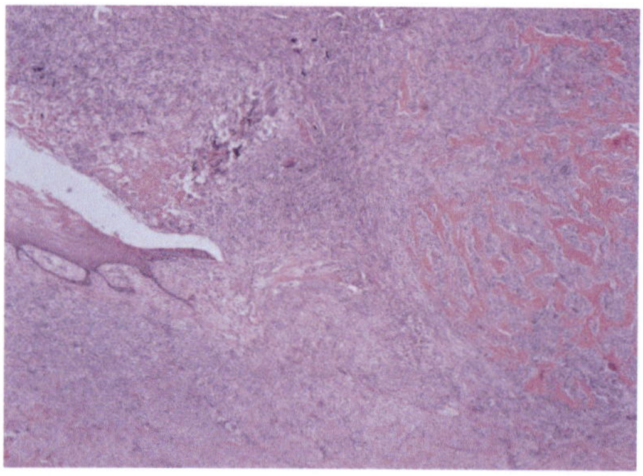

Fig. 15.43 Poorly defined infiltrating tumor with osteoid

Synonym: Extraskeletal Osteosarcoma

Histopathology (Figs. 15.43, 15.44, 15.45, and 15.46)

- Infiltrating subcutaneous tumor made of admixture of atypical spindle cells, hyperchromatic osteoblasts, and osteoid
- Matrix between spindle cells appears as unmineralized osteoid or shows mineralized trabeculae

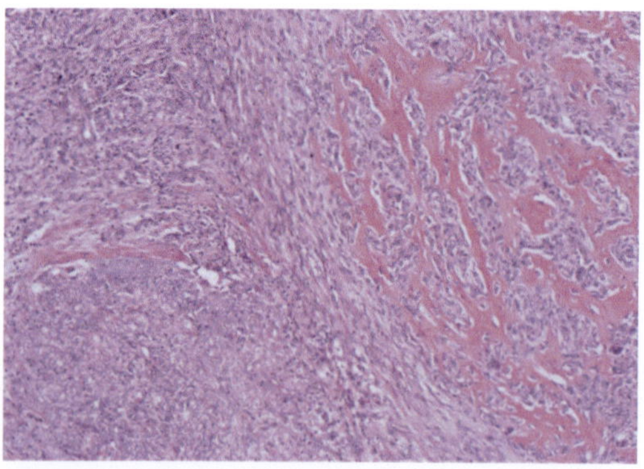

Fig. 15.44 Spindle cell proliferation surrounding pink osteoid

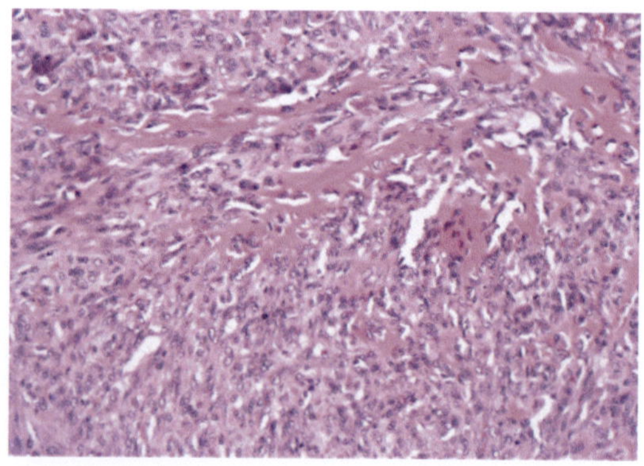

Fig. 15.45 The osteoid is rimmed by malignant osteoblasts

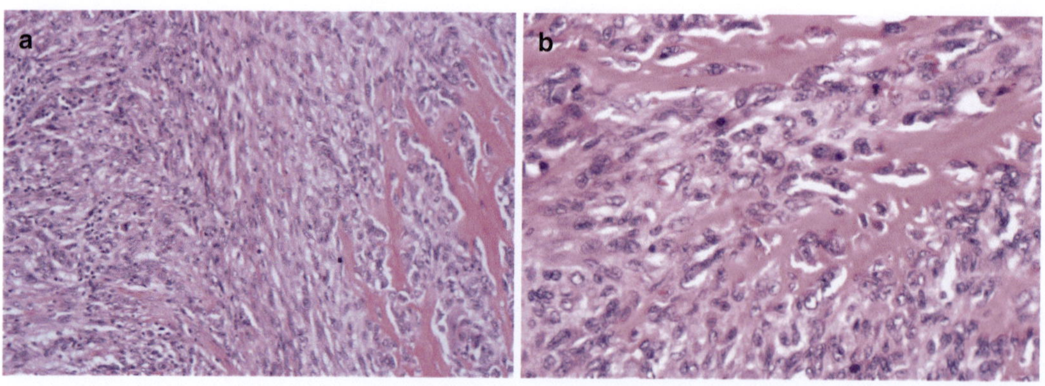

Fig. 15.46 (**a**, **b**) Spindle cells are pleomorphic and highly atypical with numerous mitoses

16 Dermatopathology P

V. Vincek, *Dermatopathology A–Z*, https://doi.org/10.1007/978-3-319-89486-7_16

Paget's Disease

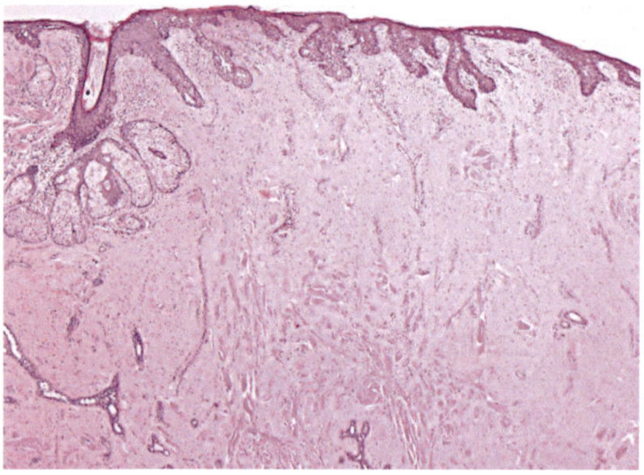

Fig. 16.1 Nipple biopsy with corrugated epidermis, mammary glands, and increased number of muscle bundles

Histopathology (Figs. 16.1, 16.2, 16.3, and 16.4)

- Epidermis infiltrated by cells with abundant pale cytoplasm
- Cells have large oval to round vesicular nuclei with occasionally prominent nucleoli
- Cells are cytokeratin 7, CEA, and EMA positive
- Mucin stains (Alcian blue, Mucicarmine) are positive in a half of the cases

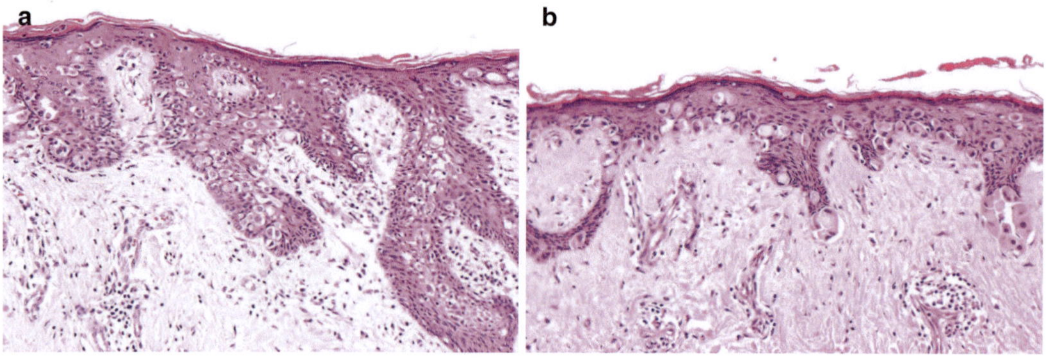

Fig. 16.2 (**a**, **b**) Epidermis is infiltrated by large pale cells

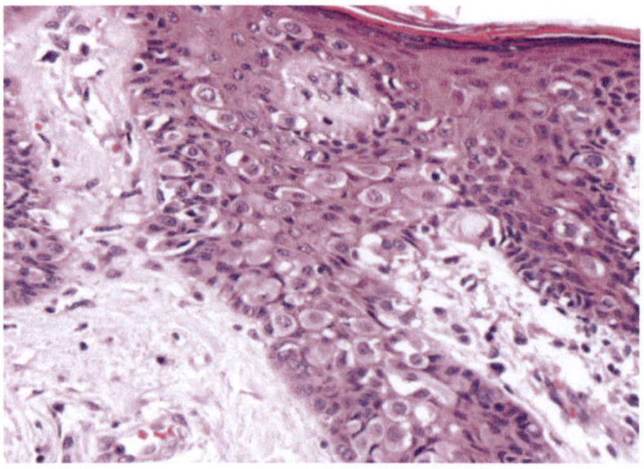

Fig. 16.3 Tumor cells vary in size and have large pale eosinophilic cytoplasm and vesicular nuclei

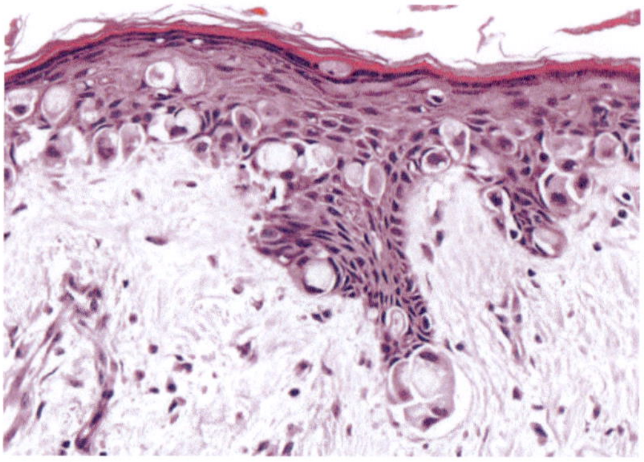

Fig. 16.4 Cytoplasm of some tumor cells has bluish hue due to the intracytoplasmic mucin

Pagetoid Reticulosis

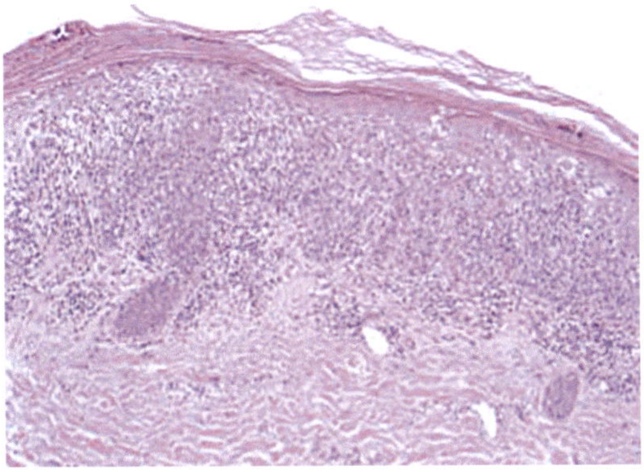

Fig. 16.5 Acanthotic epidermis with hyperkeratosis and spongiosis and no significant dermal lymphocytic infiltrate

Synonym: Woringer-Kolopp Disease

A distinct variant of mycosis fungoides with following **histopathology** (Figs. 16.5, 16.6, and 16.7)

- Acanthotic hyperkeratotic epidermis with spongiosis
- The entire epidermis is infiltrated by atypical lymphocytes
- There are no atypical lymphocytic cells in the dermis
- Dermis may contain benign lymphohistiocytic infiltrate

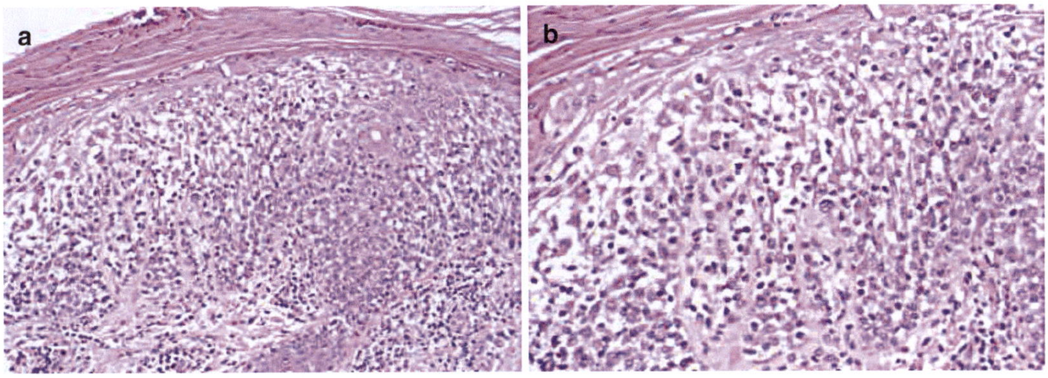

Fig. 16.6 (**a**, **b**) Lymphocytes infiltrate involving full epidermal thickness

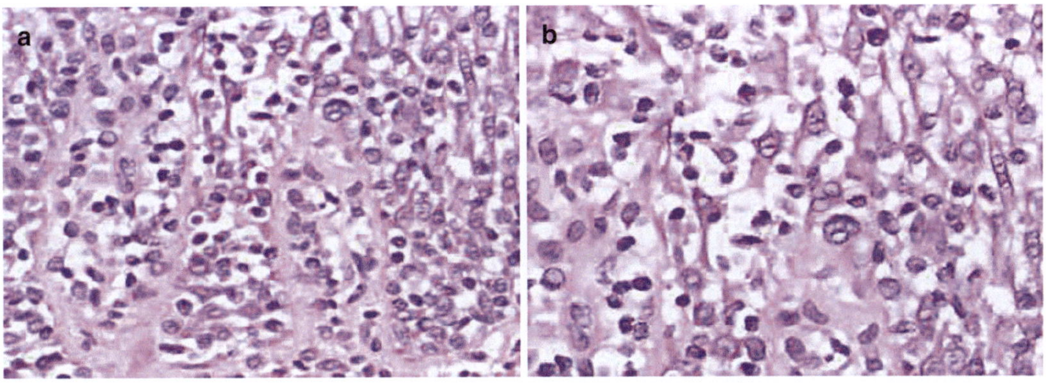

Fig. 16.7 (**a**, **b**) Epidermal spongiosis with small to medium size atypical lymphocytes

Palisaded Neutrophilic and Granulomatous Dermatitis

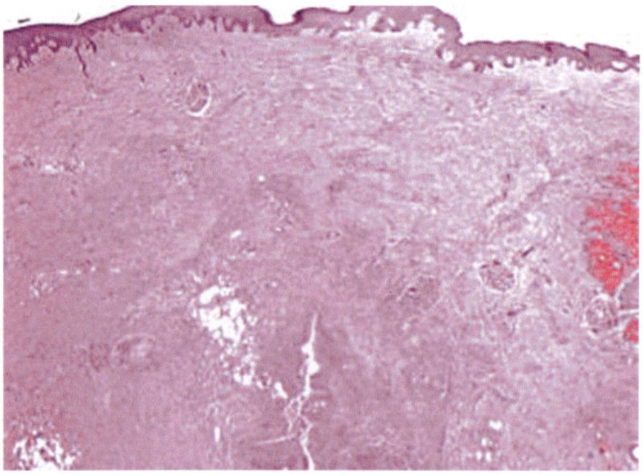

Fig. 16.8 Ill-defined subcutaneous granulomas

Synonym: Interstitial Granulomatous Dermatitis

Histopathology (Figs. 16.8, 16.9, 16.10, and 16.11)

- Superficial and deep granulomas resembling *deep granuloma annulare* but granulomas are irregular and less well defined, with minimal or no mucin
- Central necrobiosis is surrounded by histiocytes
- Neutrophilic infiltrate with karyorrhexis is scattered in between granuloma and can also be seen within necrobiotic centers

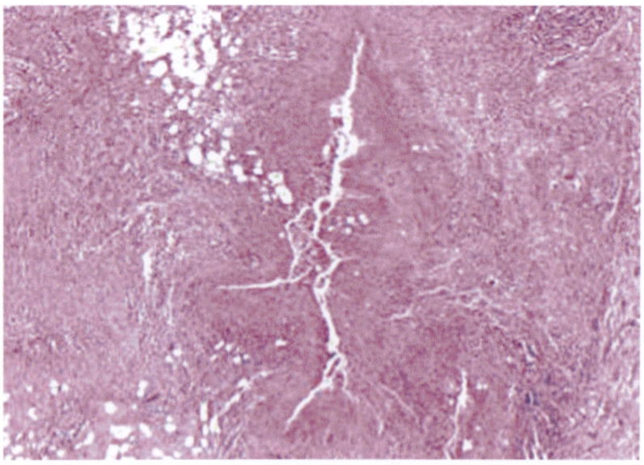

Fig. 16.9 Central irregular area of necrobiosis

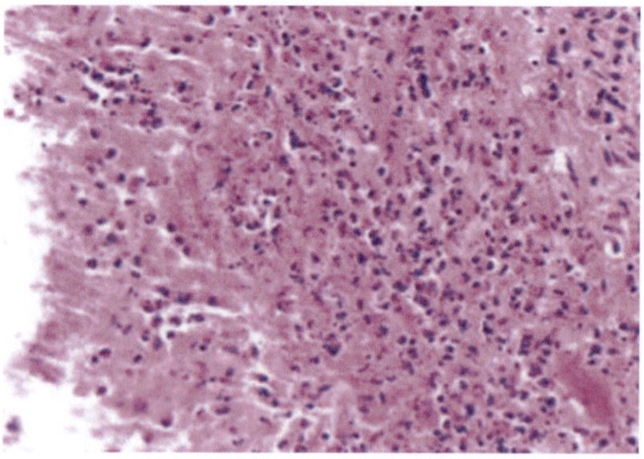

Fig. 16.10 Neutrophilic aggregates with karyorrhexis

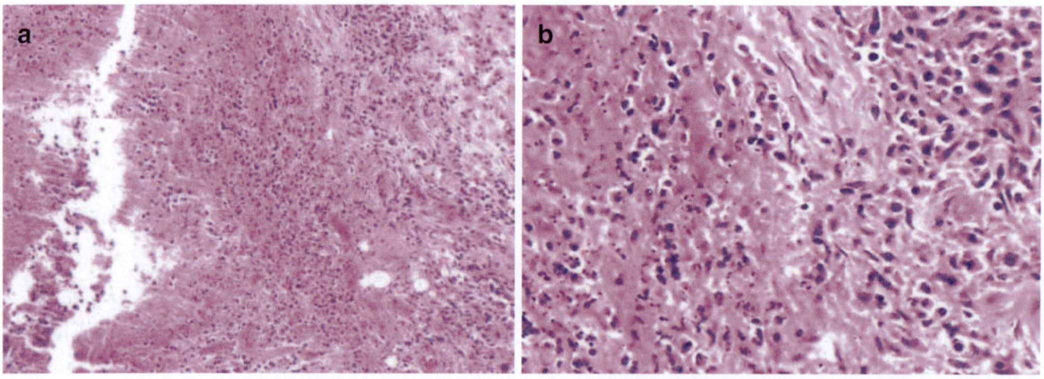

Fig. 16.11 (**a**, **b**) Central necrobiosis and karyorrhexis surrounded by histiocytes, lymphocytes, and occasional giant cells

Pancreatic Panniculitis

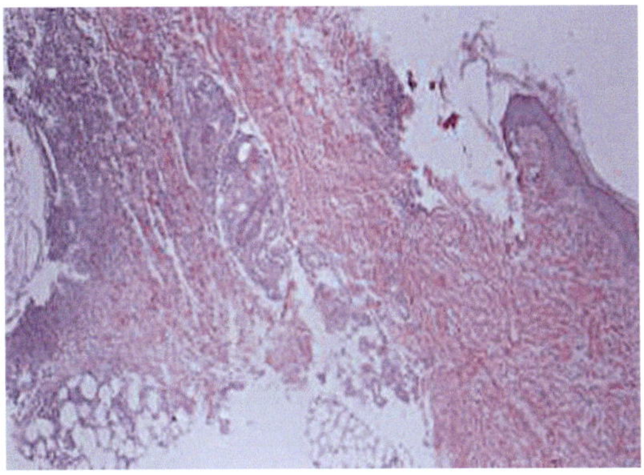

Fig. 16.12 Lobular panniculitis

Histopathology (Figs. 16.12, 16.13, 16.14, and 16.15)

- Lobular "dirty" panniculitis
- Enzymatic fat necrosis with fat "ghost" cells
- Calcification of necrotic fat is common
- Neutrophils are common at the margins of necrosis

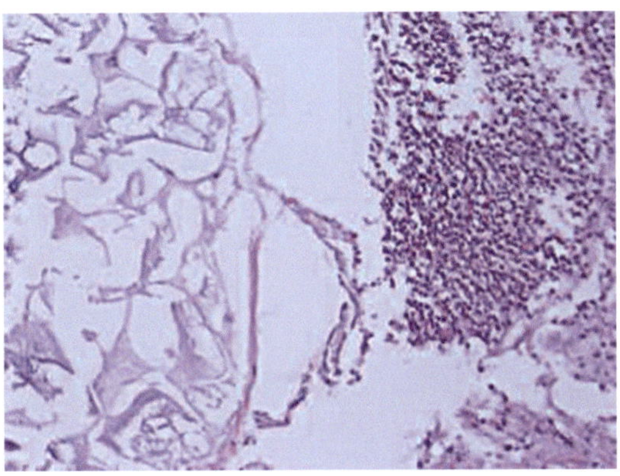

Fig. 16.13 Neutrophils are present at the edge of necrosis

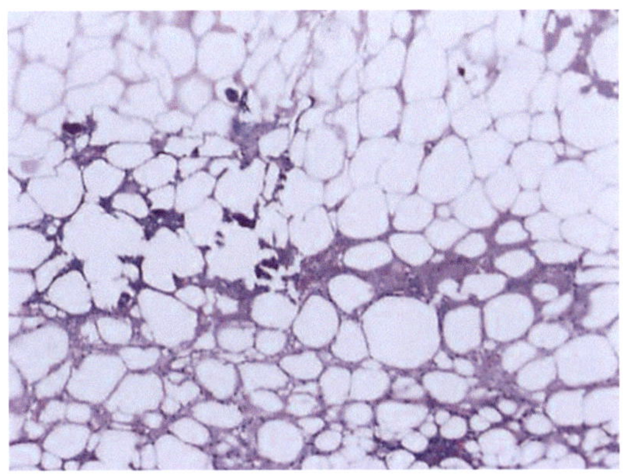

Fig. 16.14 Focal calcifications of necrotic fat

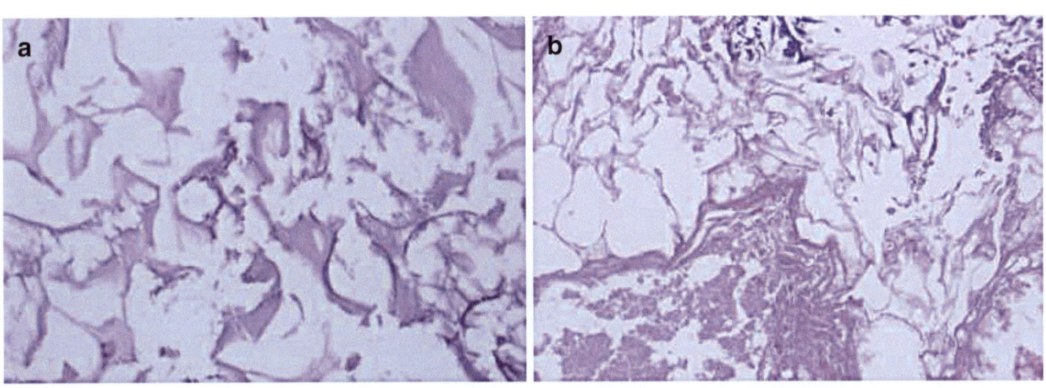

Fig. 16.15 (a, b) Fat necrosis with "ghost cells" within smudgy "dirty" pale background

Papillary Eccrine Adenoma

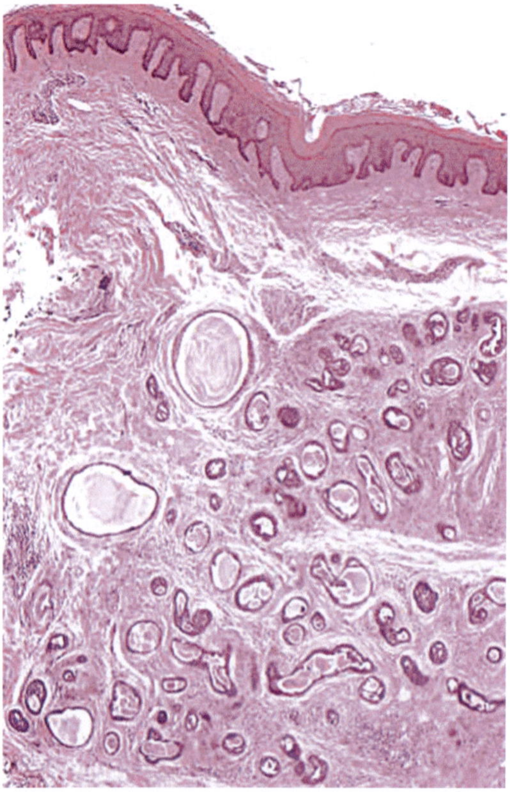

Fig. 16.16 Dilated ducts and cysts in fibrous stroma

Histopathology (Figs. 16.16, 16.17, and 16.18)
- Rare tumor predominantly on extremities and particularly affecting blacks
- Dilated ducts and cyst within fibrous stroma
- Forming vague tumor nodules without aggressive infiltrative growth
- Two layers of eosinophilic cuboidal cells that appear uniform with no cytological atypia
- Intraductal papillary projections are common
- Cribriform pattern within ducts can be seen

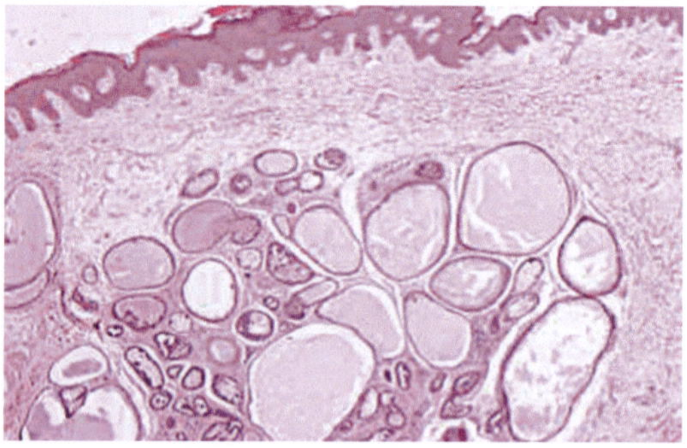

Fig. 16.17 Tumor demonstrates pushing, not infiltrating growth

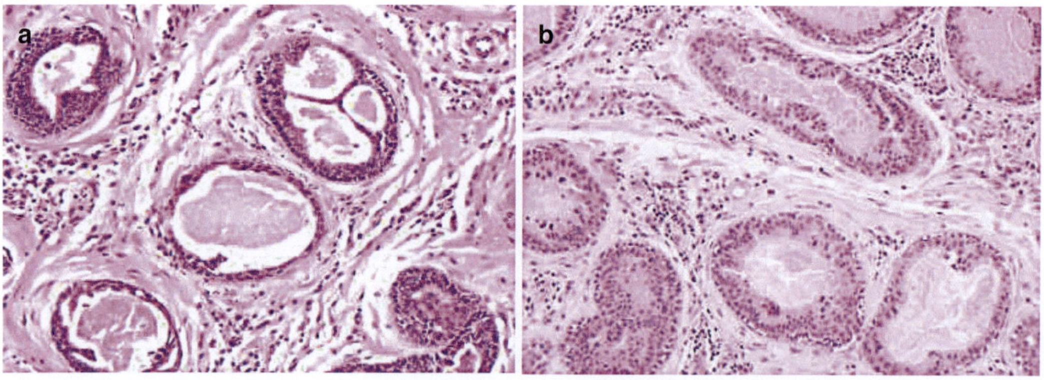

Fig. 16.18 (**a**, **b**) Ducts lined by two layers of cuboidal cells and delicate intraductal papillary projections. One duct demonstrates cribriform pattern. There is no significant cytological atypia

Papular Acrodermatitis of Childhood

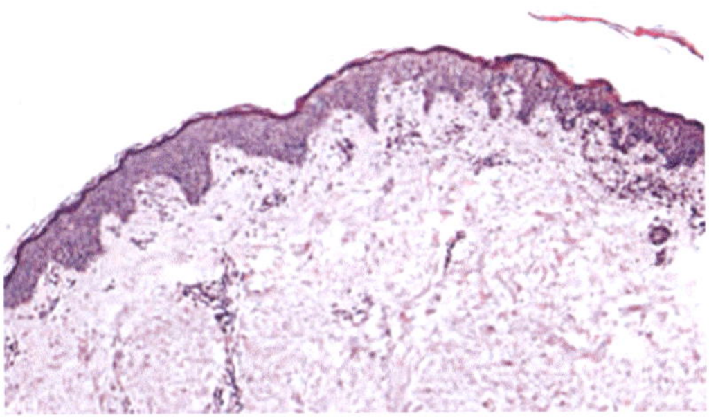

Fig. 16.19 Non-specific histopathology

Synonym: Gianotti-Crosti Disease

Histopathological changes are not specific and clinical correlation is necessary (Figs. 16.19, 16.20, and 16.21)

- Normal or mildly spongiotic epidermis
- Mild perivascular lymphocytic infiltrate
- Vacuolar interface or lichenoid inflammation is occasionally seen

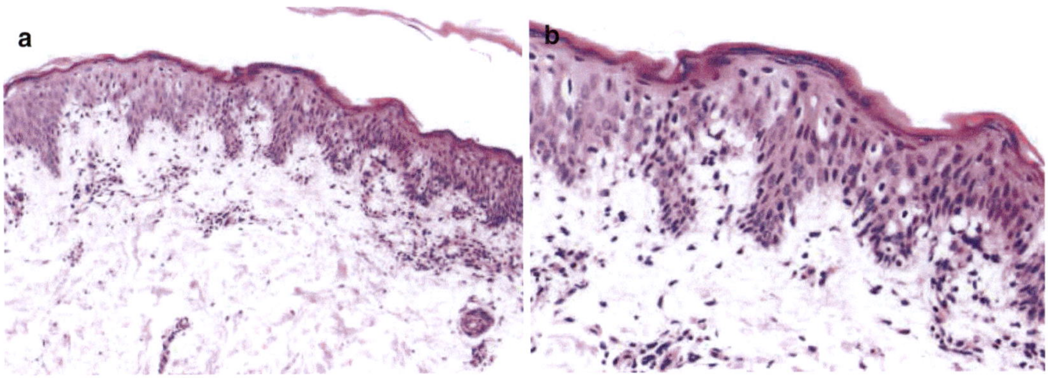

Fig. 16.20 (**a**, **b**) Mildly spongiotic epidermis with mild perivascular lymphocytic inflammation

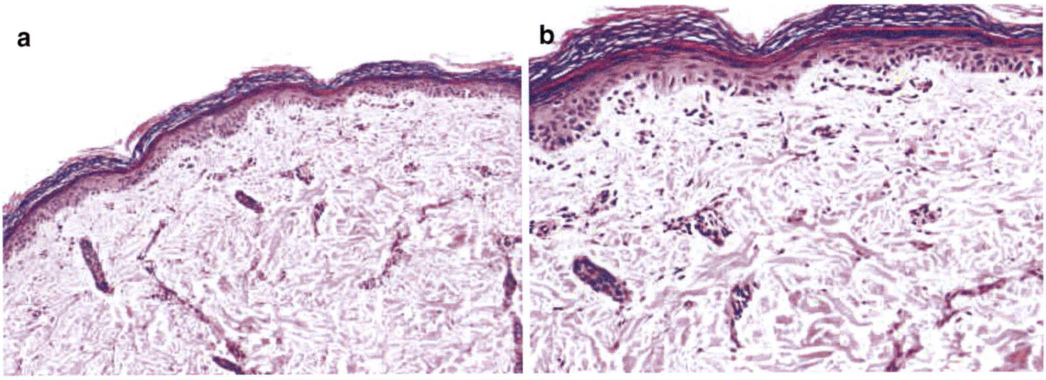

Fig. 16.21 (**a**, **b**) Unremarkable epidermis with mild perivascular lymphocytic inflammation

Papular Mucinosis

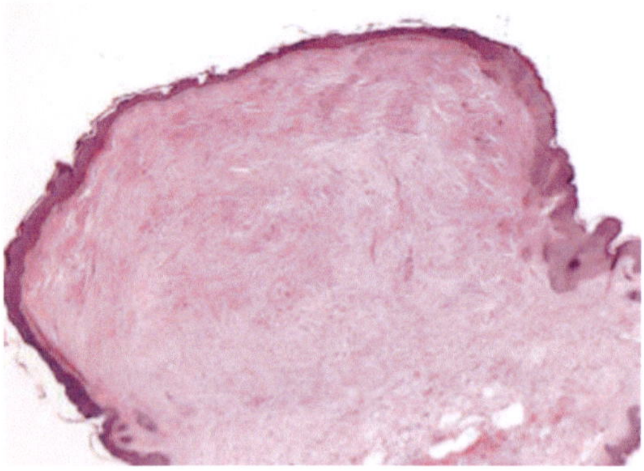

Fig. 16.22 Tag-like lesion with pale stroma

Histopathology (Figs. 16.22, 16.23, 16.24, and 16.25)

- Papillary shaped lesion
- Resembles focal dermal mucinosis
- Slight proliferation of fibroblasts with mild thickening of collagen
- Amount of mucin is variable

P.S. this is localized form of *lichen myxedematosus*

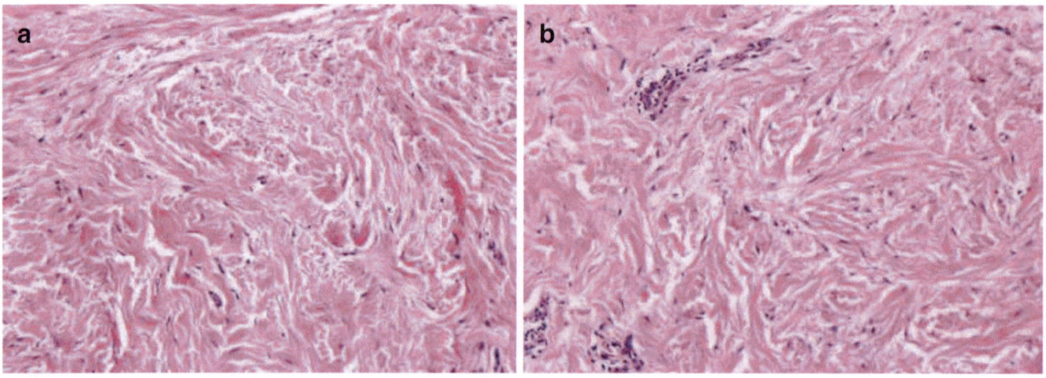

Fig. 16.23 (**a**, **b**) Thickening of collagen with pale spaces filled with mucin

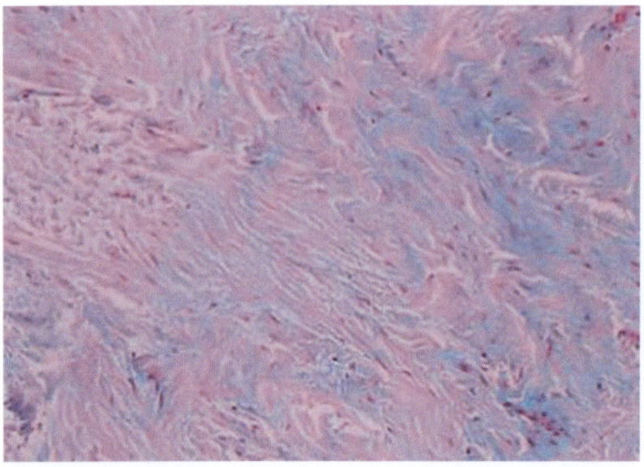

Fig. 16.24 Alcian Blue stain demonstrates variable amount of mucin (staining blue)

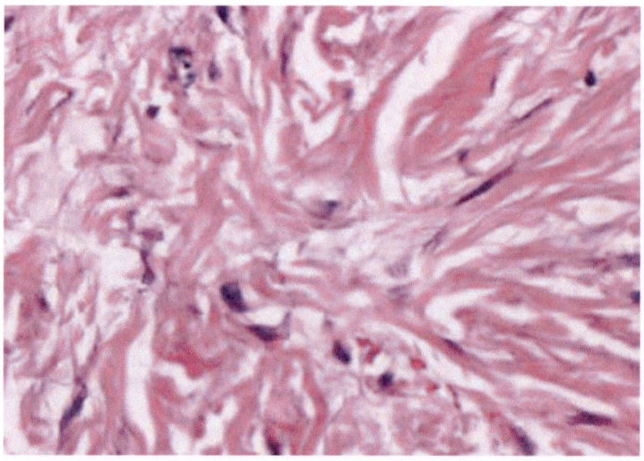

Fig. 16.25 Mild proliferation of fibroblasts among thickened collagen

Paracoccidioidomycosis

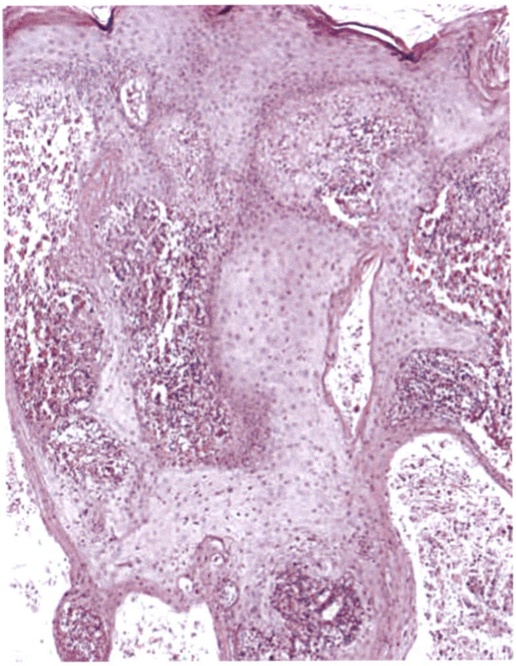

Fig. 16.26 Extensive pseudoepitheliomatous hyperplasia and exuberant inflammation with numerous neutrophils

Synonym: South American Blastomycosis

Histopathology (Figs. 16.26, 16.27, 16.28, and 16.29)

- Pseudoepitheliomatous hyperplasia with common epidermal ulceration
- Mixed inflammation with neutrophilic microabscesses
- Thick walled yeast elements of variable size (4–40 μM)
- Yeast appears as single, pairs, chains or budding yeast elements ("captain wheel")

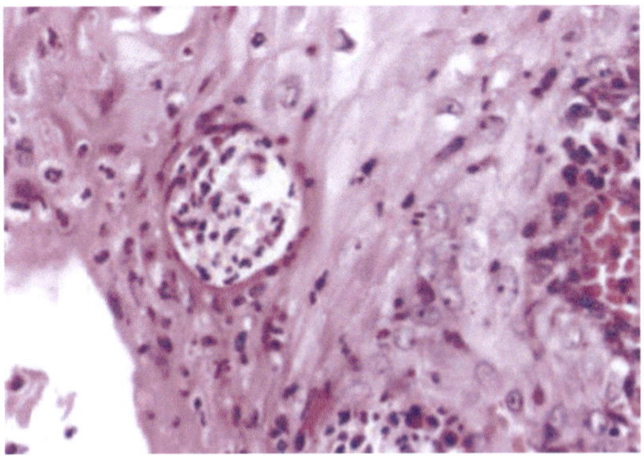

Fig. 16.27 Neutrophilic microabscess with yeast elements

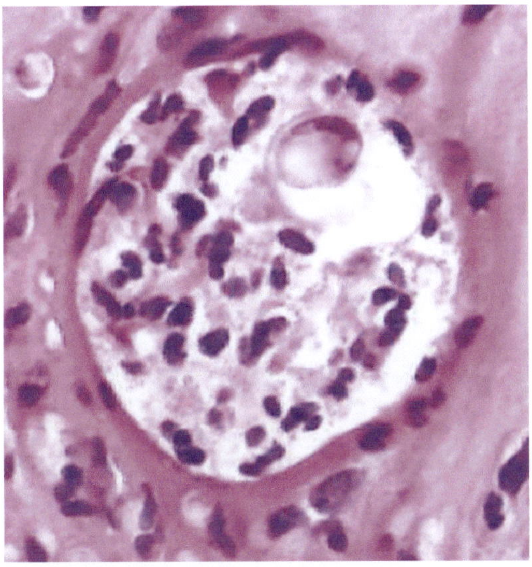

Fig. 16.28 Thick walled yeast element

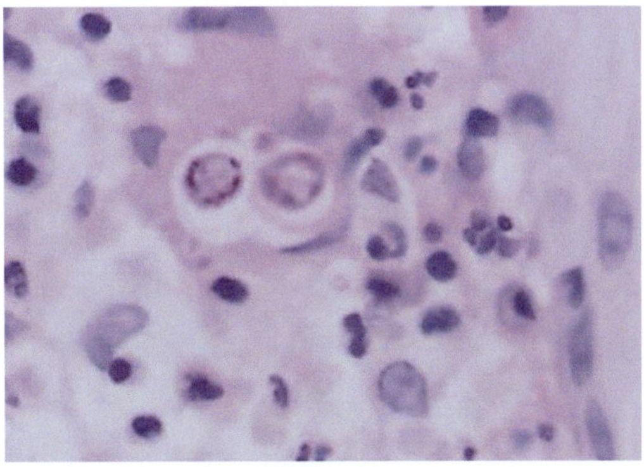

Fig. 16.29 PAS stain of yeast pair

Paraffinoma

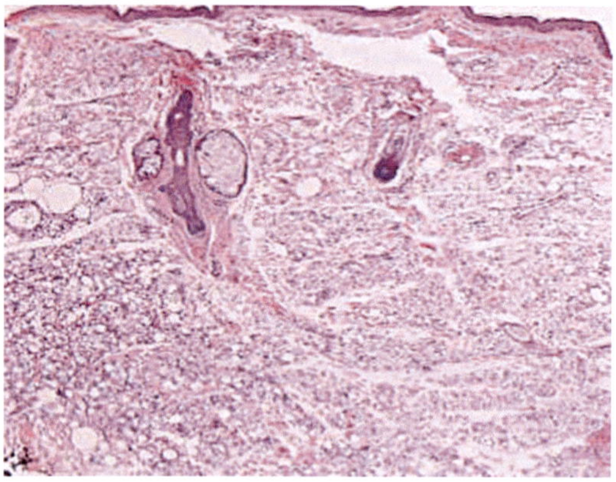

Fig. 16.30 "Swiss cheese" appearance of dermis and subcutis

Synonyms: Sclerosing Lipogranuloma, Silicoma
Reaction to various oils/silicones.

Histopathology (Figs. 16.30, 16.31, 16.32, and 16.33)
- Numerous empty round/oval spaces of variable size in the dermis and subcutis ("Swiss cheese" pattern)
- Foamy histiocytes surround empty spaces
- Reactive fibrosis is present

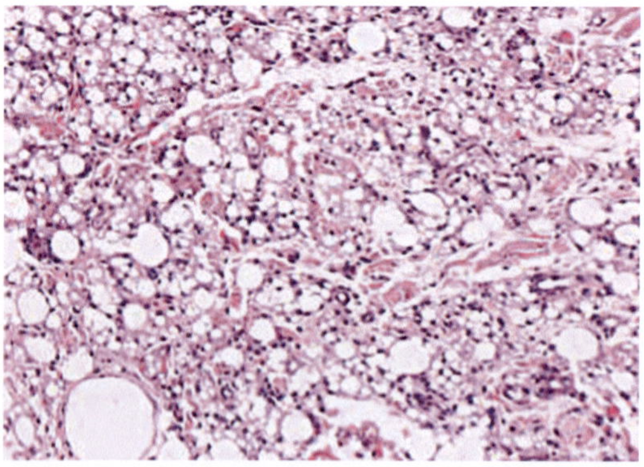

Fig. 16.31 Numerous empty, round to oval spaces in the dermis and subcutis

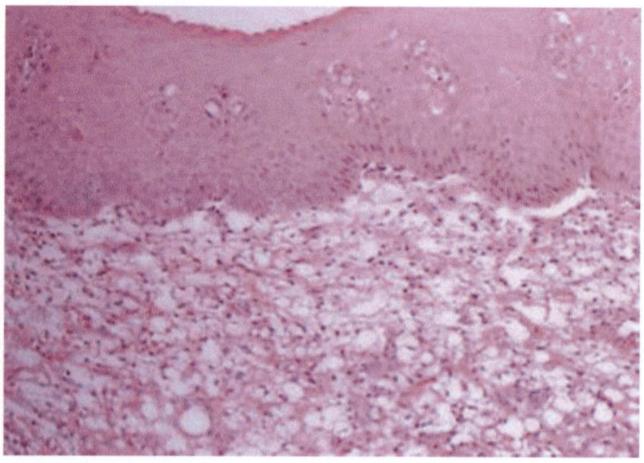

Fig. 16.32 Lip mucosa with submucosal foreign material

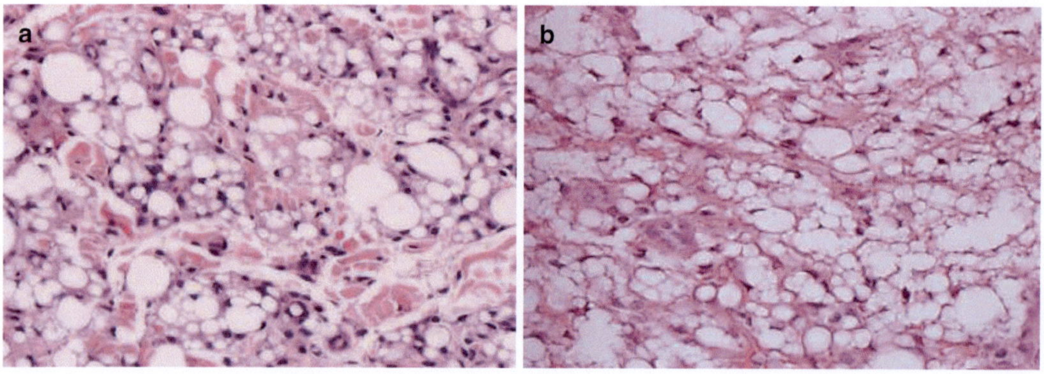

Fig. 16.33 (**a**, **b**) Histiocytes and stromal fibrosis surrounds empty spaces

Paraneoplastic Pemphigus

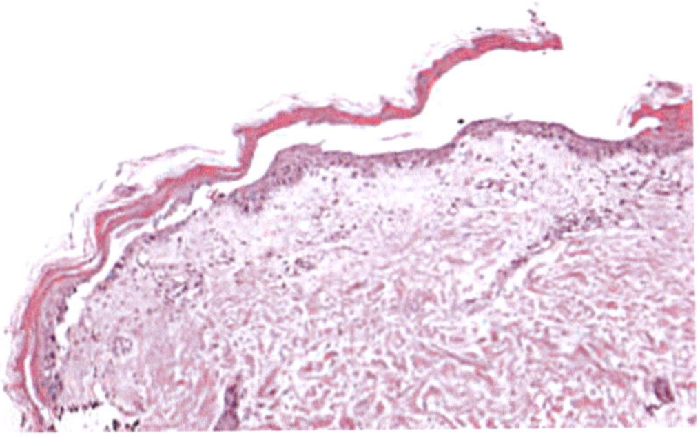

Fig. 16.34 Suprabasal acantholytic blister

Histopathology is variable reflecting polymorphic clinical presentations (Figs. 16.34, 16.35, and 16.36)

- Suprabasal acantholysis with clefting
- Variable dermal lymphocytic inflammation from very mild to significant lichen planus-like
- Interface vacuolar changes are common
- Variable number of necrotic keratinocytes

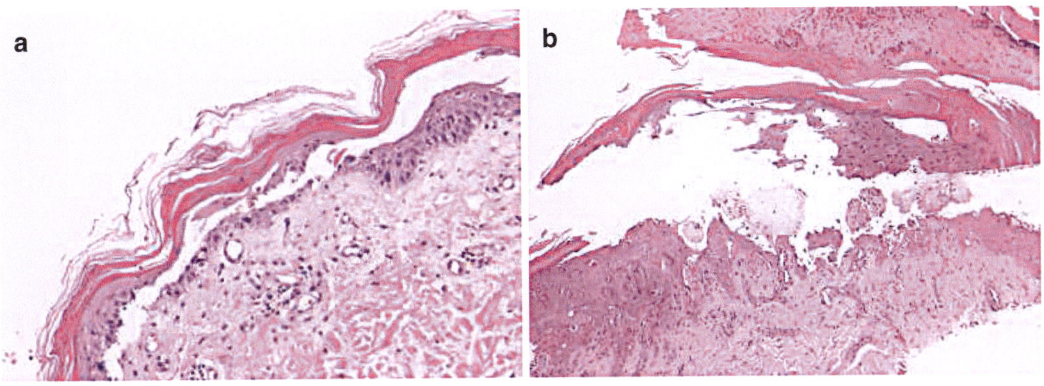

Fig. 16.35 (a, b) Interface vacuolar changes with necrotic keratinocytes and mild dermal inflammation

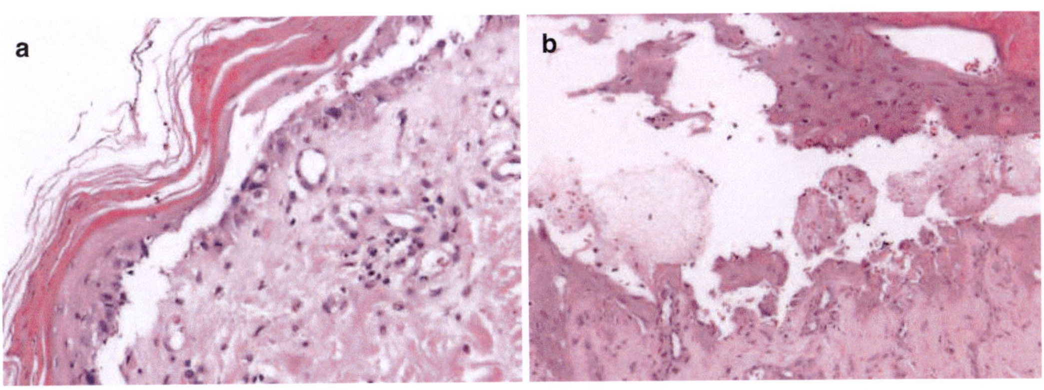

Fig. 16.36 (a, b) Suprabasal clefting and acantholysis

Parapsoriasis

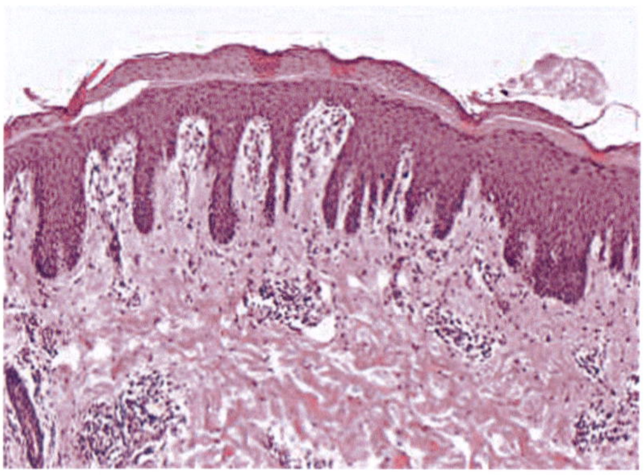

Fig. 16.37 Large plaque parapsoriasis

Histopathology

Large plaque parapsoriasis:
- Psoriasiform epidermal hyperplasia with mounds of parakeratosis, papillary dermal fibrosis, and focal lymphocytic exocytosis (Figs. 16.37, 16.38, and 16.39)

Poilkilodermic parapsoriasis:
- Atrophic epidermis with dermal telangiectasias and mild band-like dermal lymphocytic infiltrate (Fig. 16.40)

Small plaque parapsoriasis:
- *Not* specific with swavy thin epidermis and focal exocytosis (Figs. 16.41 and 16.42)

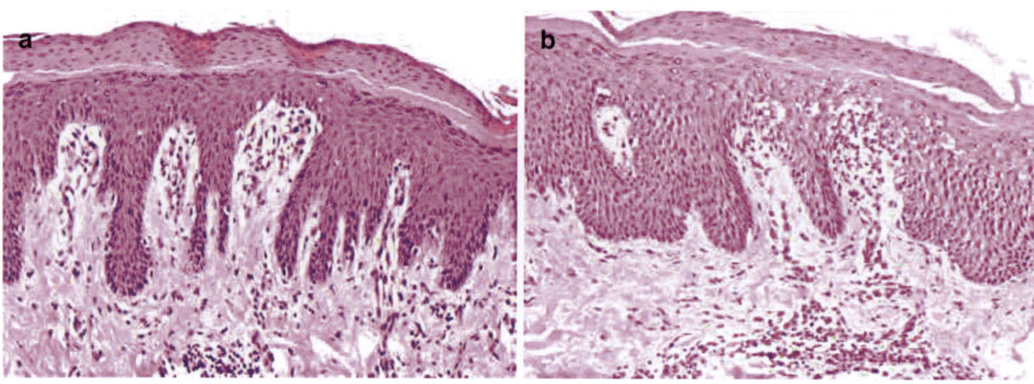

Fig. 16.38 (**a**, **b**) Psoriasiform epidermis with mounds of parakeratosis

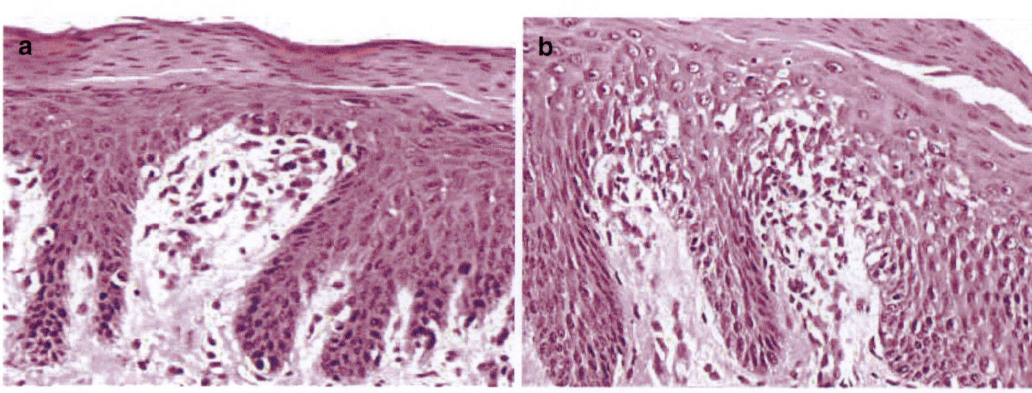

Fig. 16.39 (**a**, **b**) Focal epidermal lymphocytic exocytosis and dermal fibrosis

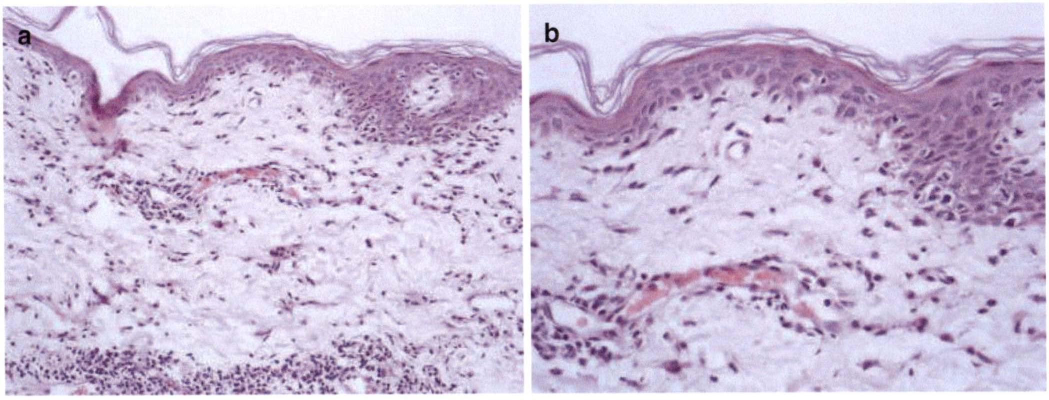

Fig. 16.40 (a, b) **Poilkilodermic parapsoriasis** with atrophic epidermis, lymphocytic exocytosis, lichenoid infiltrate and dermal telangiectasias

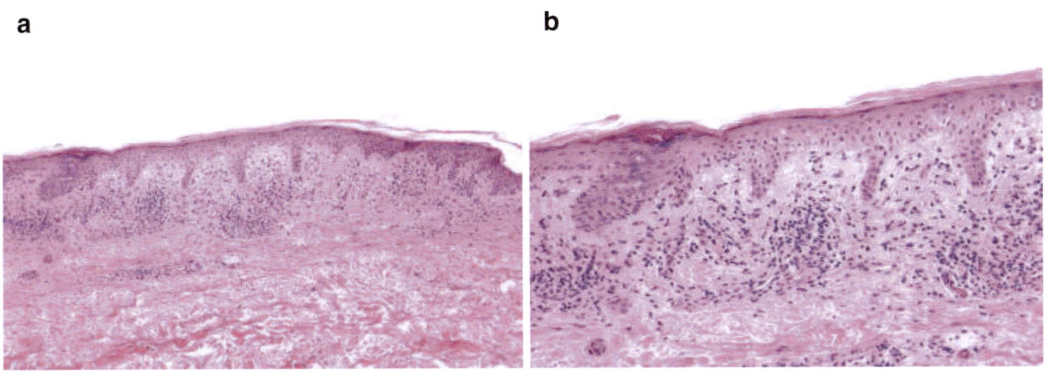

Fig. 16.41 (a, b) **Small plaque parapsoriasis** with mild perivascular lymphocytic infiltrate

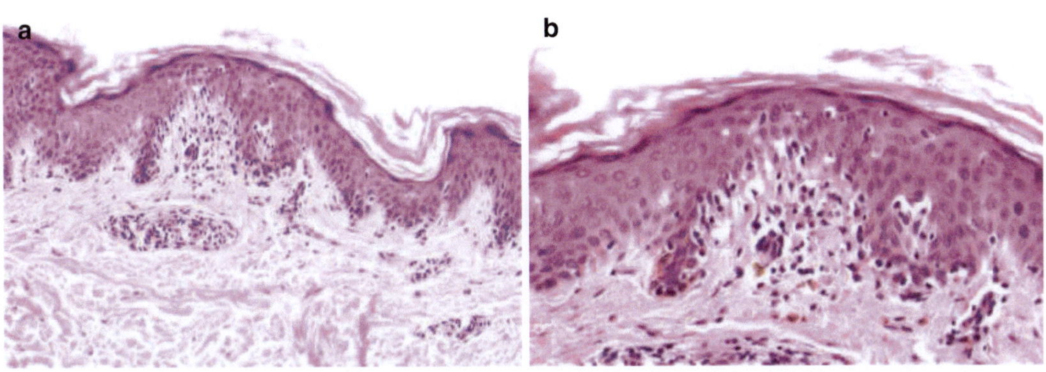

Fig. 16.42 (a, b) **Small plaque parapsoriasis** with lymphocytic exocytosis suggesting transition to mycosis fungoides

PEComa

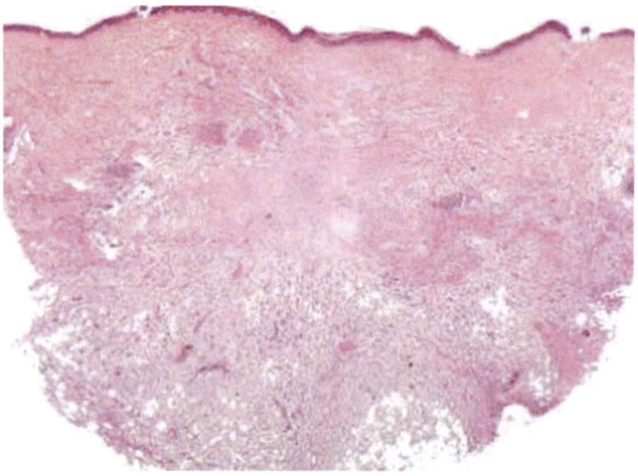

Fig. 16.43 Poorly defined dermal and subcutaneous tumor

Synonym: Perivascular Epithelioid Cell Tumor

Histopathology (Figs. 16.43, 16.44, and 16.45)

- Poorly demarcated dermal and subcutaneous tumor
- Tumor cells are arranged around thin-walled vessels
- Tumor cells have clear or pale cytoplasm with vesicular nuclei
- Tumor cells stain for some melanocytic (Melan-A, HMB45, MITF) and muscular (desmin, SMA) markers but are negative for S-100 and caldesmon

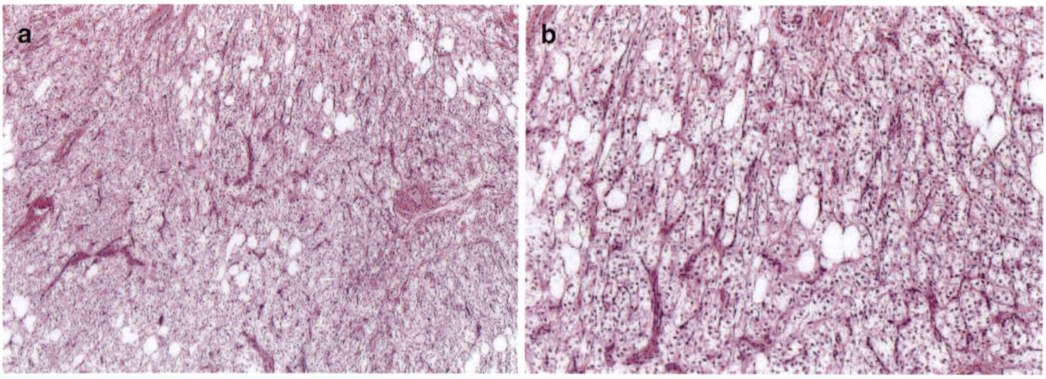

Fig. 16.44 (**a**, **b**) Vertically oriented thin vessels surrounded by pale cells

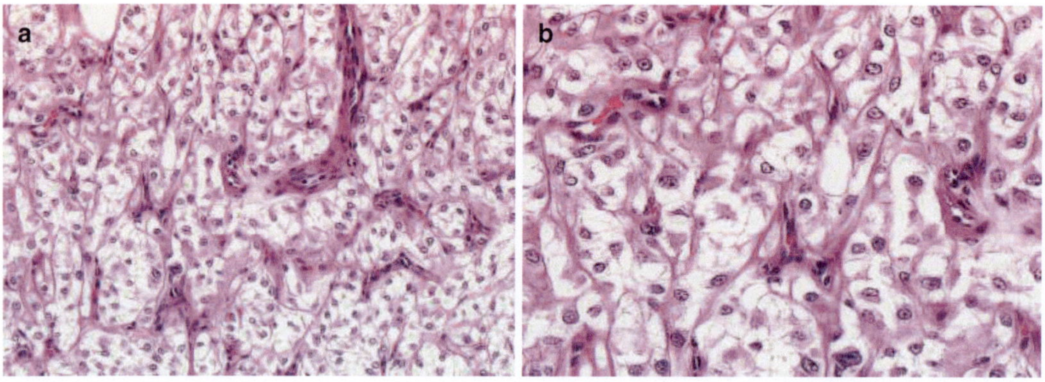

Fig. 16.45 (**a**, **b**) Cells have pale cytoplasm and vesicular nuclei with no evidence of atypia or mitoses

Pediculosis

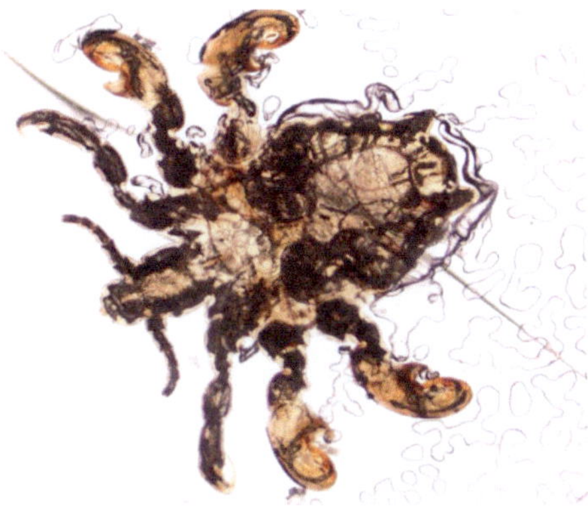

Fig. 16.46 Pubic louse (crab)

> **Synonym: Human Lice**
>
> **Histopathology** (Figs. 16.46, 16.47, 16.48, 16.49, and 16.50)
>
> – The head and pubic louse are very similar with 3 pairs of legs and 2 antennae
> – The body of head louse is slimmer comparing to pubic louse
> – The pubic louse (crab) has two front pairs of legs that resemble crab's pincher claw

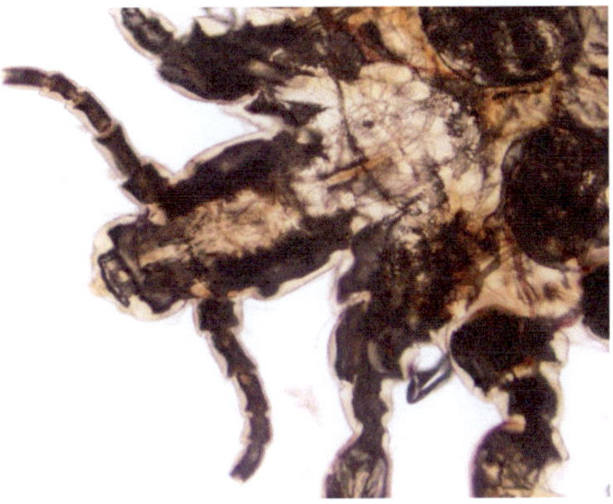

Fig. 16.47 Two antennae sticking out of the head

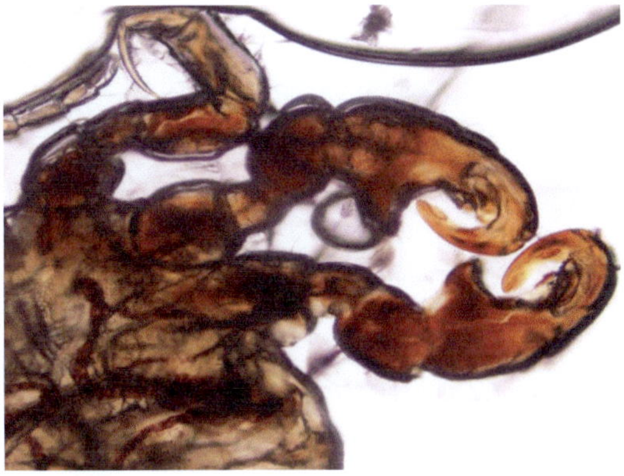

Fig. 16.48 Two front pairs of legs have pincher claws like a crab

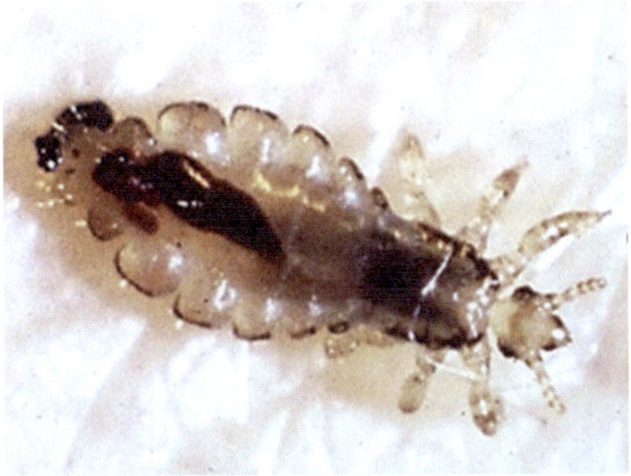

Fig. 16.49 Head louse

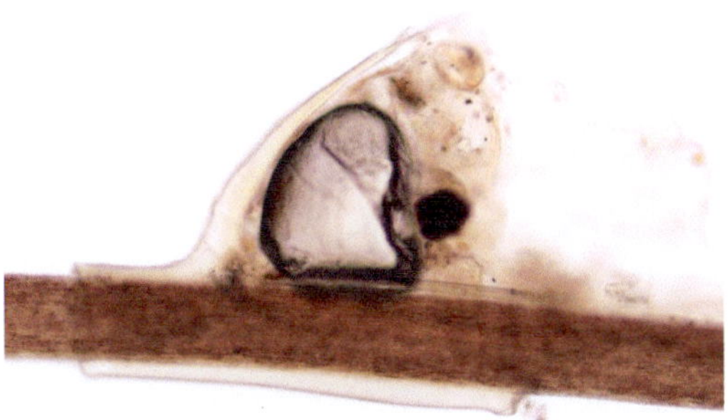

Fig. 16.50 Hair shaft with an attached egg (nit)

Pemphigus Foliaceous

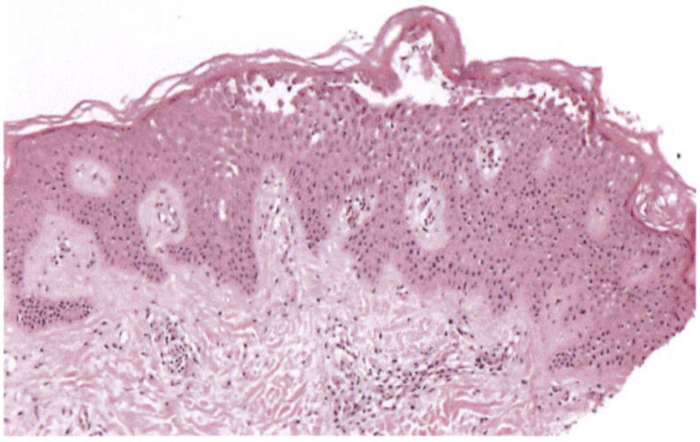

Fig. 16.51 Flacid subcorneal blister

Histopathology (Figs. 16.51, 16.52, 16.53, 16.54, and 16.55)

Early lesions:

- Subcorneal or intragranular blister with few acantholytic keratinocytes and variable number of neutrophils (vary from none to many neutrophils)

Later lesion:

- Absent roof blister with prominence of granular layer covered with serum crust with neutrophils

P.S. **Fogo Selvagem** is endemic form of disease. **Pemphigus Erythematosus** has identical histology

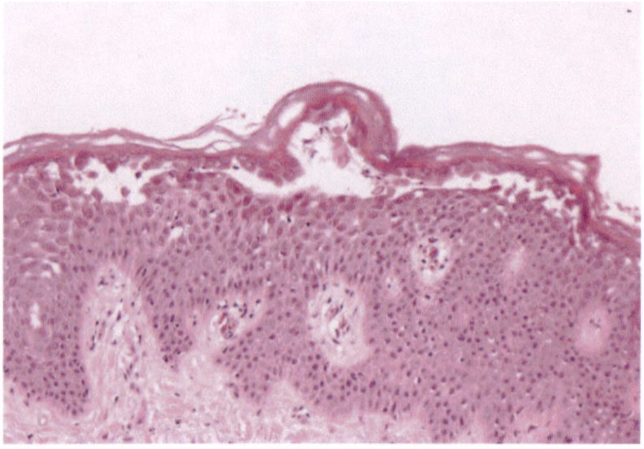

Fig. 16.52 Subcorneal blister of spongiotic epidermis

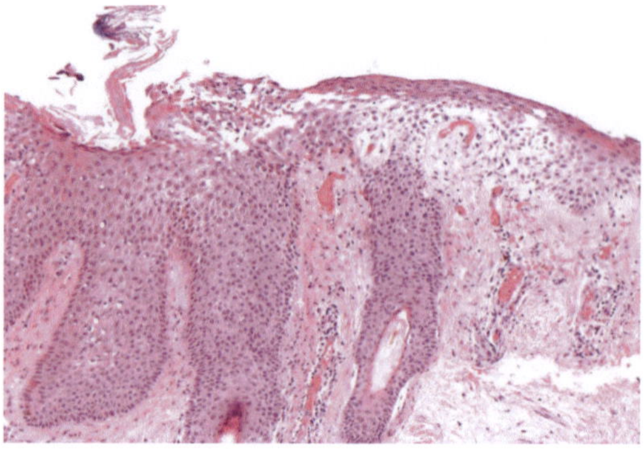

Fig. 16.53 Subcorneal blister with neutrophils

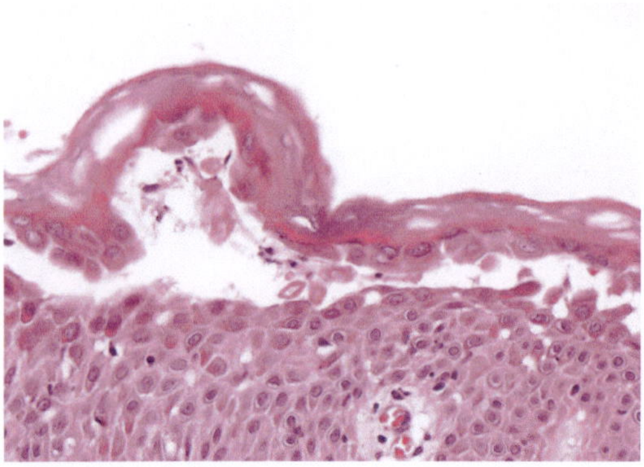

Fig. 16.54 Subcorneal blister with few acantholytic keratinocytes and no inflammatory cells; blister roof is still present

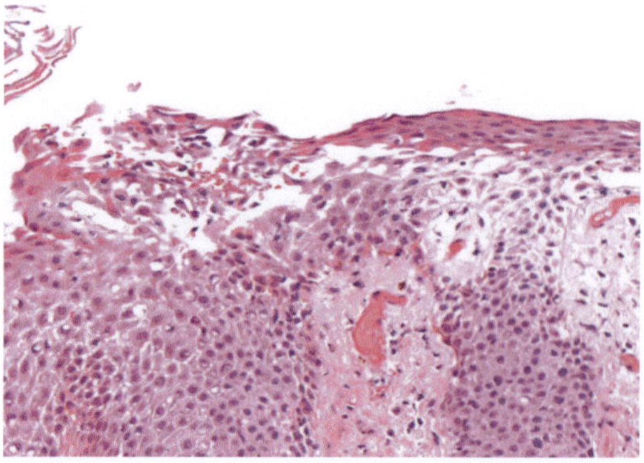

Fig. 16.55 Blister roof is missing and serum crust is forming

Pemphigus Vegetans

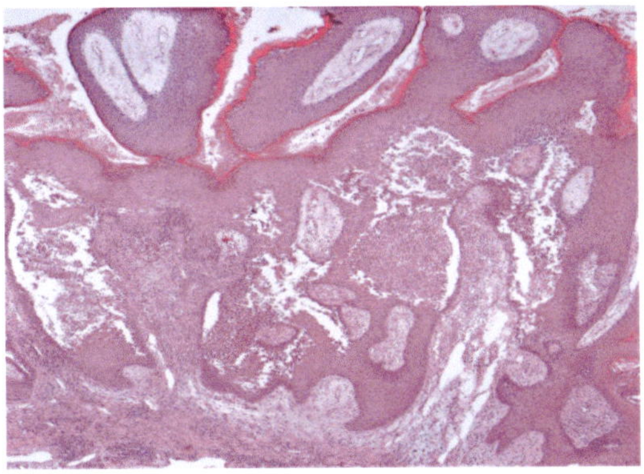

Fig. 16.56 Verruciform epidermal proliferation

Histopathology (Figs. 16.56, 16.57, and 16.58)
- Initial lesions are the same as in pemphigus vulgaris (suprabasal acantholysis with intraepidermal blister)
- Developed lesion shows verrucous epidermal hyperplasia
- Intraepidermal eosinophilic pustules are characteristic

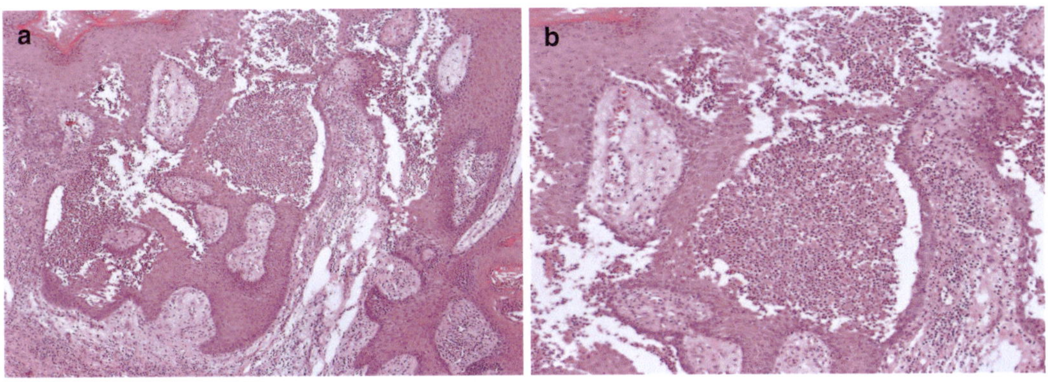

Fig. 16.57 (a, b) Intraepidermal pustules of eosinophils

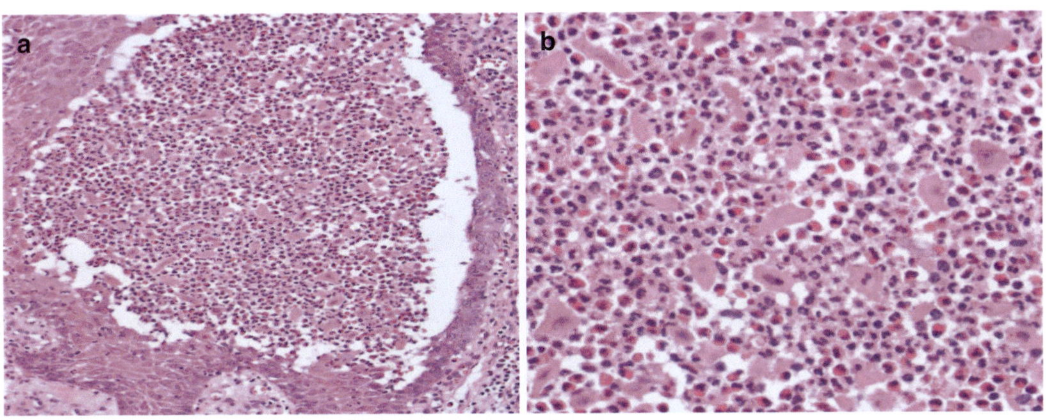

Fig. 16.58 (a, b) Eosinophils admixed with acantholytic keratinocytes

Pemphigus Vulgaris

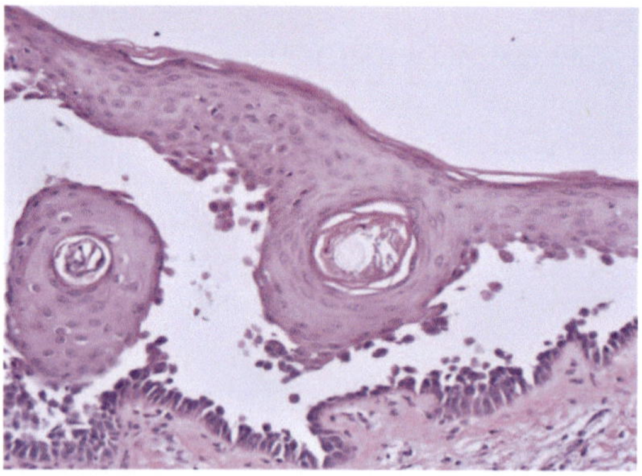

Fig. 16.59 "Cell poor" intraepidermal blister

Histopathology (Figs. 16.59, 16.60, and 16.61)

- Suprabasal acantholysis with intraepidermal blister
- Basal layer keratinocytes remain attached to the basement membrane ("row of tombstones")
- Blister contains acantholytic keratinocytes and minimal or no neutrophilic or eosinophilic inflammation
- Superficial perivascular lymphocytic inflammation

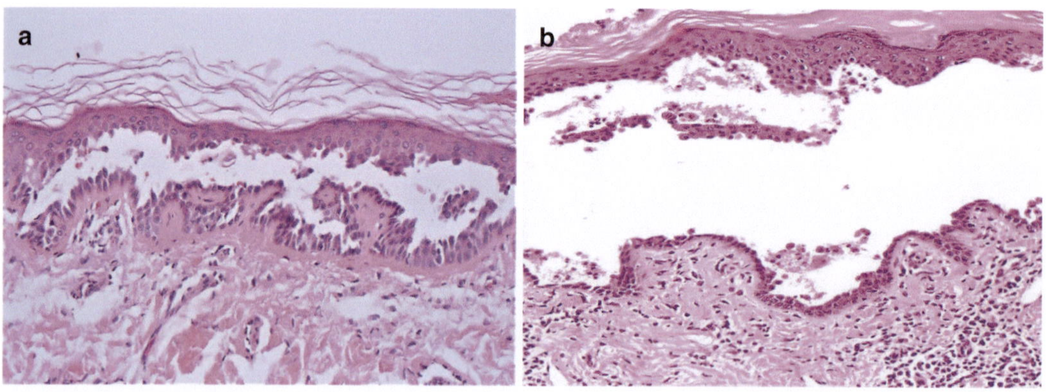

Fig. 16.60 (**a**, **b**) Suprabasal blister with basal cell keratinocytes attached to the basement membrane

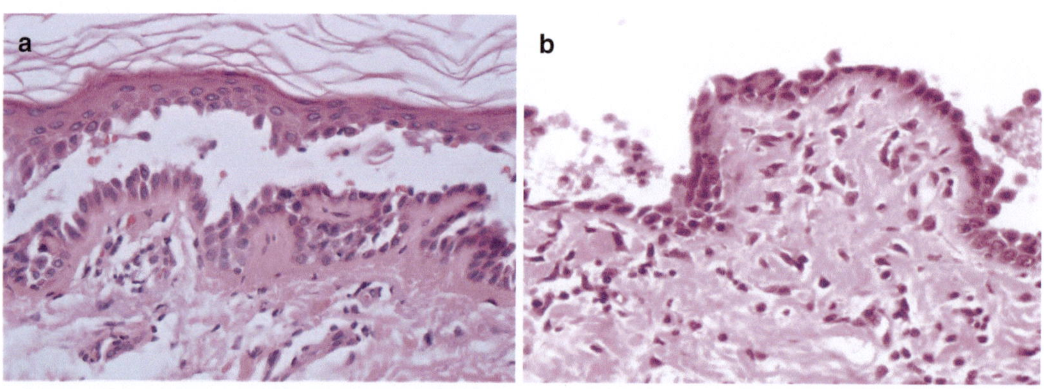

Fig. 16.61 (**a**, **b**) Blister contains few acantholytic keratinocytes; dermal lymphocytic inflammation is present

Penicillamine Dermopathy

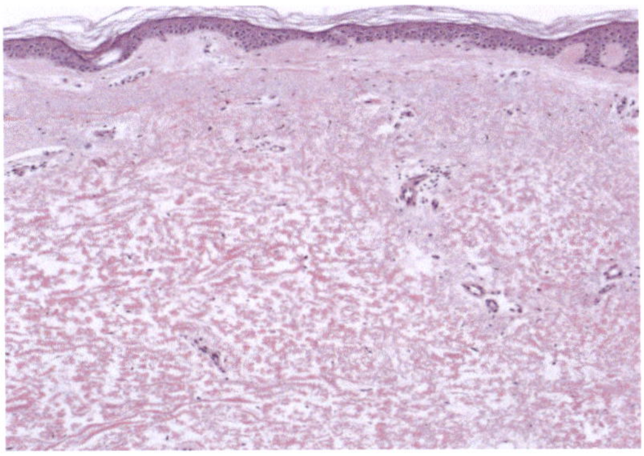

Fig. 16.62 Pale dermis with prominent elastic fibers

Histopathology (Figs. 16.62, 16.63, and 16.64)
- Increased number of abnormal elastic fibers in the dermis
- Characteristic serrated appearance of elastic fibers

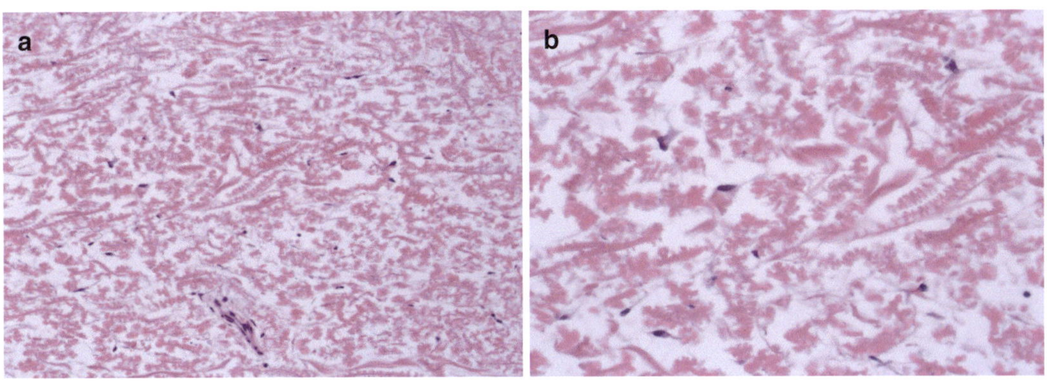

Fig. 16.63 (**a**, **b**) Increased number of abnormal dermal elastic fibers

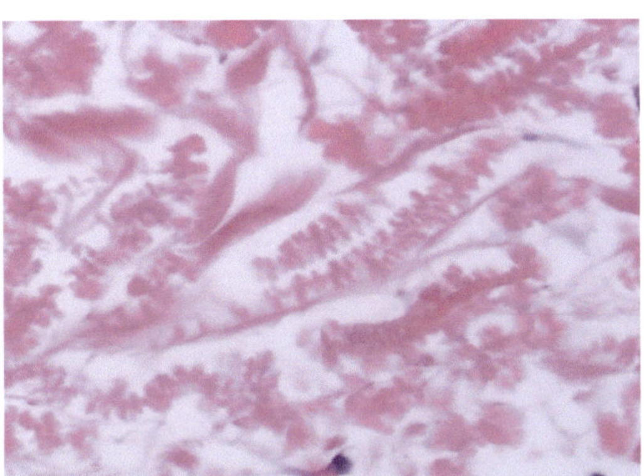

Fig. 16.64 Serrated elastic fibers are pathognomonic

Perforating Collagenosis

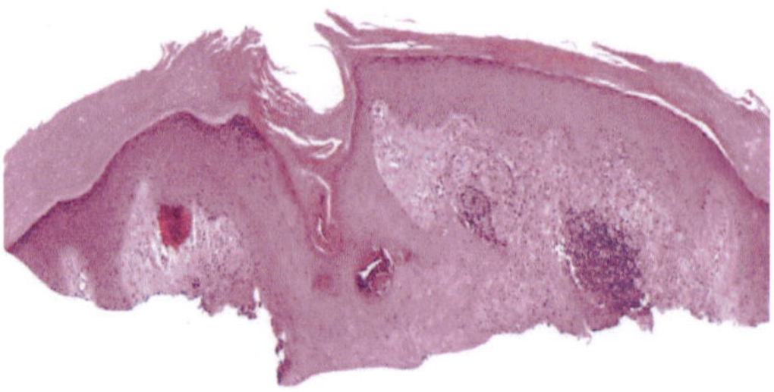

Fig. 16.65 Dome shaped lesion with central indentation

Synonym: Reactive Perforating Collagenosis

Histopathology (Figs. 16.65, 16.66, 16.67, 16.68, and 16.69)

- Umbilicated dome shaped lesion with epidermal hyperplasia and central plugging
- The plug has a basophilic appearance and is composed of degenerated collagen and acute inflammatory cells
- Elastic fibers are absent in the plug
- Dermal lymphohistiocytic infiltrate is present

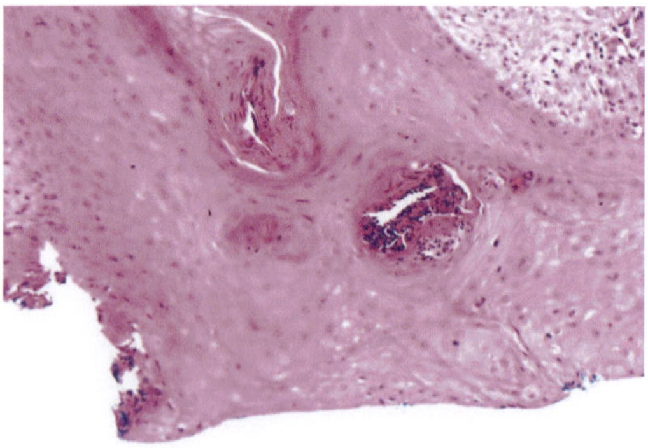

Fig. 16.66 The central basophilic plug is present

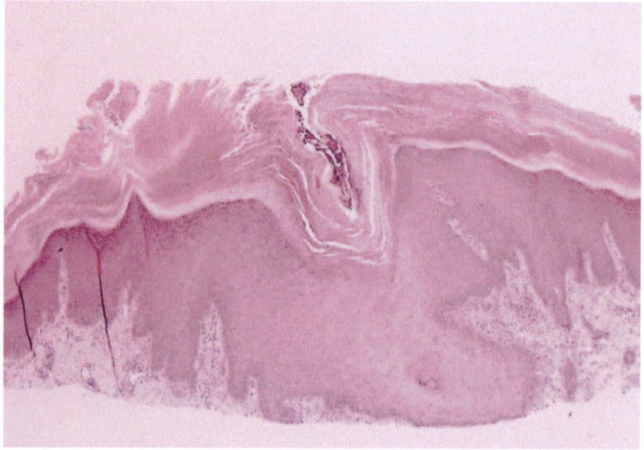

Fig. 16.67 The late stage lesion in which degenerated collagen is almost extruded

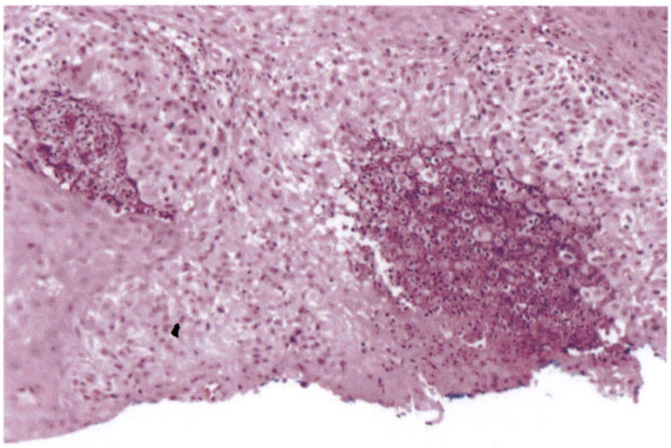

Fig. 16.68 The plug consists of degenerated collagen and inflammatory cells

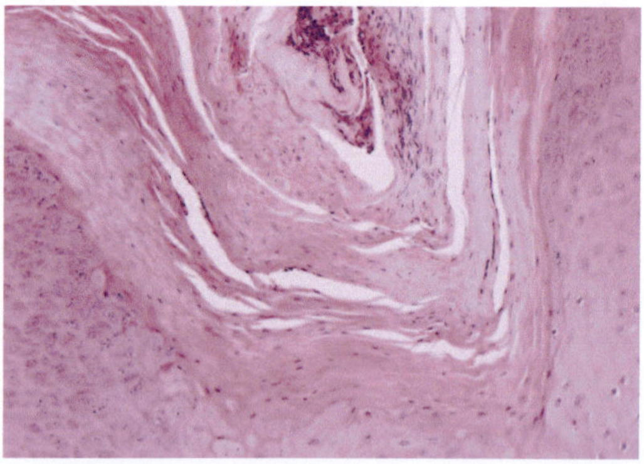

Fig. 16.69 The plug is present in the superficial portion of the stratum corneum

Perforating Dermatosis

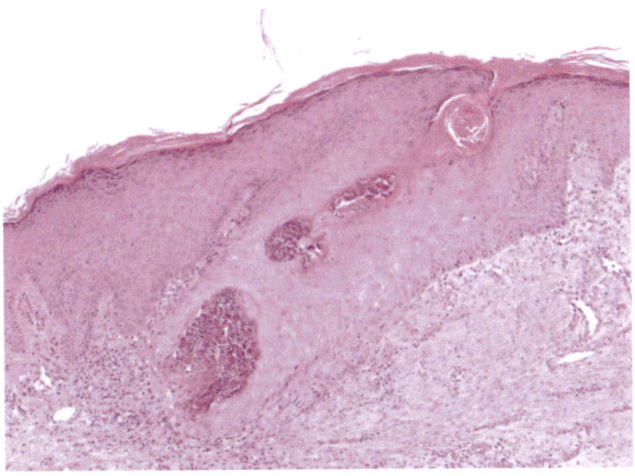

Fig. 16.70 **EPS**—Hyperplastic epidermis with central channel filled with keratin at the top

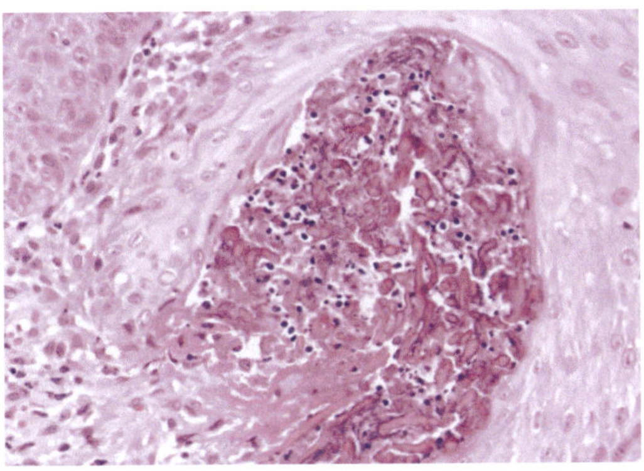

Fig. 16.71 Lower portion of channel has a plug made of degenerated elastic fibers and inflammatory debris

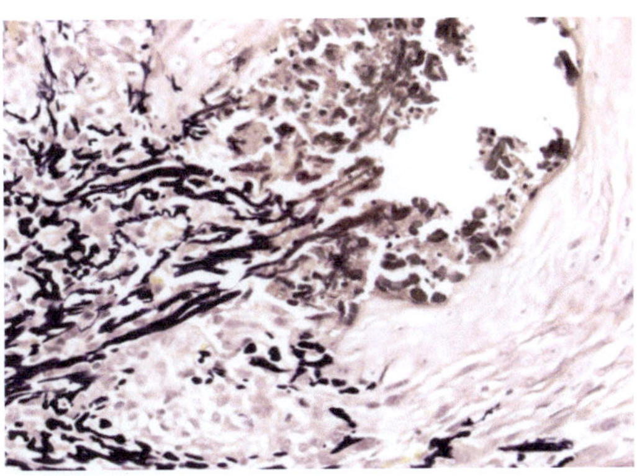

Fig. 16.72 VVG stain outlines elastic fibers

Four types of perforating dermatosis:

Elastosis perforans serpiginosa (EPS) (Figs. 16.70, 16.71, and 16.72)

- Epidermal hyperplasia with the channel through which elastic fibers are eliminated
- Superficial part of the channel is filled with keratin
- The lower portion of the channel is filled with elastic fibers and degenerated inflammatory cells

Hyperkeratosis follicularis et parafollicularis in cutem penetrans (Kyrle's disease) (Figs.16.73 and 16.74)

- Wide plug filled with laminated keratin
- There is parakeratosis in the deep part of the plug
- Lymphohistiocytic infiltrate is present in the dermis underneath the plug

Perforating collagenosis (PC) (Figs.16.75 and 16.76)

- Umbilicated dome shaped lesion with epidermal hyperplasia and central plugging
- The plug has basophilic appearance and is composed of degenerated collagen and acute inflammatory cells
- Elastic fibers are absent in the plug
- Lymphohistiocytic infiltrate is present in the dermis

Perforating folliculitis (PF) (Figs. 16.77 and 16.78)

- Dilated hair follicle
- Follicle is filled with thick keratin and degenerated, necrotic neutrophils
- Adjacent epidermis is acanthotic and hyperkeratotic
- Mild dermal lymphohistiocytic inflammation

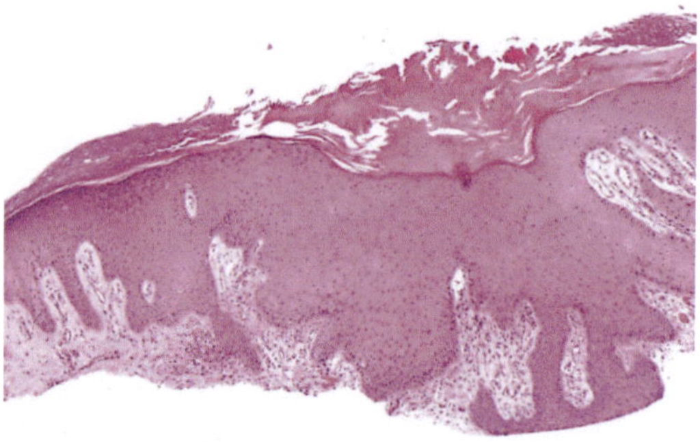

Fig. 16.73 **KD**: Wide intraepidermal invagination

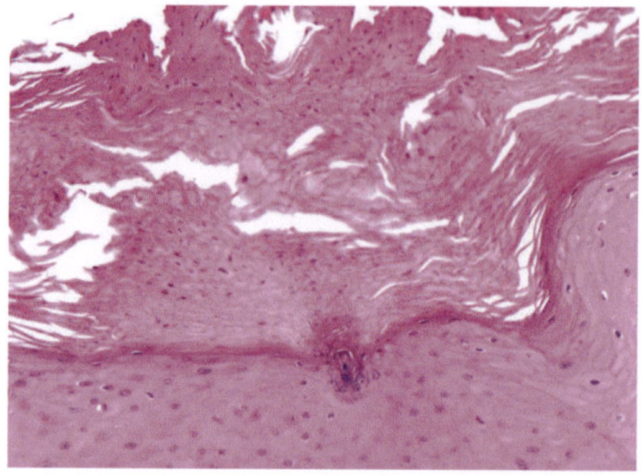

Fig. 16.74 Parakeratosis is present in the keratin plug

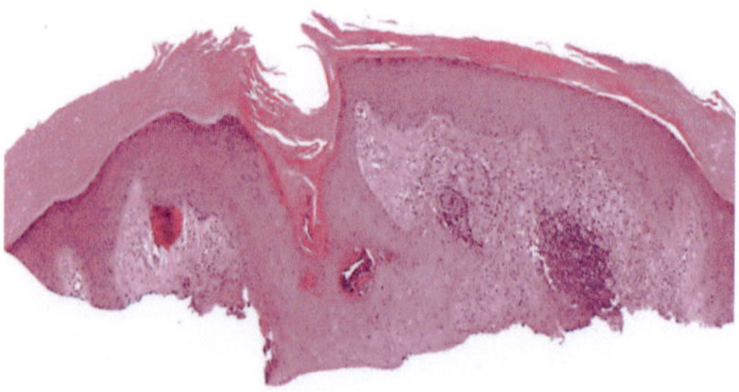

Fig. 16.75 **PF**: Dilated distorted hair follicle

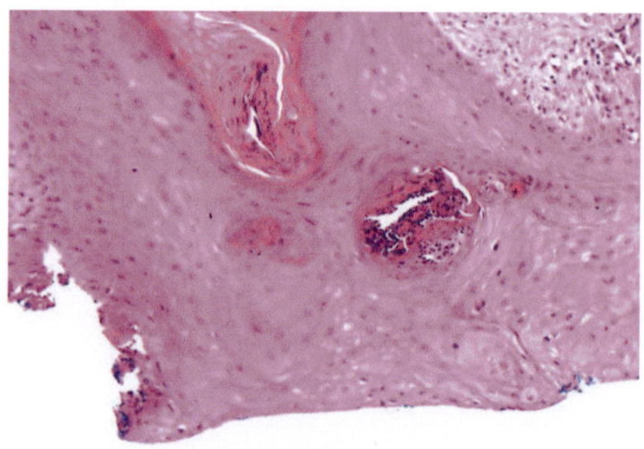

Fig. 16.76 Hair follicle is filled with orthokeratotic keratin and debris of inflammatory cells

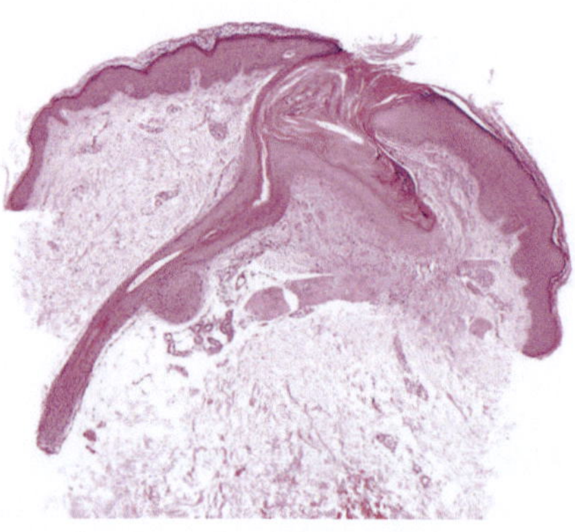

Fig. 16.77 **PC**: Dome shaped lesion with central invagination

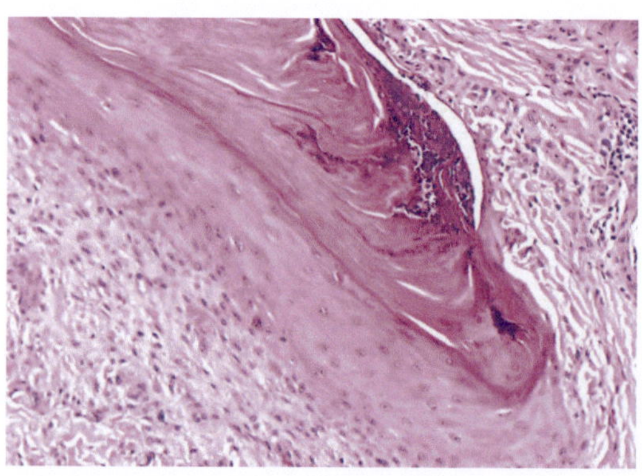

Fig. 16.78 Basophilic central plug made of degenerated collagen and inflammatory cells

Perforating Folliculitis

Histopathology (Figs. 16.79, 16.80, and 16.81)

- Dilated hair follicle
- Follicle is filled with thick keratin and degenerated, necrotic neutrophils
- Adjacent epidermis is acanthotic and hyperkeratotic
- Mild dermal lymphohistiocytic inflammation is present

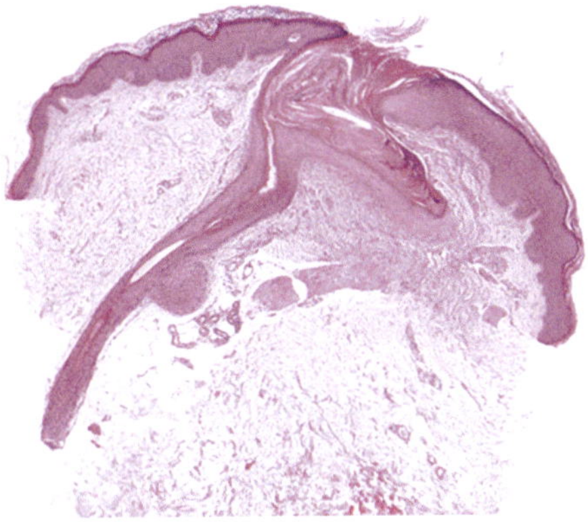

Fig. 16.79 Distorted, dilated hair follicle

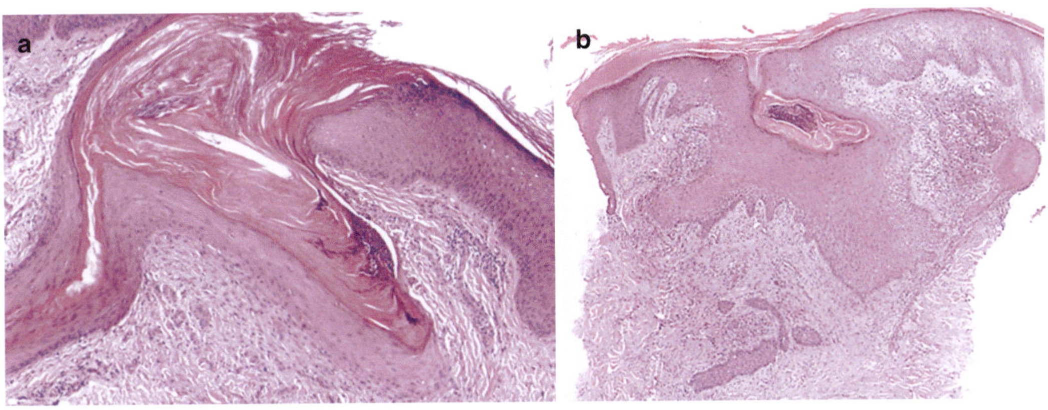

Fig. 16.80 (**a**, **b**) Dilated, plugged hair follicle with pseudoepitheliomatous hyperplasia of the adjacent epidermis

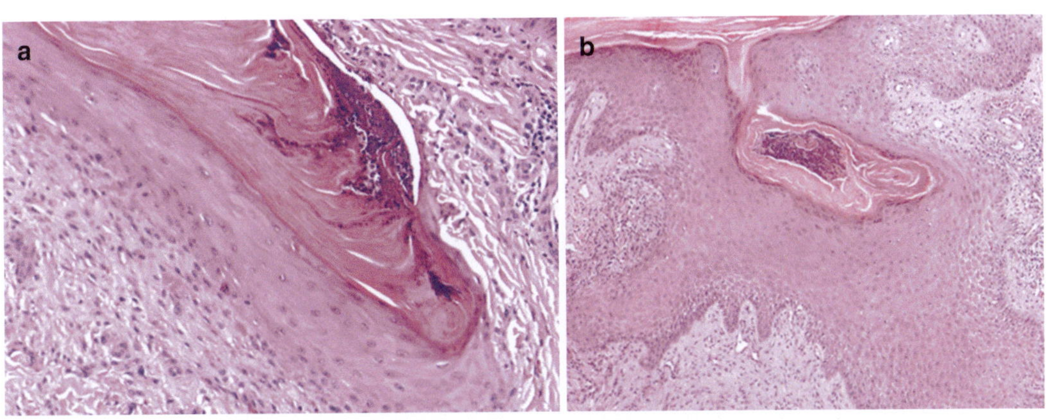

Fig. 16.81 (**a**, **b**) Follicle is filled with orthokeratotic keratin and basophilic debris of neutrophils

Perifollicular Fibroma

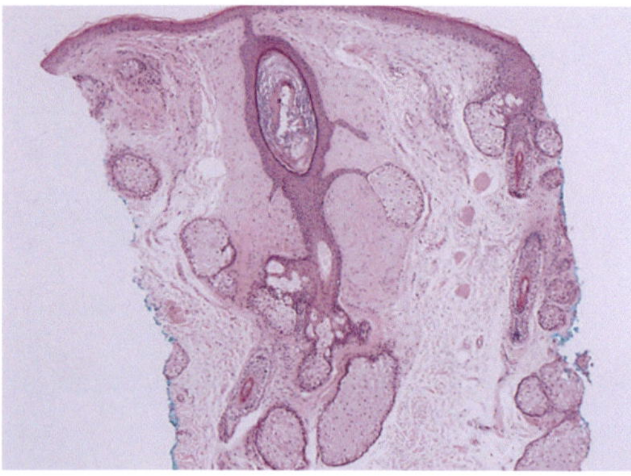

Fig. 16.82 Distorted follicle surrounded by fibrosis

Histopathology (Figs. 16.82, 16.83, and 16.84)
- Concentric cellular fibrosis encircling central follicle
- Follicle appears distorted or mildly dilated

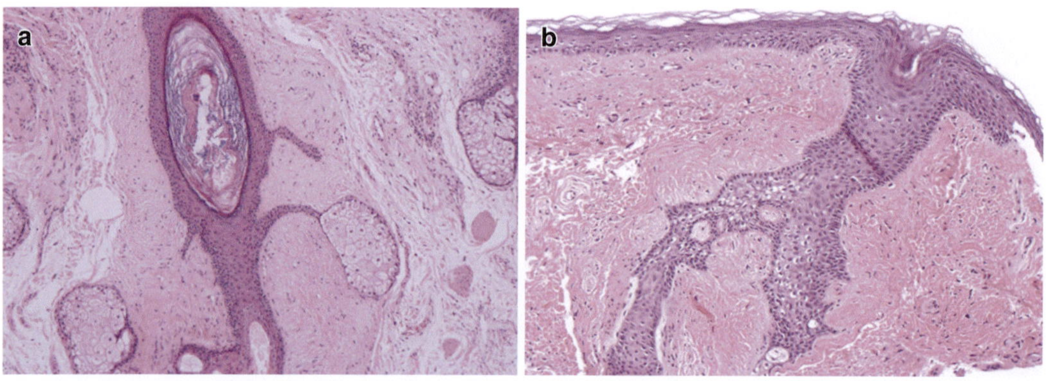

Fig. 16.83 (**a**, **b**) Central follicle with concentric perifollicular fibrosis

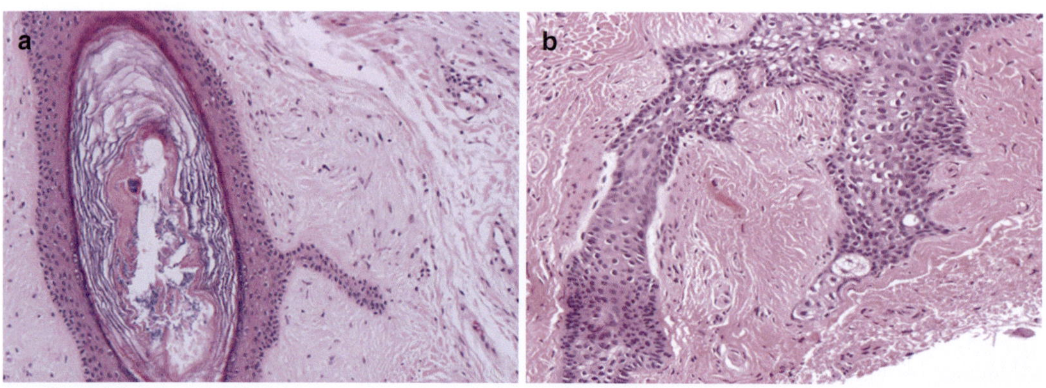

Fig. 16.84 (**a**, **b**) Perifollicular fibrous tissue is dense and cellular

Perineurioma

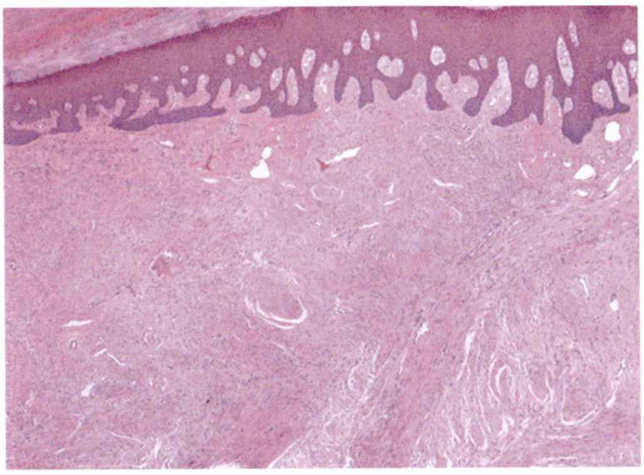

Fig. 16.85 Dermal and subcutaneous nodule

Histopathology (Figs. 16.85, 16.86, and 16.87)
- Dermal or subcutaneous non encapsulated nodule
- Tumor made of fascicles of elongated spindle cells
- Fascicles are interwoven forming storiform pattern and whorls
- Some cases show hyalinized stroma (*sclerosing perineurioma*)
- Tumor cells are EMA and Glut-1 positive and negative for neural markers

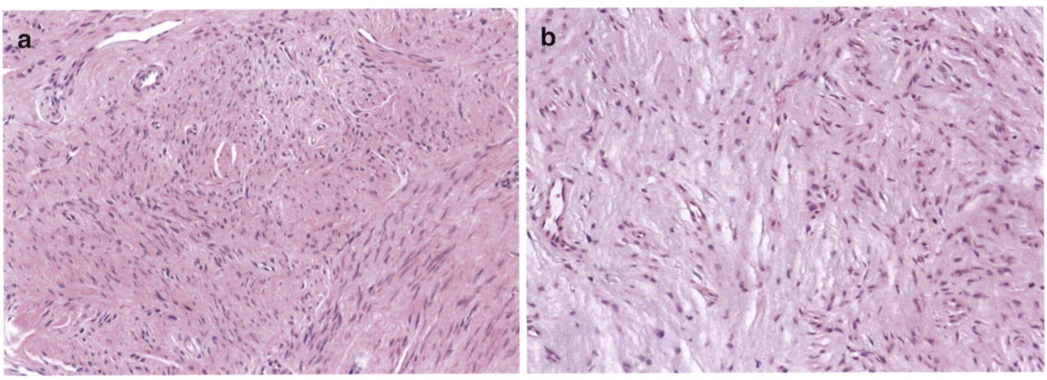

Fig. 16.86 (**a**, **b**) Interweaving fascicles and whorls

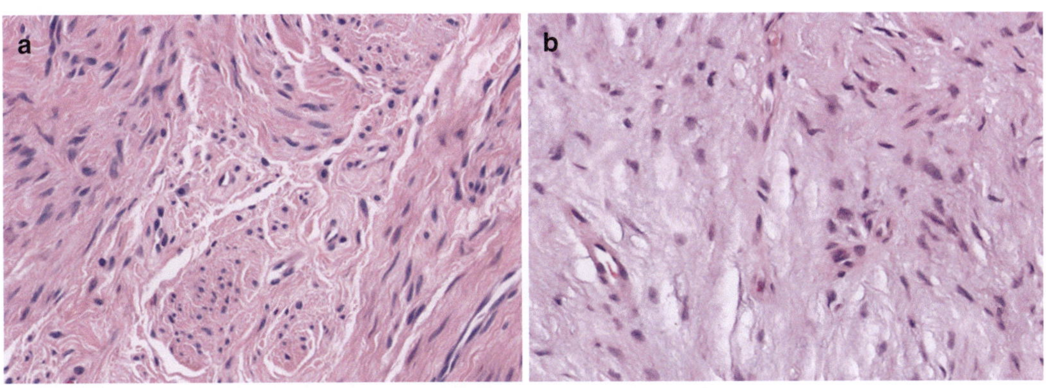

Fig. 16.87 (**a**, **b**) Fascicles are made of uniform short spindle cells with no atypia

Perioral Dermatitis

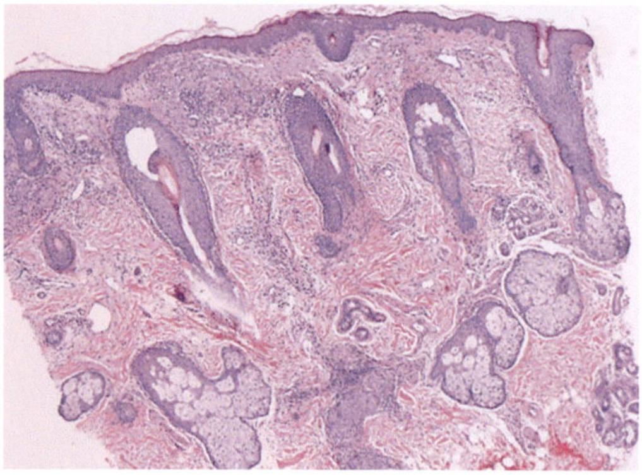

Fig. 16.88 Facial skin with vague perifollicular inflammation

Histopathology is similar to rosacea (Figs. 16.88, 16.89, 16.90, and 16.91)

- Perivascular and periadnexal lympho-histiocytic infiltrate
- Vague granulomas are present
- Giant cells can be observed
- Dermal telangiectasias are seen

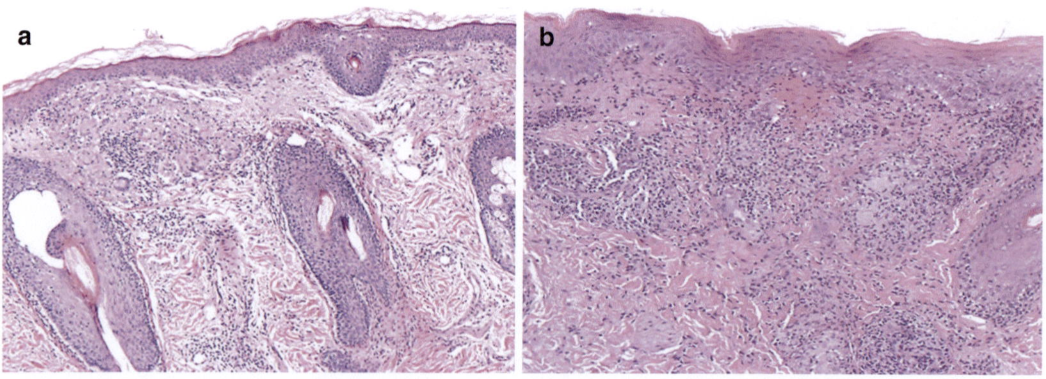

Fig. 16.89 (**a**, **b**) Perivascular and perifollicular lymphohistiocytic inflammation with vague granulomas

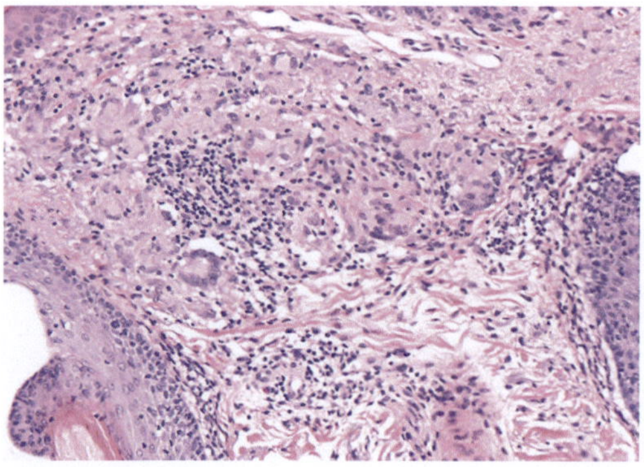

Fig. 16.90 Giant cells scattered among lymphocytes and histiocytes

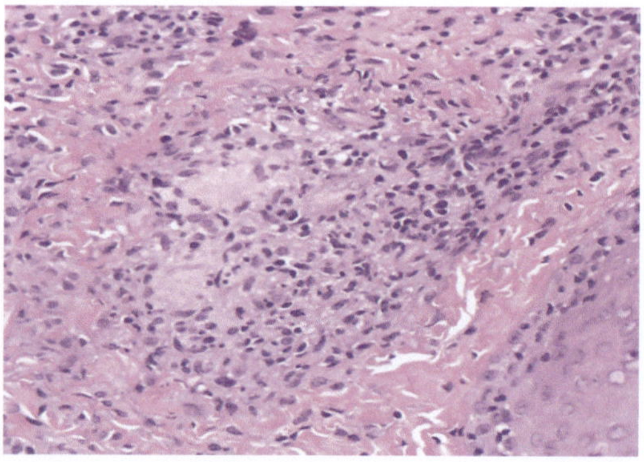

Fig. 16.91 Perifollicular granuloma

Perniosis

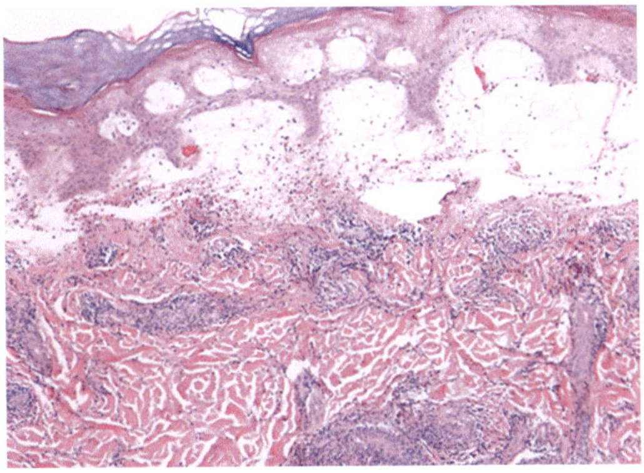

Fig. 16.92 Papillary dermal edema

Synonym: Chilblains

Histopathology (Figs. 16.92, 16.93, 16.94, and 16.95)

- Papillary dermal edema
- Superficial and deep perivascular lymphocytic infiltrate
- Dermal red blood cell extravasation
- Reactive endothelial cells ("fluffy edema")

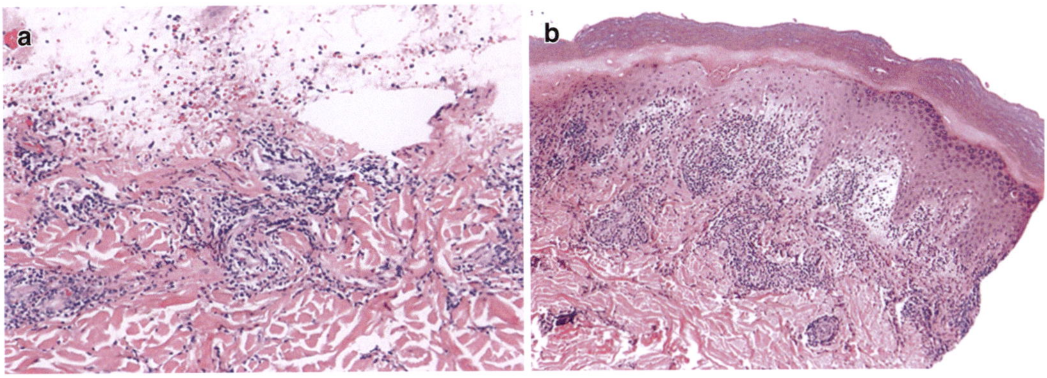

Fig. 16.93 (a, b) Superficial and deep perivascular lymphocytic infiltrate

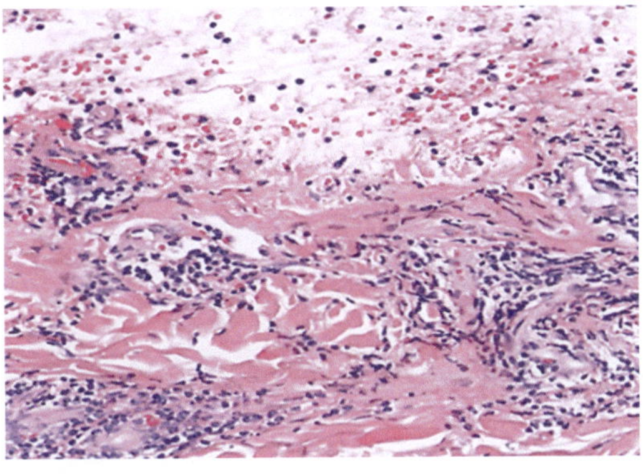

Fig. 16.94 Reactive endothelial cells and RBCs extravasation

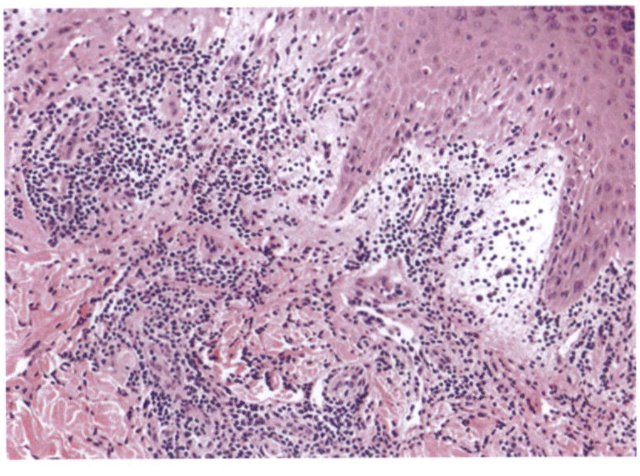

Fig. 16.95 Dermal edema and numerous dermal lymphocytes

Phaeohyphomycosis

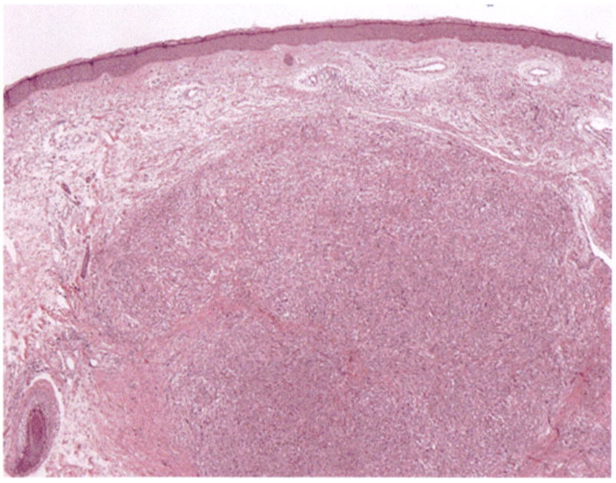

Fig. 16.96 Subcutaneous nodule

Histopathology (Figs. 16.96, 16.97, 16.98, 16.99, and 16.100)

- Normal epidermis with dermal/subcutaneous nodule(s)
- Nodule(s) consist of lymphocytes and histiocytes and in some cases extensive neutrophilic aggregates with necrosis
- Pigmented septate yeast hyphae in chains

P.S. in contrast, chromoblastomycosis has epidermal pseudoepitheliomatous hyperplasia with Medlar's bodies but no hyphae or yeast in the chains

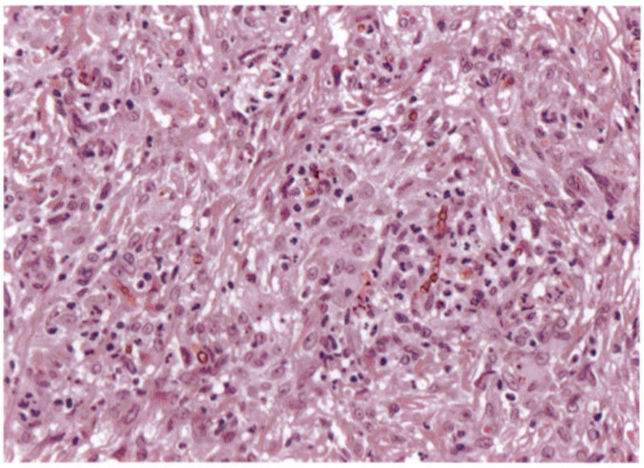

Fig. 16.97 Lymphohistiocytic inflammation with scattered neutrophils and no necrosis

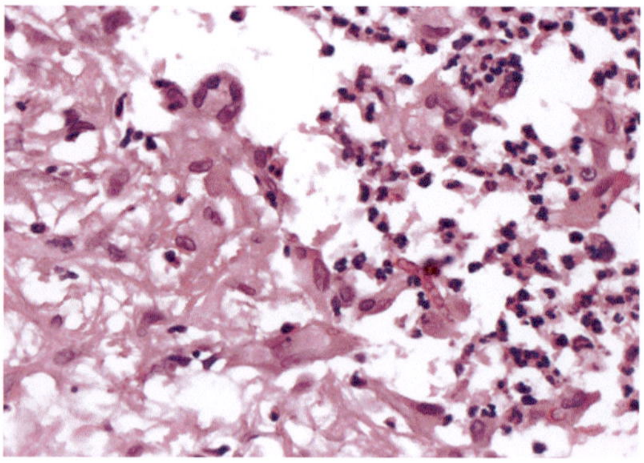

Fig. 16.98 Case with extensive neutrophilic inflammation and necrosis

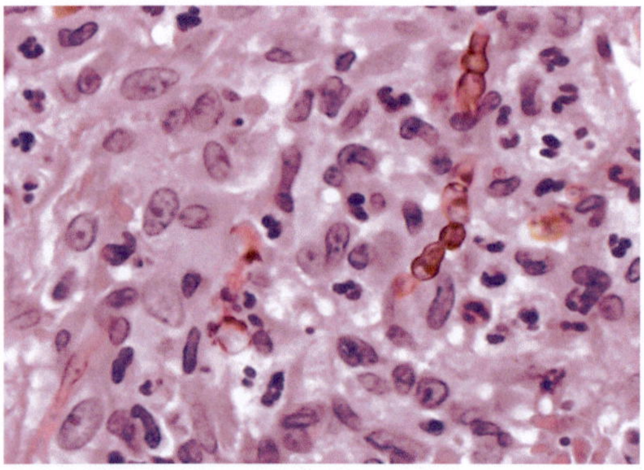

Fig. 16.99 Pigmented yeasts forming chains

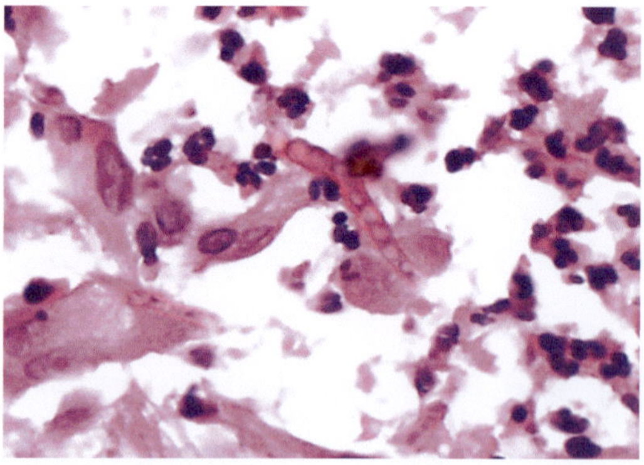

Fig. 16.100 Pigmented septate hyphae

Photoallergic Dermatitis

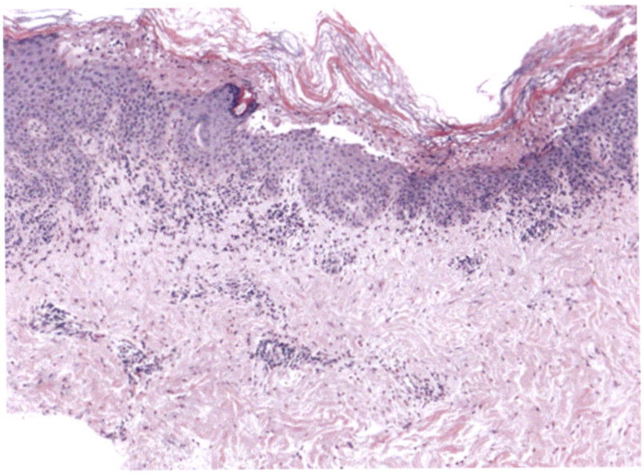

Fig. 16.101 Spongiotic dermatitis

Histopathology is akin to allergic contact dermatitis but with necrotic keratinocytes ("sunburn" cells) in the superficial epidermis (Figs. 16.101, 16.102, and 16.103)

- Variable epidermal spongiosis
- Variable number of necrotic keratinocytes with preference for the upper portion of the epidermis
- Variable number of epidermal eosinophils
- Dermal perivascular lymphocytic infiltrate with eosinophils

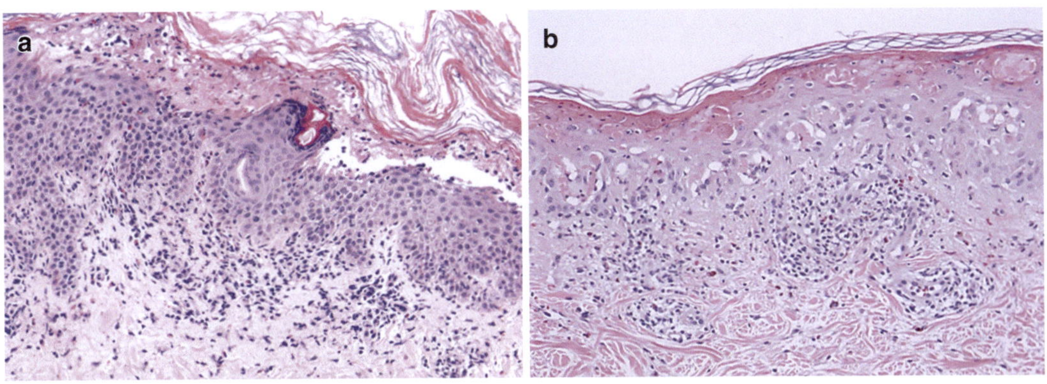

Fig. 16.102 (**a**, **b**) Necrosis of keratinocytes in the upper portion of the epidermis

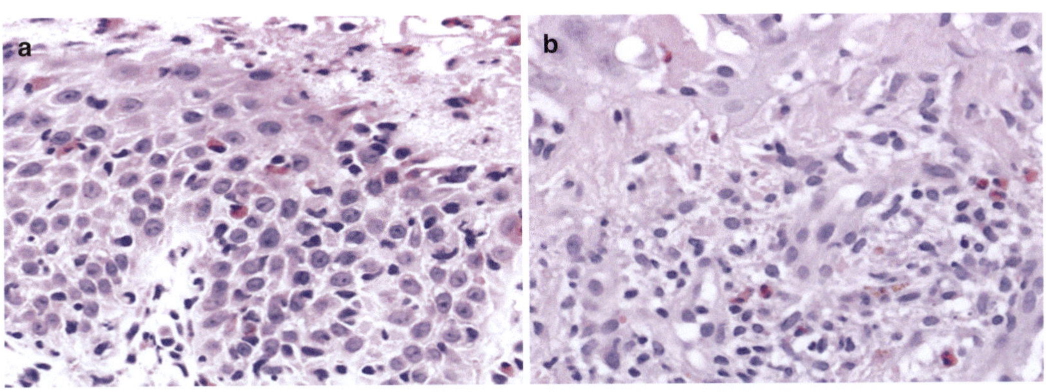

Fig. 16.103 (**a**, **b**) Epidermal spongiosis and scattered epidermal eosinophils; dermal perivascular lymphocytic infiltrate with eosinophils

Phototoxic Dermatitis

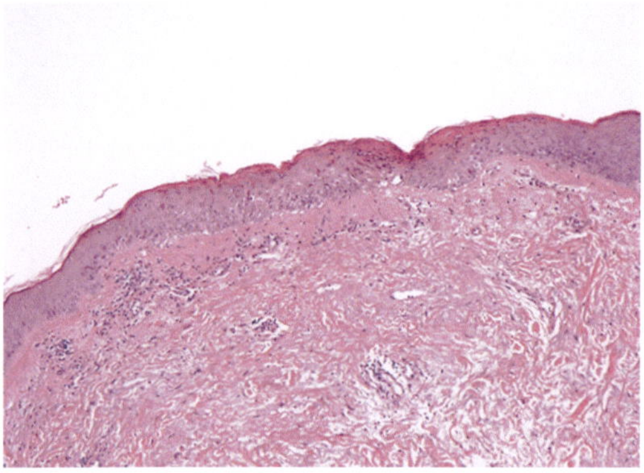

Fig. 16.104 Spongiotic dermatitis

Histopathology is akin to irritant contact dermatitis but with necrotic keratinocytes ("sunburn" cells) in the superficial epidermis (Figs. 16.104, 16.105, and 16.106)

- Variable epidermal spongiosis
- Variable number of necrotic keratinocytes with preference for the upper portion of the epidermis
- Variable number of epidermal neutrophils
- Dermal perivascular lymphocytic infiltrate with neutrophils

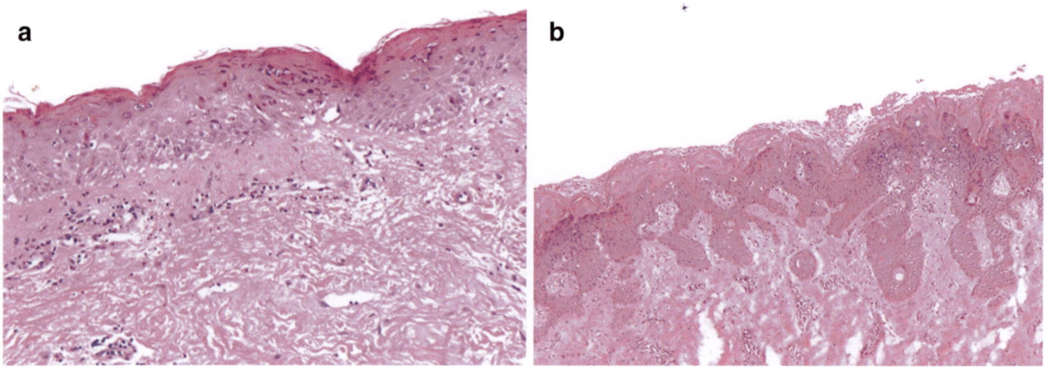

Fig. 16.105 (**a**, **b**) Necrosis of superficial epidermis with dermal perivascular lymphocytic infiltrate with neutrophils

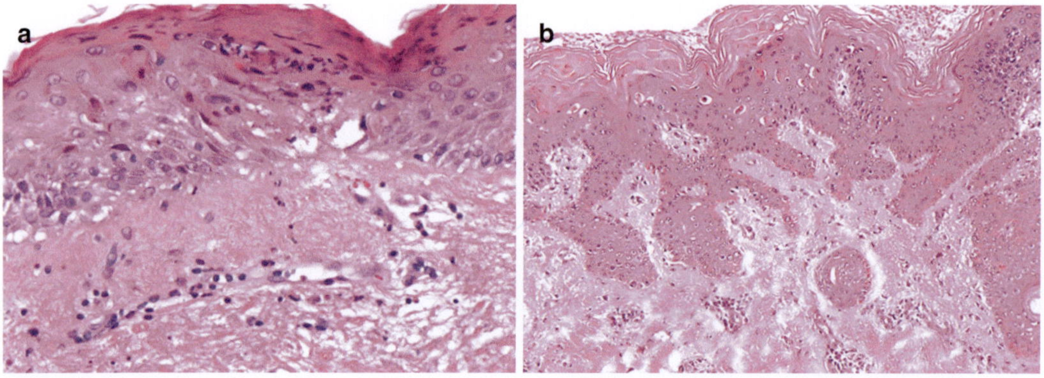

Fig. 16.106 (**a**, **b**) Necrosis of keratinocytes in the upper portion of the epidermis with neutrophilic exocytosis

Pigmented Follicular Cyst

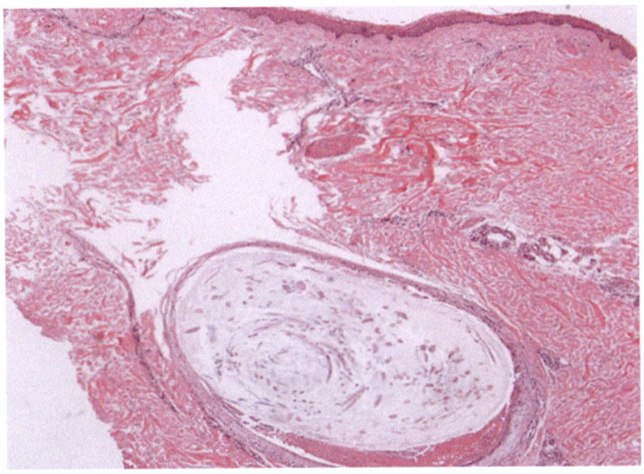

Fig. 16.107 Squamous epithelium lined cyst

Histopathology (Figs. 16.107, 16.108, and 16.109)

- Cyst lined with thin stratified squamous epithelium
- Cyst lumen filled with keratinous material
- Multiple pigmented broken hair shafts in the lumen

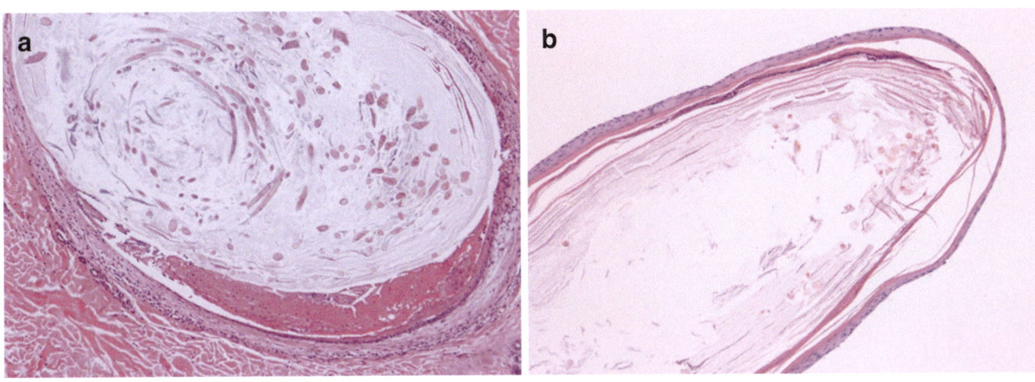

Fig. 16.108 (**a**, **b**) Cyst lined with thin keratinizing squamous epithelium

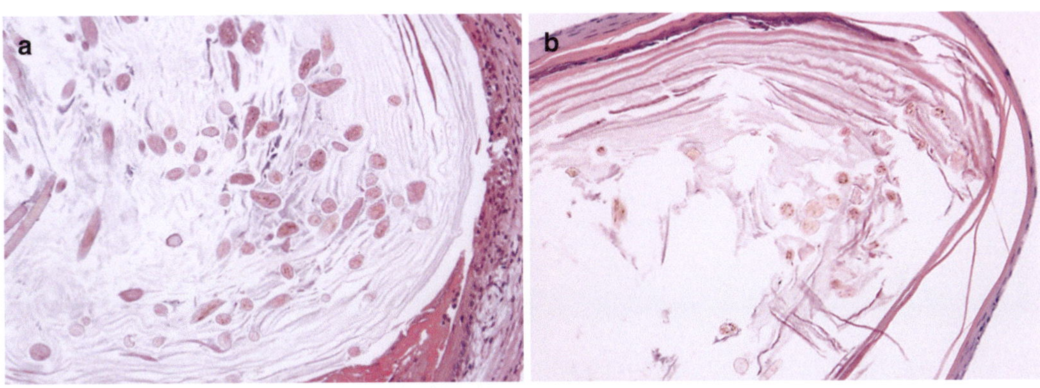

Fig. 16.109 (**a**, **b**) Cyst lumen filled with keratin and multiple fragments of broken pigmented hair shafts

Pigmented Purpuric Dermatoses

There are five **histopathological** presentations with long names (given below photos).

Schamberg's disease has prototypic histomorphology that is present in all variants (Fig. 16.110) perivascular lymphocytic infiltrate, red blood cell extravasation, and pigment incontinence in older lesions. In addition to that:

- **Purpura of Doucas and Kapetanakis** has epidermal spongiosis (Fig. 16.111)
- **Purpura of Gougerot and Blum** has lichenoid infiltrate (Fig. 16.112)
- **Purpura of Majocchi** has dermal telangiectasias (Fig. 16.113)
- **Lichen aureus** has lichenoid infiltrate as in purpura of Gougerot and Blum and clinical correlation is required to differentiate these two entities (Fig. 16.114)

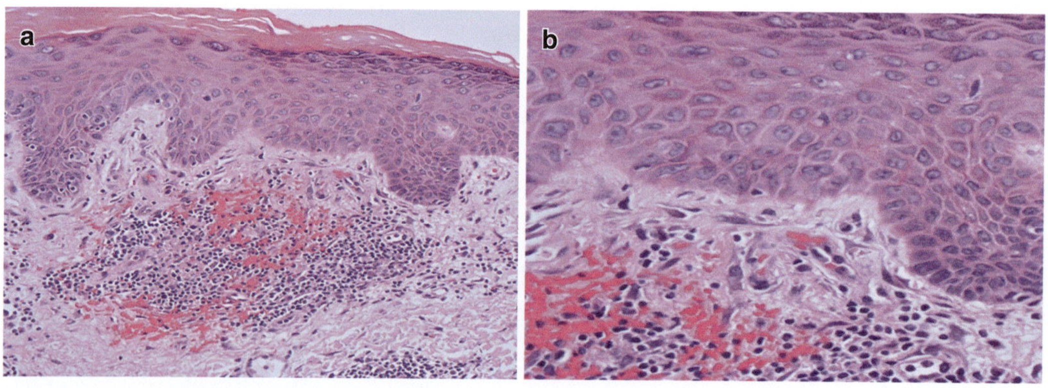

Fig. 16.110 (a, b) **Progressive pigmented dermatosis of Schamberg** with perivascular lymphocytes, red blood cell extravasation, and endothelial swelling

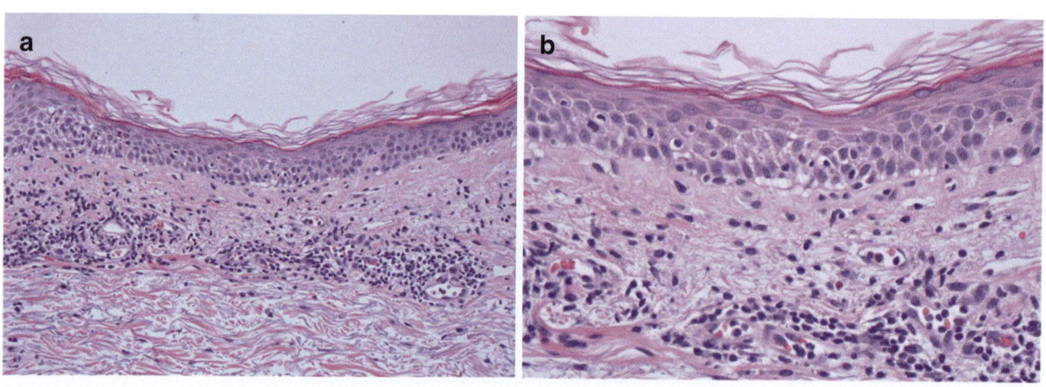

Fig. 16.111 (a, b) **Eczematoid-like purpura of Doucas and Kapetanakis** with epidermal **spongiosis**, perivascular lymphocytes, and red blood cell extravasation

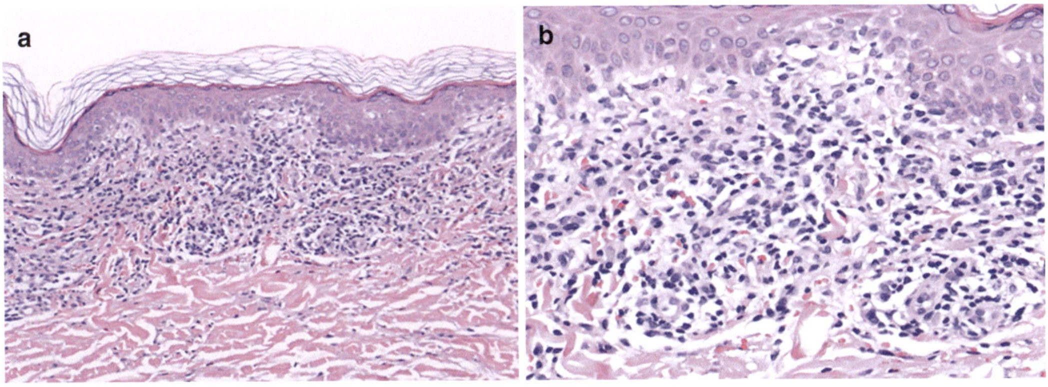

Fig. 16.112 (a, b) **Lichen aureus** with dense **lichenoid** lymphocytic infiltrate and red blood cell extravasation

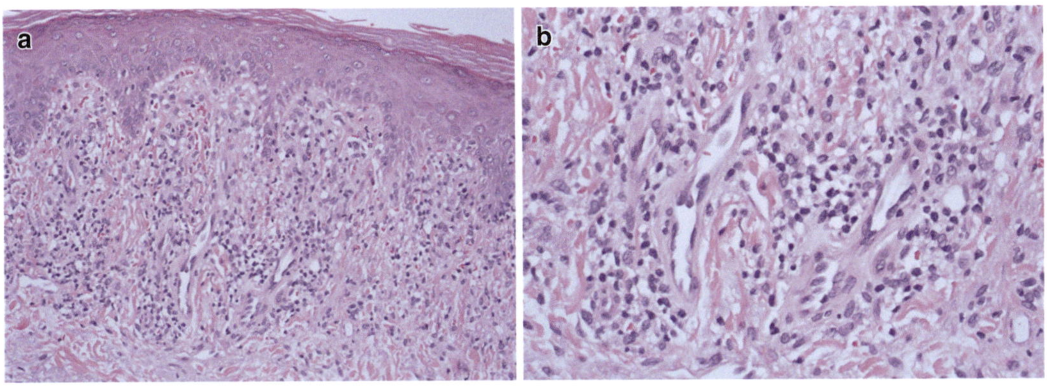

Fig. 16.113 (a, b) **Purpura annularis telangiectoides of Majocchi** with perivascular lymphocytic infiltrate and red blood cells around **dermal telangiectasias**

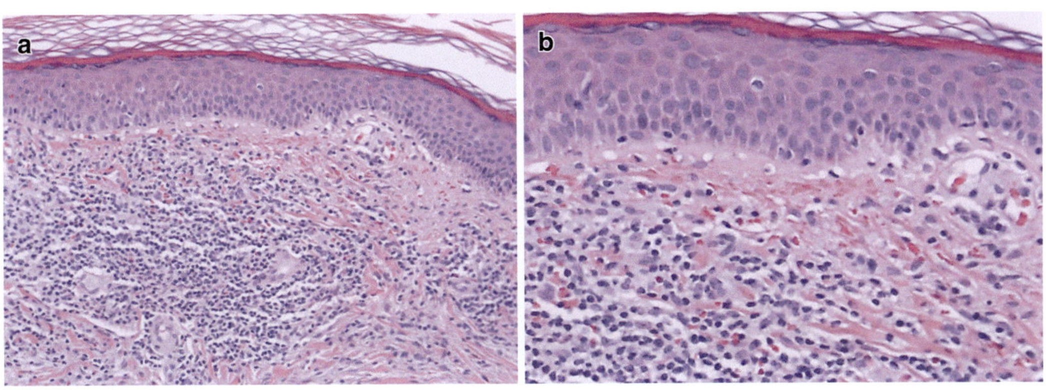

Fig. 16.114 (a, b) **Pigmented lichenoid purpuric dermatosis of Gougerot and Blum** with **lichenoid** infiltrate and dermal red blood cells

Pigmented Spindle Cell Nevus of Reed

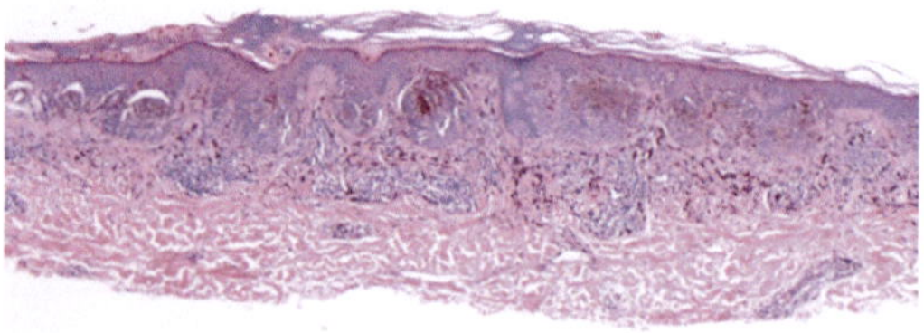

Fig. 16.115 Symmetrical pigmented melanocytic lesion

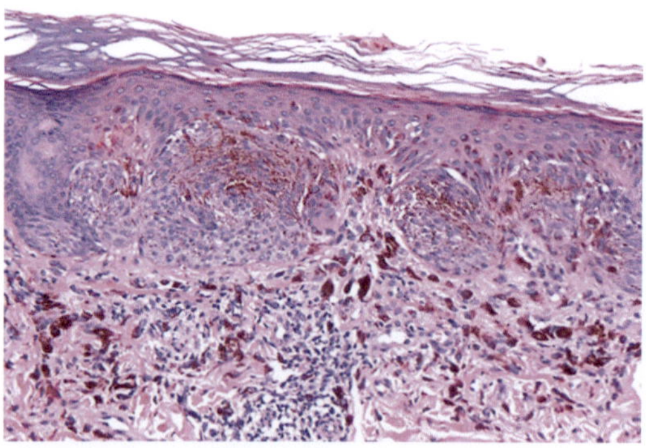

Fig. 16.116 Extensive dermal pigment incontinence

Histopathology (Figs. 16.115, 16.116, 16.117, and 16.118)

- Symmetrical, sharply demarcated melanocytic lesion that is junctional or compound but never only dermal
- Epidermis is acanthotic and hyperkeratotic
- Nests are made of spindle cells accompanied by a variable number of epithelioid cells and prominent pigmentation
- Junctional nests are "teardrop" shaped and can show clefting from the epidermis
- Camino bodies are sparse but are present
- Pagetoid melanocytic spread can be seen in the center of the lesion
- Mitoses can be seen but only in junctional component
- Dermal nests demonstrate dermal maturation and significant dermal pigment incontinence can be present

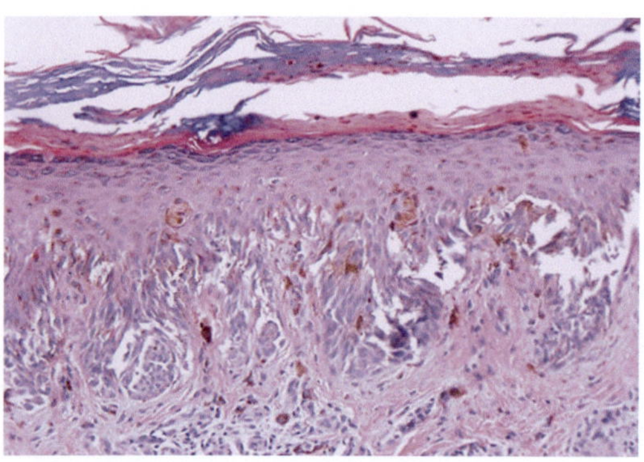

Fig. 16.117 Nests are "teardrop" shaped and consist of spindle and epithelioid cells with epidermal clefts

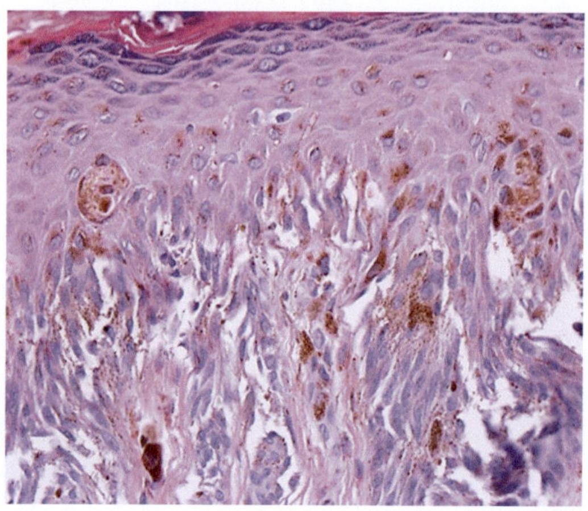

Fig. 16.118 Pagetoid melanocytic spread is common in the center of the lesion

Pilar Cyst

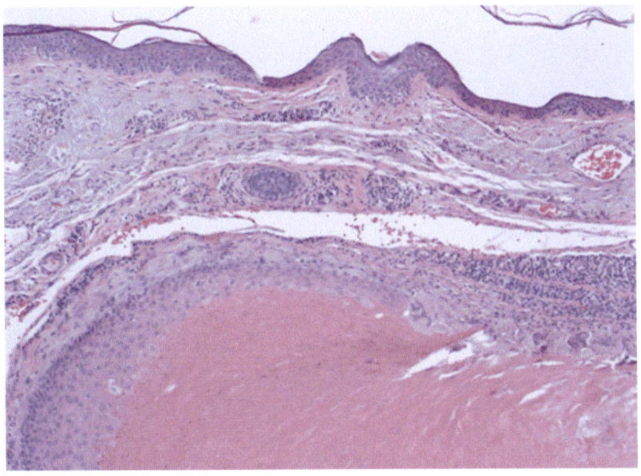

Fig. 16.119 Subcutaneous cyst

Synonym: Trichilemmal Cyst

Histopathology (Figs. 16.119, 16.120, 16.121, 16.122, and 16.123)

- Cyst lined with stratified epithelium
- Epithelium exhibit trichilemmal keratinization (no keratin granules)
- Lumen is filled with compact homogeneous keratin
- Calcifications are commonly seen

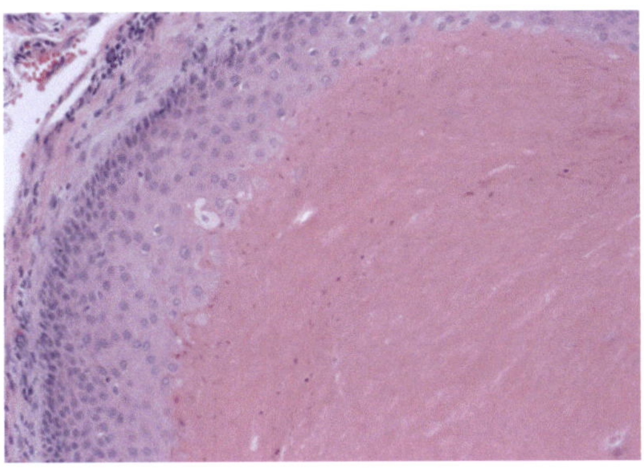

Fig. 16.120 Compact eosinophilic keratin fill the cyst lumen

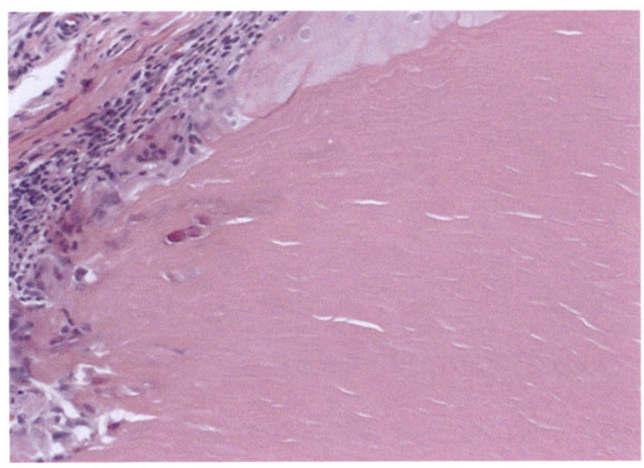

Fig. 16.121 Partially ruptured cyst

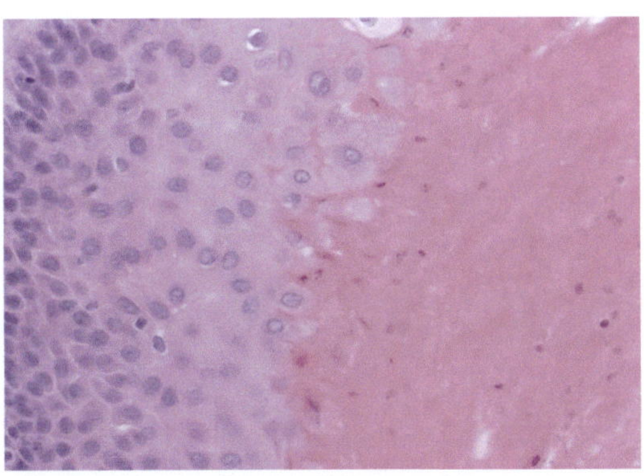

Fig. 16.122 Squamous epithelium with no granular layer

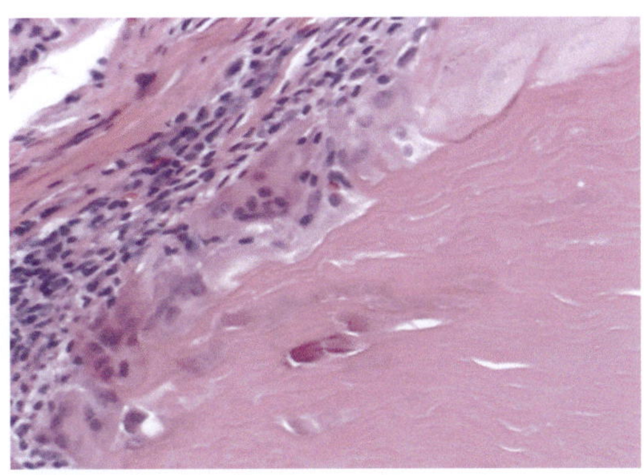

Fig. 16.123 Giant cells, lymphocytes, and focal calcification

Pilar Sheath Acanthoma

Histopathology (Figs. 16.124 and 16.125)

- Central dilated follicle filled with keratin debris
- Wall is made of acanthotic epidermis
- Wall has wide proliferating buds with pushing borders and no atypia

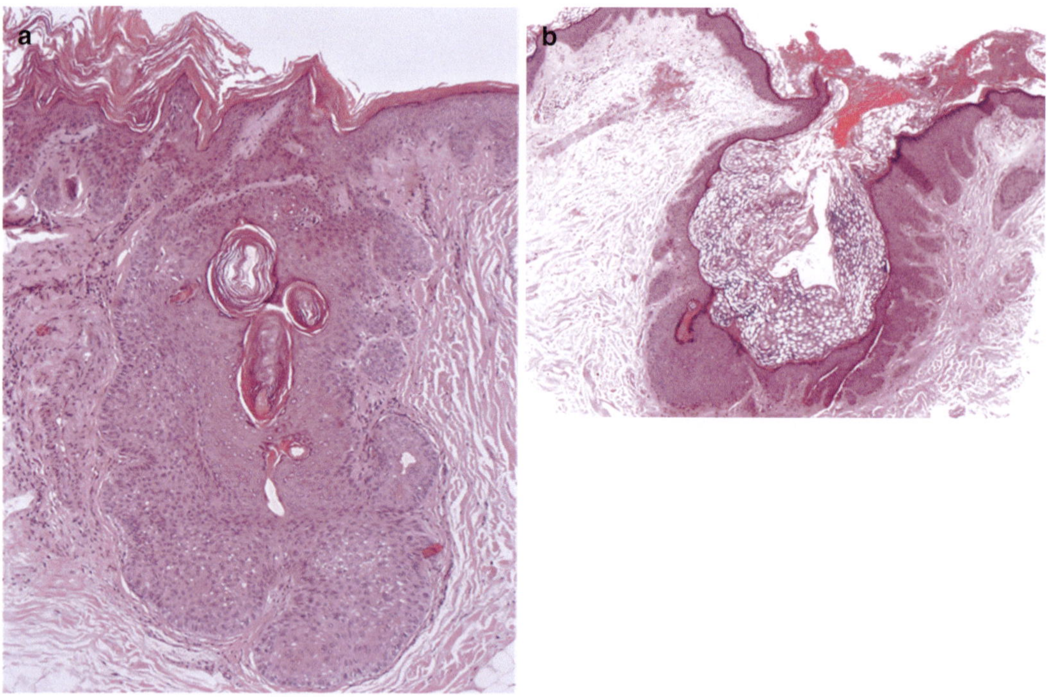

Fig. 16.124 (**a**, **b**) Dilated follicle filled with thick keratin; the wall is thickened with broad based buds

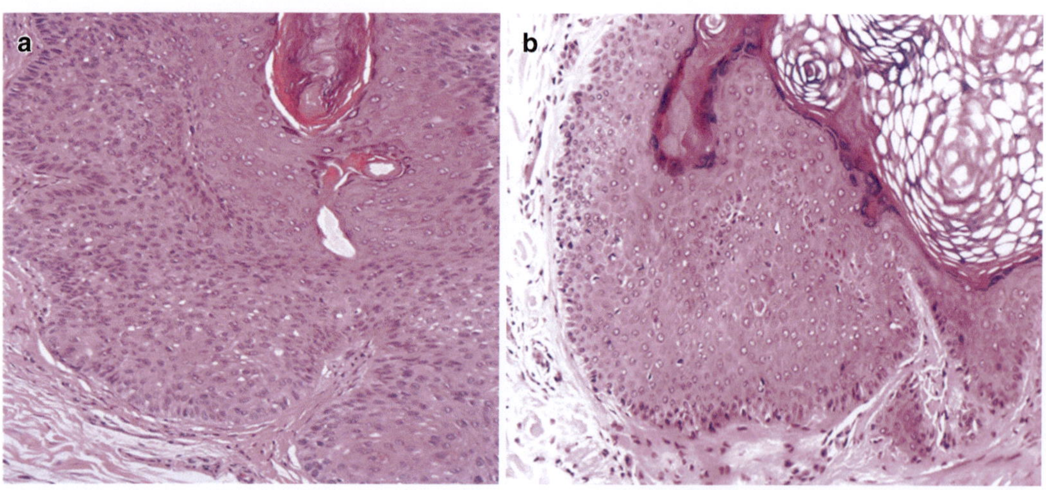

Fig. 16.125 (**a**, **b**) Proliferating buds demonstrate pushing borders with no atypia

Pilomatricoma

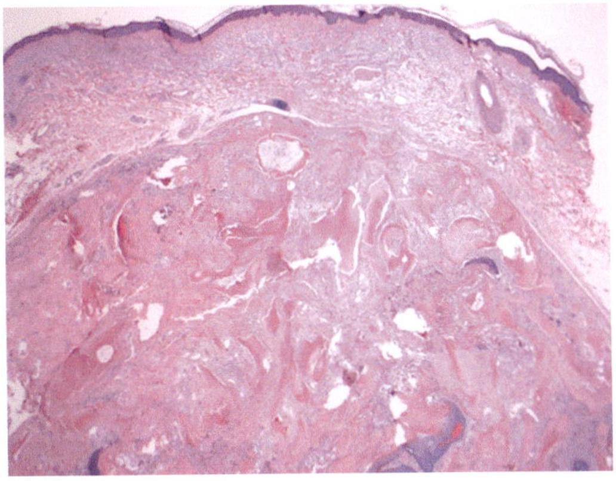

Fig. 16.126 Dermal and subcutaneous well circumscribed tumor

Synonyms: Pilomatrixoma, Calcifying Epithelioma

Histopathology (Figs. 16.126, 16.127, 16.128, and 16.129)

- Well circumscribed tumor that consists of three components in various ratio:
  - Uniform small basaloid cells with small dark nuclei
  - Eosinophilic keratin debris with "ghost" cells (nuclear shadow)
  - Keratin foreign body giant cell reaction
- Calcifications are present in over two third of cases

P.S. associated with Gardner syndrome (*APC*)

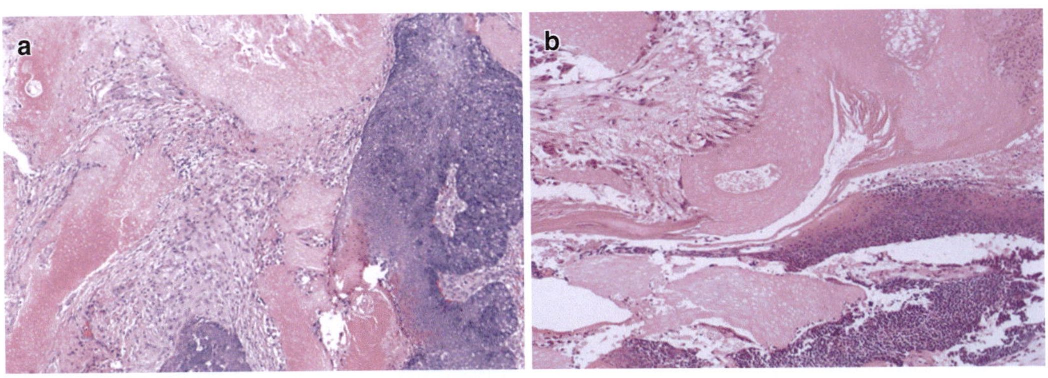

Fig. 16.127 (**a**, **b**) Three components form the tumor

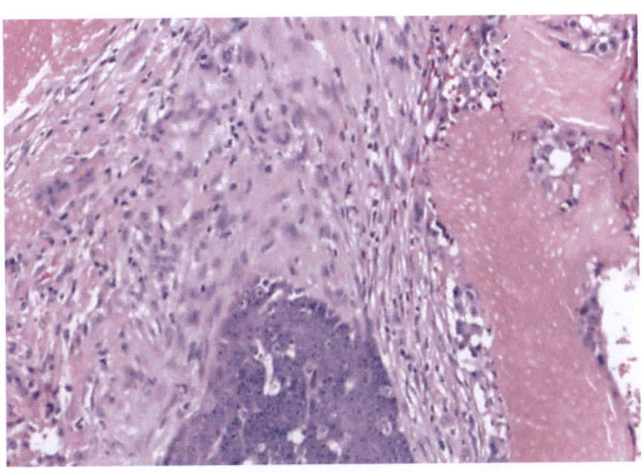

Fig. 16.128 Keratin foreign body reaction

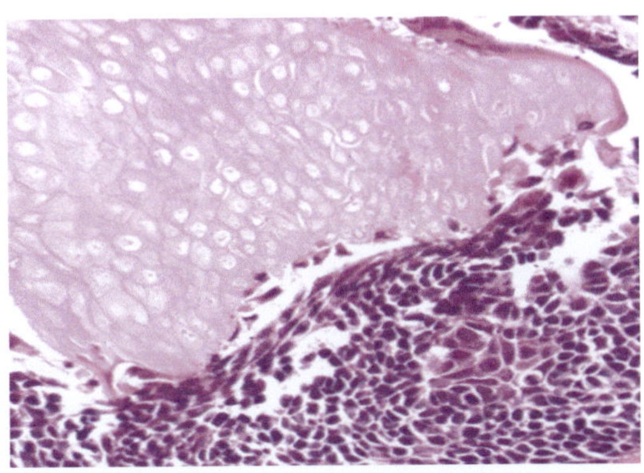

Fig. 16.129 Eosinophilic "ghost" cells and basaloid small cells

Pilomatrix Carcinoma

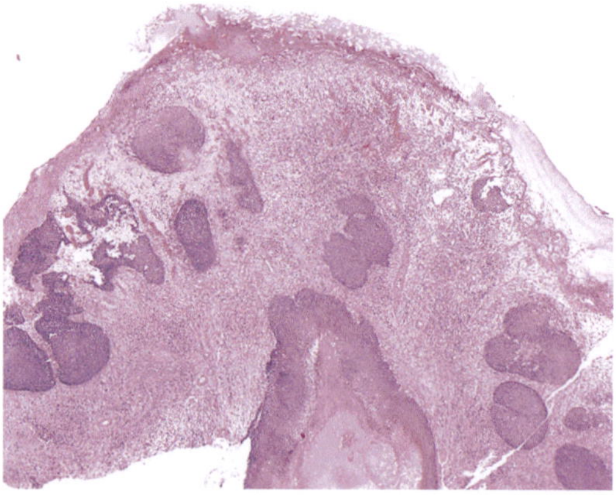

Fig. 16.130 Irregular dermal tumor with epidermal ulceration

Histopathology is similar to *pilomatricoma* but with atypia and necrosis (Figs. 16.130, 16.131, 16.132, and 16.133)

- Tumor consists of three components; basaloid cells, "ghost" cells, and inflammatory reaction
- Ulceration and necrosis are present and mitoses are easily identified
- Basaloid cells instead of small dark nuclei of basaloid cells (as seen in pilomatricoma) have irregular larger vesicular nuclei

P.S. *proliferative pilomatricoma* is histologically in between *pilomatricoma* and *pilomatrix carcinoma*

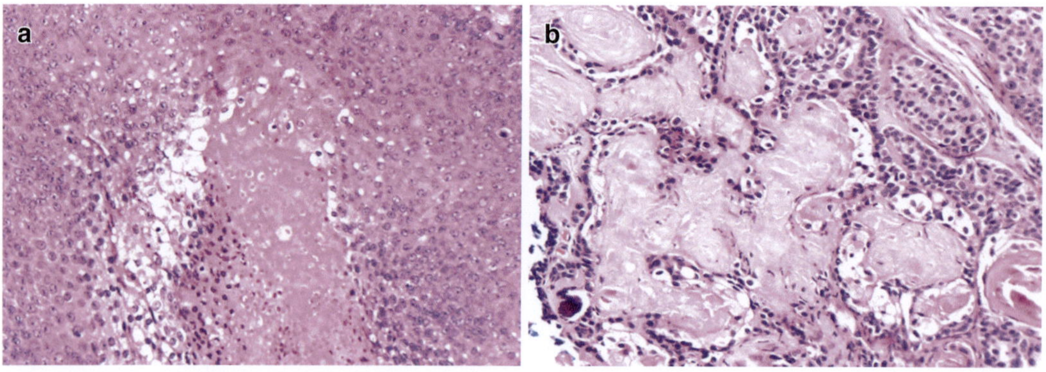

Fig. 16.131 (**a**, **b**) Basaloid cells with central "ghost" cells and surrounding inflammation

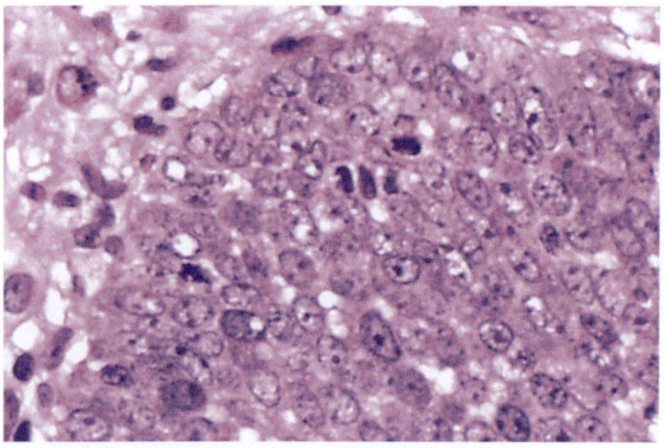

Fig. 16.132 Multiple mitoses are present

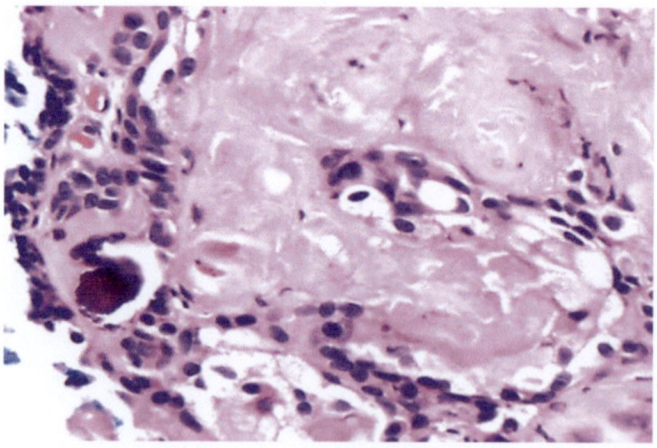

Fig. 16.133 Focal calcifications are common

Pilonidal Sinus

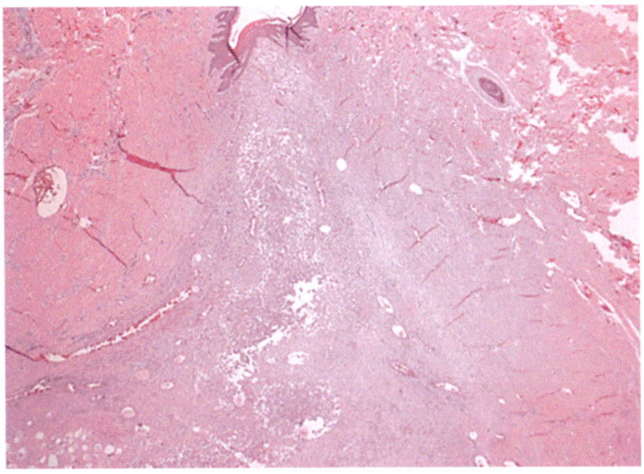

Fig. 16.134 Sinus tract at the top lined with squamous epithelium

Histopathology (Figs. 16.134, 16.135, 16.136, 16.137, and 16.138)

- Sinus tract at the top lined with squamous epithelium
- In the deeper part, the wall is made of granulation tissue
- Numerous hair shafts can be seen causing foreign body reaction
- Extensive surrounding scarring is present

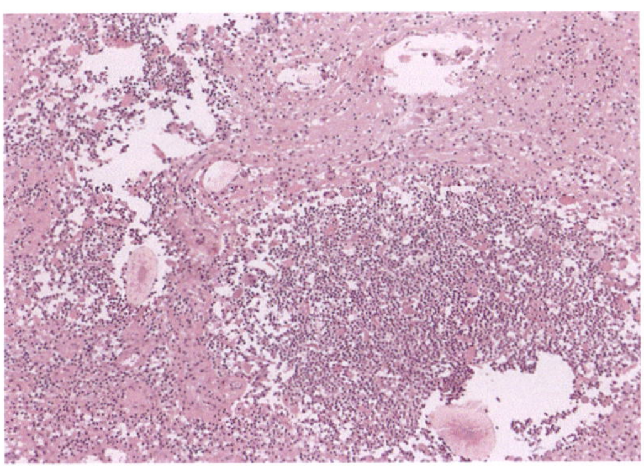

Fig. 16.135 Granulation tissue lines most of the sinus

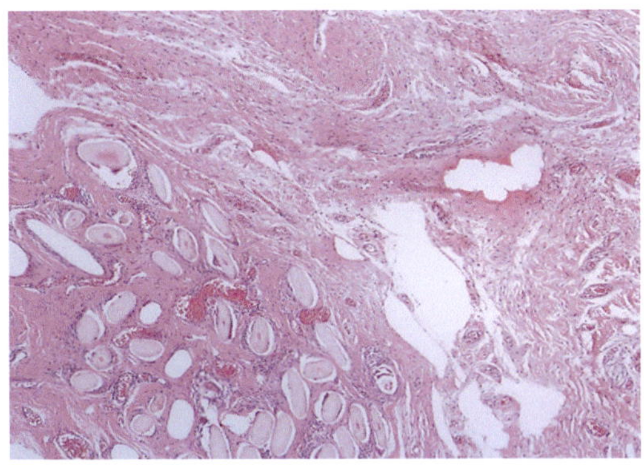

Fig. 16.136 Numerous broken hair shafts

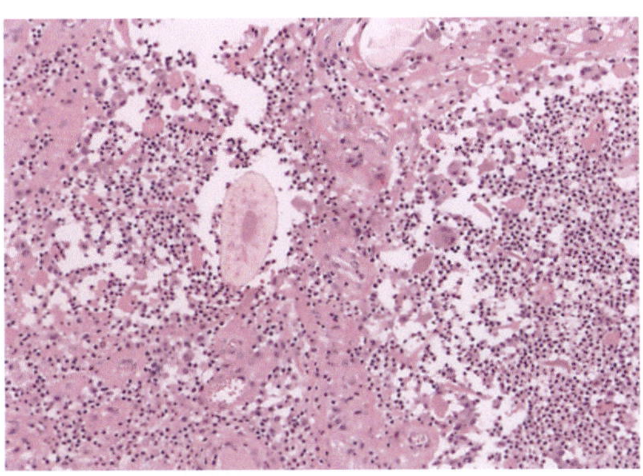

Fig. 16.137 Foreign body giant cell reaction with acute and chronic inflammation

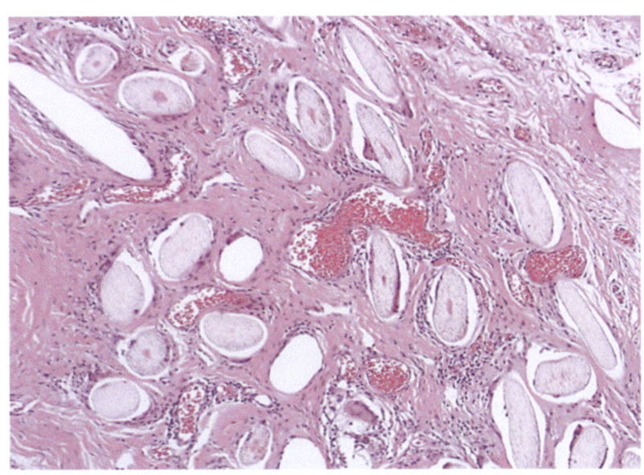

Fig. 16.138 Intensive scarring surrounds hair shafts

Pitted Keratolysis

Histopathology (Figs. 16.139, 16.140, and 16.141)

- Hyperkeratotic epidermis with formation of shallow pits filled with keratin
- Coccobacilli and/or filamentous bacteria are present in the stratum corneum
- There is no dermal inflammation

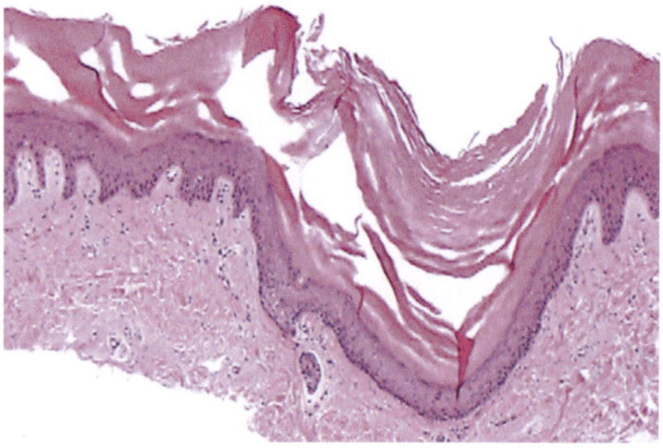

Fig. 16.139 Hyperkeratotic epidermis

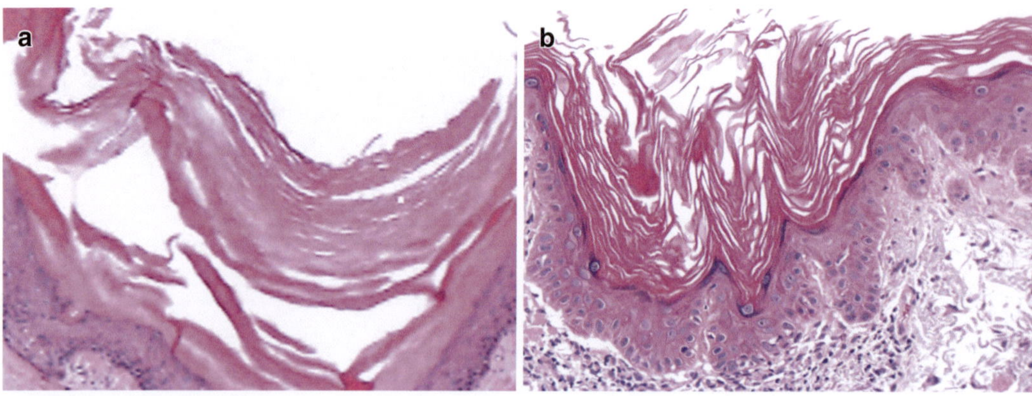

Fig. 16.140 (**a**, **b**) Shallow keratin filled pit

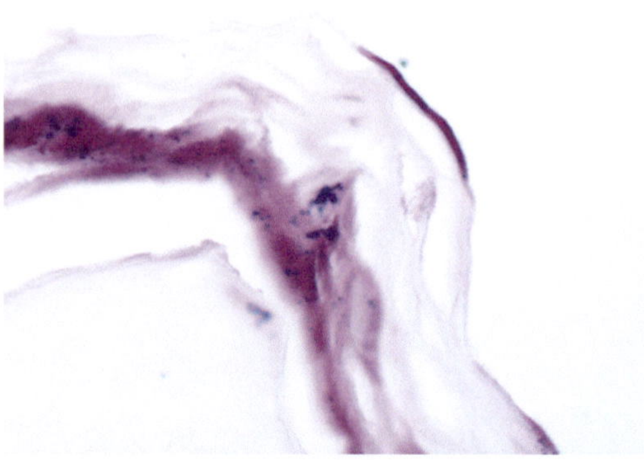

Fig. 16.141 Bacterial elements are present in the stratum corneum (Gram stain)

Pityriasis Alba

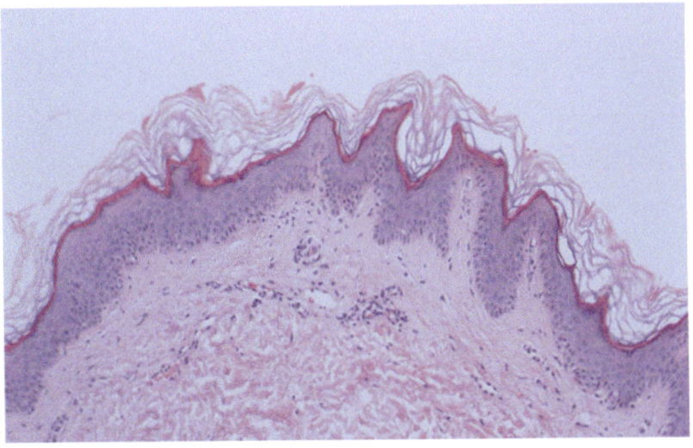

Fig. 16.142 Epidermal hyperkeratosis and acanthosis

Histopathology is nonspecific (Figs. 16.142, 16.143, and 16.144)

- Mild epidermal acanthosis, hyperkeratosis, and spongiosis
- Mild perivascular lymphocytic infiltrate
- Normal number of melanocytes with decreased melanization

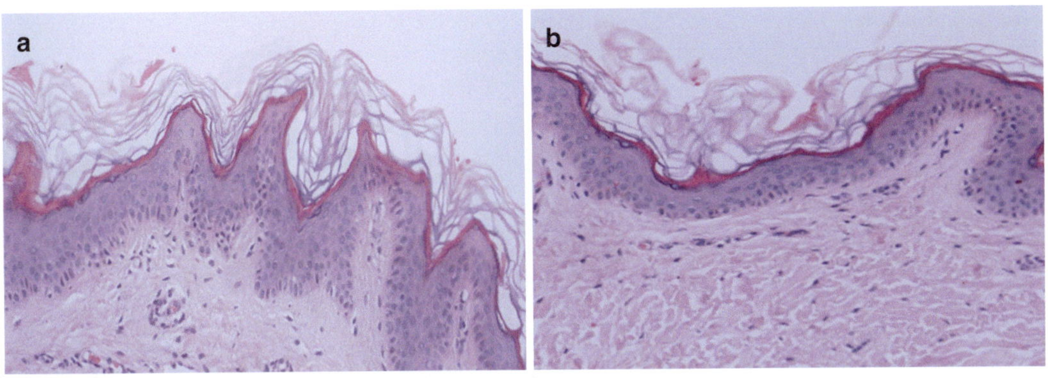

Fig. 16.143 (**a**, **b**) Mild epidermal spongiosis with mild dermal perivascular lymphocytic infiltrate

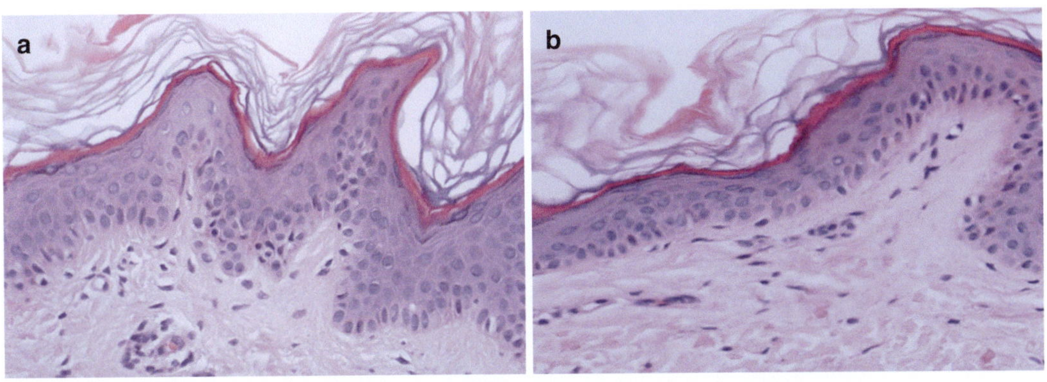

Fig. 16.144 (**a**, **b**) Epidermal melanin is decreased but number of melanocytes is normal

Pityriasis Amiantacea

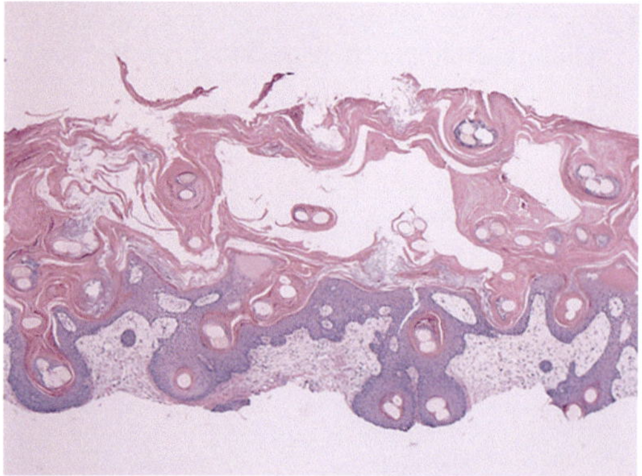

Fig. 16.145 A case of a homeless man with head lice and seborrheic dermatitis

It is a reactive process rather than a specific disease. Underlying cause can be psoriasis, seborrheic dermatosis, atopic dermatitis, tinea capitis, or head lice.

Histopathology (Figs. 16.145, 16.146, 16.147, 16.148, and 16.149)

- Extensive hyperkeratosis with epidermal acanthosis and papillomatosis
- Multiple hair shafts in stratum corneum

P.S. look for underlying disease that cause it by sampling less hyperkeratotic area

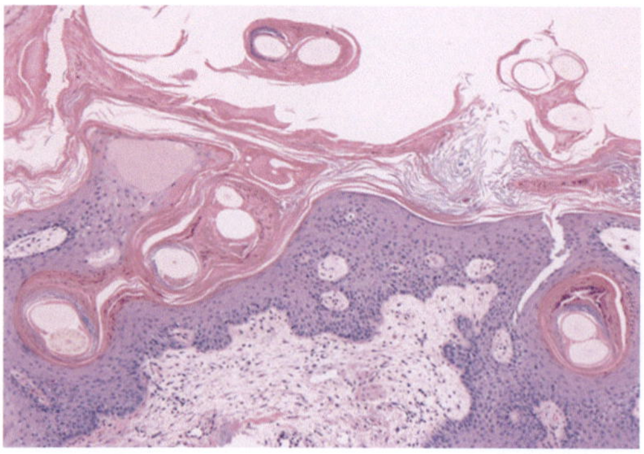

Fig. 16.146 Epidermal papillomatosis and acanthosis

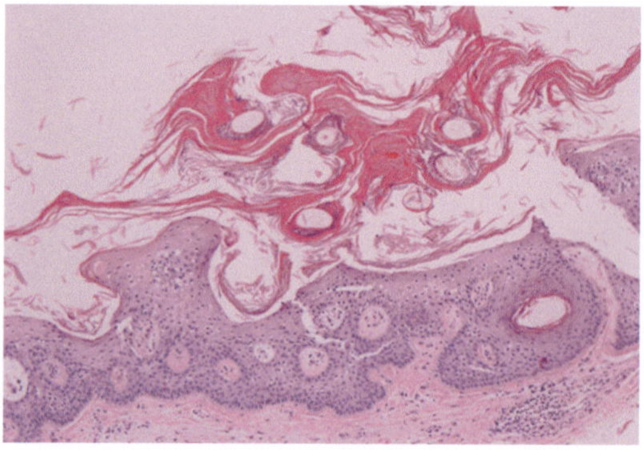

Fig. 16.147 A case of patient with atopic dermatitis

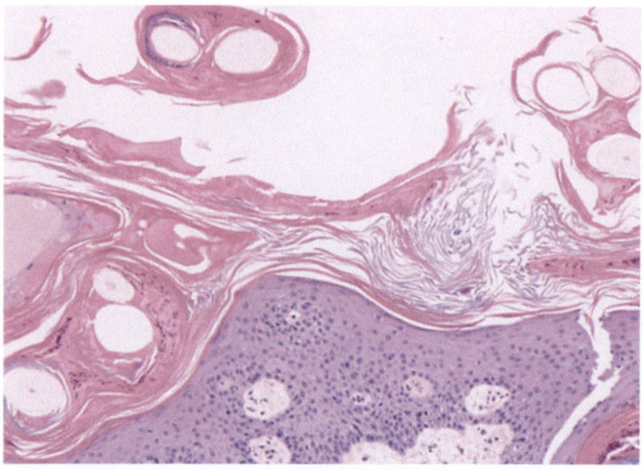

Fig. 16.148 Extensive compact hyperkeratosis

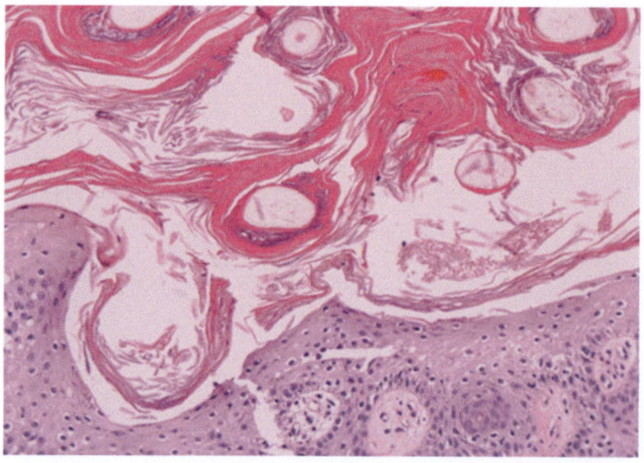

Fig. 16.149 Multiple hair shafts in stratum corneum

Pityriasis Lichenoides et Varioliformis Acuta

Synonym: Mucha-Habermann's Disease

Histopathology (Figs. 16.150, 16.151, 16.152, and 16.153)

- Superficial and deep "wedge" shaped perivascular lymphocytic infiltrate
- Interface vacuolar changes with variable lichenoid lymphocytic infiltrate
- Scattered epidermal lymphocytic exocytosis
- Necrotic keratinocytes are always seen
- Dermal red blood cell extravasation

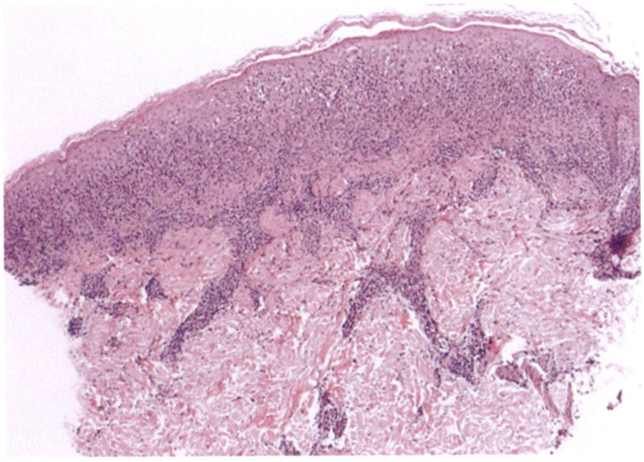

Fig. 16.150 "Wedge" shaped perivascular lymphocytic inflammation

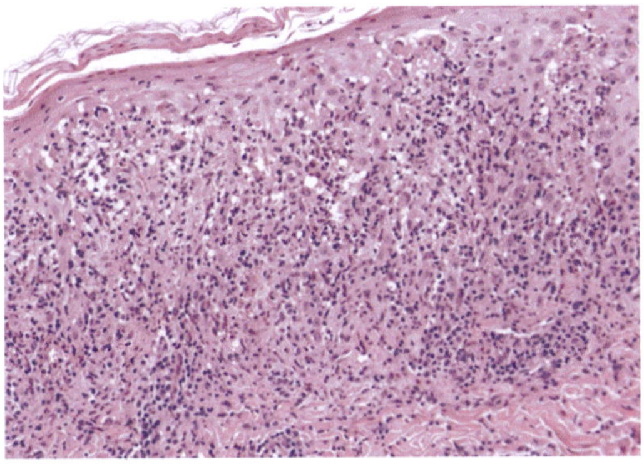

Fig. 16.151 Interface vacuolar changes with necrotic keratinocytes

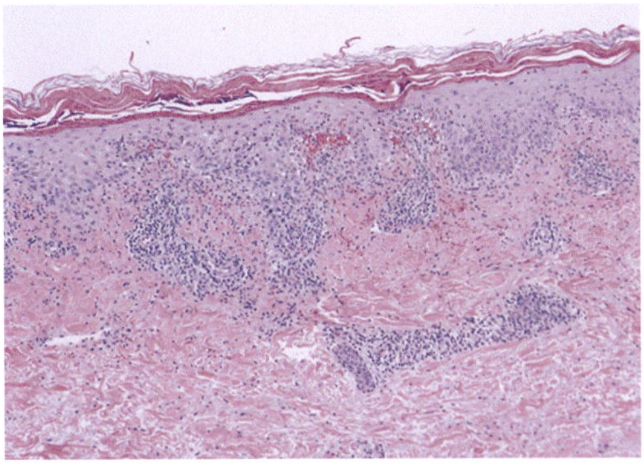

Fig. 16.152 Perivascular lymphocytic inflammation

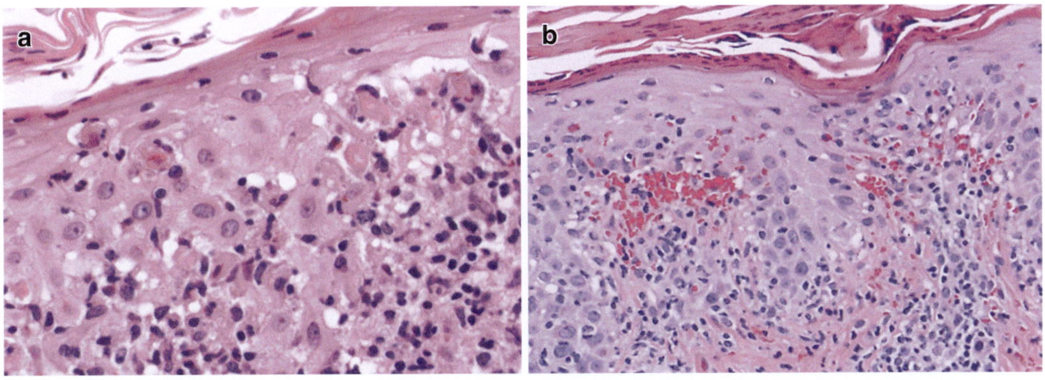

Fig. 16.153 (**a**, **b**) Necrotic keratinocytes, lymphocytic exocytosis and dermal red blood cell extravasation

Pityriasis Lichenoides Chronica

Histopathology is variable and resembles "watered down" version of PLEVA (Figs. 16.154, 16.155, 16.156, 16.157, and 16.158)

- Wavy hyperkeratotic epidermis with focal parakeratosis
- Mild interface changes and scattered necrotic keratinocytes
- Variable epidermal lymphocytic exocytosis
- Mild perivascular lymphocytic infiltrate mostly in the upper part of the dermis
- Variable dermal red blood cells

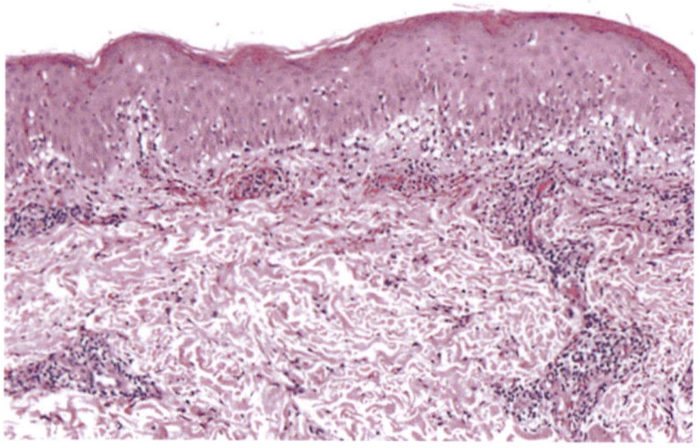

Fig. 16.154 Wavy acanthotic epidermis

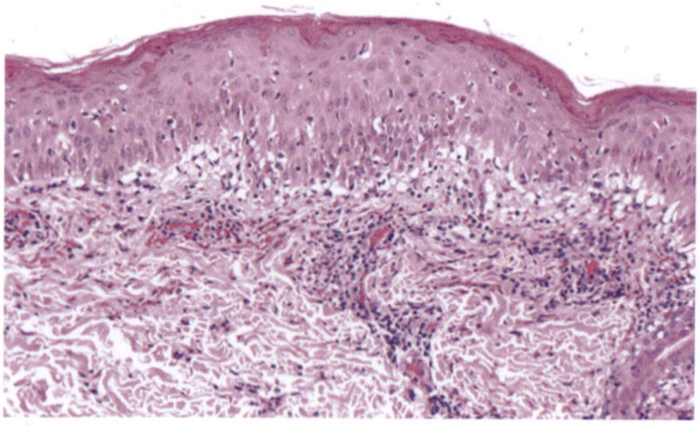

Fig. 16.155 Perivascular lymphocytic infiltrate with red blood cells

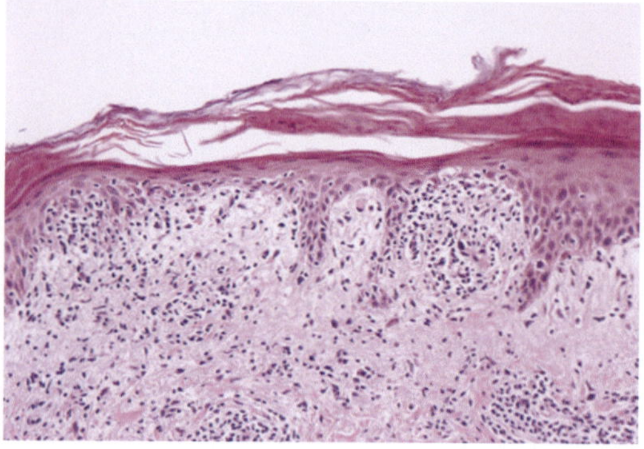

Fig. 16.156 Epidermal parakeratosis and no RBCs extravasation

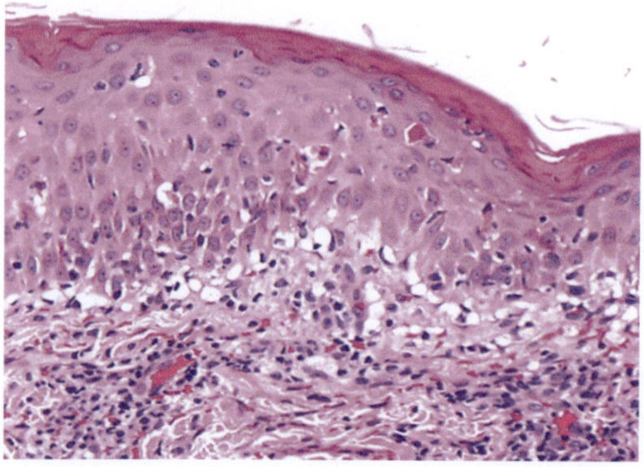

Fig. 16.157 Interface changes with scattered necrotic keratinocytes

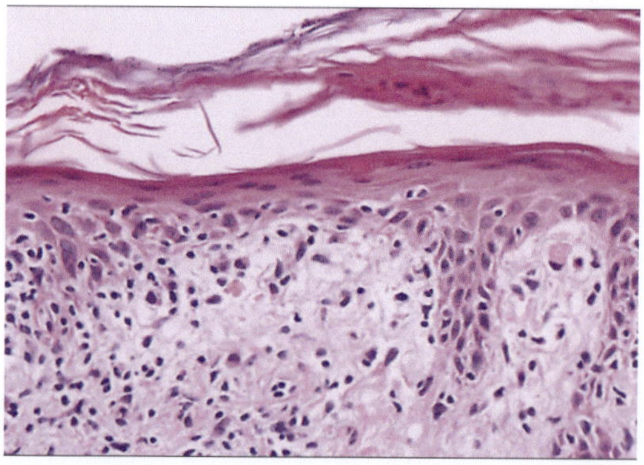

Fig. 16.158 Epidermal lymphocytic exocytosis

Pityriasis Rosea

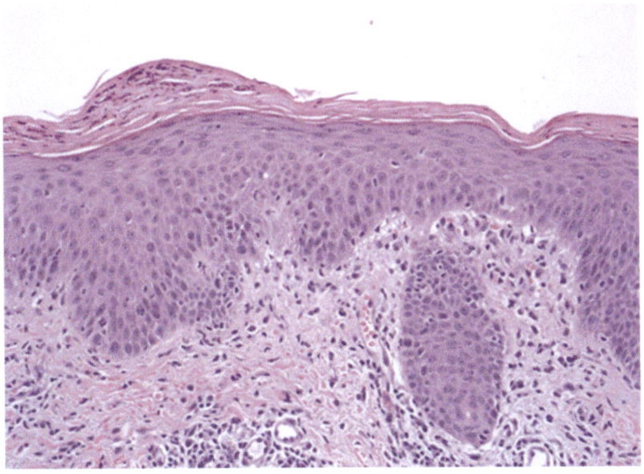

Fig. 16.159 Mild spongiotic dermatitis

Histopathology (Figs. 16.159, 16.160, 16.161, and 16.162)

- Subtle fundings with mild epidermal spongiosis
- Focal parakeratosis with "mounds" formation
- Diminished granular layer
- Red blood cell extravasation
- Mild to moderate perivascular lymphocytic infiltrate
- Sometimes small epidermal vesicles with lymphocytes

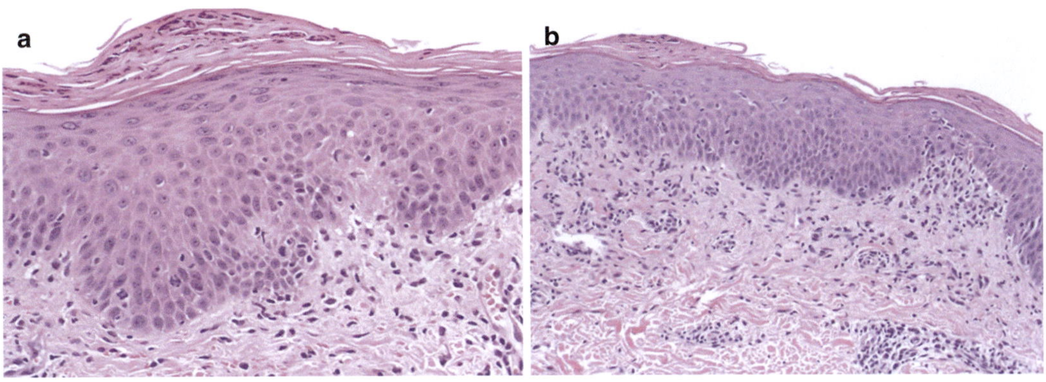

Fig. 16.160 (**a**, **b**) Focal epidermal parakeratosis with dermal perivascular lymphocytic inflammation and focal red blood cells

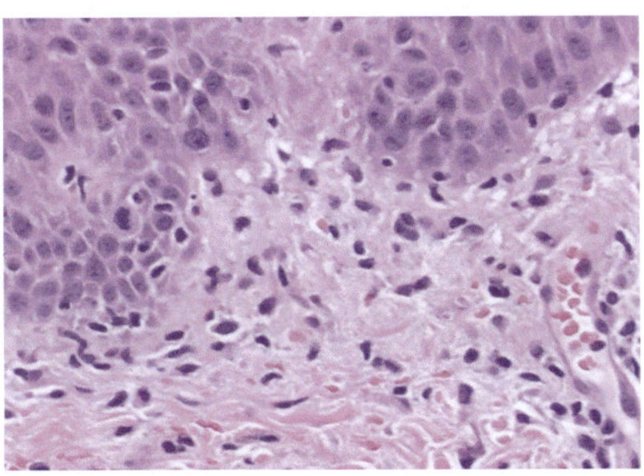

Fig. 16.161 Dermal RBCs extravasation

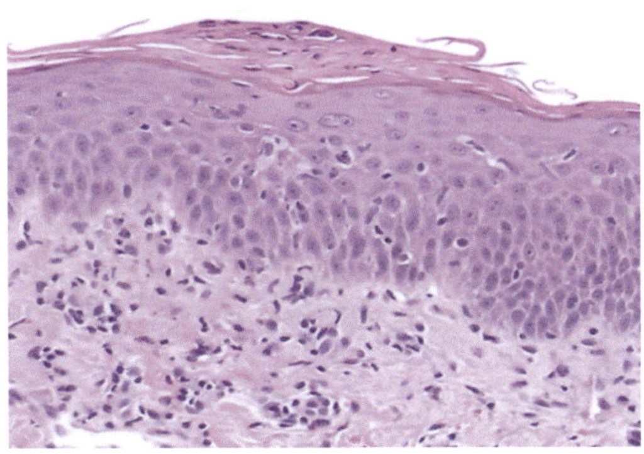

Fig. 16.162 Mound of parakeratosis with diminished granular layer

Pityriasis Rubra Pilaris

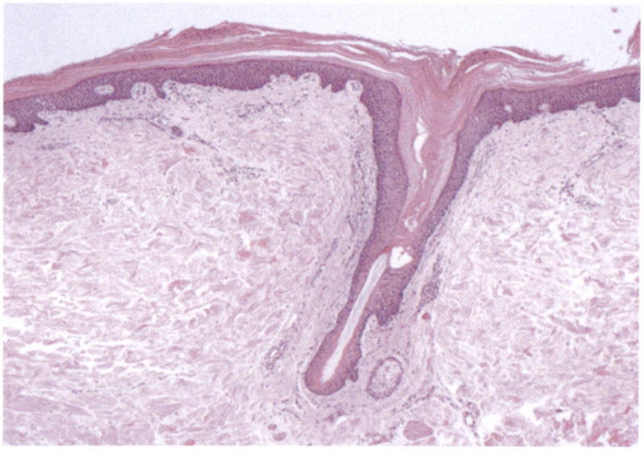

Fig. 16.163 Epidermal acanthosis with broad rete ridges and plugged dilated hair follicle

Histopathology (Figs. 16.163, 16.164, 16.165, 16.166, and 16.167)

- Psoriasiform epidermis or epidermal acanthosis with broad rete ridges
- Hyperkeratotic epidermis with alternating orthokeratosis and parakeratosis horizontally and vertically
- Follicular plugging with shoulder parakeratosis
- Mild perivascular lymphocytic infiltrate

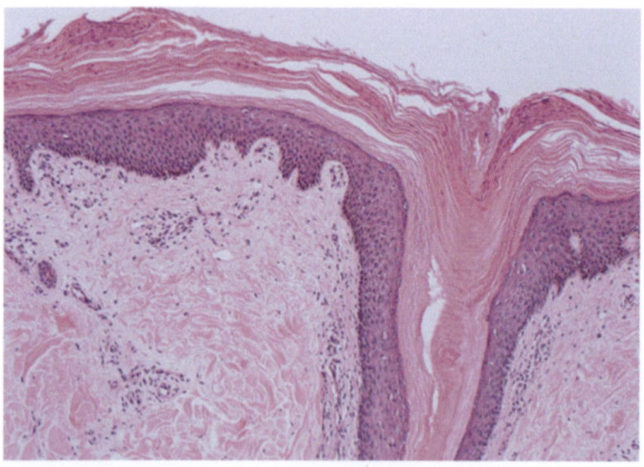

Fig. 16.164 Follicular plugging

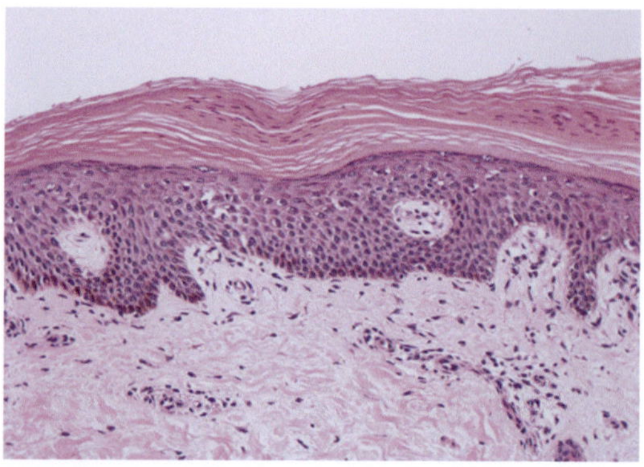

Fig. 16.165 Mild dermal perivascular inflammation

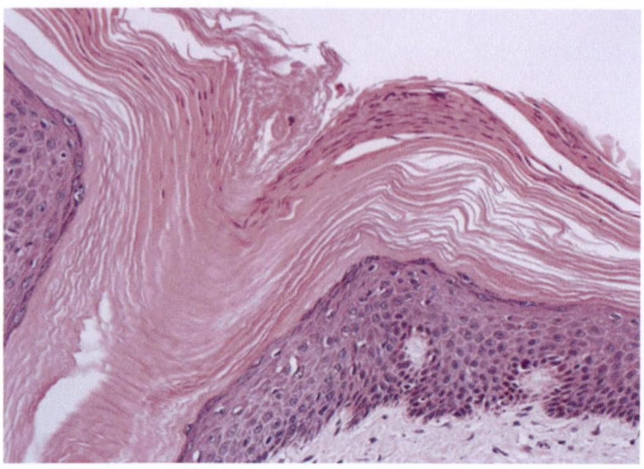

Fig. 16.166 Shoulder parakeratosis

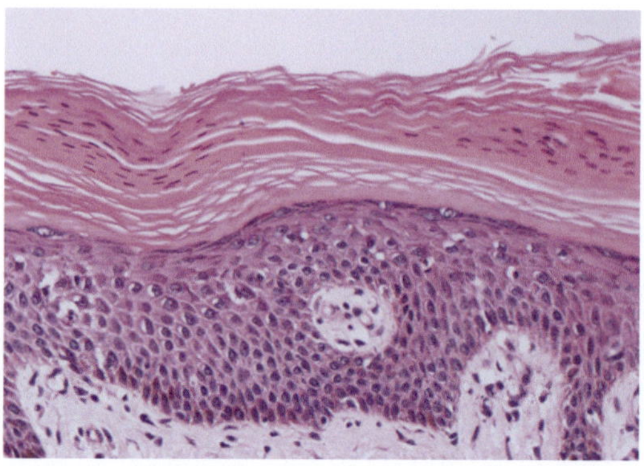

Fig. 16.167 Horizontal and vertical alternation of ortho and parakeratosis

Pityriasis Versicolor

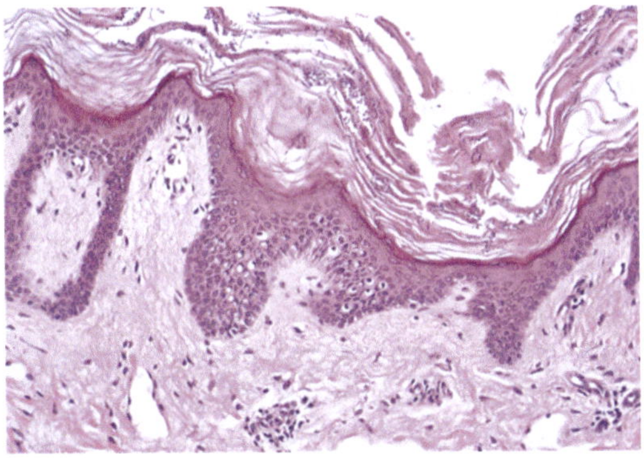

Fig. 16.168 Hyperkeratotic epidermis

Synonym: Tinea Versicolor

Histopathology (Figs. 16.168, 16.169, 16.170, 16.171, and 16.172)

- Epidermal hyperkeratosis
- Mild perivascular lymphocytic infiltrate
- Minimal epidermal spongiosis
- Presence of elongated hyphae and spores of *Malassezia furfur* or *M. ovalis* in the stratum corneum in "spaghetti and meatballs" pattern

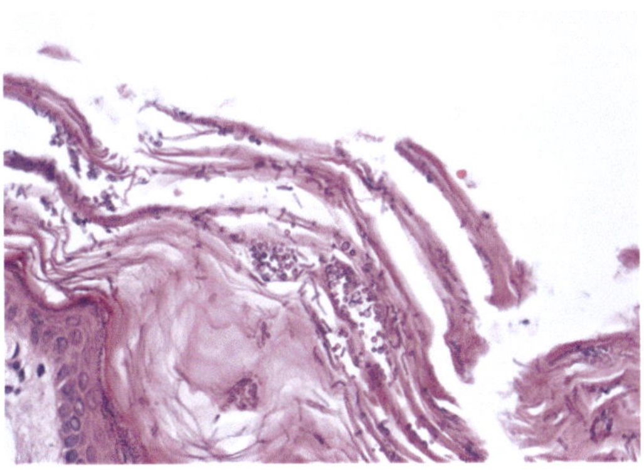

Fig. 16.169 Elongated hyphae and spores in the stratum corneum

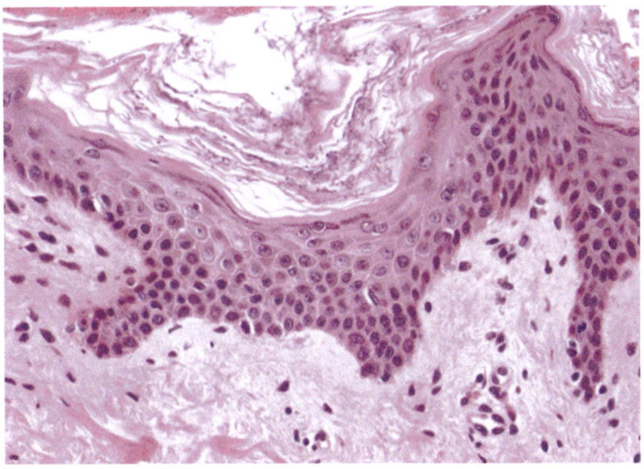

Fig. 16.170 Mild spongiosis and perivascular lymphocytic infiltrate

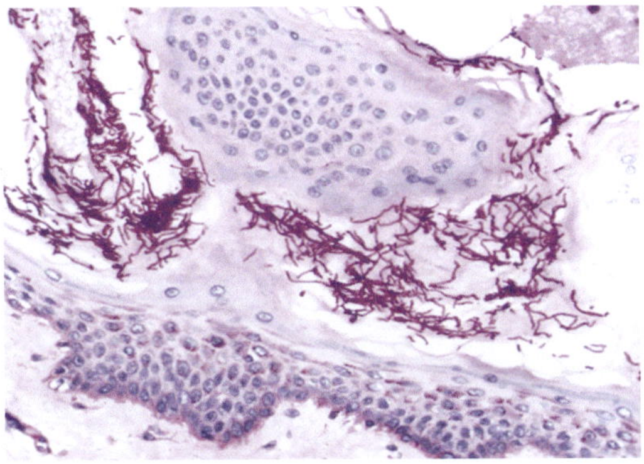

Fig. 16.171 "Spaghetti and meatballs" of *Malassezia* on PAS slide

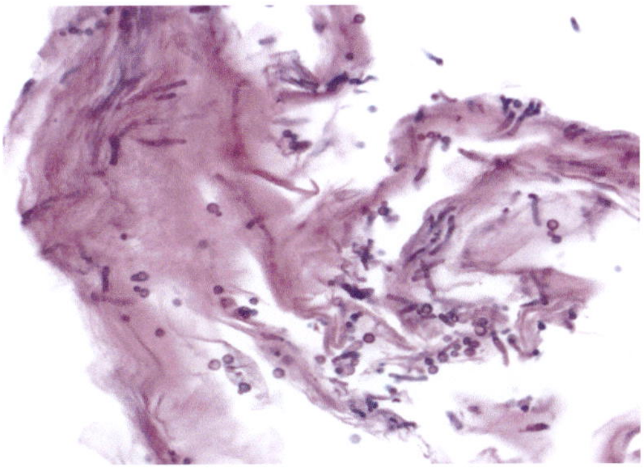

Fig. 16.172 "Spaghetti and meatballs" of *Malassezia* on H&E slide

Plasmacytoma

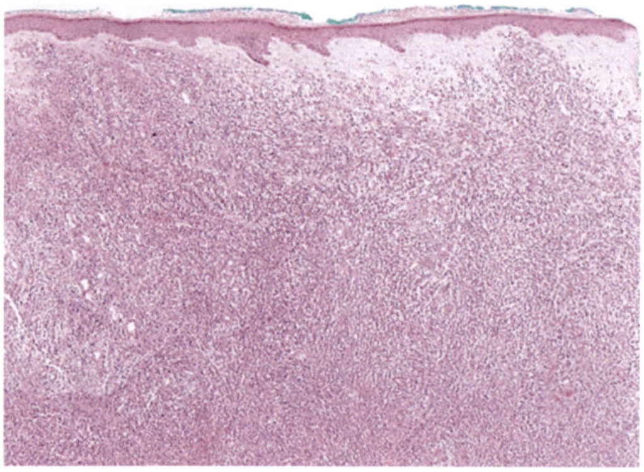

Fig. 16.173 Diffuse subcutaneous infiltrate with Grenz zone

Histopathology (Figs. 16.173, 16.174, 16.175, 16.176, and 16.177)

- Diffuse or nodular subcutaneous infiltrate
- Grenz zone is frequently present
- Cytology of the cells varies from well-differentiated cell with typical plasma cell features to poorly-differentiated with pleomorphic cells
- Tumor cells are CD38, CD79a, and CD138 positive

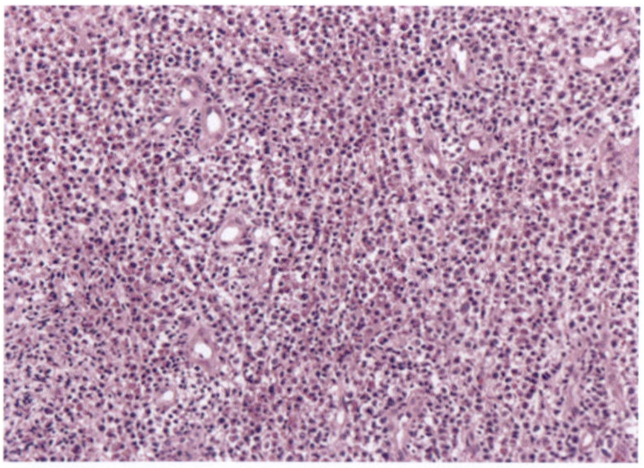

Fig. 16.174 Well-differentiated plasmacytoma

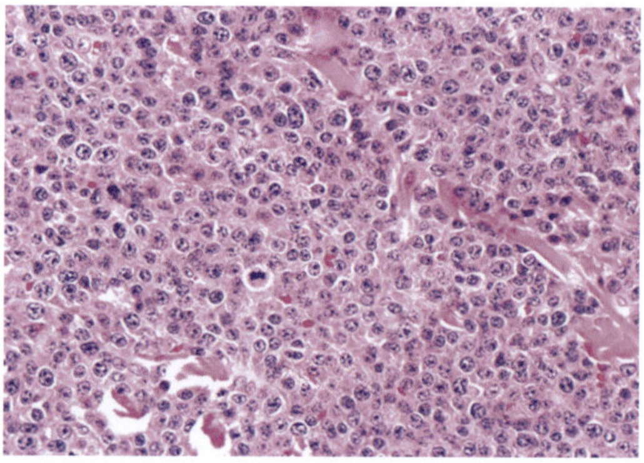

Fig. 16.175 Poorly-differentiated plasmacytoma

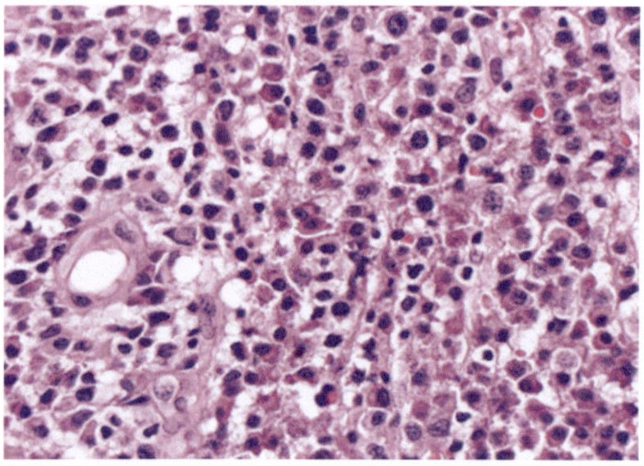

Fig. 16.176 Easily recognized plasma cells with peripheral nuclei and intracytoplasmic inclusions (Russell bodies)

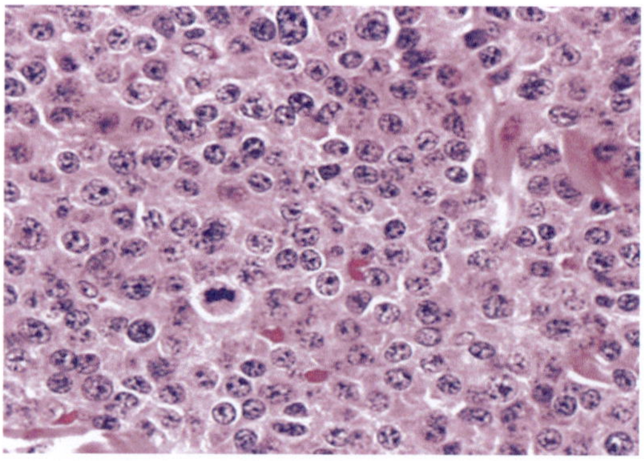

Fig. 16.177 Speckled nuclei and mitosis. Special stains are needed to confirm cell origin

Pleomorphic Fibroma

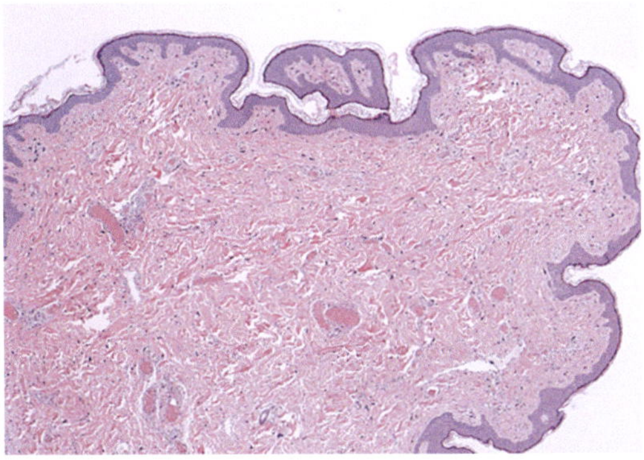

Fig. 16.178 Polypoid lesion with sclerotic stroma

Histopathology (Figs. 16.178, 16.179, and 16.180)

- Polypoid or dome-shaped fibrous lesion
- Sparse fibroblasts
- Scattered between collagen bundle are large irregular cells (CD68+) with dark irregular nucleus and scant cytoplasm ("monster cells")

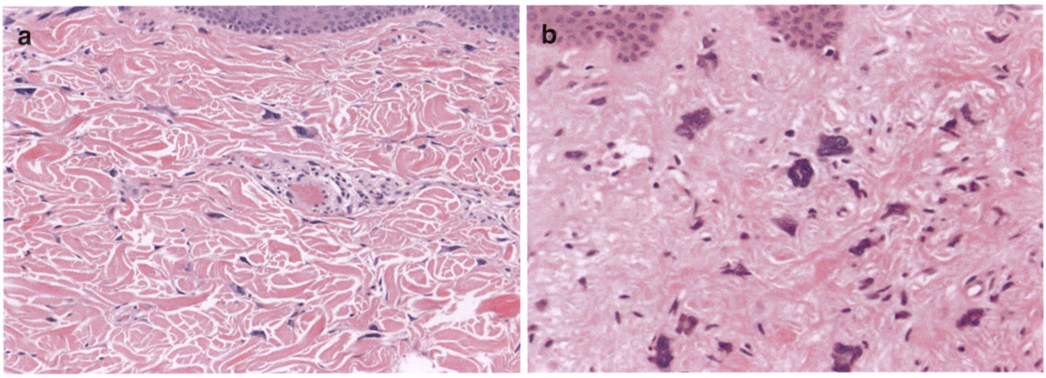

Fig. 16.179 (**a**, **b**) Hypocellular fibrotic stroma and scattered dark irregular cells

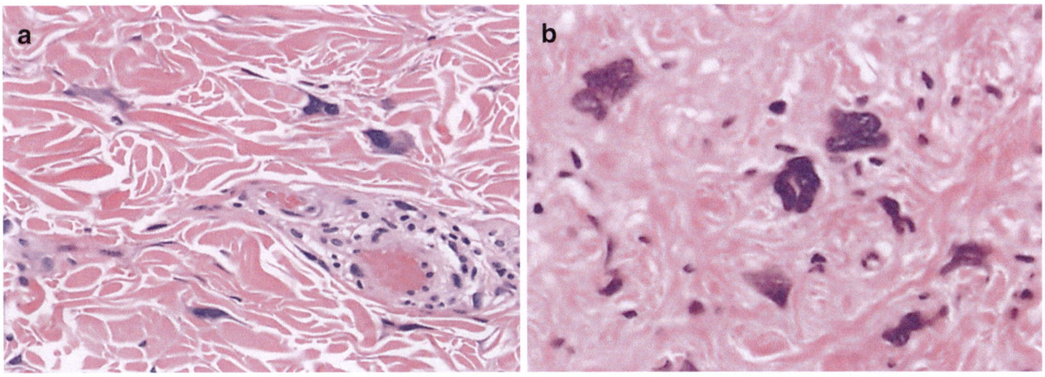

Fig. 16.180 (**a**, **b**) "Monster cells" are large irregular cells with dark nuclei and scant cytoplasm embedded in sclerotic stroma

Poikiloderma

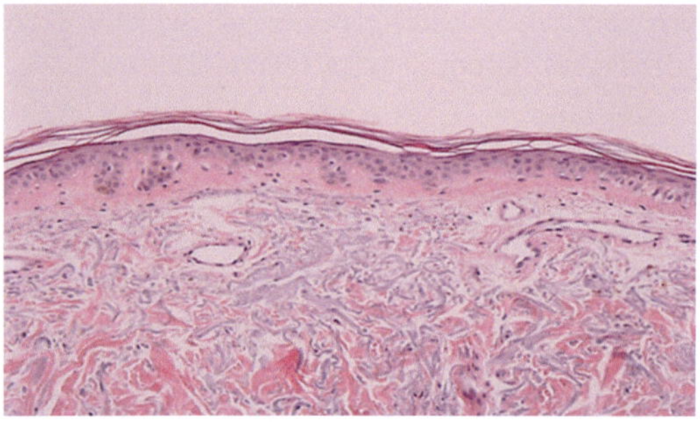

Fig. 16.181 Atrophic epidermis with dermal telangiectasias

Histopathology (Figs. 16.181, 16.182, 16.183, and 16.184)

- Atrophic epidermis with hyperkeratosis
- Focal interface vacuolar changes can be seen
- Dermal telangiectasias
- Variable dermal pigment incontinence
- Minimal inflammation

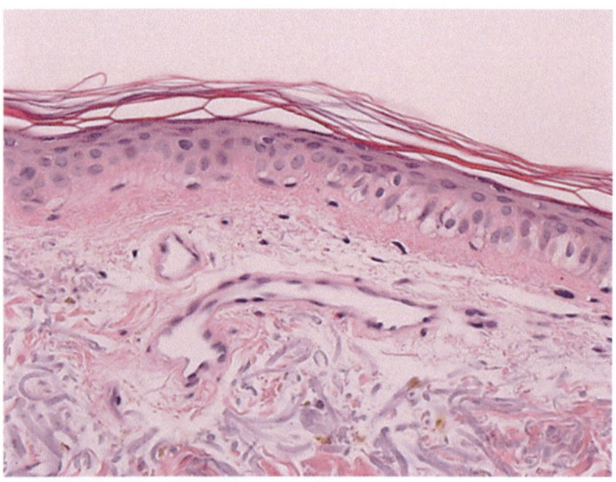

Fig. 16.182 Focal vacuolar changes at the interface are present. Dermal telangiectasias and pigment incontinence

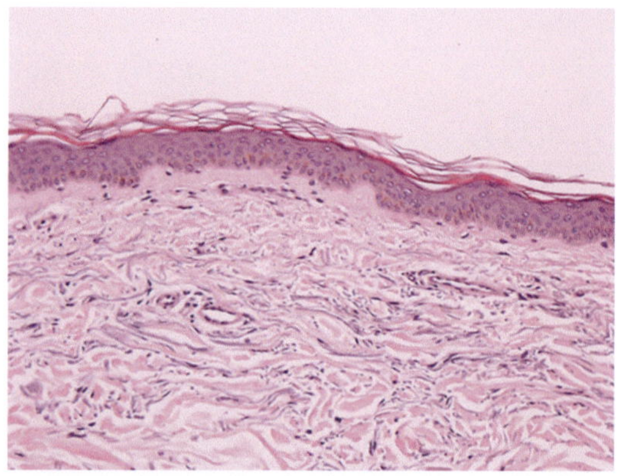

Fig. 16.183 Atrophic epidermis with hyperkeratosis, dermal dilated capillaries, and no pigment incontinence

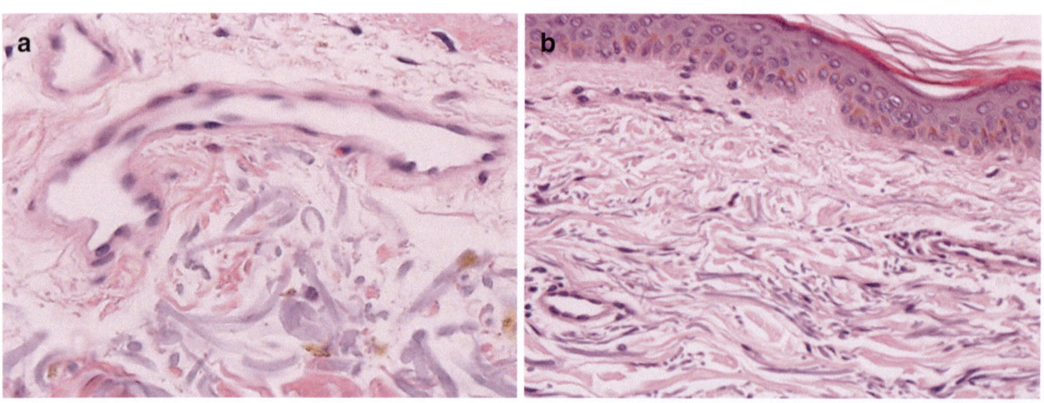

Fig. 16.184 (**a**, **b**) In *poikiloderma of Civatte,* in addition to typical features, prominent solar elastosis is present

Polyarteritis Nodosa

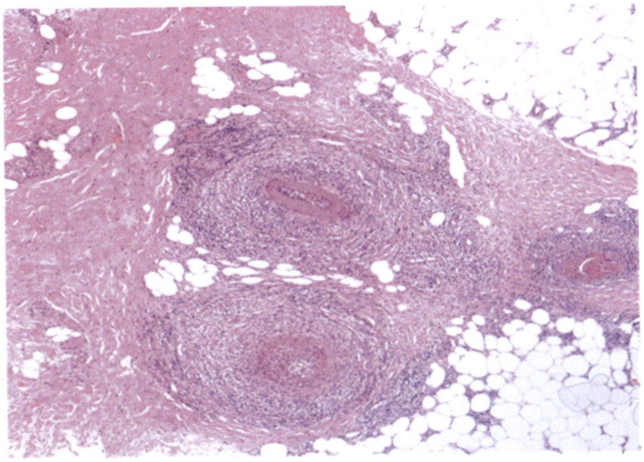

Fig. 16.185 Vasculitis of small and medium size dermal and subcutaneous vessels

Histopathology (Figs. 16.185, 16.186, and 16.187)

- Necrotizing vasculitis of medium-sized arteries
- Smaller vessels can also be involved
- Destruction of vessel wall with fibrinoid deposition
- Neutrophilic infiltrate around the vessel and in the vessel wall
- Luminal thrombi might form

P.S. keep in mind that some cases have only features of leukocytoclastic vasculitis

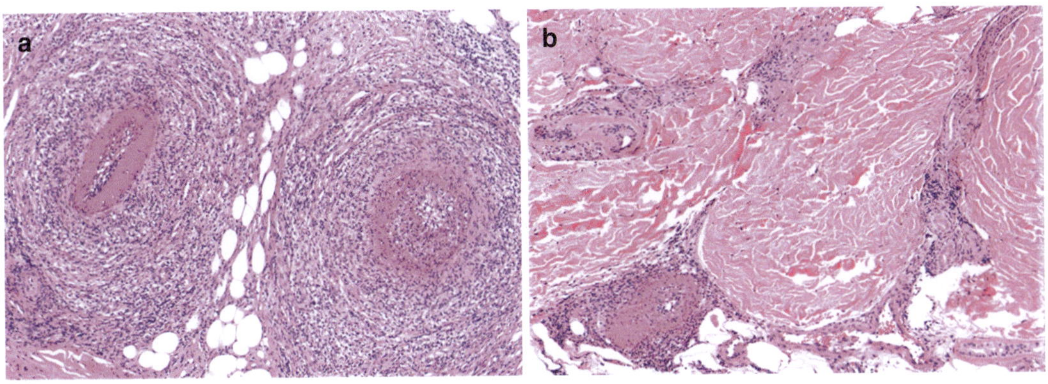

Fig. 16.186 (**a**, **b**) Fibrinoid necrosis of medium size vessels wall with perivascular and intravascular neutrophilic infiltrate

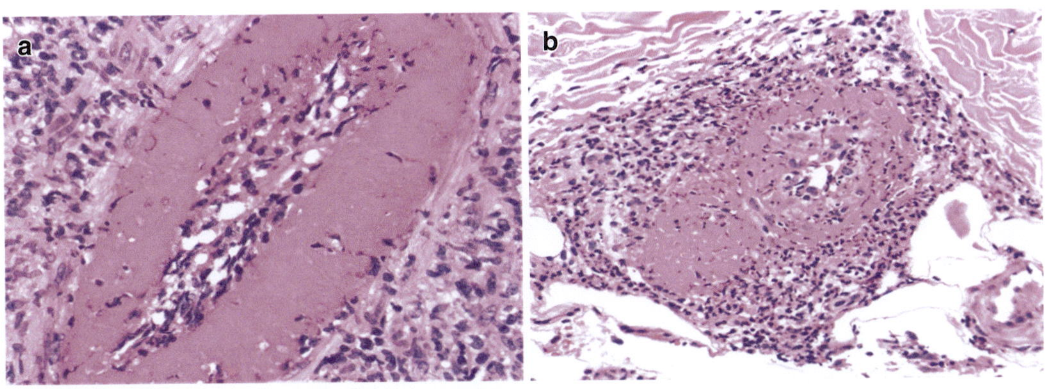

Fig. 16.187 (**a**, **b**) Neutrophils surround vessels and infiltrate into the wall; endothelial cells are reactive

Polymorphous Light Eruption

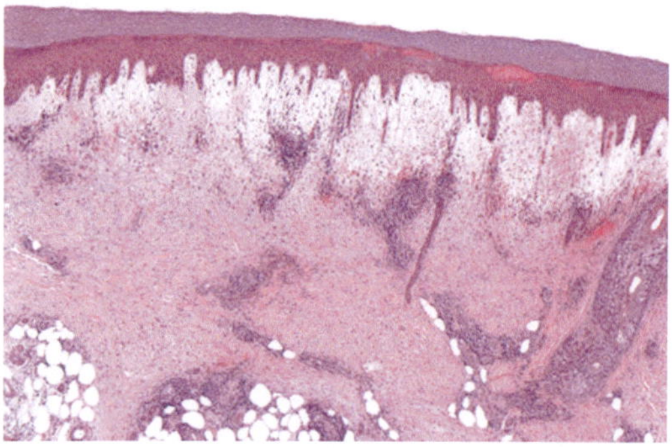

Fig. 16.188 Hyperkeratotic epidermis and dermal edema

Histopathology (Figs. 16.188, 16.189, and 16.190)

- Hyperkeratotic epidermis
- Superficial dermal edema that can lead to blister formation
- Superficial and deep perivascular and interstitial lymphocytic inflammation
- Some eosinophils and neutrophils can be seen

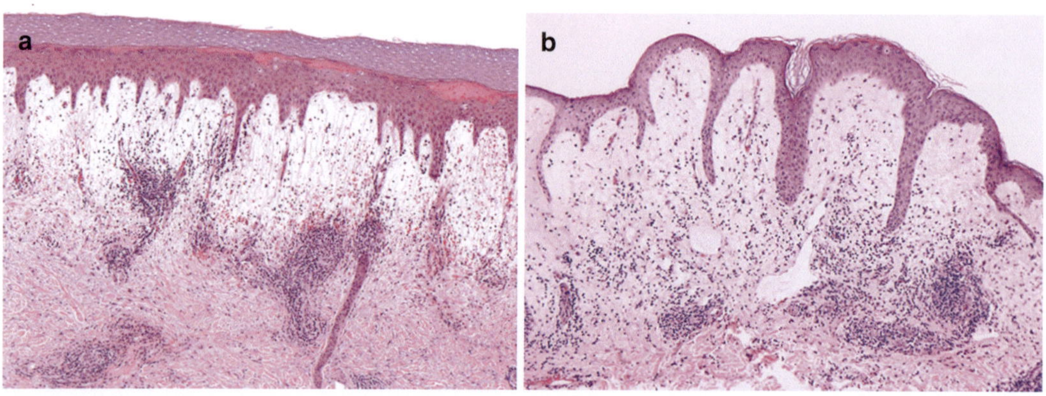

Fig. 16.189 (**a**, **b**) Extensive edema of the papillary dermis

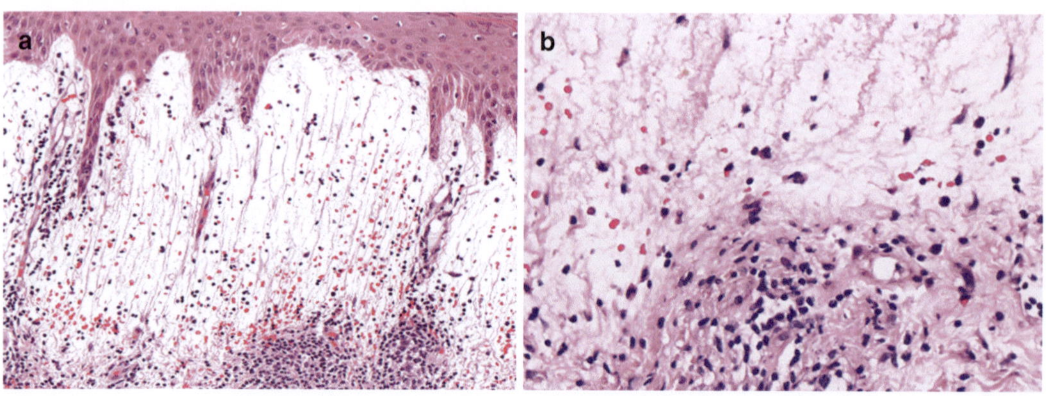

Fig. 16.190 (**a**, **b**) Perivascular and interstitial lymphocytic inflammation and RBCs extravasation

Porocarcinoma

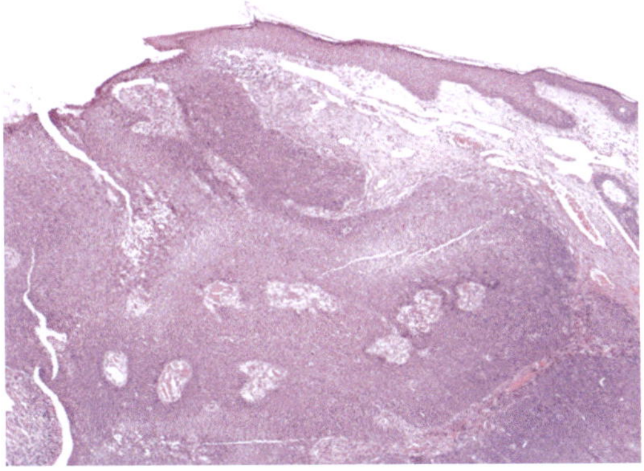

Fig. 16.191 Tumor with multiple attachments to the epidermis infiltrates subcutis

Histopathology could be summarized as "poroma-like" tumor with atypia (Figs. 16.191, 16.192, 16.193, and 16.194)

- Tumor demonstrates multiple attachments to the epidermis
- Infiltrate the dermis with broad pushing front or is more infiltrative
- Tumor cells demonstrate atypia with mitosis
- Areas of necrosis are common
- Focal squamous feature can be seen (squamous variant of porocarcinoma)

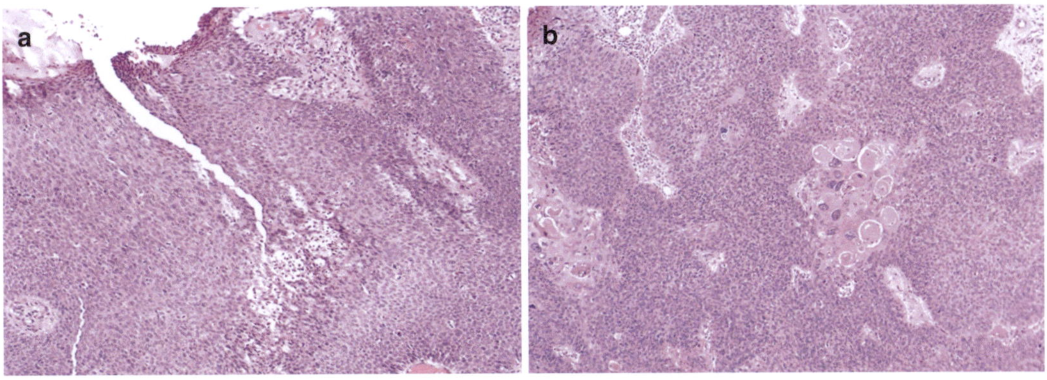

Fig. 16.192 (**a**, **b**) Tumor cells appear cuboidal relatively uniform "poroma-like"

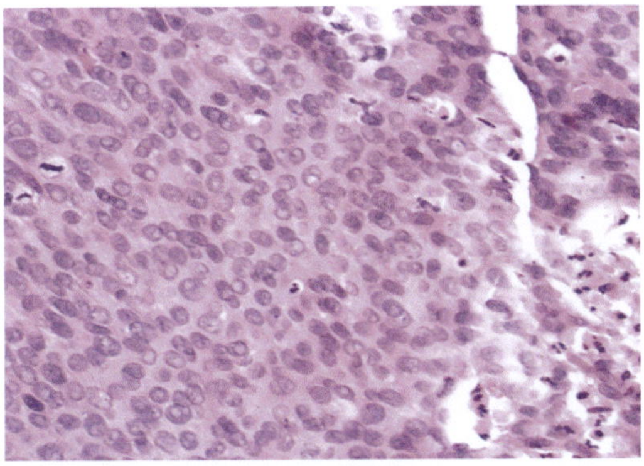

Fig. 16.193 On higher magnification cytological atypia, mitoses, and focal necrosis are apparent

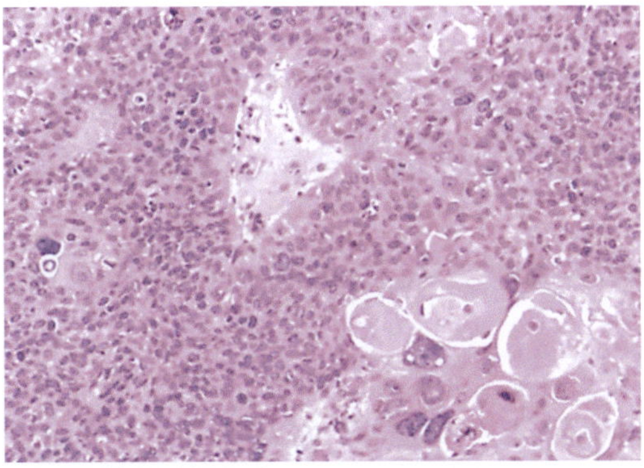

Fig. 16.194 Atypical squamous area is present

Poroma

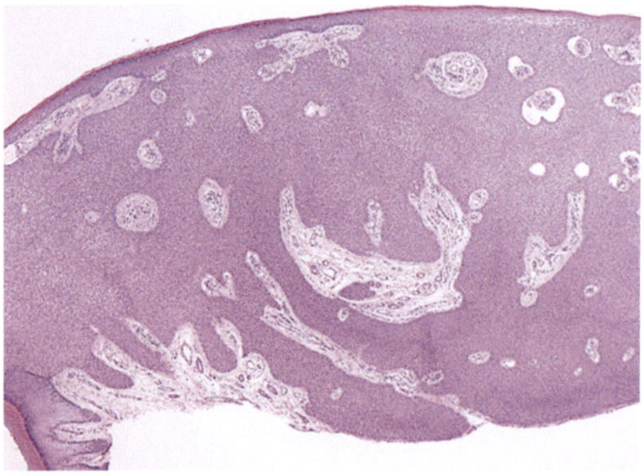

Fig. 16.195 Tumor with multiple attachments to the epidermis

Synonym: Eccrine Poroma

Histopathology (Figs. 16.195, 16.196, and 16.197)

- Cords and broad columns of uniform basaloid cells extending into the dermis from the normal epidermis
- There are multiple tumor attachments to the epidermis
- Tumor cells are uniform and slightly cuboidal with darker uniform nuclei (CK7+)
- Ducts (CEA+) are commonly formed within tumor

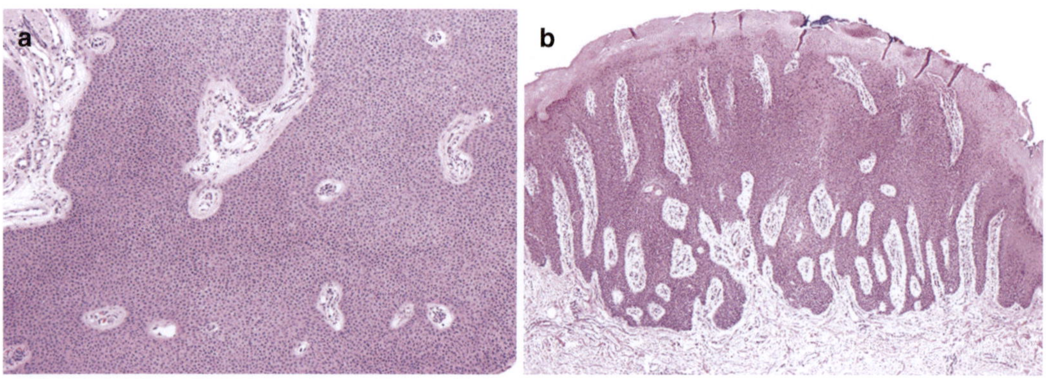

Fig. 16.196 (**a**, **b**) Cords and broad tumor columns infiltrate into the dermis

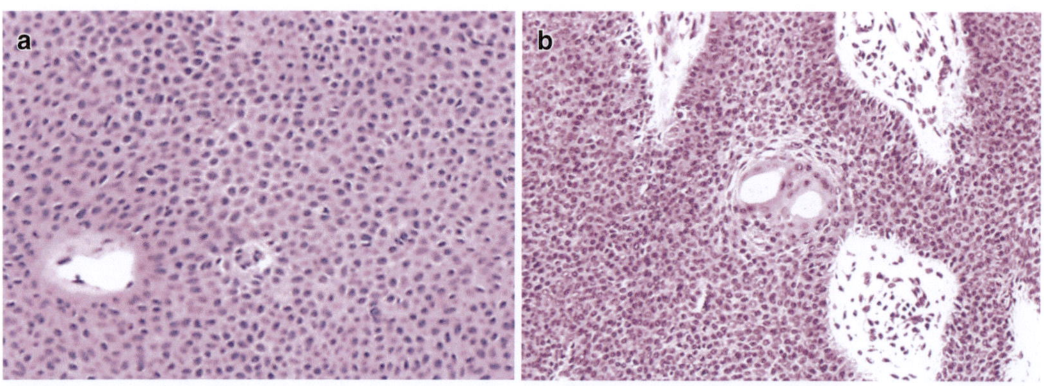

Fig. 16.197 (**a**, **b**) Uniform cells with no atypia. Darker nuclei with no mitoses. Ductal structures are present within the tumor

Porokeratosis

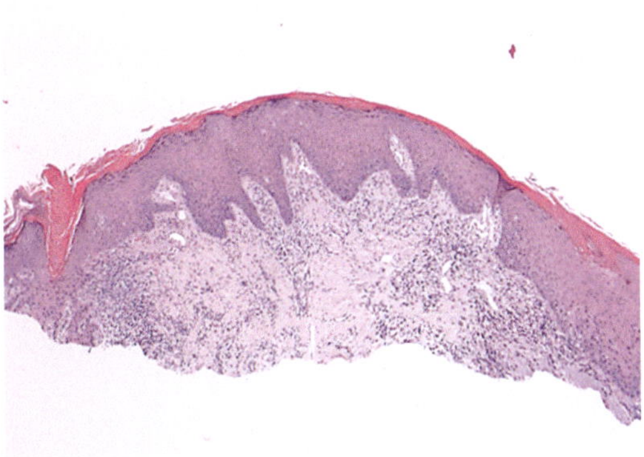

Fig. 16.198 Hyperkeratotic epidermis with two "cornoid" lamellae facing each other

Heterogeneous group of clinical entities with similar histopathology but pathognomonic sign in all forms is "cornoid" lamella (Figs. 16.198, 16.199, and 16.200)

- "Cornoid" lamella is a narrow leaning lamella of parakeratosis
- If entire lesion is sampled two "cornoid" lamellae are leaning toward each other
- The epidermis in between lamellas can vary from atrophic to acanthotic and hyperkeratotic
- Beneath "cornoid" lamellae the granular layer is diminished

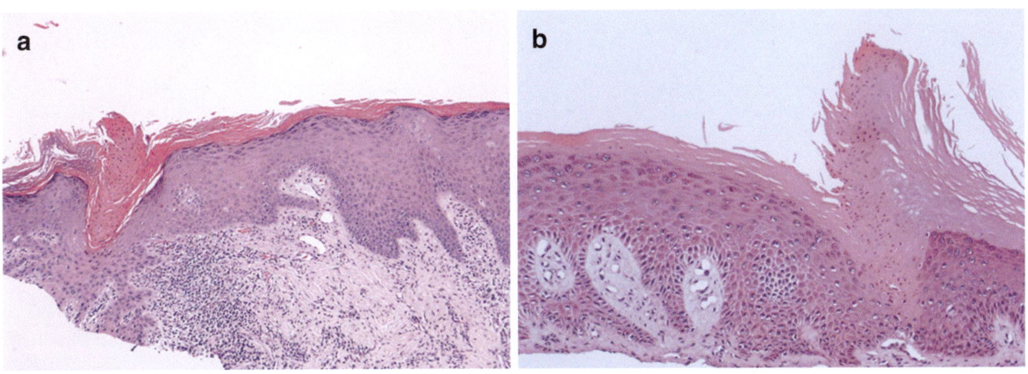

Fig. 16.199 (**a**, **b**) Keratin filled epidermal depression with column of parakeratosis leaning toward the opposite side of the lesion

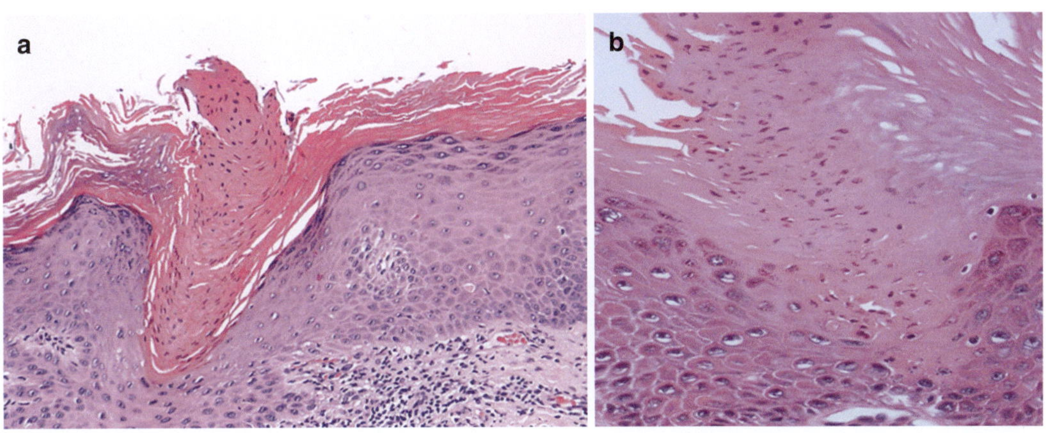

Fig. 16.200 (**a**, **b**) Granular layer is diminished below the lamella

Porphyria

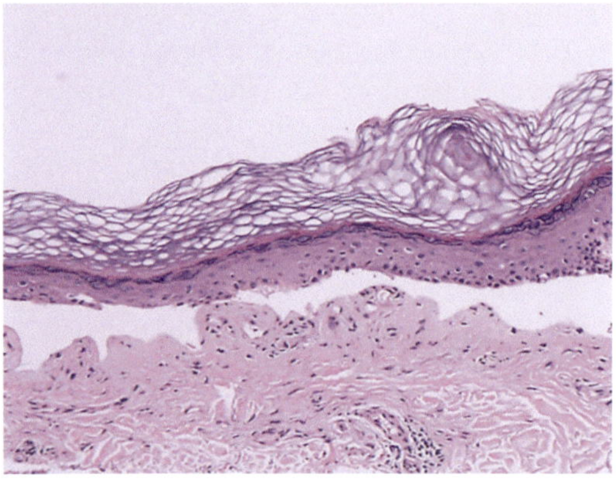

Fig. 16.201 Subepidermal blister without inflammatory cells

There are various clinical presentations of porphyria but **histopathology** of cutaneous lesions is similar in all of them (Figs. 16.201, 16.202, 16.203, and 16.204)

- Subepidermal "cell poor" blister
- Minimal inflammation
- Hyalinized dermal papillae with "festooning"
- Mildly thickened wall of blood vessels
- Dermal solar elastosis

P.S. *pseudoporhyria* show similar features

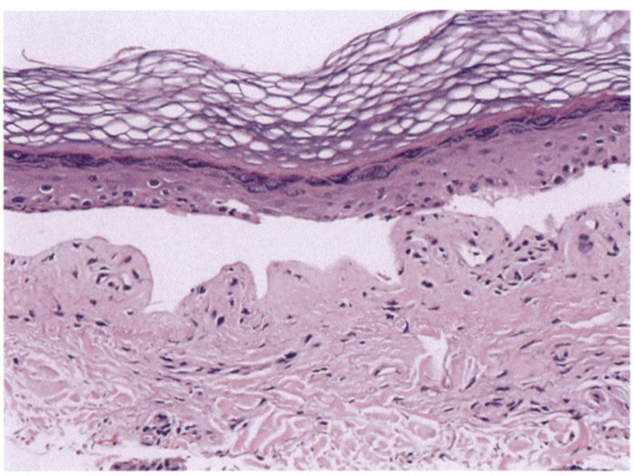

Fig. 16.202 Hyalinized dermal papillae

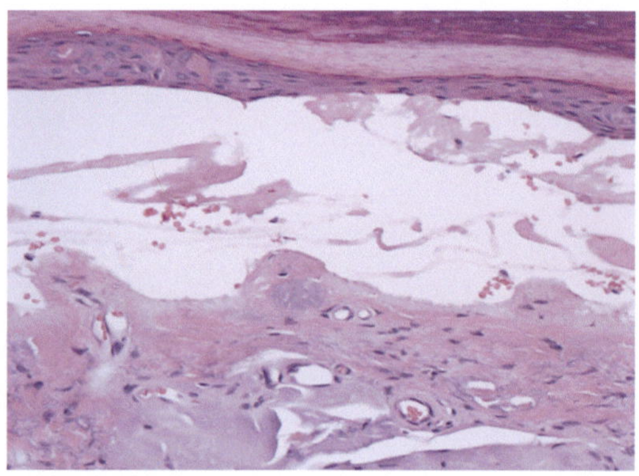

Fig. 16.203 Solar elastosis and prominent dermal vessels

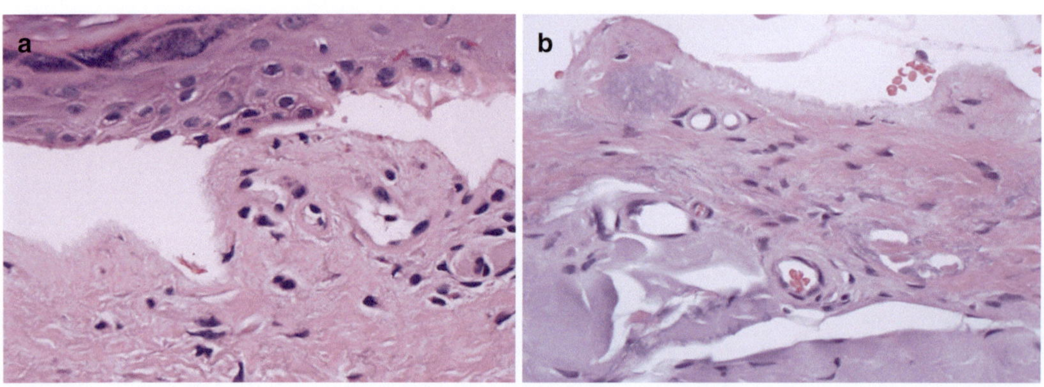

Fig. 16.204 (**a**, **b**) Dermal papillae with "festooning"

Postinflammatory Pigment Alteration

This entity may represent the end stage of almost any inflammatory skin disorder.

Histopathology (Figs. 16.205, 16.206, and 16.207)
- Normal epidermis and variable dermal pigment incontinence with dermal melanophages
- Variable perivascular lymphocytic infiltrate and occasional interface vacuolar changes

P.S. **Notalgia Paresthetica** and **Melasma (Chloasma)** show similar H&E histopathology but dermal pigment incontinence is less abundant. Also in *Melasma* epidermal melanin is slightly increased

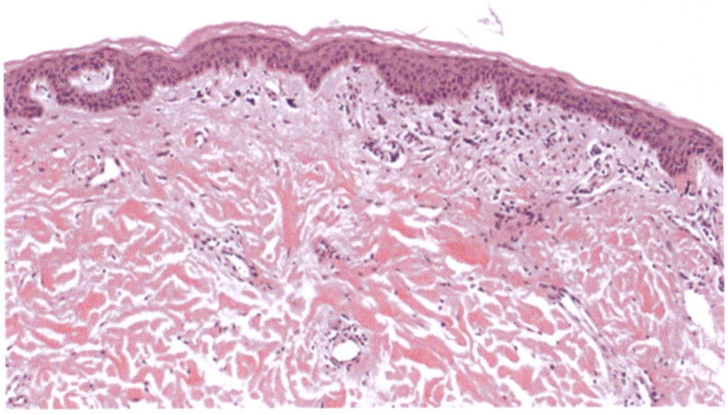

Fig. 16.205 Normal appearing epidermis and dermal pigment

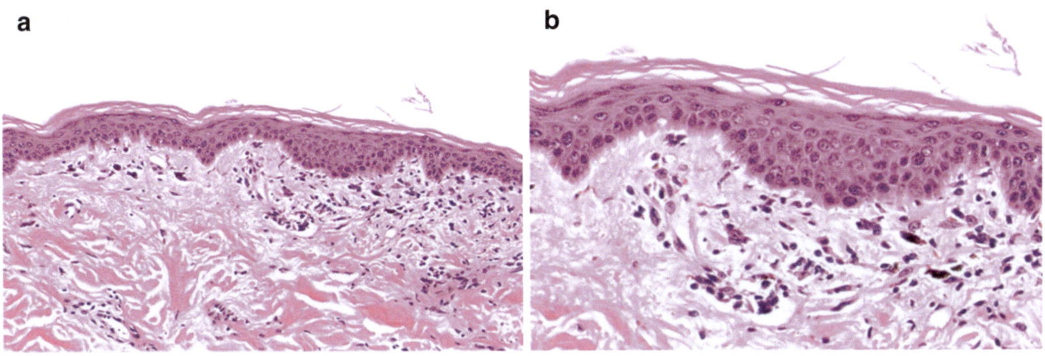

Fig. 16.206 (**a**, **b**) Mild case with normal epidermis, dermal pigment incontinence, and mild lymphocytic inflammation

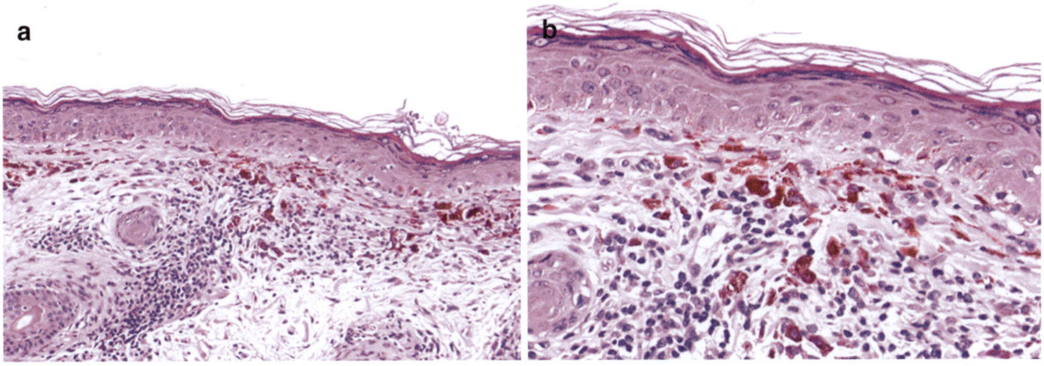

Fig. 16.207 (**a**, **b**) A case with more dermal melanophages and moderate lymphocytic inflammation

Pretibial Myxedema

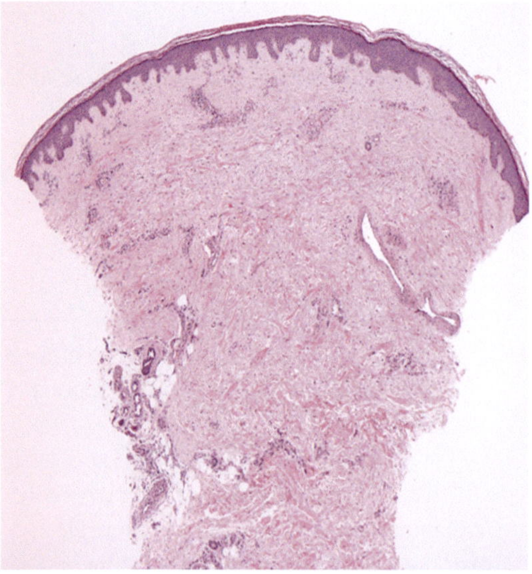

Fig. 16.208 Dermis and subcutis appears pale with bluish hue

Synonym: Localized Myxedema

Histopathology (Figs. 16.208, 16.209, 16.210, and 16.211)
- Epidermis is normal
- Collagen fibers are separated by prominent mucin
- Scattered stellate fibroblast can be seen
- Number of fibroblasts is not increased

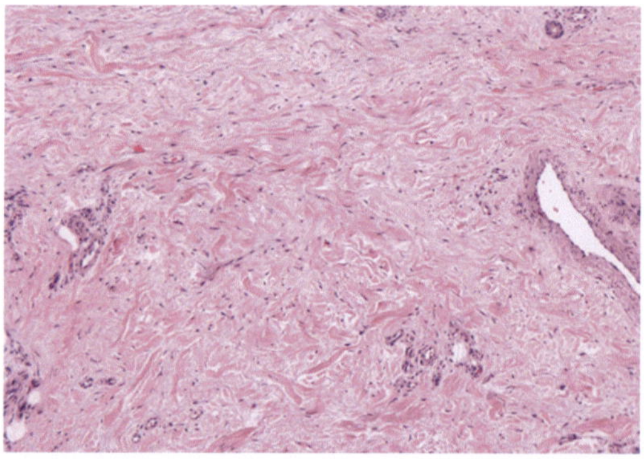

Fig. 16.209 Stroma with gray bluish hue coming from dermal mucin

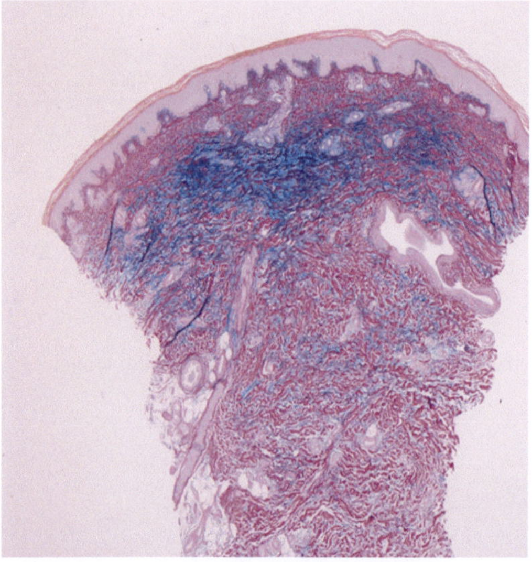

Fig. 16.210 Alcian Blue stain (blue) outlines prominent dermal and subcutaneous mucin

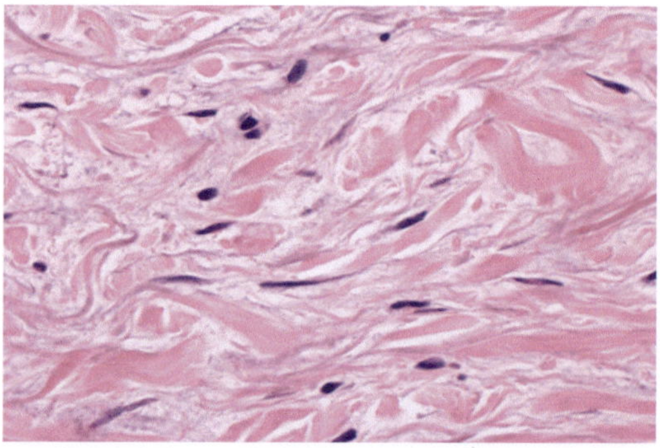

Fig. 16.211 Collagen fibers are separated by the mucin. Stellate fibroblasts are present but are not increased in the number

Primary Cutaneous Anaplastic Large Cell T-Cell Lymphoma

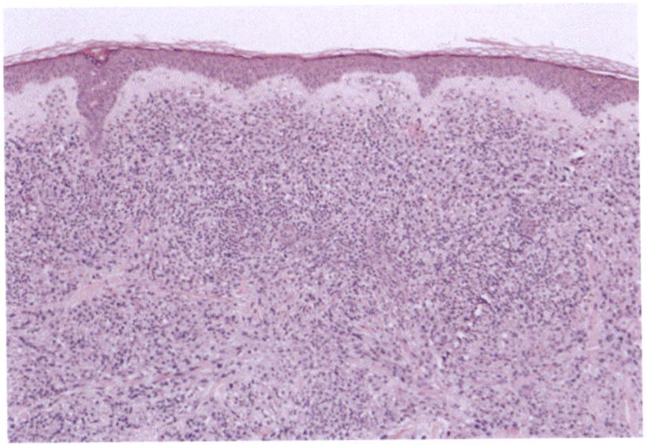

Fig. 16.212 Diffuse dermal infiltrate, lacking epidermal infiltrate

Histopathology (Figs. 16.212, 16.213, 16.214, 16.215, and 16.216)

- Diffuse, dermal T-cell lymphocytic infiltrate with usually lack of epidermotropism
- Most cases have large morphology with prominent anaplasia
- Reactive small lymphocytes can be admixed but more commonly with variable presence of neutrophils and/or eosinophils
- Most of atypical cells (>70%) are CD30+ with a T-helper phenotype (CD2+, CD3+, CD4+, CD8−, CD15−)

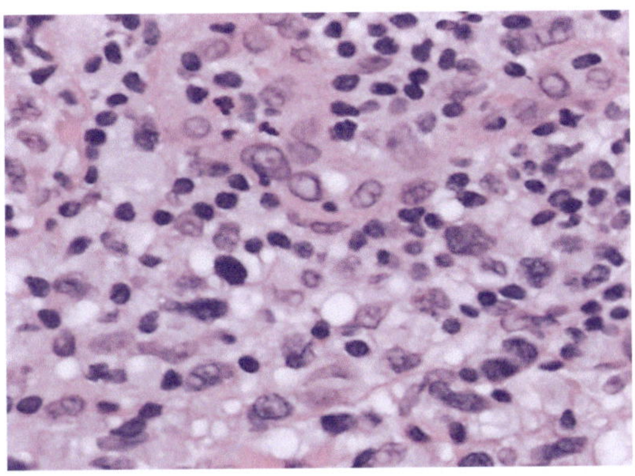

Fig. 16.213 Highly irregular cells with multiple atypical mitoses

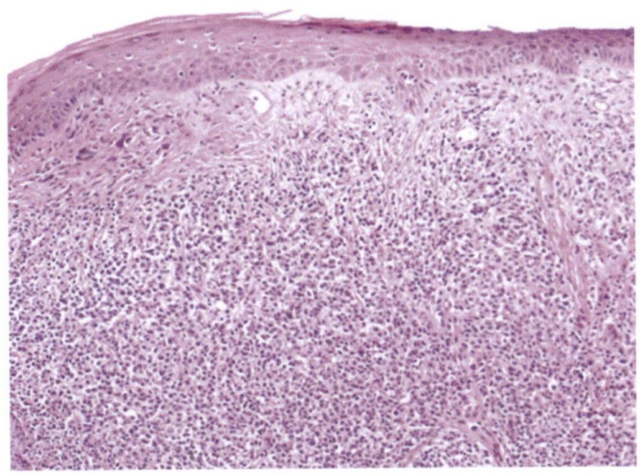

Fig. 16.214 Mixed infiltrate with prominent, large cell infiltrate

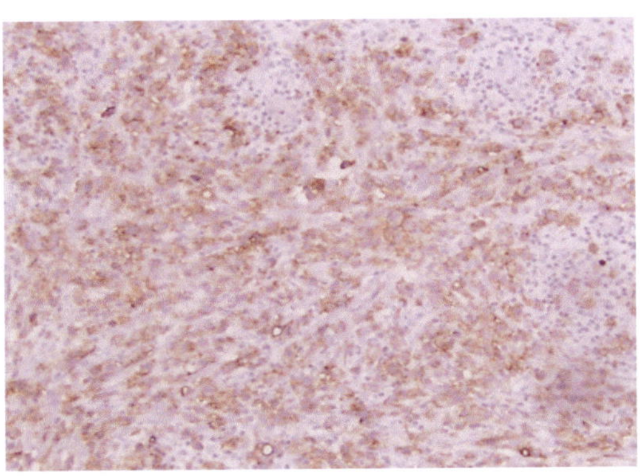

Fig. 16.215 CD30 highlights majority of large atypical cells

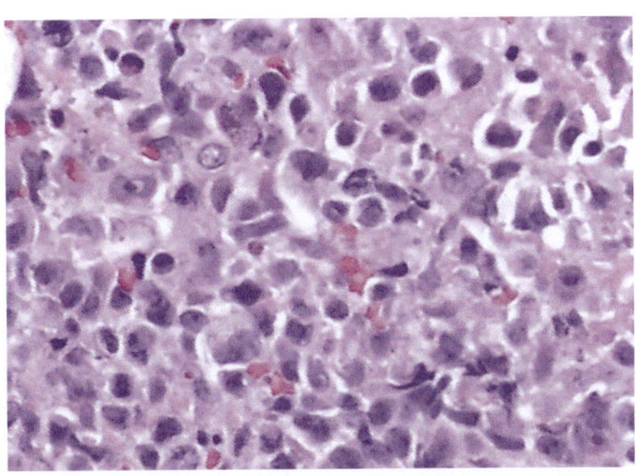

Fig. 16.216 Cells have irregular, hyperchromatic nuclei

Primary Cutaneous Diffuse Large B-Cell Lymphoma-Leg Type

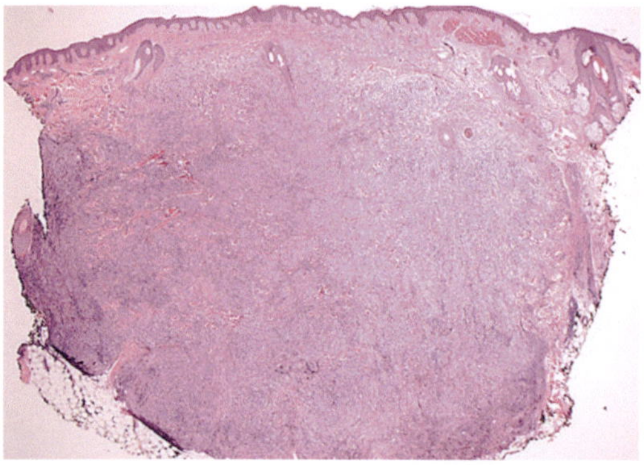

Fig. 16.217 Dense dermal and subcutaneous infiltrate

Histopathology (Figs. 16.217, 16.218, 16.219, and 16.220)
- Diffuse dense dermal and subcutaneous infiltrate
- Large cells with irregular nuclei
- Reactive small lymphocytes are sparse
- Mitoses are easily identified
- Tumor cells are CD20+, CD79a+, Bcl-2+, MUM1+, FOX-P1+, Bcl-6+

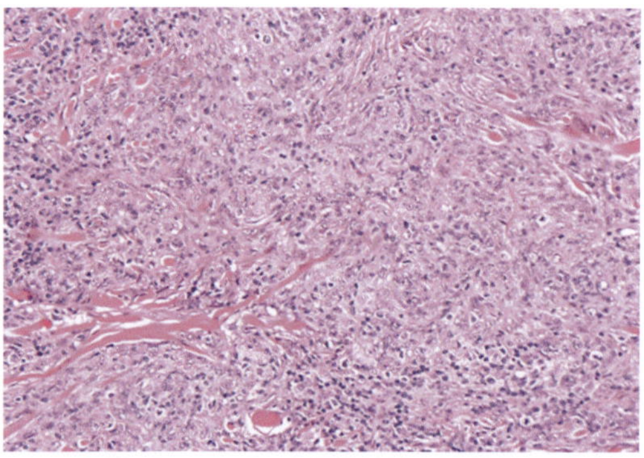

Fig. 16.218 Tumor consists almost completely of large tumor cells

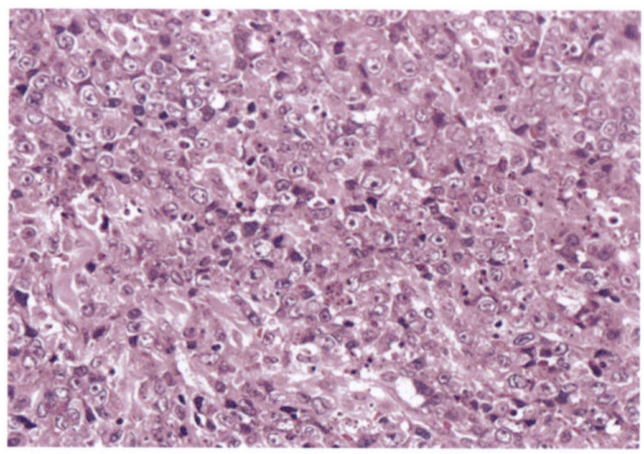

Fig. 16.219 Numerous scattered mitosis and apoptotic cells

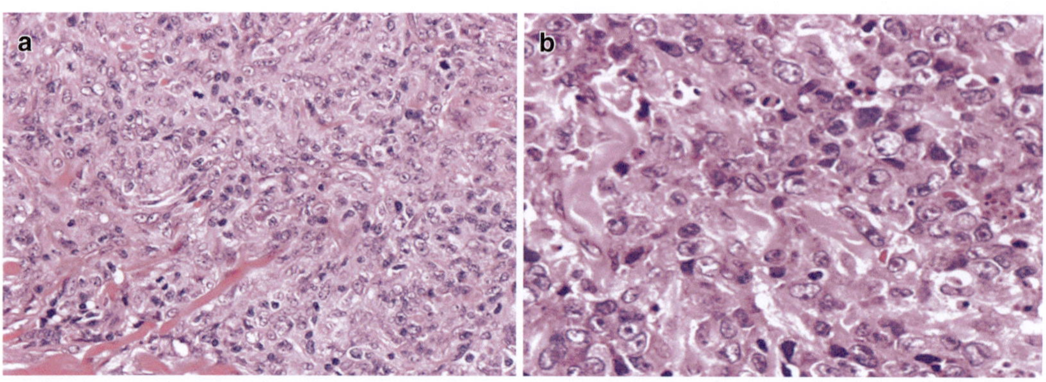

Fig. 16.220 (a, b) Large cells with atypical nuclei and only sparse reactive small lymphocytes

Primary Cutaneous Follicle Center Lymphoma

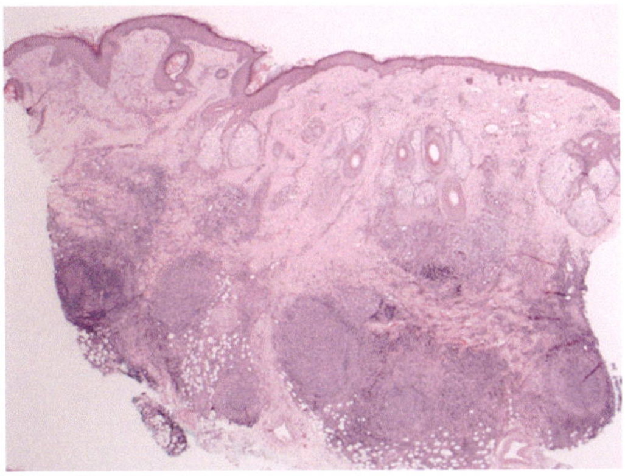

Fig. 16.221 Dermal and subcutaneous follicular lymphocytic infiltrate with sparing of the epidermis

Histopathology (Figs. 16.221, 16.222, and 16.223)

- Dermal and subcutaneous lymphocytic infiltrate
- Follicular pattern with follicles missing the mantle zone
- The diffuse pattern also exists but is much less common
- Composed of two cell types normally found in the follicular center: small to medium cells (centrocytes) and large lymphocytes (centroblasts) admixed with some normal small lymphocytes
- CD20+, CD79a+, CD10+, Bcl-6+, CD5−, CD43−, Bcl2−

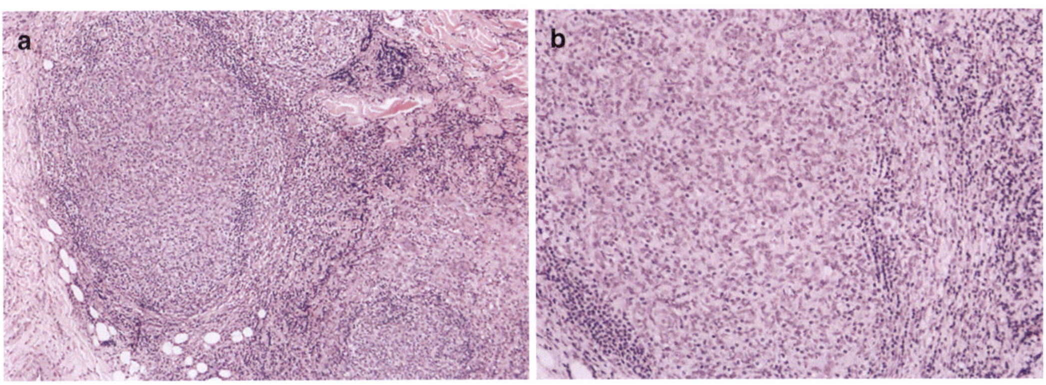

Fig. 16.222 (**a**, **b**) Follicles have reduced mantle zone. Centers are made of monomorphic cells with no tangible body macrophages. These are all atypical findings that are not seen in reactive lymphoid follicles

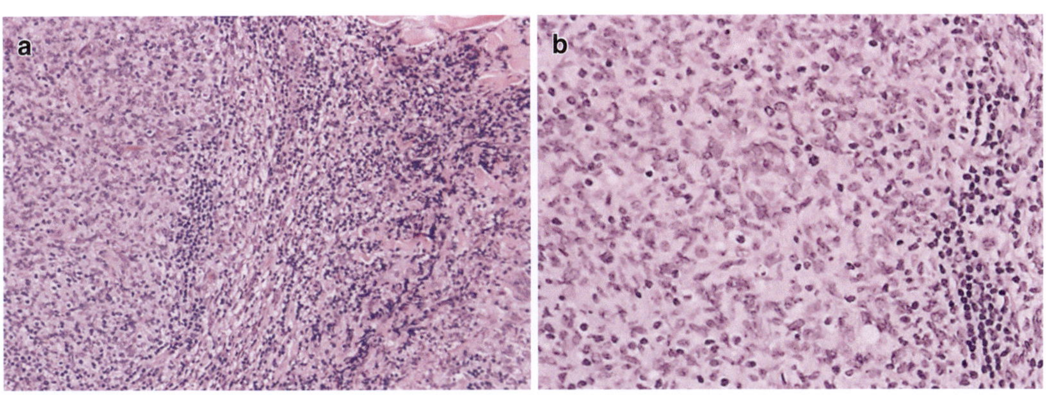

Fig. 16.223 (**a**, **b**) Small to medium cells (centrocytes) and large lymphocytes (centroblasts)

Primary Cutaneous Mantle Cell Lymphoma

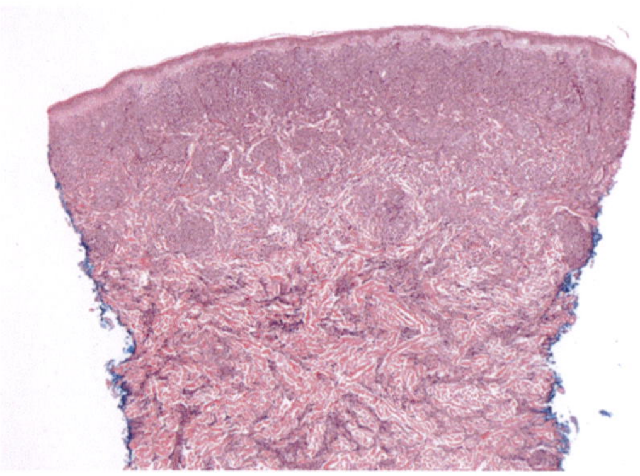

Fig. 16.224 Diffuse infiltrate of dermis and subcutis

Very rarely primary and mostly secondary skin involvement.

Histopathology (Figs. 16.224, 16.225, and 16.226)

- Diffuse lymphocytic infiltrate of dermis and subcutis
- Small to medium sized lymphocytes with irregular nuclei
- IHC is required to confirm diagnosis
- The cells are CD5+, CD20+, cyclin D1 +, Bcl6−, CD10−, CD23−

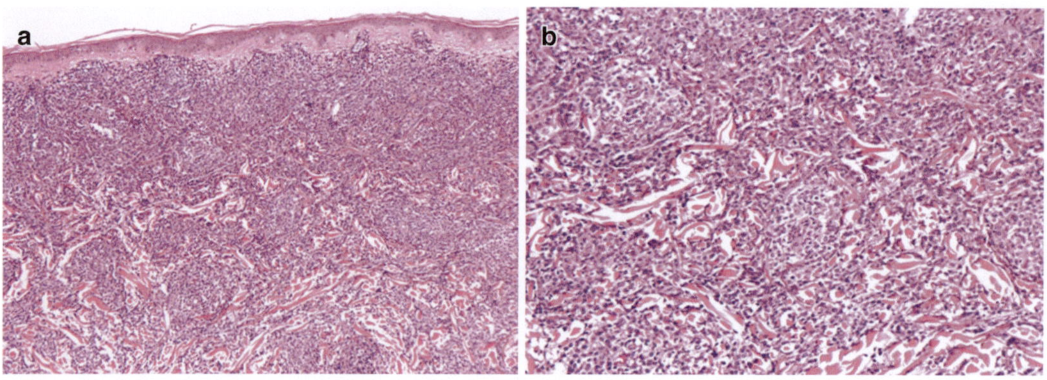

Fig. 16.225 (**a**, **b**) Monotonous infiltrate completely destroys adnexal structures but does not infiltrate the epidermis

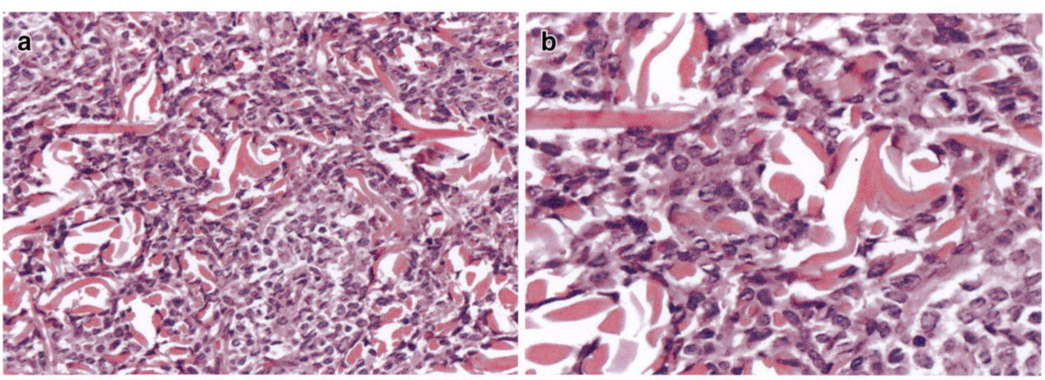

Fig. 16.226 (**a**, **b**) Cells are small to medium sized with irregular nuclei and scattered mitoses

Primary Cutaneous Marginal Zone Lymphoma

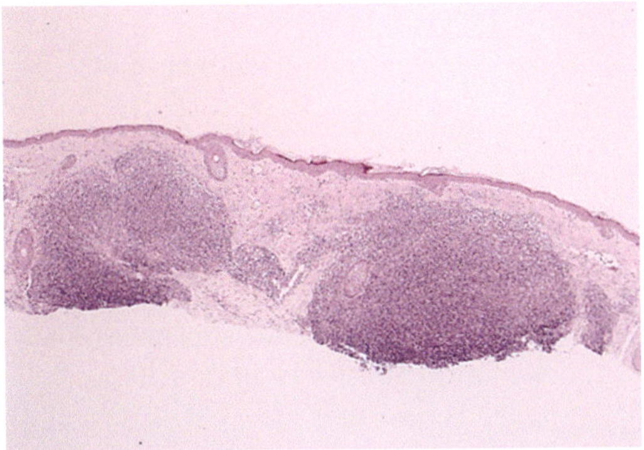

Fig. 16.227 Multinodular dermal infiltrate

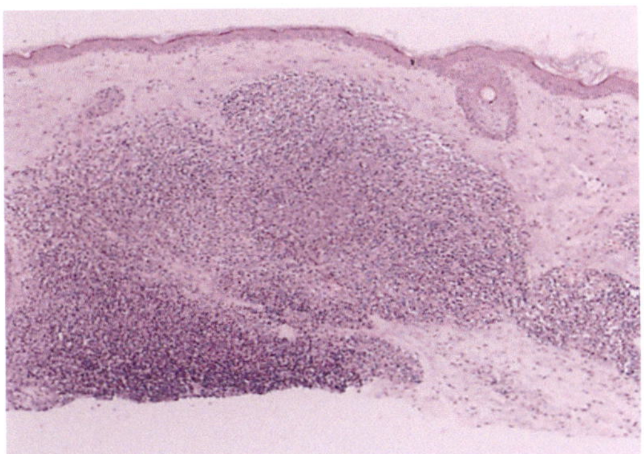

Fig. 16.228 Vague germinal center is present in the central nodule

Histopathology (Figs. 16.227, 16.228, and 16.229)

- Dense dermal nodular infiltrate
- Infiltrate with vague pale germinal centers surrounded by dark small lymphocytes and, more peripherally, with pale neoplastic marginal zone lymphocytes
- Neoplastic cells are atypical and mitoses can be seen
- Germinal centers can be present within the nodule
- The marginal zone cells are CD20+, CD79a+, Bcl6−, CD5−, CD10−, CD23−

P.S. in lymphoplasmocytic variant (primary cutaneous plasmacytoma), associated with *Borrelia burgdorferi* infection, neoplastic plasma cells are admixed with marginal zone cells

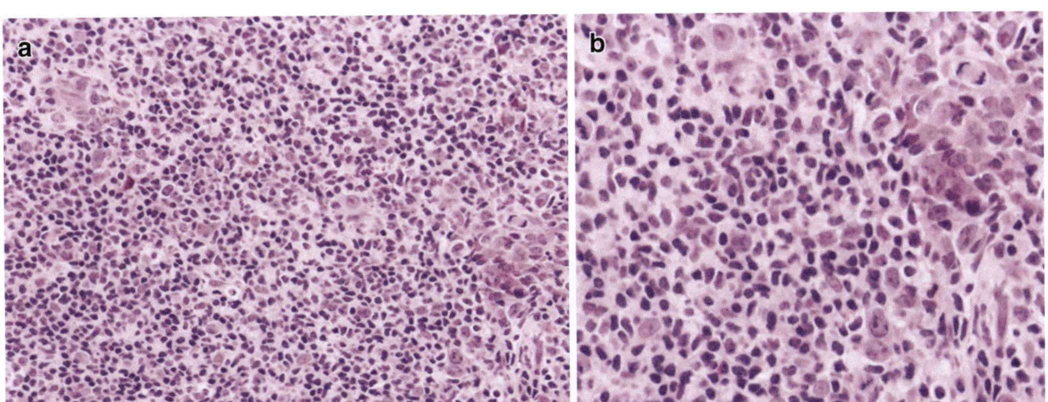

Fig. 16.229 (**a**, **b**) Dark cells of the follicular mantle surrounded with neoplastic large pale marginal zone cells. Neoplastic cells are pleomorphic with scattered mitosis

Proliferating Epidermal Inclusion Cyst

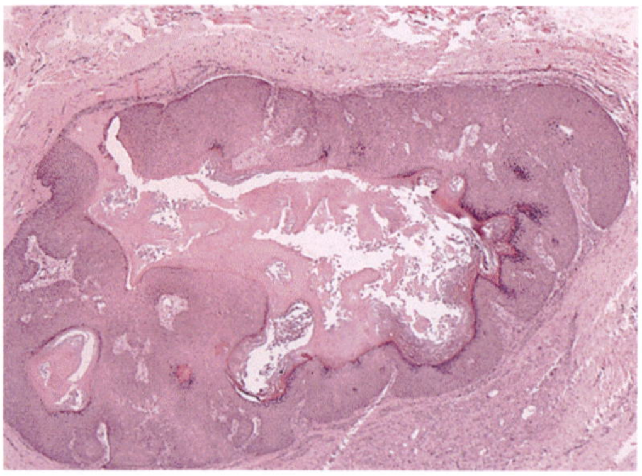

Fig. 16.230 Cyst lined with squamous epithelium

Synonym: Proliferating Epidermoid Cyst

Histopathology (Figs. 16.230, 16.231, and 16.232)

- Epidermal inclusion cyst lined with squamous epithelium with granular layer
- Proliferating sheaths of squamous epithelium grow mostly inward into cyst lumen but can also grow outward pushing into surrounding connective tissue
- No cytological atypia, necrosis, or mitoses

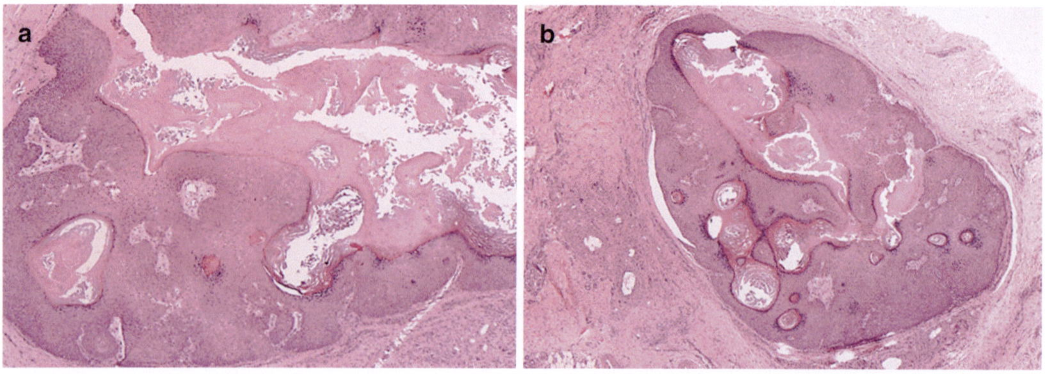

Fig. 16.231 (**a**, **b**) Epidermal inclusion cyst with squamous epithelium growing into the lumen of the cyst

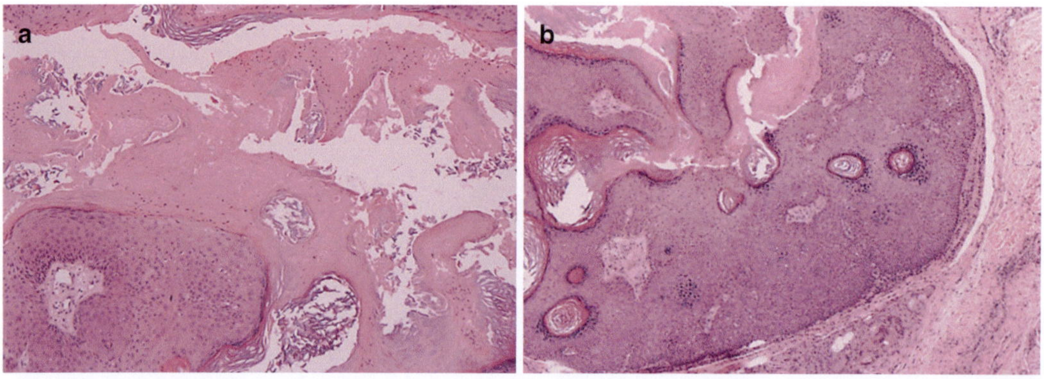

Fig. 16.232 (**a**, **b**) Epithelium has granular layer and there is no evidence of atypia

Proliferating Pilar Cyst

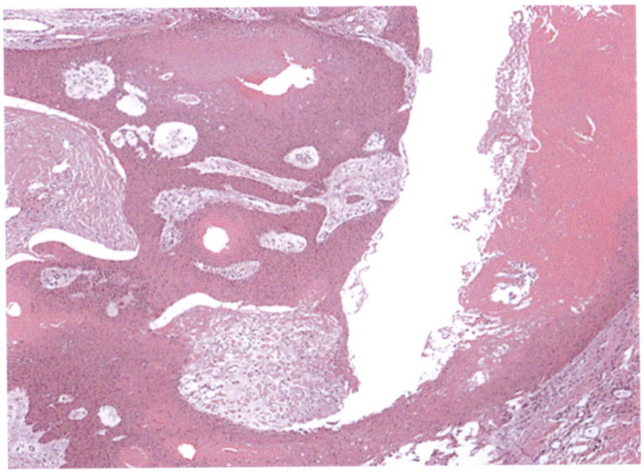

Fig. 16.233 Pilar cyst with proliferating sheaths of squamous epithelium showing pushing borders

Synonym: Proliferating Trichilemmal Cyst

Histopathology (Figs. 16.233, 16.234, 16.235, 16.236, and 16.237)

- Arising from pilar cyst
- Nests of squamous epithelium extending into the adjacent connective tissue and inward into the cyst lumen
- Areas of trichilemmal keratinization characterized by absence of the granular layer can be easily identified
- Cytological atypia vary from minimal to severe

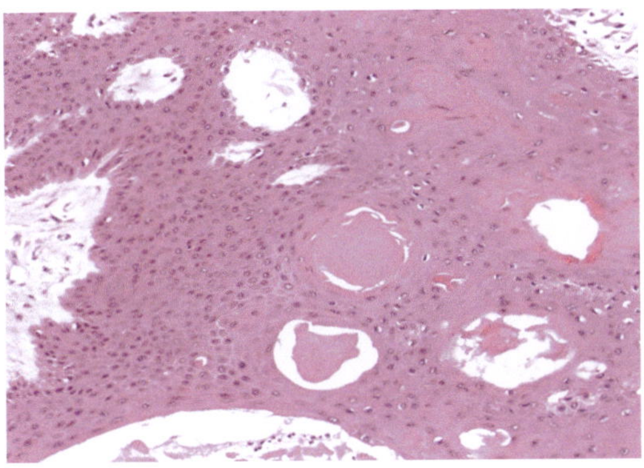

Fig. 16.234 Benign proliferating pilar cyst

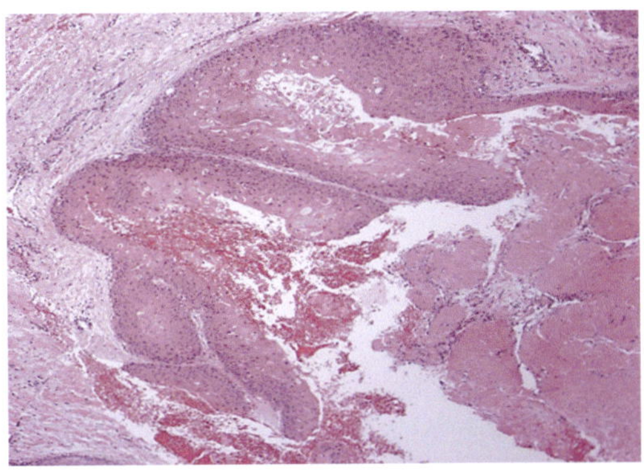

Fig. 16.235 Malignant proliferating pilar tumor with central necrosis

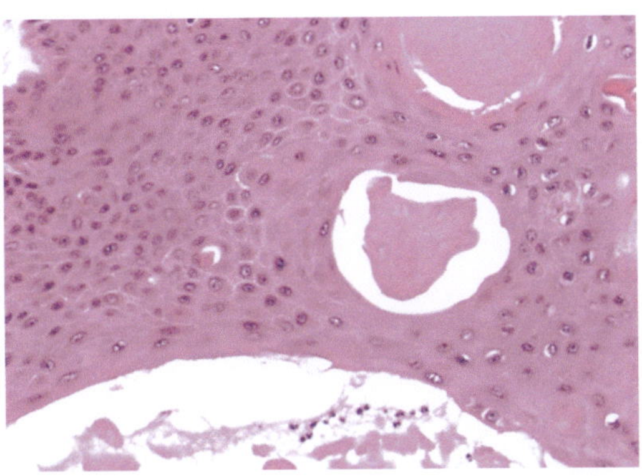

Fig. 16.236 Uniform cells with no atypia or mitoses; easily identified trichilemmal keratinization

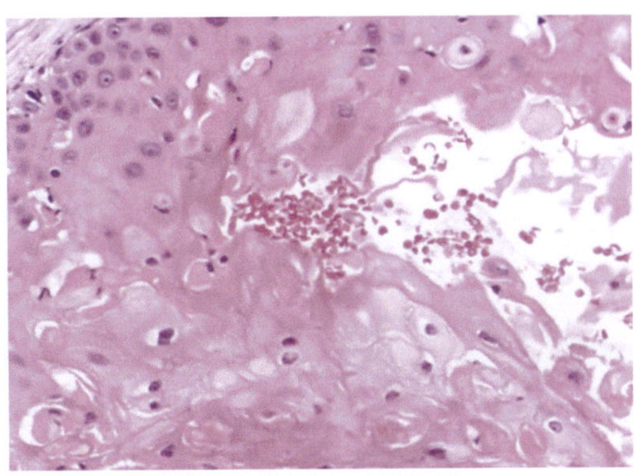

Fig. 16.237 Cytological atypia and mitoses

Progressive Nodular Histiocytosis

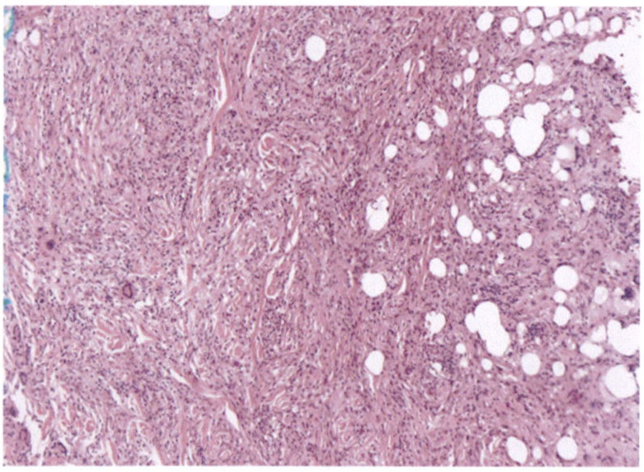

Fig. 16.238 Poorly defined infiltrating tumor

Histopathological findings are between *cellular dermatofibroma* and *xanthogranuloma* (Figs. 16.238, 16.239, 16.240, 16.241, and 16.242)

- Dermal and subcutaneous dense tumor
- Areas made of spindle cell histiocytes organized in vague storiform pattern resembling *cellular dermatofibroma*
- Areas made of vacuolated and anthomatized cells, giant cells and histiocytes resembling *xanthogranuloma*

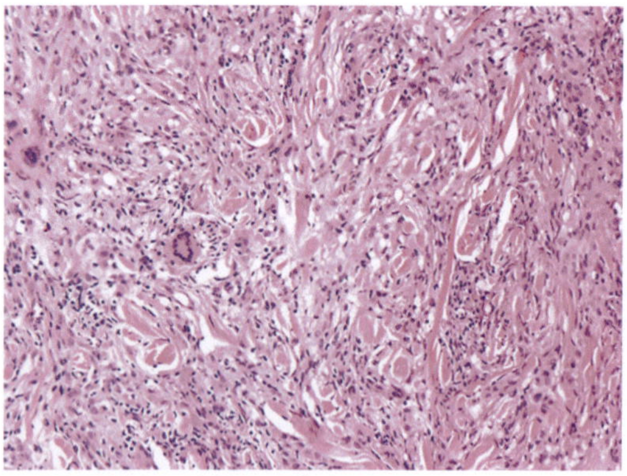

Fig. 16.239 Xanthogranuloma-like area

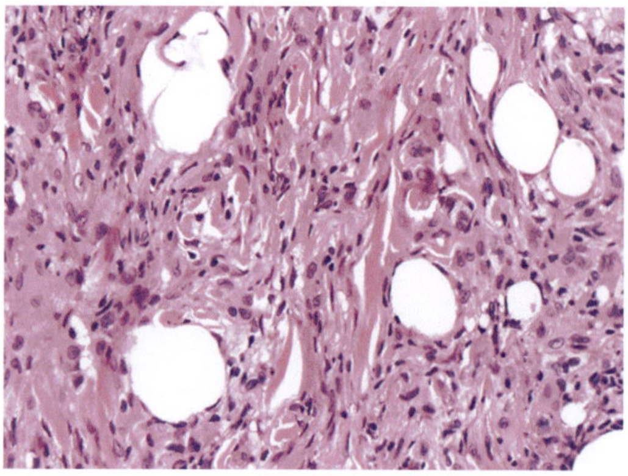

Fig. 16.240 Cellular dermatofibroma-like area

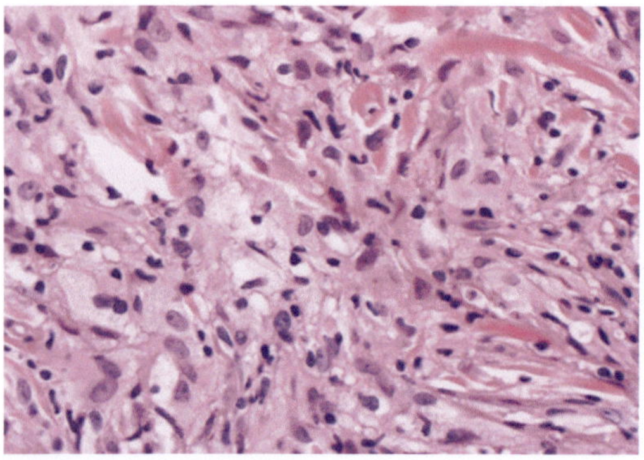

Fig. 16.241 Xanthoma cells, vacuolated histiocytes and giant cells

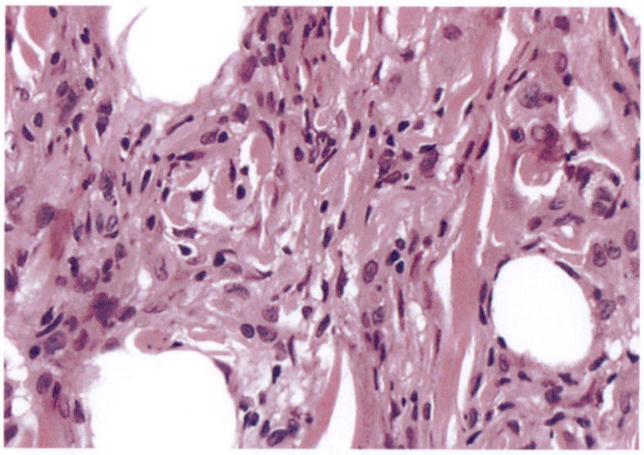

Fig. 16.242 Spindle and epithelioid foamy histiocytes with trapped collagen

Protothecosis

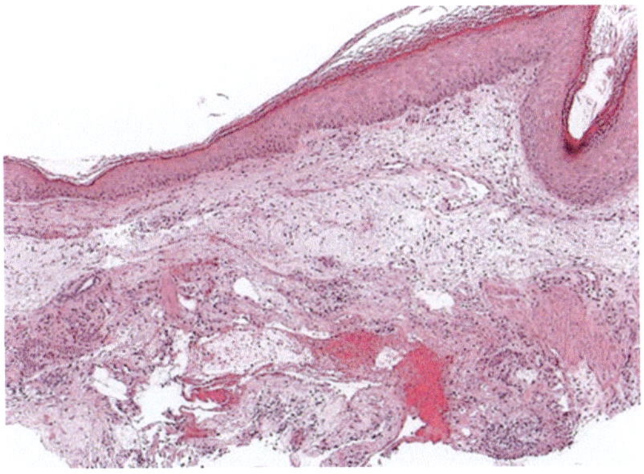

Fig. 16.243 Subcutanous inflammation

Histopathology (Figs. 16.243, 16.244, 16.245, and 16.246)

- Cutaneous inflammation vary from minimal to granulomatous inflammation with admixed lymphocytes, plasma cells, and some neutrophils
- Focal necrosis can be seen
- Pleomorphic *Prototheca* algae organisms are present
- Septation and morula formation in "daisy" form

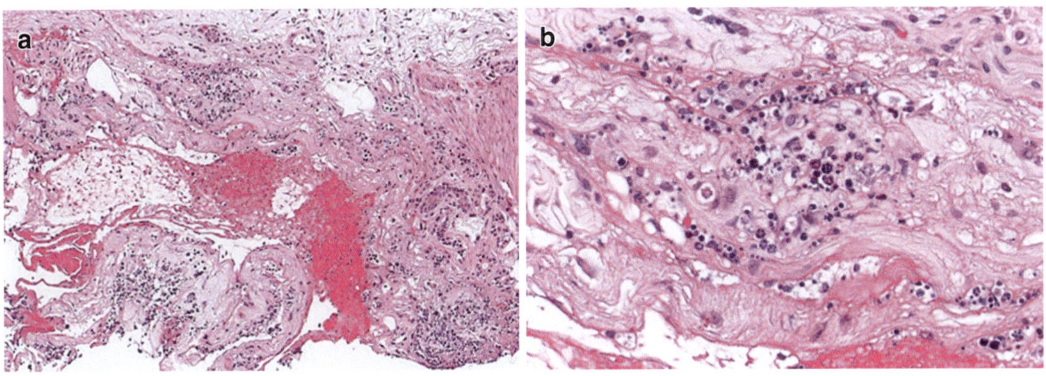

Fig. 16.244 (**a**, **b**) Necrosis with mixed inflammation

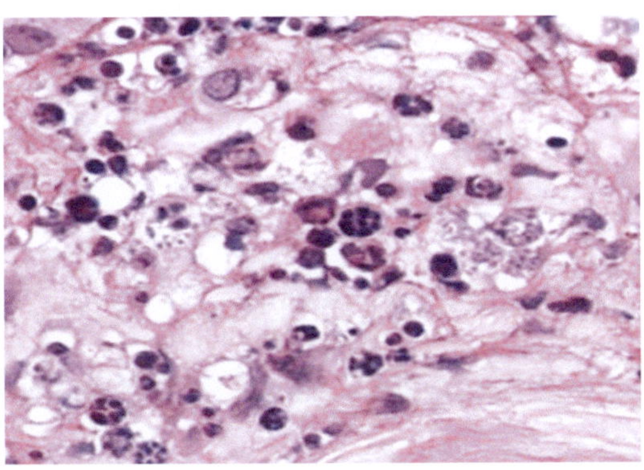

Fig. 16.245 Spherical *Prototheca* bodies are present

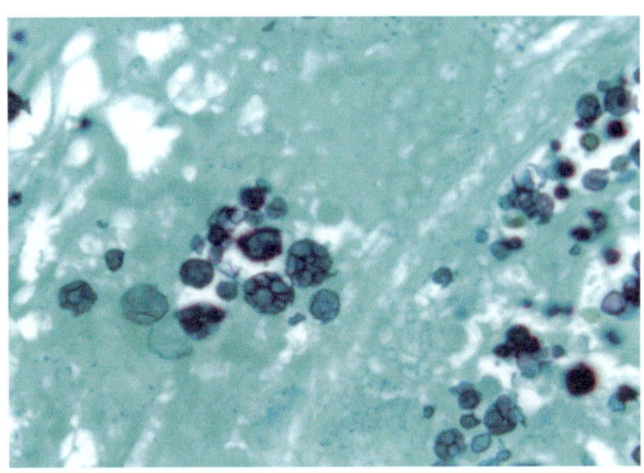

Fig. 16.246 GMS stain highlights morula formations in "daisy" shape

Prurigo Nodularis

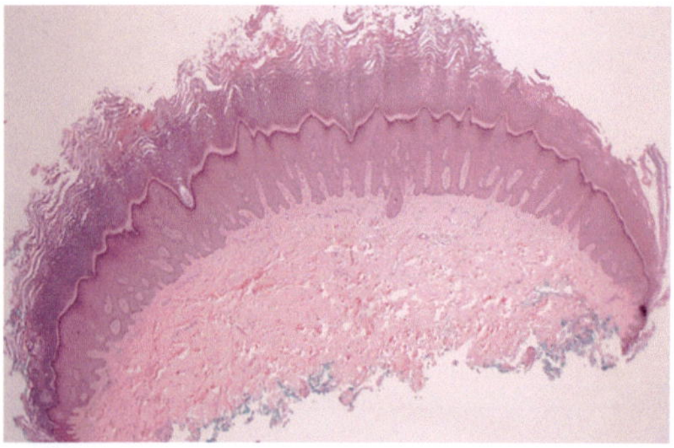

Fig. 16.247 Dome shaped lesion

Synonym: Picker's Nodule

Histopathology (Figs. 16.247, 16.248, 16.249, 16.250, and 16.251)

- Dome shaped lesion
- Architecture varies from regular acanthotic epidermis with hyperkeratosis and hypergranulosis to irregular epidermis with pseudoepitheliomatous hyperplasia
- Papillary dermal fibrosis and mild perivascular lymphocytic infiltrate

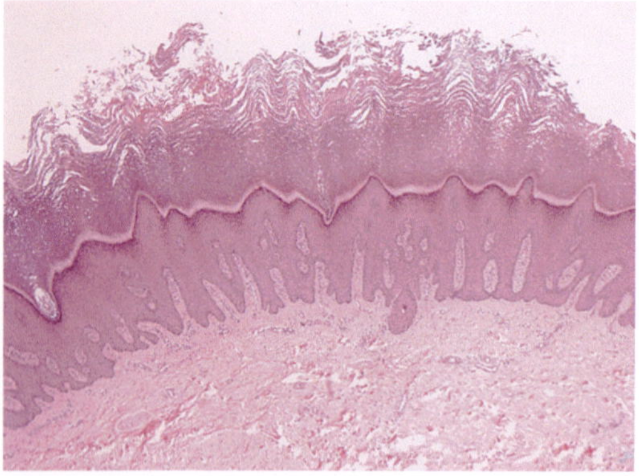

Fig. 16.248 Epidermal papillomatosis and hyperkeratosis

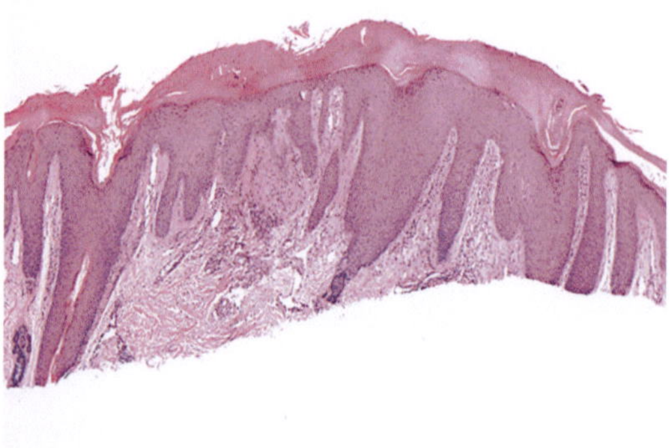

Fig. 16.249 Irregular pseudoepitheliomatous hyperplasia

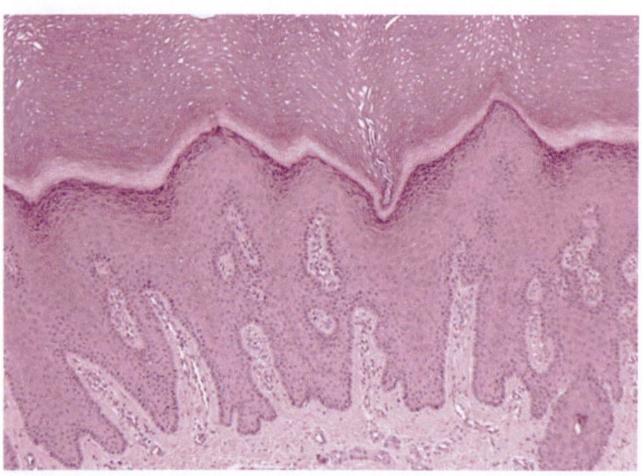

Fig. 16.250 Epidermal hypergranulosis and dermal fibrosis

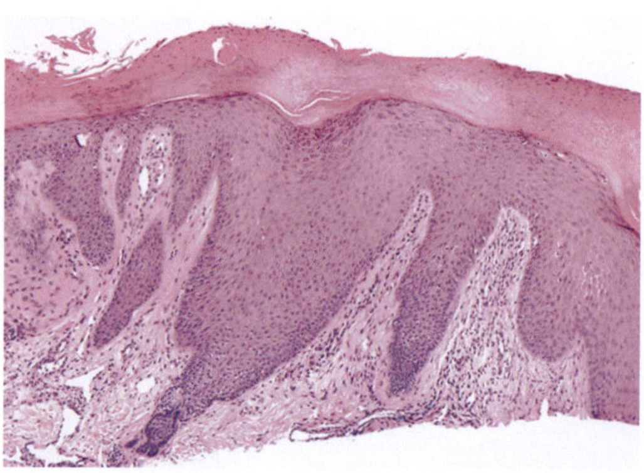

Fig. 16.251 Dermal fibrosis and mild inflammation

Pruritic Papules of HIV

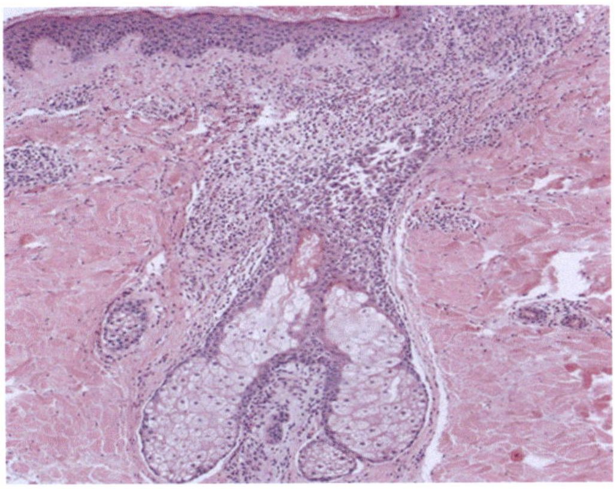

Fig. 16.252 HIV associated eosinophilic folliculitis

Synonym: Papular Eruption of HIV

Histopathological finding are not specific (Figs. 16.252, 16.253, 16.254, 16.255, and 16.256)

- Epidermal spongiosis
- Epidermal hyperkeratosis and parakeratosis in older lesions
- Perivascular lymphocytic infiltrate with variable number of eosinophils
- Commonly accompanied by eosinophilic folliculitis

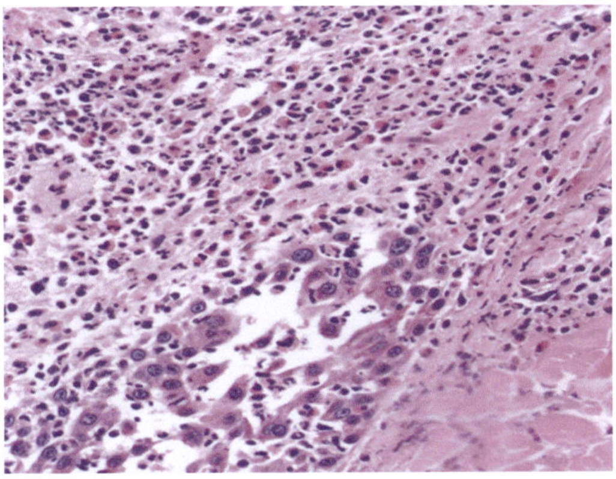

Fig. 16.253 Dense perifollicular inflammation

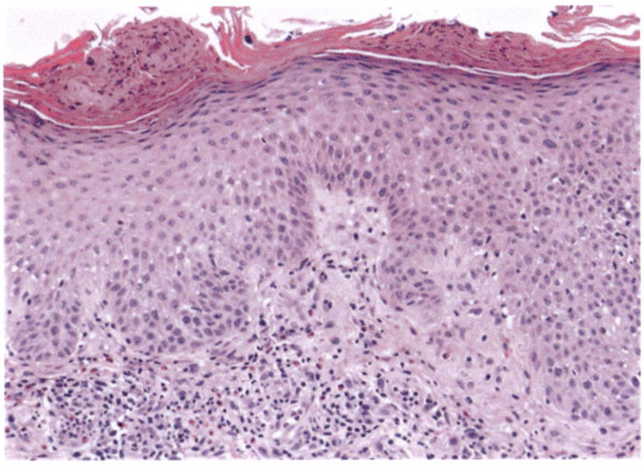

Fig. 16.254 Hyperkeratotic spongiotic epidermis with parakeratosis

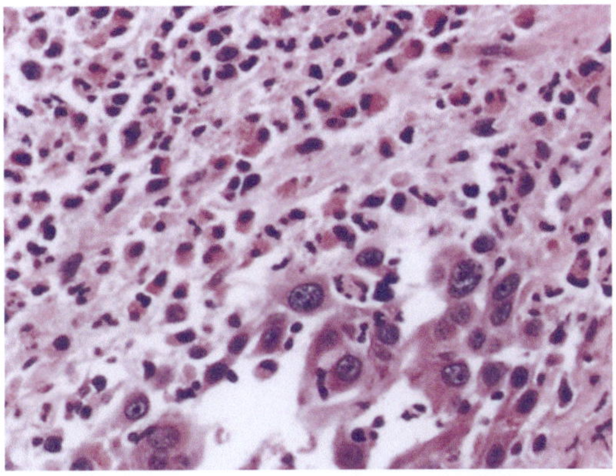

Fig. 16.255 Numerous perifollicular eosinophils

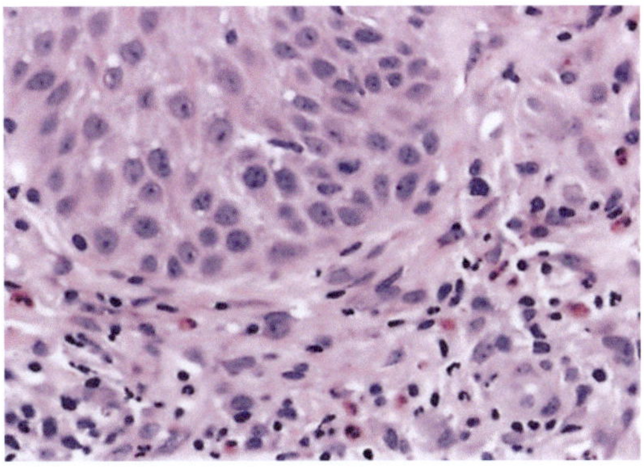

Fig. 16.256 Perivascular lymphocytic infiltrate with eosinophils

Pruritic Urticarial Papules and Plaques of Pregnancy

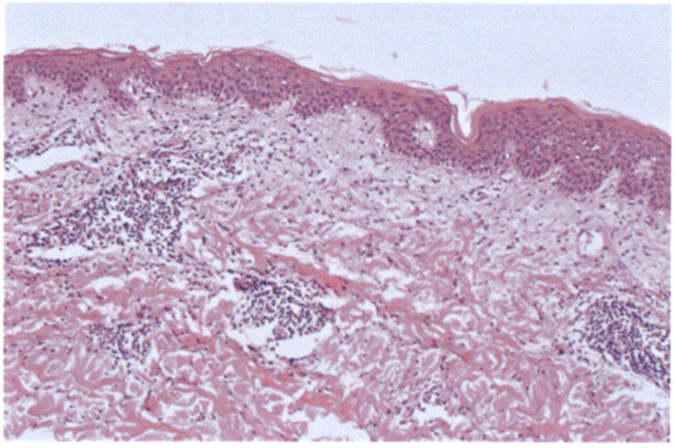

Fig. 16.257 Dermal edema and inflammation

Synonyms: Toxic Erythema of Pregnancy, Polymorphous Eruption of Pregnancy, Late Onset Prurigo of Pregnancy

Histopathology is not specific (Figs. 16.257, 16.258, and 16.259)

- Mild epidermal spongiosis that can form vesicles
- Mild dermal edema with mild perivascular lymphocytic infiltrate
- Perivascular and interstitial dermal eosinophils

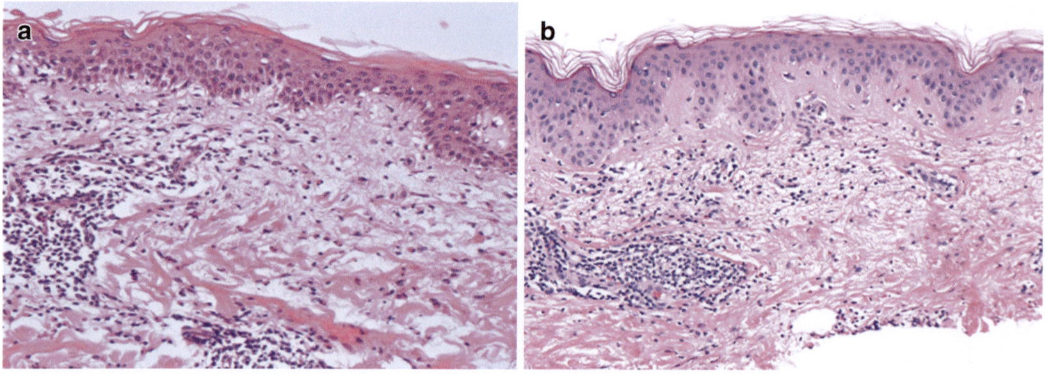

Fig. 16.258 (**a**, **b**) Mild epidermal spongiosis with mild dermal edema and perivascular lymphocytic infiltrate

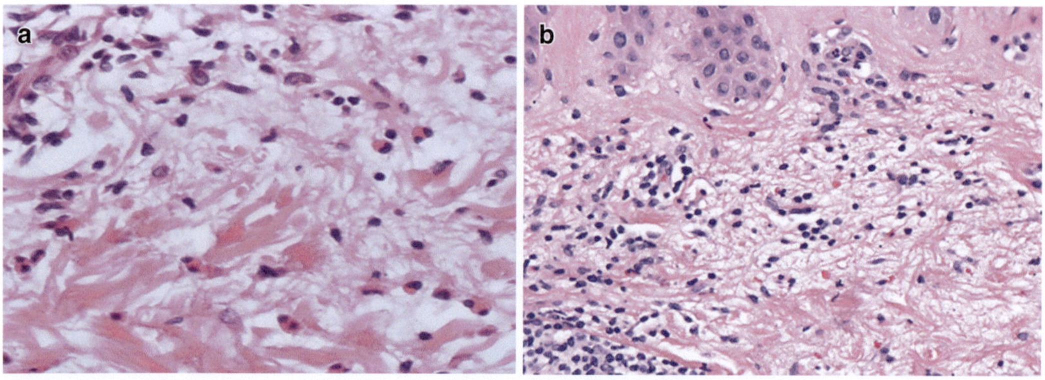

Fig. 16.259 (**a**, **b**) Perivascular and interstitial eosinophils are present

Pseudocyst of Auricle

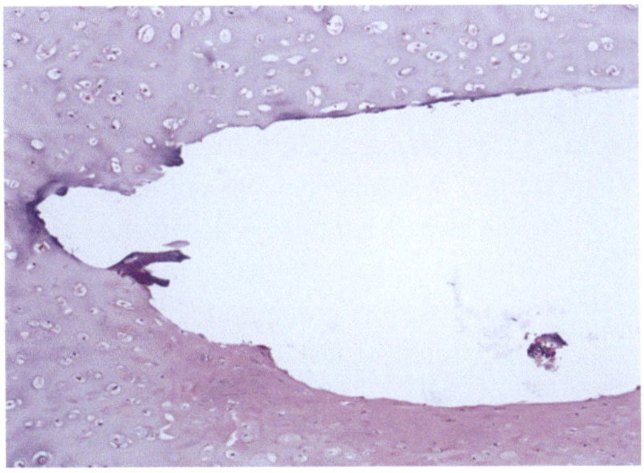

Fig. 16.260 Empty space within cartilage

Histopathology (Figs. 16.260, 16.261, and 16.262)

- Pseudocyst with no epithelial lining within the ear cartilage
- No inflammation
- Adjacent chondrocytes are focally degenerated
- The lumen is empty or filled with serous pink fluid

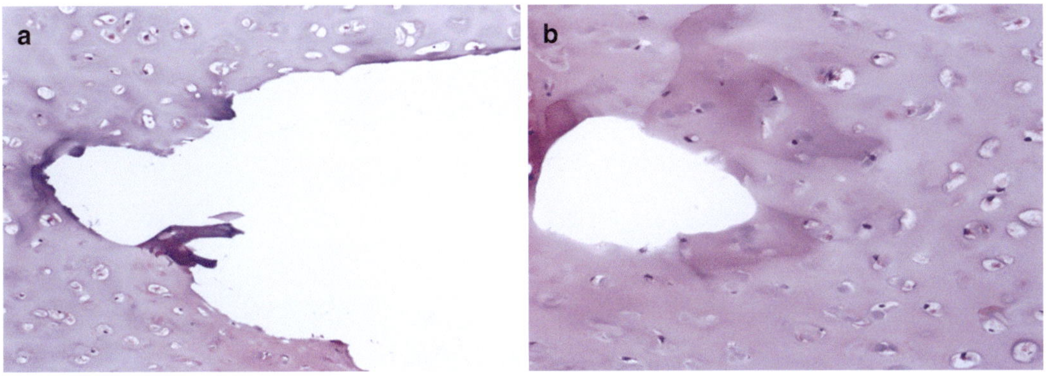

Fig. 16.261 (**a**, **b**) Intracartilaginous empty space with no epithelial lining

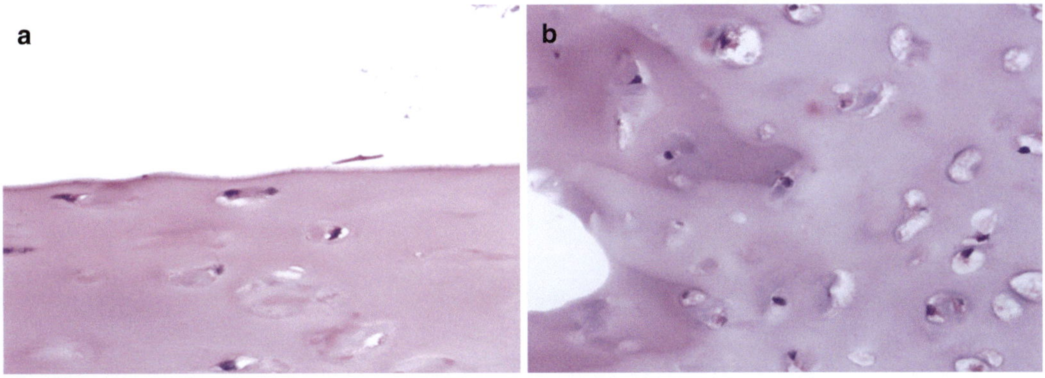

Fig. 16.262 (**a**, **b**) Chondrocytes appears degenerated with dark nuclei

Pseudolymphoma

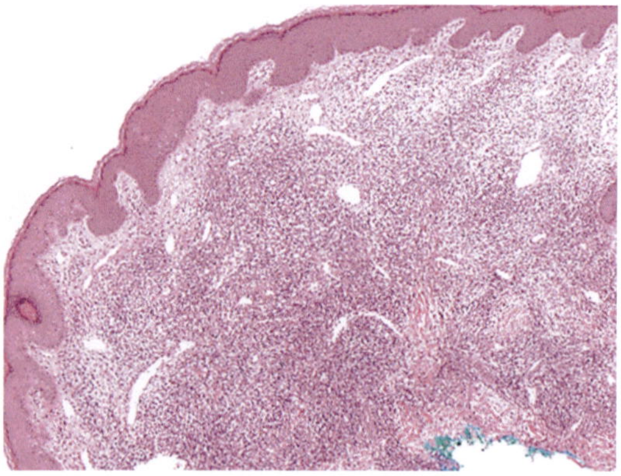

Fig. 16.263 Dense dermal and subcutaneous inflammation without epidermotropism

Synonym: Cutaneous Lymphoid Hyperplasia

Histopathology (Figs. 16.263, 16.264, 16.265, 16.266, and 16.267)

- Dermal and subcutaneous admixture of T and B cell lymphocytes with no epidermal involvement
- Additional cells give a hint to the cause
- Eosinophils suggest drug reaction
- Neutrophils and loose keratin flakes suggest a reaction to ruptured follicle/cyst
- Eosinophils and neutrophils suggest insect bite
- Plasma cells suggest *Borrelia* infection

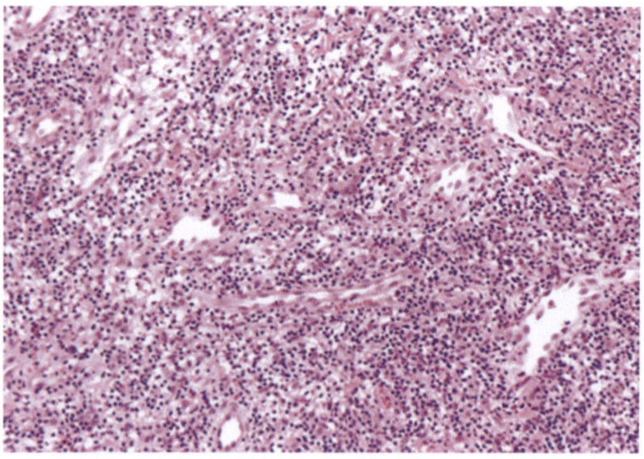

Fig. 16.264 Numerous eosinophils are admixed with lymphocytes, histiocytes, and reactive endothelial cells

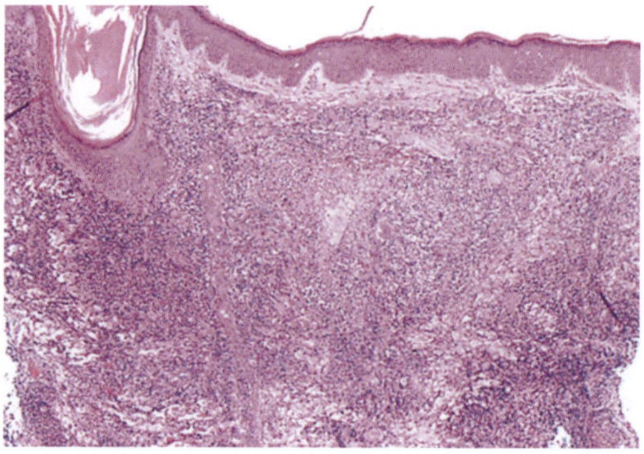

Fig. 16.265 Dense perifollicular lymphocytic infiltrate with neutrophils and few giants cells around dilated follicle

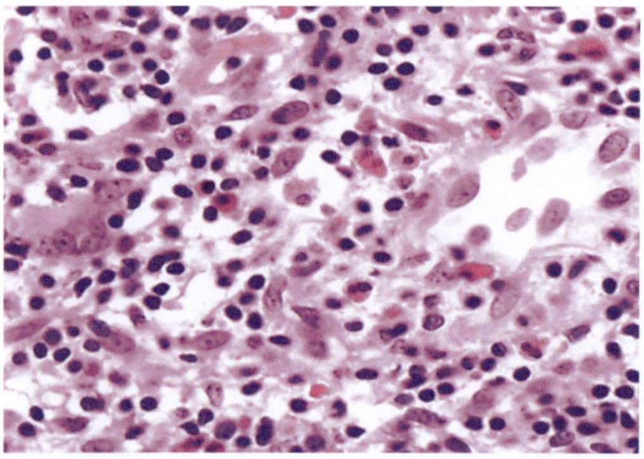

Fig. 16.266 Eosinophils are suggesting drug reaction or insect bite

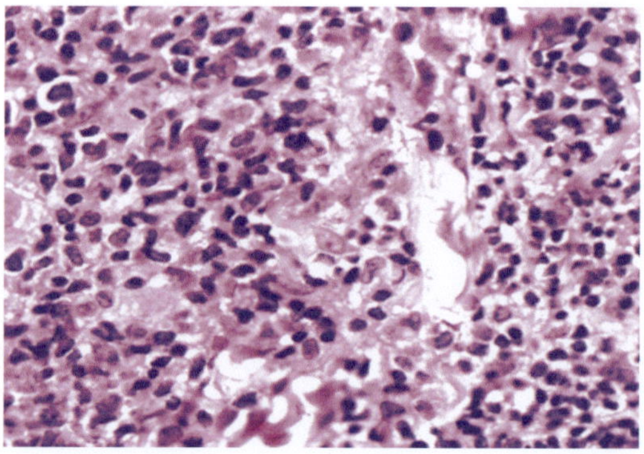

Fig. 16.267 Keratin flakes suggest a reaction to a ruptured follicle

Pseudopelade of Brocq

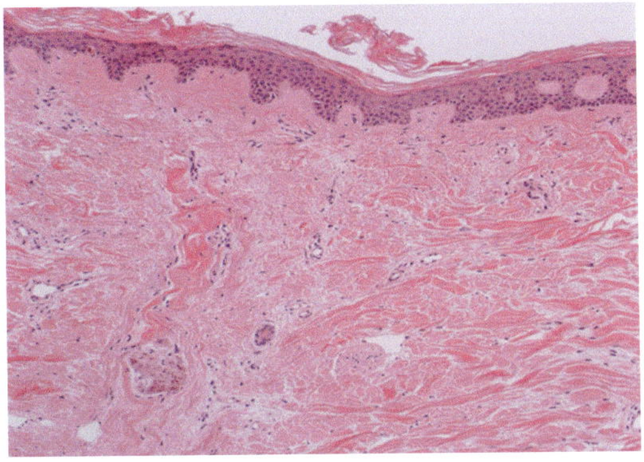

Fig. 16.268 Established lesion presents as scarring alopecia with absence of hair follicles and sebaceous glands

Synonym: Idiopathic Scarring Alopecia

Histopathology (Figs. 16.268, 16.269, 16.270, 16.271, and 16.272)

- Early lesions: mild perifollicular lymphocytic infiltrate in the upper portion of the follicle
- Concentric fibrosis surrounds hair follicle
- Established lesions: loss of hair follicle and sebaceous glands
- Fibrous stellae extend above and below pilar muscle

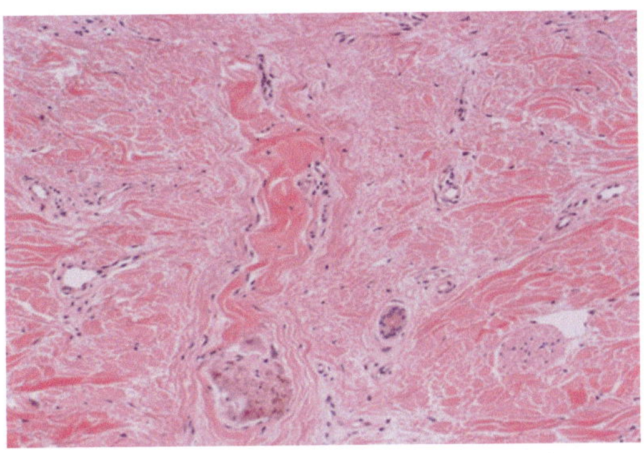

Fig. 16.269 Fibrous stella has replaced hair follicle

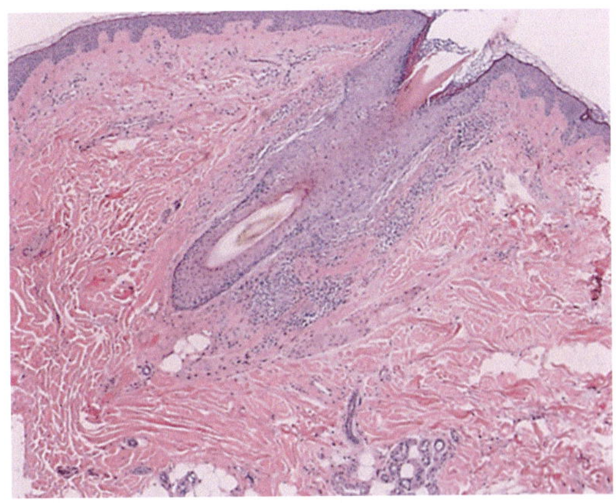

Fig. 16.270 Early lesion with inflammation

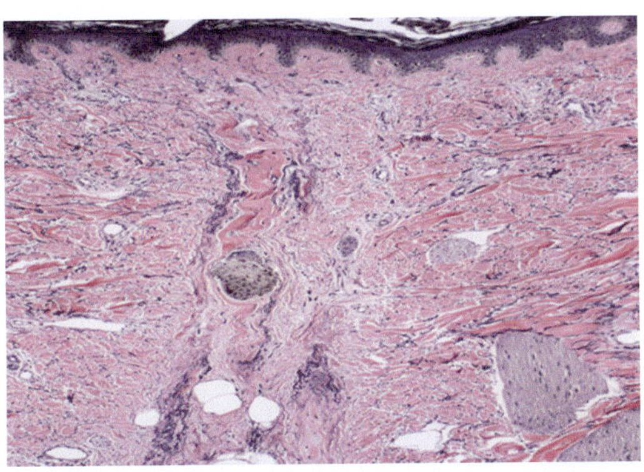

Fig. 16.271 VVG stain outlines elastic fibers that are preserved and thickened around the fibrous band

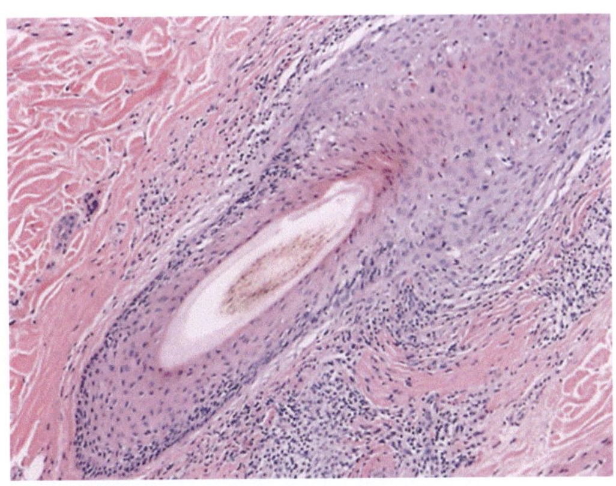

Fig. 16.272 Perifollicular lymphocytic infiltrate with formation of concentric fibrosis

Pseudoporhyria

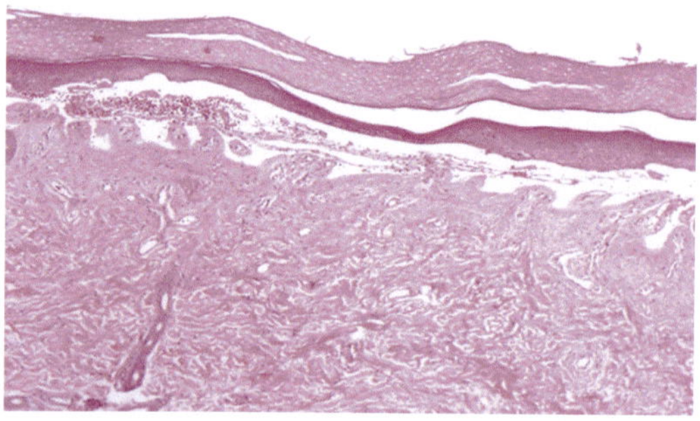

Fig. 16.273 Subepidermal "cell poor" blister

Synonym: Bullous Dermatosis of Hemodialysis

Histopathology is indistinguishable from *porphyria cutanea tarda* (Figs. 16.273, 16.274, 16.275, 16.276, and 16.277)

- Subepidermal blister with no inflammatory cells
- The bottom of the blister has dermal papillae in "festooning" pattern
- Dermal vessels are thickened
- Dermal solar elastosis is present

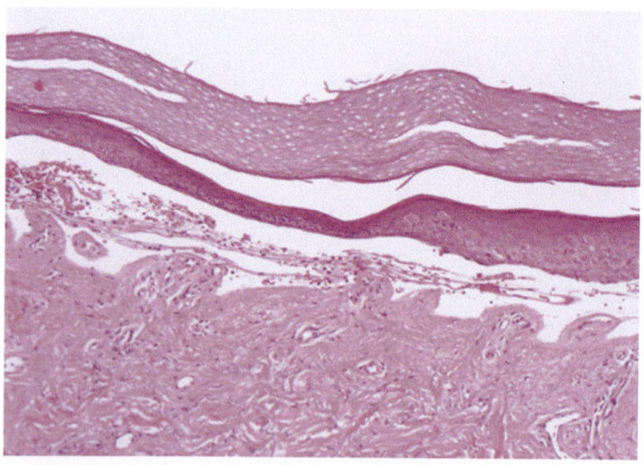

Fig. 16.274 Some fibrin and red blood cells are present within the blister wall

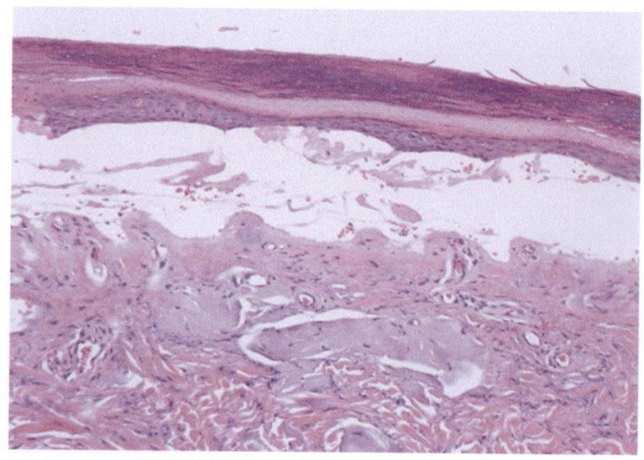

Fig. 16.275 Extensive dermal solar elastosis

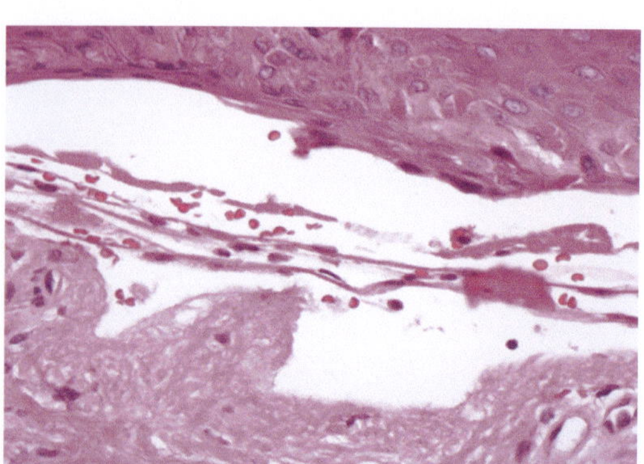

Fig. 16.276 Dermal papillae in "festooning" pattern

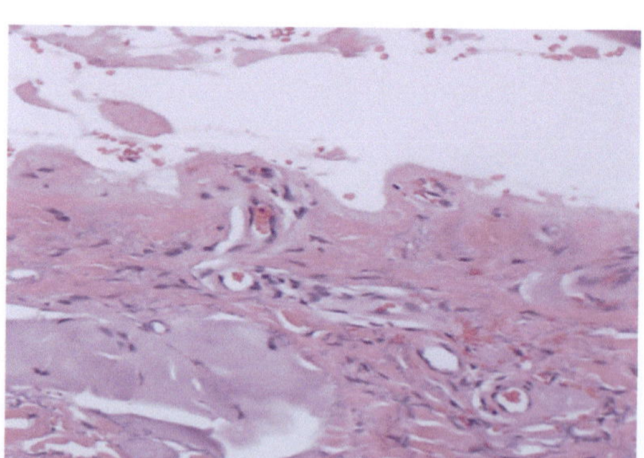

Fig. 16.277 Dermal blood vessels with thickened wall

Pseudoxanthoma Elasticum

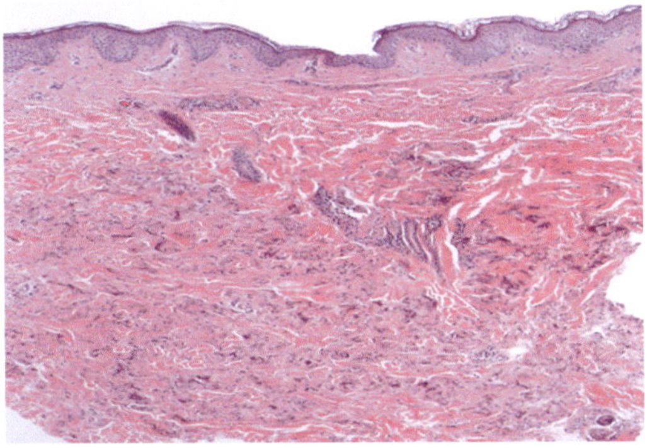

Fig. 16.278 Eosinophilic granular material in the middle and lower dermis

Synonym: Grönblad-Strandberg Syndrome

Histopathology (Figs. 16.278, 16.279, and 16.280)

- Numerous dermal fragmented purple elastic fibers in the middle and lower dermis
- Elastic fibers are short, thickened, curled, irregular, and haphazardly organized
- Calcium deposits are present on elastic fibers (Von Kossa stain)

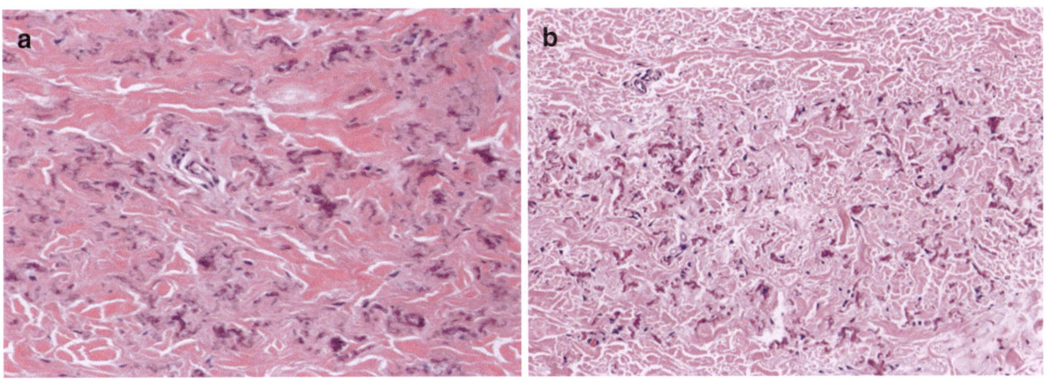

Fig. 16.279 (**a**, **b**) Haphazardly organized irregular, fragmented and thickened elastic fibers

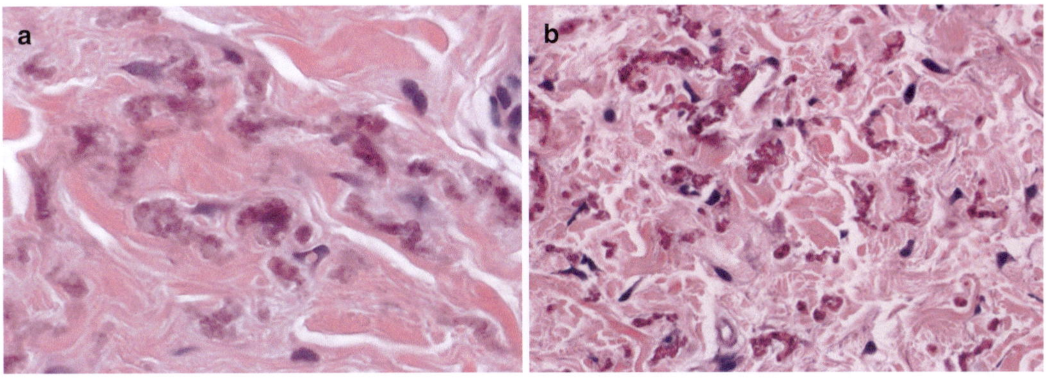

Fig. 16.280 (**a**, **b**) Calcium deposits (dark purple) are present on the top of elastic fibers

Psoriasis

Histopathology of Psoriasis Vulgaris (Figs. 16.281 and 16.282)

- Regular epidermal psoriasiform hyperplasia
- Hyperkeratosis with mounds of parakeratosis (early lesions) or confluent parakeratosis (established lesions)
- Loss of granular layer with thinning of suprapapillary epidermis
- Neutrophils within stratum corneum (Munro's microabscess) and within stratum spinosum (Kogoj's pustules)
- Dilated capillaries in the papillary dermis

Histopathology of Pustular Psoriasis (Figs. 16.283, 16.284, and 16.285)

- Intraepidermal pustules of Kogoj
- In early lesions pustule is surrounded with spongiotic epidermis
- In established lesion pustule is surrounded with psoriasiform epidermis with hypogranulosis

Histopathology of Guttate Psoriasis: (Figs. 16.286, 16.287, and 16.288)

- Epidermal mound of parakeratosis with admixed neutrophils
- Epidermis is less psoriasiform and more spongiotic

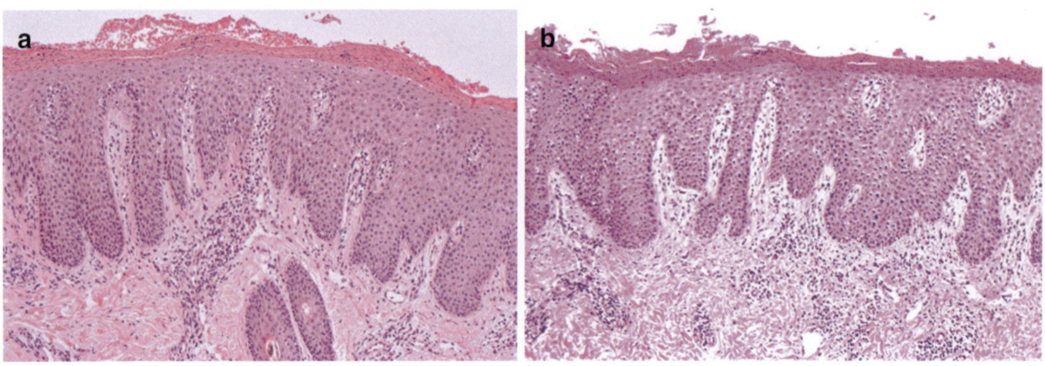

Fig. 16.281 (**a**, **b**) **Psoriasis Vulgaris** with regular epidermal psoriasiform papillomatosis with thin suprapapillary epidermis

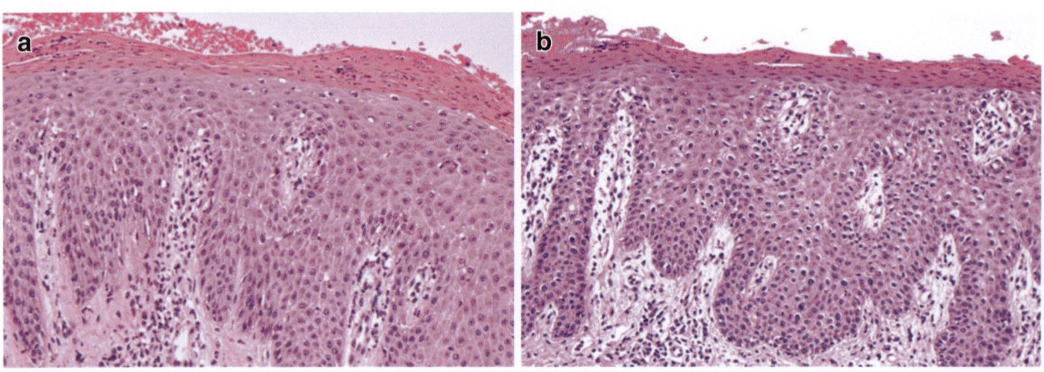

Fig. 16.282 (**a**, **b**) Epidermal parakeratosis with intracorneal neutrophils. Stratum granulosum is absent. Papillary dermal capillaries are dilated

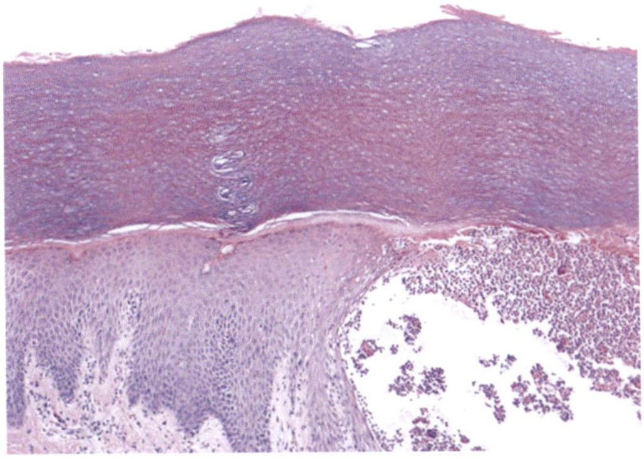

Fig. 16.283 **Palmo-plantar pustular psoriasis**: pustule arising in psoriasiform acral skin

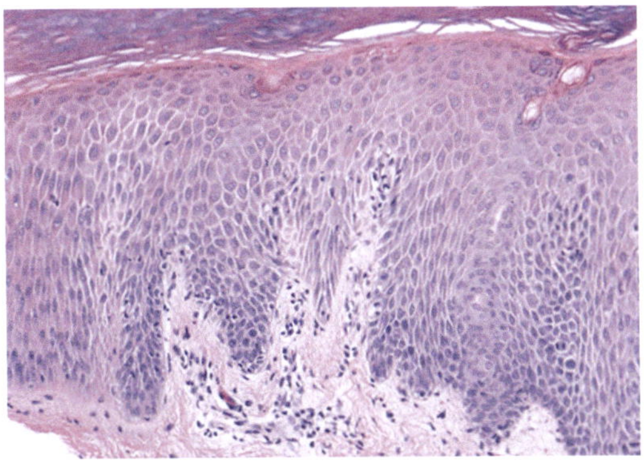

Fig. 16.284 At the lateral edge of the pustule the epidermis is psoriasiform with an absence of granular layer

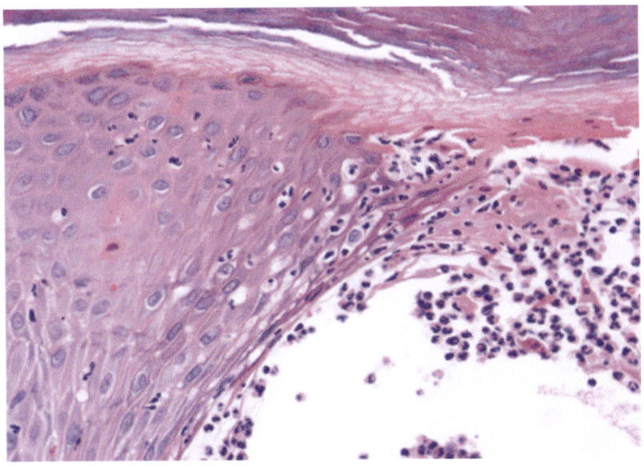

Fig. 16.285 Intraepidermal neutrophilic pustule

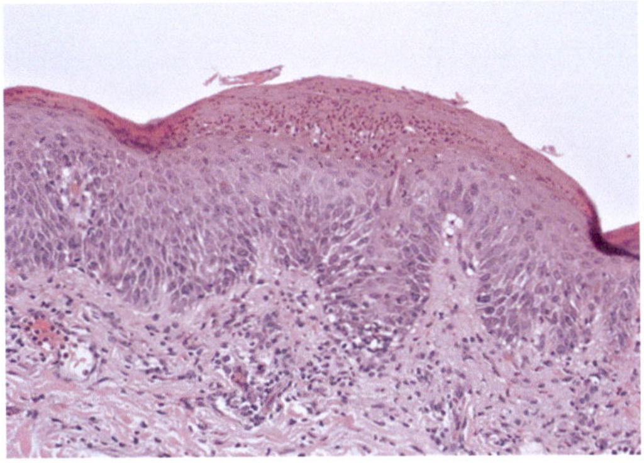

Fig. 16.286 **Guttate psoriasis**: mild psoriasiform hyperplasia

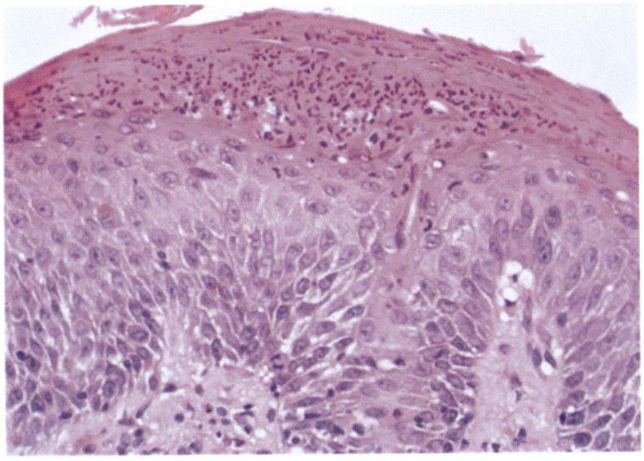

Fig. 16.287 Intraepidermal neutrophilic aggregate

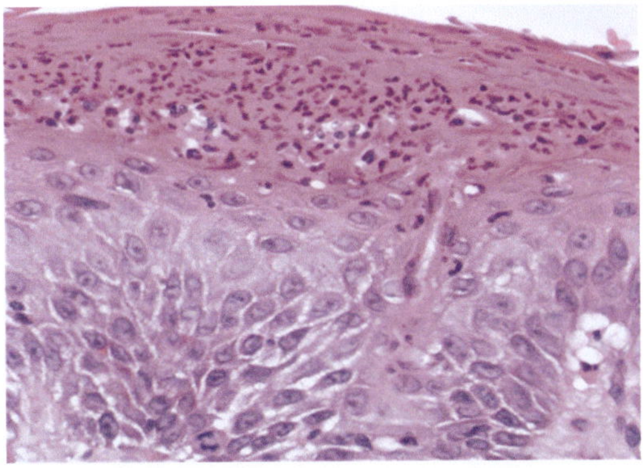

Fig. 16.288 Neutrophilic pustule within parakeratosis

Purpura Fulminans

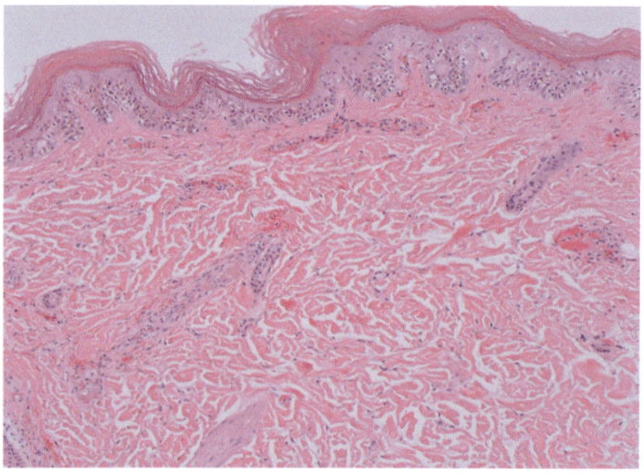

Fig. 16.289 Dermal and subcutaneous thrombi

Synonym: Disseminated Intravascular Coagulation

Histopathology (Figs. 16.289, 16.290, 16.291, 16.292, and 16.293)

- Numerous dermal and subcutaneous thrombi
- Mild perivascular lymphocytic infiltrate
- Dermal red blood cell extravasation
- Epidermal necrosis varying from occasional necrotic keratinocytes to full thickness necrosis

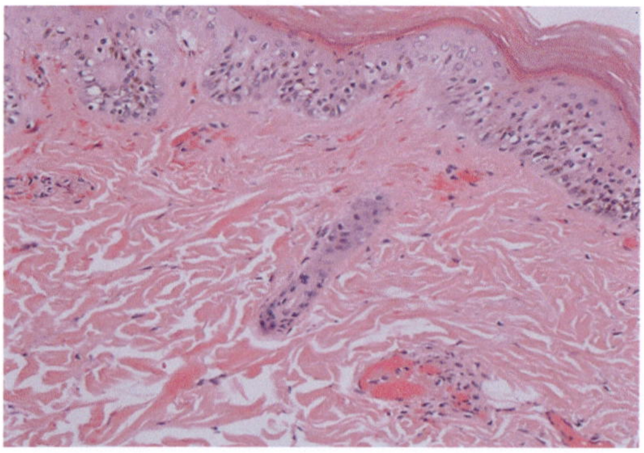

Fig. 16.290 Mildly spongiotic epidermis with occasional necrotic keratinocytes

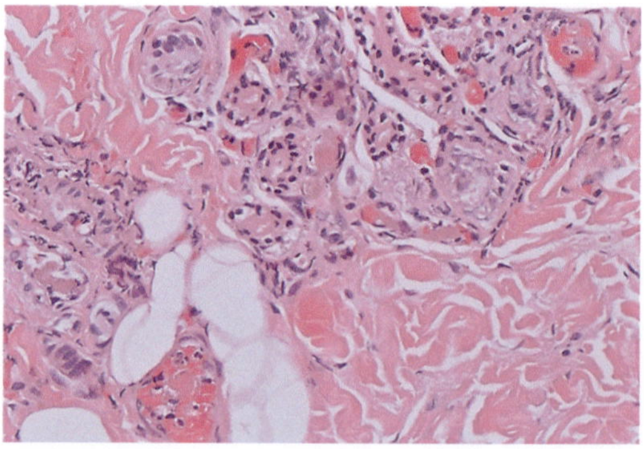

Fig. 16.292 Congested, thrombosed vessels with RBCs extravasation

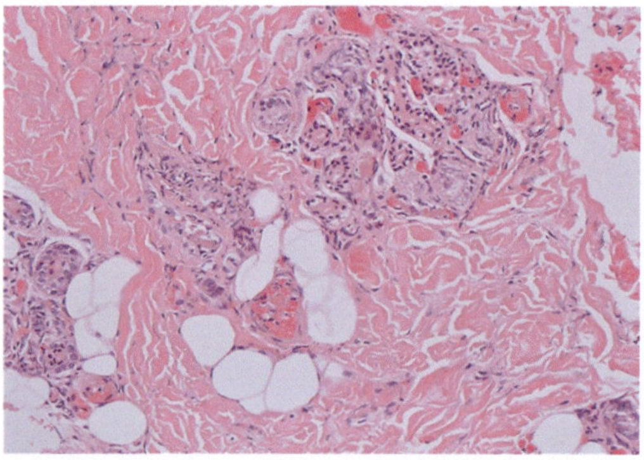

Fig. 16.291 Numerous thrombi in capillaries with mild perivascular lymphocytic inflammation

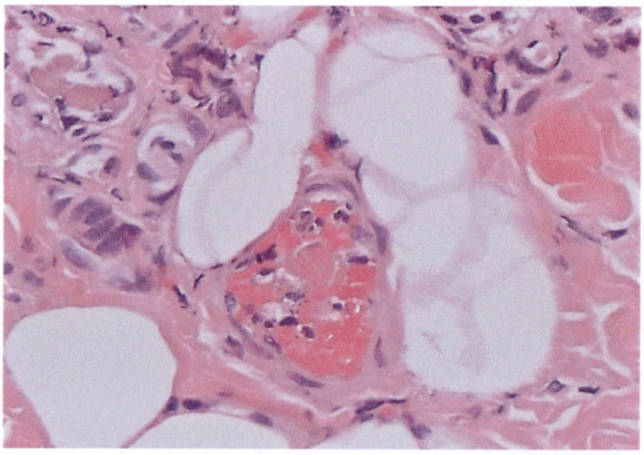

Fig. 16.293 Congested capillary with thrombus formation

Purpura Senilis

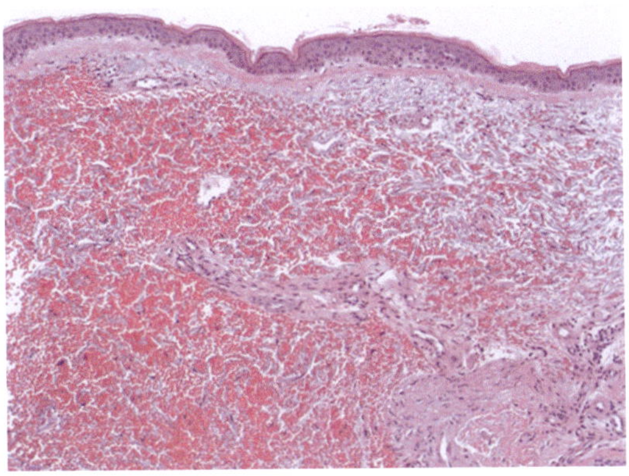

Fig. 16.294 Extensive dermal and subcutaneous purpura

Synonyms: Solar Purpura, Senile Purpura

Histopathology (Figs. 16.294, 16.295, 16.296, 16.297, and 16.298)

- Atrophic epidermis
- Extensive dermal solar elastosis
- Dermal and subcutaneous red blood cell extravasation that varies from mild to severe

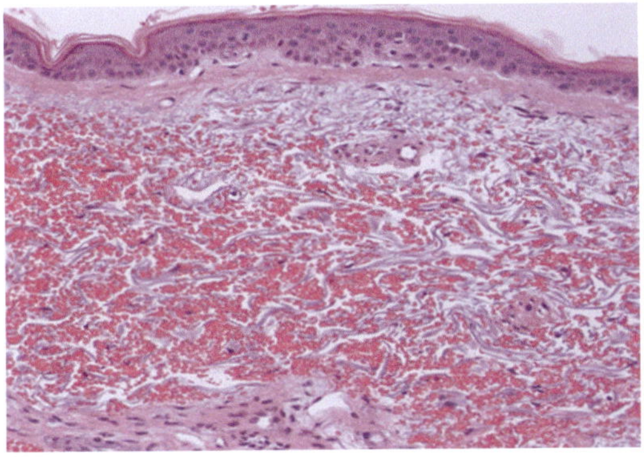

Fig. 16.295 Extensive dermal solar elastosis

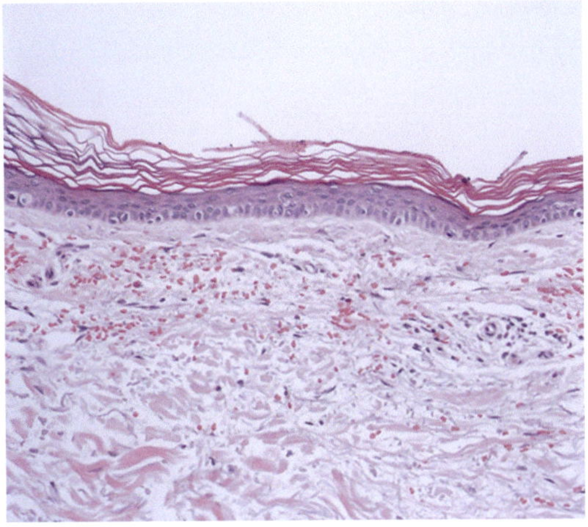

Fig. 16.296 Atrophic epidermis with solar elastosis

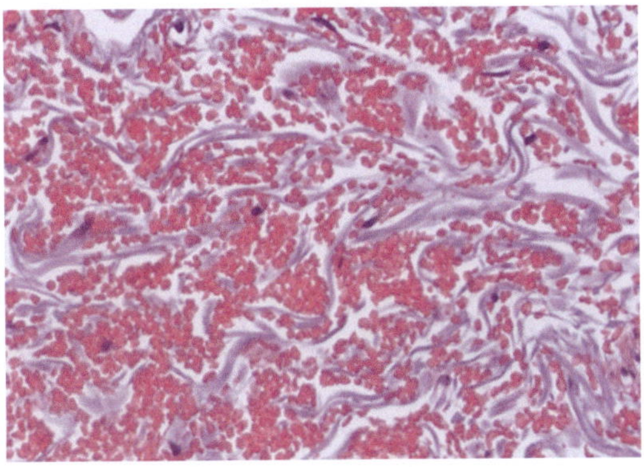

Fig. 16.297 Extensive red blood cell extravasation

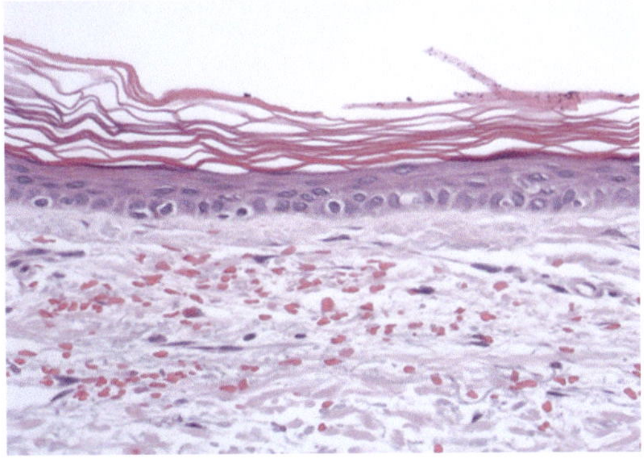

Fig. 16.298 Moderate red blood cell extravasation

Pyoderma Faciale

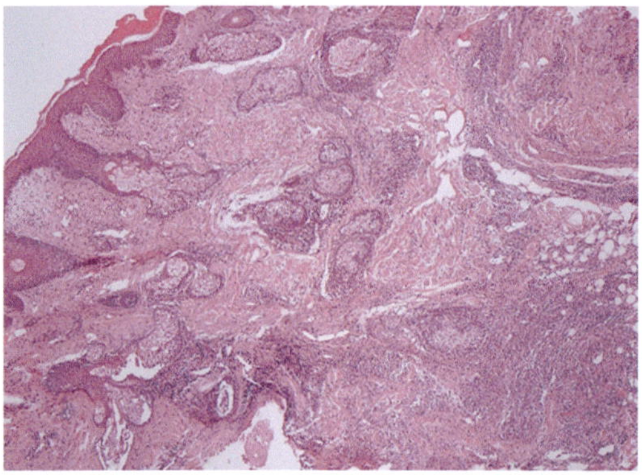

Fig. 16.299 Dermal and subcutaneous inflammation with panniculitis

Synonym: Rosacea Fulminans

Histopathology (Figs. 16.299, 16.300, and 16.301)
- Dense dermal infiltrate of neutrophils, lymphocytes, and histiocytes
- Follicular abscesses are present
- Lobular and septal panniculitis can be present

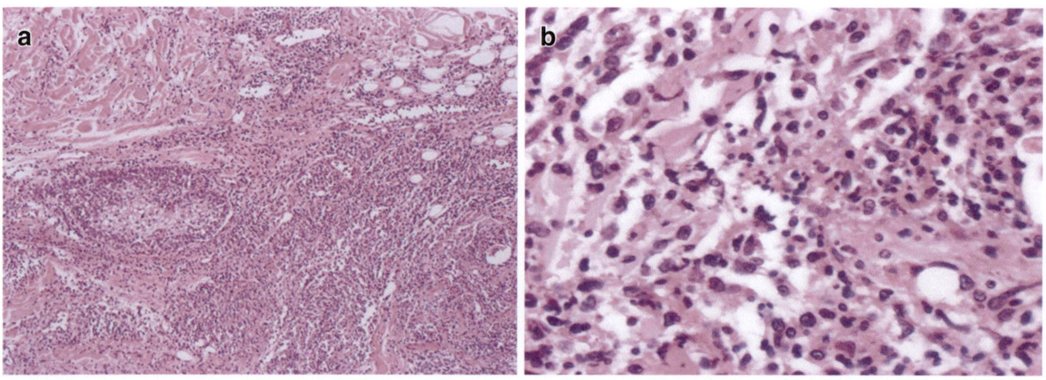

Fig. 16.300 (**a**, **b**) Dense mixed dermal inflammation with lymphocytes, histiocytes, and numerous neutrophils

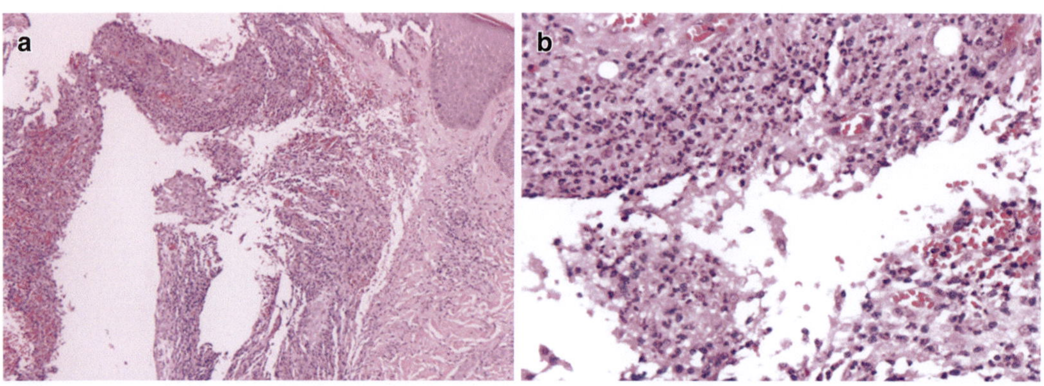

Fig. 16.301 (**a**, **b**) Follicular neutrophilic abscess with destruction of the follicle

Pyoderma Gangrenosum

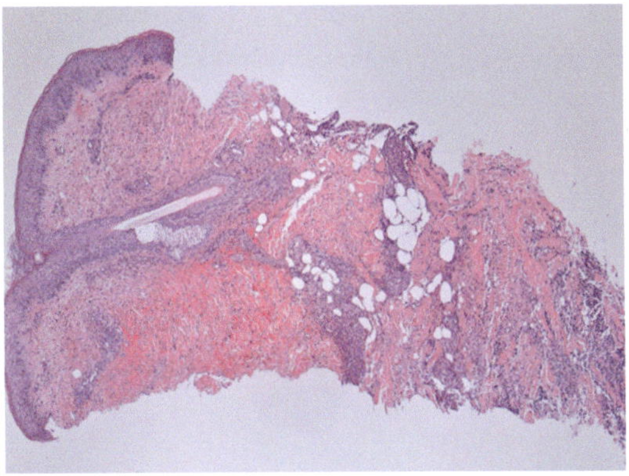

Fig. 16.302 The biopsy from the edge of the lesion

Histopathology is variable and not specific, characterized by ulceration with abscess formation:

Early lesions: (Figs. 16.302, 16.303, and 16.304)
- Perifollicular inflammation with abscess formation

Established lesions (Figs. 16.305 and 16.306)
- Necrosis with ulcer formation
- Mixed inflammatory response with neutrophils and abscess formation
- Vascular damage and variable vasculitis are probably present secondary to the surrounding inflammation

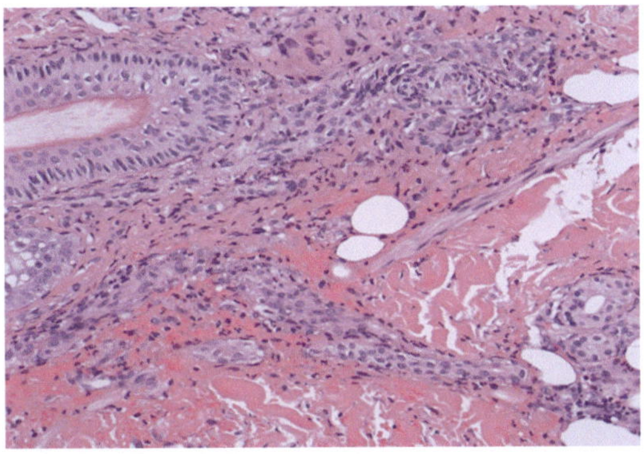

Fig. 16.303 Perifollicular inflammation with numerous neutrophils

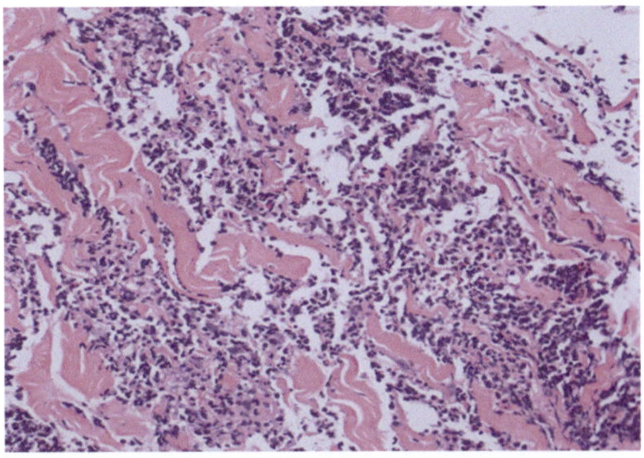

Fig. 16.304 Necrosis and neutrophilic inflammation

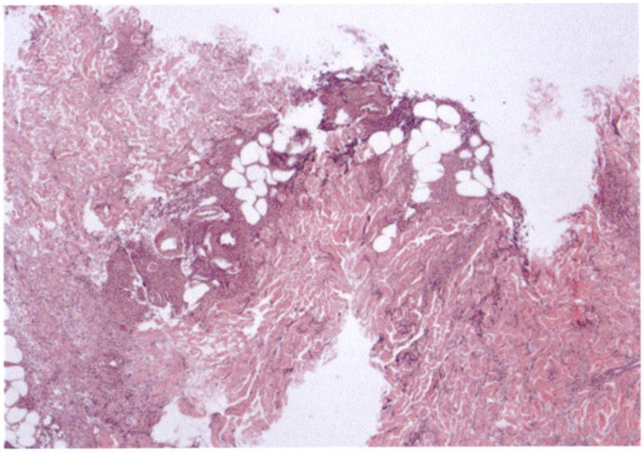

Fig. 16.305 Neutrophilic aggregate forming an abscess

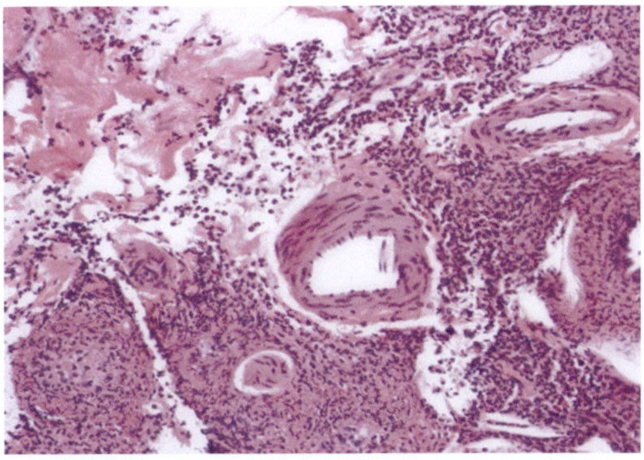

Fig. 16.306 Vascular damage is present but most likely due to the surrounding inflammation

Pyogenic Granuloma

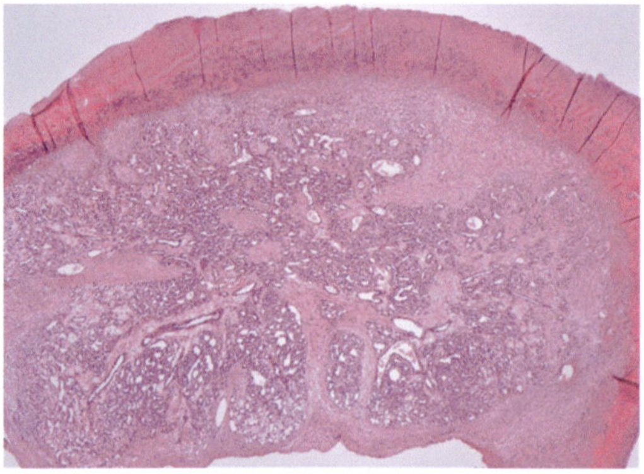

Fig. 16.307 Dome shaped vascular lesion with excoriated epidermis

Synonyms: Granuloma Telangiectaticum, Lobular Capillary Hemangioma

Histopathology (Figs. 16.307, 16.308, and 16.309)
- Dome shaped vascular lesion
- Atrophic epidermis is frequently eroded
- Common peripheral epidermal collarette
- Dermal and subcutaneous capillary vascular proliferation in lobular pattern
- Endothelial cells are plump, moderately pleomorphic, and mitoses can be seen

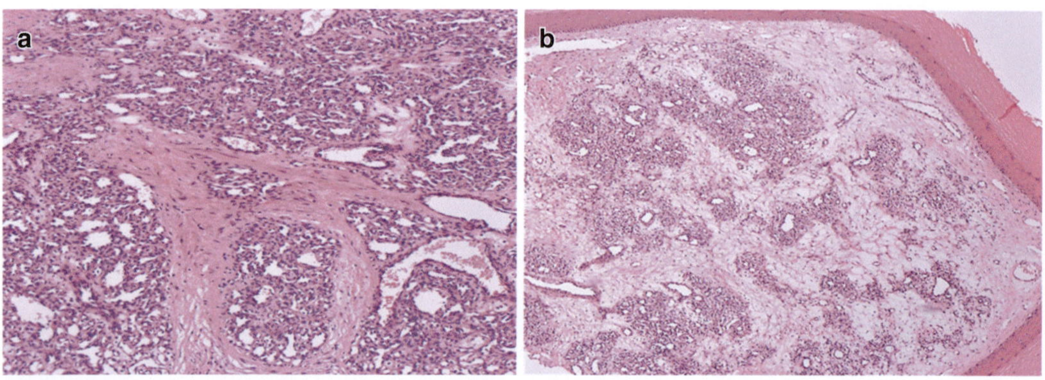

Fig. 16.308 (**a**, **b**) Vascular proliferation of small blood vessels organized in a lobular pattern

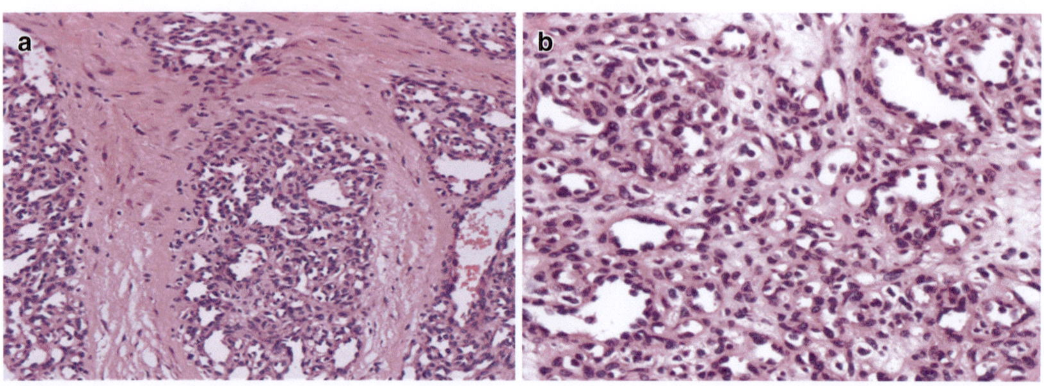

Fig. 16.309 (**a**, **b**) Endothelial cells lining small capillaries demonstrate nuclear polymorphism but no atypia

Dermatopathology R

17

V. Vincek, *Dermatopathology A–Z*, https://doi.org/10.1007/978-3-319-89486-7_17

Radiation Dermatitis

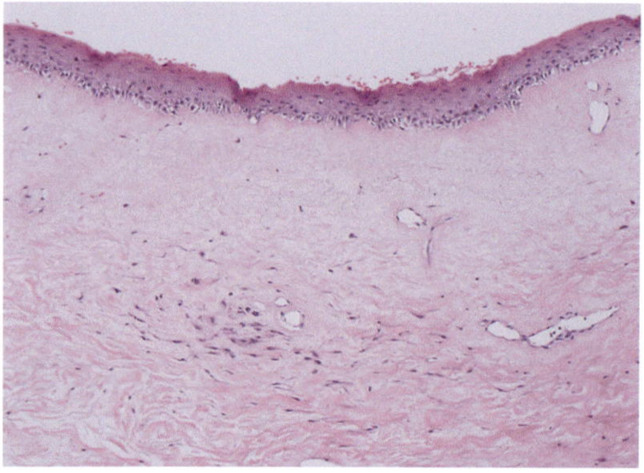

Fig. 17.1 Atrophic epidermis, with dermal sclerosis and absence of adnexal structures

Acute radiation dermatitis is not biopsied as it is an obvious clinical diagnosis.

Histopathology of chronic radiation dermatitis (Figs. 17.1, 17.2, 17.3, and 17.4)

- Dermal smudgy fibrosis with telangiectasias
- Atypical stellate fibroblasts
- Absence of adnexal structures
- Reactive endothelial cells

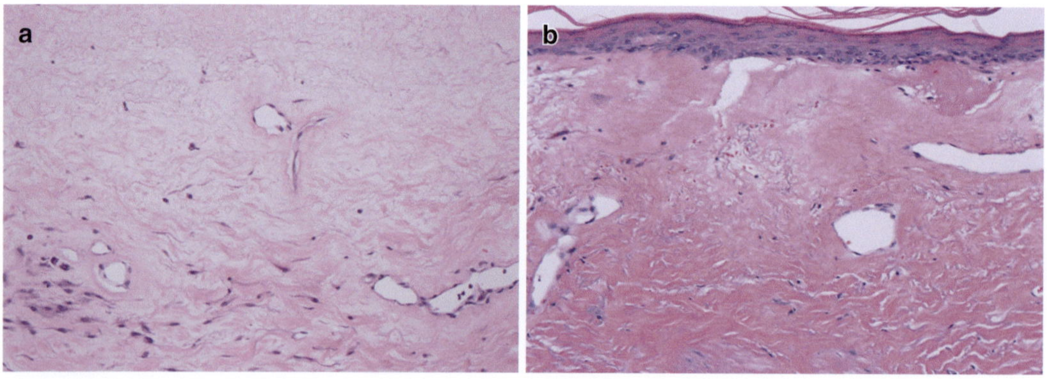

Fig. 17.2 (a, b) Dermal telangiectasias in sclerotic, smudgy dermis

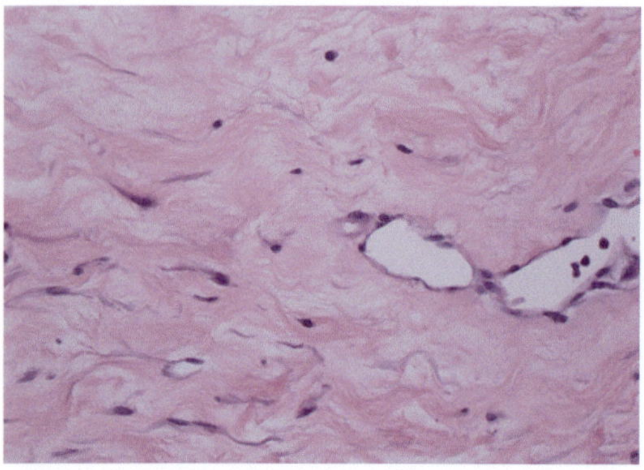

Fig. 17.3 Stellate fibroblasts

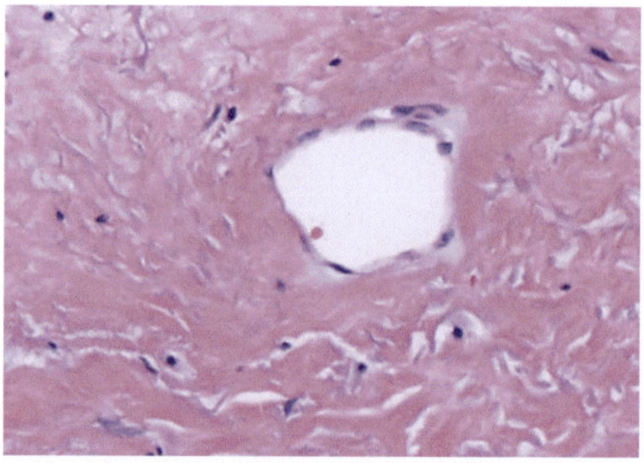

Fig. 17.4 Dilated capillary in fibrotic dermis

Recurrent Nevus

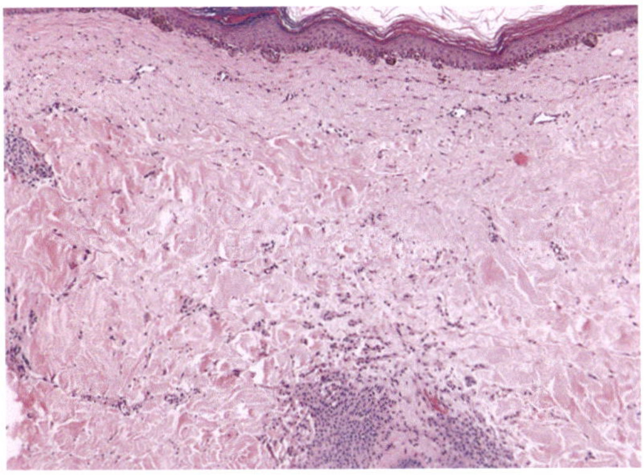

Fig. 17.5 Atrophic epidermis with junctional melanocytes and dermal scar with underlying dermal nevus

Synonym: Nevus Recurrence

Histopathology (Figs. 17.5, 17.6, 17.7, and 17.8)

- Flat epidermis with diminished rete ridges
- Dermal scar
- Melanocytic proliferation in epidermis limited to area above the scar
- Dermal nevus underneath the scar
- Sometimes cytological atypia of junctional melanocytes

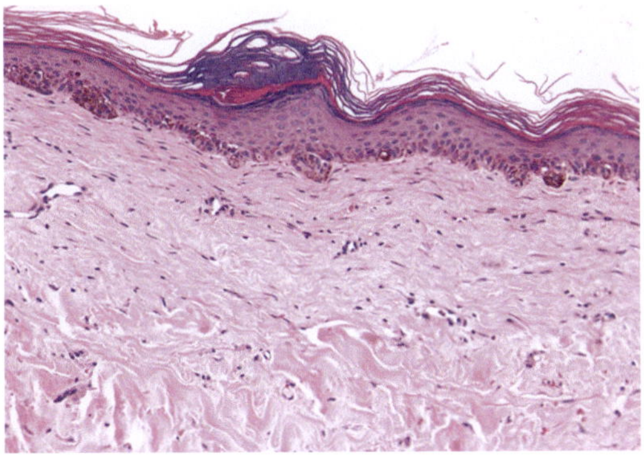

Fig. 17.6 Mild atypia of junctional melanocytes

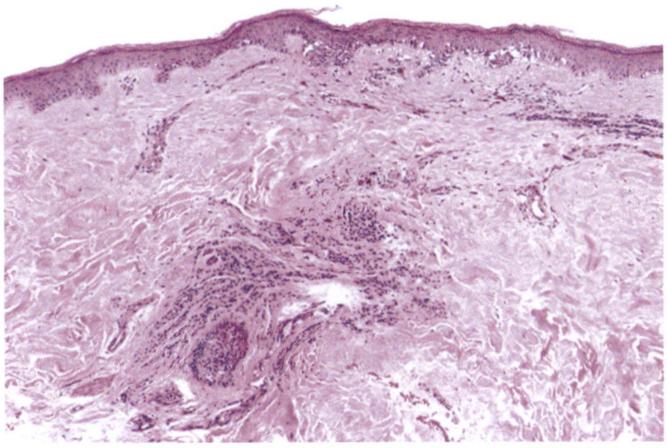

Fig. 17.7 Lesion with three layers: junctional nevus, scar in the upper dermis, and dermal nevus in the lower dermis

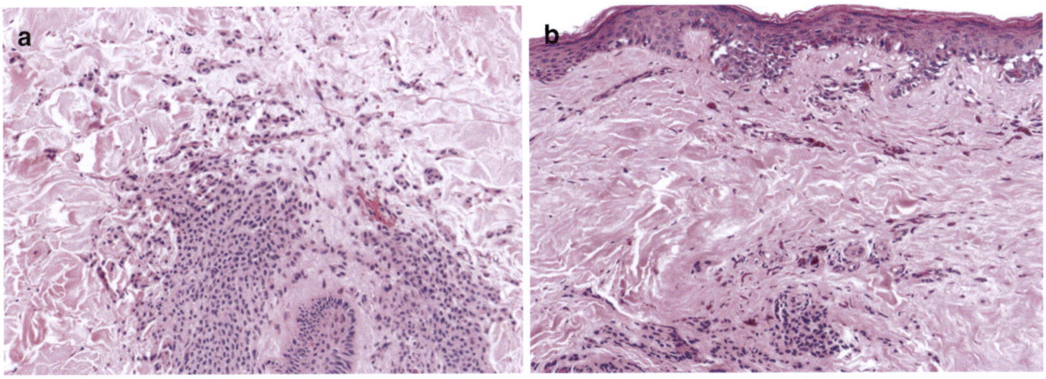

Fig. 17.8 (a, b) Dermal scar with underlying maturing dermal nevus cells with no atypia

Relapsing Polychondritis

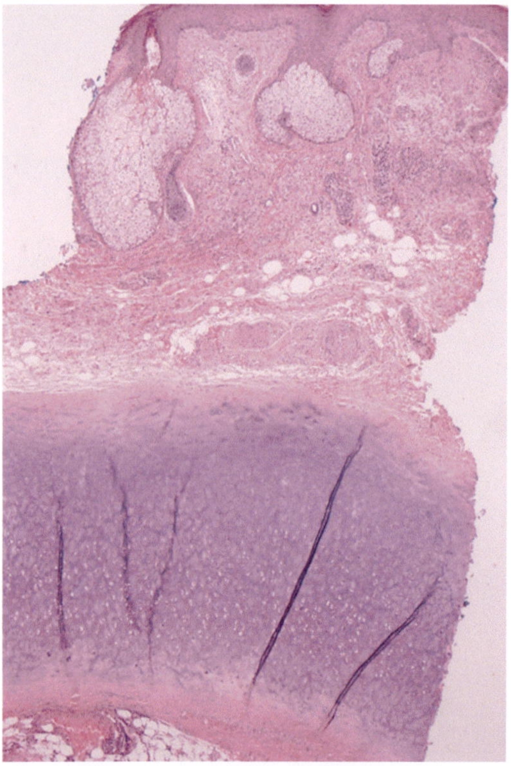

Fig. 17.9 Inflammation abuts the cartilage

Histopathology (Figs. 17.9, 17.10, and 17.11)
- Mixed inflammatory infiltrate in the perichondrial tissue
- Vacuolization and pyknosis of focal chondrocytes

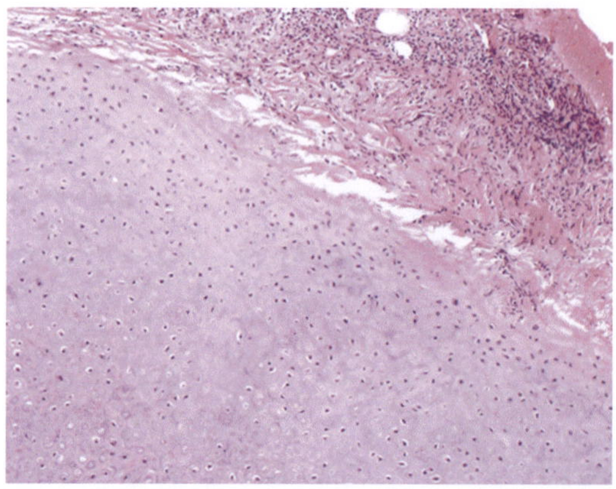

Fig. 17.10 Mixed inflammation adjacent to the cartilage

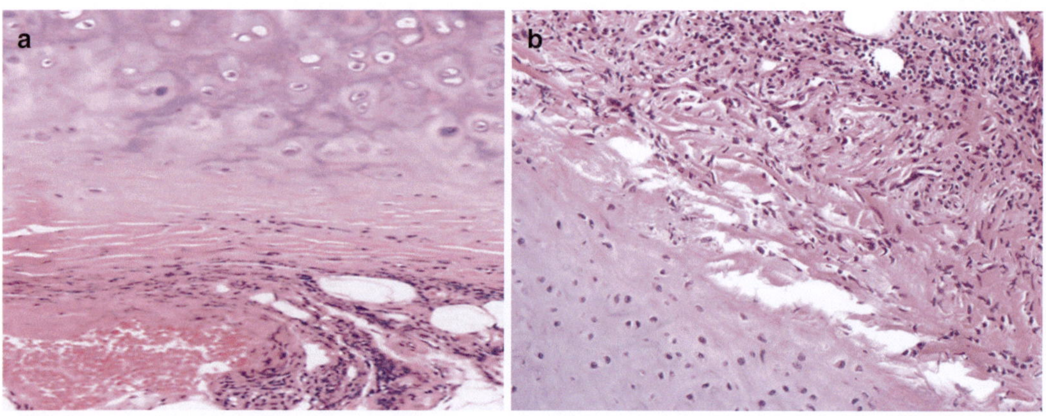

Fig. 17.11 (**a**, **b**) Some chondrocytes are vacuolated and pyknotic

Reticular Erythematous Mucinosis

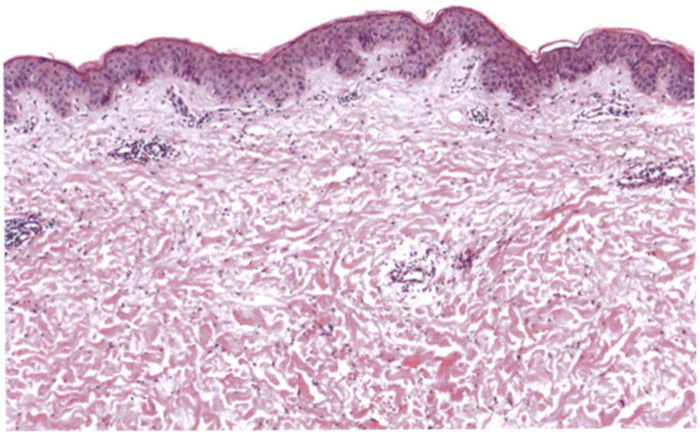

Fig. 17.12 Dermis with slightly separated collagen fibers

Histopathology (Figs. 17.12, 17.13, 17.14, and 17.15)

- Perivascular lymphocytic infiltrate
- Separated collagen fibers
- Variable amount of dermal mucin
- Occasional stellate fibroblasts

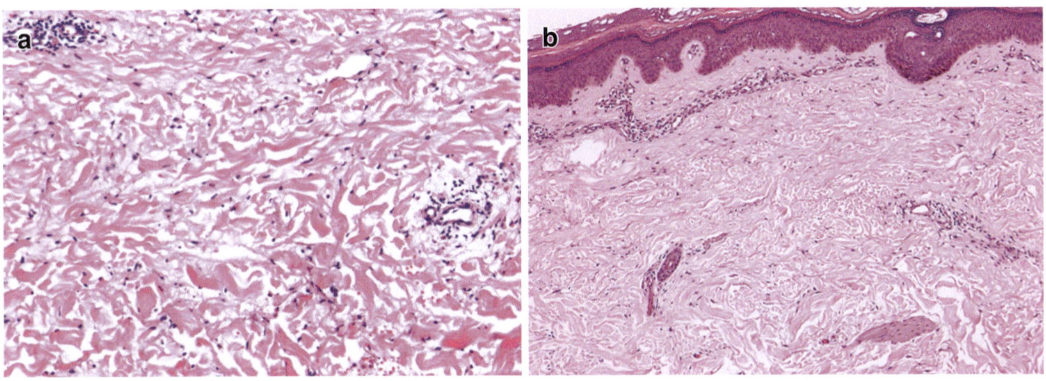

Fig. 17.13 (**a**, **b**) Perivascular lymphocytic infiltrate with separated collagen fibers; bluish mucin material is present in between collagen

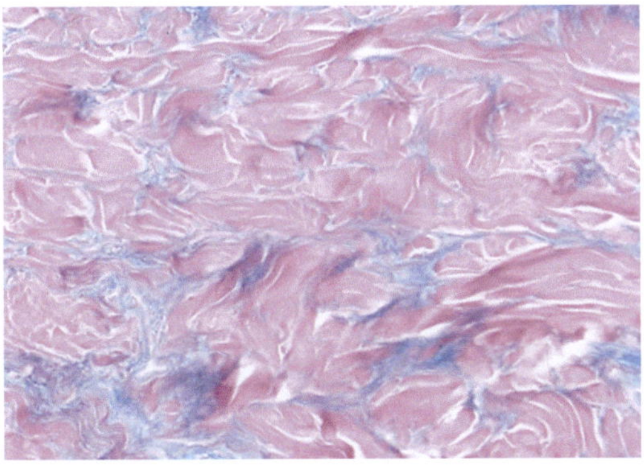

Fig. 17.14 Dermal mucin within collagen bundles (Alcian Blue stain)

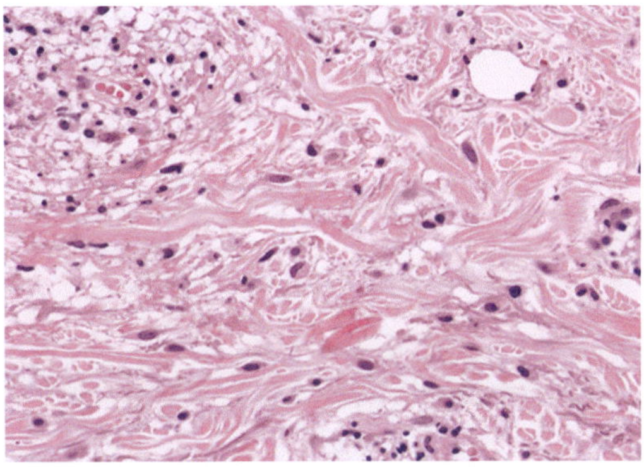

Fig. 17.15 Perivascular lymphocytes and some stellate fibroblasts

Reticulohistiocytoma

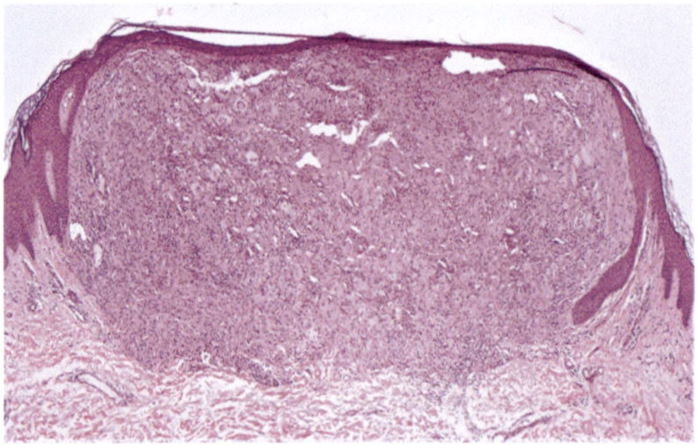

Fig. 17.16 Non encapsulated dermal nodule with epidermal collarette

Synonym: Lipoid Dermatoarthritis

Histopathology (Figs. 17.16, 17.17, 17.18, 17.19, and 17.20)

- Circumscribed, un-encapsulated dermal nodule made of histiocytes and large multinucleated giant cells (CD68+)
- Giant cells have central glassy dark eosinophilic cytoplasm that is PAS positive
- Small number of lymphocytes and neutrophils and absence of xanthoma cells (unlike in xanthogranuloma)

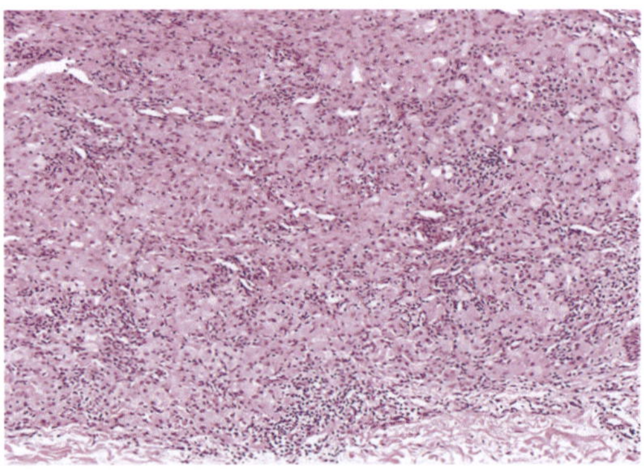

Fig. 17.17 Mixture of pale histiocytes, giant cells, and some lymphocytes

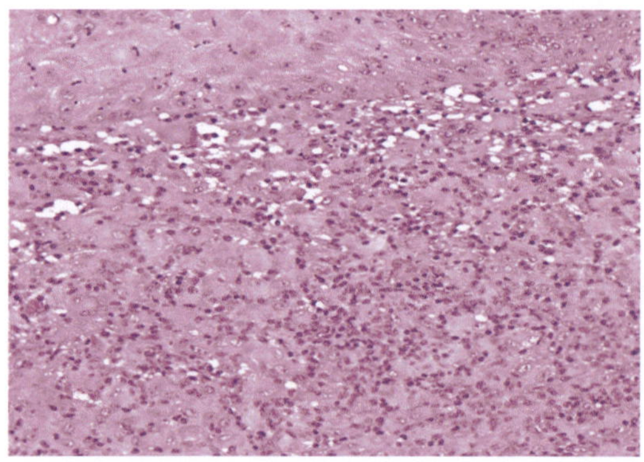

Fig. 17.18 Tumor pushes against the epidermis but it doesn't erode it

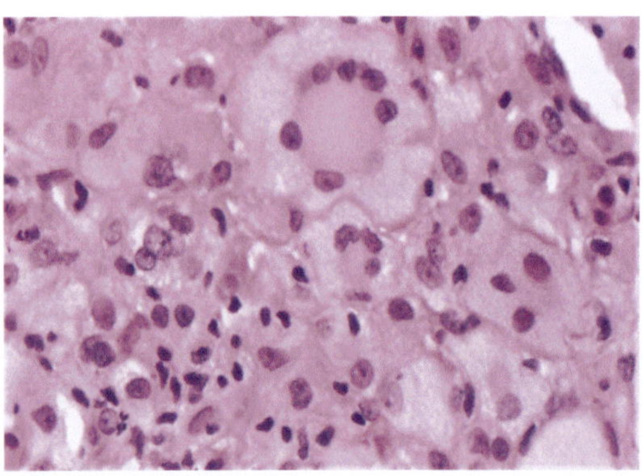

Fig. 17.19 Multinucleated giant cells with central ground glass cytoplasm

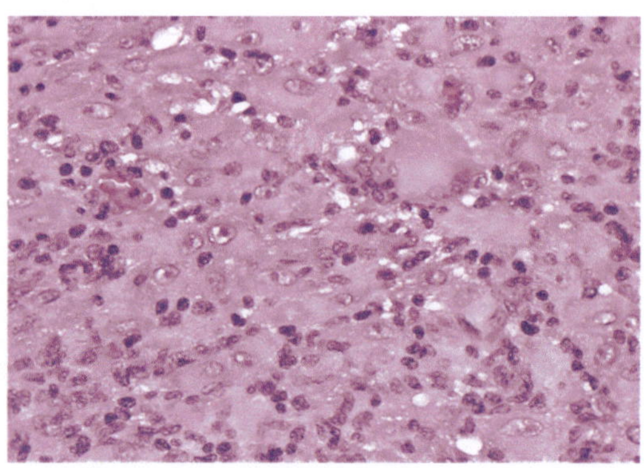

Fig. 17.20 Xanthoma cells are not seen

Rhabdomyoma

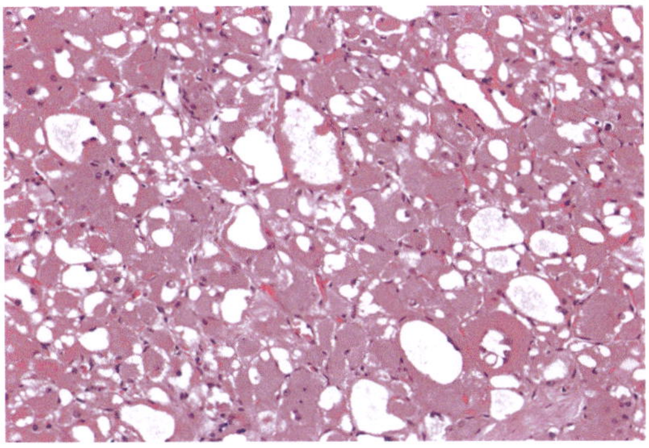

Fig. 17.21 Adult type rhabdomyoma presenting as subcutaneous tumor

Histopathology

Adult type (Figs. 17.21, 17.22, 17.23, and 17.24)

- Round to polygonal cells with small peripherally placed nuclei (muscle specific actin+, desmin+, myoglobin+)
- Eosinophilic finely granular cytoplasm
- Variable cross striation

Fetal type:

- Undifferentiated spindle cells
- Scattered immature trap-shaped muscle fibers

P.S. very rare cutaneous tumor

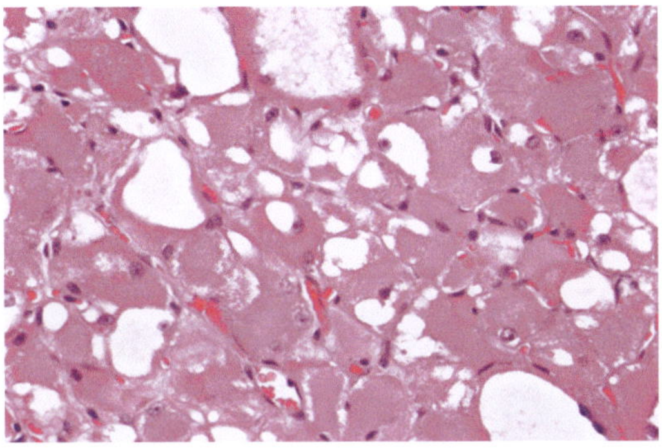

Fig. 17.22 Round and polygonal cells with finely granular pink cytoplasm

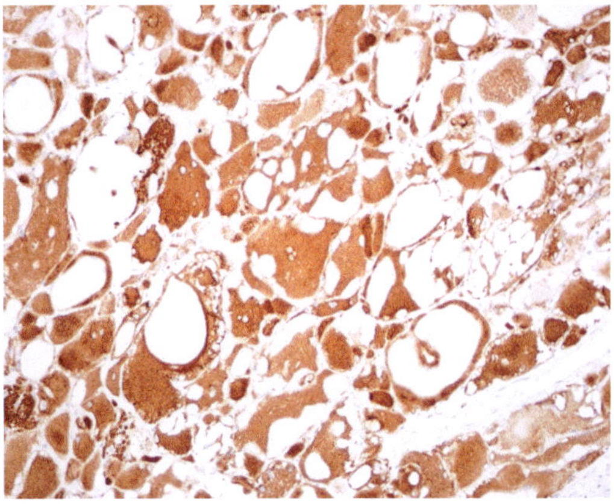

Fig. 17.23 Desmin stains striated muscle cells

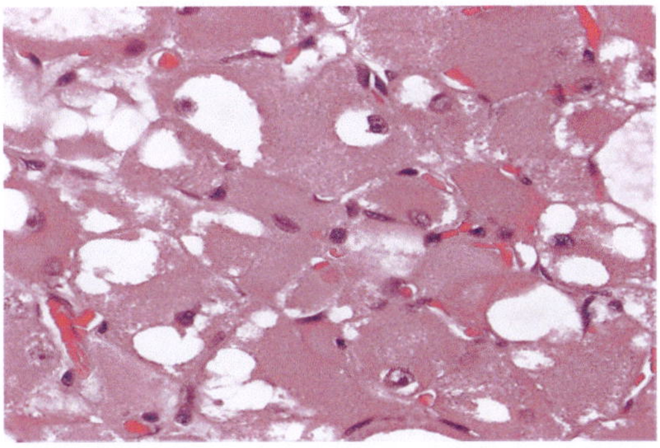

Fig. 17.24 Peripherally placed dark nuclei

Rhabdomyosarcoma

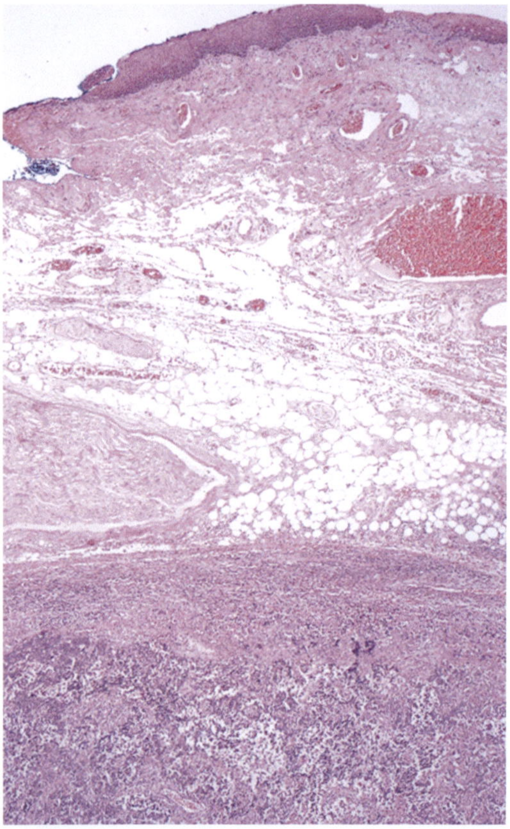

Fig. 17.25 Subcutaneous tumor with large areas of necrosis

There are several types of rhabdomyosarcoma.

Embryonal type accounts for 75% of all tumors (Figs. 17.25 and 17.26)

- Tumor made of undifferentiated small, round, blue cells alternating in hyper and hypocellular areas
- Scattered "strap-shaped" rhabdomyoblasts
- Scattered necrosis and mitoses

Alveolar type:

- Prominent fibrous septa
- Small blue cells are lining septa forming structures similar to pulmonary alveoli

Pleomorphic type:

- Disorderly arranged small blue cells
- Admixed large atypical eosinophilic pleomorphic cells
- Extensive necrosis

P.S. tumor cells are desmin+, myoglobin+, myogenin+

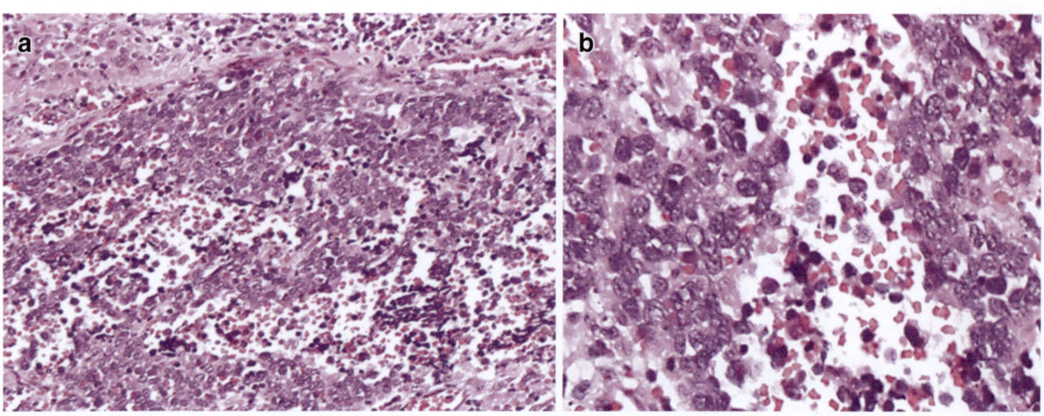

Fig. 17.26 (**a**, **b**) Sheath of atypical round blue cells surrounds area of necrosis; scattered mitotic figures are present

Rheumatoid Nodule

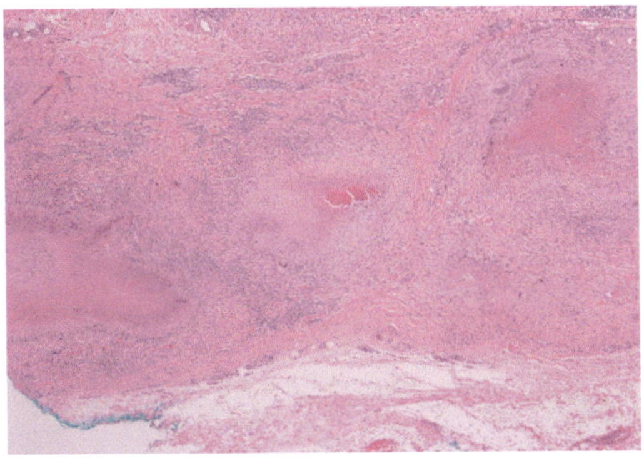

Fig. 17.27 Multiple granulomas in the subcutaneous fibroadipose tissue

Histopathology (Figs. 17.27, 17.28, 17.29, and 17.30)

- Large irregular granulomas with central necrobiosis but no mucin
- Sometimes neutrophils can be seen in the center
- Nodules mostly located in deeper dermis and subcutis although they can also be more superficial (particularly elbow lesions) and even perforate the epidermis
- Necrobiotic center surrounded by histiocytes and lymphocytes

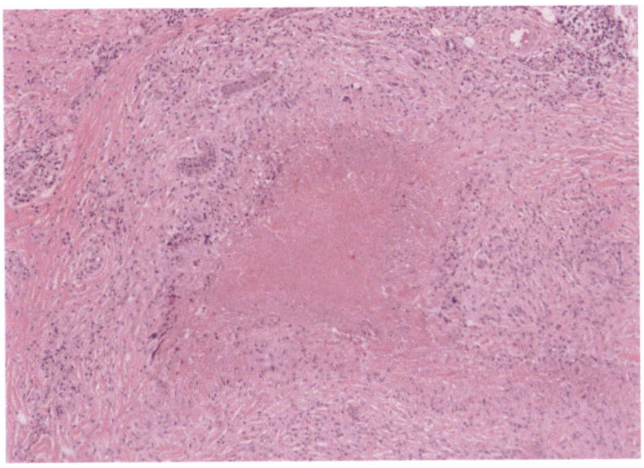

Fig. 17.28 Stellar shaped granuloma with surrounding lymphocytes and histiocytes

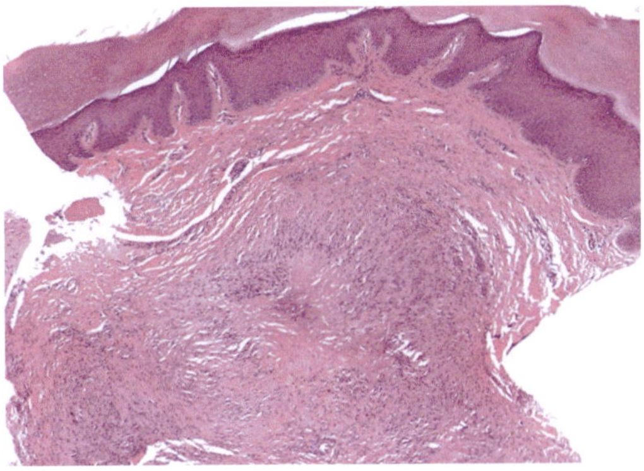

Fig. 17.29 Irregular granuloma in lower dermis and subcutis

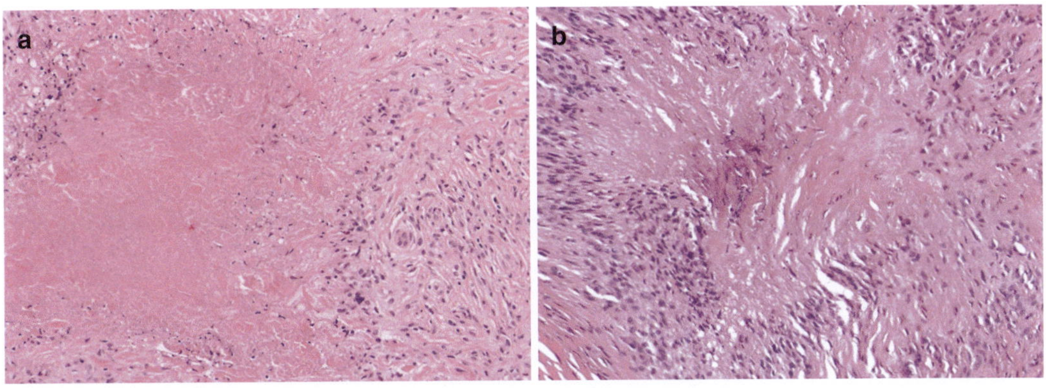

Fig. 17.30 (**a**, **b**) Granuloma with necrobiosis and neutrophilic debris in the center

Rhinophyma

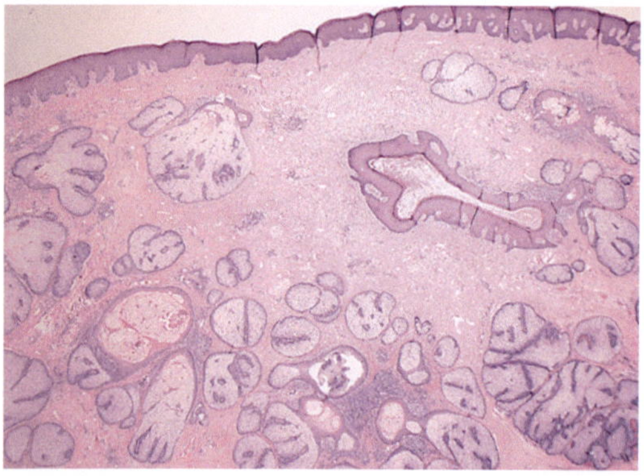

Fig. 17.31 Numerous sebaceous glands and dilated follicles

Histopathology (Figs. 17.31, 17.32, 17.33, 17.34, and 17.35)
- Extensive proliferation of benign sebaceous glands
- Dermal fibrosis and dermal telangiectasias
- Multiple dilated hair follicles forming "milia-like" cysts

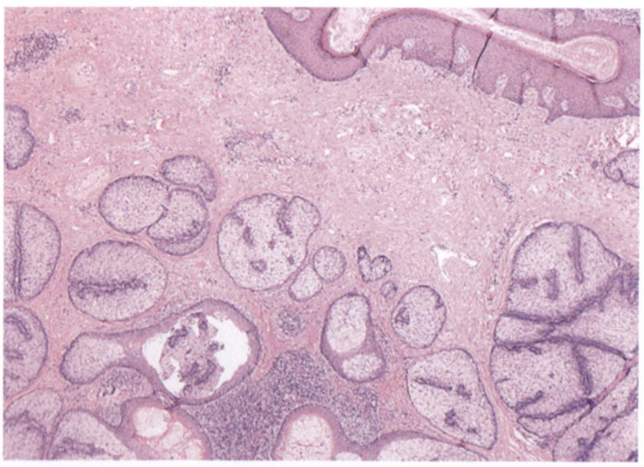

Fig. 17.32 Mild focal lymphocytic inflammation is present

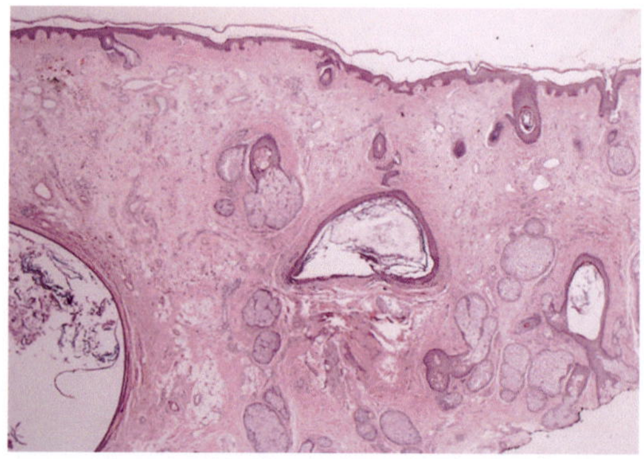

Fig. 17.33 Dilated hair follicles forming multiple cysts

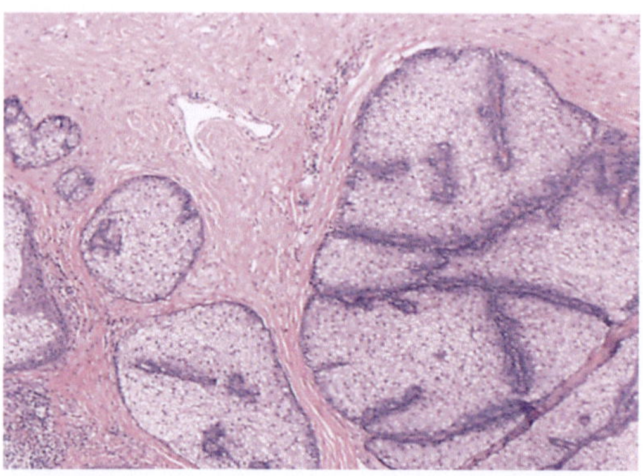

Fig. 17.34 Dermal fibrosis surrounds hyperplastic sebaceous glands

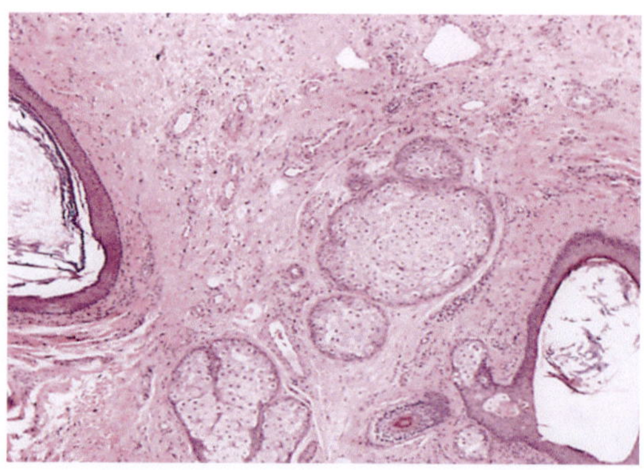

Fig. 17.35 Multiple telangiectasias are present in sclerotic stroma

Rhinoscleroma

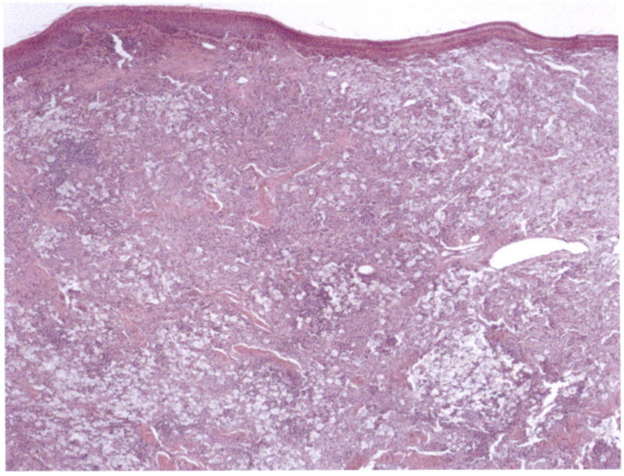

Fig. 17.36 Dense dermal and subcutaneous infiltrate

Histopathology (Figs. 17.36, 17.37, 17.38, and 17.39)

- Dense infiltrate of histiocytes, lymphocytes, and plasma cells
- Many foamy histiocytes (Mikulicz cells) and scattered Russell bodies (plasma cells with proteinaceous material)
- GIEMSA, Warthin-Starry, and PAS stains demonstrate *Klebsiella rhinoscleromatis* within foamy histiocytes

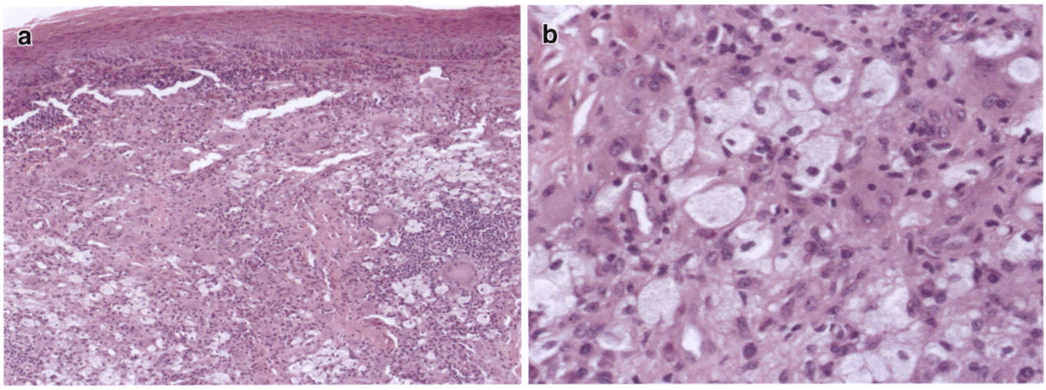

Fig. 17.37 (**a**, **b**) Mixed inflammation consisting of foamy histiocytes, lymphocytes, and some plasma cells

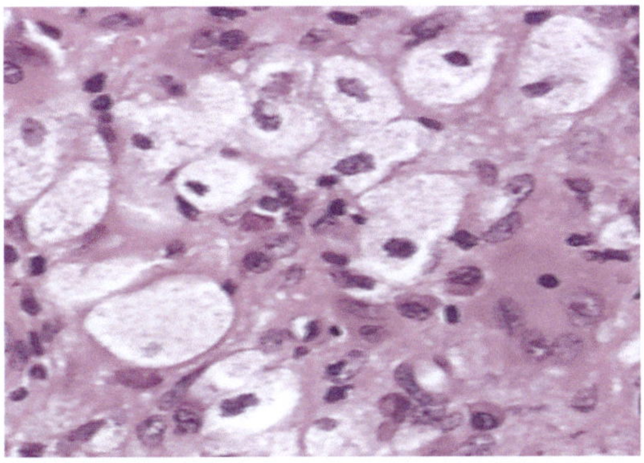

Fig. 17.38 Mikulicz cells (foamy histiocytes) are numerous

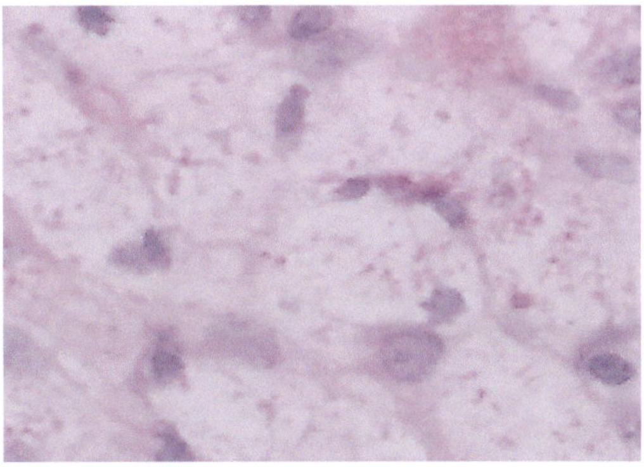

Fig. 17.39 Faint bacterial elements within histiocytes (PAS)

Rhinosporidiosis

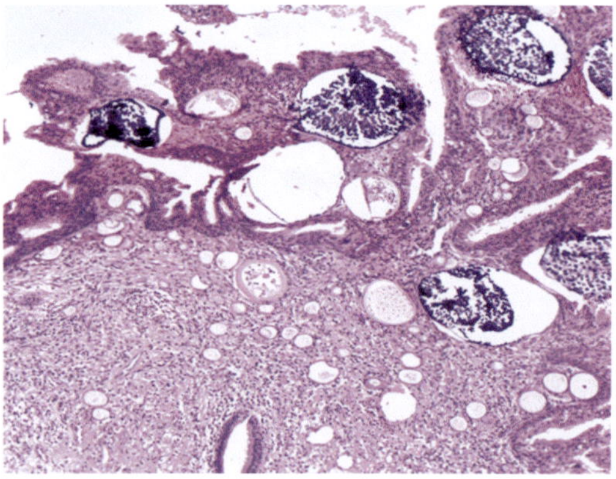

Fig. 17.40 Polypoid nasal lesion with mixed inflammation

Histopathology (Figs. 17.40, 17.41, and 17.42)

- Mostly nasal polypoid lesions covered with respiratory mucosa
- Submucosa with large sporangias (30–350 μm) filled with numerous endospores (7–9 μm)
- Spores mature to form thick walled trophic cysts
- Dense mixed submucosal inflammation

P.S. conjunctiva is a common site of infection in dry climate and the nose in humid climate

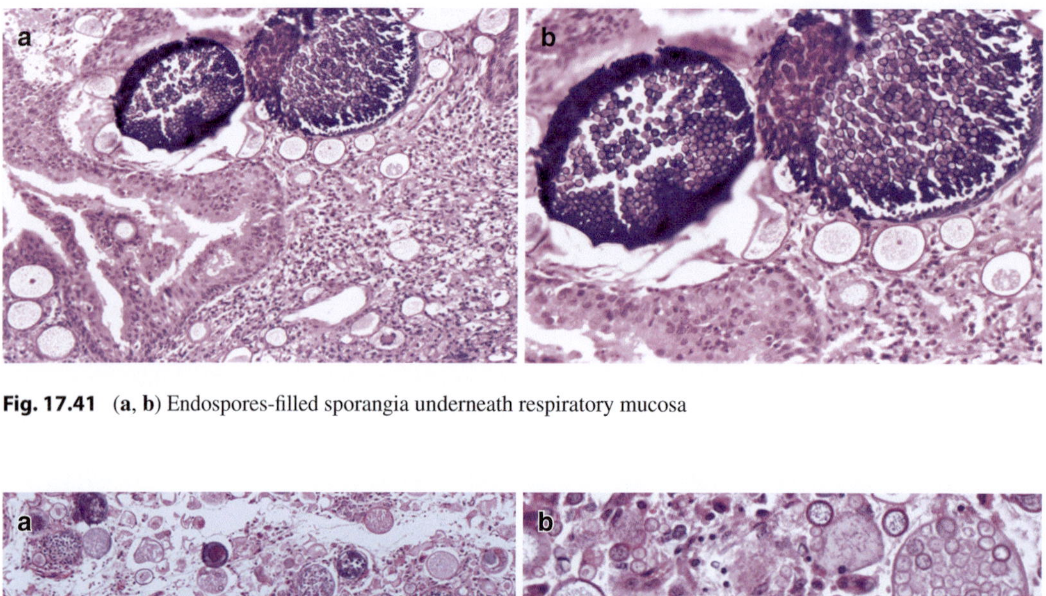

Fig. 17.41 (**a**, **b**) Endospores-filled sporangia underneath respiratory mucosa

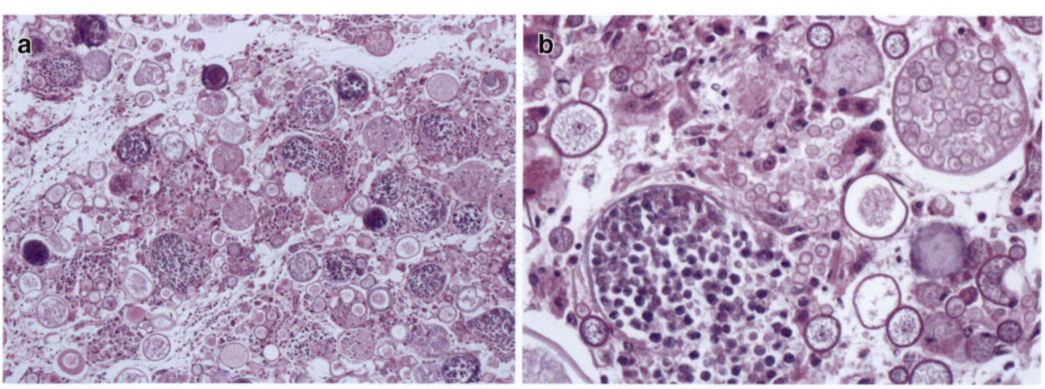

Fig. 17.42 (**a**, **b**) Multiple trophic cysts with thick wall

Rosacea

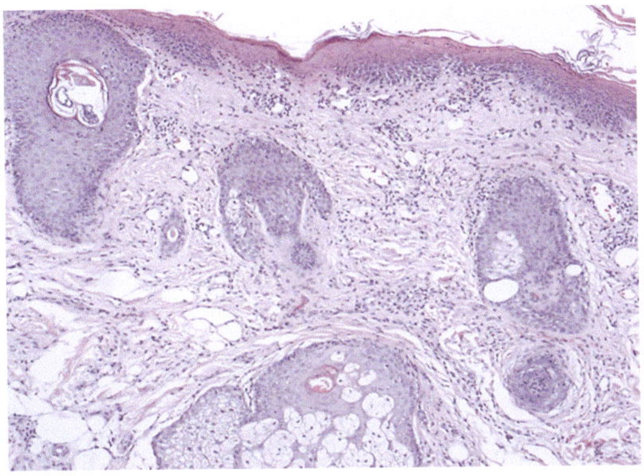

Fig. 17.43 Mild perivascular and perifollicular lymphocytic infiltrate

Synonym: Acne Rosacea

Histopathology varies with severity and type (Figs. 17.43, 17.44, 17.45, 17.46, and 17.47)

- Starts with non-specific histology with mild perifollicular and perivascular lymphocytic inflammation and dermal telangiectasias
- As the disease progresses, perifollicular and perivascular infiltrate is denser with perifollicular epithelioid non necrotizing granuloma. *Demodex* mites are commonly present within follicles.
- In pustular rosacea neutrophilic folliculitis is seen

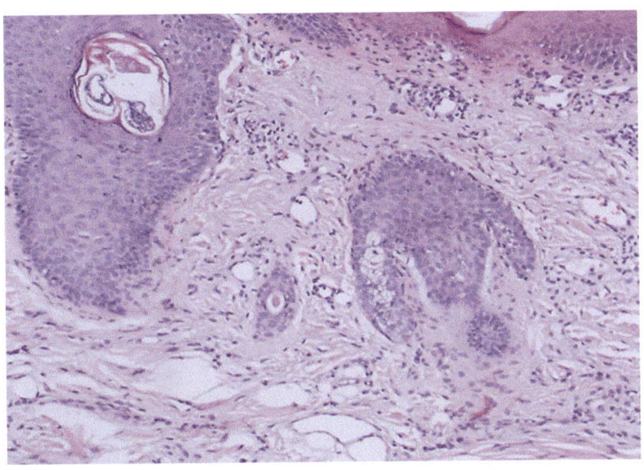

Fig. 17.44 Dilated hair follicle with *Demodex* mite

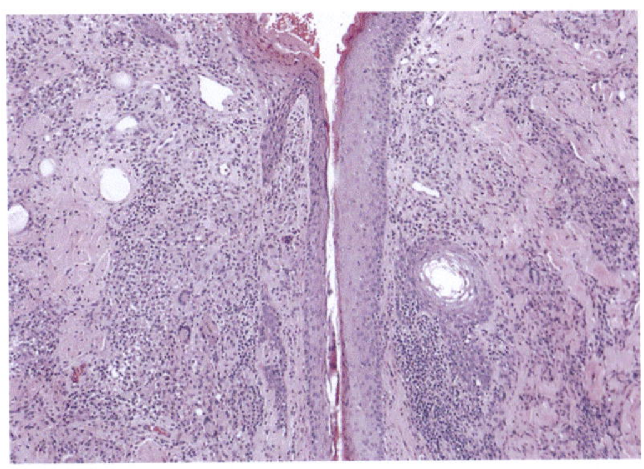

Fig. 17.45 Perifollicular non necrotizing vague granulomas

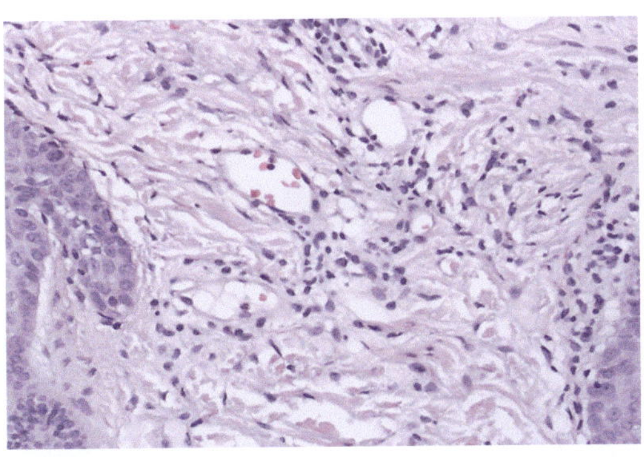

Fig. 17.46 Dermal telangiectasias with mild perivascular lymphocytic infiltrate

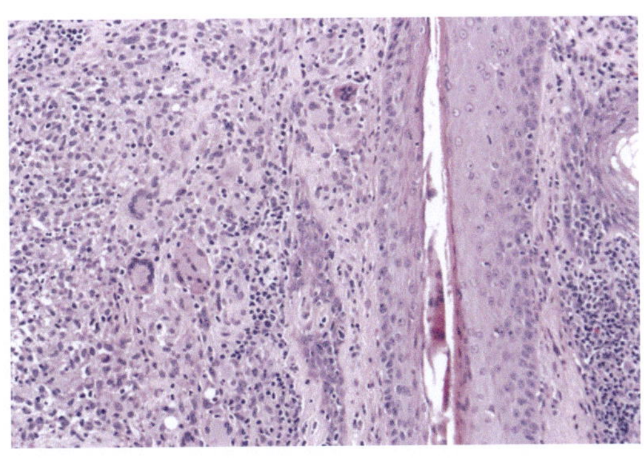

Fig. 17.47 Occasional giant cells are present within granuloma

Rosai Dorfman Disease

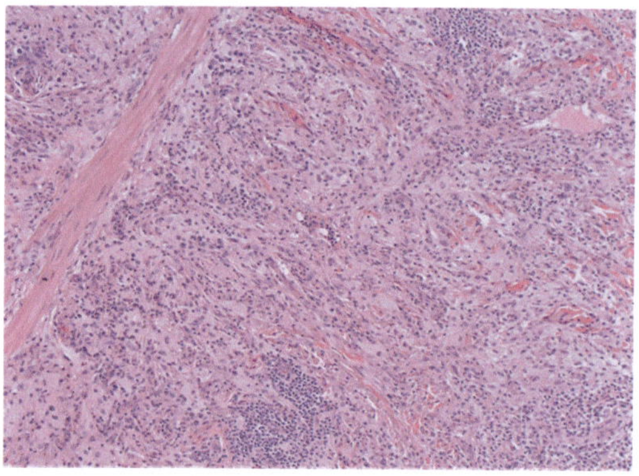

Fig. 17.48 Dense dermal cellular infiltrate

Histopathology (Figs. 17.48, 17.49, 17.50, and 17.51)

- Dense dermal infiltrate
- Large histiocytes with abundant eosinophilic cytoplasm with admixed lymphocytes and occasional plasma cells with no cytological atypia
- Lymphocytes, plasma cells, and red blood cells are engulfed by histiocytes (emperipolesis) forming "bean bag" histiocytes
- Histiocytes are CD68+, S100+, and CD1a−

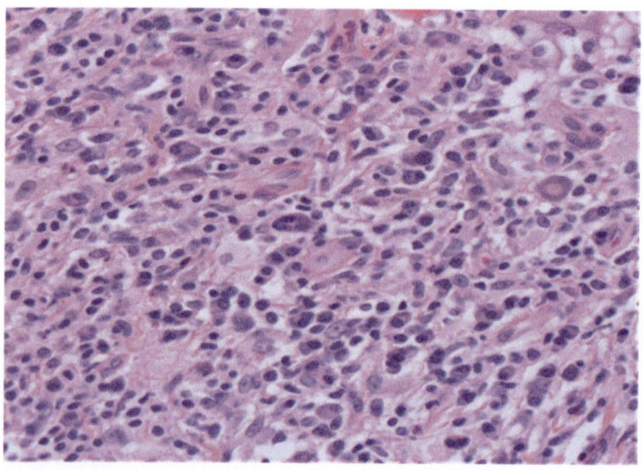

Fig. 17.49 Histiocytes admixed with lymphocytes and plasma cells

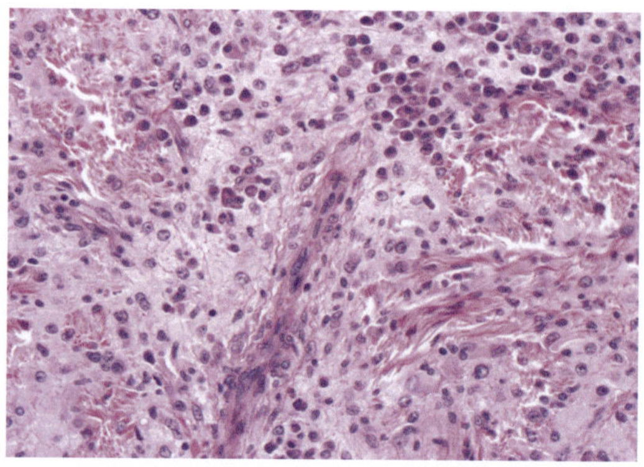

Fig. 17.50 Histiocyte rich areas stand out as pale areas

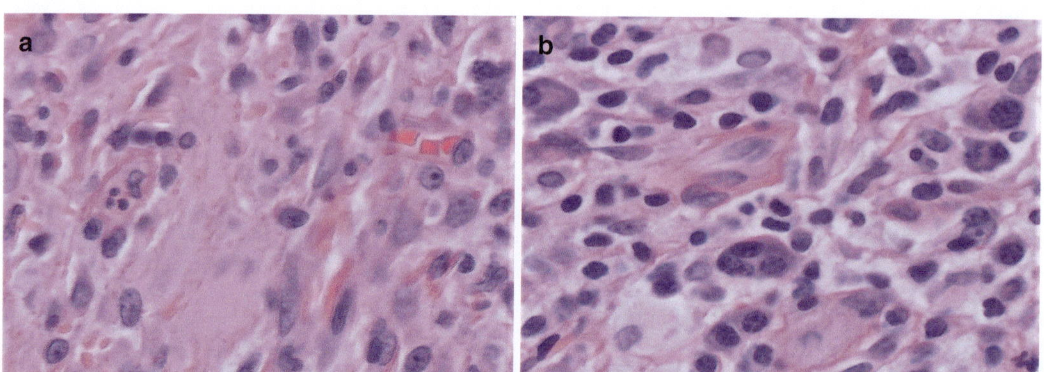

Fig. 17.51 (**a**, **b**) "Bean bag" histiocytes that contain lymphocytes, plasma cell and RBCs in the cytoplasm

18 Dermatopathology S

V. Vincek, *Dermatopathology A–Z*, https://doi.org/10.1007/978-3-319-89486-7_18

Sarcoidosis

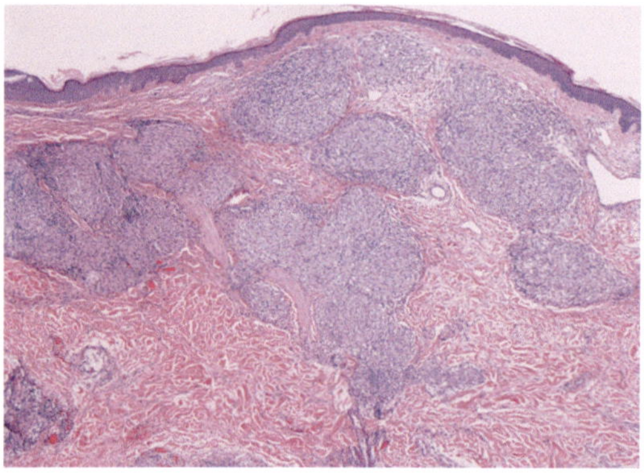

Fig. 18.1 Dermal and subcutaneous granulomas

Histopathology (Figs. 18.1, 18.2, 18.3, 18.4, and 18.5)

- Dermal and subcutaneous non-necrotizing granulomas
- Granulomas composed of epithelioid histiocytes with sparse lymphocytic infiltrate, so called "naked granuloma"
- Asteroid and Schumann bodies can be present

P.S. sarcoidosis is a diagnosis of exclusion and infection should always be excluded

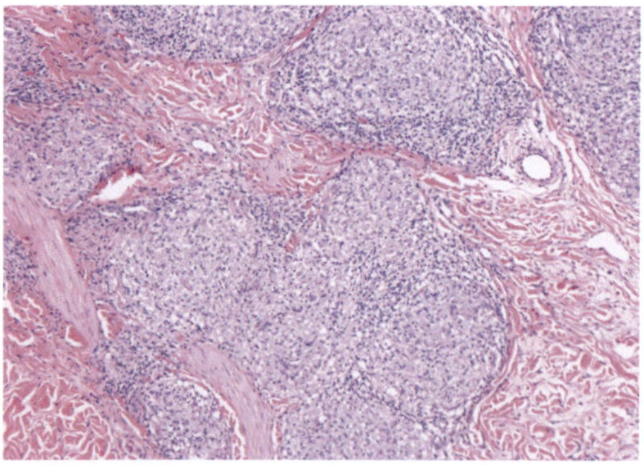

Fig. 18.2 Rounded granulomas made of pale (epithelioid) histiocytes with a paucity of surrounding lymphocytes

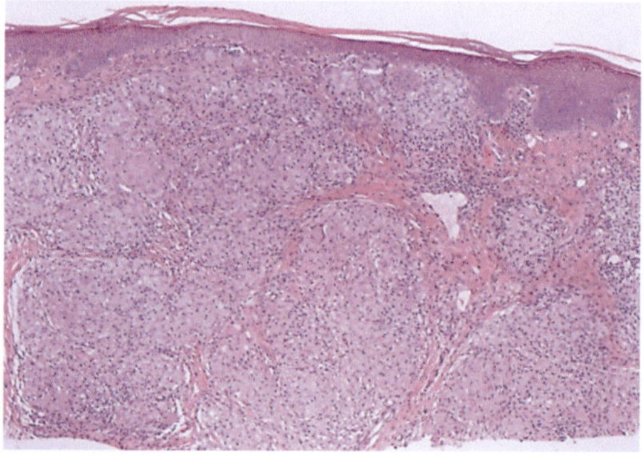

Fig. 18.3 Granulomas, without central necrosis, are naked without surrounding lymphocytes

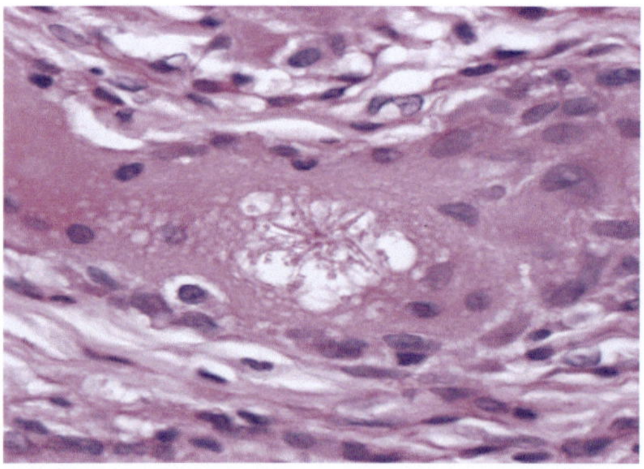

Fig. 18.4 Asteroid body

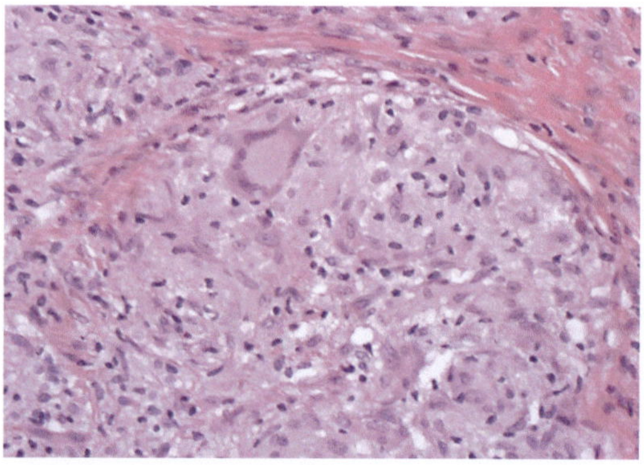

Fig. 18.5 Giant cells can be seen but are not numerous

Scabies

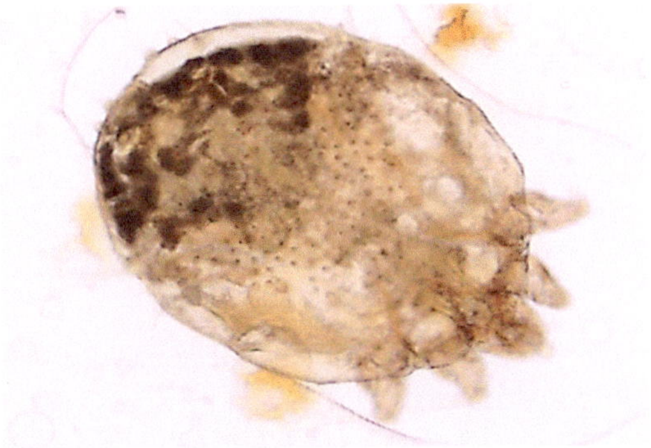

Fig. 18.6 Intact scabies mite

Histopathology (Figs. 18.6, 18.7, 18.8, 18.9, and 18.10)

- Acanthotic, spongiotic and hyperkeratotic epidermis
- Intraepidermal burrow with scabies mite
- Dermal perivascular lymphocytic infiltrate with numerous eosinophils
- Epidermal eosinophils can be present
- In Norwegian scabies, mites are numerous and epidermis is markedly hyperkeratotic

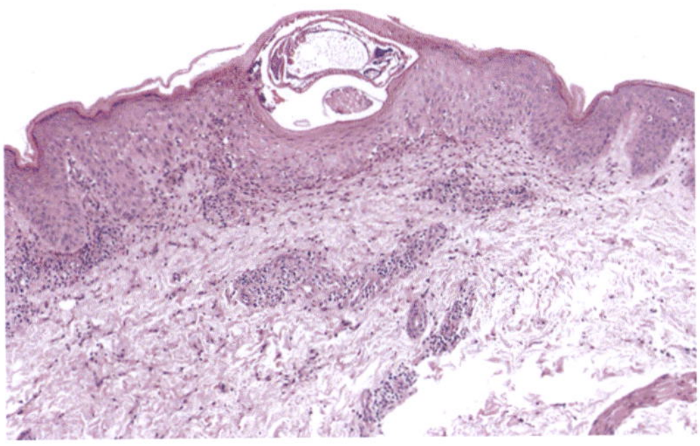

Fig. 18.7 The mite is located underneath stratum corneum

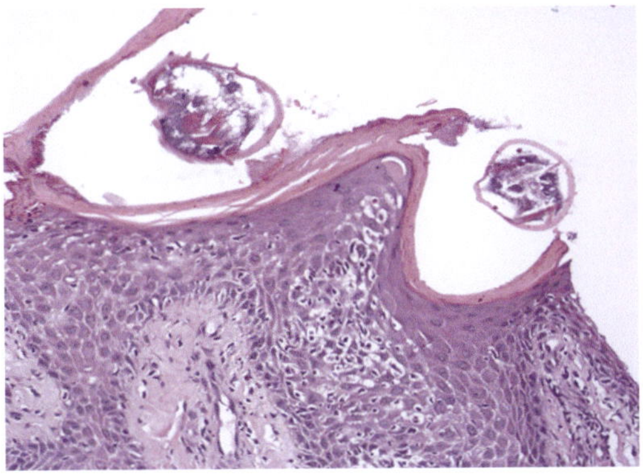

Fig. 18.8 Two mites in acanthotic epidermis with spongiosis

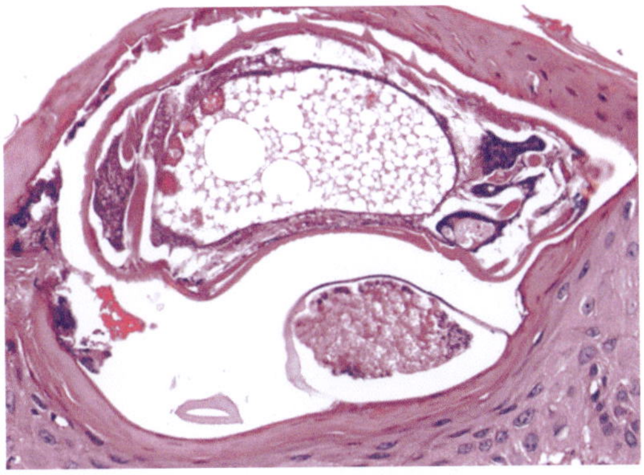

Fig. 18.9 Mite with characteristic barbed cuticle projections

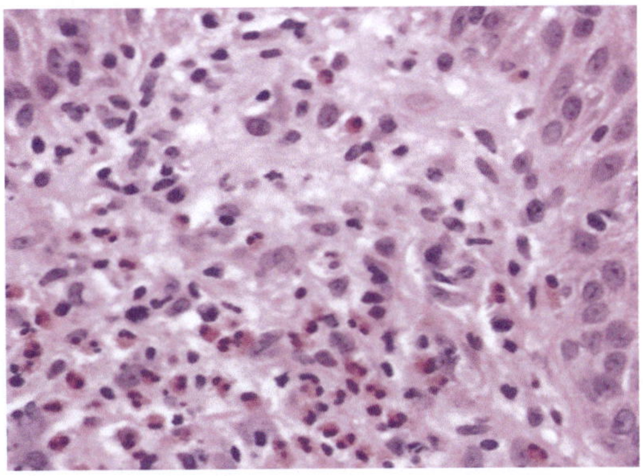

Fig. 18.10 Dermis contains numerous eosinophils

Scar

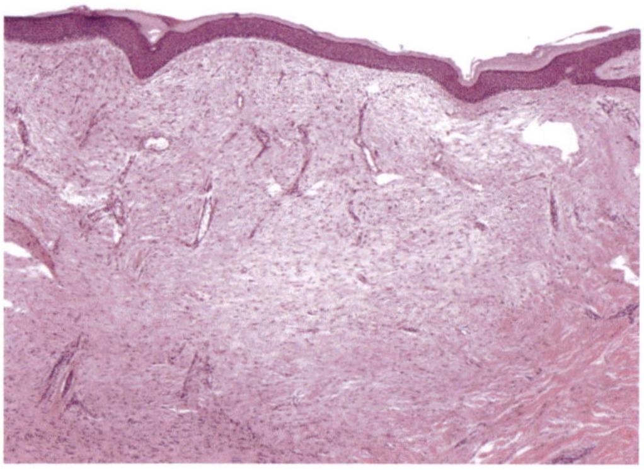

Fig. 18.11 **5 weeks old** scar with dermal fibrosis and vertically oriented blood vessels

Synonym: Cicatrix

Histopathology depends on the time since injury (Figs. 18.11, 18.12, 18.13, 18.14, and 18.15)

- In 24 h neutrophils appear at the edge of the blood clot
- By day 3 neutrophils are replaced by macrophages
- By day 5 the wound is filled with granulation tissue
- By second week fibroblasts proliferate, collagen increases and inflammation diminishes
- By a month fibrotic scar is formed with minimal inflammation left

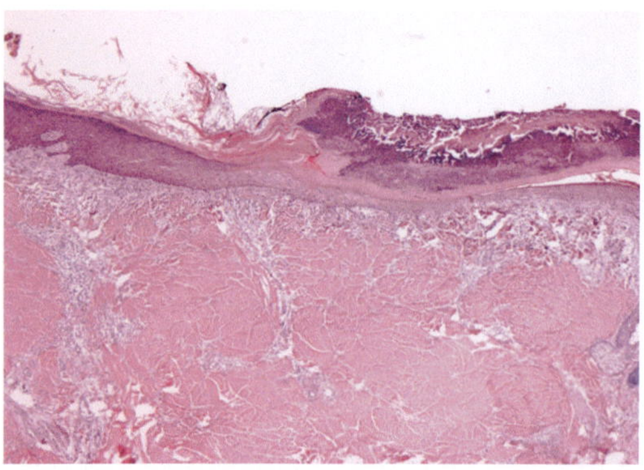

Fig. 18.12 **2 weeks old** scar

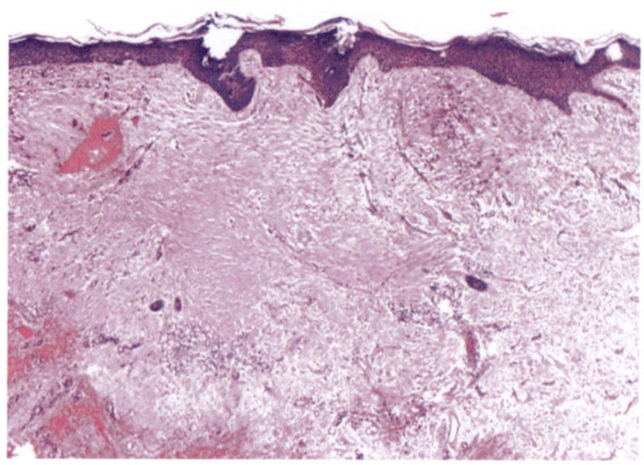

Fig. 18.13 **3 weeks old** scar

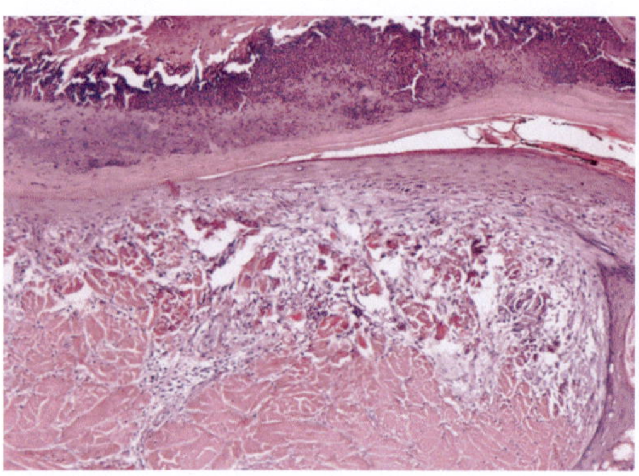

Fig. 18.14 Serum crust, pseudoepitheliomatous hyperplasia, and dermal granulation tissue

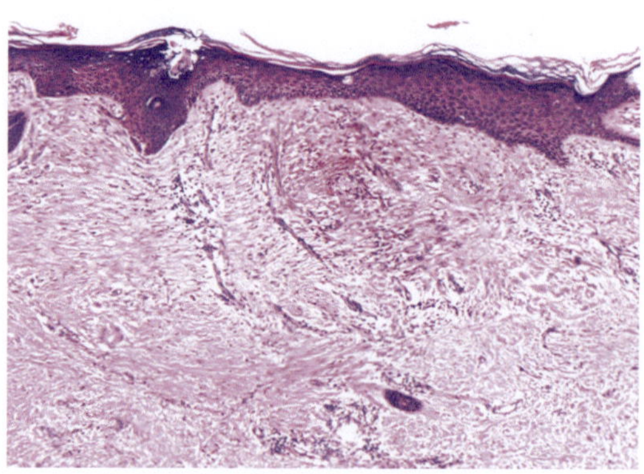

Fig. 18.15 Granulation tissue including hemosiderin laden macrophages (center) and organized scar around

Scarring Alopecia

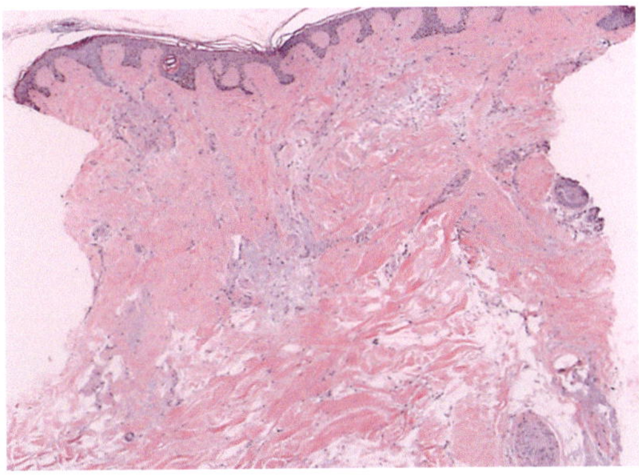

Fig. 18.16 Dermal scarring with absence of hair follicles

Primary scarring alopecia can be **lymphocytes associated** and caused by *central centrifugal cicatricial alopecia, follicular mucinosios, lupus erythematosus, lichen planopilaris, or pseudopelade of Brocq*

or **neutrophils associated** and caused by *dissecting cellulitis, folliculitis decalvans, acne keloidalis, or tinea capitis.*

Histopathology of end stage scarring alopecia of any cause looks very similar with dermal fibrosis, absence of hair follicles, and minimal inflammation (Figs. 18.16, 18.17, 18.18, 18.19, and 18.20).

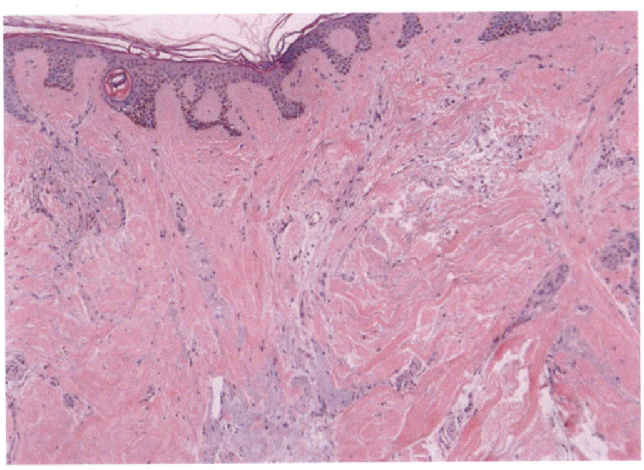

Fig. 18.17 End stage pseudopelade of Brocq

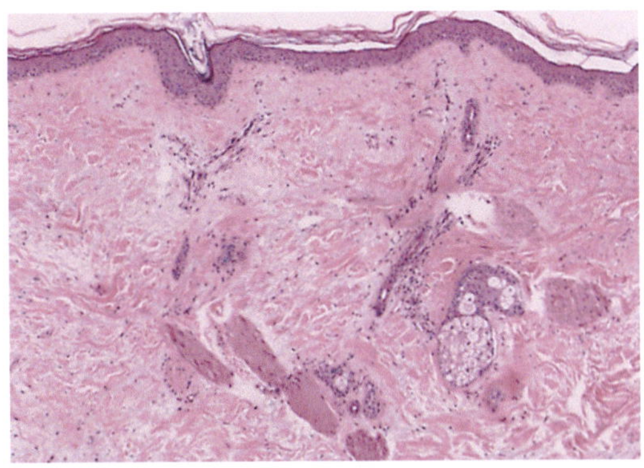

Fig. 18.18 End stage scarring alopecia due to lupus

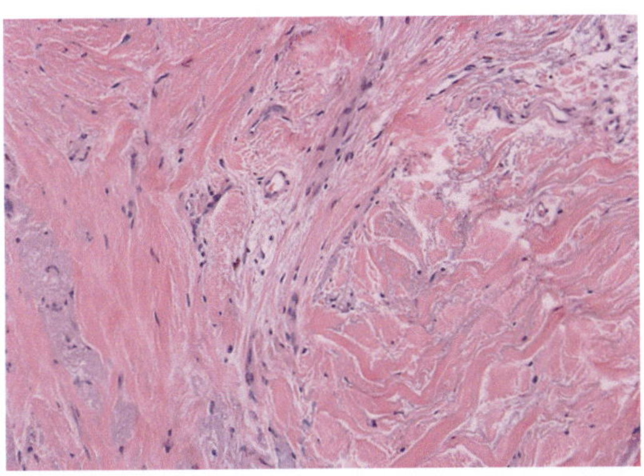

Fig. 18.19 Dense dermal scar with sparse inflammation

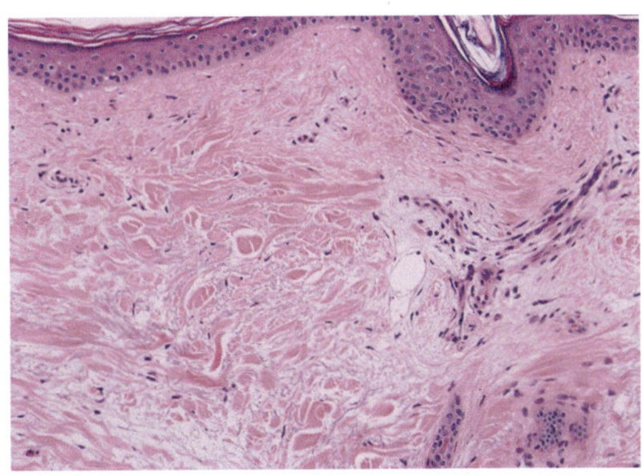

Fig. 18.20 Dermal fibrosis with increased amount of mucin and mild inflammation

Scleredema

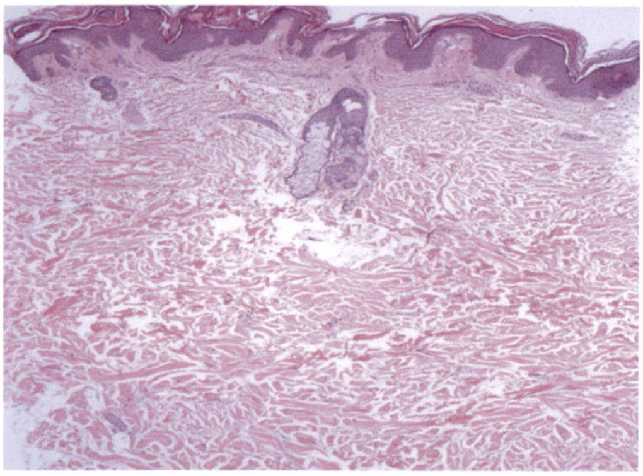

Fig. 18.21 Dermal and subcutaneous sclerosis

Histopathology (Figs. 18.21, 18.22, 18.23, 18.24, and 18.25)

- Thick, sclerotic collagen bundles with no increase in the number of fibroblasts
- Separation of collagen bundles with "empty" spaces
- Minimal amount of mucin which decreases as the lesion matures
- Up to 1/3 of established cases have no mucin
- Inflammation is usually minimal but if present mast cells can be seen

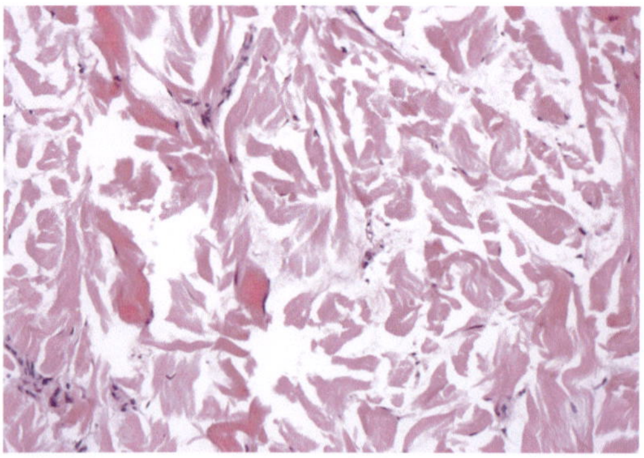

Fig. 18.22 Thickened collagen bundle with "empty" spaces

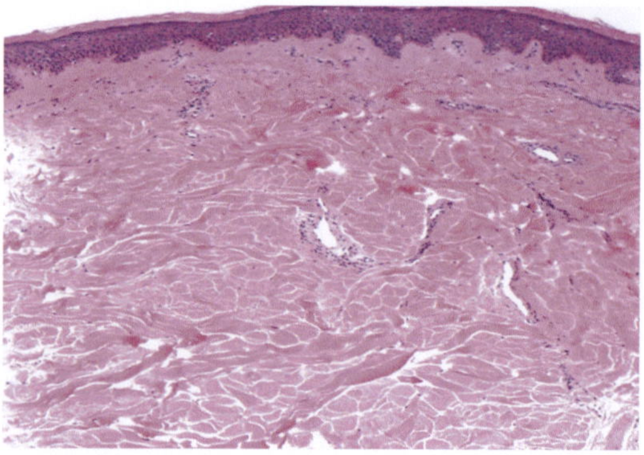

Fig. 18.23 Established lesion

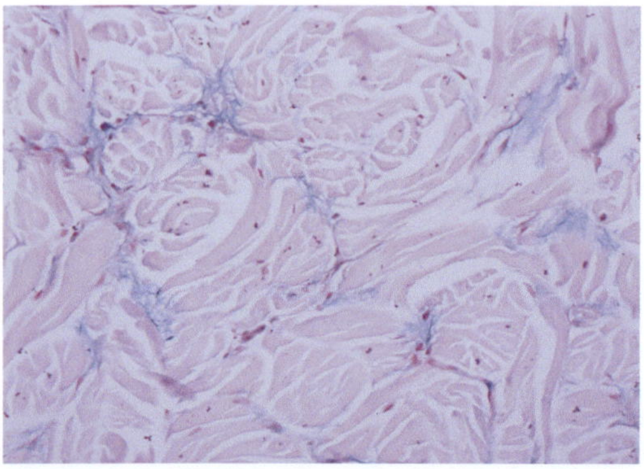

Fig. 18.24 Alcian Blue stain (dark blue) outlines small amount of mucin in early lesion

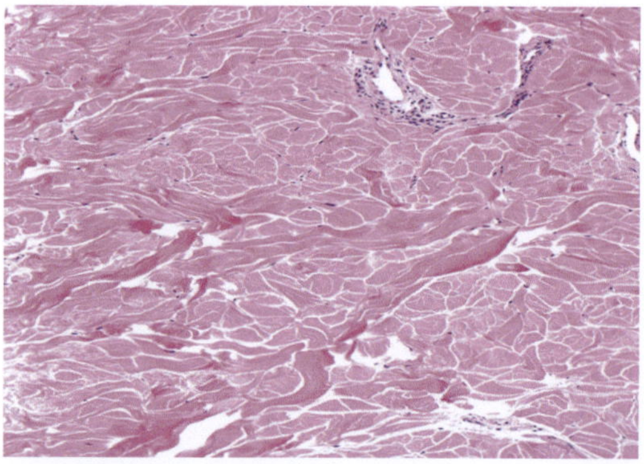

Fig. 18.25 Sclerotic collagen separated by "empty" spaces and minimal or no mucin

Sclerema Neonatorum

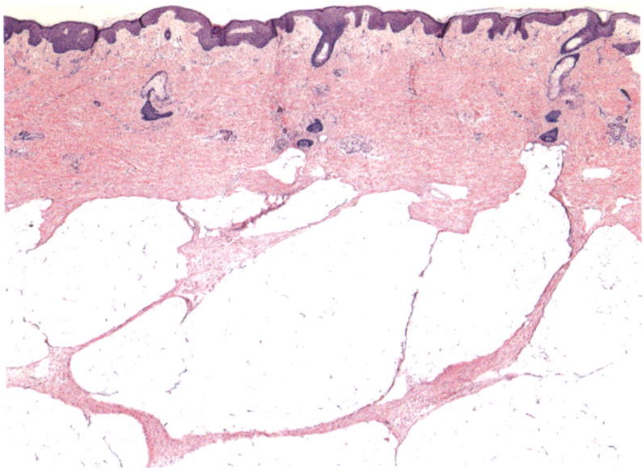

Fig. 18.26 Thickened dermis and subcutis

Histopathology (Figs. 18.26, 18.27, 18.28, and 18.29)

- Thickened fibrotic dermis
- Thickened fat septae with edema
- Very little or no inflammation
- No calcification
- Fine, needle-shaped clefts in the adipocytes

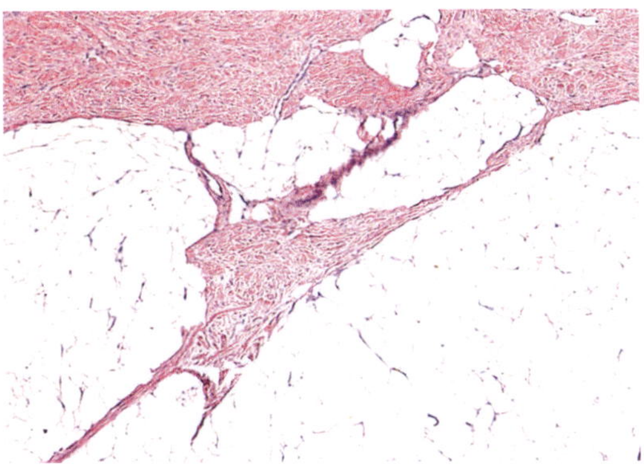

Fig. 18.27 Thick fibrous septa

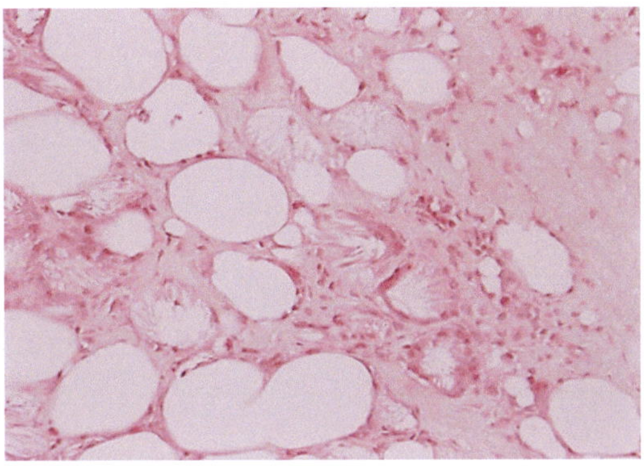

Fig. 18.28 Minimal inflammation

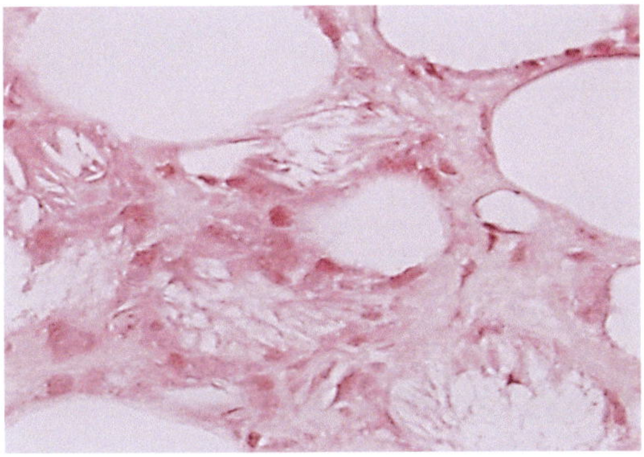

Fig. 18.29 Needle-shaped cholesterol clefts

Scleromyxedema

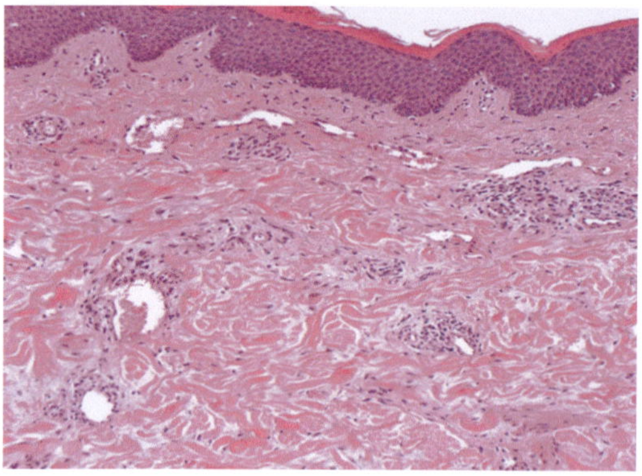

Fig. 18.30 Established lesion of scleromyxedema

Histopathology is different in early and established lesions (Figs. 18.30, 18.31, 18.32, 18.33, and 18.34)

Early lesion—disorganized collagen with increased number of fibroblasts and easily found mucin separating collagen

Established lesion—increased number of fibroblasts with significant fibrosis

- Mucin is less evident or even absent
- Perivascular lymphocytic inflammation is present

P.S. it is a subtype of diffuse *lichen myxedematosus*

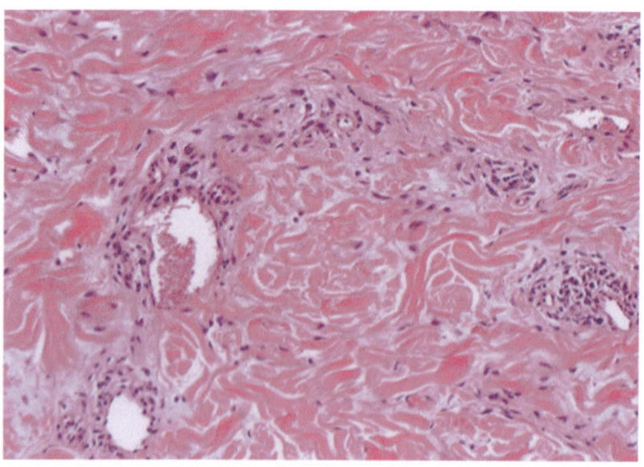

Fig. 18.31 Increased number of fibroblasts with dermal fibrosis

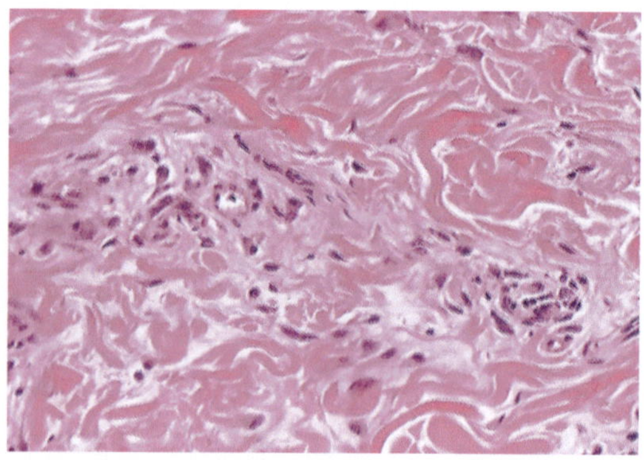

Fig. 18.32 Mild perivascular lymphocytic infiltrate is present

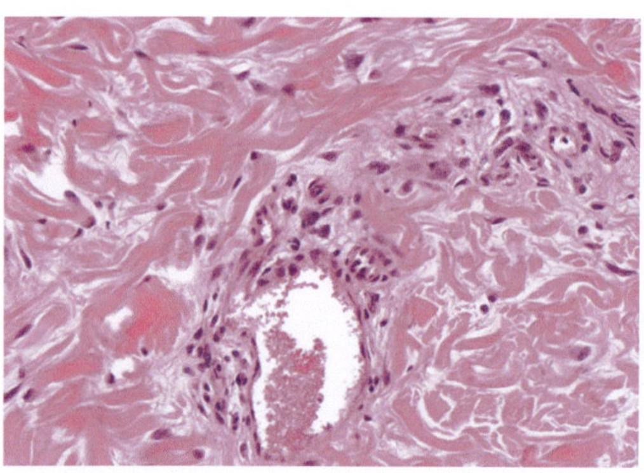

Fig. 18.33 Bluish dermal mucin between collagen

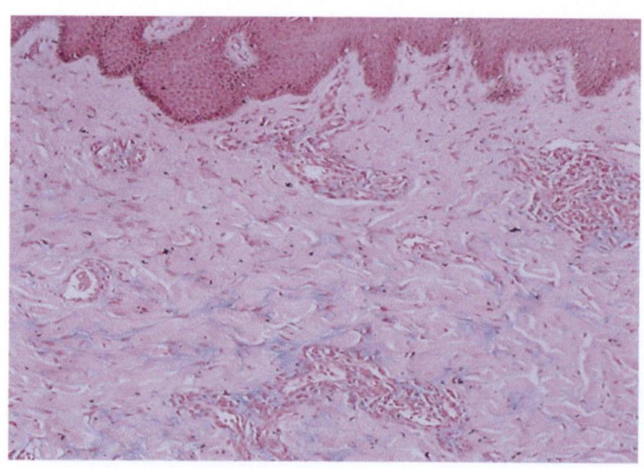

Fig. 18.34 Scattered dermal mucin (Alcian Blue)

Sclerotic Fibroma

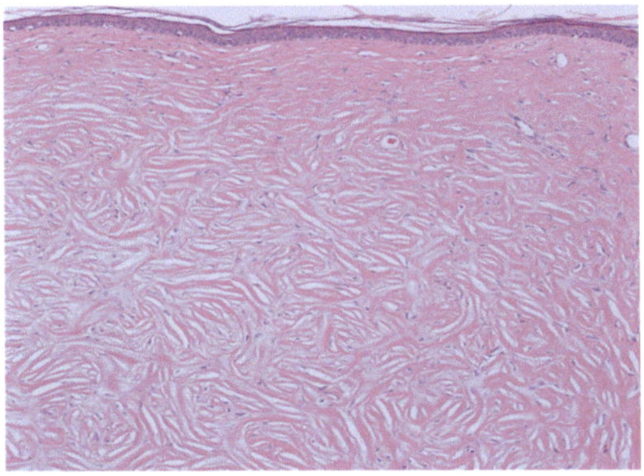

Fig. 18.35 Dermal sclerotic nodule

Synonym: Storiform Collagenoma

Histopathology (Figs. 18.35, 18.36, and 18.37)

- Circumscribed non-encapsulated lesion
- Hypocellular hyalinized stroma
- Cleft-like spaces formed between collagen
- "Wood grain" like appearance
- Cells are CD34+

P.S. may be associated with Cowden syndrome (*PTEN*)

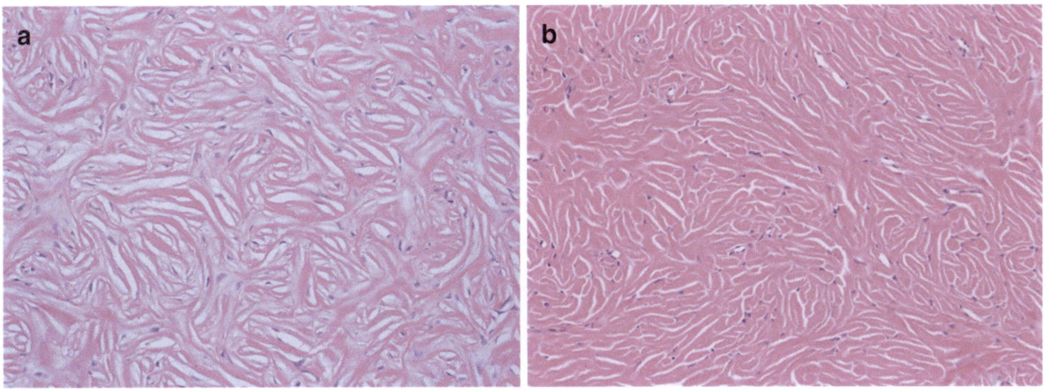

Fig. 18.36 (**a**, **b**) Hypocellular collagen bundles in storiform pattern

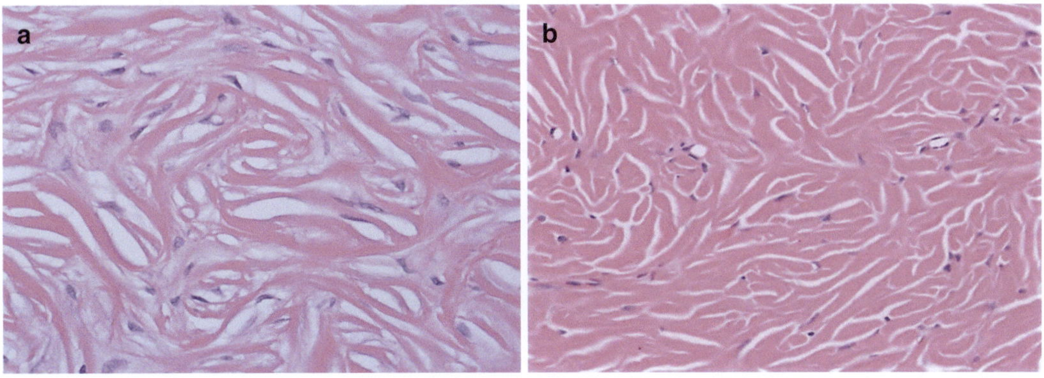

Fig. 18.37 (**a**, **b**) "Wood grain" appearance of collagen bundles separated with clefts

Schistosomiasis

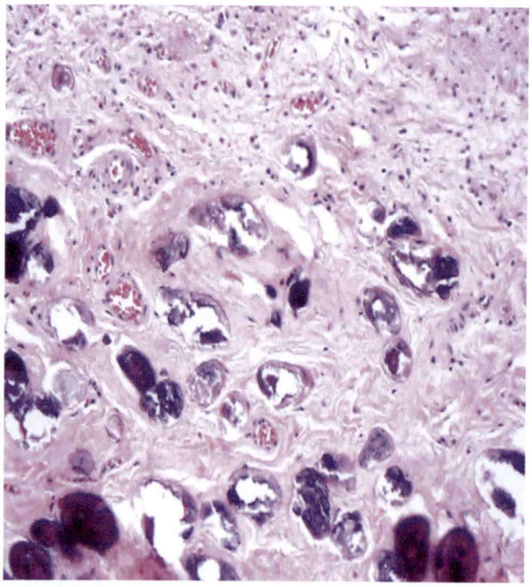

Fig. 18.38 Dense scar with calcified *Schistosoma* eggs

Synonyms: Bilharziasis, Swimmer's Itch

Histopathology (Figs. 18.38 and 18.39)

- Dermal and subcutaneous mixed inflammation that varies from abscess with variable number of eosinophils to chronic scarring response with minimal inflammation
- Dead ova frequently calcify

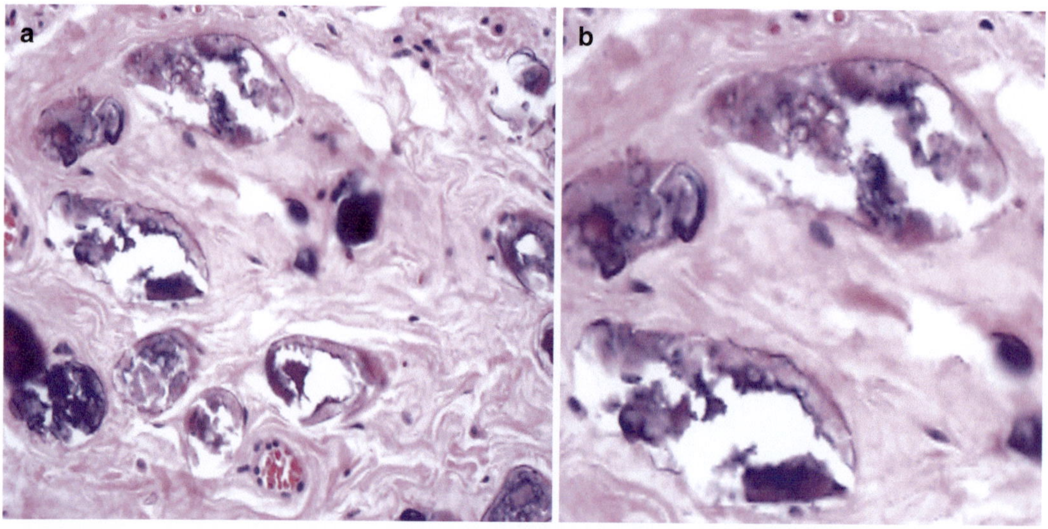

Fig. 18.39 (**a, b**) Numerous dead calcified ova with mild chronic inflammation and fibrosis

Schwannoma

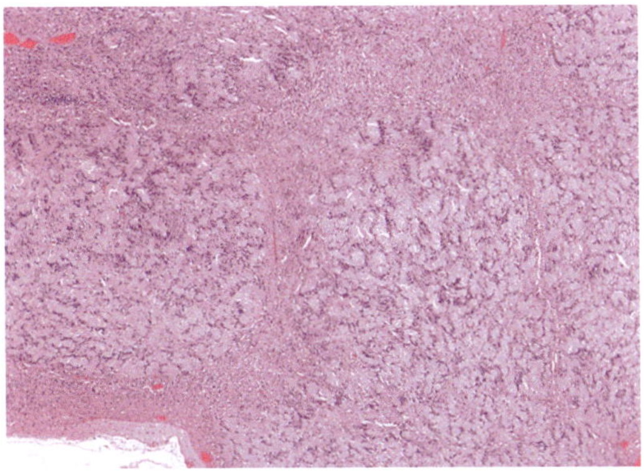

Fig. 18.40 Subcutaneous non encapsulated nodular tumor

Histopathology (Figs. 18.40, 18.41, 18.42, and 18.43)

- Well circumscribed subcutaneous tumor of elongated spindle cells in hyalinized stroma
- Cells (S100+) demonstrate nuclear palisading (Verocay bodies)
- Alternating hypercellular (Antoni A) and hypocellular (Antoni B) areas
- Nuclear hyperchromasia and mild nuclear polymorphism

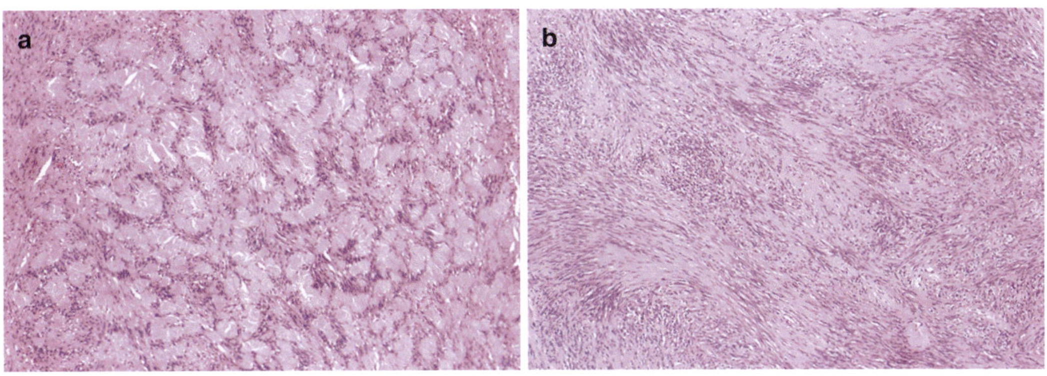

Fig. 18.41 (**a**, **b**) Spindle cells with alternating hypercellular and hypocellular areas

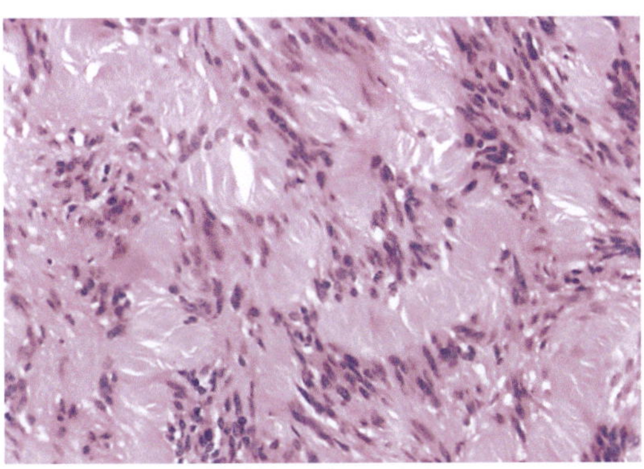

Fig. 18.42 Antoni A and Antoni B areas

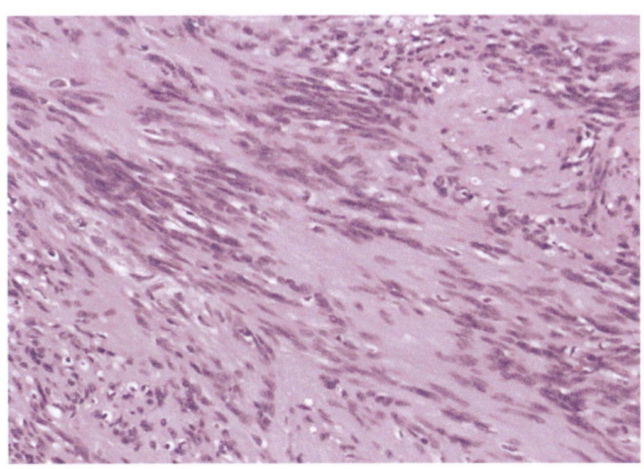

Fig. 18.43 Dark elongated nuclei in hyalinized stroma

Sebaceoma

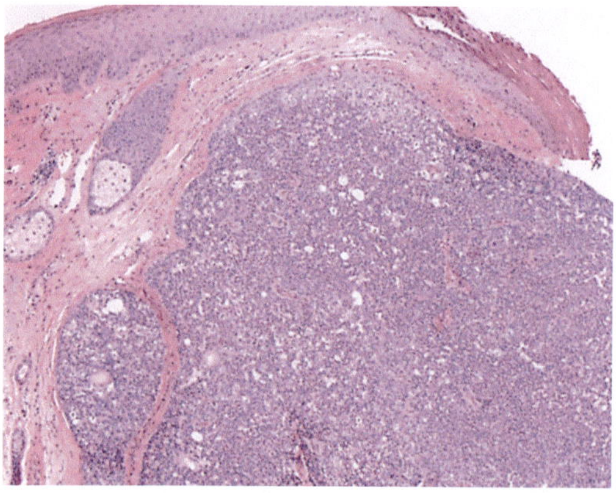

Fig. 18.44 Basaloid dermal tumor with no significant infiltration

Histopathology (Figs. 18.44, 18.45, and 18.46)

- Dermal nodule with no significant infiltration of the subcutis and frequent epidermal involvement
- Variable mixture of basaloid and mature sebocytes (EMA+) lacking well defined lobular structure
- Peripheral palisading and myxoid stroma is missing, distinguishing it from basal cell carcinoma
- Basaloid cells are small and uniform with sparse mitoses whereas mature sebocytes are scattered, not organized, like in sebaceous adenoma
- Common ducts and cysts with sebaceous debris

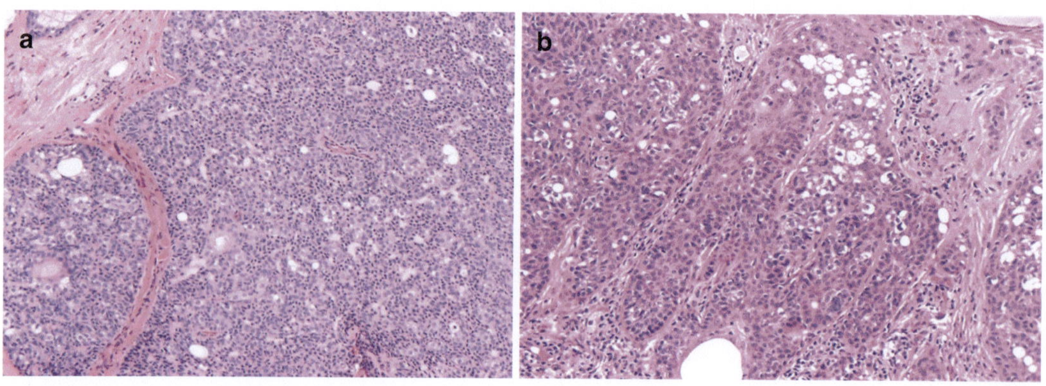

Fig. 18.45 (**a**, **b**) No peripheral palisading, stromal retraction, or well defined lobular structure; ducts and cyst are present within the tumor

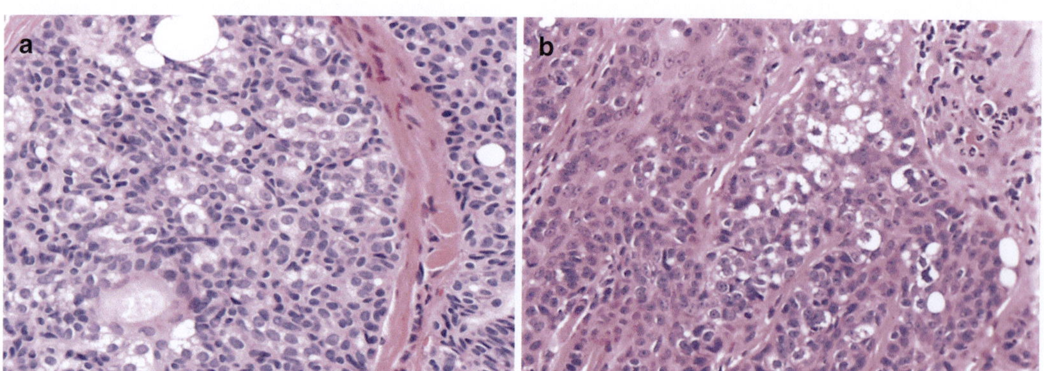

Fig. 18.46 (**a**, **b**) Mature sebocytes are randomly scattered among basaloid cells; no evidence of cytological atypia

Sebaceous Adenoma

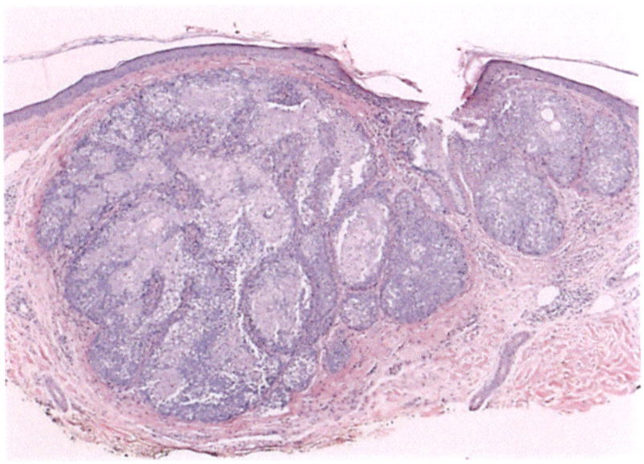

Fig. 18.47 Nodular sebaceous lesion attached to the epidermis

Histopathology (Figs. 18.47, 18.48, 18.49, and 18.50)

- Well defined sebaceous lesion attached to atrophic epidermis
- Lobular pale tumor structure
- Lobules are composed of small basaloid cells at the periphery, mature sebaceous cells in the center, and transitional cells in between
- Mature sebaceous cells outnumber basaloid cells

P.S. associated with Muir-Torre syndrome

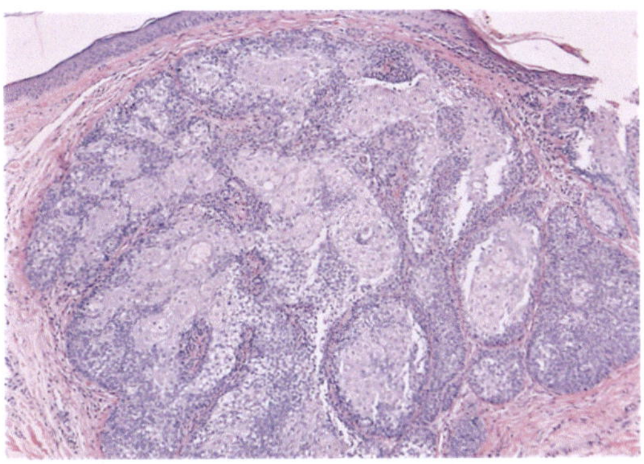

Fig. 18.48 Basaloid, transitional, and mature sebaceous cells form lobules

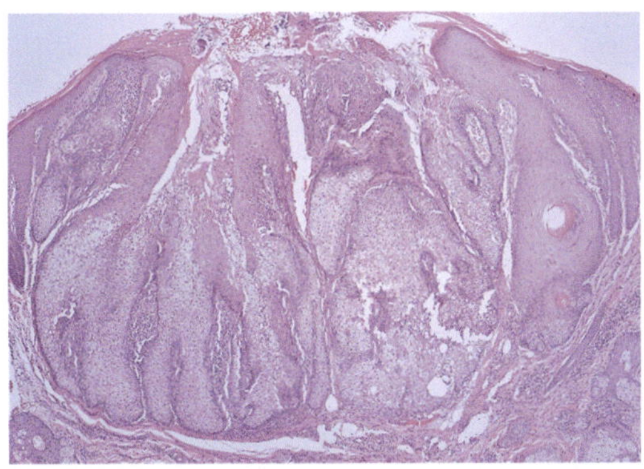

Fig. 18.49 Well defined lobular structures

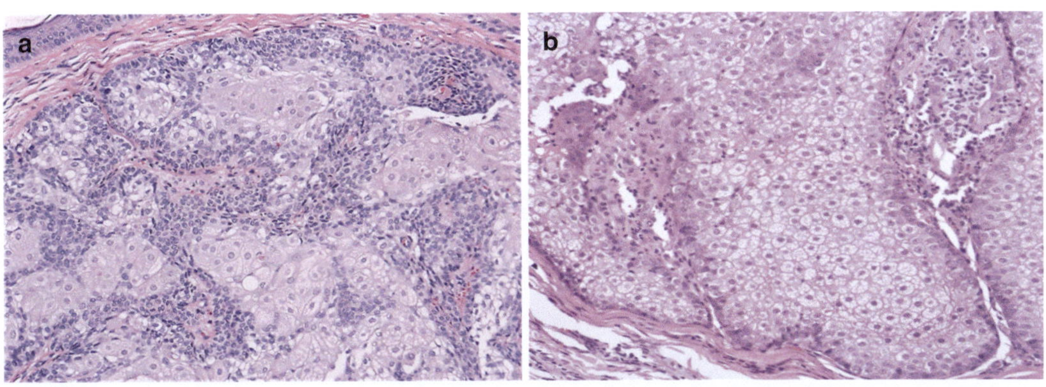

Fig. 18.50 (**a**, **b**) Mature sebaceous cells, with no atypia or mitoses, form the majority of tumor cells

Sebaceous Carcinoma

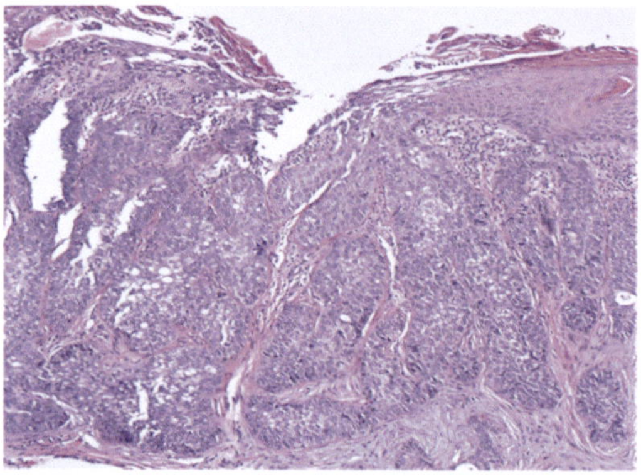

Fig. 18.51 Multilobular tumor infiltrating dermis

Histopathology (Figs. 18.51, 18.52, 18.53, 18.54, and 18.55)

- Multilobular infiltrating dermal tumor with a spectrum of lesions
  - **Well differentiated** with easily found "sebaceous-like" pale cells with multivacuolated cytoplasm and vesicular nuclei
  - **Poorly differentiated** with atypical cells that don't have obvious sebaceous features and have large atypical nuclei and vaguely vacuolated cytoplasm
- Cells are EMA+, androgen receptor+, Ber-ep4−

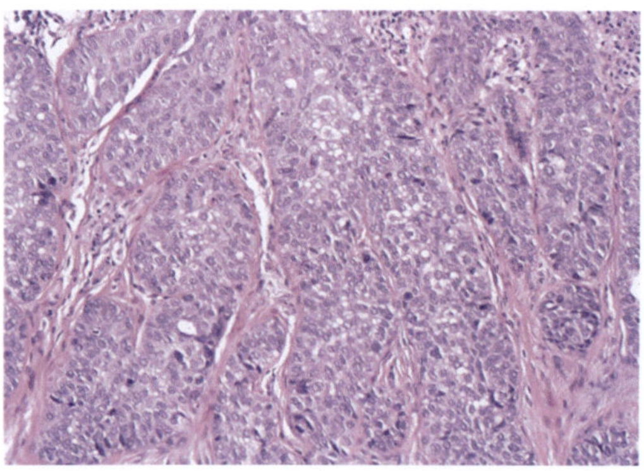

Fig. 18.52 Cells with multivacuolated cytoplasm and vesicular nuclei

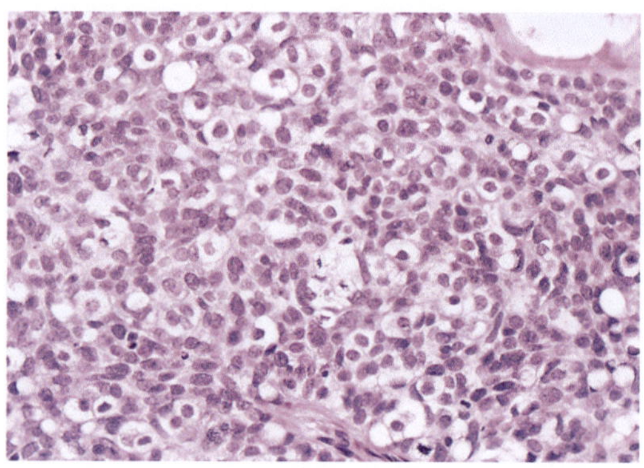

Fig. 18.53 Cells with dark nuclei and sparse cytoplasm are admixed with pale multivacuolated cells

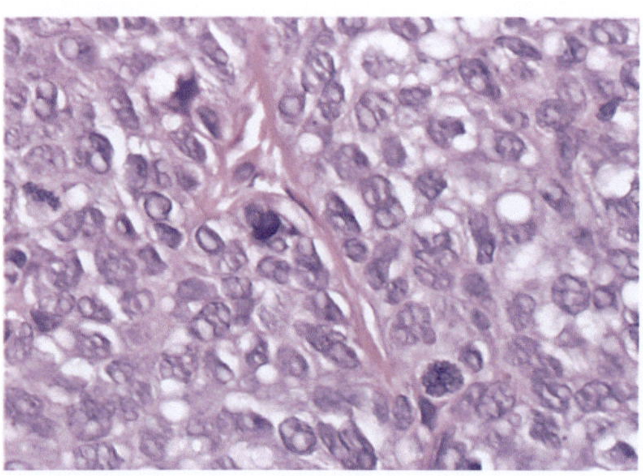

Fig. 18.54 Mitoses and apoptotic cells are present

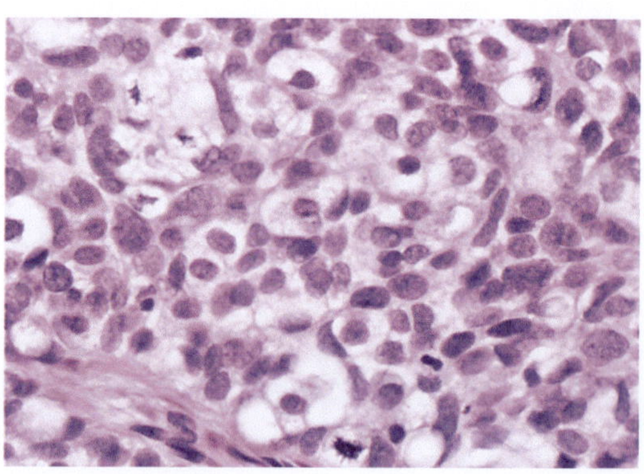

Fig. 18.55 Pale multivacuolated cells with multiple mitoses

Sebaceous Hyperplasia

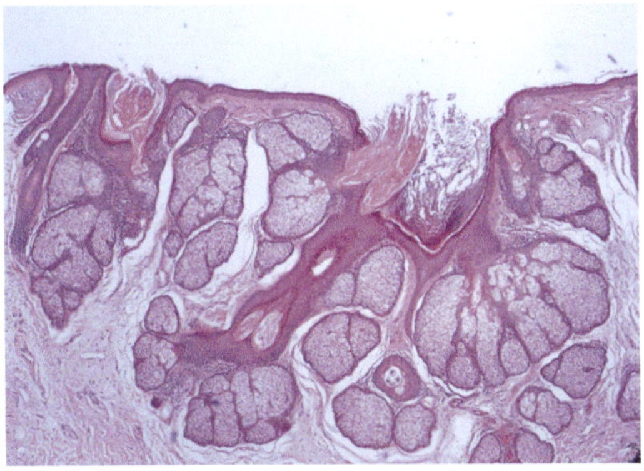

Fig. 18.56 Dilated and keratin plugged follicular infundibulum with attached multiple sebaceous glands

Histopathology (Figs. 18.56, 18.57, and 18.58)
- Hyperplasia of mature sebaceous glands
- Four or more sebaceous glands attached to central infundibulum
- Normal ration of basaloid and mature sebaceous cells
- Central infundibulum is usually dilated and filled with keratin

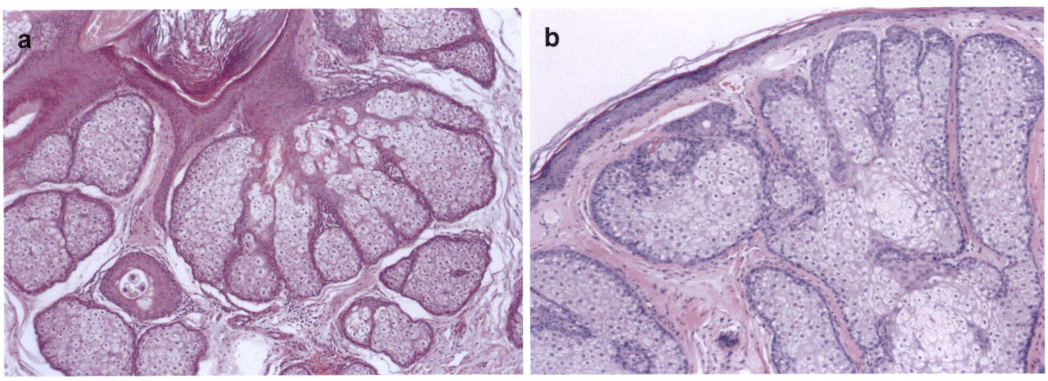

Fig. 18.57 (**a**, **b**) Normal ratio of basaloid and mature sebaceous glands

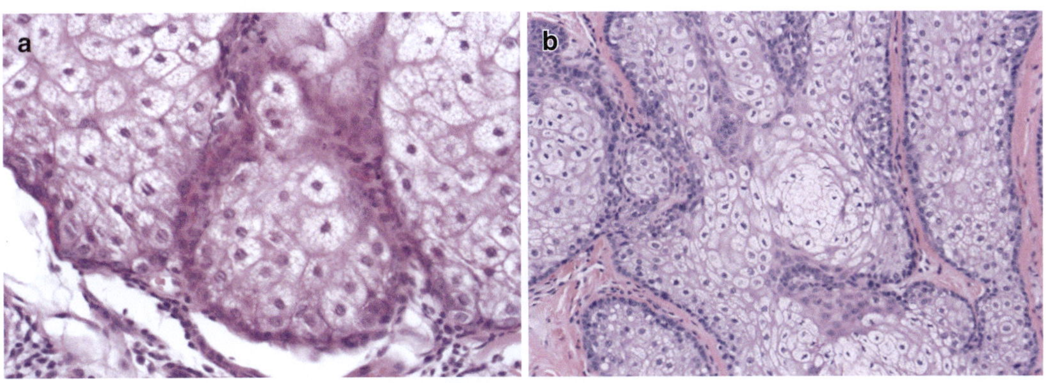

Fig. 18.58 (**a**, **b**) Sebaceous cells with no cytological atypia

Seborrheic Dermatitis

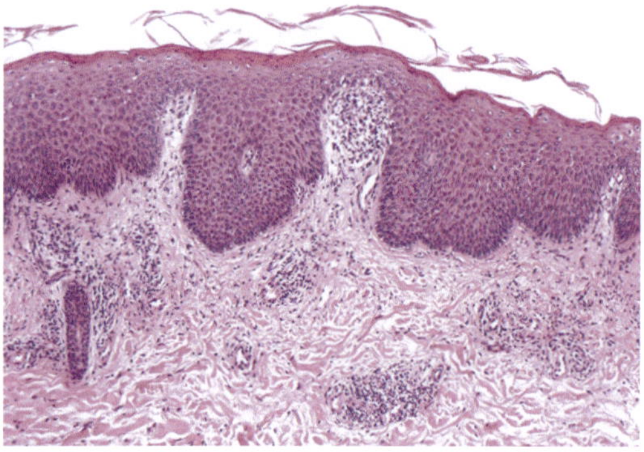

Fig. 18.59 Irregular epidermal psoriasiform hyperplasia

Histopathology is subtle and frequently not specific (Figs. 18.59, 18.60, 18.61, 18.62, and 18.63)

- Irregular psoriasiform hyperplasia
- Variable epidermal spongiosis with lymphocytic exocytosis
- Focal parakeratosis commonly associated with neutrophils
- Mild perivascular lymphocytic infiltrate

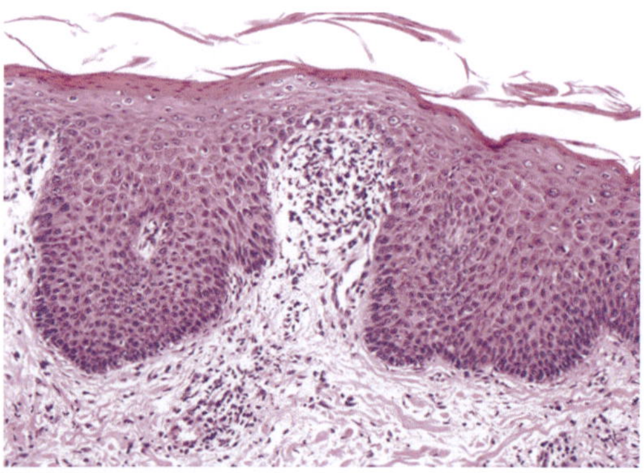

Fig. 18.60 Mild epidermal spongiosis

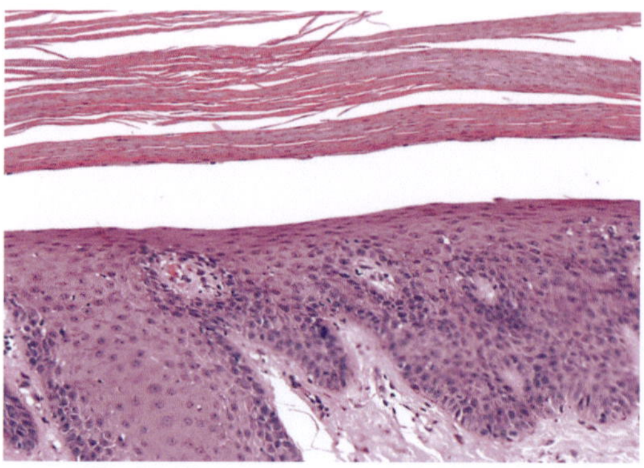

Fig. 18.61 Compact stratum corneum

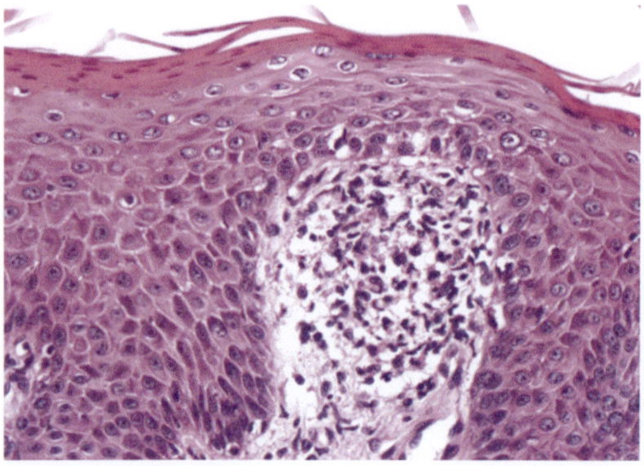

Fig. 18.62 Epidermal parakeratosis and dermal perivascular lymphocytic inflammation

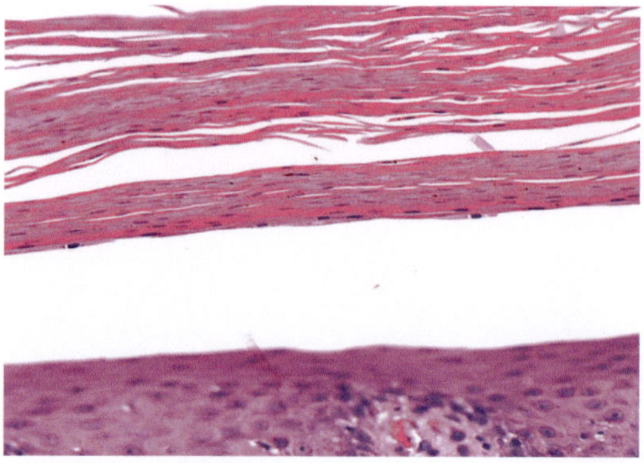

Fig. 18.63 Epidermal parakeratosis

Seborrheic Keratosis

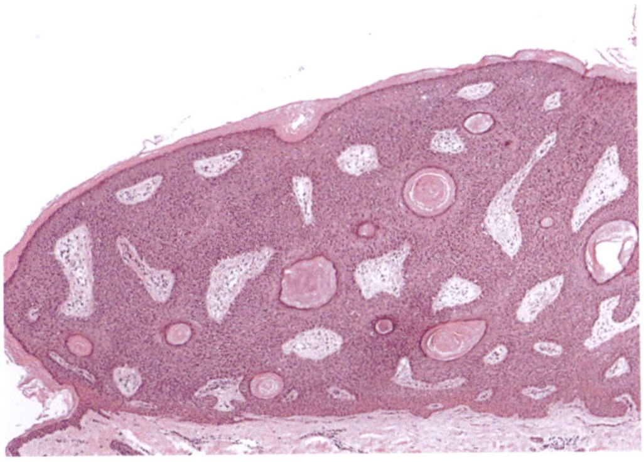

Fig. 18.64 **Acanthotic SK** with uniform proliferation of keratinocytes and horn pseudocysts

Histopathology (Figs. 18.64, 18.65, 18.66, 18.67, 18.68, 18.69, 18.70, 18.71)

- Multiple variants but all are composed of small uniform keratinocytes
- All types have variable acanthosis and hyperkeratosis
- Horn pseudocysts are present in all variants but not in macular/flat and clonal variant

P.S. *Leser-Trélat* is sudden appearance of multiple seborrheic keratosis in association with internal malignancy

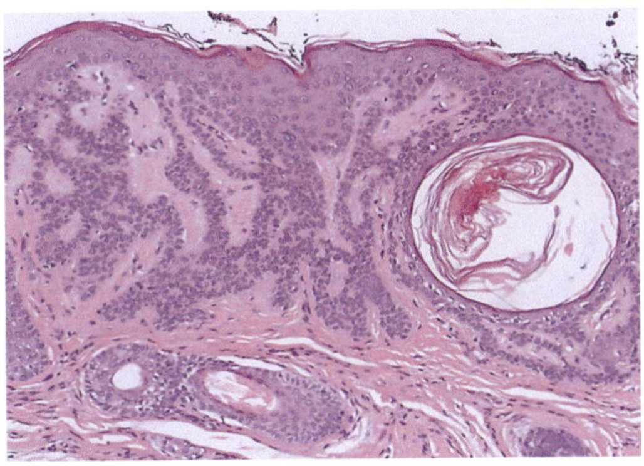

Fig. 18.65 **Reticulated/adenoid SK** with "net like" pattern

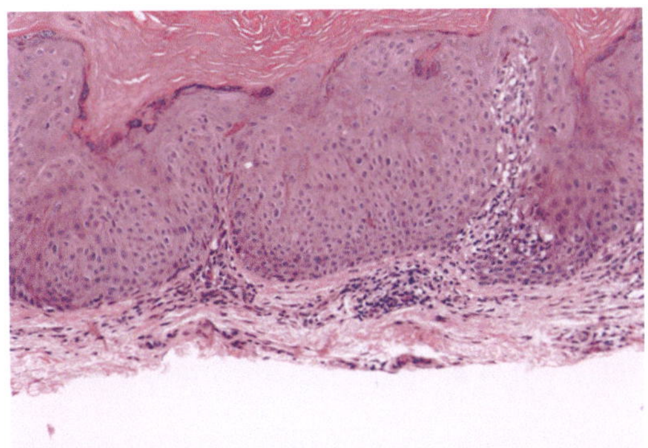

Fig. 18.66 **Clonal SK** with uniform epidermal nests

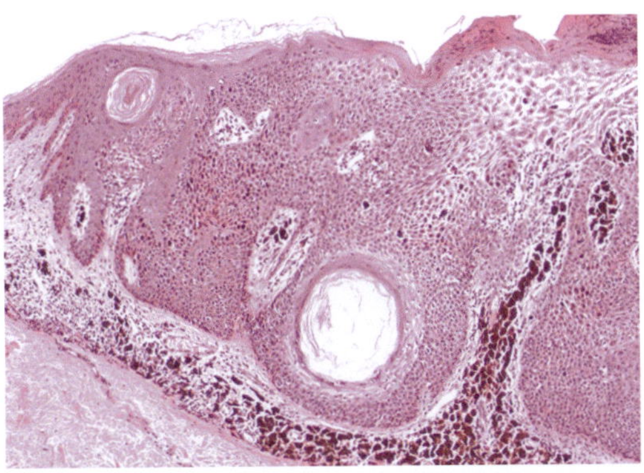

Fig. 18.67 **Pigmented SK** with melanin pigment within and outside of proliferating keratinocytes

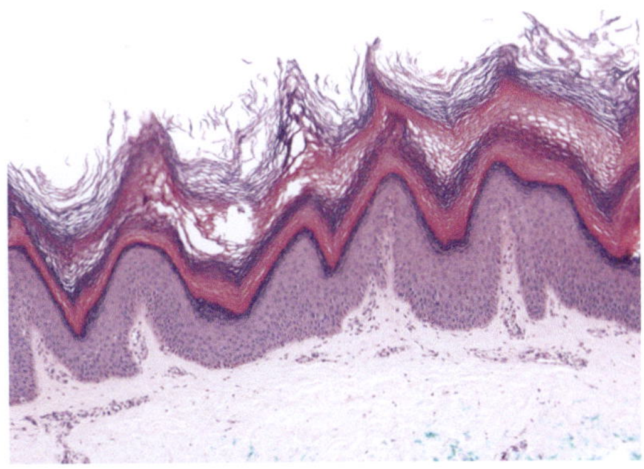

Fig. 18.68 **Macular/flat SK** with uniform proliferating keratinocytes

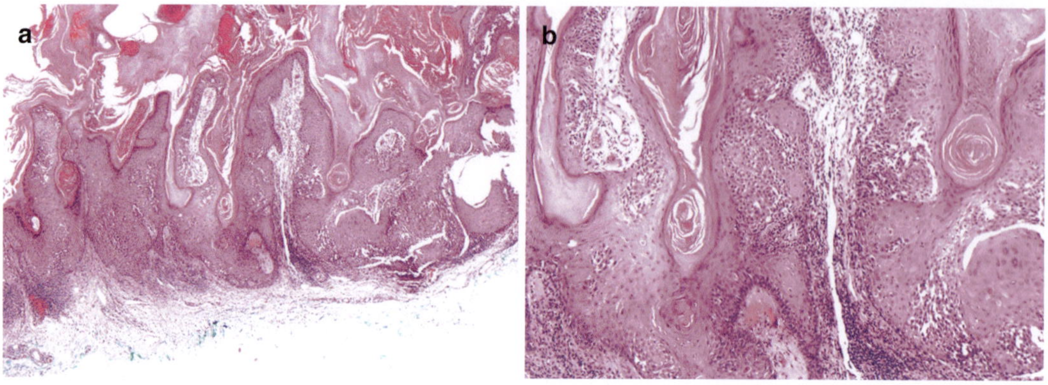

Fig. 18.69 (**a**, **b**) **Irritated SK** with irregular papillomatosis and squamous eddies

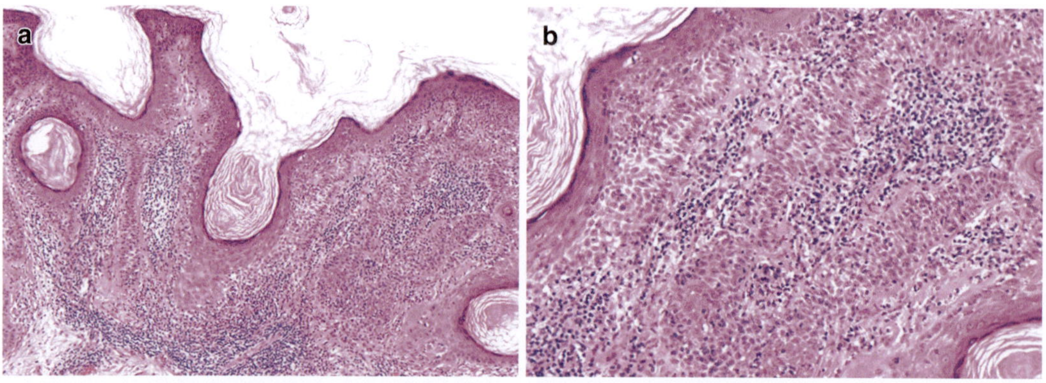

Fig. 18.70 (**a**, **b**) **Inflamed SK** with numerous lymphocytes

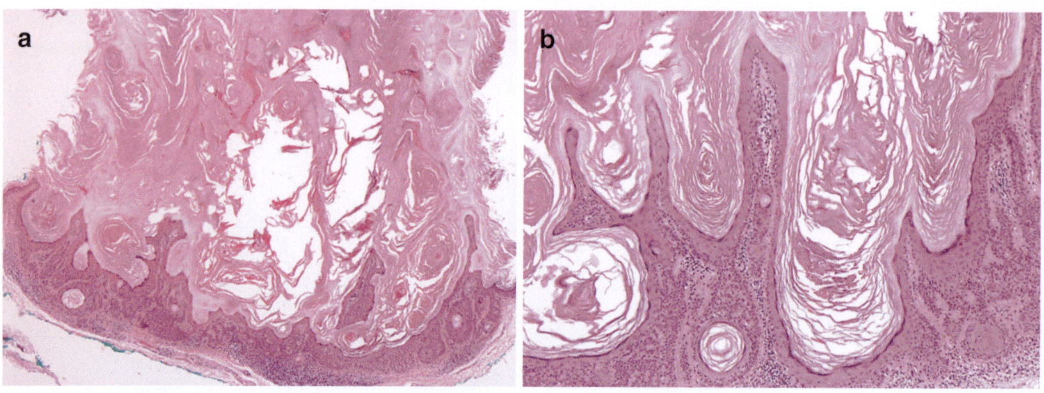

Fig. 18.71 (**a**, **b**) **SK with cutaneous horn**

Solar Elastosis

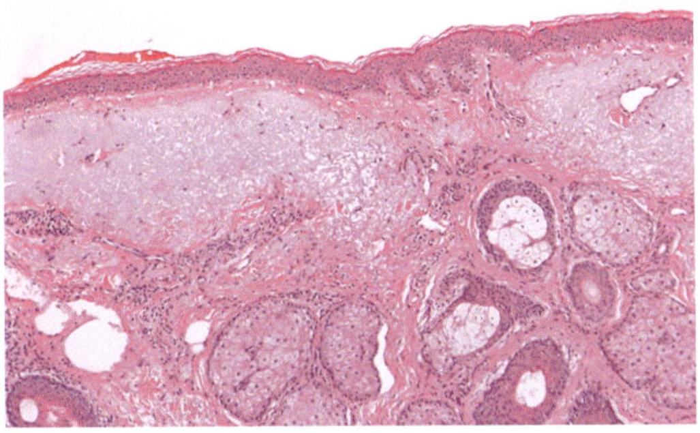

Fig. 18.72 Irregular amorphous nodules in the upper dermis

Synonym: Actinic Elastosis

Histopathology (Figs. 18.72, 18.73, 18.74, 18.75, and 18.76)

- Fragmented, irregular elastic fibers
- Elastic fibers have gray blue appearance
- In more extensive solar damage elastic fibers form gray bluish amorphous nodules in the upper dermis
- Irregular cracks are present within aggregates

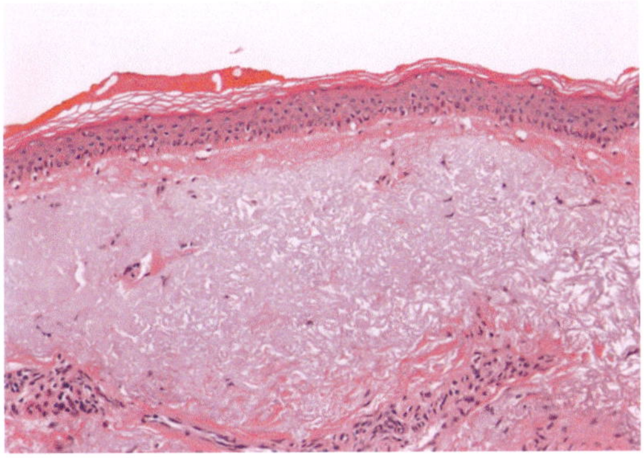

Fig. 18.73 Irregular nodules formed by damaged elastic fibers

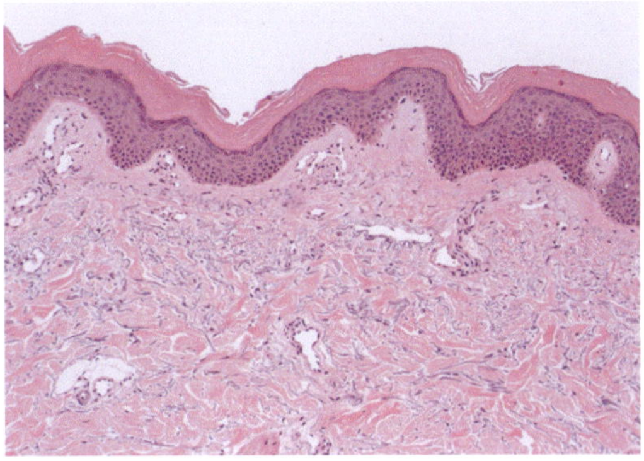

Fig. 18.74 Pale dermis with no inflammation

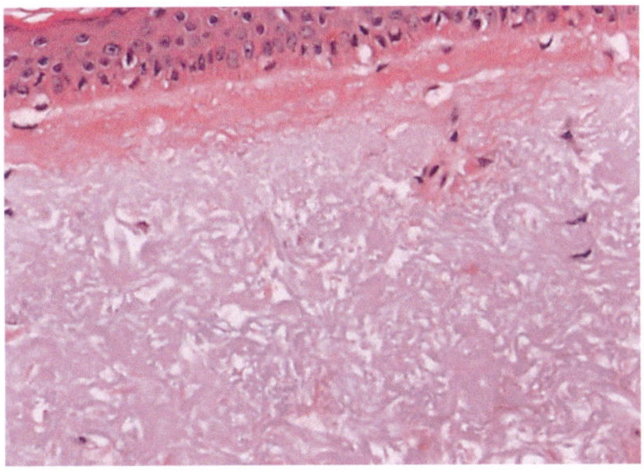

Fig. 18.75 Irregular cracks are present within dermal aggregates

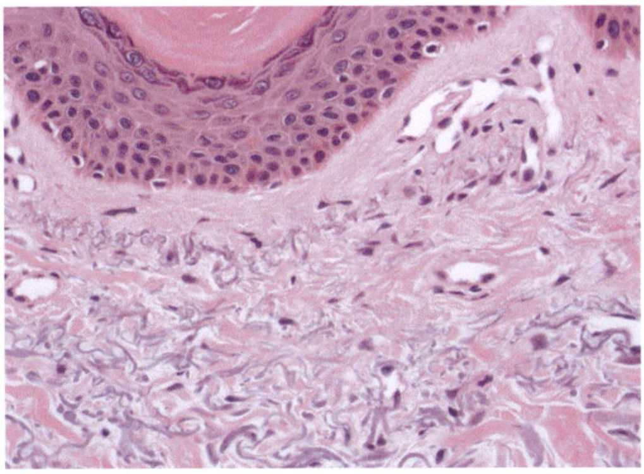

Fig. 18.76 Fragmented, irregular gray bluish elastic fibers

Solar Lentigo

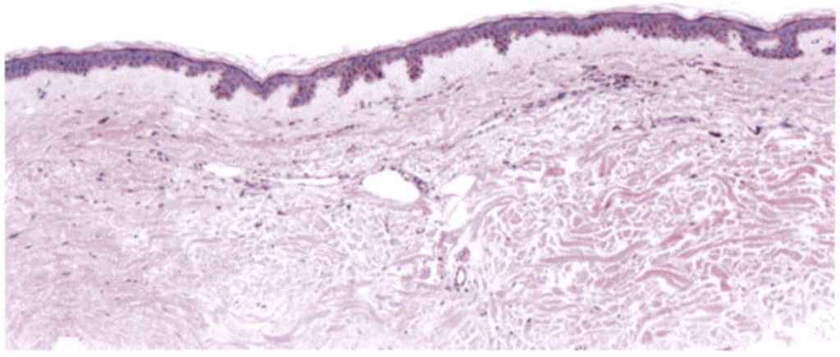

Fig. 18.77 Atrophic epidermis with finger-like projections

Synonym: Actinic Lentigo

Histopathology (Figs. 18.77, 18.78, and 18.79)

- Elongation of club-shaped rete ridges
- Basal hyperpigmentation of keratinocytes
- Number of melanocytes is normal or slightly increased
- Variable number of dermal melanophages
- Dermal solar elastosis

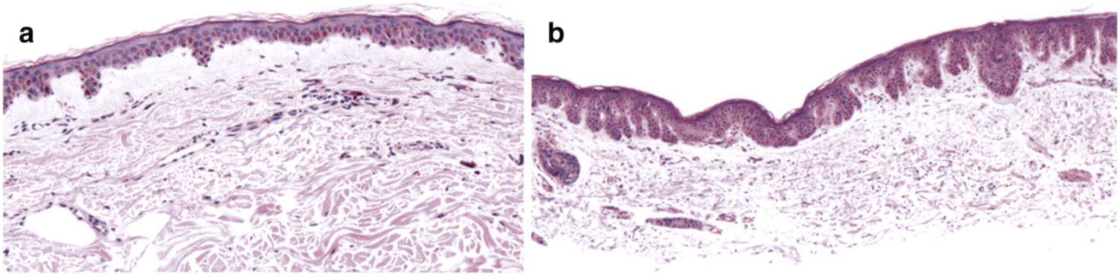

Fig. 18.78 (**a**, **b**) Elongation of club-shaped hyperpigmented rete-ridges with no significant increase of melanocytes

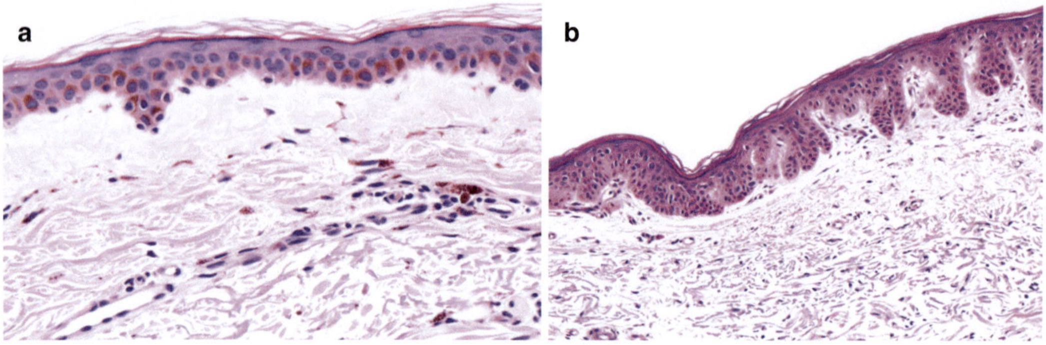

Fig. 18.79 (**a**, **b**) Extensive solar elastosis with dermal pigment incontinence

Special Site Nevus

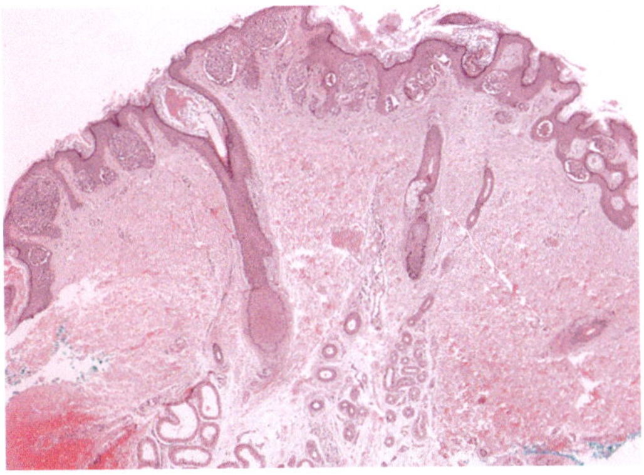

Fig. 18.80 Special site junctional nevus of axilla

Synonym: Nevus of the Special Site (NOSS)
Special sites are along the embryonic milk line, flexural sites, genitalia, palms/soles, ear, and scalp.

Not *all* nevi at special sites have features of NOSS.

Histopathology vary between different sites but they have in common the following (Figs. 18.80, 18.81, 18.82, 18.83, and 18.84)

- Enlarged junctional nests
- Common split of nests from keratinocytes
- Common epidermal pagetoid spread

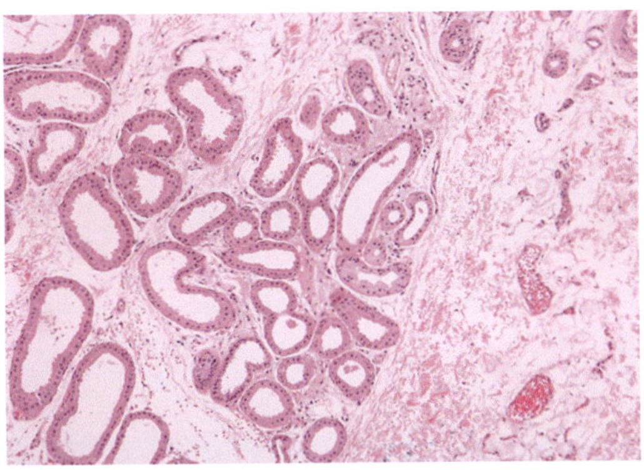

Fig. 18.81 Apocrine glands confirm axillary location

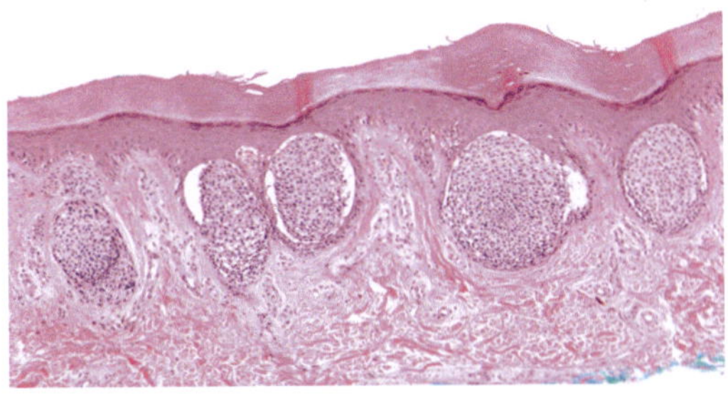

Fig. 18.82 Enlarged junctional nests of acral site

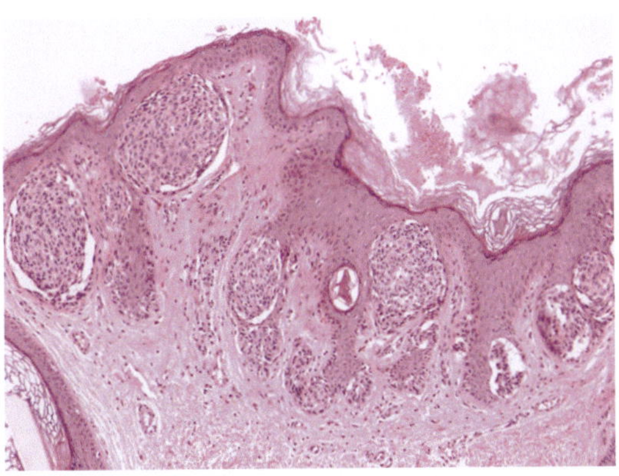

Fig. 18.83 Nests retract from keratinocytes

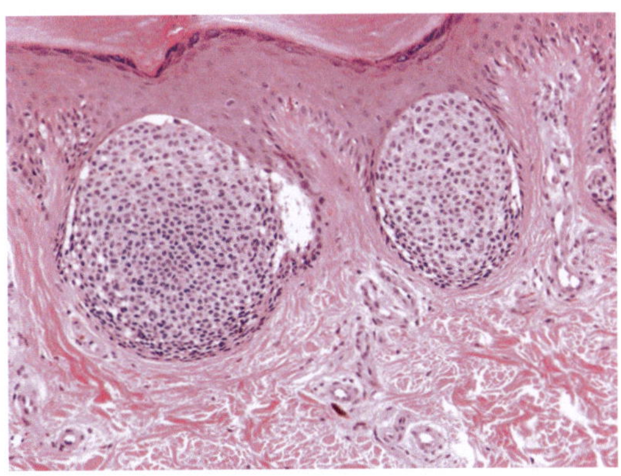

Fig. 18.84 Melanocytes show maturation within nests

Spider Angioma

Synonyms: Nevus Araneous, Arterial Spider

Histopathology (Figs. 18.85, 18.86, 18.87, and 18.88)
- Central vertical arteriole in the dermis
- Smaller vascular channels are branching from the central arteriole

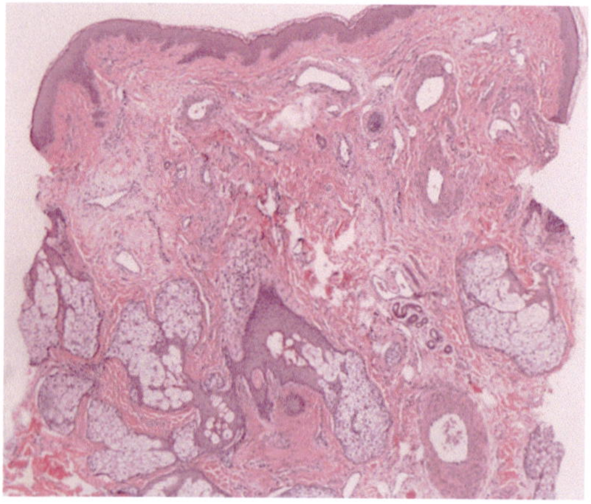

Fig. 18.85 Arteriole that is vertical to the epidermis

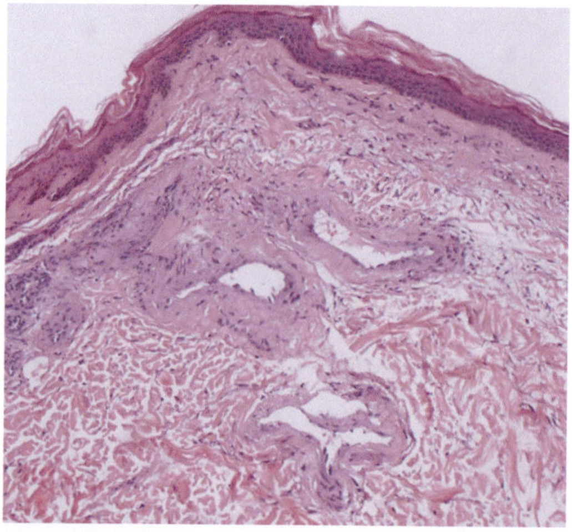

Fig. 18.86 Smaller vessels are branching from the central arteriole

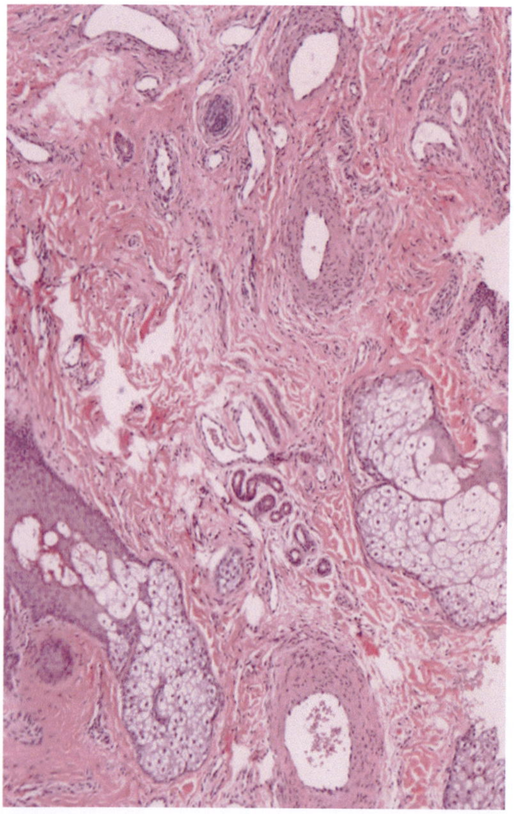

Fig. 18.87 Vertical arteriole starts to branch in the dermis

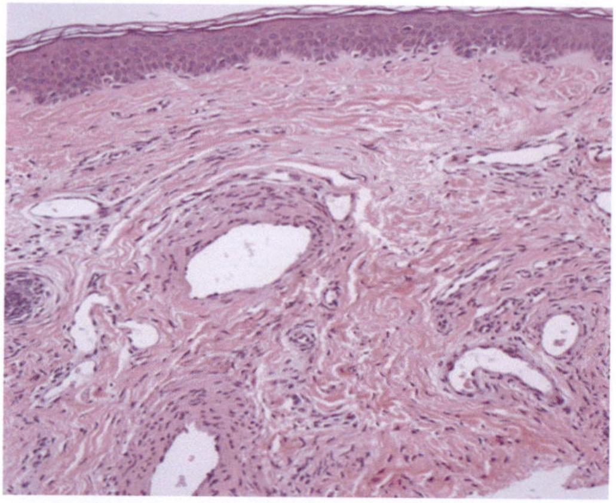

Fig. 18.88 Vessels are lined by flat endothelial cells

Spiradenoma

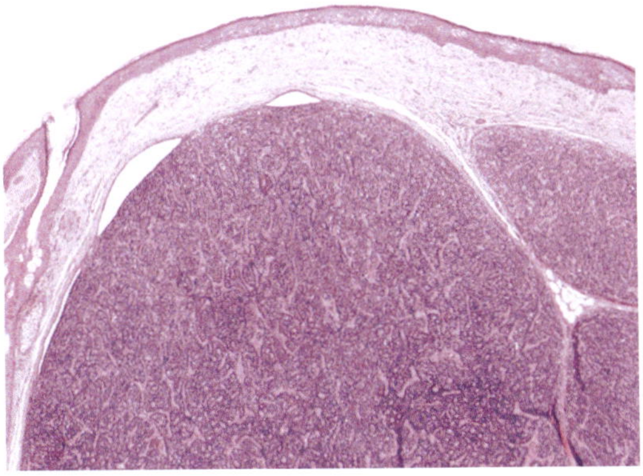

Fig. 18.89 Rounded nodules in subcutis

Synonym: Eccrine Spiradenoma

Histopathology (Figs. 18.89, 18.90, 18.91, and 18.92)

- One or multiple rounded nodules in dermis and subcutis with no epidermal connection
- Nodules are made of smaller darker outside cells and larger paler inner cells with small duct-like structures present
- Lymphocytes are scattered throughout the tumor
- Stroma around and inside nodules is hyalinized
- Peripheral vascular channels can be prominent

P.S associated with Brooke-Spiegler syndrome

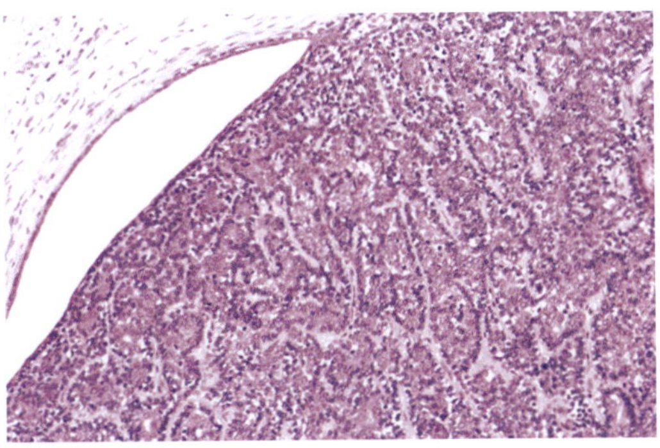

Fig. 18.90 Tumor with peripheral dilated vascular channel

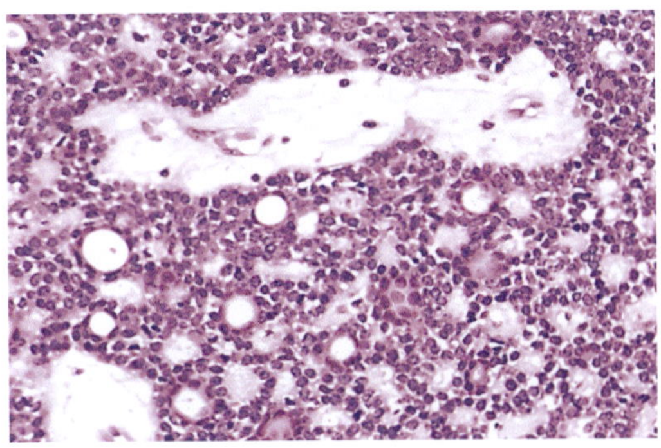

Fig. 18.91 Tumor with small ducts and hyalinized stroma

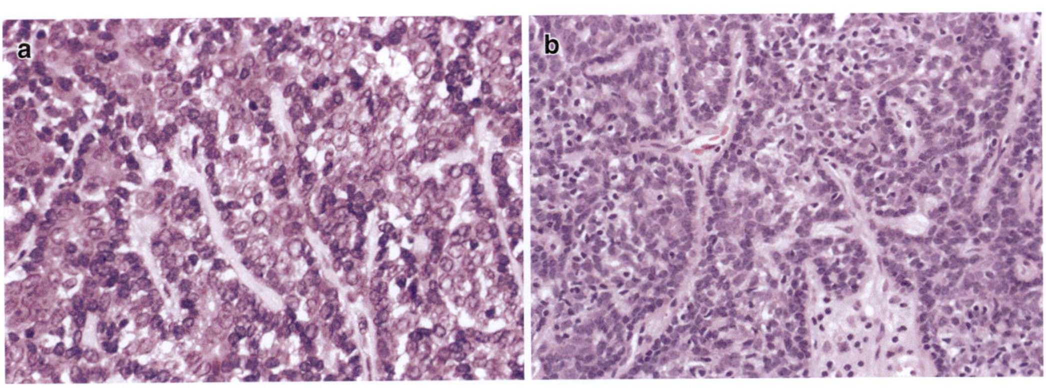

Fig. 18.92 (**a**, **b**) Darker outside cells and paler inner cells peppered with lymphocytes on the top

Spiradenocarcinoma

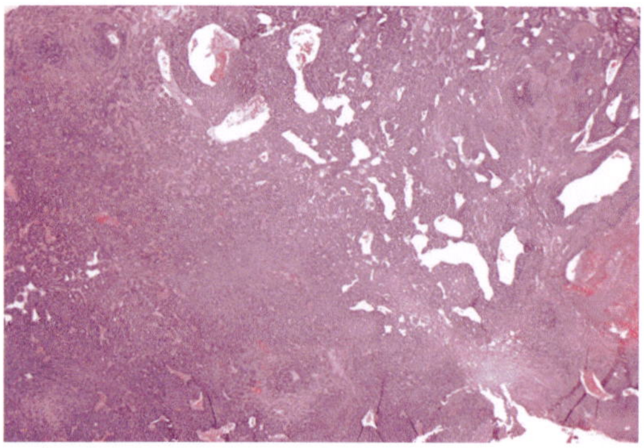

Fig. 18.93 Large tumor nodule with spiradenoma on the left, necrosis in right lower corner, and squamous changes in the right upper corner

Synonym: Carcinoma Ex Eccrine Spiradenoma

Histopathology (Figs. 18.93, 18.94, 18.95, 18.96, and 18.97)

- Large dermal/subcutaneous nodules with remnants of benign spiradenoma
- Presence of necrosis and easily found mitoses
- Frequent atypical squamous areas

P.S. tumor develops in long standing spiradenoma. Associated with Brooke-Spiegler syndrome (*CYLD1*)

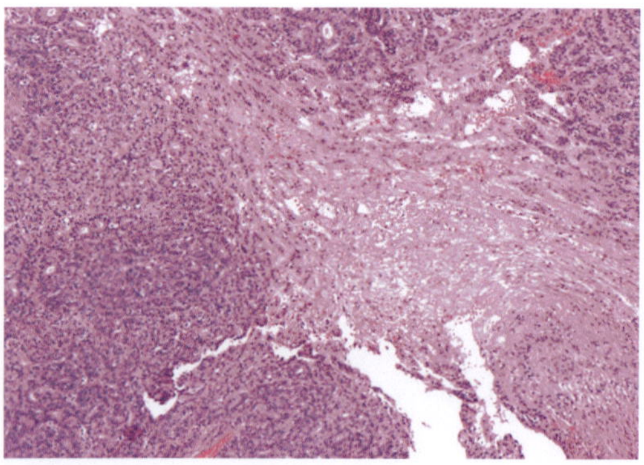

Fig. 18.94 Central necrosis

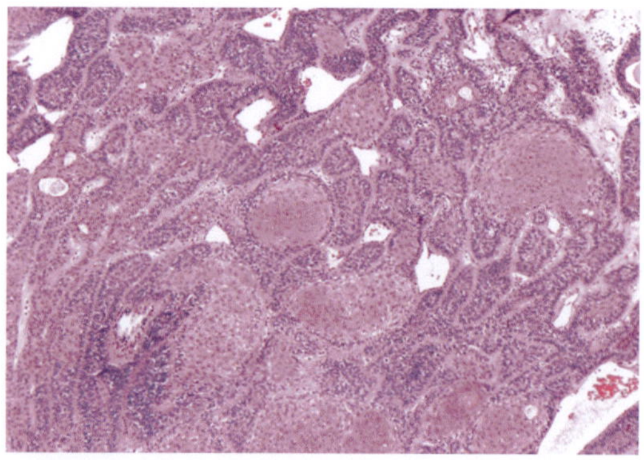

Fig. 18.95 Squamous area resembling squamous cell carcinoma

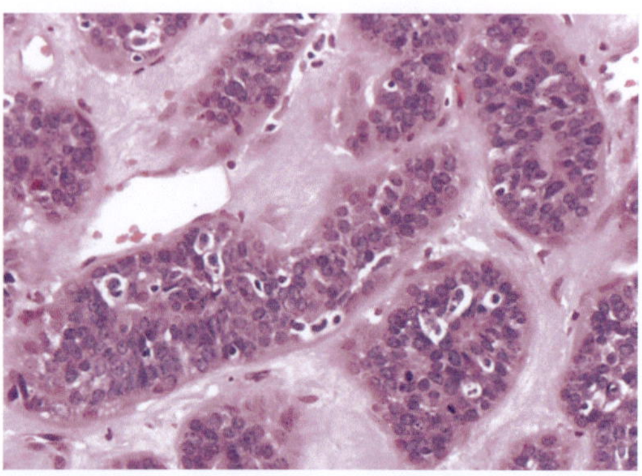

Fig. 18.96 Cytological atypia of "spiradenoma-like" islands with hyalinized stroma and "peppered on" lymphocytes

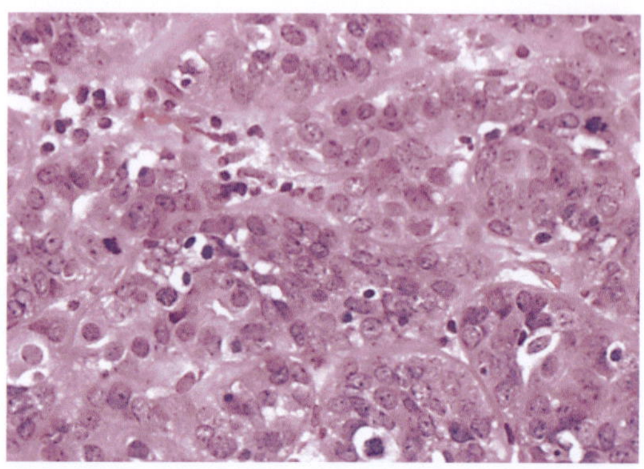

Fig. 18.97 Numerous mitoses are present

Spitz Nevus

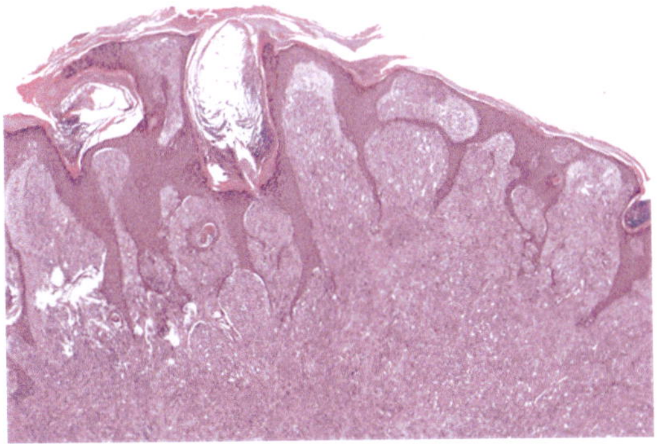

Fig. 18.98 Epidermal hyperkeratosis and papillomatosis with maturing melanocytic lesion

Histopathology (Figs. 18.98, 18.99, 18.100, 18.101, and 18.102)

- Horizontally and vertically symmetric lesion with no consumption of the hyperkeratotic papillomatous epidermis
- Epithelioid and/or spindle uniformly pleomorphic cells forming junctional nests and dermal maturing nests
- Junctional nests cleft from the epidermis
- Pale, pink hyaline globules (Kamino's bodies) and multinucleated nevus cells at epidermo-dermal junction
- Pagetoid spread common in the center of the lesion and mitoses can be present in the superficial part

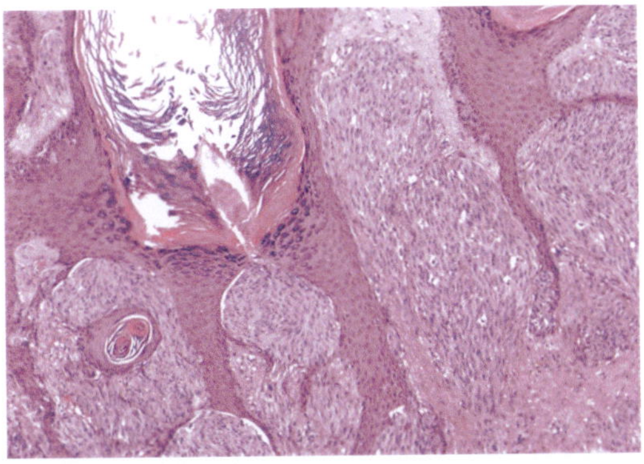

Fig. 18.99 Spindle cell variant forming "tear dropping" fascicles

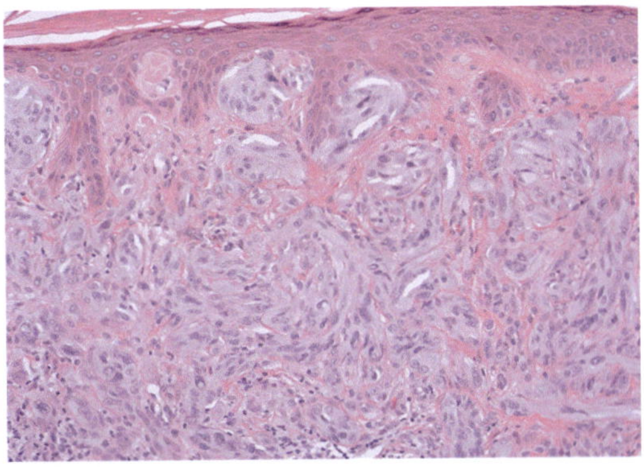

Fig. 18.100 Epithelioid variant with pleomorphic cells that mature

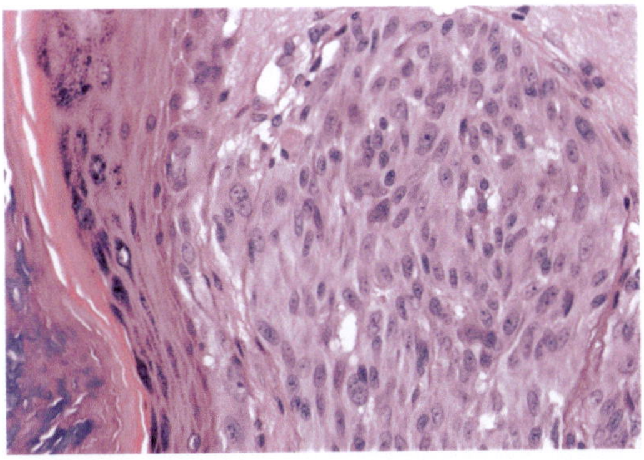

Fig. 18.101 Junctional nests with clefts and Kamino bodies

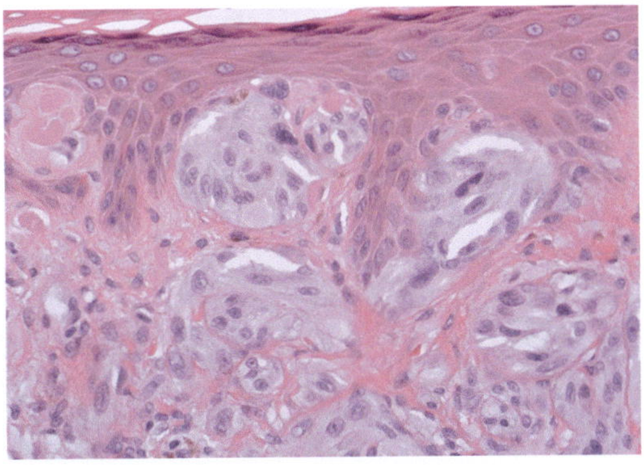

Fig. 18.102 Mild cellular pleomorphism but no significant atypia

Splinter

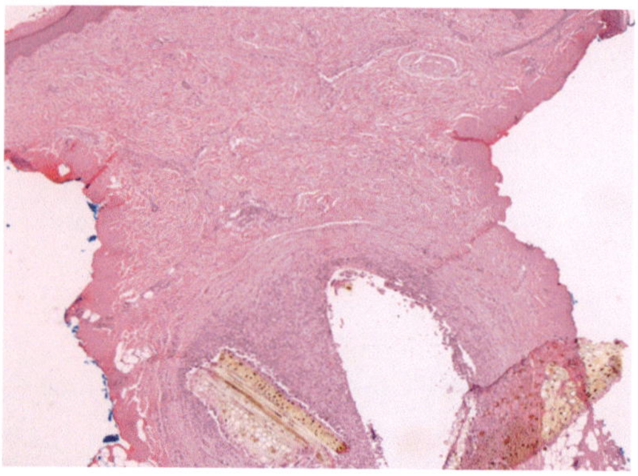

Fig. 18.103 **Splinter** embedded in the deep dermis

Histopathology (Figs. 18.103, 18.104, 18.105, and 18.106)

- Plant material usually causes strong neutrophilic inflammation with admixed lymphocytes and histiocytes
- Surrounding fibrosis and scarring is present
- Pigmented fungi are commonly found

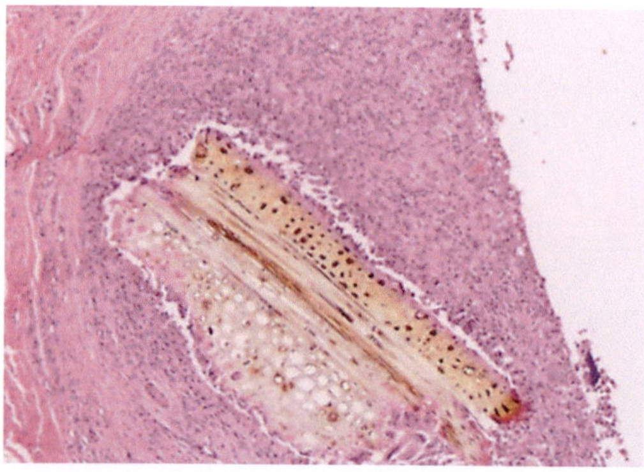

Fig. 18.104 Plant material is darkly pigmented with pigmented rectangular plant cells

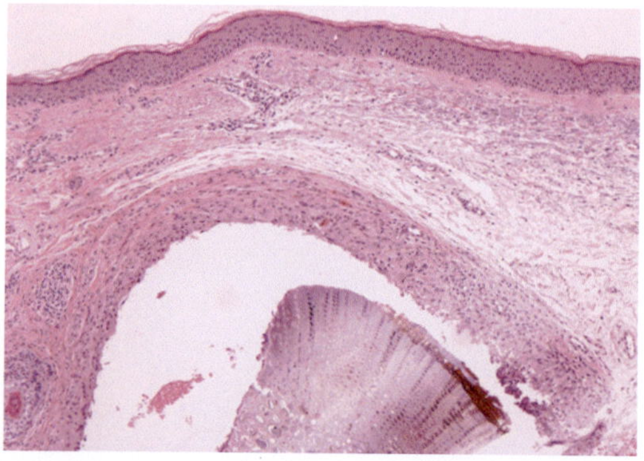

Fig. 18.105 Plant material surrounded by pseudocapsule made of lymphocytes and histiocytes

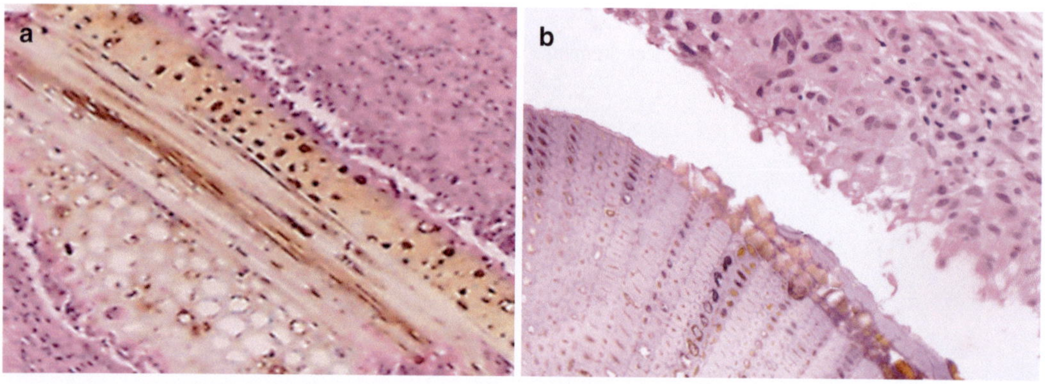

Fig. 18.106 (**a**, **b**) Plant material surrounded by mixed inflammation

Sporotrichosis

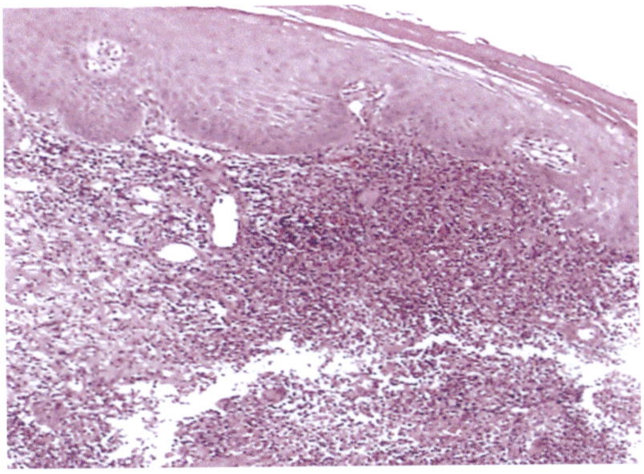

Fig. 18.107 Acanthotic epidermis with dermal inflammation

Histopathology (Figs. 18.107, 18.108, 18.109, and 18.110)

- Acanthotic epidermis with common pseudoepitheliomatous hyperplasia
- Dermal suppurative granulomas
- Asteroid bodies may be present
- Round/oval spores (4–6 μm) that are usually difficult to find in the tissue
- Single or less commonly multiple buds

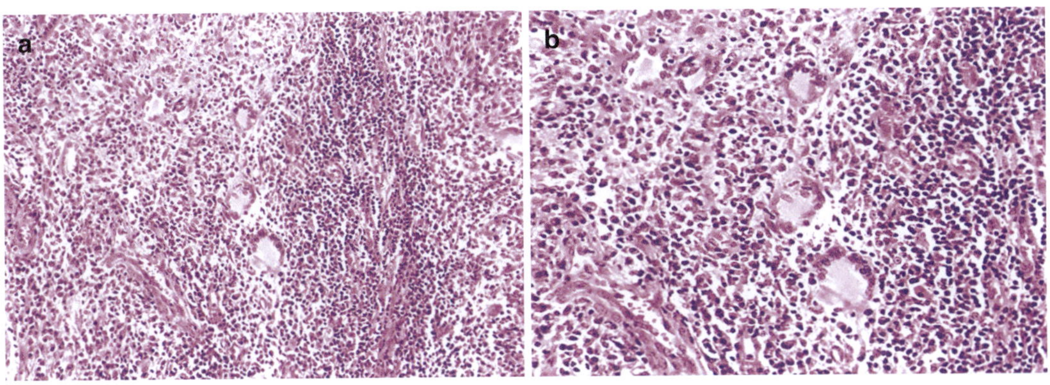

Fig. 18.108 (**a**, **b**) Suppurative granulomas with cuff of histiocytes, giant cells, and neutrophils

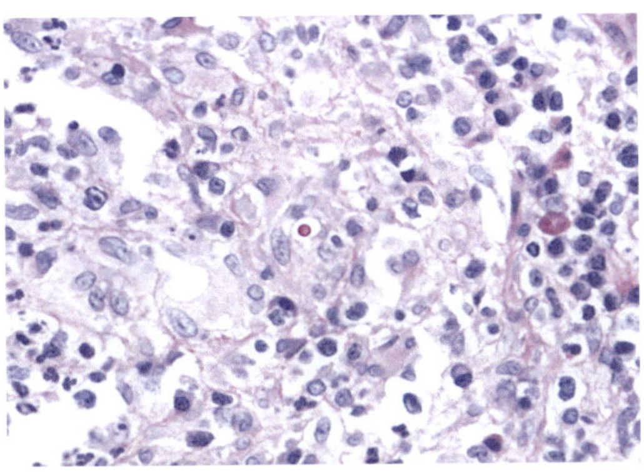

Fig. 18.109 PAS stain spore within the histiocyte

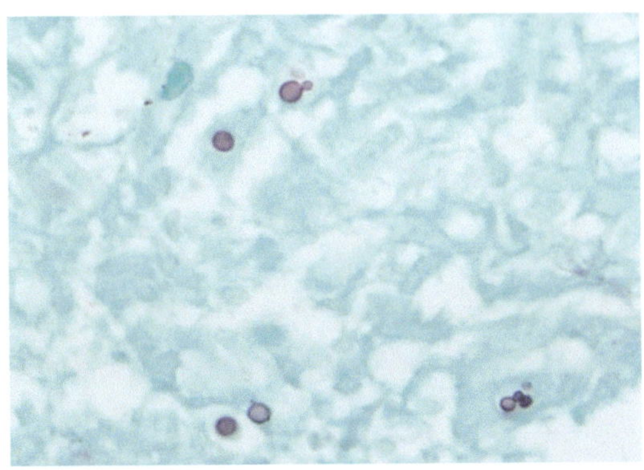

Fig. 18.110 GMS stains round/oval spores with single buds

Squamous Cell Carcinoma

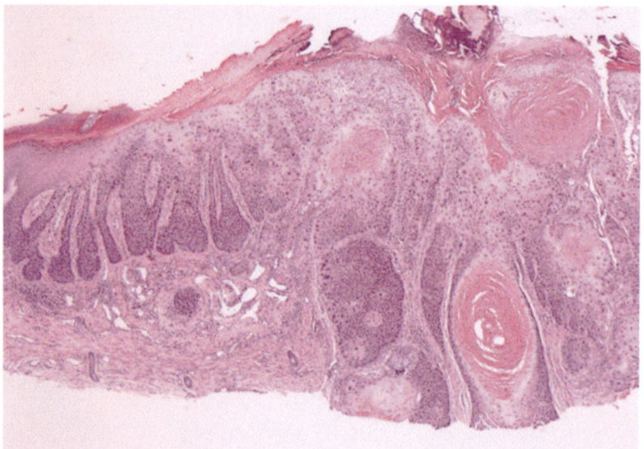

Fig. 18.111 SCC arising in the epidermis and invading the dermis

Histopathology (Figs. 18.111, 18.112, 18.113, 18.114, 18.115, 18.116, 18.117, 18.118, 18.119, 18.120, and 18.121)

- Nests of atypical keratinocytes (AE1/AE3+, CK5/6+, EMA+, BerEP4−)
- Tumor arises in epidermis and invades dermis
- Cells are pleomorphic with abundant eosinophilic cytoplasm and large irregular nuclei
- Necrosis and mitoses are easily identified

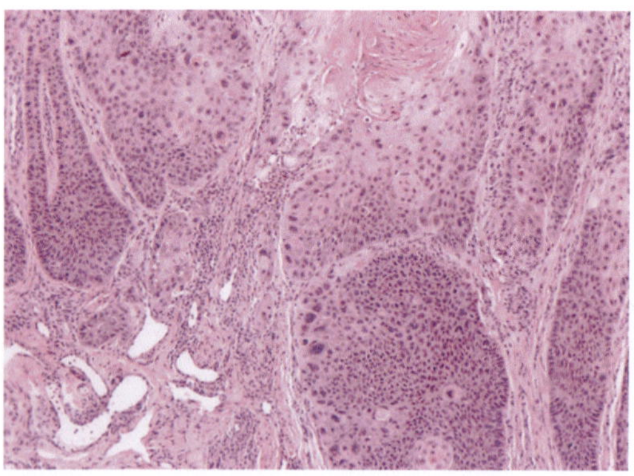

Fig. 18.112 Tumor nests invading into stroma

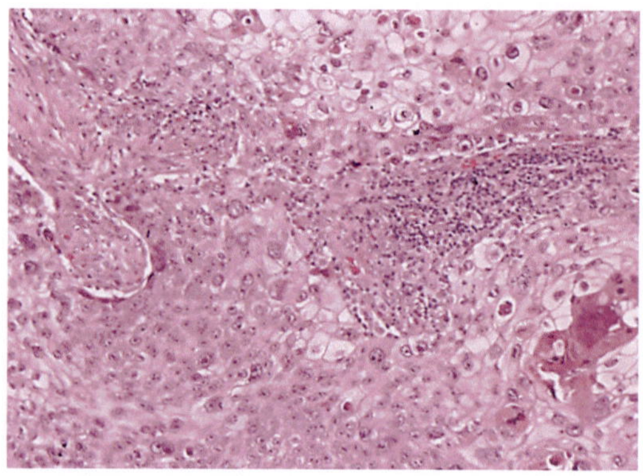

Fig. 18.113 Tumor with irregular islands of keratinization

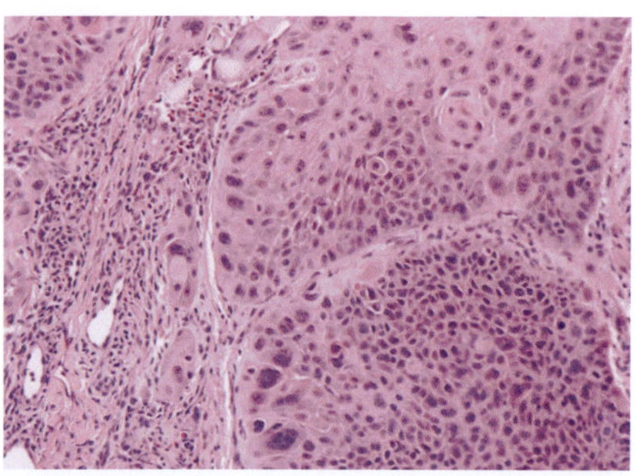

Fig. 18.114 Smaller nests are breaking away from the tumor (left)

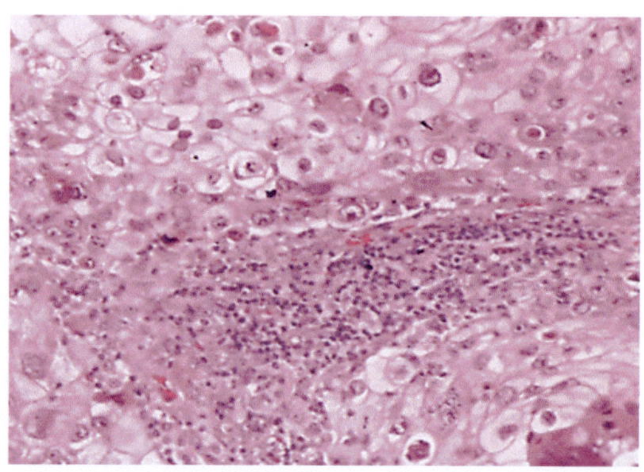

Fig. 18.115 Scattered numerous apoptotic keratinocytes

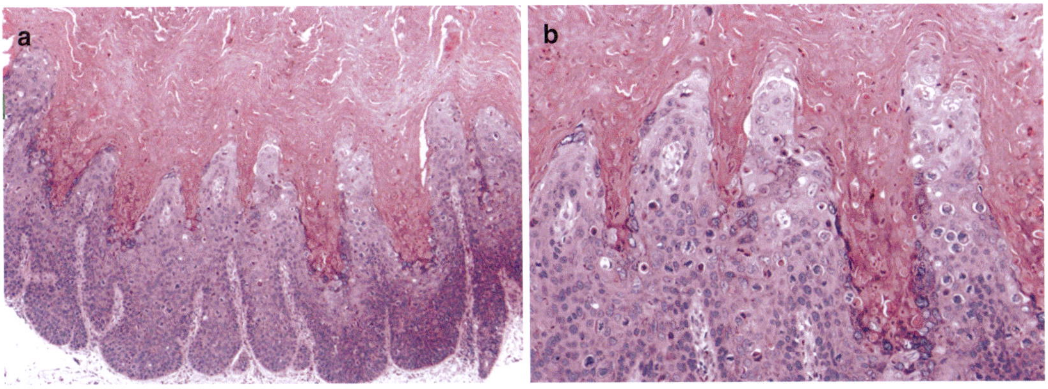

Fig. 18.116 (**a**, **b**) **In situ SCC** with verruciform shape and full thickness epidermal atypia of keratinocytes

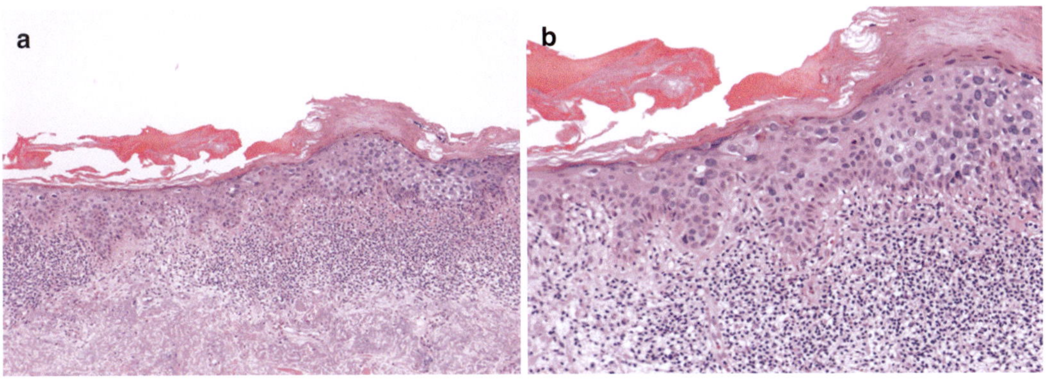

Fig. 18.117 (**a**, **b**) **In situ SCC** with pagetoid features

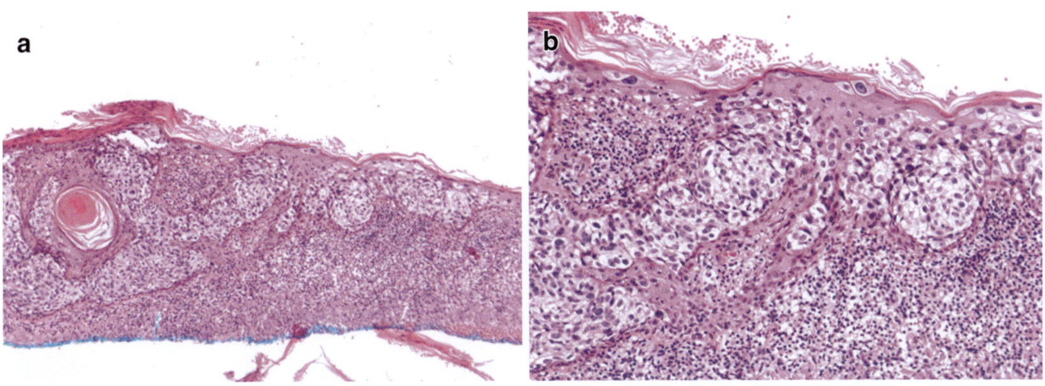

Fig. 18.118 (**a**, **b**) **In situ SCC** with clear cell features

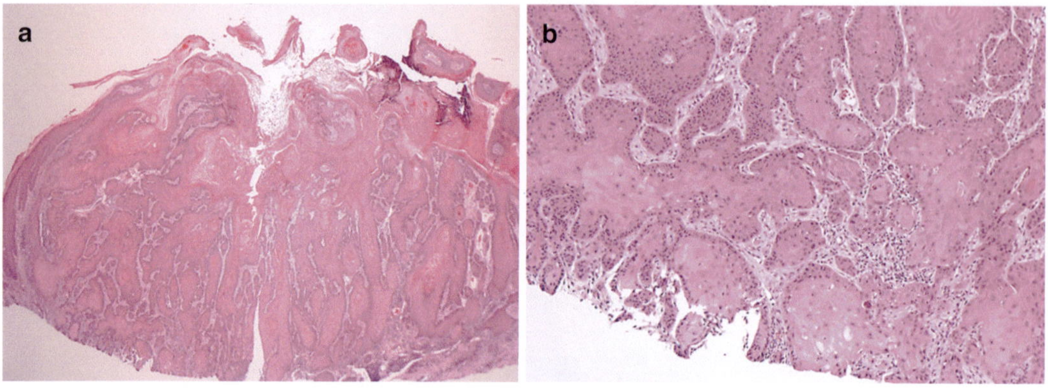

Fig. 18.119 (**a**, **b**) **Keratoacanthoma-like SCC** with crater shape and dermal invasion

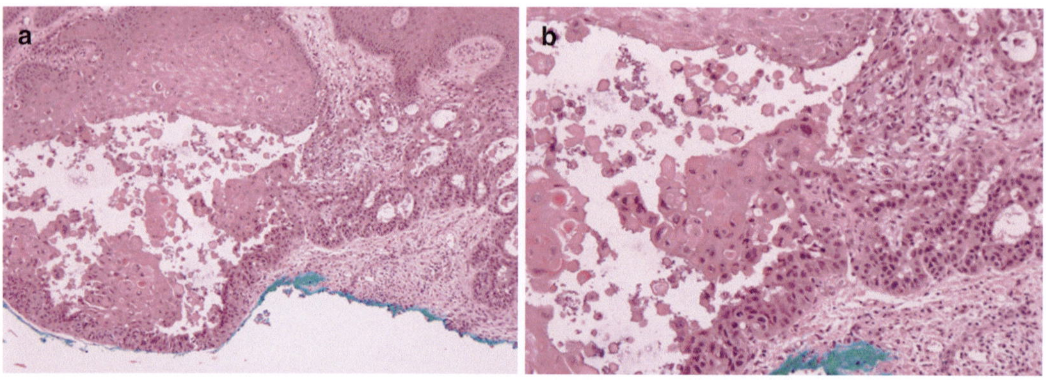

Fig. 18.120 (**a**, **b**) **Acantholytic SCC** with atypical keratinocytes separated by acantholysis

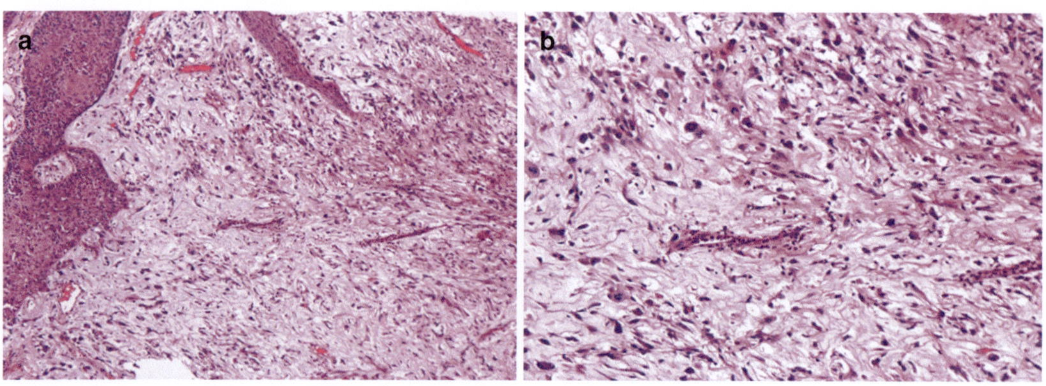

Fig. 18.121 (**a**, **b**) **Spindle cell SCC** with elongated irregular cells

Staphylococcal Scalded Skin Syndrome

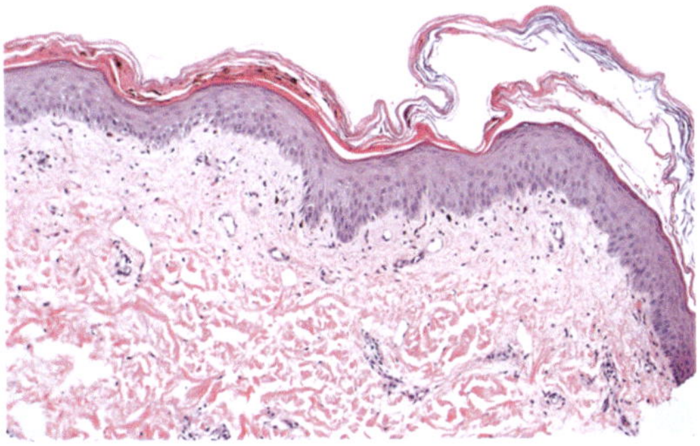

Fig. 18.122 Subcorneal clefting

Synonyms: Ritter's disease, Pemphigus Neonatorum

Histopathology (Figs. 18.122, 18.123, and 18.124)
- Cleft through the granular layer of the stratum corneum
- Dyskeratosis and inflammation is usually minimal although not always
- Epidermis below the split appears normal or mildly spongiotic

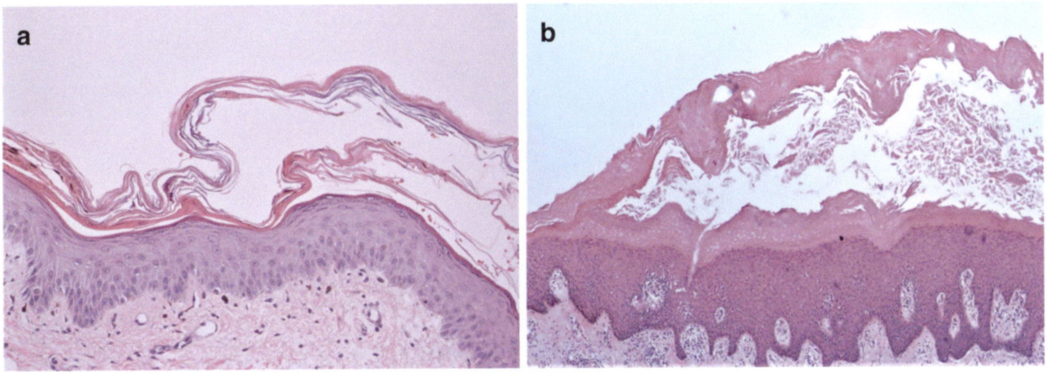

Fig. 18.123 (**a**, **b**) Subcorneal separation with no dyskeratosis or inflammation

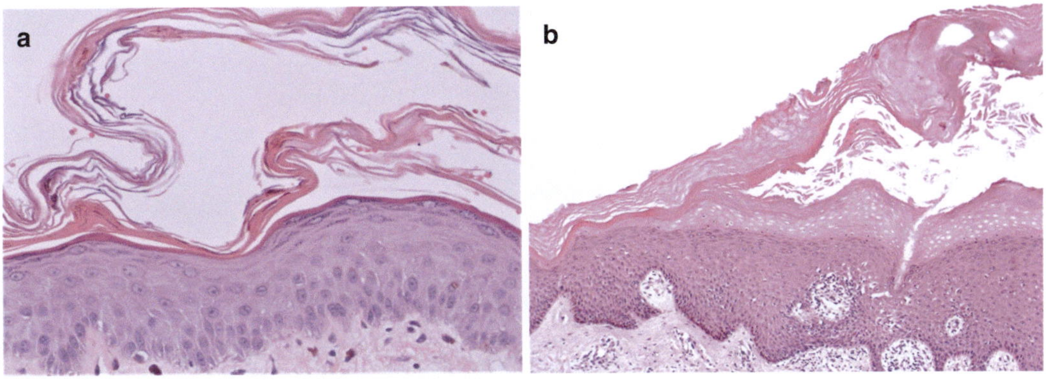

Fig. 18.124 (**a**, **b**) Epidermis is normal below the split

Steatocystoma

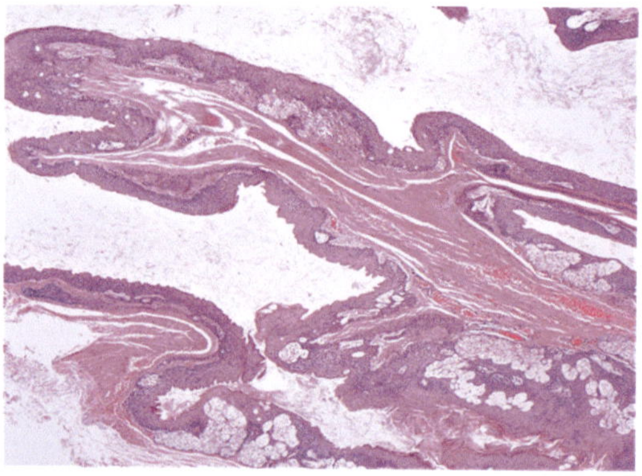

Fig. 18.125 Irregularly shaped cyst

Synonym: Sebocystomatosis

Histopathology (Figs. 18.125, 18.126, and 18.127)

- Irregular cyst lined with stratified squamous epithelium
- Wavy compact pink cuticle on the surface of the epidermis
- Sebaceous glands arise from the cyst wall

P.S. rare cases associated with Gardner's syndrome, pachyonychia congenita, ectodermal dysplasia

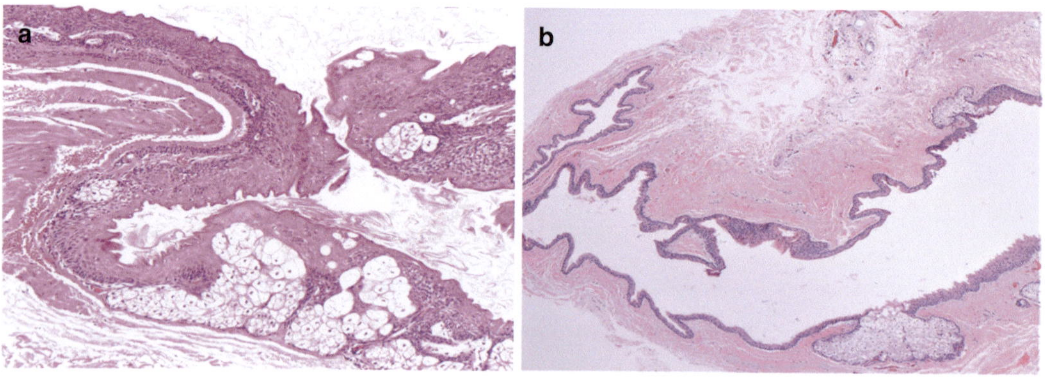

Fig. 18.126 (a, b) Cyst wall made of squamous epithelium with attached sebaceous glands

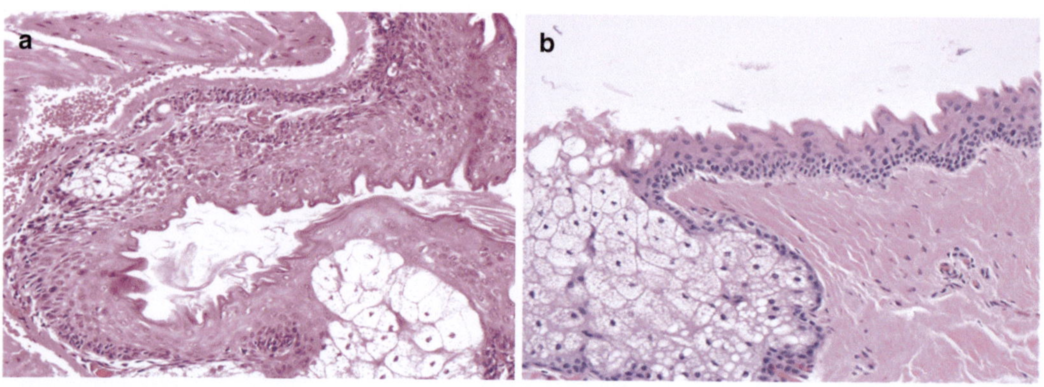

Fig. 18.127 (a, b) Wavy compact pink cuticle on the epidermal surface

Striae Distansae

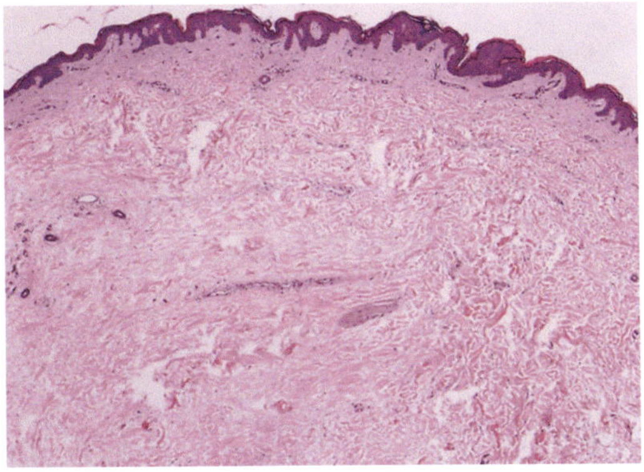

Fig. 18.128 Author's own biopsy of **stria alba** with normal dermis to the right and stretch mark dermis to the left

Synonym: Stretch Marks

Histopathology of **stria rubra** (early lesion):

- Reduction and reorganization of elastic fibers and fibrillin fibers
- Fine elastic fibers in the dermis with thicker fibers at the periphery

Histopathology of **stria alba** (established lesion):

- Atrophic epidermis and loss of skin appendages (Fig. 18.128)
- Collagen packed parallel to the epidermis with decreased and broken elastic fibers (Figs. 18.129, 18.130, 18.131, and 18.132)

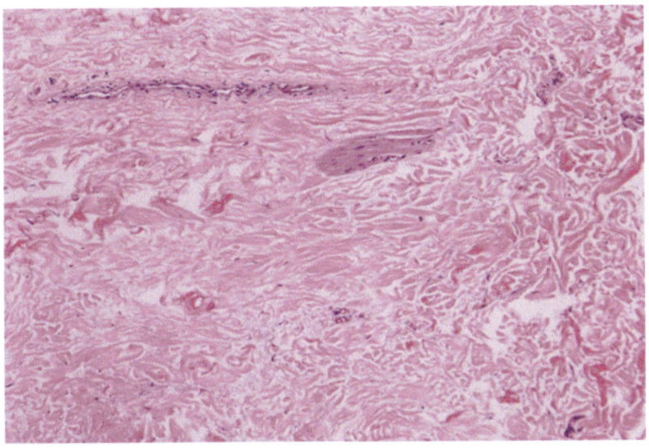

Fig. 18.129 Normal randomly arranged collagen on the right (normal) and parallelly organized collagen on the left (stria)

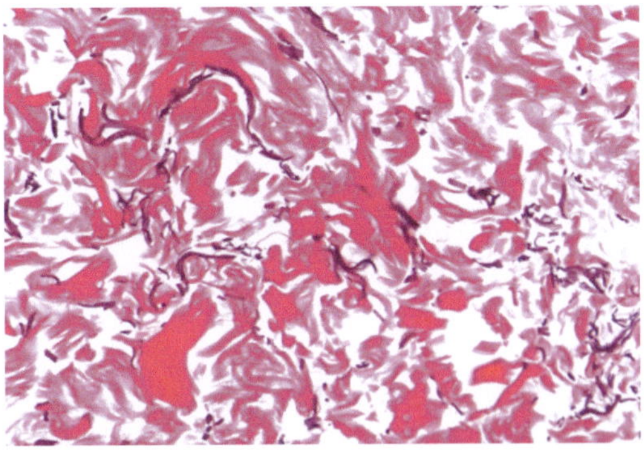

Fig. 18.130 Elastic fibers and collagen bundles in normal skin (VVG stain)

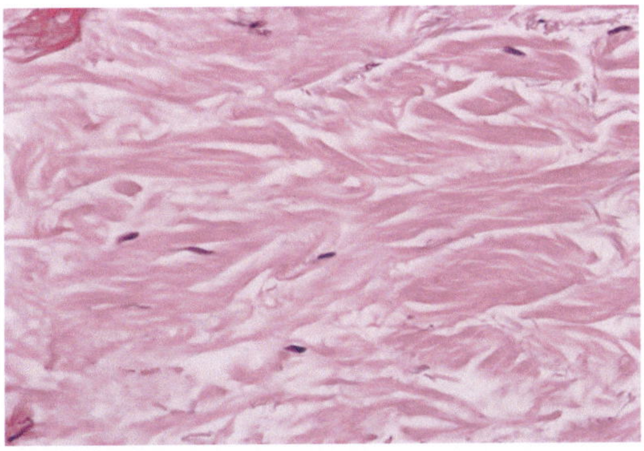

Fig. 18.131 Collagen bundles are parallel to the epidermis

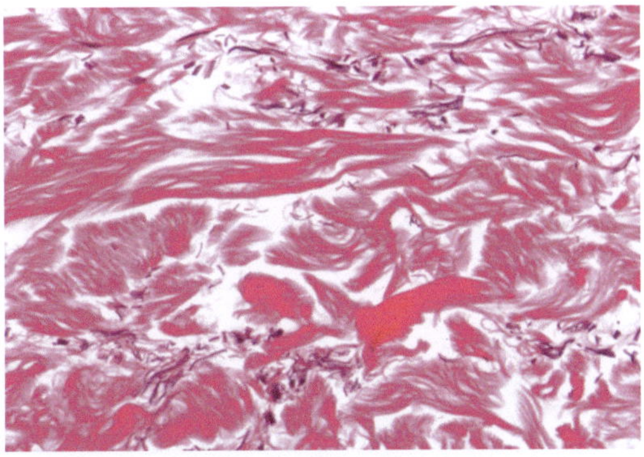

Fig. 18.132 In stria elastic fibers are broken and focally missing among parallelly laid collagen (VVG stain)

Strongyloidiasis

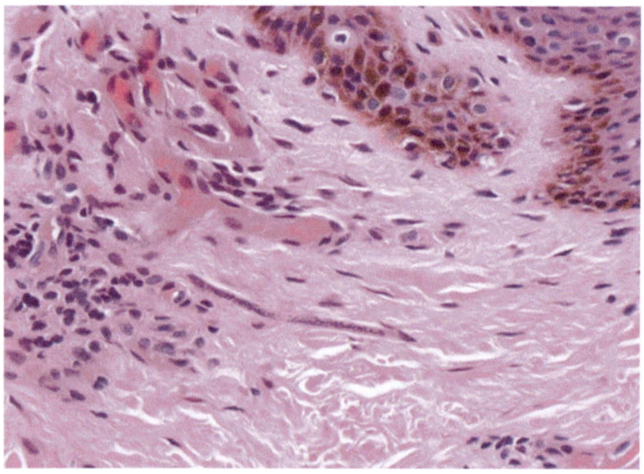

Fig. 18.133 Elongated larva with mixed dermal

Synonyms: Larva Currens, Creeping Infection

Histopathology in *cutaneous larva currens*:

- Wavy filariform larva in the dermis with mild perivascular lymphocytic inflammation and admixed eosinophils (Figs. 18.133 and 18.134)

Histopathology in *systemic strongyloidiasis*:

- Nematode worms and eggs within small intestine in hyperinfection syndrome (Figs. 18.135, 18.136, and 18.137)

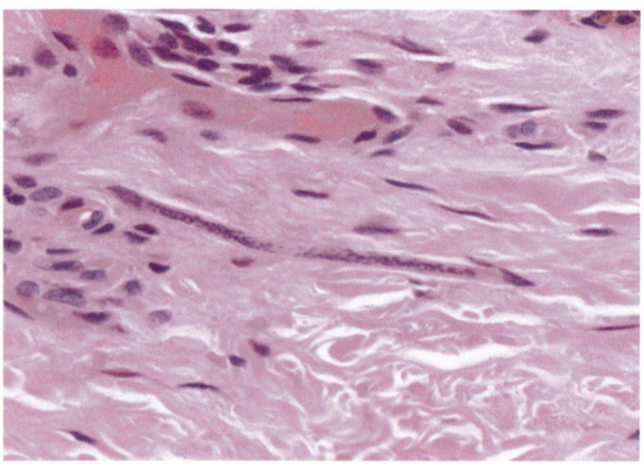

Fig. 18.134 Lancet shaped stippled

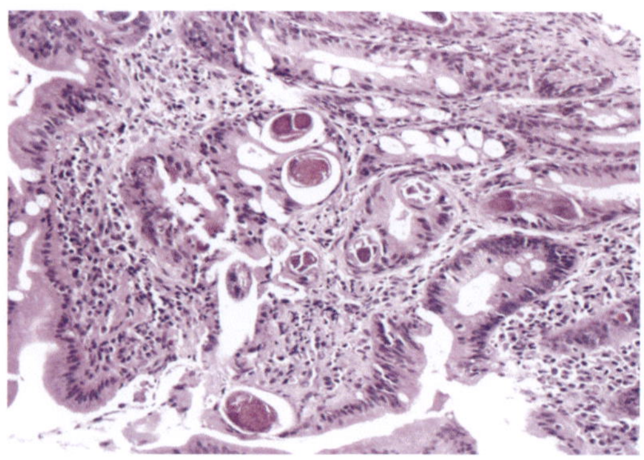

Fig. 18.135 A case of hyperinfection syndrome of strongyloidiasis with excessive worm burden within the small intestine

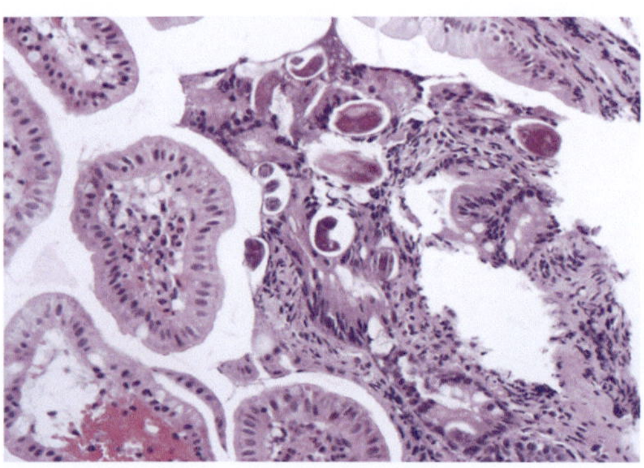

Fig. 18.136 *S. stercoralis* in the small intestine

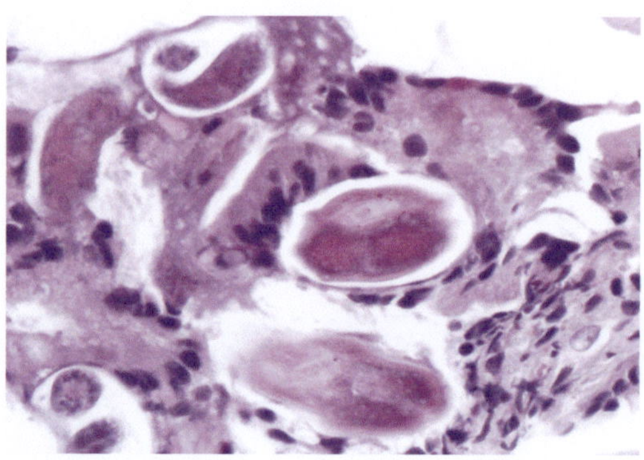

Fig. 18.137 *S. stercoralis* eggs

Stucco Keratosis

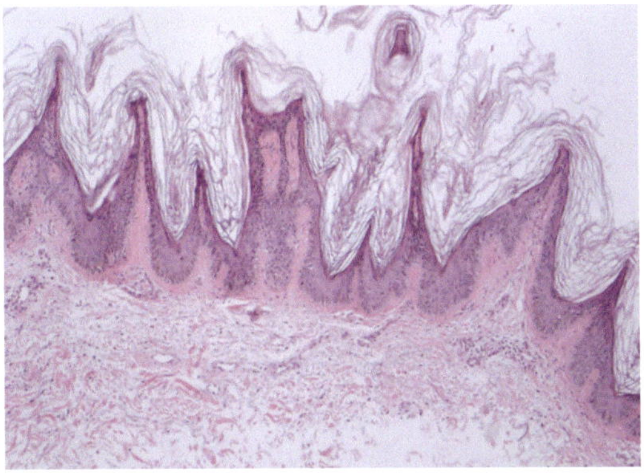

Fig. 18.138 Epidermal with "church spire" pattern

Synonyms: Keratosis Alba, Digitate Seborrheic Keratosis

Histopathology (Figs. 18.138, 18.139, and 18.140)

- Hyperkeratosis and regular papillomatosis of the epidermis ("church spire" pattern)
- No epidermal acanthosis
- No presence of horn pseudocysts
- No inflammatory changes

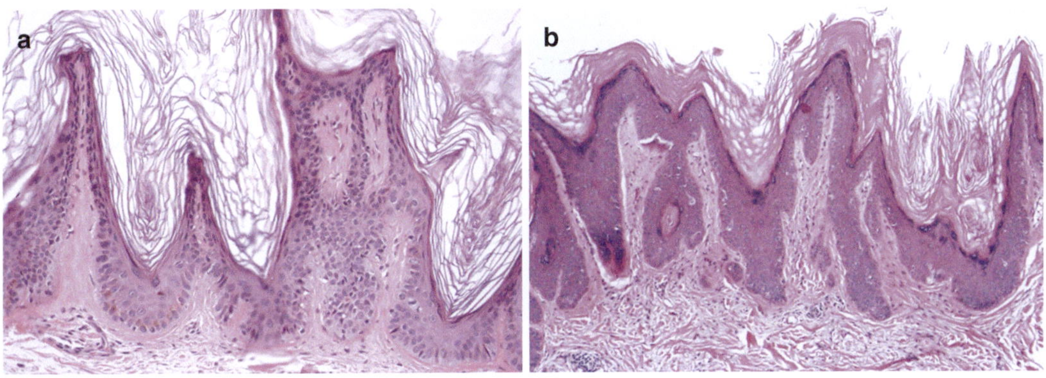

Fig. 18.139 (a, b) Epidermal hyperkeratosis and papillomatosis

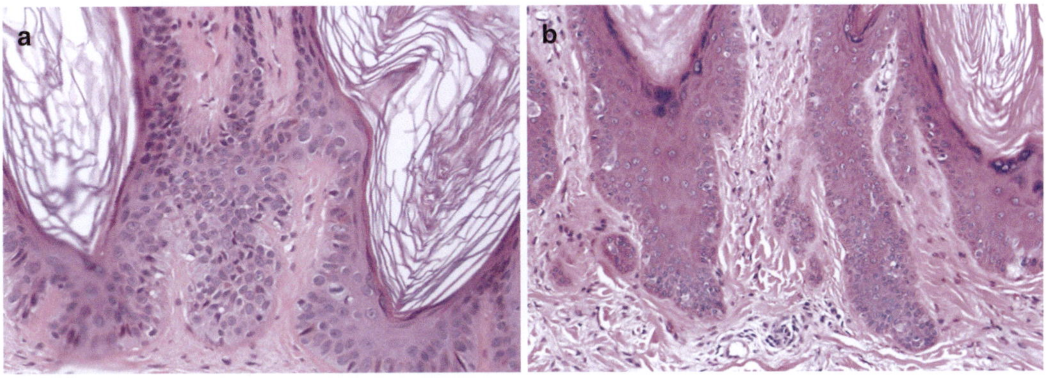

Fig. 18.140 (a, b) Absence of epidermal acanthosis and absence of pseudocysts

Subacute Cutaneous Lupus Erythematosus

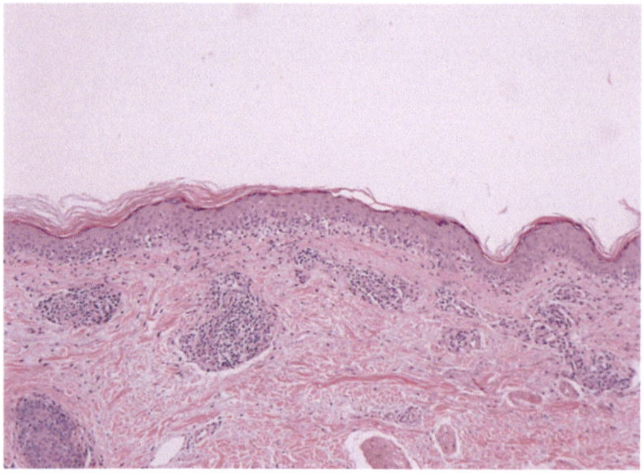

Fig. 18.141 Interface vacuoles with dermal inflammation

Histopathology (Figs. 18.141, 18.142, and 18.143)
- Atrophic epidermis with hyperkeratosis and effaced epidermal rete ridges
- Interface vacuolar changes with apoptotic keratinocytes
- Perivascular mild lymphocytic infiltrate
- Dermal mucin is mildly increased

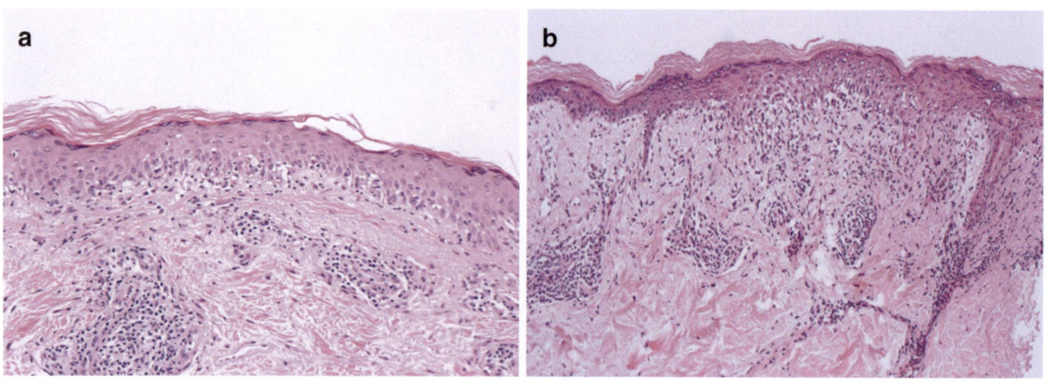

Fig. 18.142 (**a**, **b**) Flattened epidermis with hyperkeratosis; interface changes and mild dermal perivascular lymphocytic inflammation

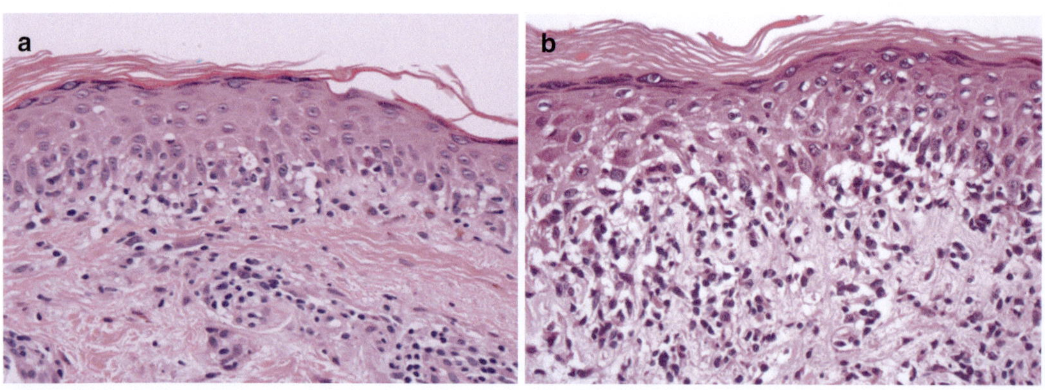

Fig. 18.143 (**a**, **b**) Hydropic degeneration of basal layer keratinocytes with vacuolar changes and scattered cytoid bodies

Subcorneal Neutrophilic Pustulosis

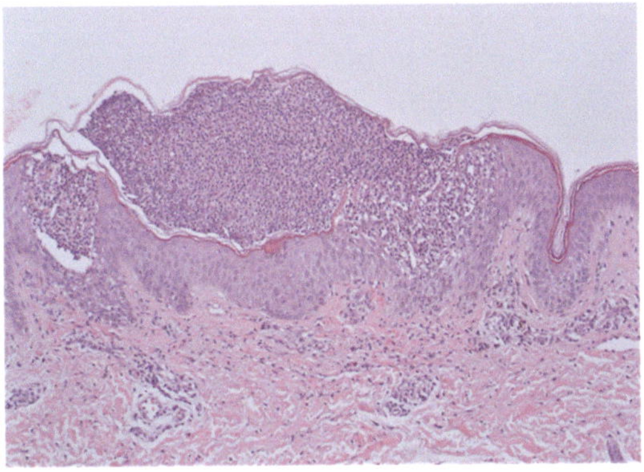

Fig. 18.144 Subcorneal pustule with mild mixed dermal perivascular inflammation

Synonym: Sneddon-Wilkinson Disease

Histopathology (Figs. 18.144, 18.145, and 18.146)

- Tense subcorneal neutrophilic pustule
- Epidermis underneath the pustule is unremarkable
- Perivascular dermal mixed inflammation

P.S. subcorneal neutrophilic pustules of bullous impetigo are flaccid

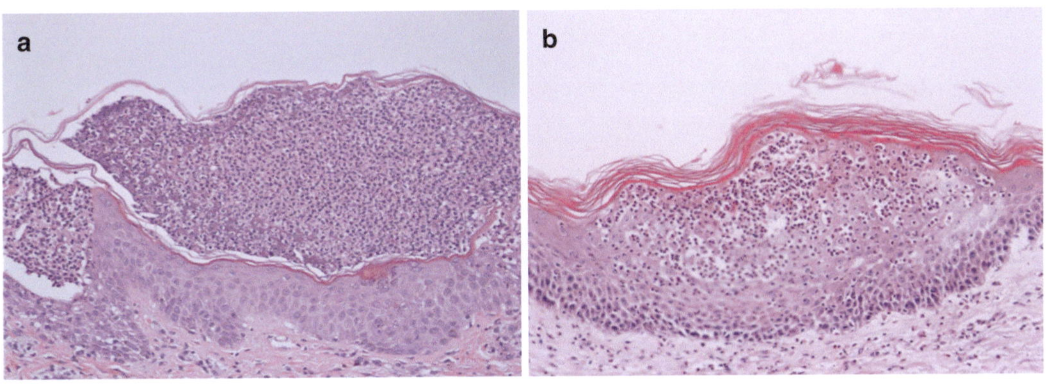

Fig. 18.145 (**a**, **b**) Epidermis underneath the pustule appears unremarkable

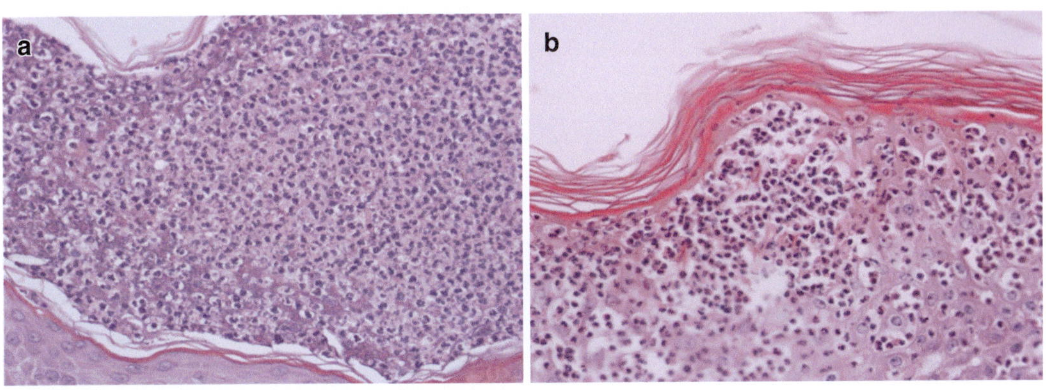

Fig. 18.146 (**a**, **b**) Tense subcorneal neutrophilic pustule

Subcutaneous Fat Necrosis of the Newborn

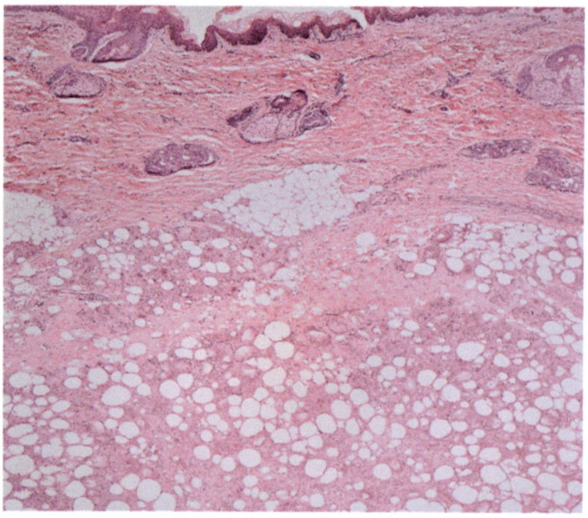

Fig. 18.147 Unremarkable epidermis and dermis with patchy fat necrosis

Poststeroidal panniculitis shows identical histopathology (Figs. 18.147, 18.148, 18.149, and 18.150)

- Normal epidermis and dermis
- Patchy lobular fat necrosis
- Crystallization of fat with stellate clefting
- Mixed inflammatory response
- Giant cells can be present

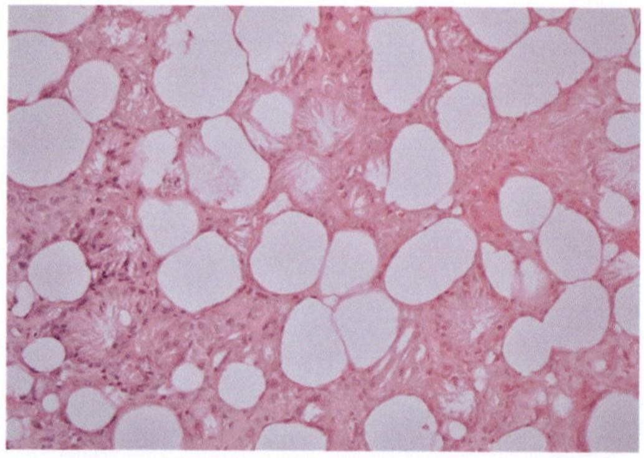

Fig. 18.148 Mild patchy mixed inflammatory reaction

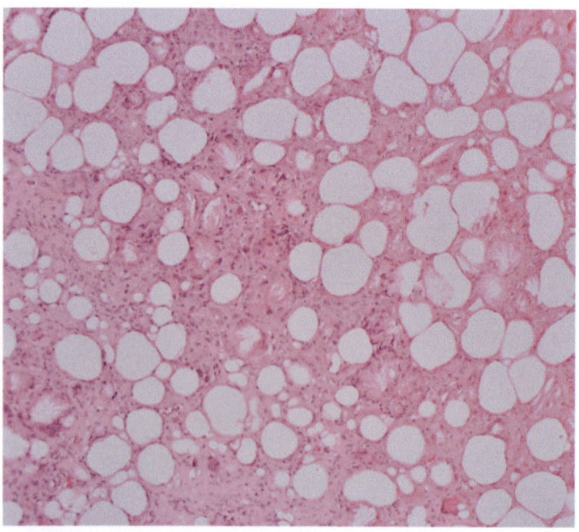

Fig. 18.149 Patchy fat necrosis with adipocytes of various sizes

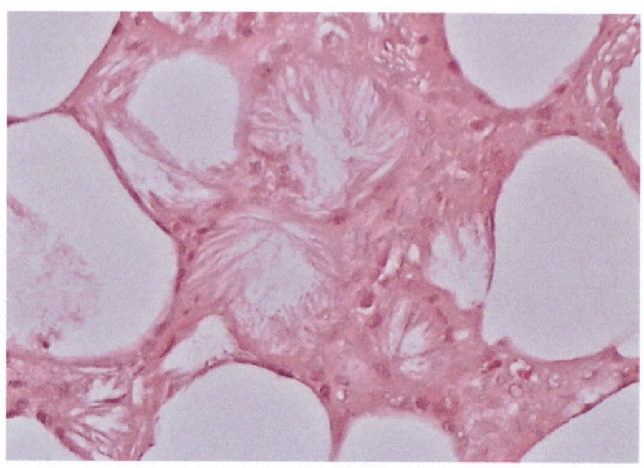

Fig. 18.150 Eosinophilic feathery crystals within adipocytes

Subcutaneous Panniculitis-Like T-Cell Lymphoma

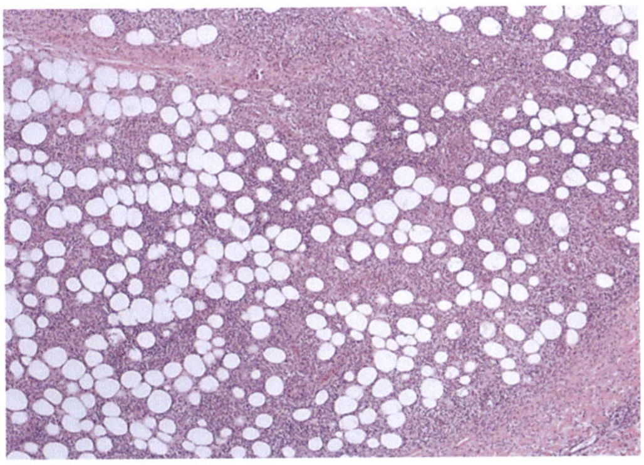

Fig. 18.151 Lobular lymphocytic infiltrate with septal spillover

Synonym: Panniculitis-like T-cell Lymphoma

Histopathology (Figs. 18.151, 18.152, and 18.153)

- Diffuse infiltrate of subcutaneous adipose tissue by atypical lymphocytes in "lace-like" pattern
- Primary lobular distribution with some septal spillover
- Lymphocytes are CD3+, CD4−, CD8+, granzyme B+, perforin+ consistent with a cytotoxic/suppressor phenotype

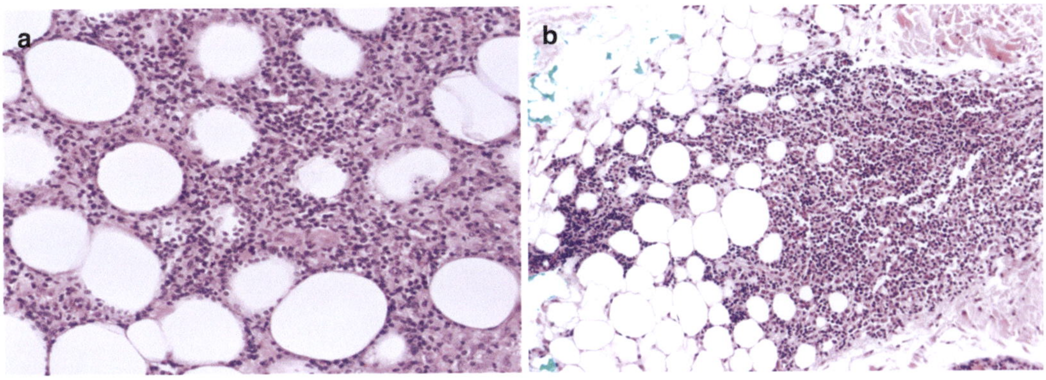

Fig. 18.152 (**a**, **b**) Dense lymphocytic infiltrate creating "lace-like" appearance

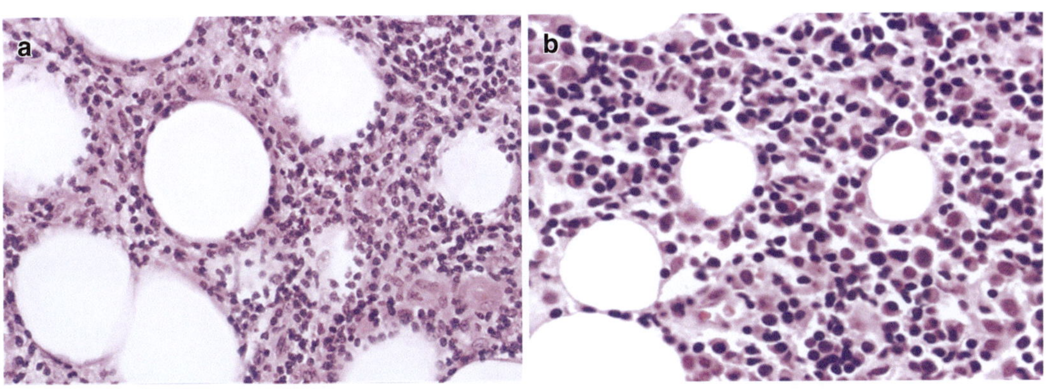

Fig. 18.153 (**a**, **b**) Atypical lymphocytes with some histiocytes

Sunburn

Histopathology varies depending on the severity (Figs. 18.154, 18.155, and 18.156)

- Scattered necrotic pyknotic keratinocytes particularly in the upper portion of the epidermis ("sunburn" cells)
- Vacuolar changes at the epidermodermal interface
- Dermal perivascular lymphocytic inflammation
- Dermal edema and red blood cell extravasation present in more severe sun burn
- Full thickness epidermal necrosis with subepidermal blister present in most severe burns

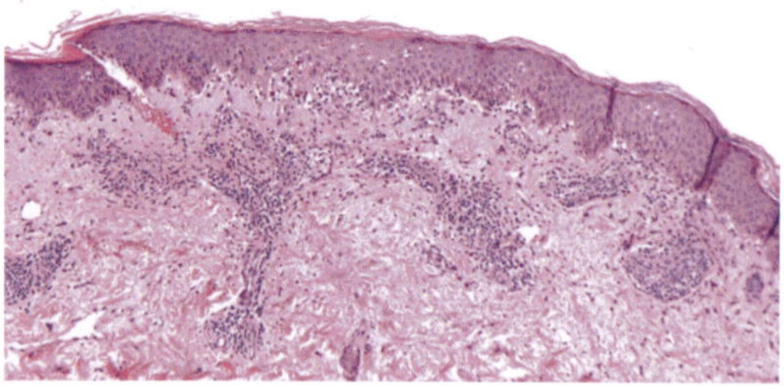

Fig. 18.154 Moderate sunburn

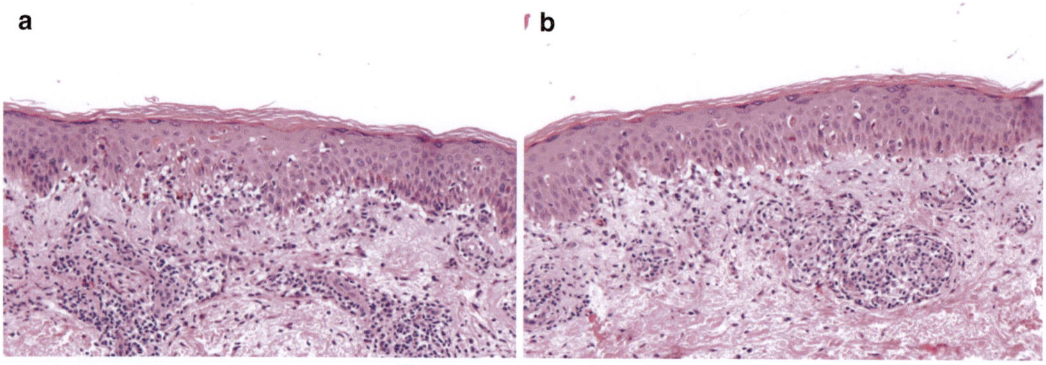

Fig. 18.155 (**a**, **b**) Perivascular lymphocytic inflammation and mild red blood cell extravasation

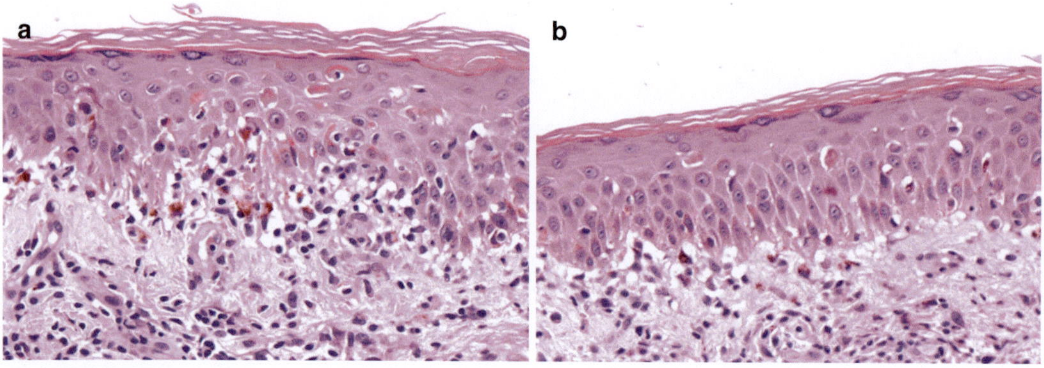

Fig. 18.156 (**a**, **b**) Scattered necrotic keratinocytes ("sunburn" cells) with interface vacuolar changes

Supernumerary Digit

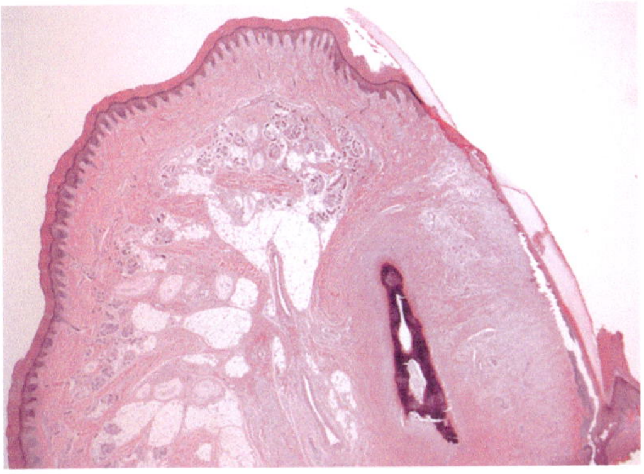

Fig. 18.157 Polypoid lesion with bone

Synonym: Accessory Digit

Can present as miniaturized finger (shown here) or as amputation neuroma (see traumatic neuroma)

Histopathology (Figs. 18.157, 18.158, 18.159, 18.160, and 18.161)

- Polypoid structure with central bone or cartilage depending on the patient age
- Epidermis with the features of acral skin
- Nail can be present
- Not oriented neural elements are usually present

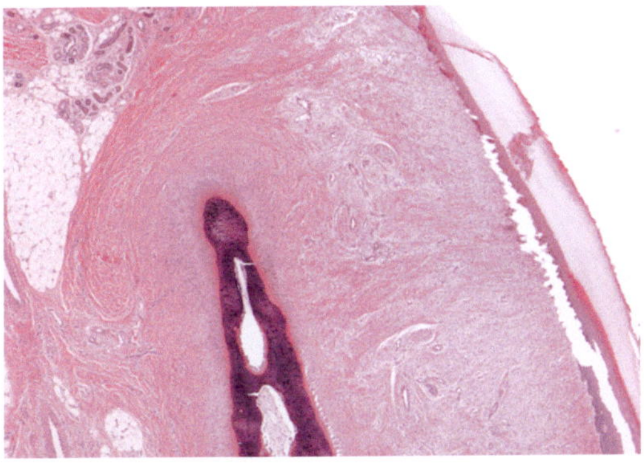

Fig. 18.158 Nail with nail bed and underlying fibroconnective stroma and bone

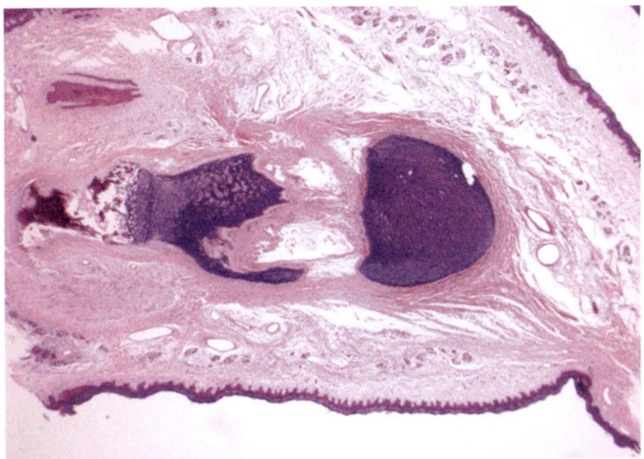

Fig. 18.159 Polypoid lesion with central bone forming cartilage

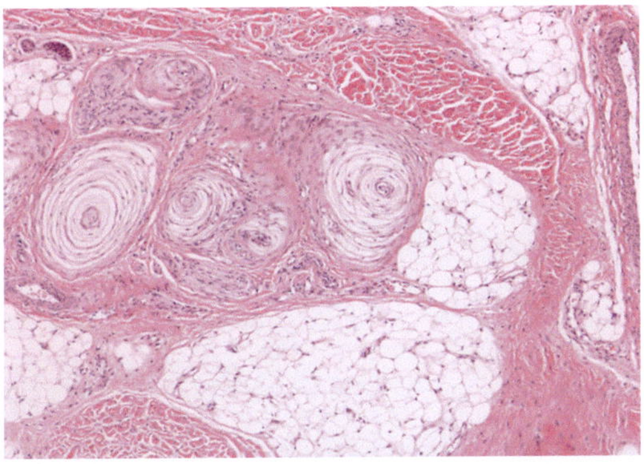

Fig. 18.160 Large neural elements

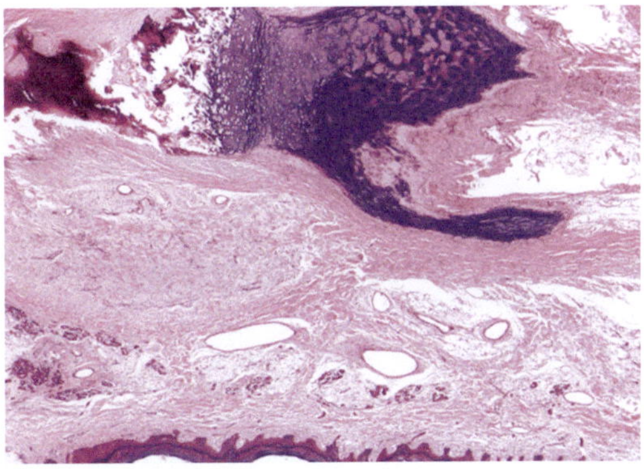

Fig. 18.161 Neural elements between epidermis and bone

Supernumerary Nipple

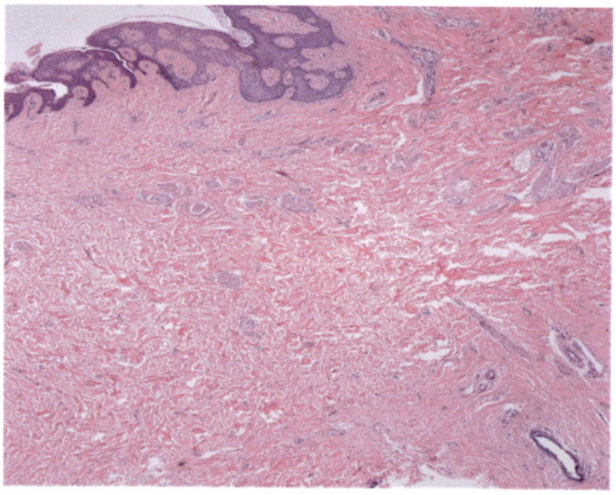

Fig. 18.162 Breast-like tissue

Synonym: Accessory Nipple

Histopathology (Figs. 18.162, 18.163, 18.164, and 18.165)
- Resembles normal nipple
- Mild epidermal hyperplasia and hyperpigmentation
- Increased number of dermal smooth muscles
- Dermal mammary ducts and subcutaneous mammary glands

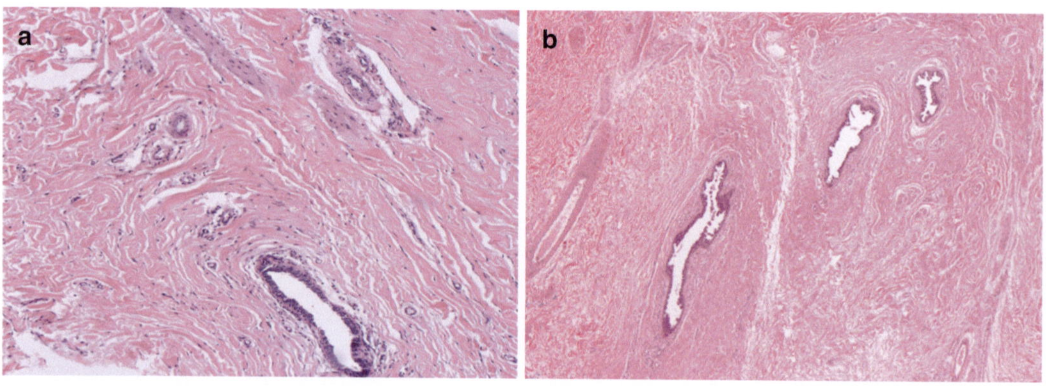

Fig. 18.163 (**a**, **b**) Mammary ducts surrounded by muscle bundles

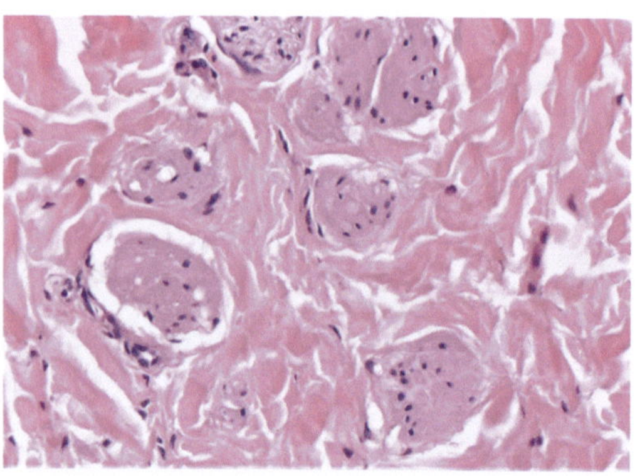

Fig. 18.164 Numerous smooth muscle bundles

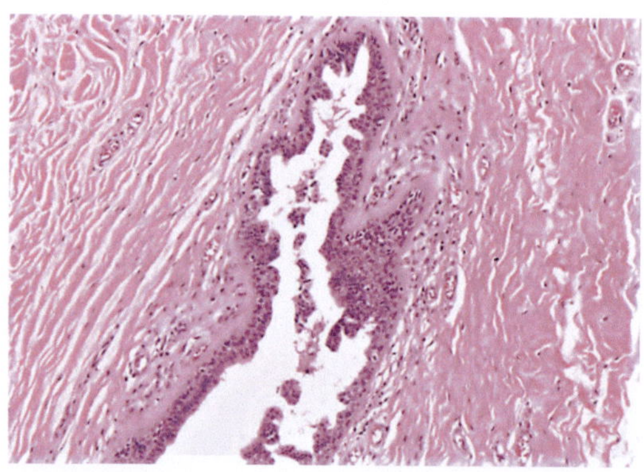

Fig. 18.165 Mammary ducts lined with two cell layers

Suture Granuloma

Histopathology (Figs. 18.166, 18.167, and 18.168)

- Foreign body granuloma
- Multiple suture fragments with histiocytes, lymphocytes, and giant cells
- Surrounding fibrosis and scarring

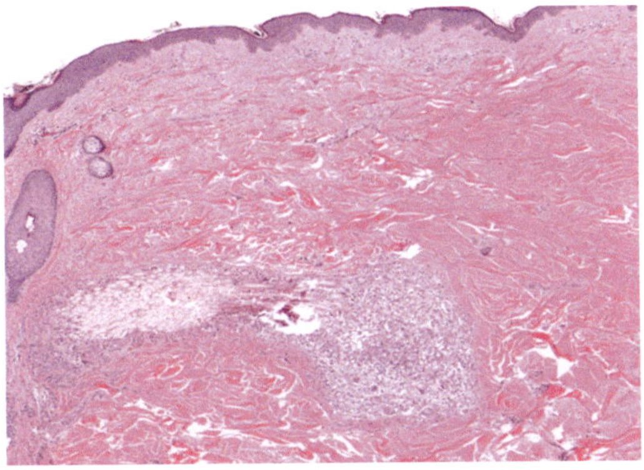

Fig. 18.166 Foreign material in the dermis

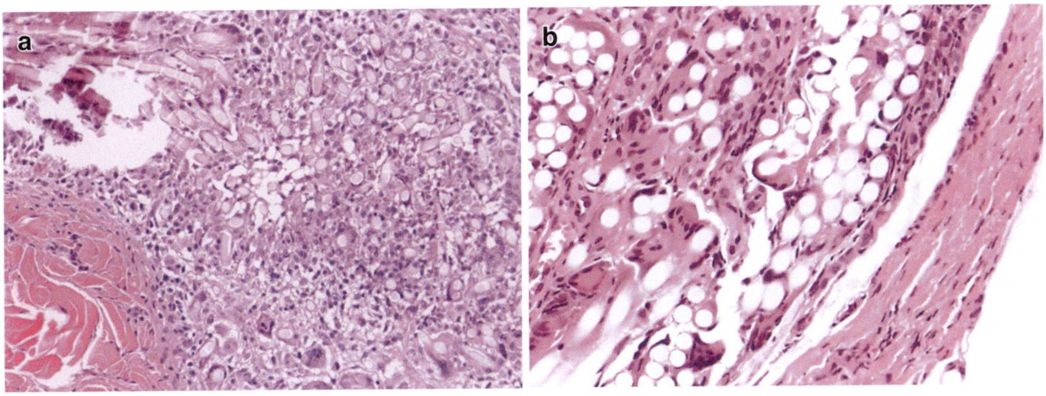

Fig. 18.167 (**a**, **b**) Multiple suture fragments grouped together and surrounded by scar

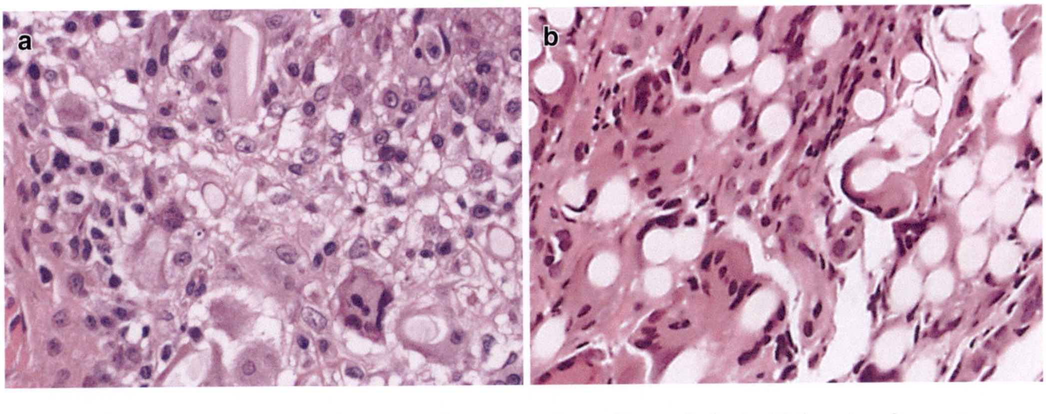

Fig. 18.168 (**a**, **b**) Histiocytes, lymphocytes, and numerous giant cells are admixed with the suture fragments

Sweet's Syndrome

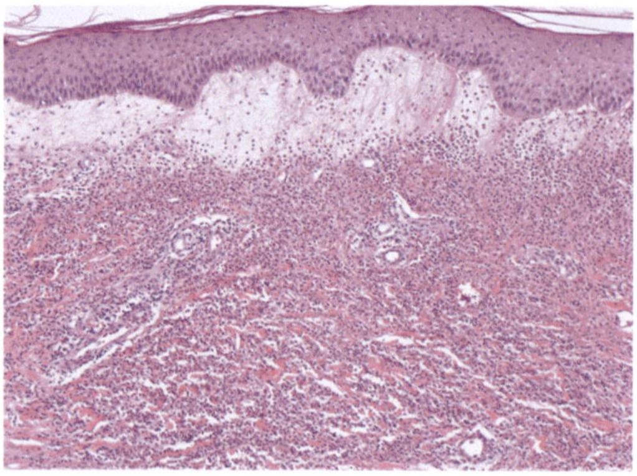

Fig. 18.169 Normal epidermis with papillary dermal edema and dense underlying neutrophilic infiltrate

Synonym: Acute Febrile Neutrophilic Dermatosis

Histopathology (Figs. 18.169, 18.170, and 18.171)

- Papillary dermal edema and dermal neutrophilic inflammation with sparing of the epidermis
- Vascular damage can be mild, characterized by plump reactive endothelial cells, to more severe, characterized by diffuse neutrophilic leukocytoclasia

P.S. *Rheumatoid Neutrophilic Dermatosis* and *Bowel-associated Dermatosis-arthritis Syndrome (BADAS)* have identical histopathology to *Sweet's*

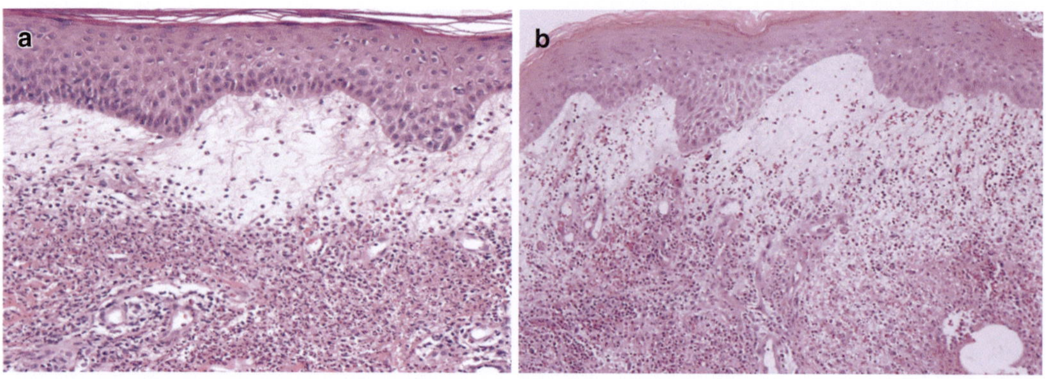

Fig. 18.170 (**a**, **b**) Diffuse dermal neutrophilic infiltrate and papillary dermal edema

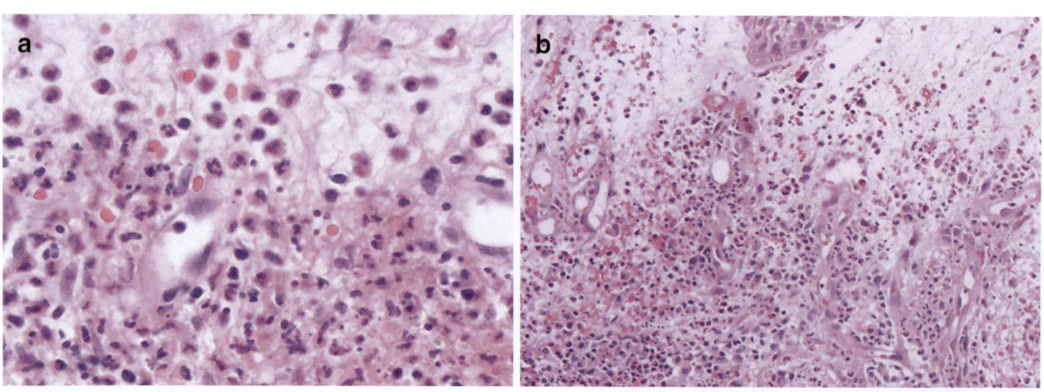

Fig. 18.171 (**a**, **b**) Plump endothelial cells with neutrophilic leukocytoclasia and red blood cell extravasation

Synovial Cyst

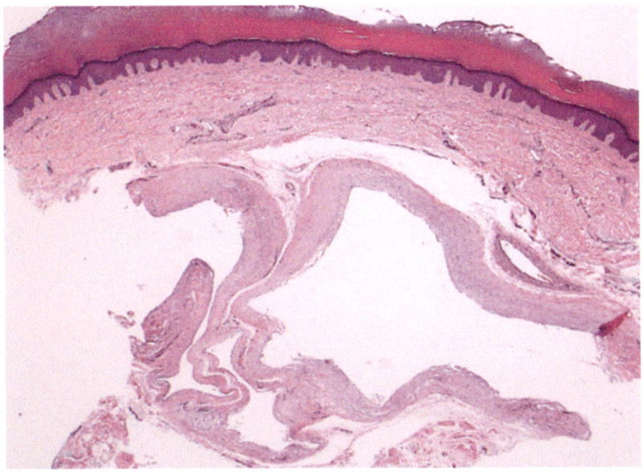

Fig. 18.172 Irregular cyst with corrugated wall

Synonyms: Metaplastic Synovial Cyst, Ganglion Cyst

Histopathology (Figs. 18.172, 18.173, and 18.174)

- Large irregular cyst formed of synovium-like tissue that can communicate with the surface
- Cyst wall is synovial-like, made of thickened, fibrotic, scar-like tissue
- The cyst lining is made of histiocytes and flattened fibrotic cells

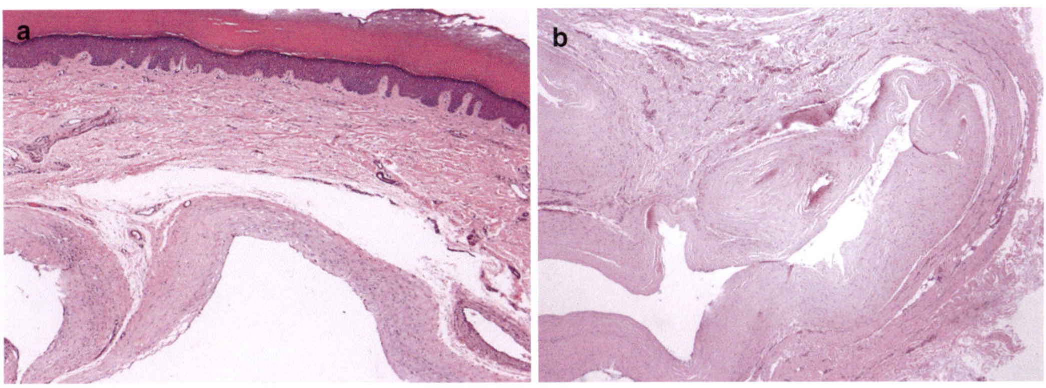

Fig. 18.173 (**a**, **b**) Cyst wall resembles normal synovium

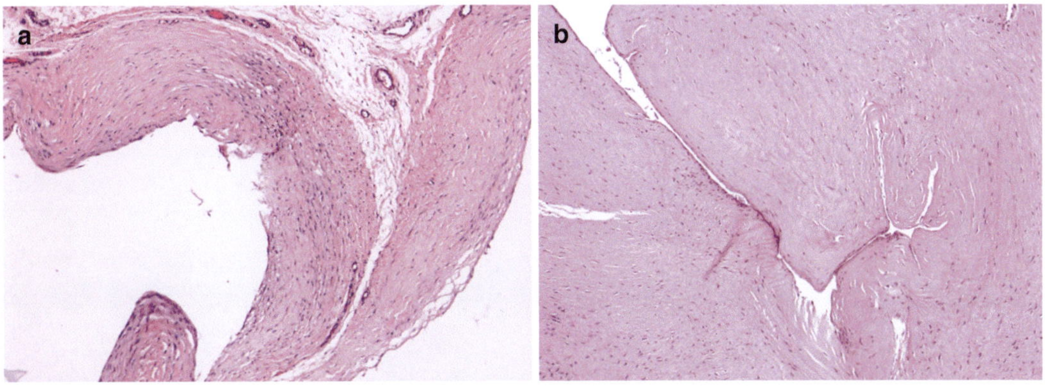

Fig. 18.174 (**a**, **b**) Wall is made of "scar-like" tissue and the lining is made of histiocytes and/or flattened fibroblasts

Syphilis

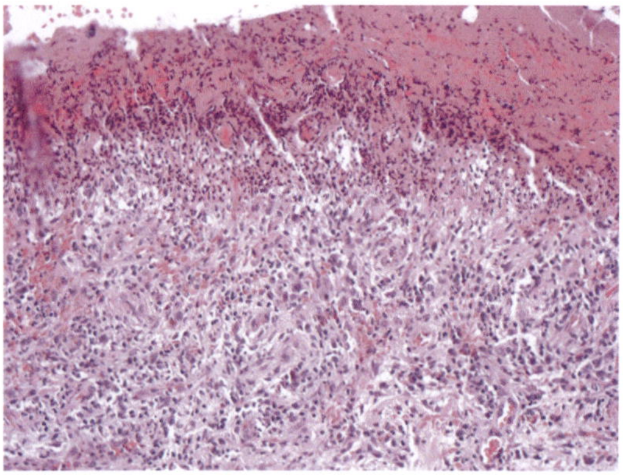

Fig. 18.175 **Primary syphilitic chancre** with excoriated epidermis

Histopathology

Primary (Figs. 18.175, 18.176, and 18.177)—ulcerated epidermis in the center and epidermal hyperplasia at the edges

- Dense lymphoplasmocytic infiltrate with reactive endothelial cells

Secondary—macular lesion has subtle histomorphology with normal epidermis and sparse perivascular lymphoplasmocytic infiltrate (Figs. 18.178 and 18.179)

- As lesions become papular (condyloma lata) the epidermis becomes hypertrophic with lymphoplasmocytic inflammation and epidermal neutrophils (Figs. 18.180, 18.181, 18.182, and 18.183)

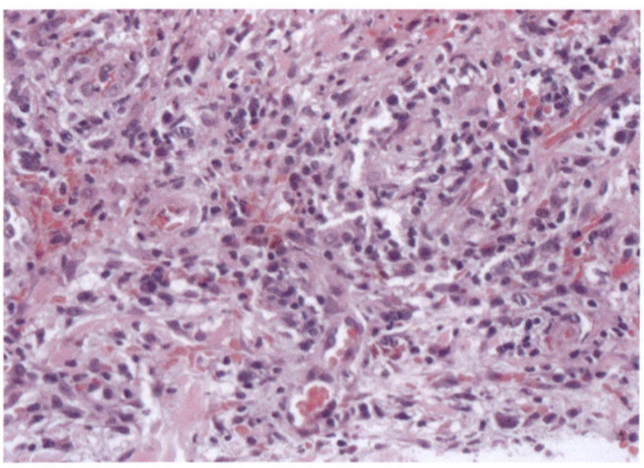

Fig. 18.176 Reactive endothelial cells and RBCs extravasation

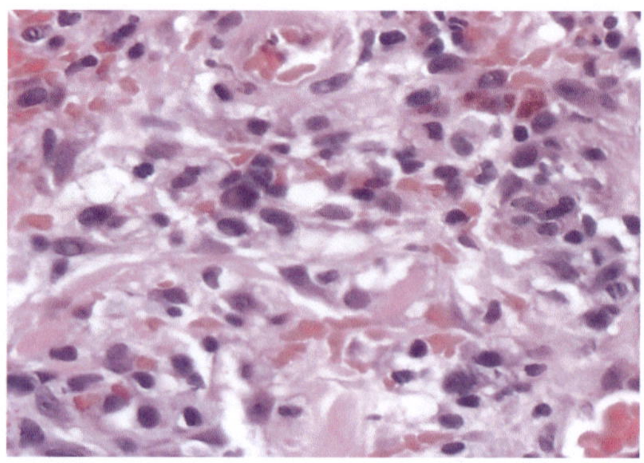

Fig. 18.177 Numerous lymphocytes and plasma cells

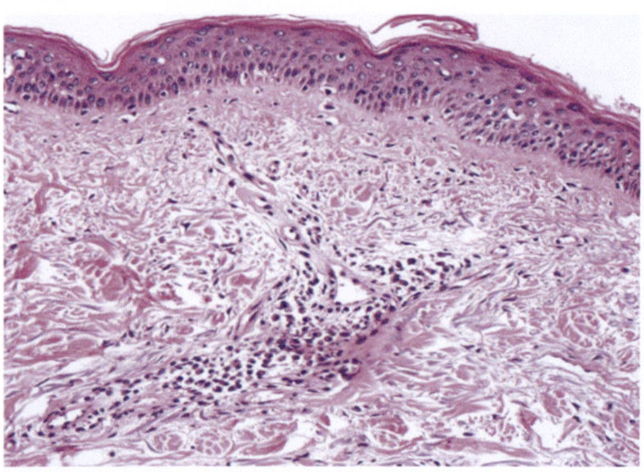

Fig. 18.178 **Macular secondary syphilis** with normal epidermis

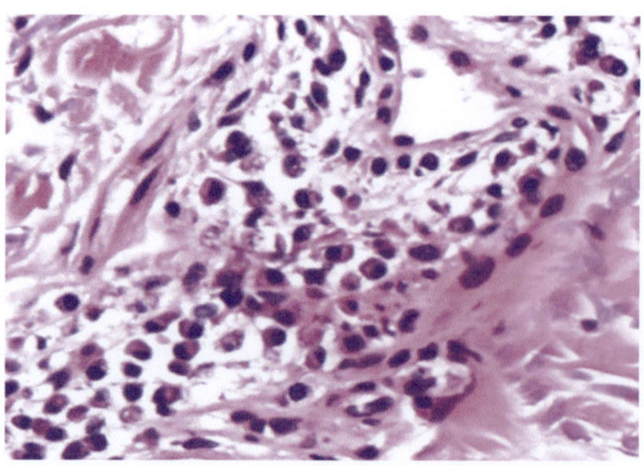

Fig. 18.179 Perivascular lymphoplasmocytic infiltrate

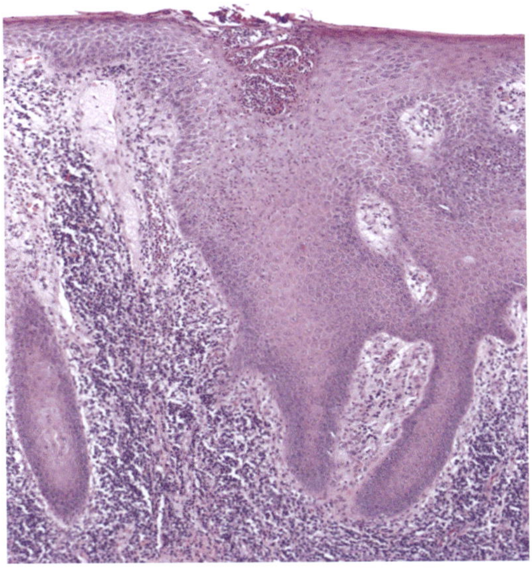

Fig. 18.180 **Condyloma lata** case of secondary syphilis with pseudoepitheliomatous hyperplasia

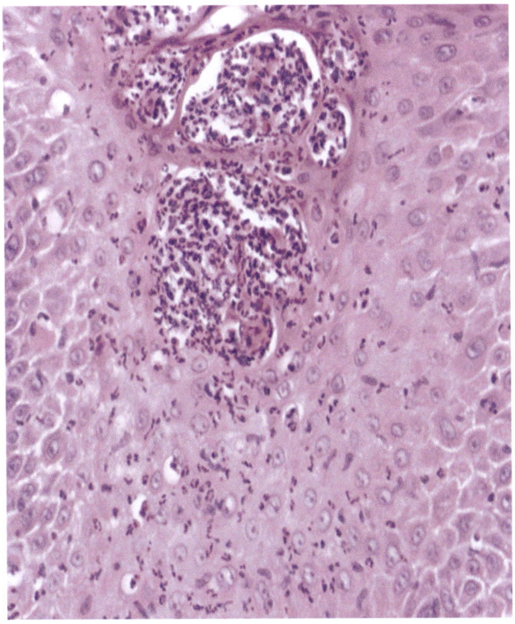

Fig. 18.181 Characteristic intraepidermal microabscess

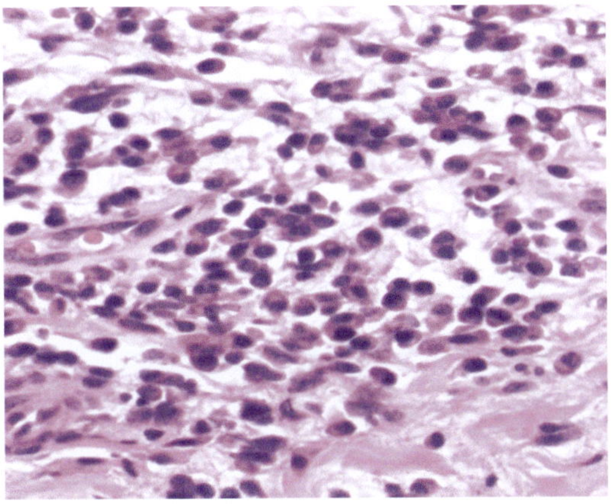

Fig. 18.182 Dense dermal inflammation with numerous plasma cells

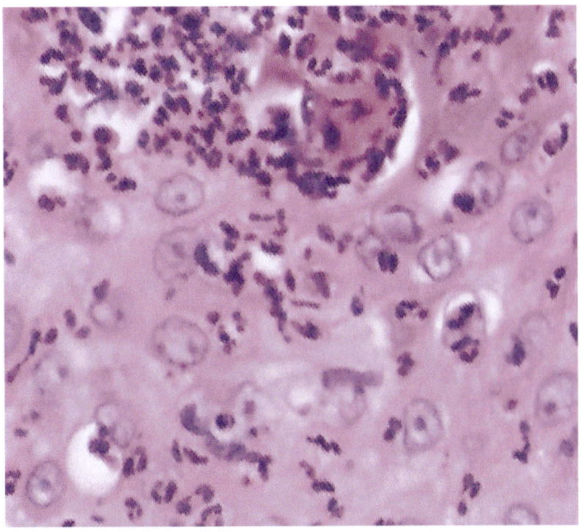

Fig. 18.183 Intraepidermal neutrophilic aggregate

Syringocystadenoma Papilliferum

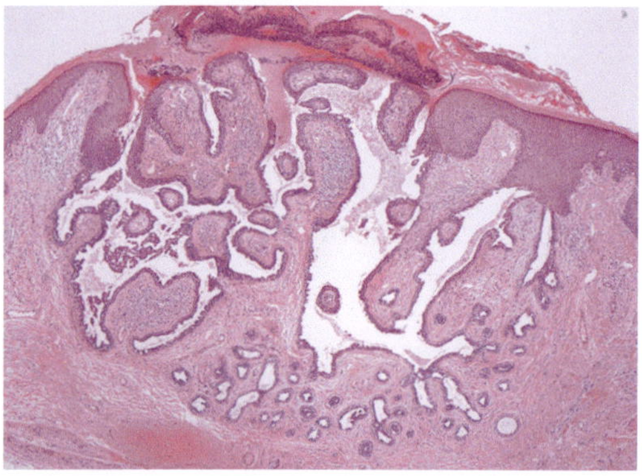

Fig. 18.184 Invaginated tumor connected to the epidermis

Histopathology (Figs. 18.184, 18.185, and 18.186)

- Tumor is connected to the epidermis
- Cystic invagination with papillary proliferations
- Papillae lined by two layers of cuboidal/columnar cells
- Outer layer shows focal apocrine secretions
- Papillae are broad based
- Papillary stroma contains numerous plasma cells

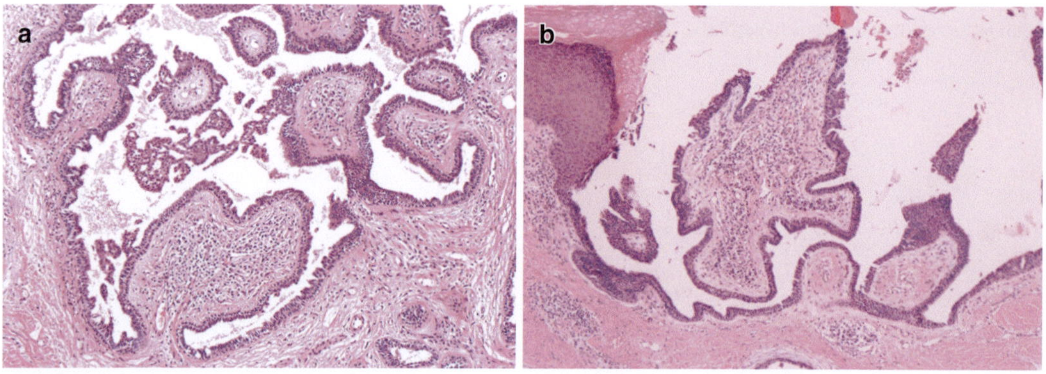

Fig. 18.185 (**a**, **b**) Broad based papillae with fibrovascular core and numerous plasma cells

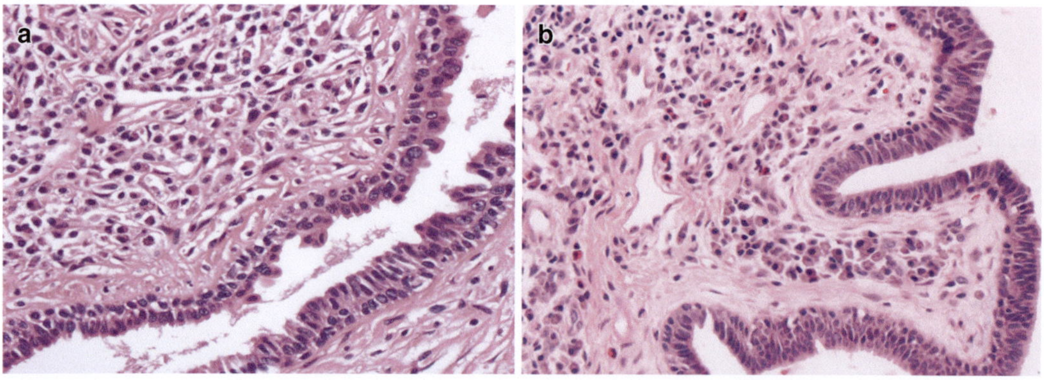

Fig. 18.186 (**a**, **b**) Papillae covered with two layers of cuboidal/columnar cells with apocrine snouts and plasma cells in the stroma

Syringofibroadenoma

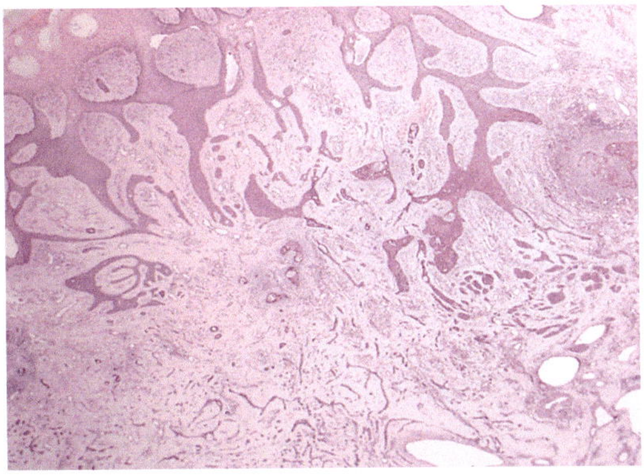

Fig. 18.187 Tumor with multiple epidermal connection points

Histopathology (Figs. 18.187, 18.188, 18.189, and 18.190)
- Tumor arises from epidermis at multiple points
- Smaller sheets and thin anastomosing strands of epithelial cells
- Fibrovascular stroma that can be myxoid
- Epithelial strands contain small ducts (CEA)

P.S. multiple palmoplantar syringofibroadenomas associated with Schöpf-Schulz-Passarge syndrome

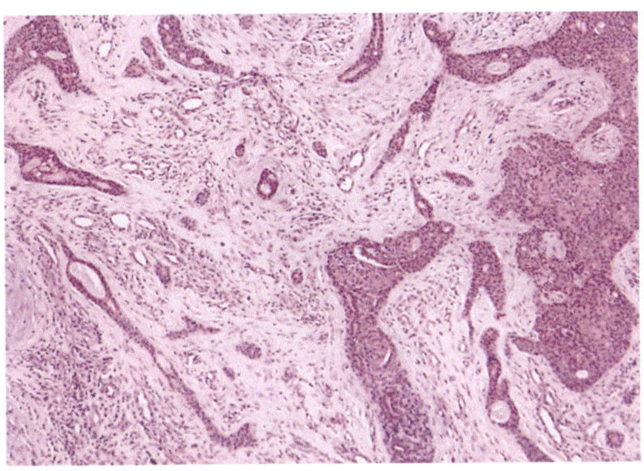

Fig. 18.188 Smaller clusters and strands of epithelial cells

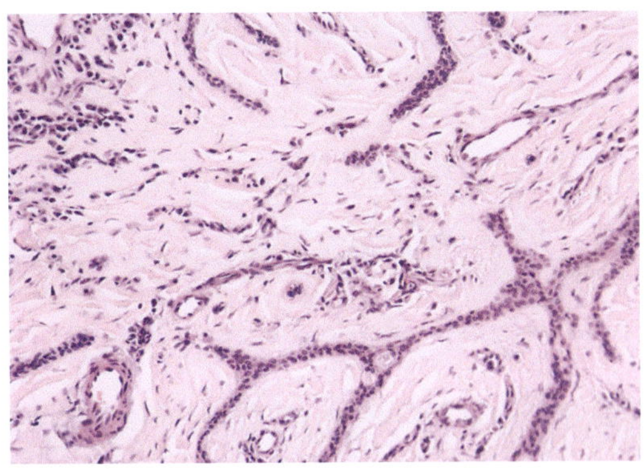

Fig. 18.189 Strands form delicate network in bluish myxoid stroma

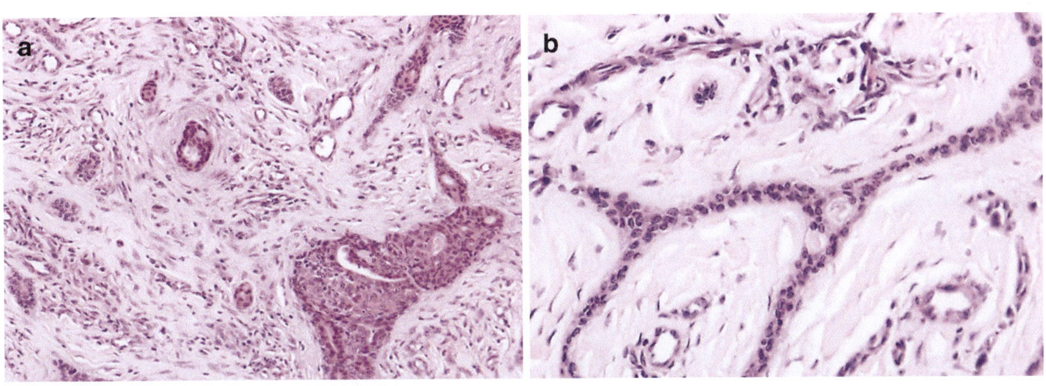

Fig. 18.190 (**a**, **b**) Small ducts are present within epithelial clusters and strands

Syringoma

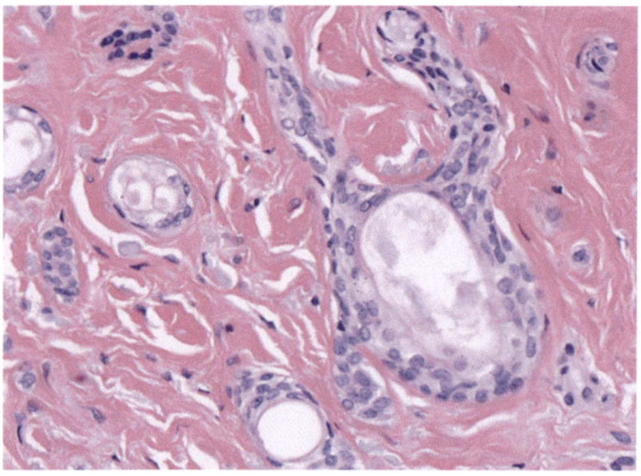

Fig. 18.191 Characteristic "tadpole" appearing duct

Histopathology (Figs. 18.191, 18.192, 18.193, and 18.194)

- Dermal tumor with small irregular ducts (CEA+) and tubules in dense stroma
- Some ducts have "tadpole" appearance
- Ducts are lined with two layers of flattened cuboidal cells
- In clear cell variant duct lining cells have clear cytoplasm
- Absence of infiltrative growth or atypia

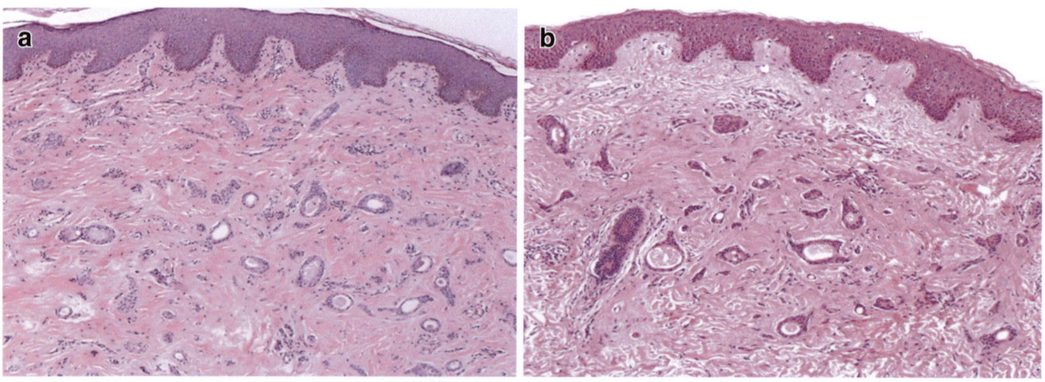

Fig. 18.192 (**a**, **b**) Small irregular ducts and tubules in dense dermal stoma

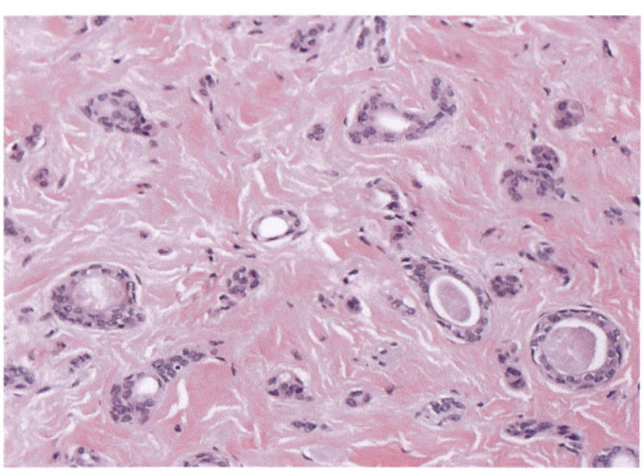

Fig. 18.193 Ducts are lined with two layers of cuboidal cells

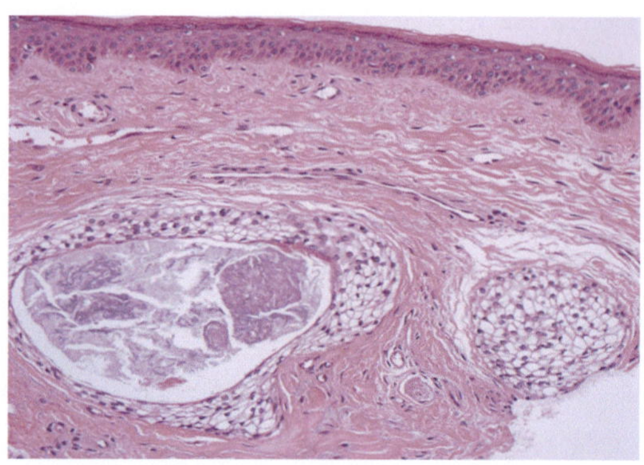

Fig. 18.194 In clear cell variant, ducts are lined with cells that have clear cell cytoplasm

19 Dermatopathology T

V. Vincek, *Dermatopathology A–Z*, https://doi.org/10.1007/978-3-319-89486-7_19

Takayasu Arteritis

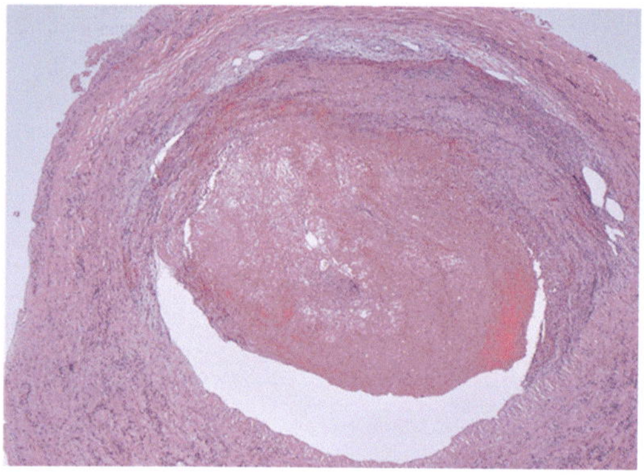

Fig. 19.1 Thrombosis of large vessel

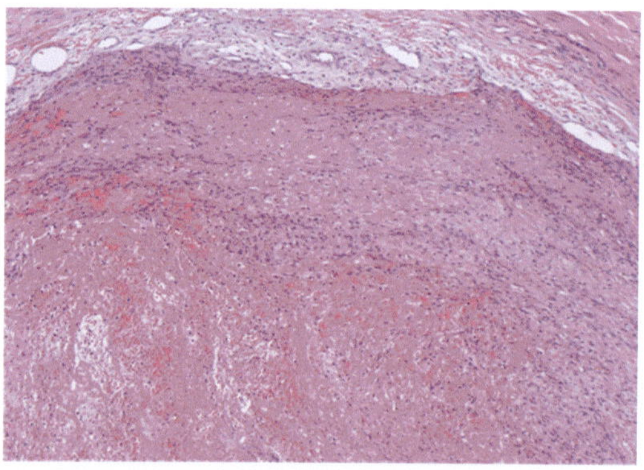

Fig. 19.2 Full thickness necrosis of vascular wall

Synonym: Pulseless Disease

Major pathology involves aorta and its main branches and histology is indistinguishable from giant cell arteritis. Skin lesions were described in only half of patients.

Skin lesions are nonspecific and can present as *pyoderma gangrenosum-like lesion, erythema nodosum-like lesion, erythema induratum-like lesion,* and/or *dermal purpura.*

Occasionally cutaneous necrotizing vasculitis can be present. It is identical to giant cell vasculitis but usually with fewer giant cells.

Histopathology demonstrates (Figs. 19.1, 19.2, and 19.3)

- Thrombosis of large vessels
- Full thickness necrosis
- Mixed inflammation consisting of lymphocytes, histiocytes, and occasional giant cells

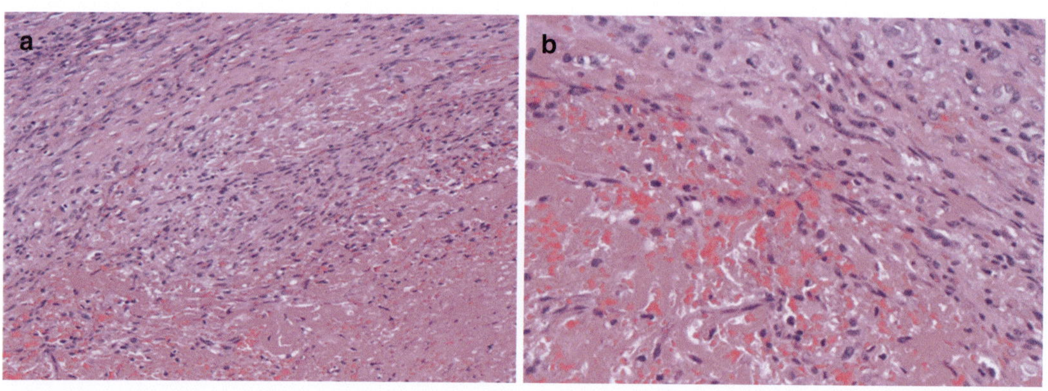

Fig. 19.3 (**a**, **b**) Fibrinoid necrosis with mixture of lymphocytes, histiocytes, and occasional giant cells

Talon Noir

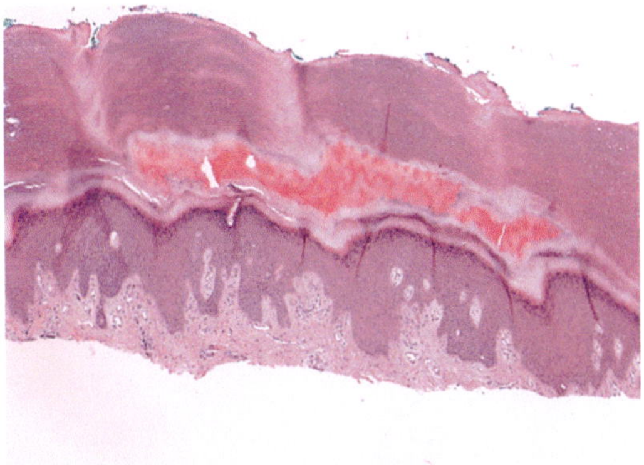

Fig. 19.4 Acral skin with hemorrhage

Synonym: Black Heel

Histopathology (Figs. 19.4, 19.5, and 19.6)

- Acral skin with hyperkeratosis and acanthosis
- Intraepidermal hemorrhage and red blood cell lysis
- Mild dermal inflammation and mild dermal red blood cell extravasation can be present

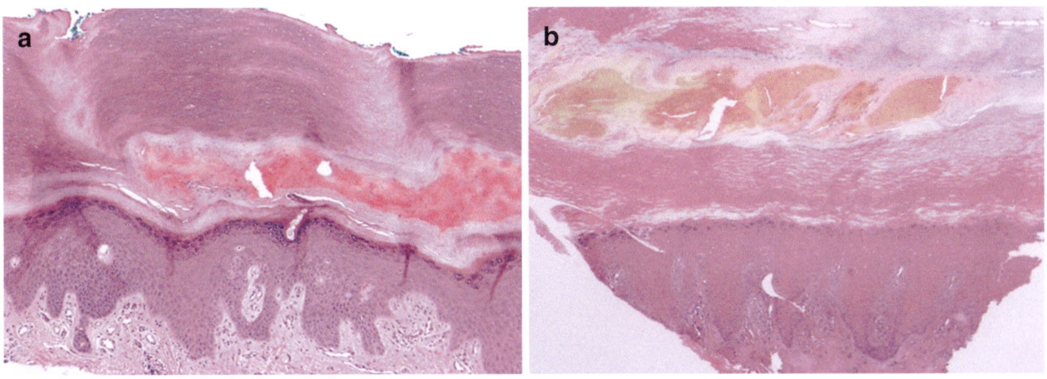

Fig. 19.5 (**a**, **b**) Hyperkeratotic, acanthotic epidermis with intraepidermal hemorrhage

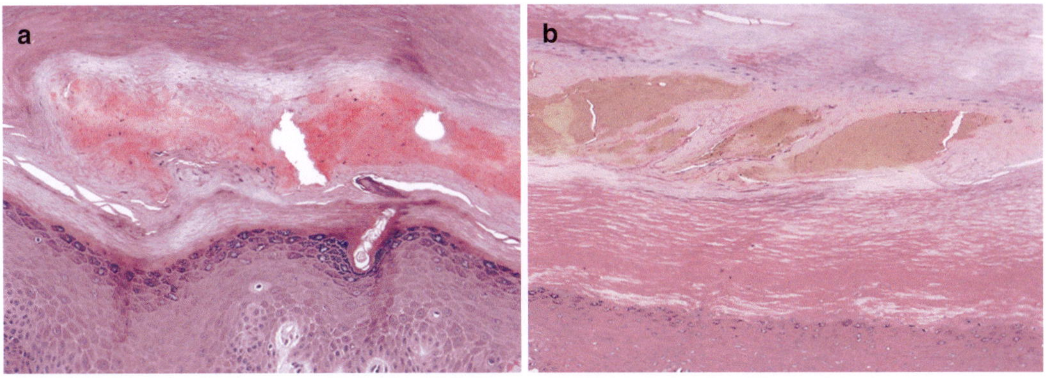

Fig. 19.6 (**a**, **b**) Red blood cells can be at various stages of lysis

Tattoo

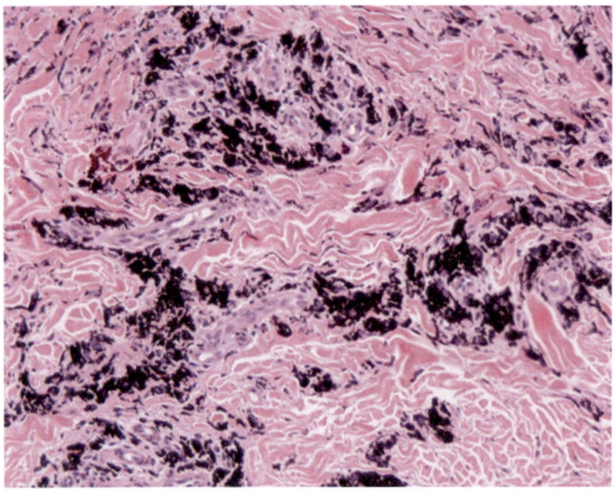

Fig. 19.7 Dermal deposits of black foreign material

Histopathology (Figs. 19.7, 19.8, 19.9, 19.10, and 19.11)

- Pigmented foreign body material scattered in the upper part of the dermis
- The pigment is more concentrated around dermal blood vessels
- No inflammation present in the majority of tattoos but granulomatous reaction can develop
- Regardless the color of the tattoo, majority of them show black color on H&E slides. Recently, red tattoo dies were introduced that stay red on the H&E slides

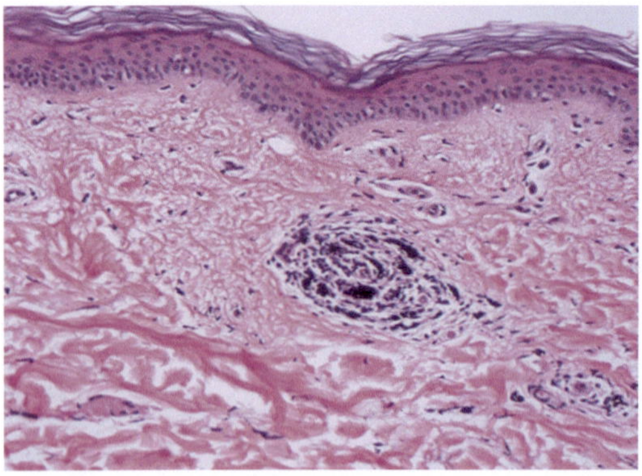

Fig. 19.8 Perivascular black pigment

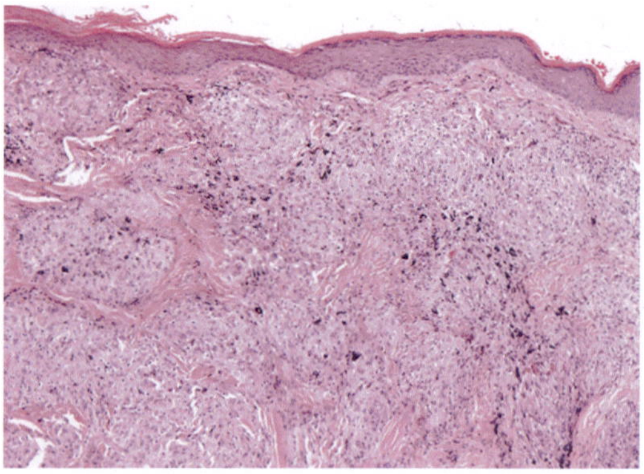

Fig. 19.9 Exuberant histiocytic infiltrate with granulomas

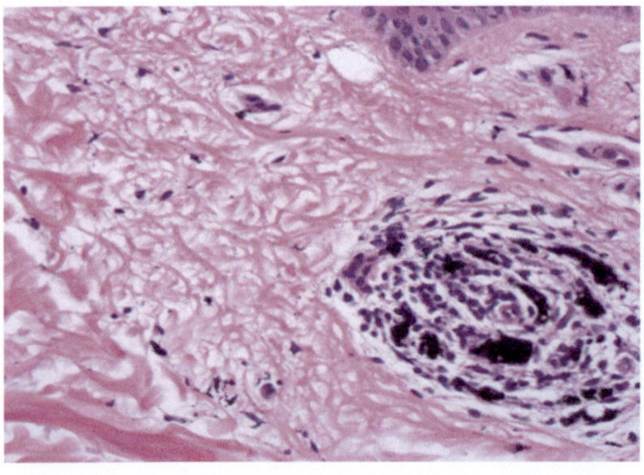

Fig. 19.10 Minimal inflammation around the foreign material

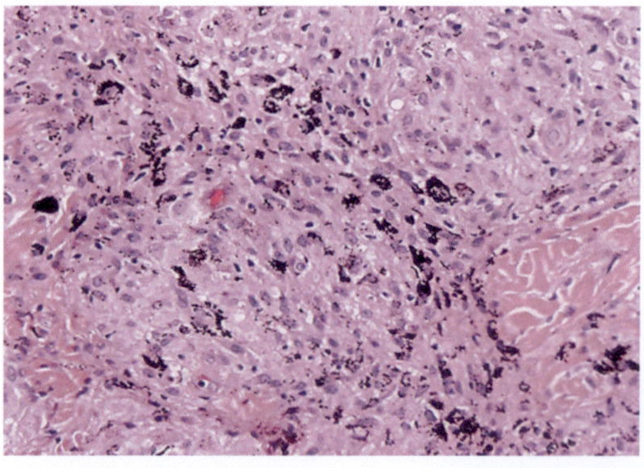

Fig. 19.11 Histiocytic infiltrate surrounds tattoo material

Telangiectasias

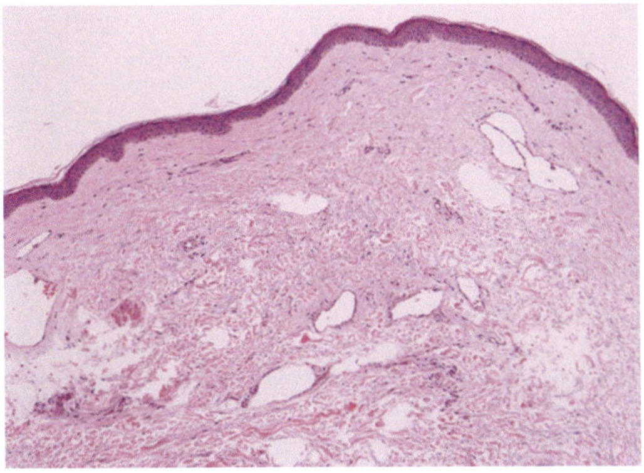

Fig. 19.12 Dilated dermal vascular channels

Histopathology (Figs. 19.12, 19.13, and 19.14)
- Dilated small capillaries in the dermis
- Most of the time, the lumen is empty or it contains a few erythrocytes
- Mild dermal edema is usually present

P.S. telangiectasias are part of many skin diseases including rosacea and basal cell carcinoma or are a disease by itself such in generalized essential telangiectasias

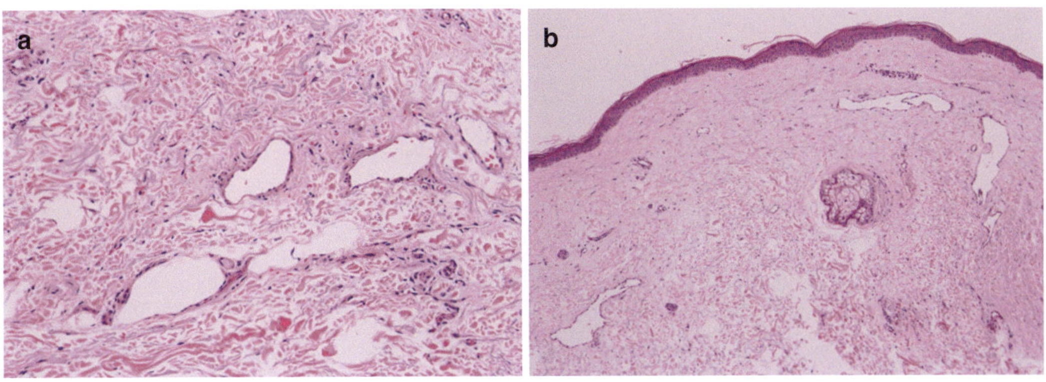

Fig. 19.13 (**a**, **b**) Dilated capillaries randomly scattered in the dermis. The wall is made of single layer of endothelial cells

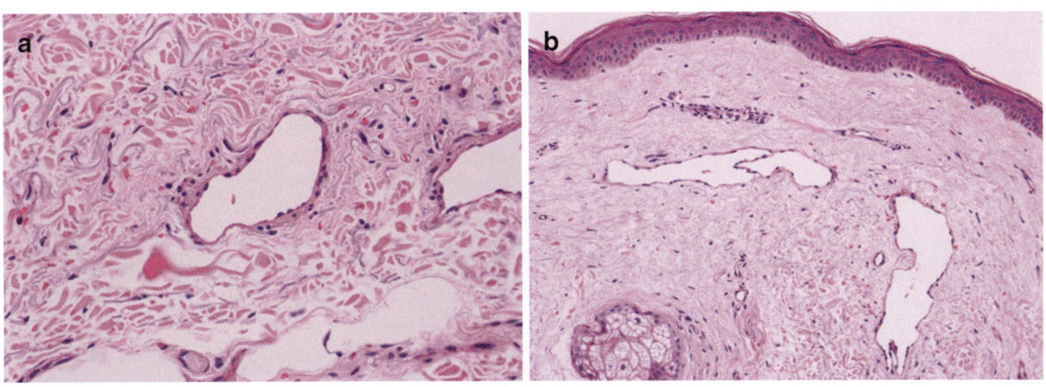

Fig. 19.14 (**a**, **b**) The lumen of telangiectasias is usually empty. Mild surrounding dermal edema is present

Telangiectasia Macularis Eruptiva Perstans

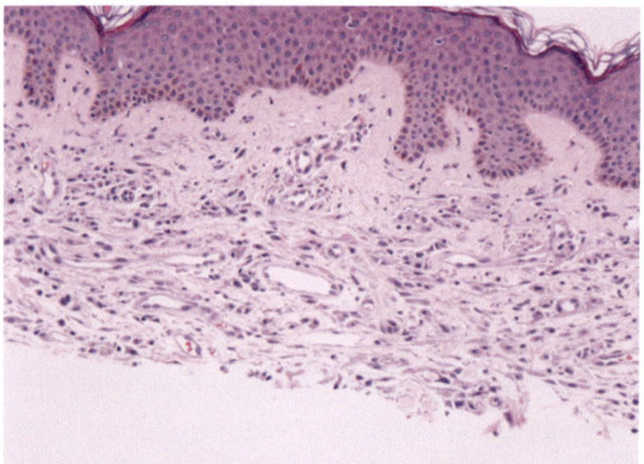

Fig. 19.15 Dermal telangiectasias

Histopathology (Figs. 19.15, 19.16, 19.17, and 19.18)

- Findings can be very subtle
- Dermal telangiectasias with increased number of perivascular mast cells (>20 mast cells on 40× magnification)
- Mast cells have "fried egg" appearance
- Mast cell tryptase and CD117 immunostains are very useful to better visualize and count number of mast cells

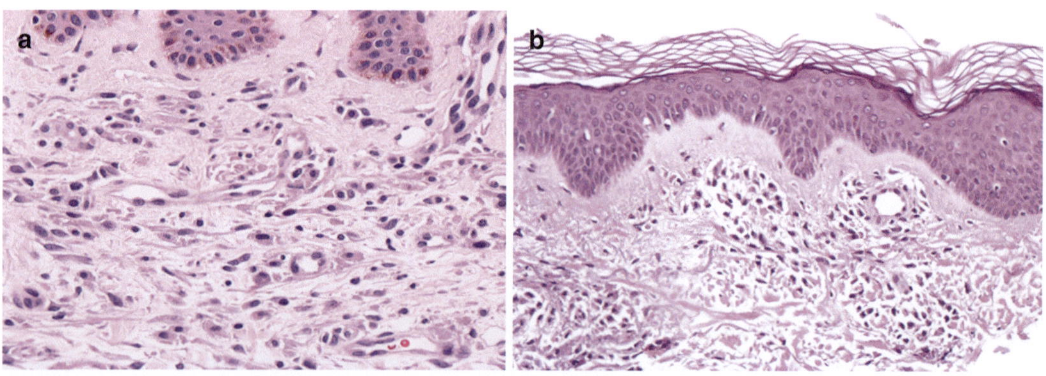

Fig. 19.16 (**a**, **b**) Dermal telangiectasias with perivascular and interstitial mast cells

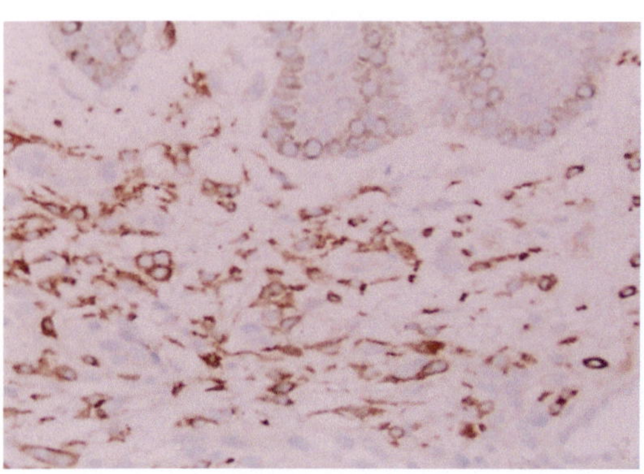

Fig. 19.17 Mast cell tryptase stain highlights mast cells

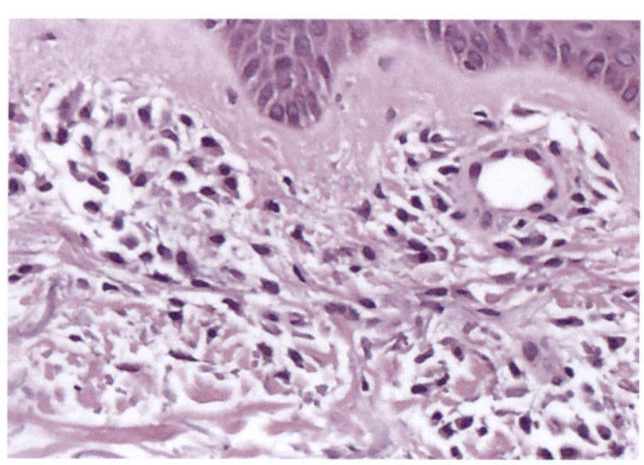

Fig. 19.18 Mast cells surround dermal capillaries

Telogen Effluvium

Histopathology (Figs. 19.19, 19.20, and 19.21)

- Similar to normal scalp with the exception during the active phase of hair shedding
- All follicles are terminal follicles
- Most follicles are in anagen stage
- In active stage of hair loss there is an increased number of catagen/telogen hairs, approximately by 20–30%
- No or minimal inflammation and no scarring

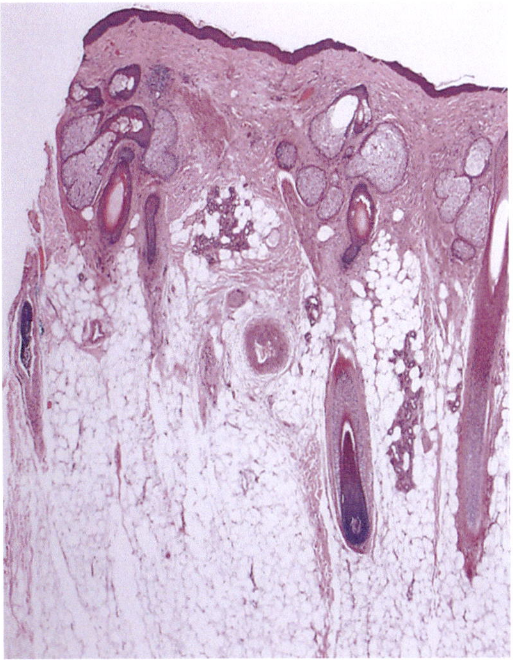

Fig. 19.19 A biopsy during the shedding stage of telogen effluvium with two anagen hairs on the right and two catagen hairs on the left

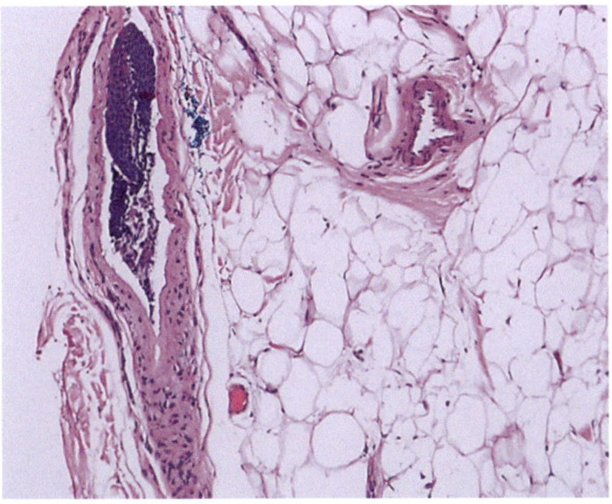

Fig. 19.20 Fibrous streamers of catagen follicles

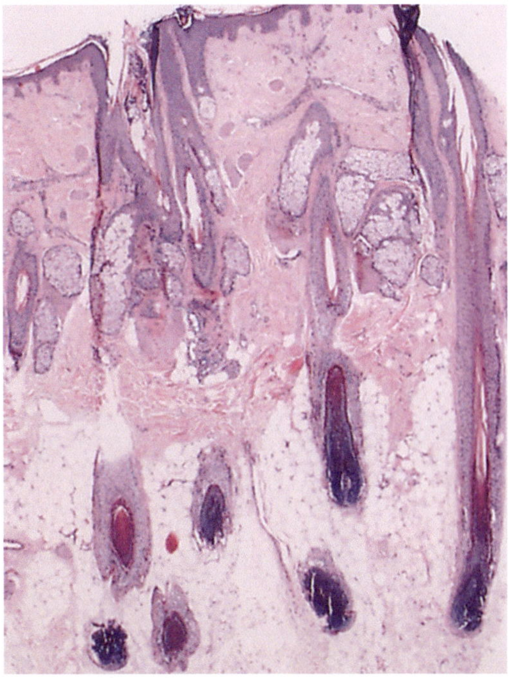

Fig. 19.21 A biopsy from chronic telogen effluvium that appears like normal scalp. Anagen hairs with no inflammation

Temporal Arteritis

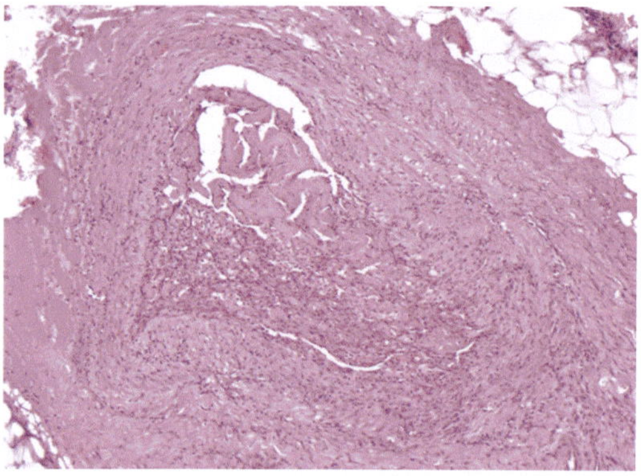

Fig. 19.22 Large vessel with inflamed wall and occluded lumen

Synonym: Giant Cell Arteritis

Histopathology (Figs. 19.22, 19.23, and 19.24)

- Granulomatous vasculitis of large vessels
- The entire vessel circumference or a portion is affected
- Infiltrate is made of lymphocytes, histiocytes, and variable number of giant cells
- Intima and media are affected the most

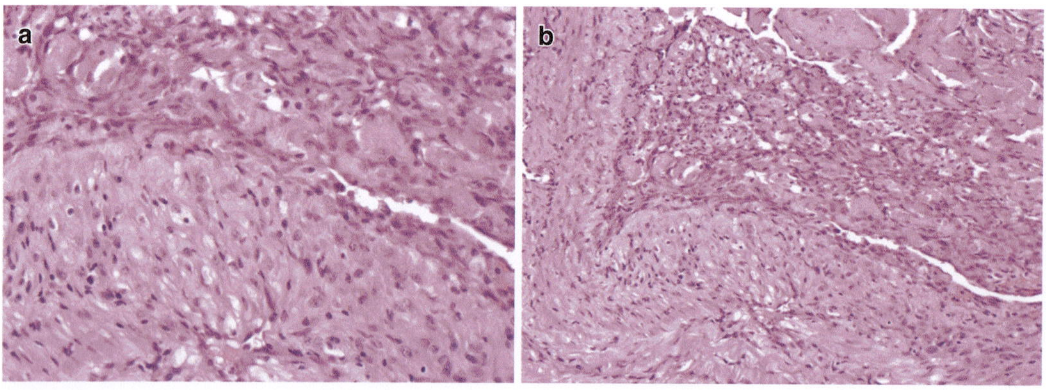

Fig. 19.23 (**a**, **b**) Intima and media of vessel is infiltrated by lymphocytes, histiocytes, and giant cells

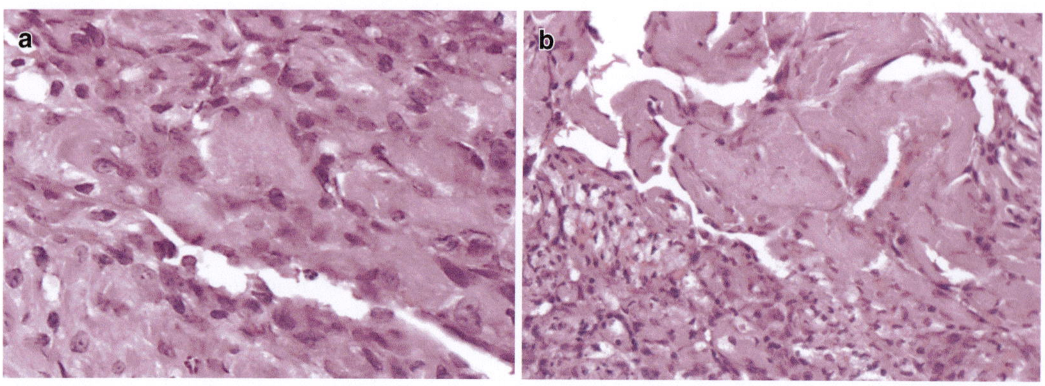

Fig. 19.24 (**a**, **b**) Langerhans giant cells scattered among chronic inflammatory cells and fibrinoid background

Tick

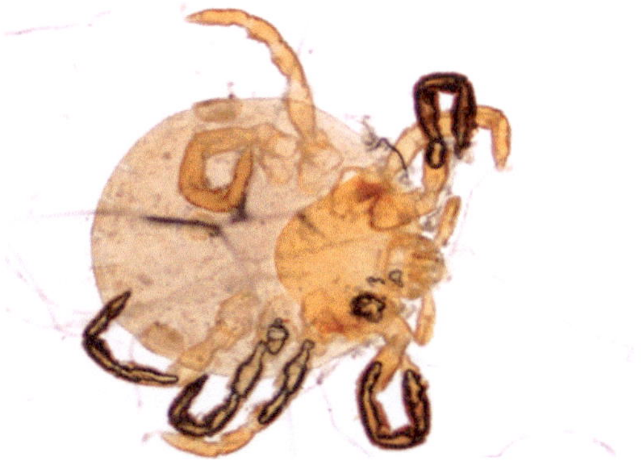

Fig. 19.25 The size and shape depends on tick species and feeding status. All species have four pair of legs

Histopathology (Figs. 19.25, 19.26, and 19.27)

- Usually a portion of the acellular cuticle or mouth piece are embedded within ulcerated skin
- Mixed inflammation made of neutrophils, lymphocytes, histiocytes, and occasional eosinophils
- Fibrotic pseudocapsule surrounds tick material

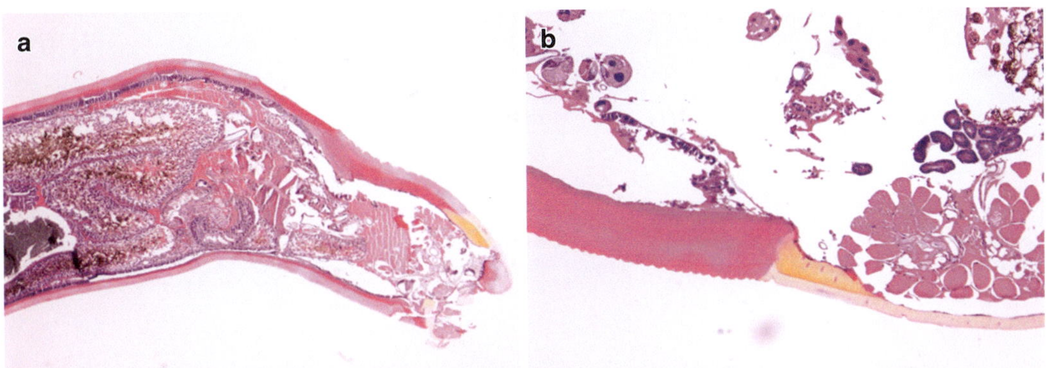

Fig. 19.26 (**a**, **b**) Thick acellular cuticle with barb like projections. The jaw portion of the tick with striated muscle

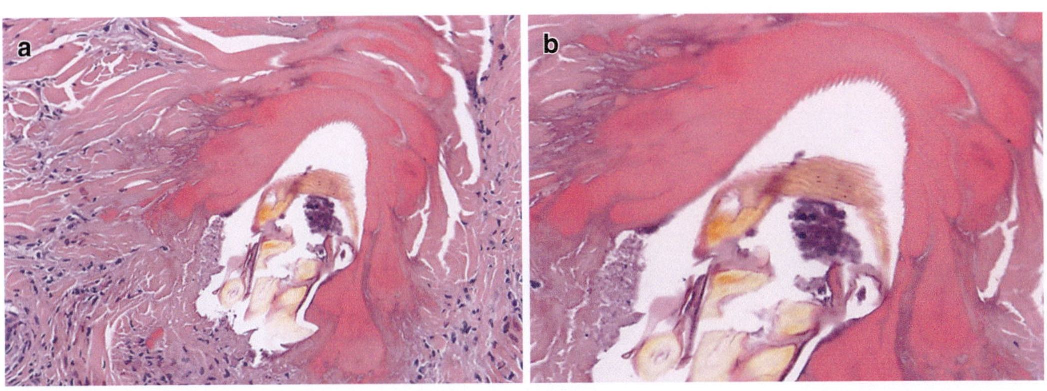

Fig. 19.27 (**a**, **b**) Thick hyaline structure representing tick cuticle is embedded in the dermis and surrounded by acute and chronic inflammation and scarring. Cuticle has barb like projections that serve as anchors during feeding

Tinea

Synonyms: Dermatophytoses, Ringworm

- Caused by Microsporum, Trichophyton, or Epidermophyton
- Multiple locations
  T. barbae—beard
  T. capitis/T. favosa—scalp
  T. corporis—trunk and extremities
  T. cruris—groin
  T. manum—hand
  T. pedis—feet
  T. unguium—nails

Histopathology depends on the site:

In dry skin areas

- Normal appearing skin with compact stratum corneum, so called "invisible dermatosis". PAS outlines fungal hyphae in the stratum corneum (Figs. 19.28, 19.29, 19.30, and 19.31) *or*
- Mild dermal inflammation with compact orthokeratosis and a "mound" of neutrophils and parakeratosis. Fungal elements are "sandwiched" in between orthokeratosis and neutrophils/parakeratosis (Figs. 19.32, 19.33, 19.34, and 19.35)

In wet skin areas

- Spongiotic acanthotic epidermis with vesicles that contains neutrophilic aggregates and fungal hyphae (Figs. 19.36 and 19.37)

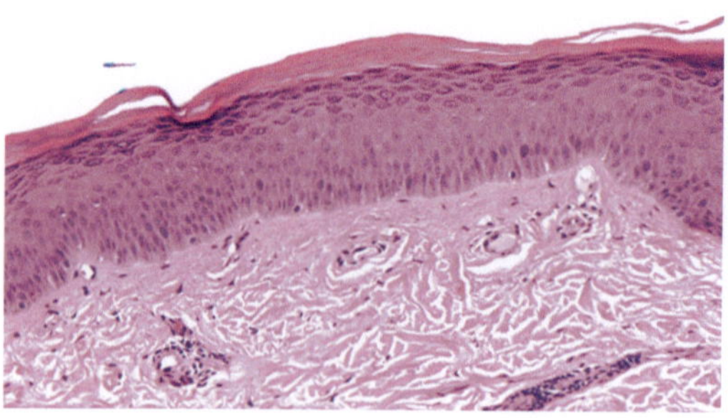

Fig. 19.28 Normal appearing skin with compact orthokeratosis

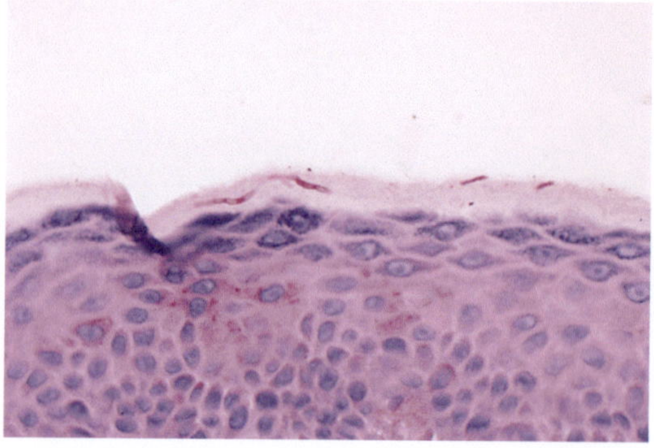

Fig. 19.29 Periodic acid-Schiff (PAS) outline hyphae

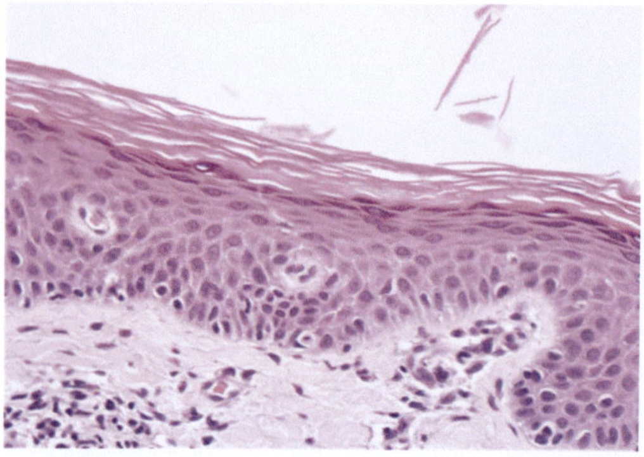

Fig. 19.30 "Invisible dermatosis" with mild epidermal spongiosis and very mild perivascular lymphocytic infiltrate

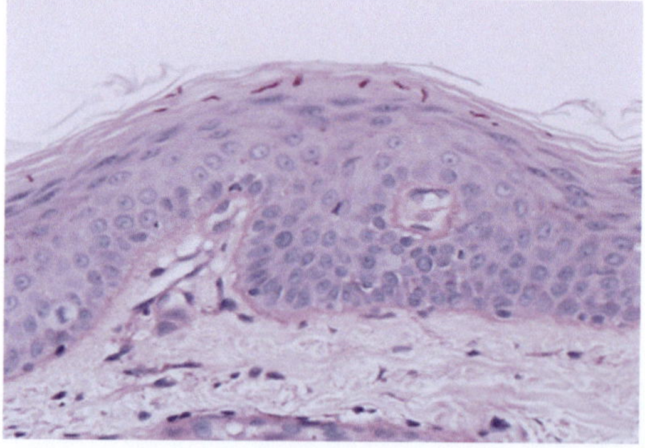

Fig. 19.31 PAS stain demonstrates hyphae in the stratum corneum

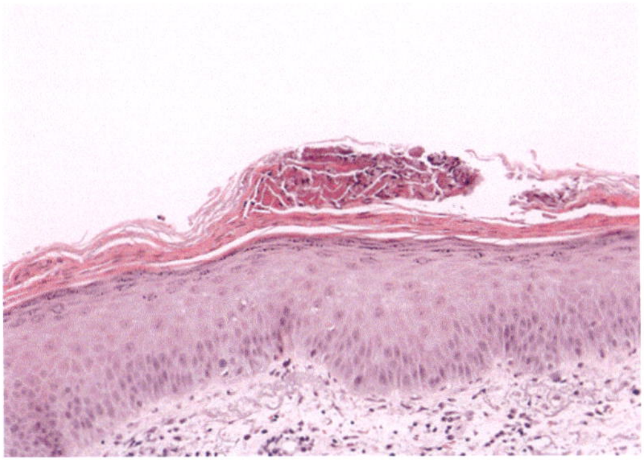

Fig. 19.32 "Mound" of neutrophils and parakeratosis within compact stratum corneum. Mild dermal inflammation

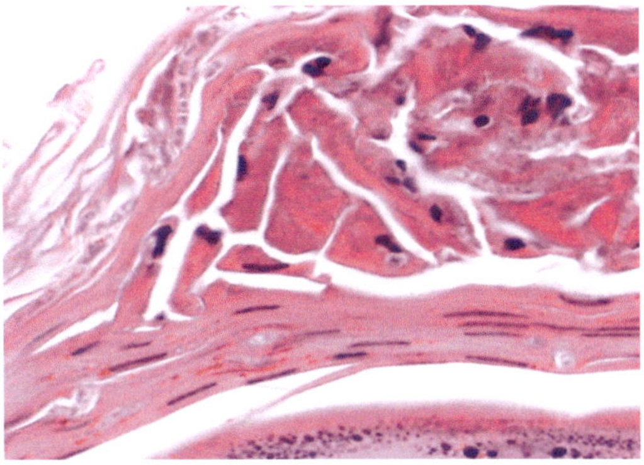

Fig. 19.33 On H&E slide hyphae appears as pale elements sandwiched below and around neutrophilic aggregate

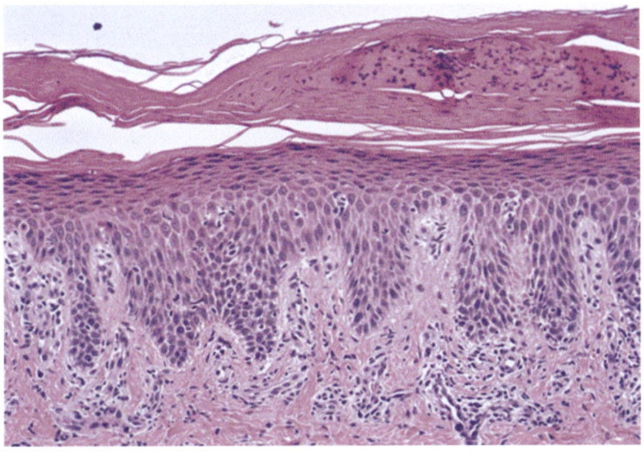

Fig. 19.34 Acanthotic epidermis with spongiosis and papillomatosis. Focal parakeratosis and neutrophils in the stratum corneum

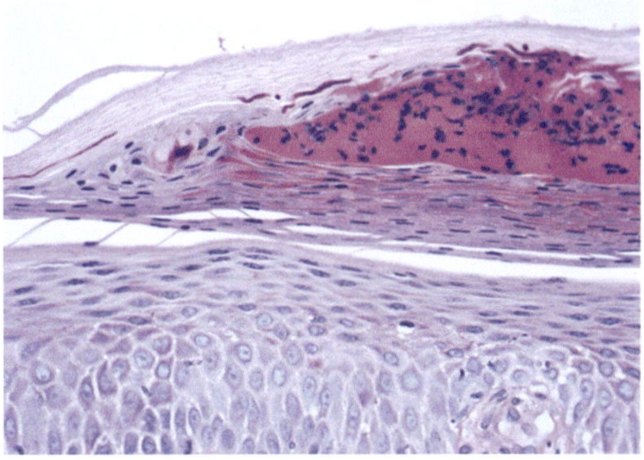

Fig. 19.35 Hyphae are outlined with PAS stain adjacent to the neutrophilic aggregate

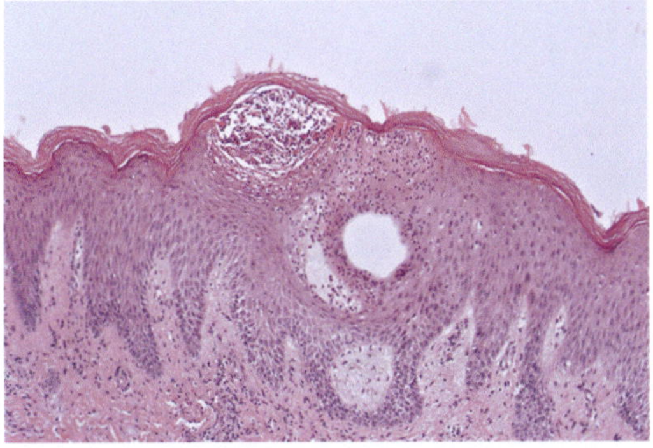

Fig. 19.36 Acanthotic epidermis with irregular papillomatosis and intracorneal neutrophilic pustule

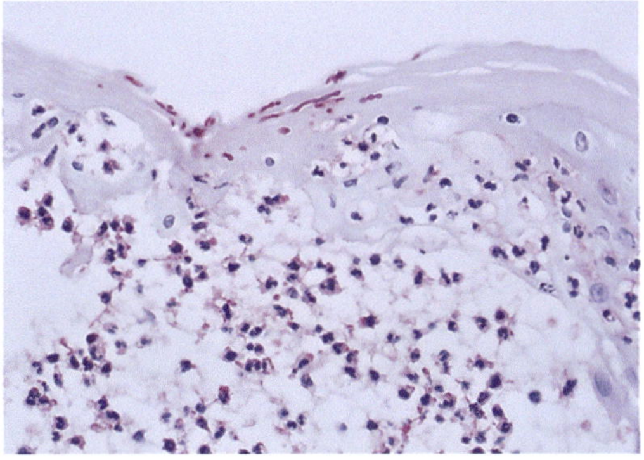

Fig. 19.37 PAS stain demonstrates hyphae in the stratum corneum above neutrophilic pustule

Tinea Nigra

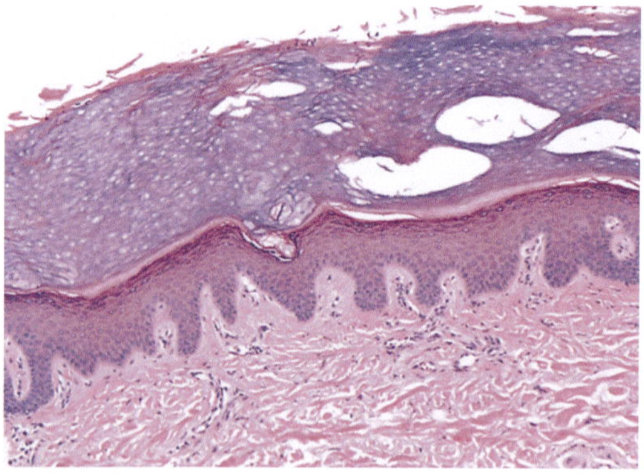

Fig. 19.38 Acral skin that appears normal on low magnification

Despite name, **tinea nigra** is not a dermatophyte. It is caused by *Hortaea werneckii.*

Histopathology (Figs. 19.38, 19.39, 19.40, and 19.41)

- Acral skin with thick stratum corneum
- Branching gray/brown fungal hyphae in the superficial portion of stratum corneum
- Minimal or no dermal inflammation

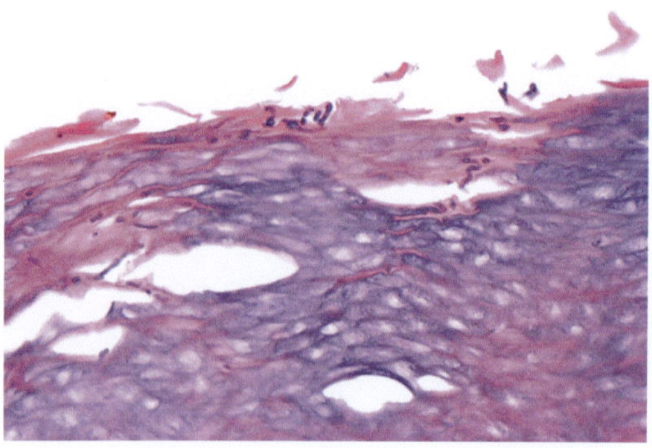

Fig. 19.39 Pigmented hyphae stand out in the epidermis

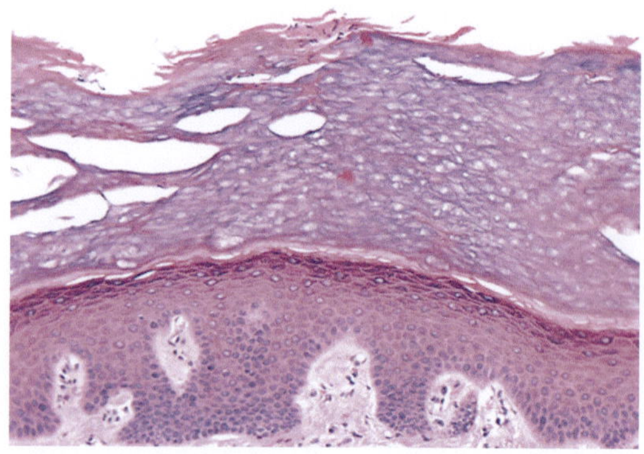

Fig. 19.40 No inflammation is present in the dermis

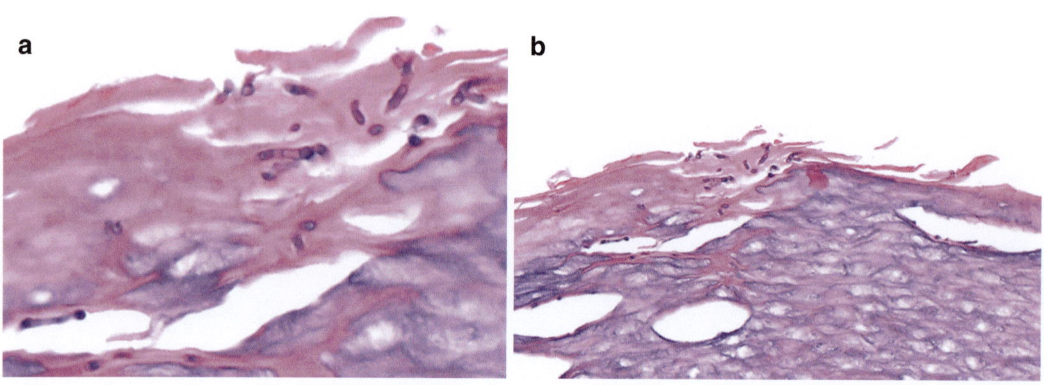

Fig. 19.41 (**a**, **b**) Pigmented branching septated fungal hyphae in the superficial portion of the stratum corneum

Thromboangiitis Obliterans

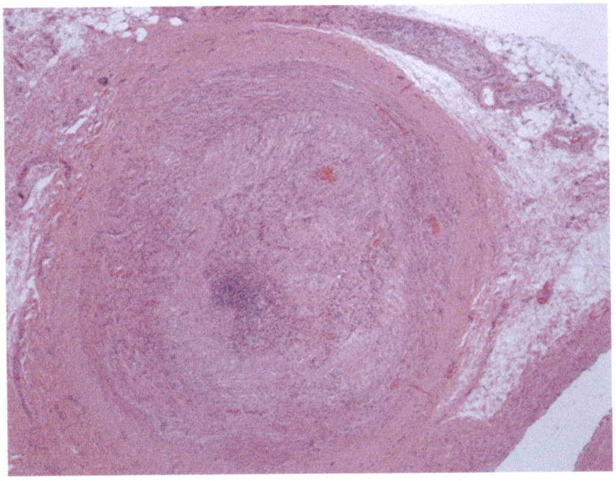

Fig. 19.42 Thrombosed medium size artery

Synonym: Buerger's Disease

Histopathology (Figs. 19.42, 19.43, and 19.44)

- Thrombosis of medium and large size arteries and sometimes veins
- Mixed inflammation made of lymphocytes, histiocytes, neutrophils, and occasional giant cells
- Intraluminal organizing thrombus with microabscess

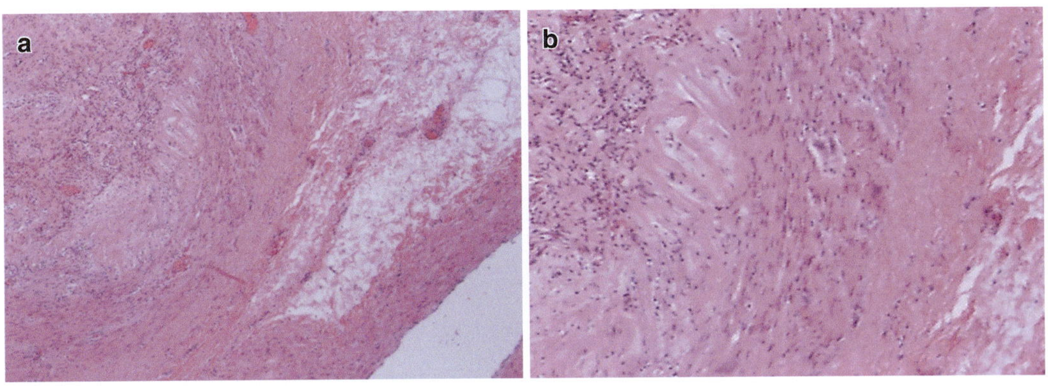

Fig. 19.43 (**a**, **b**) Vessel wall infiltrated with lymphocytes, histiocytes, and few giant cells

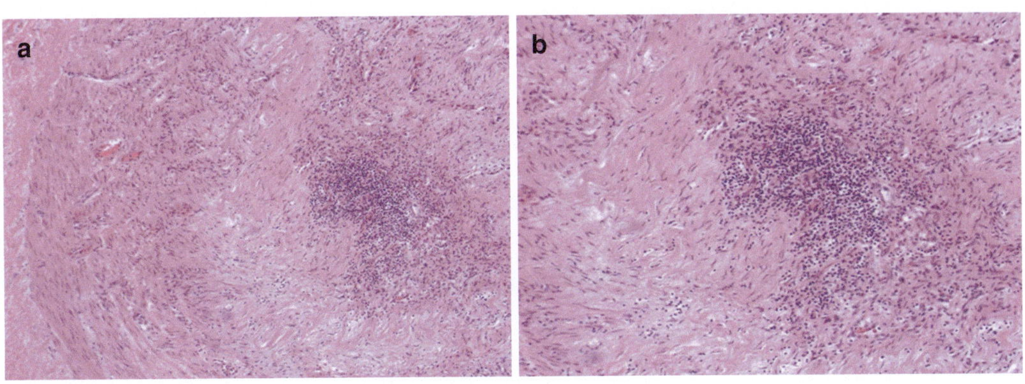

Fig. 19.44 (**a**, **b**) Lumen filled with organizing thrombus and inflammation

Thrombophlebitis

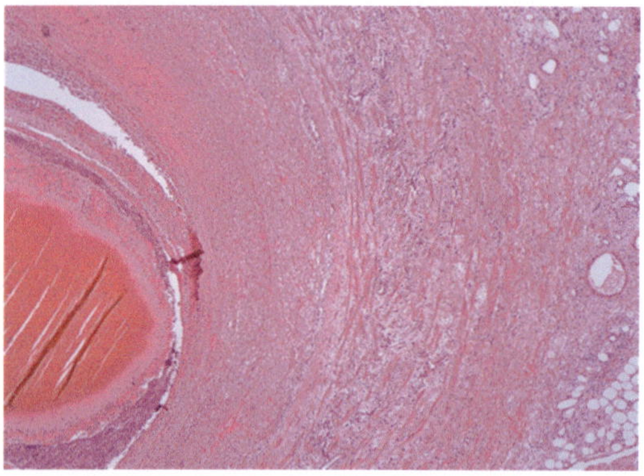

Fig. 19.45 Thrombosis of medium size vein

Histopathology (Figs. 19.45, 19.46, and 19.47)

- Involves medium size veins
- Early lesions demonstrate vascular thrombosis with neutrophilic infiltrate in the vessel wall
- Established lesions demonstrate organizing thrombus with chronic inflammation within the vessel wall

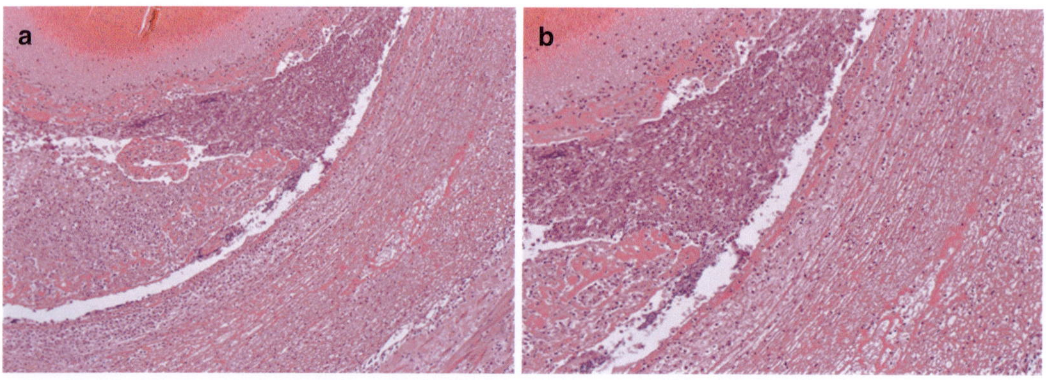

Fig. 19.46 (**a**, **b**) Early lesion showing intravascular thrombus that is starting to be organized

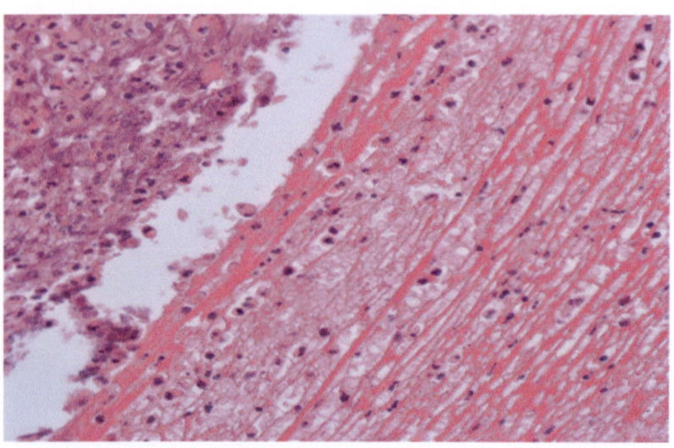

Fig. 19.47 Neutrophils are present in the wall of the vessel

Thymic Cyst

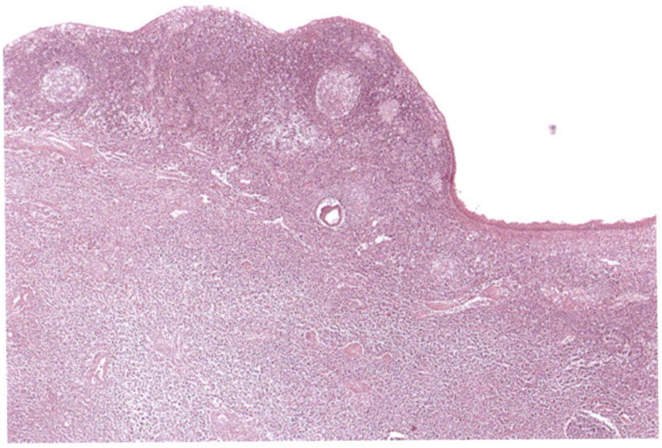

Fig. 19.48 Cyst with abundant lymphocytes in the wall

Histopathology (Figs. 19.48, 19.49, and 19.50)

- The cyst wall is variably lined with stratified squamous, cuboidal, or ciliated epidermis
- Cyst wall is made of thymic tissue that is composed of abundant lymphocytes and lymphoid follicles with scattered Hassall's corpuscles

P.S. branchial cleft cyst is similar but without Hassall's corpuscles

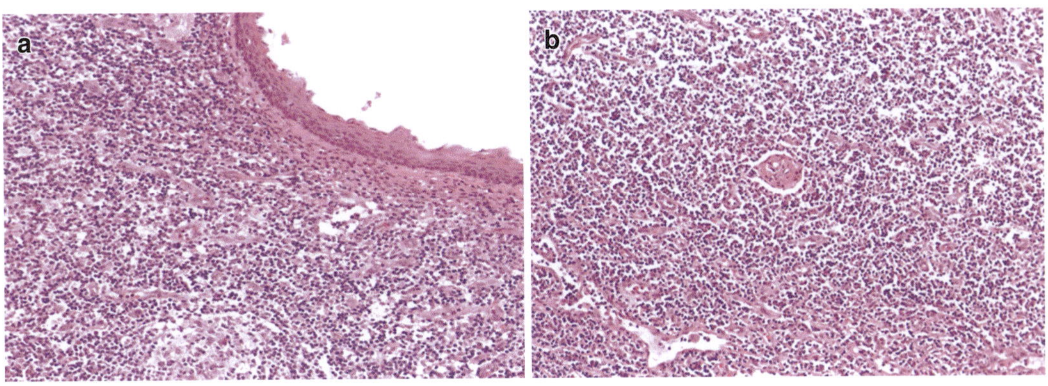

Fig. 19.49 (**a**, **b**) Cyst wall made of stratified squamous epithelium surrounded by dense lymphocytic infiltrate with Hassall's corpuscles

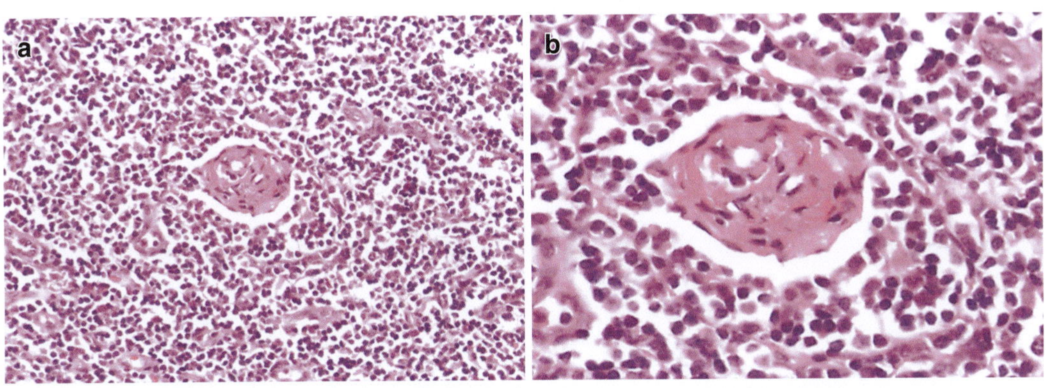

Fig. 19.50 (**a**, **b**) Hassall's corpuscles made of epithelioid cells forming round pink laminated structures

Thyroglossal Cyst

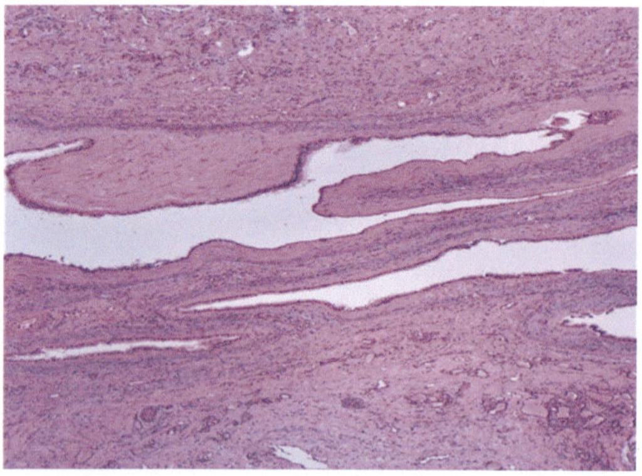

Fig. 19.51 Cyst lined with thin lining

Histopathology (Figs. 19.51, 19.52, 19.53, and 19.54)

- Cyst lined with cuboidal ciliated cells
- Thyroid follicles filled with eosinophilic colloid are present in the cyst wall and in between cysts
- Lymphocytes are scattered between thyroid follicles

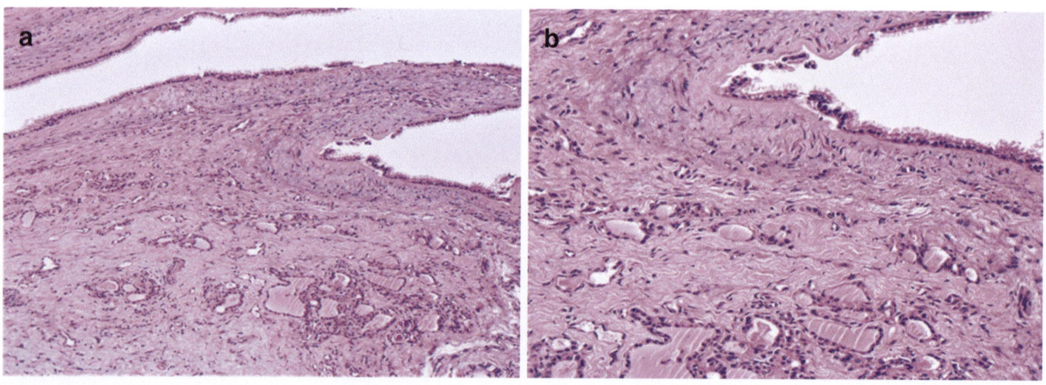

Fig. 19.52 (**a**, **b**) Colloid containing thyroid follicles are present in the cyst wall. Mild scattered lymphocytic inflammation is present

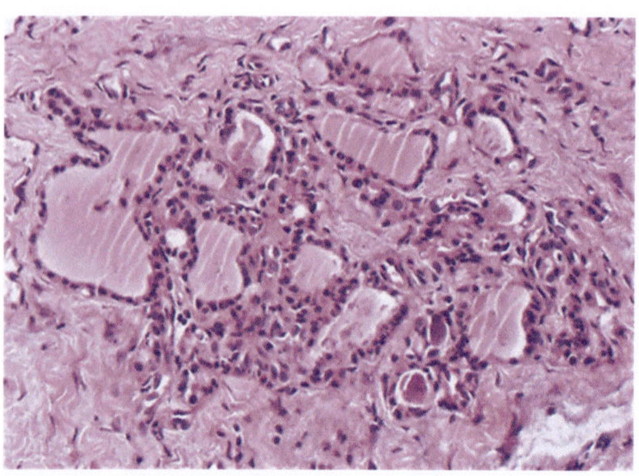

Fig. 19.53 Thyroid follicles vary in size

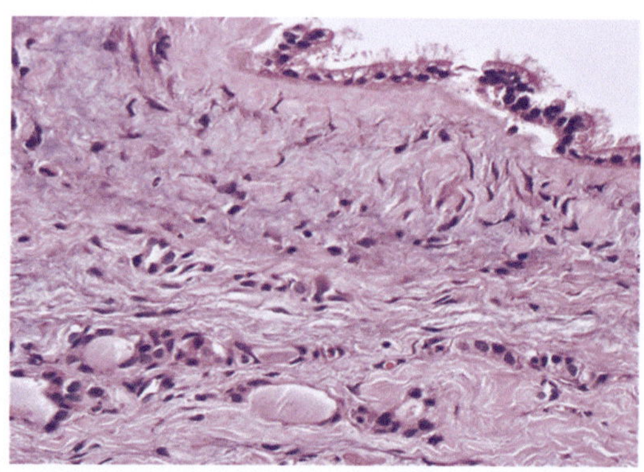

Fig. 19.54 Ciliated cuboidal cells and thyroid follicles

Toxic Epidermal Necrolysis

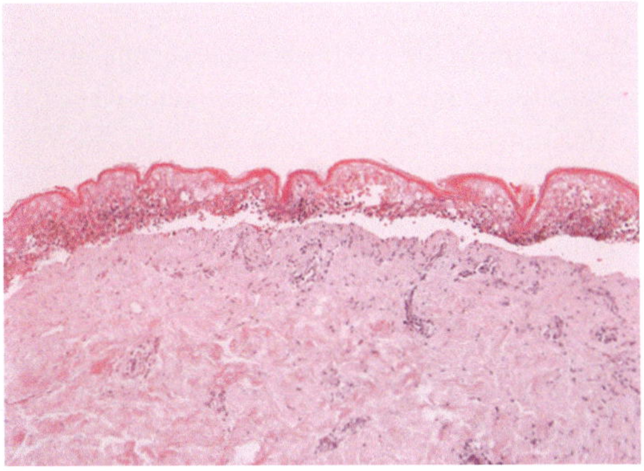

Fig. 19.55 Necrotic epidermis with minimal inflammation

Synonyms: Lyell's disease, Stevens-Johnson Syndrome

Histopathology (Figs. 19.55, 19.56, and 19.57)

- Full thickness epidermal necrosis
- Minimal dermal inflammation
- Subepidermal blister with epidermo-dermal separation
- Individual single cell keratinocytic necrosis can be seen at the edge of the lesion

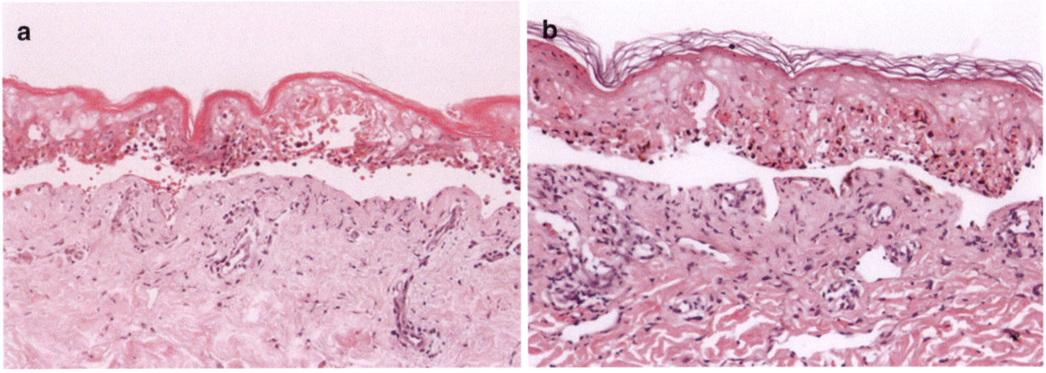

Fig. 19.56 (**a**, **b**) Full thickness epidermal necrosis with subepidermal separation

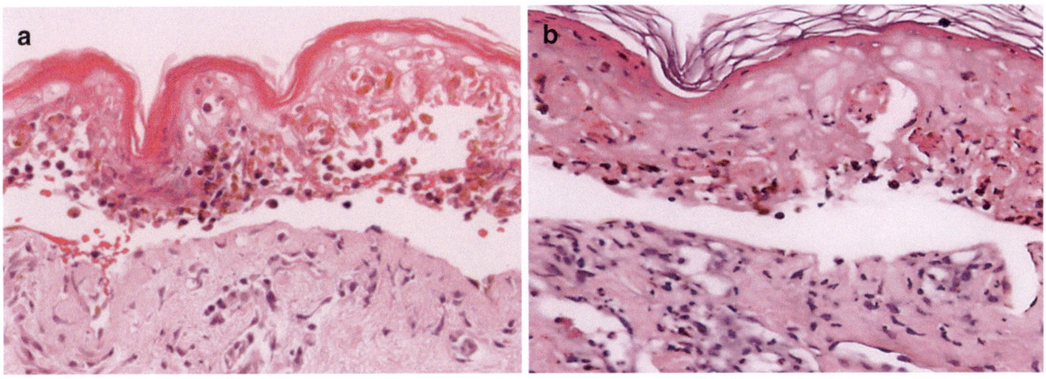

Fig. 19.57 (**a**, **b**) Minimal dermal inflammation with accumulation of pigment at the bottom of the necrotic epidermis

Traction Alopecia/Pressure Alopecia

Histopathology of traction alopecia and pressure alopecia appears like a milder version of trichotillomania (Figs. 19.58, 19.59, 19.60, 19.61)
- Number of anagen hairs is decreased and number of telogen/catagen hairs is increased reducing anagen/telogen ratio
- Minimal or no inflammation
- Follicular plugging and dermal pigment cast
- In addition, in *pressure alopecia* vascular thrombosis and necrosis can be seen and in *traction alopecia* there is fibrosis present around hair follicle

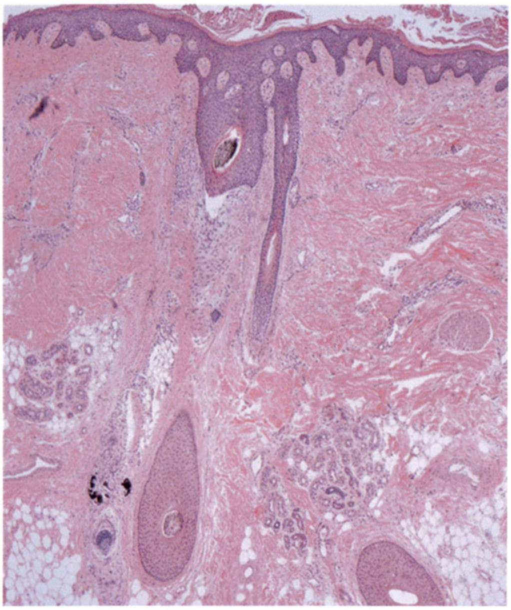

Fig. 19.58 Damaged anagen hair

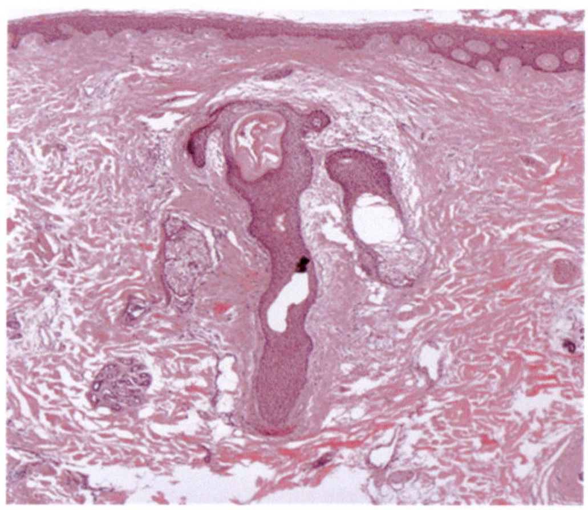

Fig. 19.59 Follicular plugging and perifollicular fibrosis

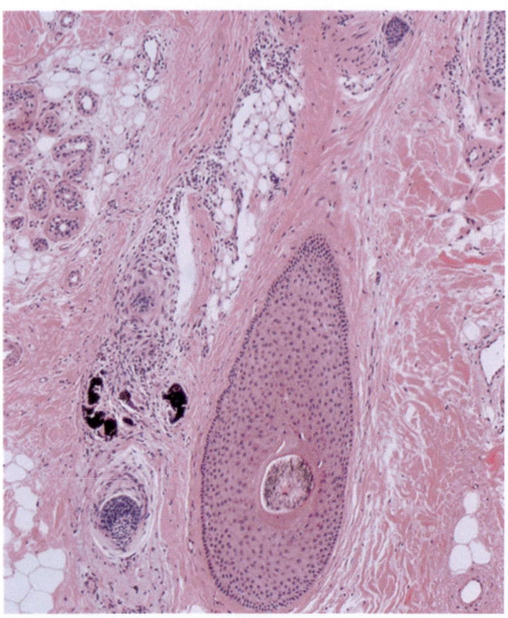

Fig. 19.60 Dermal pigment cast and minimal inflammation

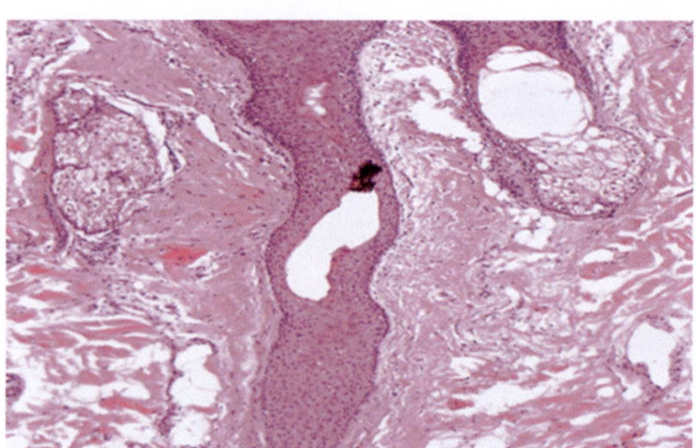

Fig. 19.61 Distorted follicle with perifollicular fibrosis

Transient Neonatal Pustular Melanosis

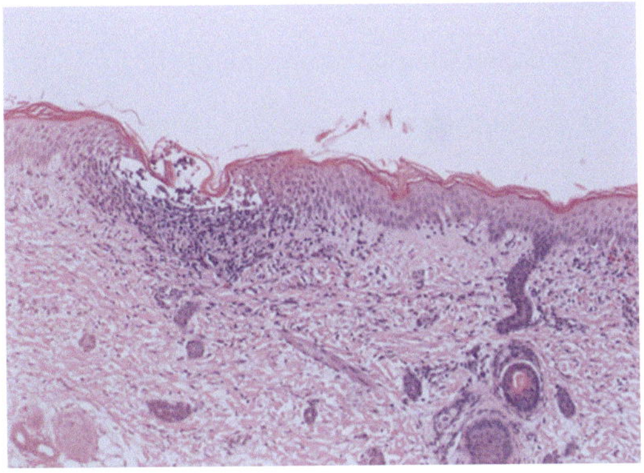

Fig. 19.62 Subcorneal pustule

Histopathology (Figs. 19.62, 19.63, and 19.64)

- Subcorneal or intraepidermal neutrophilic pustule
- Variable number of eosinophils
- Variable number of neutrophils and eosinophils present in the dermis underneath epidermal pustule

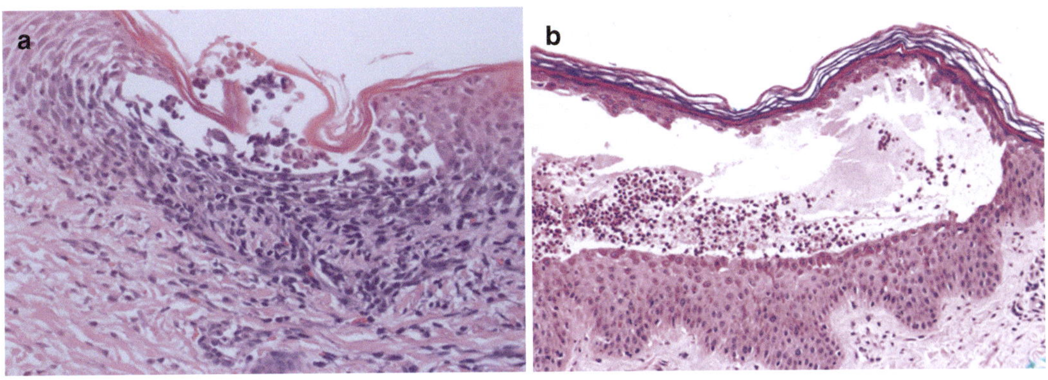

Fig. 19.63 (**a**, **b**) Neutrophils and few eosinophils present in the dermis underneath the epidermal neutrophilic pustule

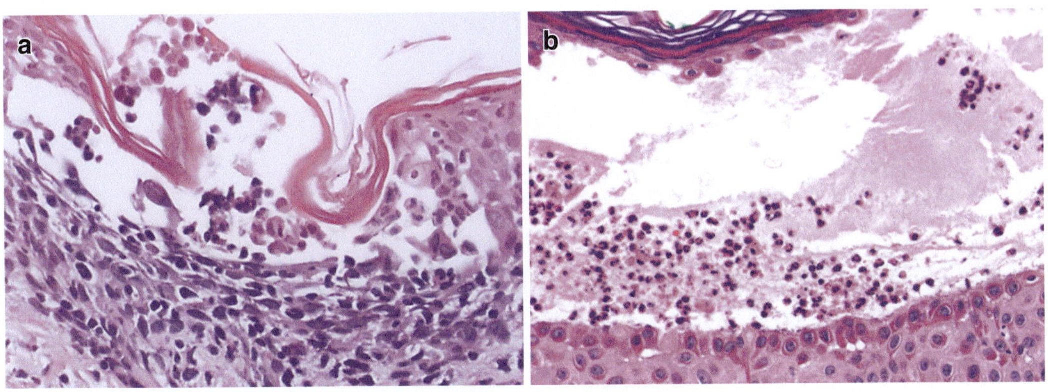

Fig. 19.64 (**a**, **b**) Subcorneal neutrophilic pustule with few eosinophils

Traumatic Fat Necrosis

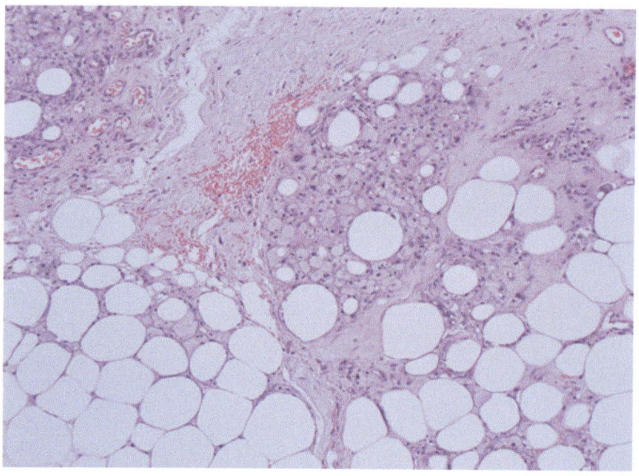

Fig. 19.65 Traumatized adipose tissue and RBCs extravasation

Synonym: Traumatic Panniculitis

Histopathology (Figs. 19.65, 19.66, 19.67, 19.68, and 19.69)

- Adipocytes of various size with admixed lymphocytes, lipophages (foamy histiocytes), and giant cells
- Focal necrosis and red blood cell extravasation
- Common dystrophic calcification and scarring

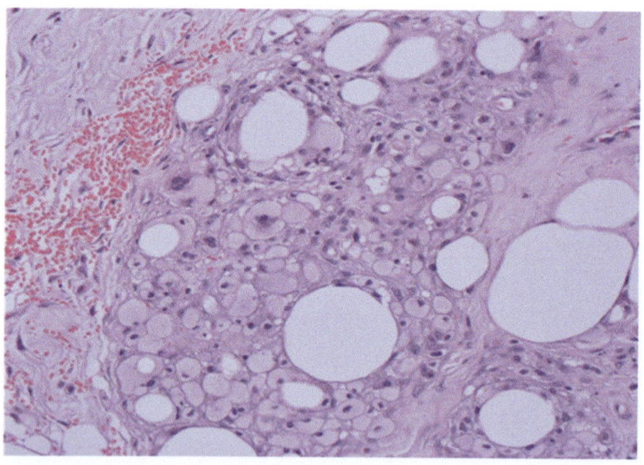

Fig. 19.66 Adipocytes with lipophages, lymphocytes, and giant cells

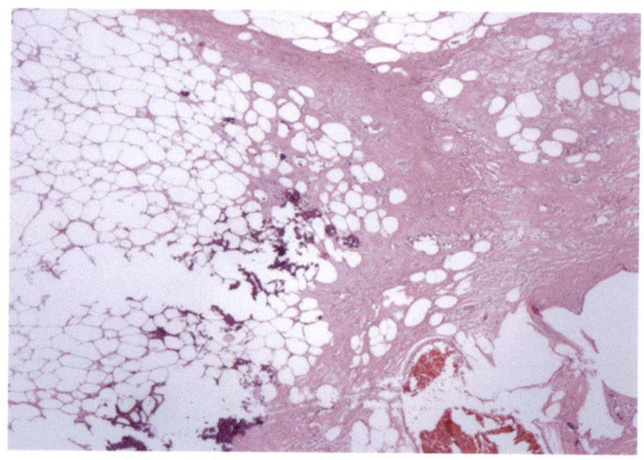

Fig. 19.67 Fat necrosis and scarring

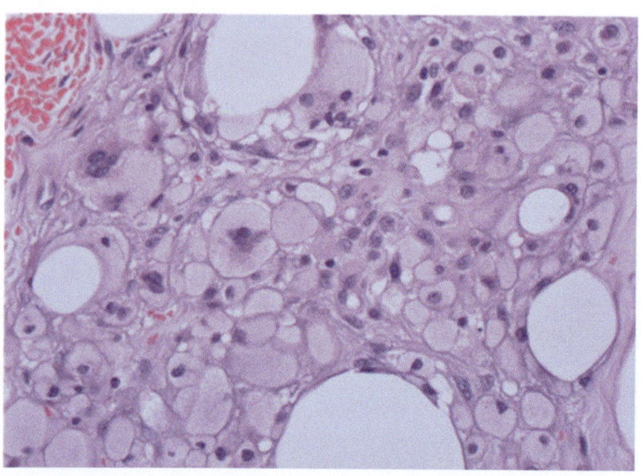

Fig. 19.68 Numerous lipophages of variable size

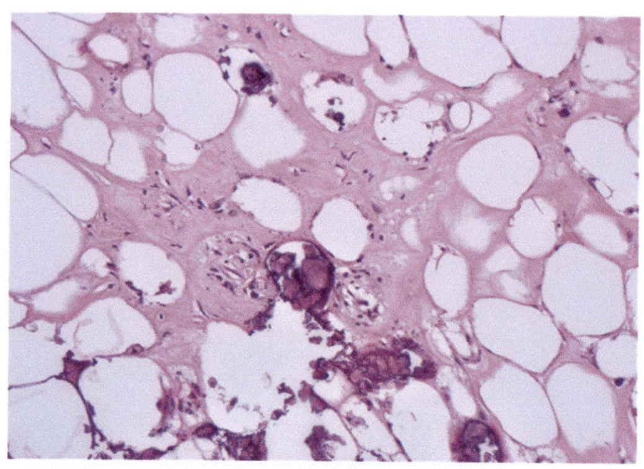

Fig. 19.69 Dystrophic calcifications

Traumatic Neuroma/Amputation Neuroma

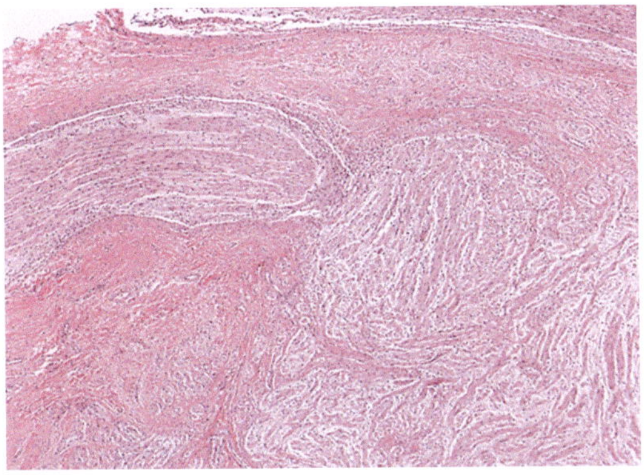

Fig. 19.70 Large neural elements haphazardly arranged

Present at the site of limb amputation.

Histopathology (Figs. 19.70, 19.71, 19.72, 19.73, and 19.74)

- Numerous irregularly oriented large neural elements (S100+) characterized by elongated wavy cells
- Surrounding scarring and smaller spindle shaped neural elements

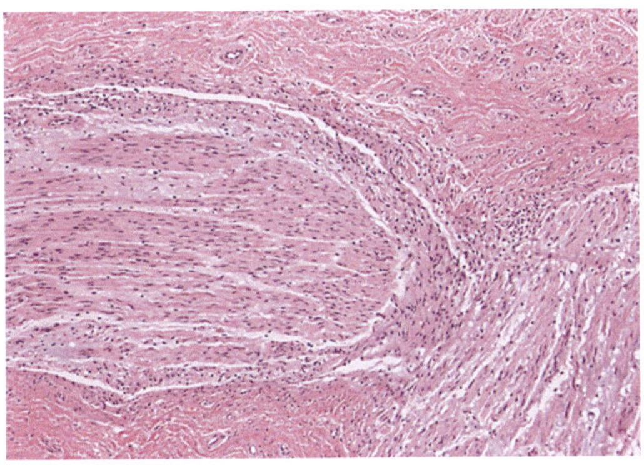

Fig. 19.71 Neural elements are oriented in various directions

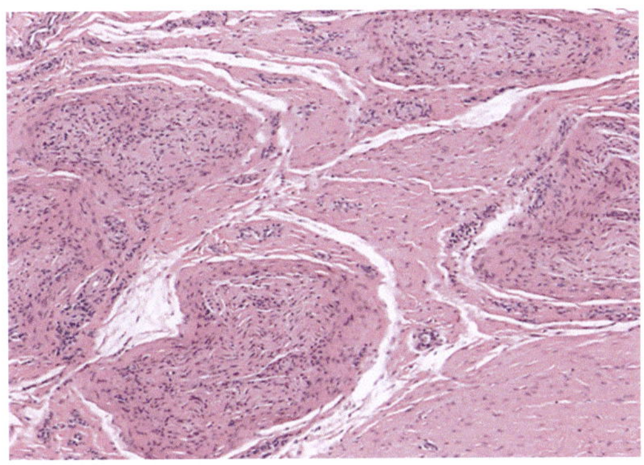

Fig. 19.72 Extensive scarring surrounds neural elements

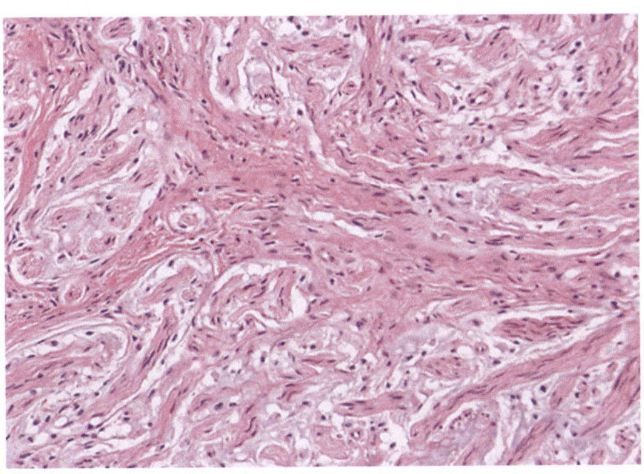

Fig. 19.73 Smaller spindle neural cells are present in the scar

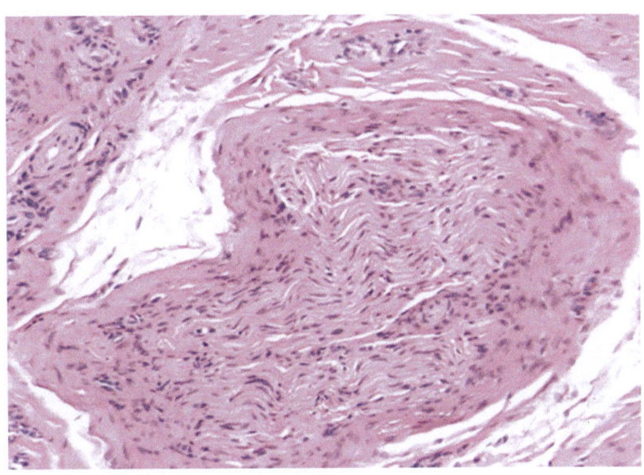

Fig. 19.74 Neural elements made of wavy elongated cells

Traumatic Neuroma/Rudimentary Digit

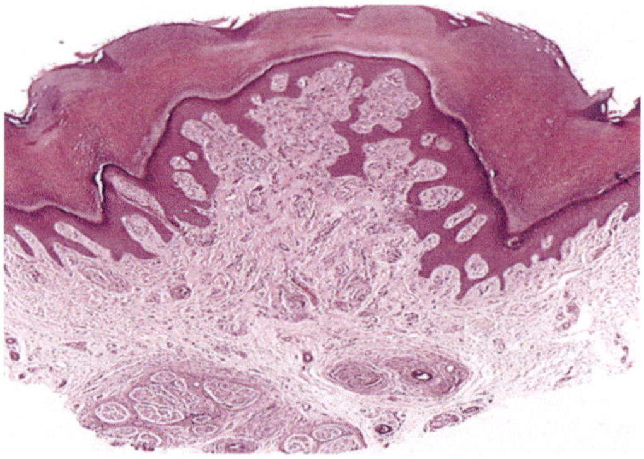

Fig. 19.75 Acral skin with dermal and subcutaneous neural elements

Present at the site of supernumerary digit.

Histopathology (Figs. 19.75, 19.76, and 19.77)

- Acral skin
- Small nerve fascicles (S100+) made of elongated wavy cells oriented in different directions
- Neural elements haphazardly orientated
- Surrounding fibrosis

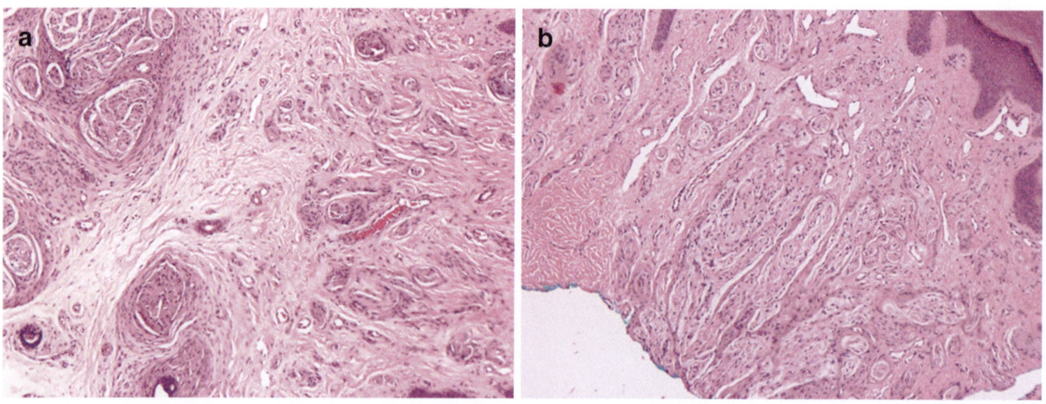

Fig. 19.76 (**a**, **b**) Small nerve fascicle haphazardly embedded in fibrous stroma

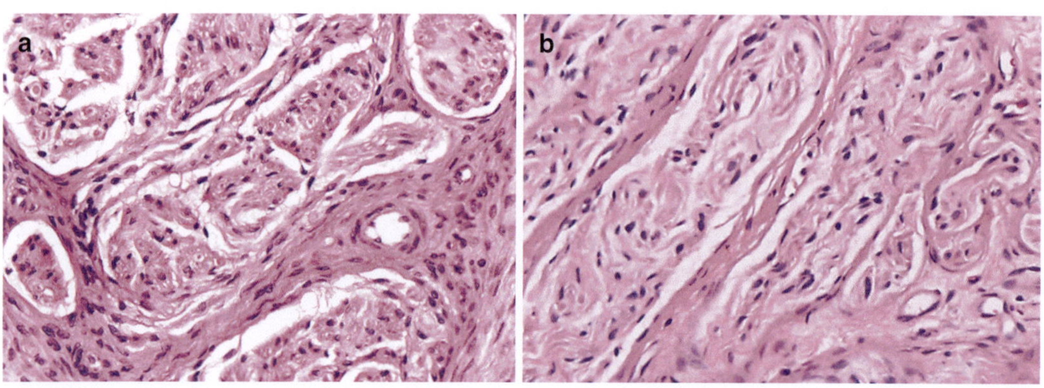

Fig. 19.77 (**a**, **b**) Neural elements with wavy nuclei surrounded by perineural loose stroma

Trichilemmal Carcinoma

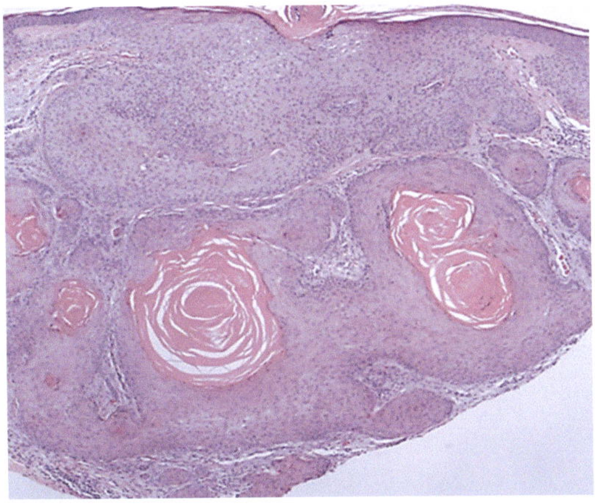

Fig. 19.78 Well differentiated multinodular tumor with superficial portion resembling trichilemmoma

Histopathology (Figs. 19.78, 19.79, 19.80, 19.81, and 19.82)

- Well differentiated tumors have focal resemblance to trichilemmoma and focal resemblance to squamous cell carcinoma but with the presence of trichilemmal keratinization (absence of a granular layer)
- Less differentiated tumors show invasion with multiple lobules pushing into dermis and subcutis
- Lobules are made of central pale cells and peripheral palisading of darker cells with cytological atypia and scattered mitoses
- Lobules are surrounded by prominent basement membrane

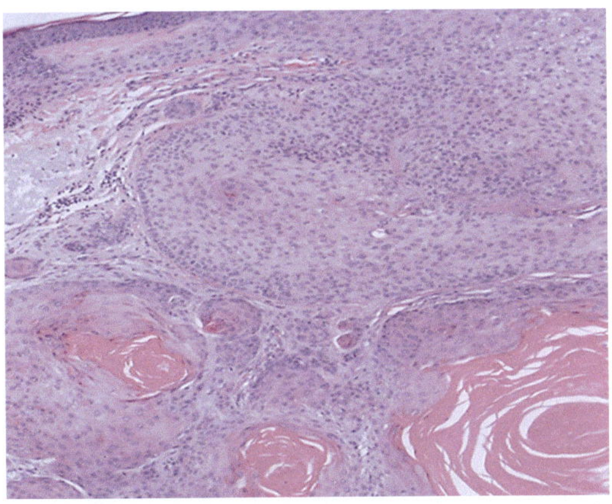

Fig. 19.79 Cytological atypia with trichilemmal keratinization

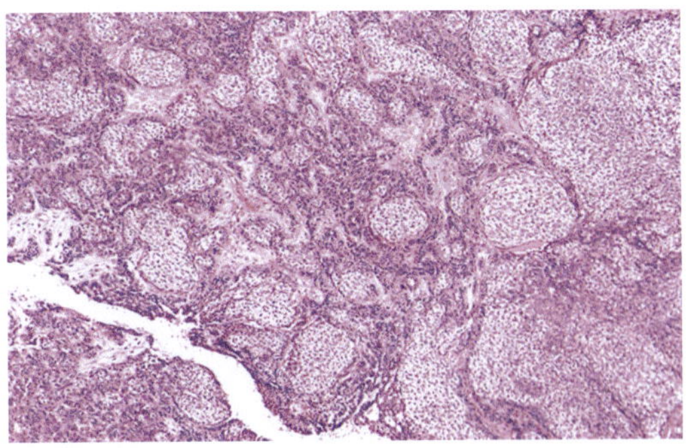

Fig. 19.80 Infiltrating pale lobules of less differentiated tumor

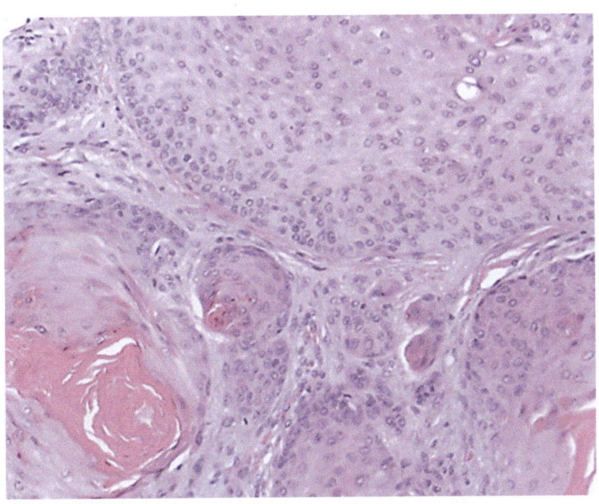

Fig. 19.81 Peripheral palisading of darker cells

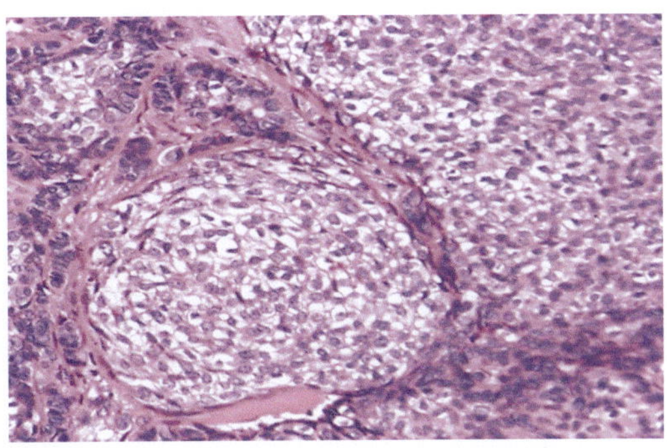

Fig. 19.82 Central pale cells surrounded by palisading dark cells

Trichilemmoma

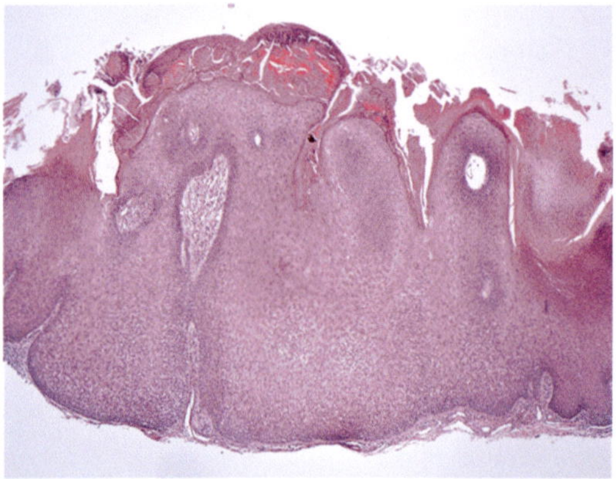

Fig. 19.83 Multilobular folliculocentric tumor

Histopathology (Figs. 19.83, 19.84, 19.85, 19.86, and 19.87)

- Lobular proliferation centered around hair follicle with pushing borders
- Uniform PAS positive cells with clear cell cytoplasm and peripheral palisading and no cytological atypia or mitoses
- Accentuated pink basement membrane
- *Desmoplastic* variant with biphasic appearance of peripheral conventional trichilemmoma and central smaller pale cells with desmoplastic stroma

P.S. associated with Cowden syndrome (*PTEN*)

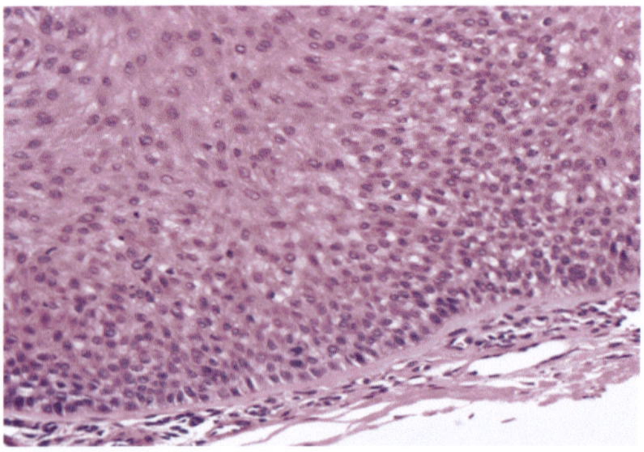

Fig. 19.84 Peripheral palisading of tumor cells

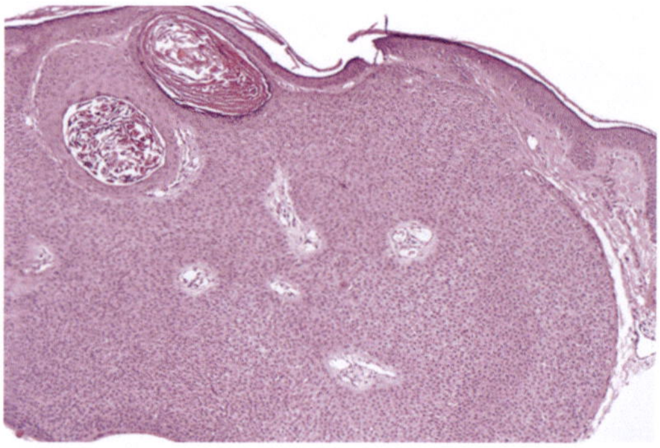

Fig. 19.85 Pushing tumor borders

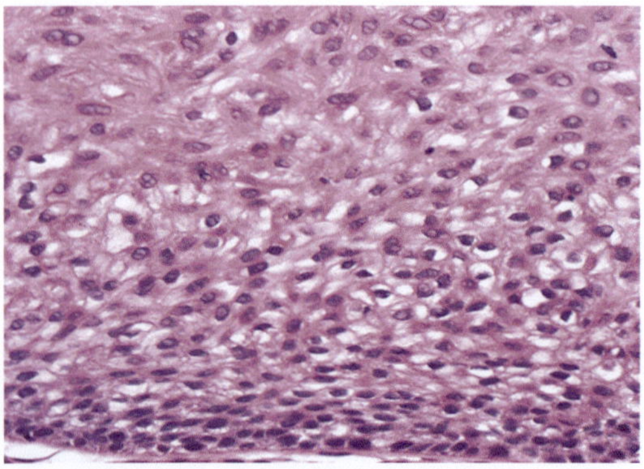

Fig. 19.86 Pale uniform polygonal cells

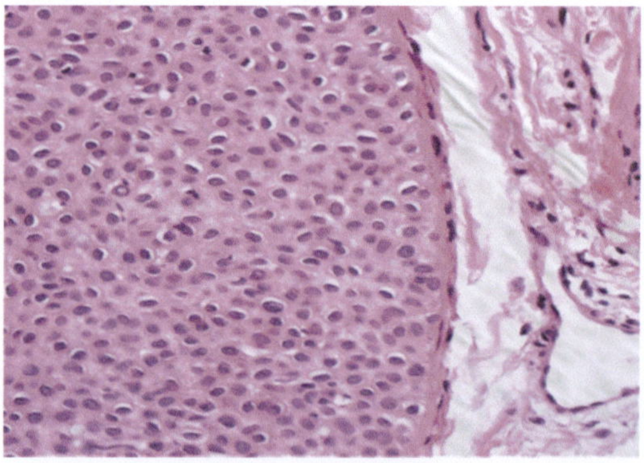

Fig. 19.87 Eosinophilic basement membrane

Trichilemmoma Desmoplastic

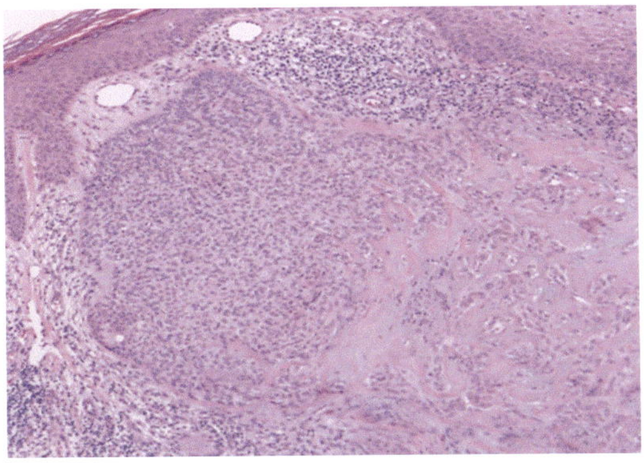

Fig. 19.88 Lobular tumor with pushing borders

Histopathology (Figs. 19.88, 19.89, 19.90, 19.91, and 19.92)

- Folliculocentric lobular dermal proliferation with pushing borders
- Central uniform pale cells
- Peripheral darker cells forming palisade
- Prominent basement membrane surround lobules
- Central stroma is hyalinized or desmoplastic
- Tumor cells are entrapped in hyalinized stroma forming smaller irregular groups and strands

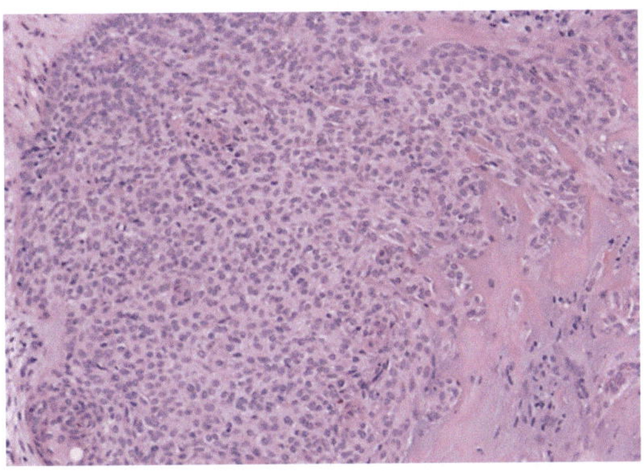

Fig. 19.89 Lobule made of uniform central pale cells with no atypia or mitoses

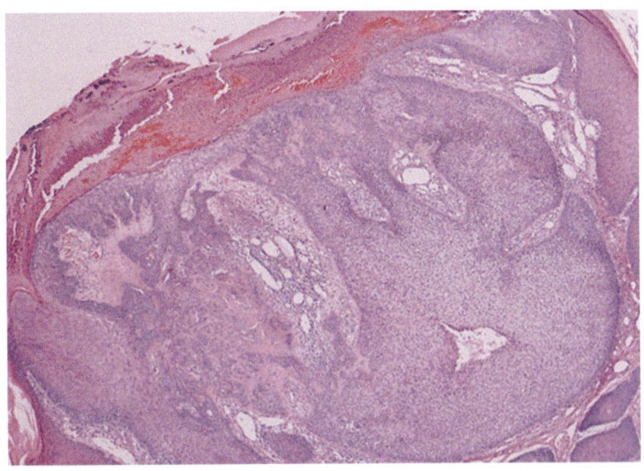

Fig. 19.90 Tumor centered around hair follicle with central pale and peripheral darker palisading cells

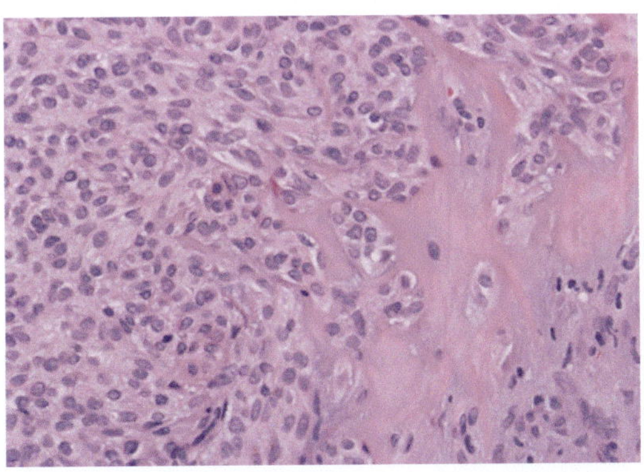

Fig. 19.91 Hyalinized stroma in the center of the lobule

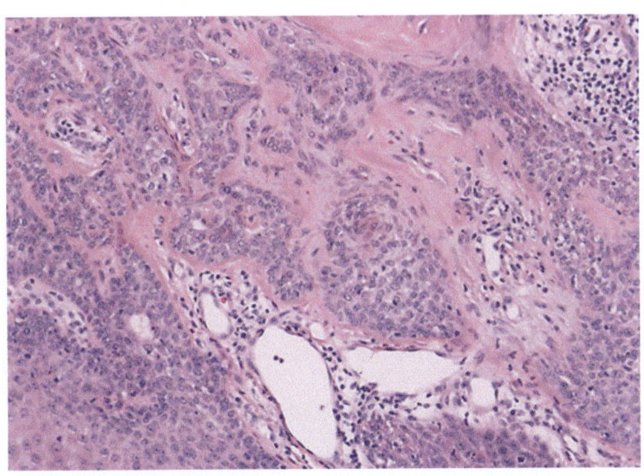

Fig. 19.92 Tumor strands are entrapped in desmoplastic stroma

Trichoadenoma of Nikolowski

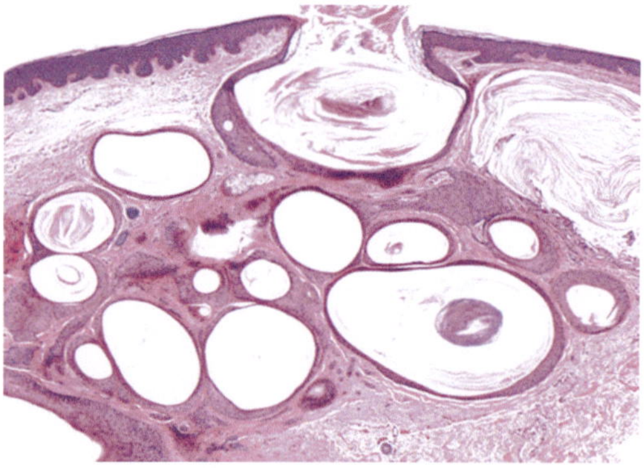

Fig. 19.93 Tumor made of numerous dermal cysts

Histopathology (Figs. 19.93, 19.94, 19.95, 19.96, and 19.97)

- Dermal tumor composed of numerous cysts
- Tumor is folliculocentric and not connected to the epidermis
- Cysts are lined by squamous epithelium with granular layer
- Solid epithelial islands can be seen but are only a minor component

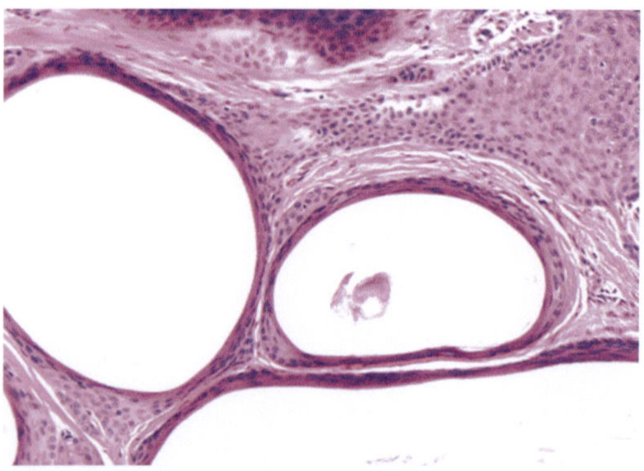

Fig. 19.94 Multiple cysts with squamous epithelial lining

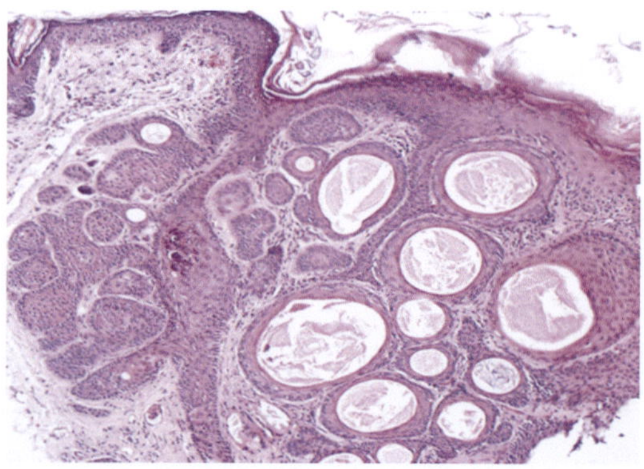

Fig. 19.95 Folliculocentric dermal tumor

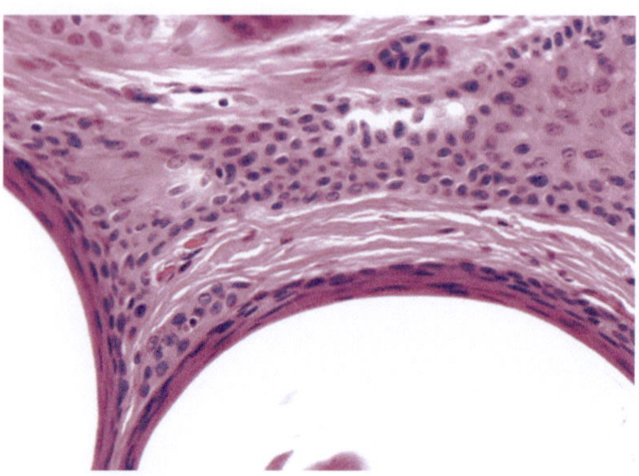

Fig. 19.96 Cysts are filled with laminated keratin

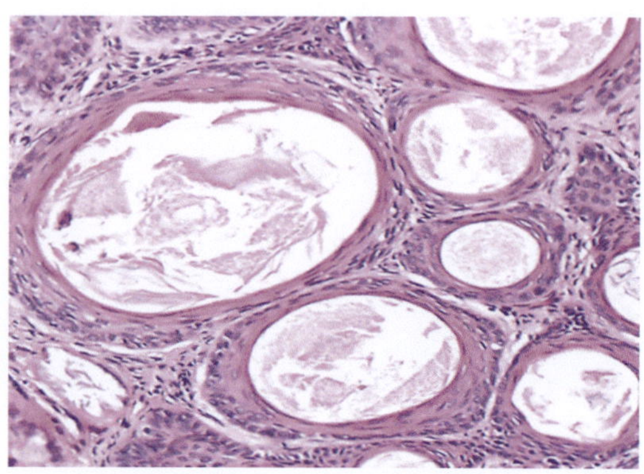

Fig. 19.97 No evidence of cytological atypia or mitoses

Trichoblastoma

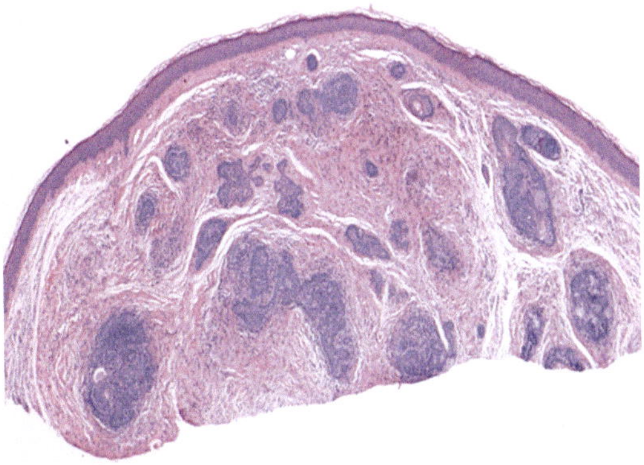

Fig. 19.98 Non-encapsulated dermal and subcutaneous tumor

Histopathology is similar to trichoepithelioma (TE) with highlighted difference (Figs. 19.98, 19.99, and 19.100)

- TB present as nodular tumor in deeper dermis and subcutis with no epidermal connection (1/3rd of TE have epidermal connection)
- Nests, sheets, or cluster of basaloid cells with peripheral palisading and no stromal retraction (like TE)
- Keratin cysts and calcification are present rarely unlike in TE
- Papillary mesenchymal body present like in TE
- Conspicuous dense stroma

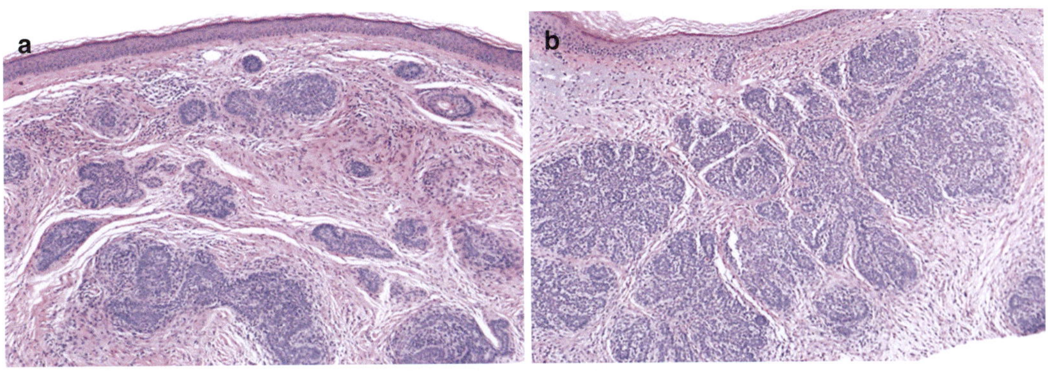

Fig. 19.99 (**a**, **b**) Cluster and nests of basaloid cells with no stromal retraction

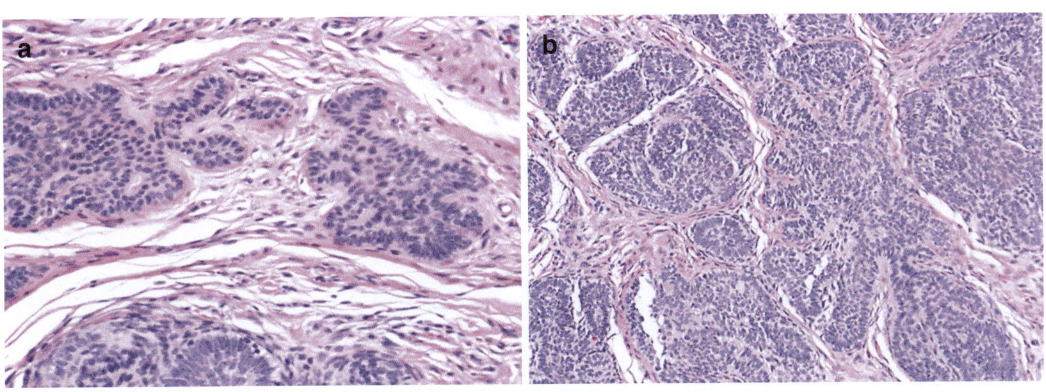

Fig. 19.100 (**a**, **b**) Papillary mesenchymal bodies with peripheral palisading embedded in dense stroma

Trichodiscoma

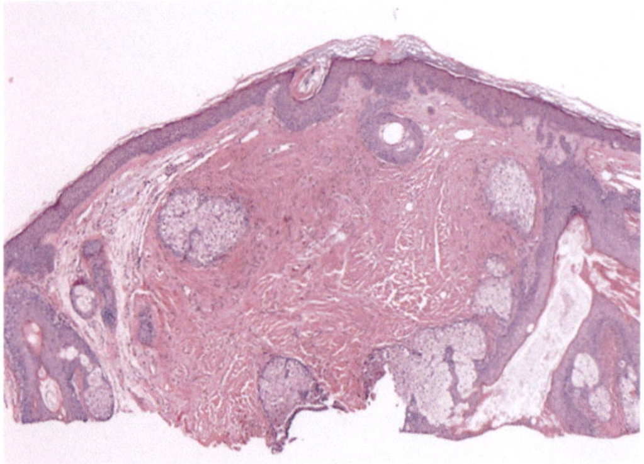

Fig. 19.101 Superficial dermal fibrous plate

Histopathology (Figs. 19.101, 19.102, 19.103, 19.104, and 19.105)
- Atrophic epidermis with epidermal collarette
- Dermal plate of fibroconnective tissue
- Spindle fibroblasts in the stoma that vary from loose to focally hyalinized
- Discoid fibrous plate bordered by hair follicle
- Thin wall vessels are present within discoid plate

P.S. associated with Birt-Hogg-Dubé syndrome (*FLCN*)

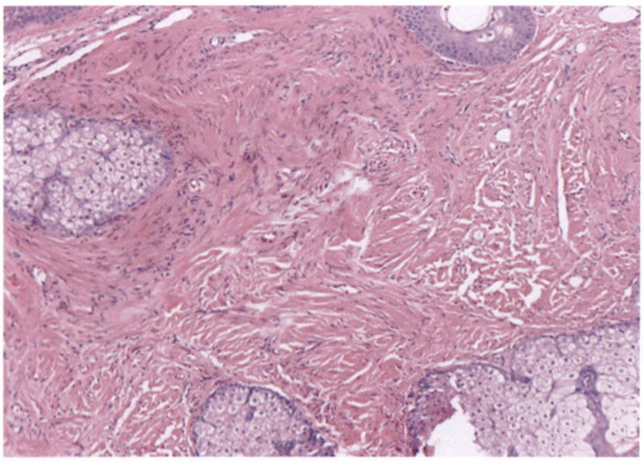

Fig. 19.102 Spindle cells fibroblasts with no atypia

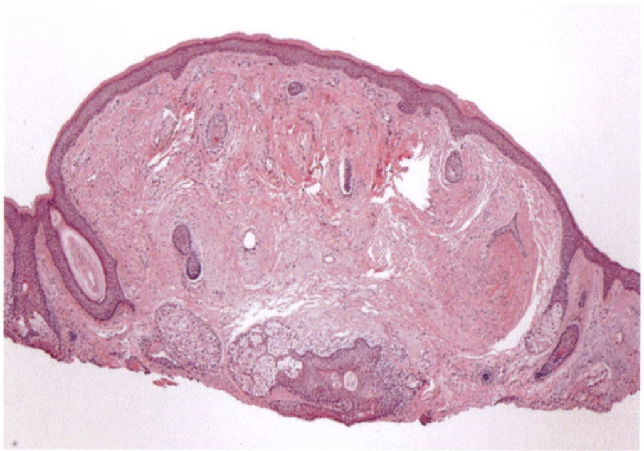

Fig. 19.103 Dermal plate of fibrous tissue in between two hair follicles

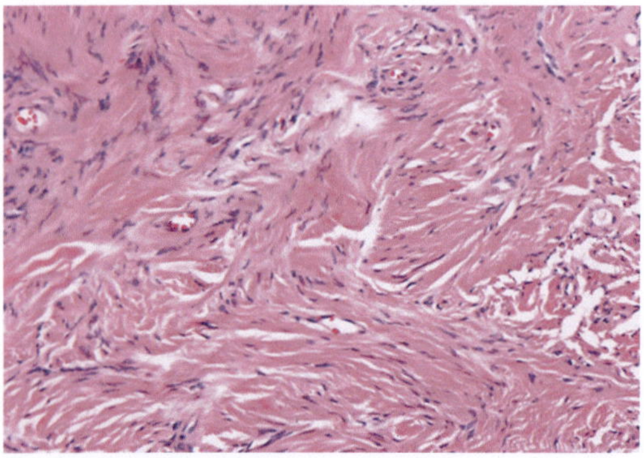

Fig. 19.104 Dense hyalinized stroma

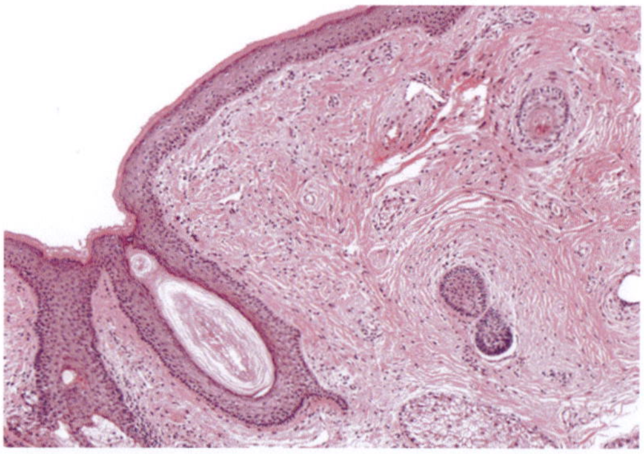

Fig. 19.105 Irregular thin vessels are present within the discoid plate

Trichoepithelioma

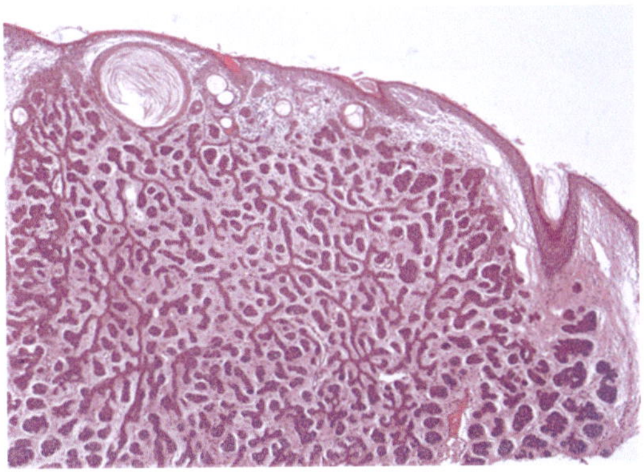

Fig. 19.106 Cords of basaloid cells connected to the epidermis

Histopathology (Figs. 19.106, 19.107, 19.108, 19.109, and 19.110)

- Dermal basaloid tumor occasionally (1/3 of cases) connected to epidermis
- Nests, lobules, and cords of basaloid cells with peripheral palisading and no stromal retraction
- Papillary mesenchymal bodies of primitive hair follicles are present
- Keratin cysts are observed
- Dense to loose stroma that is not retracted

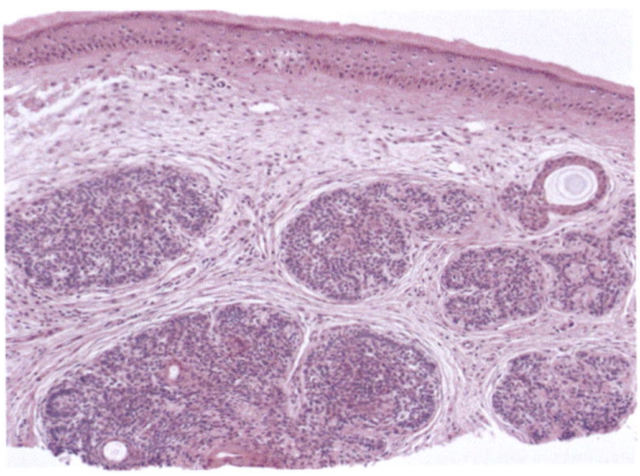

Fig. 19.107 Basaloid dermal lobules of different sizes

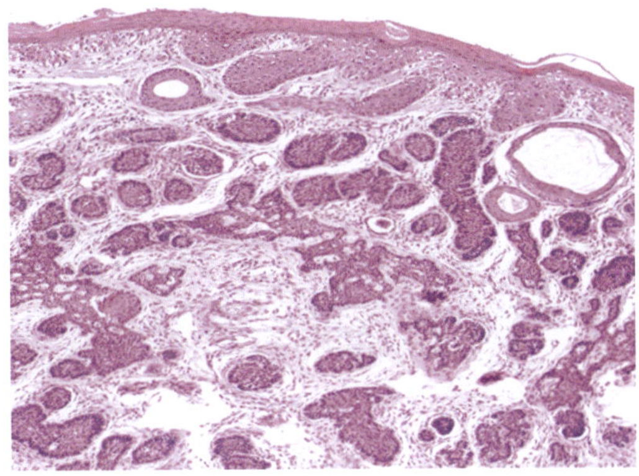

Fig. 19.108 Multiple keratin cysts with tumor lobules in loose stroma

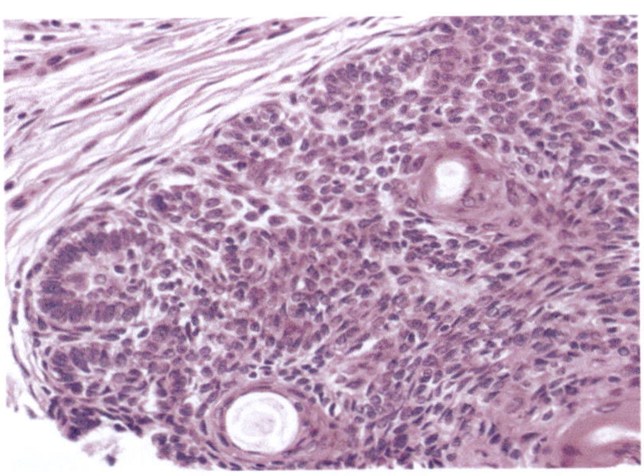

Fig. 19.109 Peripheral palisading and no stromal retraction

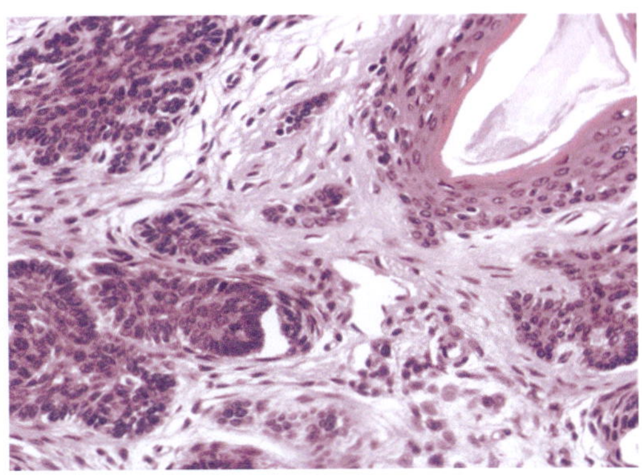

Fig. 19.110 Papillary mesenchymal bodies and keratin cysts

Trichoepithelioma Desmoplastic

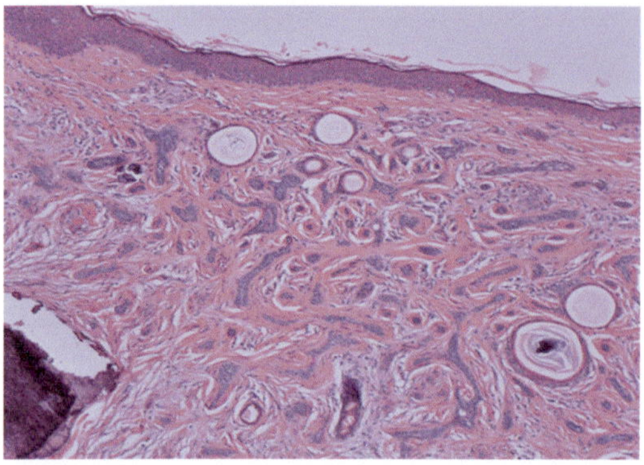

Fig. 19.111 Irregular dermal cords of basaloid cells

Histopathology (Figs. 19.111, 19.112, 19.113, 19.114, and 19.115)

- Cords and small nests of basaloid cells in dermis
- Cords usually made of two cell layers
- Desmoplastic hyalinized stroma
- No stromal retraction or basaloid palisading
- Many keratinous cysts and focal calcifications

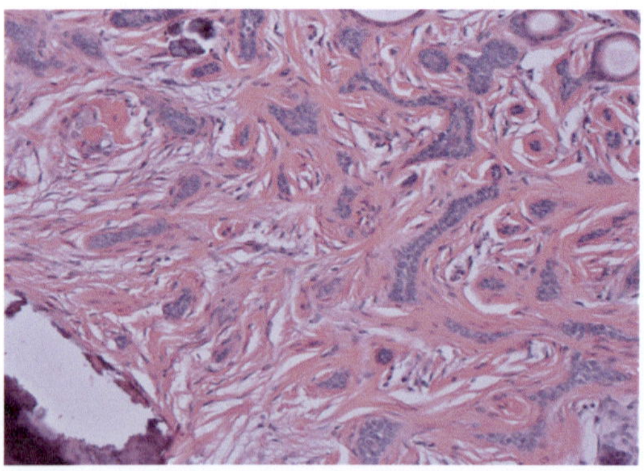

Fig. 19.112 Multiple cysts and calcifications

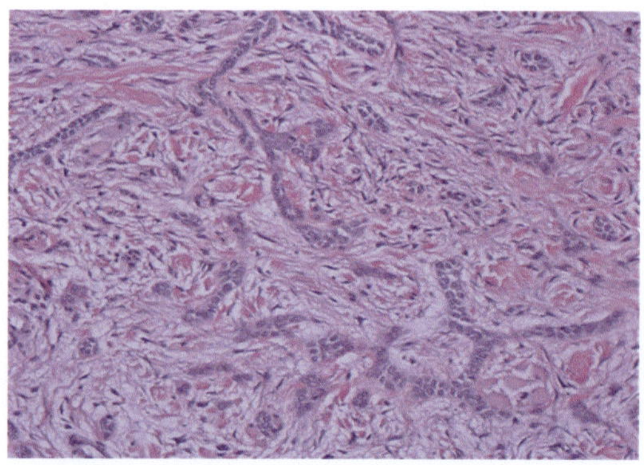

Fig. 19.113 Cords made of two cell layers

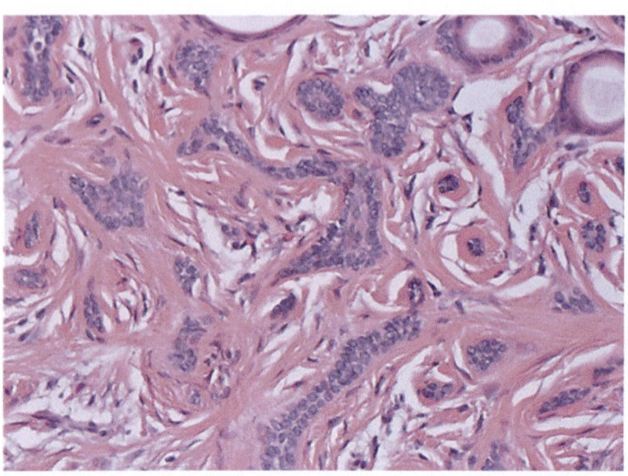

Fig. 19.114 Dense stroma with no stromal retraction

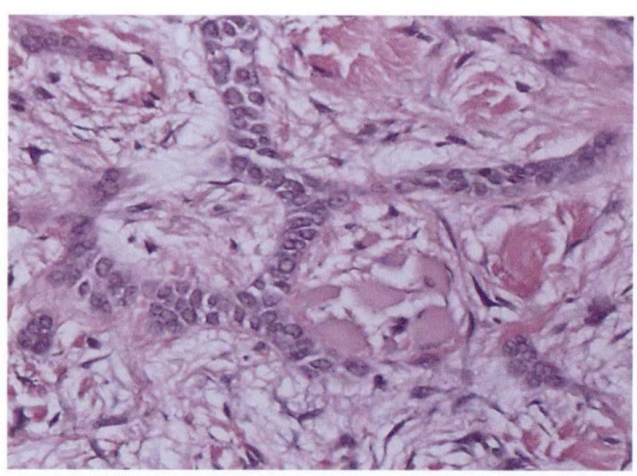

Fig. 19.115 No evidence of cytological atypia

Trichofolliculoma

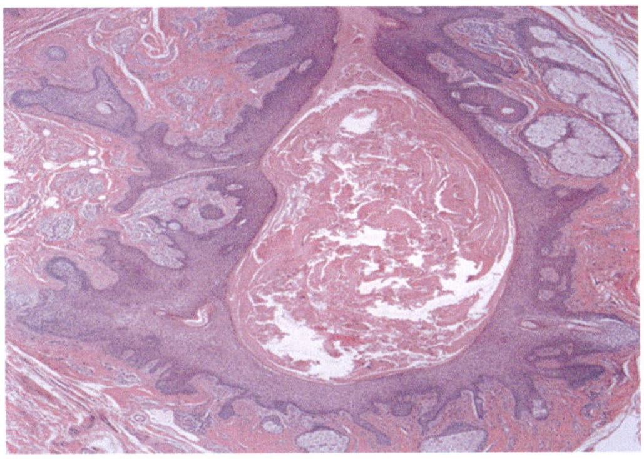

Fig. 19.116 Widely dilated hair follicle

Histopathology (Figs. 19.116, 19.117, and 19.118)

- One or more dilated hair follicles connected to the epidermis and filled with keratin
- Multiple secondary hair follicles branching out from the central follicle
- Secondary hair follicles can be in various stages of maturation from germinative to mature hairs

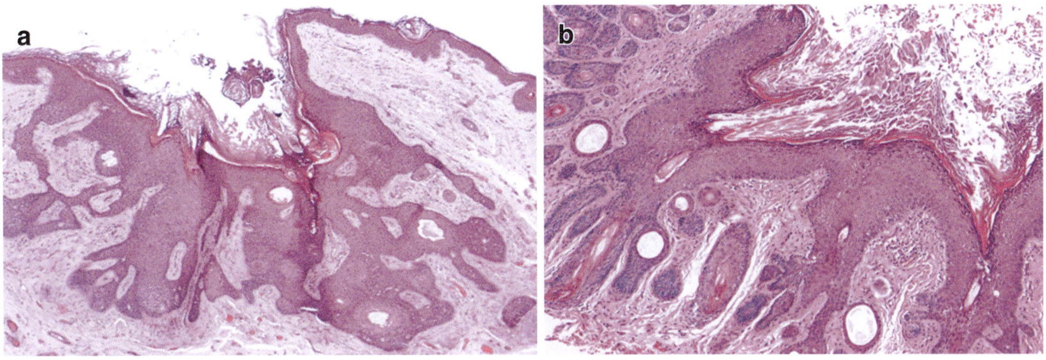

Fig. 19.117 (**a**, **b**) Dilated hair follicle opened to the surface and filled with keratin

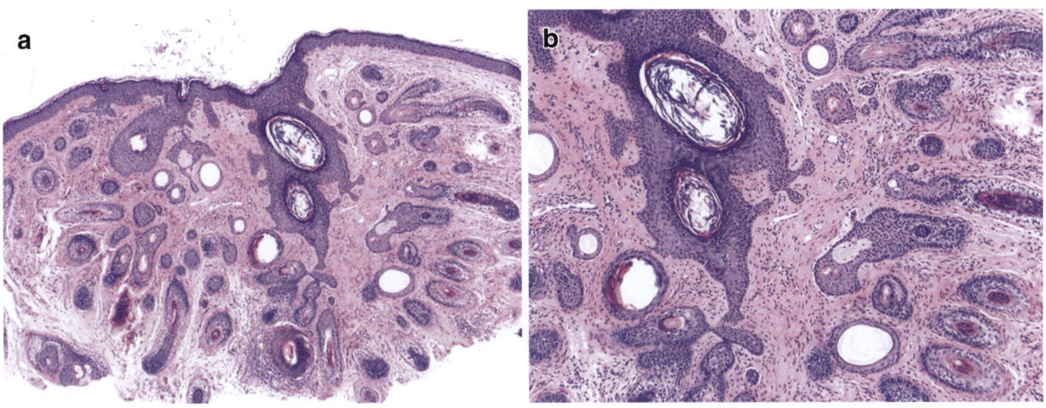

Fig. 19.118 (**a**, **b**) Multiple secondary hair follicles connected to the central follicle

Trichogerminoma

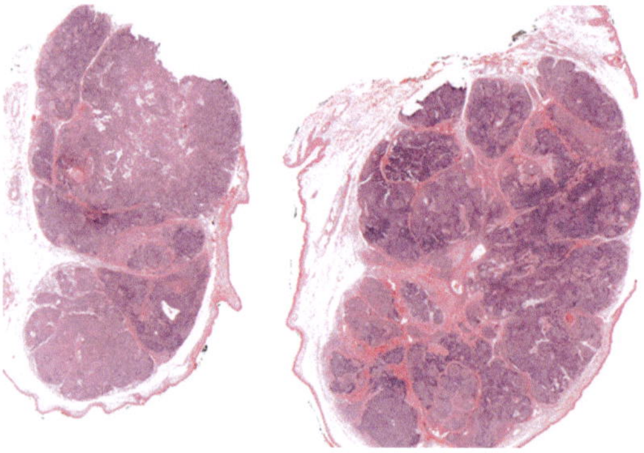

Fig. 19.119 Well demarcated subcutaneous nodules

Histopathology (Figs. 19.119, 19.120, and 19.121)
- Well demarcated dermal and subcutaneous nodules
- Basaloid densely packed "cell balls" with peripheral condensation forming palisading
- "Cell balls" have pale center and are separated by thin fibrous strands with no stromal retraction

P.S. tumor is probably a variant of trichoblastoma

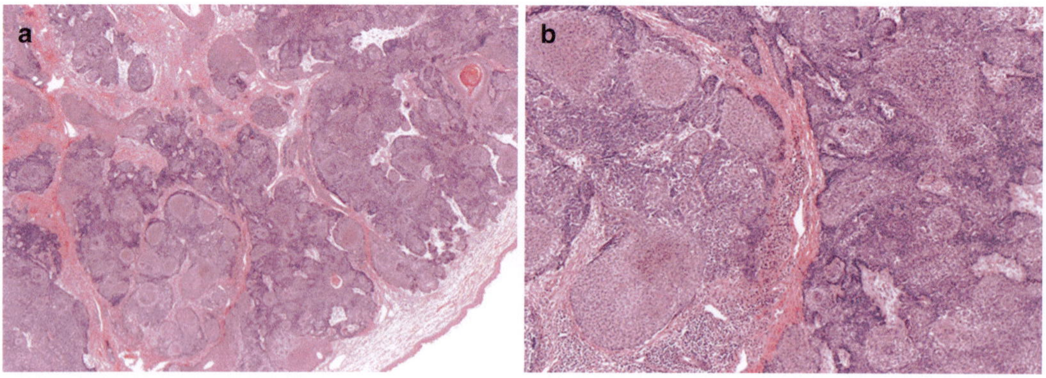

Fig. 19.120 (**a**, **b**) Densely packed basaloid nodule with pale center separated by dense thin stromal strands

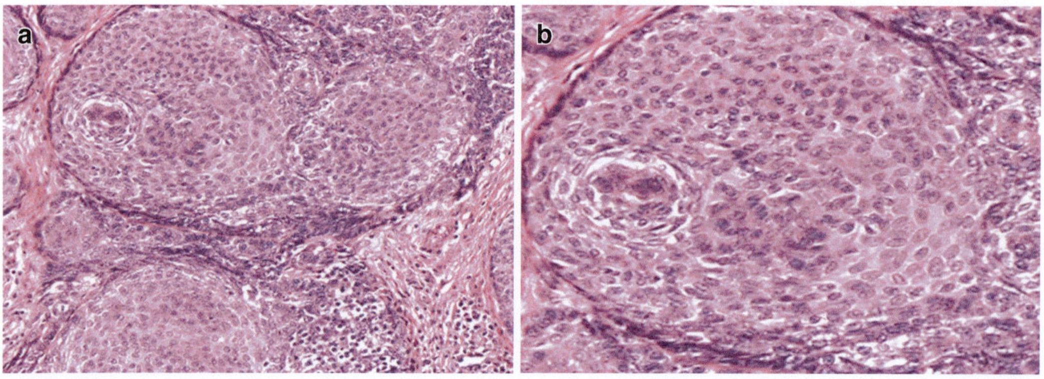

Fig. 19.121 (**a**, **b**) Germinative tumor with central pale micronodule surrounded by palisading basaloid cells

Trichostasis Spinulosa

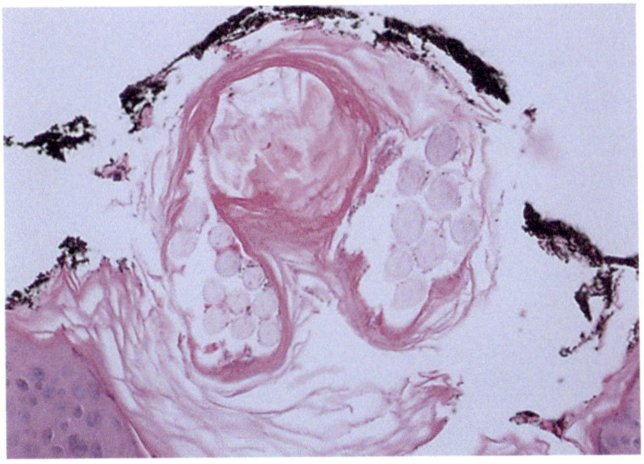

Fig. 19.122 Multiple hair shafts

Histopathology (Figs. 19.122, 19.123, and 19.124)

- Dilated hair follicle with keratin plug
- Multiple hair shafts are present within the follicle

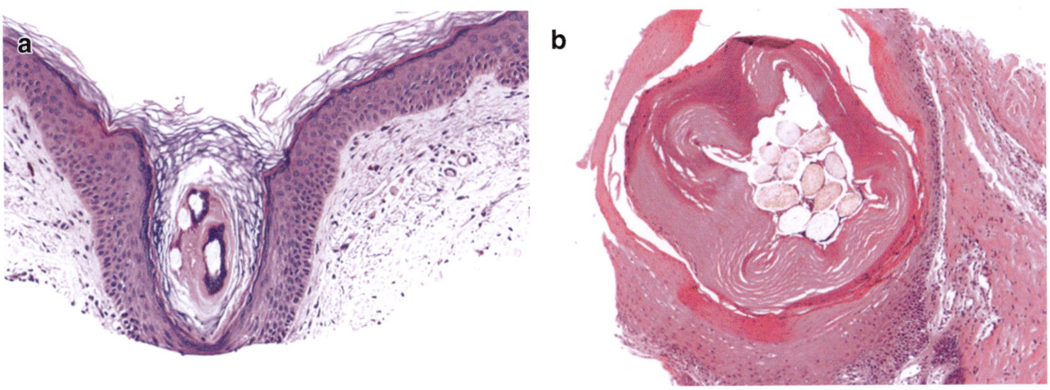

Fig. 19.123 (a, b) Keratin plugged dilated follicle

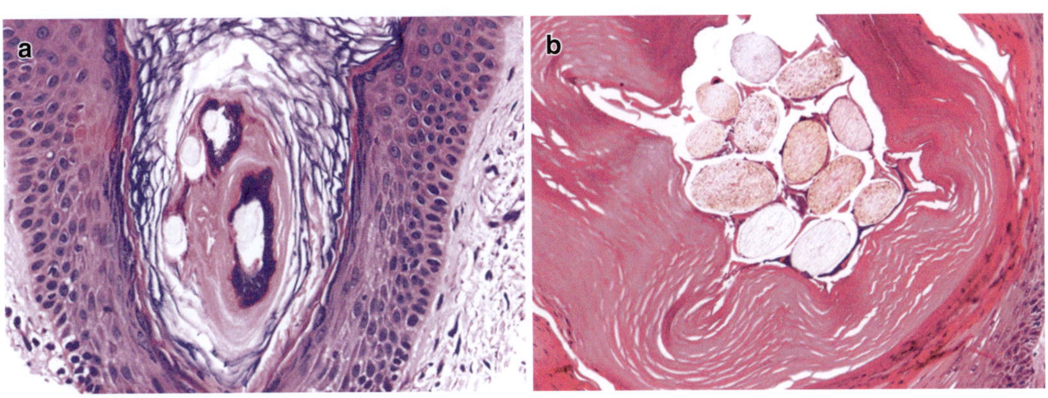

Fig. 19.124 (a, b) Multiple hair shafts present within the follicle

Trichotillomania

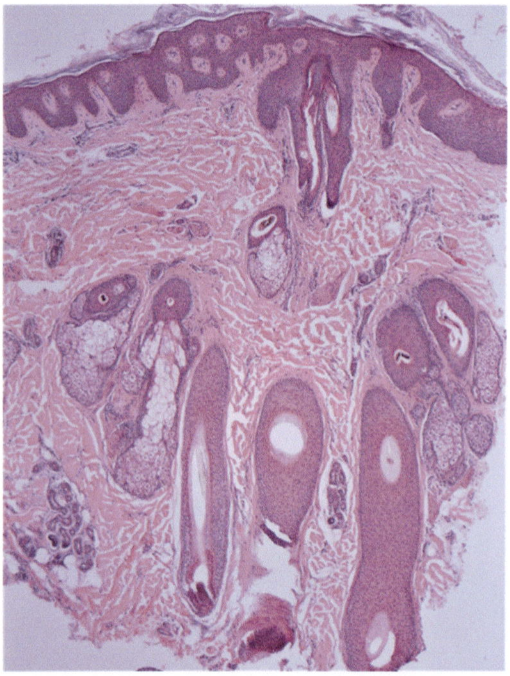

Fig. 19.125 Distorted hair follicles and broken shafts

Histopathology (Figs. 19.125, 19.126, and 19.127)
- Increased number of catagen and telogen hairs
- Distortion of hair follicle bulbs
- Melanin cast present in dilated follicles
- Presence of empty hair follicles
- Follicular stellae can be present

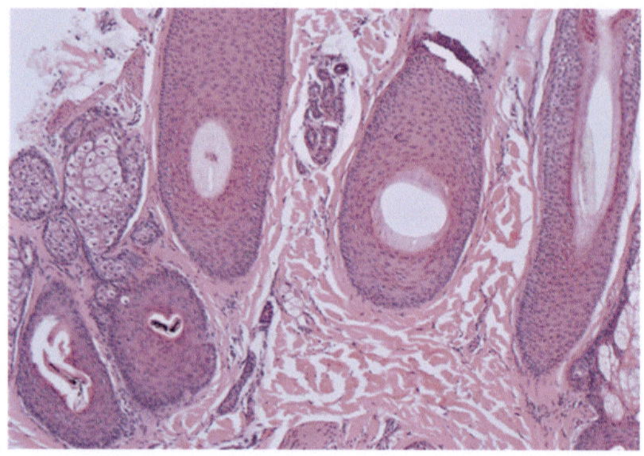

Fig. 19.126 Some hair follicles are empty

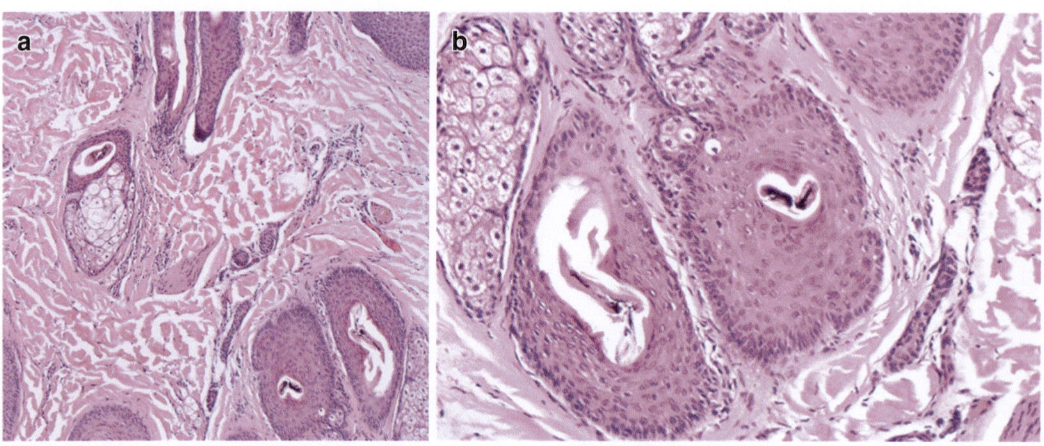

Fig. 19.127 (a, b) Melanin cast and distorted shafts within hair follicles

Tuberculosis

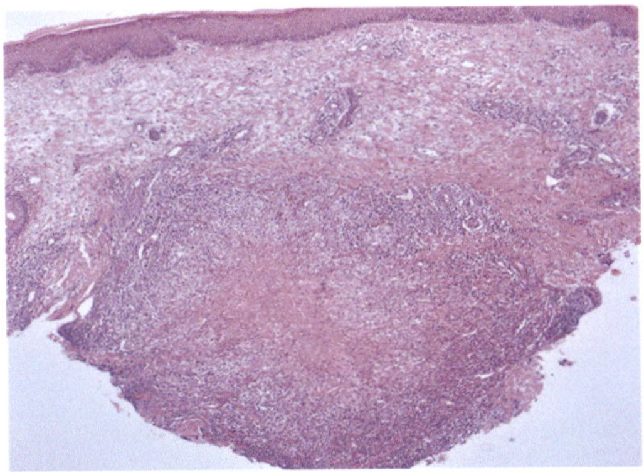

Fig. 19.128 A case of **scrofuloderma**

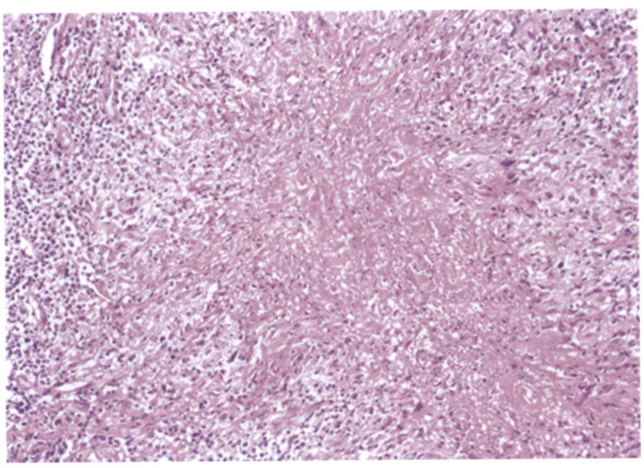

Fig. 19.129 Granuloma with central caseating necrosis and peripheral mixed inflammation eventually forming abscess

Histopathology is variable depending on the clinical presentation. It can be simplified and divided into 3 groups based on the presence and extent of caseous necrosis.

Granulomas with intense caseous necrosis: ***Scrofuloderma*** with extensive necrosis and abscess formation; ***gumma (metastatic TB abscess)*** with central ulceration and abundant caseous necrosis (Figs. 19.128, 19.129, 19.130, and 19.131)

Granulomas with absence of caseous necrosis: ***lichen scrofulosurum*** with granulomas adjacent to adnexa

Granulomas with variable caseous necrosis: ***TB verrucose cutis*** with prominent epidermal acanthosis and hyperkeratosis; (Figs. 19.132, 19.133, 19.134) ***primary cutaneous TB*** with variable necrotizing neutrophilic infiltrate; ***acute military TB*** with lymphoplasmocytic infiltrate; ***TB orificialis*** with superficial ulcer and underlying caseous necrosis; ***papulonecrotic TB*** accompanied with leukocytoclastic vasculitis. (Figs. 19.135, 19.136, and 19.137)

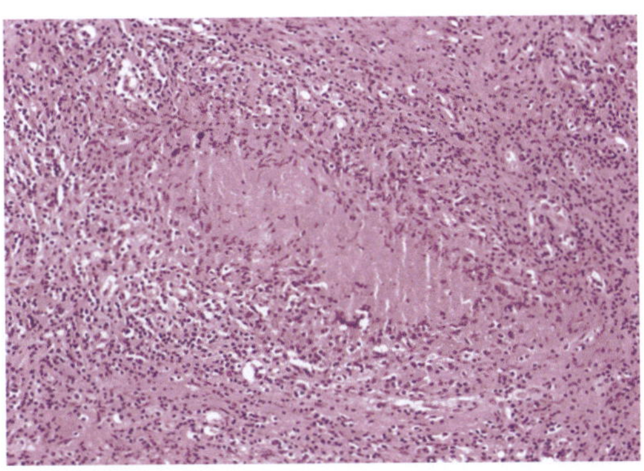

Fig. 19.130 A case of **gumma** with abundant caseous necrosis

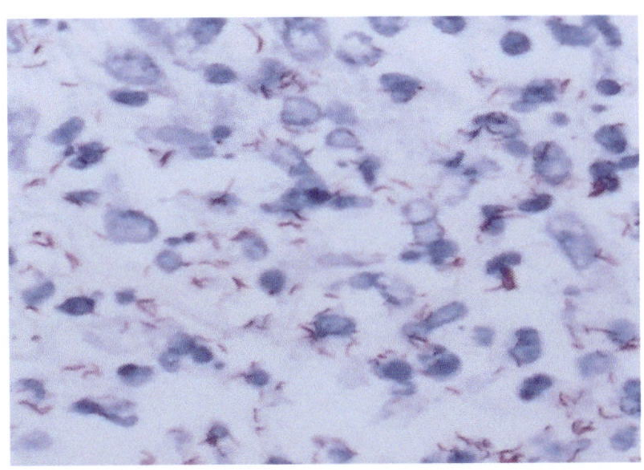

Fig. 19.131 **AFB** stain detects mycobacterias (purple)

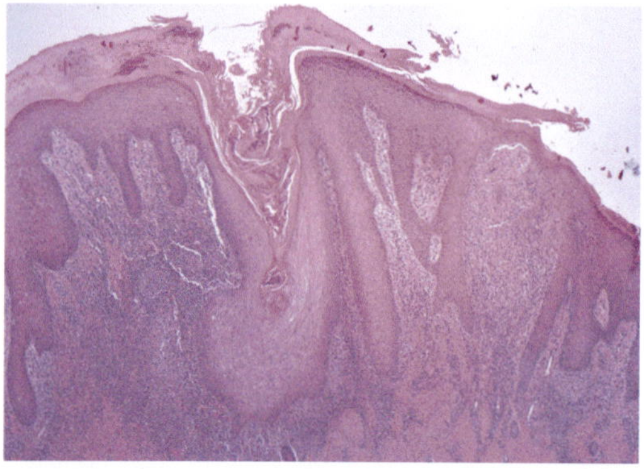

Fig. 19.132 Case of **TB verrucose cutis** with epidermal hyperplasia

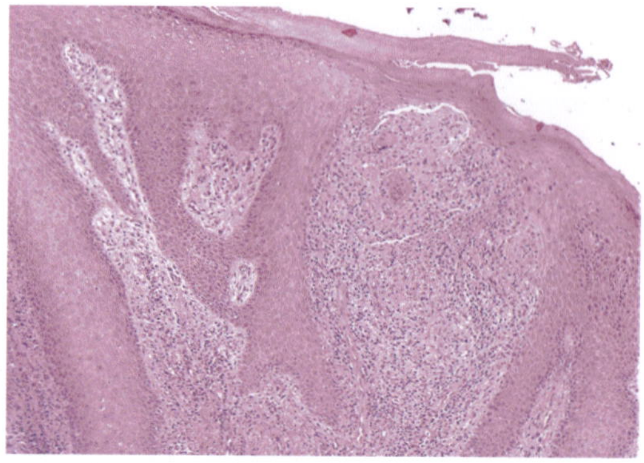

Fig. 19.133 Granuloma in the superficial dermis

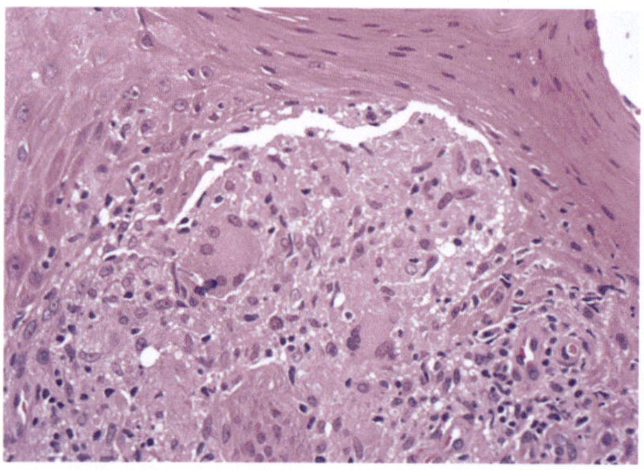

Fig. 19.134 Granuloma with Langerhans-type giant cells and no caseation

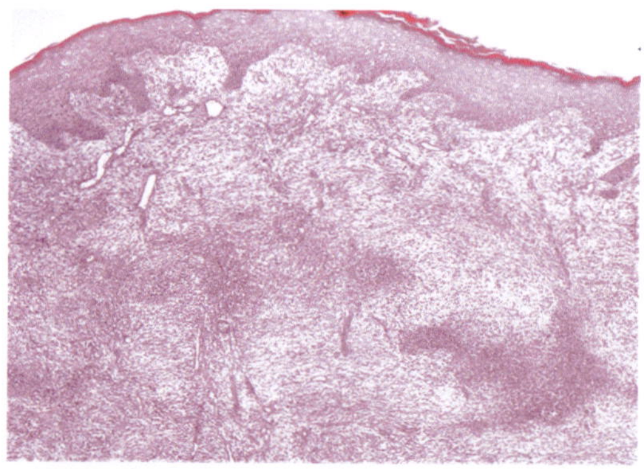

Fig. 19.135 Primary **inoculation TB, miliary TB, TB orificialis,** have variable caseous necrosis

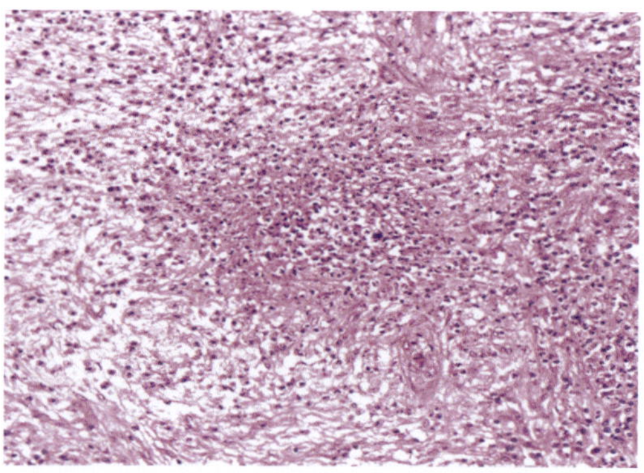

Fig. 19.136 Necrotizing neutrophilic infiltrate

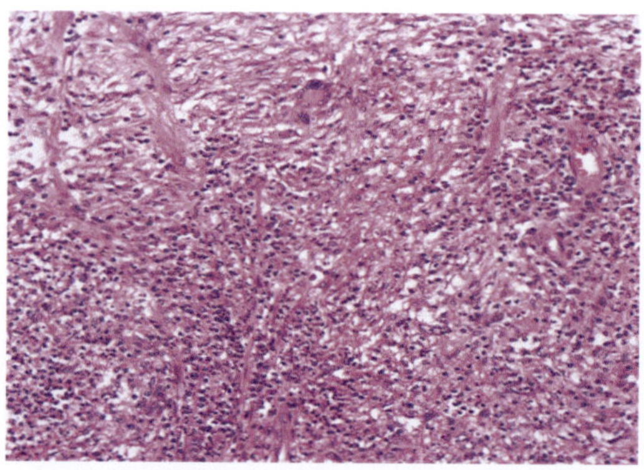

Fig. 19.137 Granulomas with variable caseous necrosis

Tubular Apocrine Adenoma

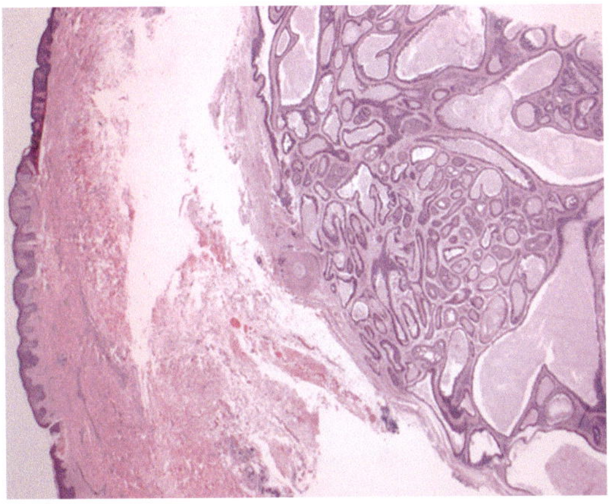

Fig. 19.138 Tumor nodule with no infiltrative growth

Synonyms: Apocrine Adenoma, Papillary Tubular Adenoma, Tubulopapillary Hidradenoma

Histopathology (Figs. 19.138, 19.139, and 19.140)

- Deep dermal nodular tumor composed of tubules and cysts of variable size in hyalinized stroma
- Tubular lining consisting of two or multilayer of cuboidal cells with inner cells demonstrating apocrine secretion with no cytological atypia or necrosis; papillae can be present within tubules but devoid of central stroma

P.S. associated with nevus sebaceous and syringocystadenoma papilliferum

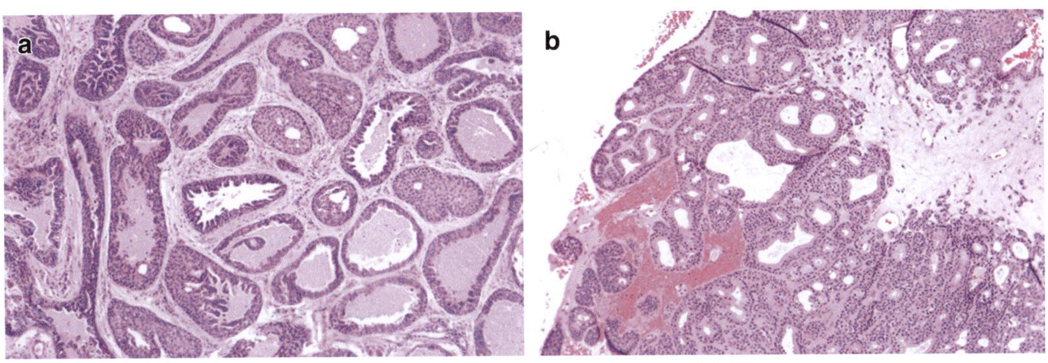

Fig. 19.139 (**a**, **b**) Tubules and cysts of variable size filled with eosinophilic apocrine secretion embedded in hyalinized stroma

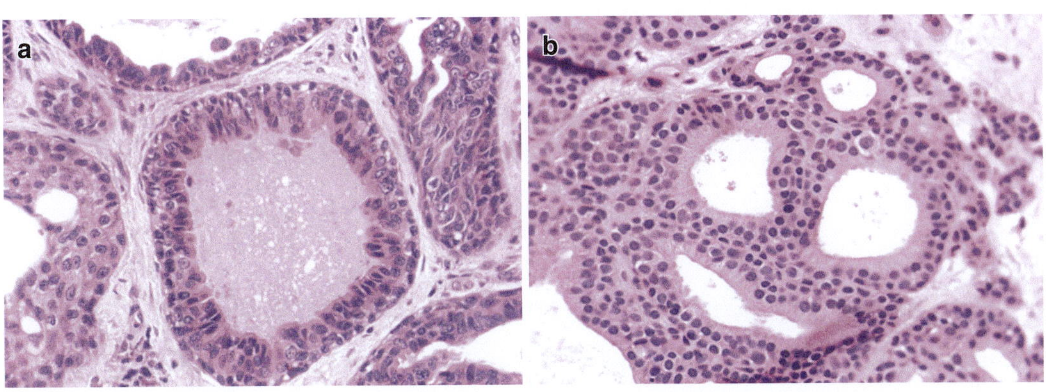

Fig. 19.140 (**a**, **b**) Multilayers or two layers of uniform cuboidal cells with inner layer showing apocrine secretion

Tufted Hemangioma

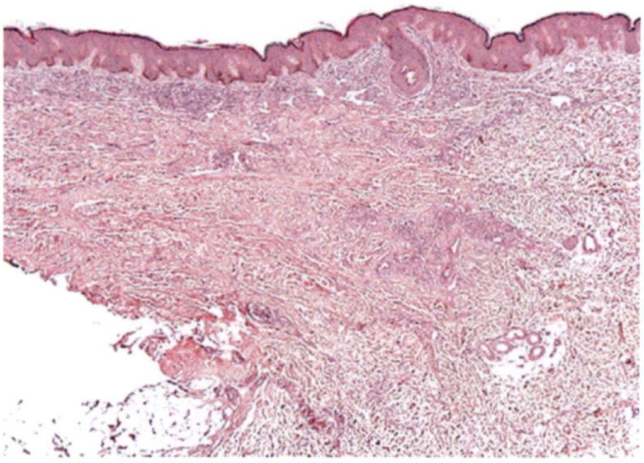

Fig. 19.141 Poorly defined dermal vascular proliferation

Histopathology (Figs. 19.141, 19.142, 19.143, 19.144, and 19.145)

- Ill-defined dermal vascular proliferation in sclerotic stroma
- Vessels are organized in small tufts with "cannonball" distribution
- Tufts are made of epithelioid and spindle endothelial cells
- Tufts are surrounded by "slit-like" vascular lumina and hyaline globules can be seen within the tufts

P.S. associated with Kasabach-Merritt syndrome

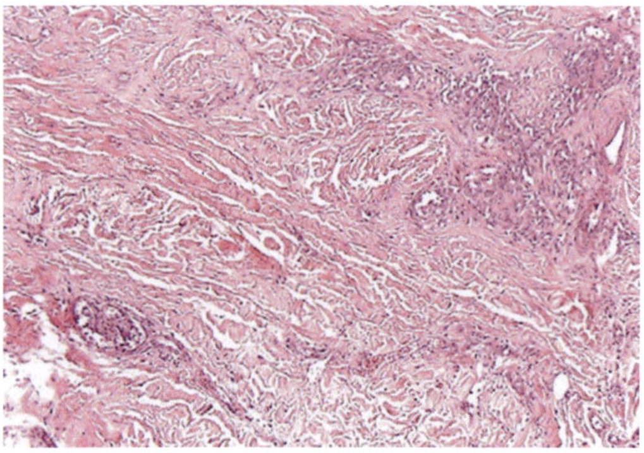

Fig. 19.142 "Cannonball" distribution of vascular tufts

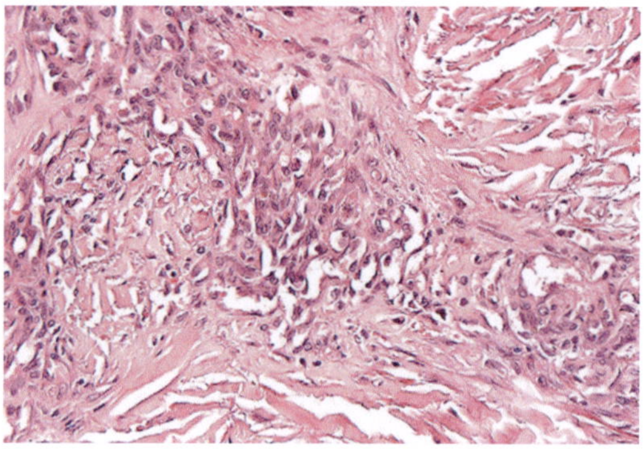

Fig. 19.143 Epitheliod endothelial cells forming "slit-like" spaces

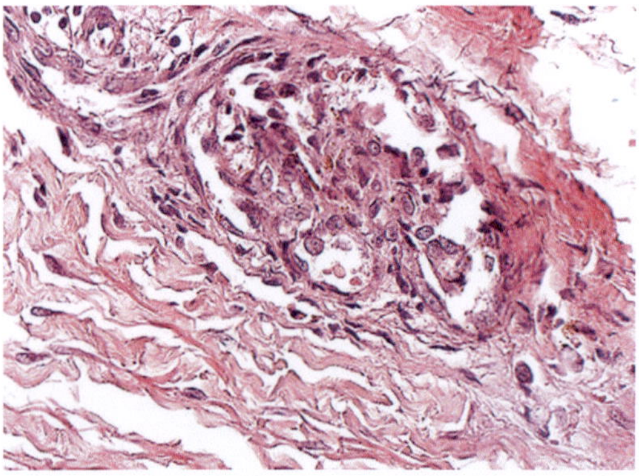

Fig. 19.144 Rounded collection of epithelioid endothelial cells

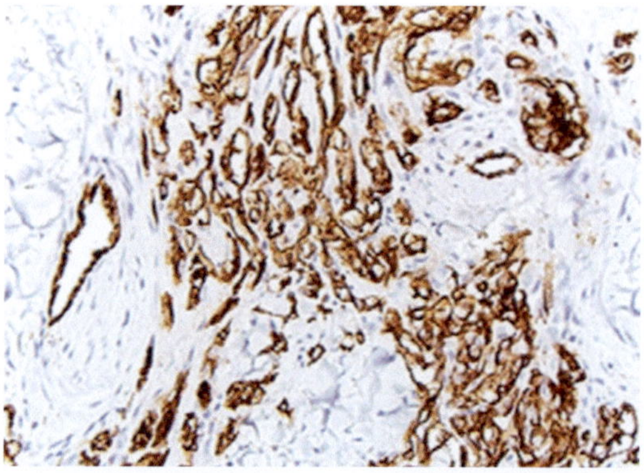

Fig. 19.145 CD31 stain outlines endothelial cells

Tumid Lupus

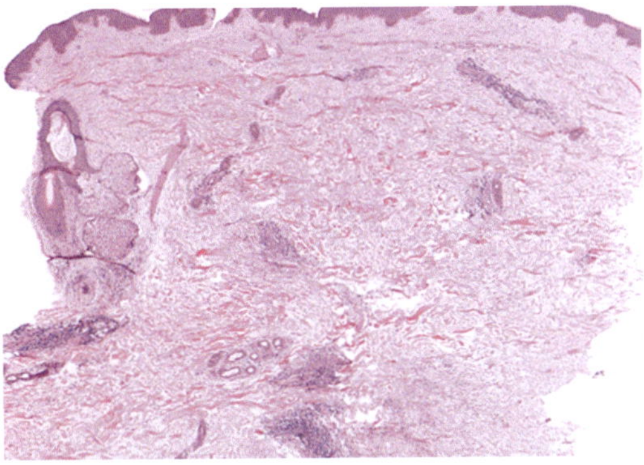

Fig. 19.146 Normal appearing epidermis with superficial and deep perivascular inflammation

Histopathology (Figs. 19.146, 19.147, 19.148, and 19.149)

- Epidermal changes are absent
- Follicular plugging is absent
- Superficial and deep perivascular lymphocytic infiltrate
- Collagen fibers are separated by bluish dermal mucin (Alcian Blue and Colloidal Iron positive)

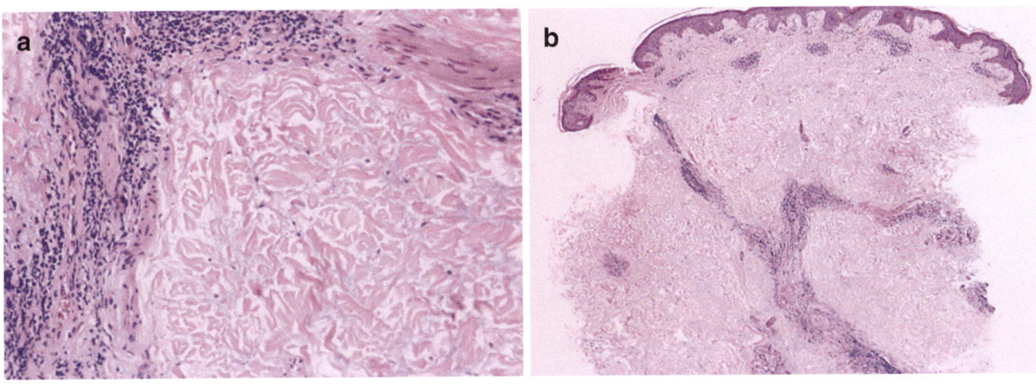

Fig. 19.147 (**a**, **b**) Perivascular inflammation consists mostly of lymphocytes

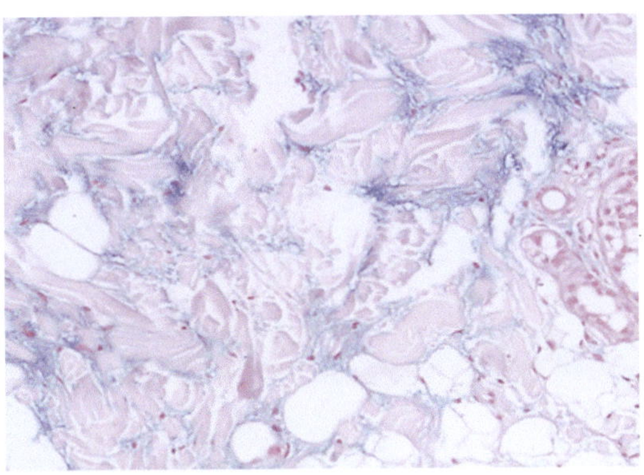

Fig. 19.148 Alcian Blue stains mucin as blue material in between collagen fibers

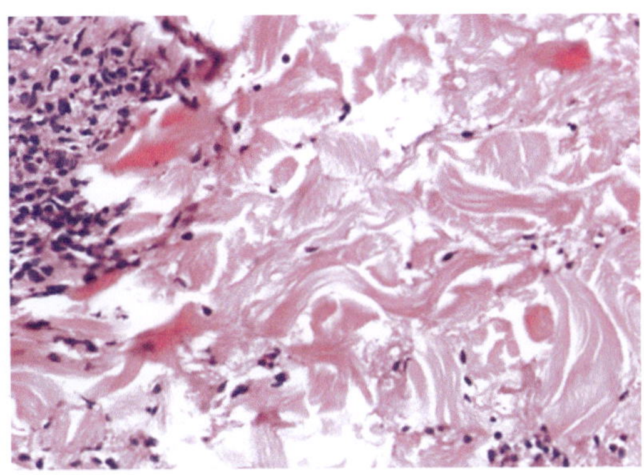

Fig. 19.149 Collagen fibers are separated by mucin

Tumor of Follicular Infundibulum

Many dermatopathologists, including myself, believe that this is a variant of basal cell carcinoma.

Histopathology (Figs. 19.150, 19.151, and 19.152)

- Tumor made of strands of basaloid cells
- Tumor has multiple connections to the epidermis
- Strands run parallel to the epidermis and form network

P.S. associated with Cowden's disease and nevus sebaceous

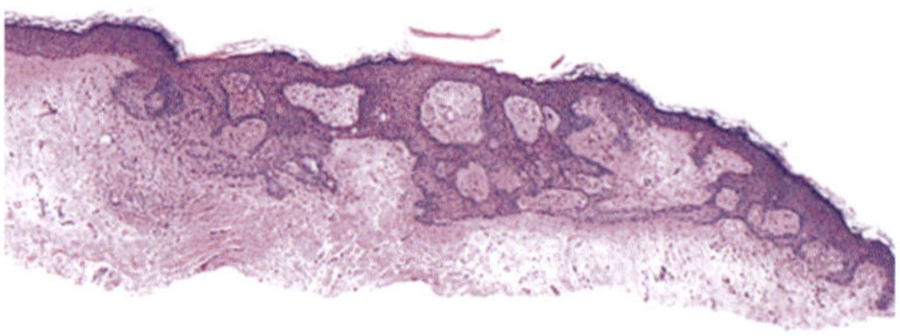

Fig. 19.150 Multiple tumor connections to the epidermis

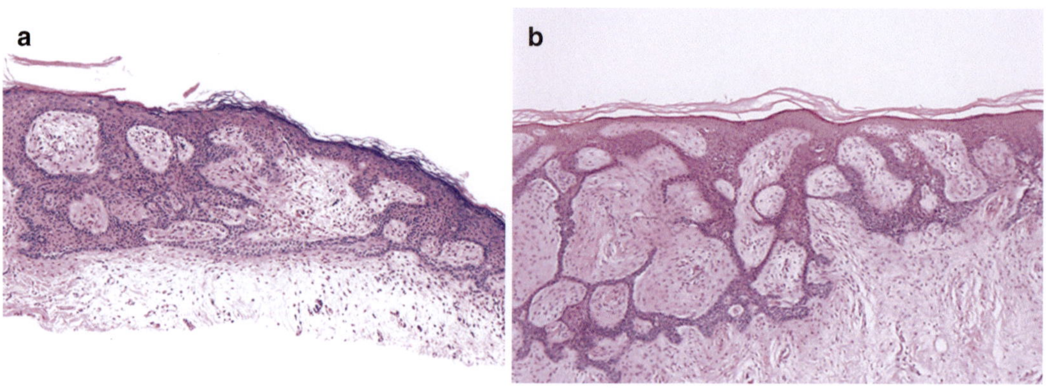

Fig. 19.151 (**a**, **b**) Tumor strands run parallel to the epidermis and form plate parallel with the epidermis

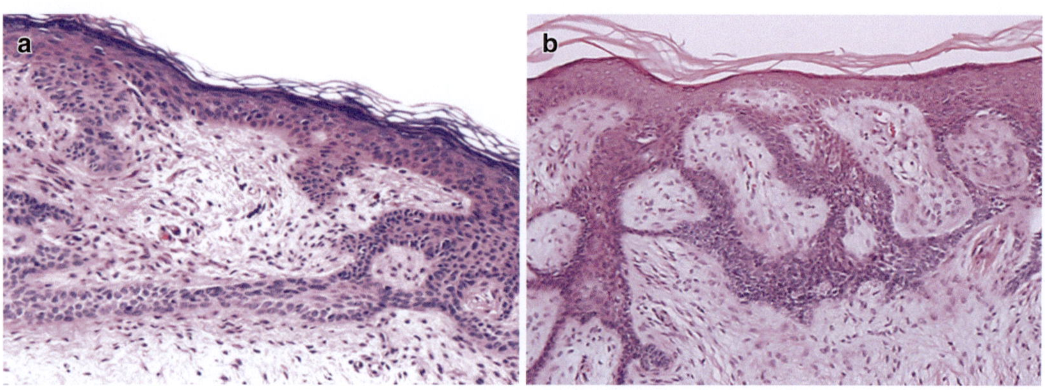

Fig. 19.152 (**a**, **b**) Basaloid tumor cells demonstrate vague palisading in myxoid stroma

Tungiasis

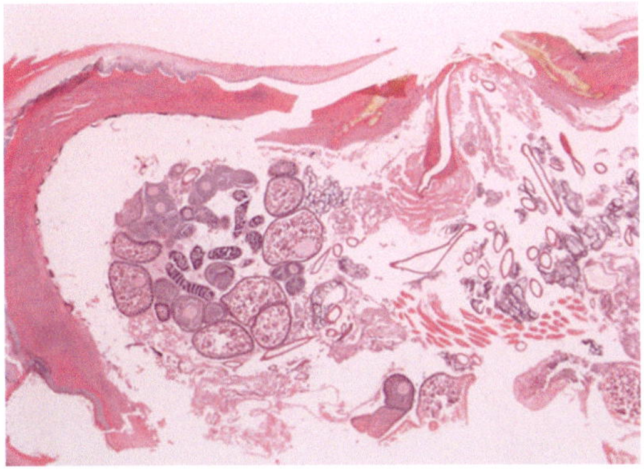

Fig. 19.153 Chitinous exoskeleton encircles internal organs

Infestation by female sand flea, *Tunga penetrans.*

Histopathology (Figs. 19.153, 19.154, 19.155, 19.156, and 19.157)

- The bulk of flea is intraepidermal and superficial dermis
- Surrounding pseudoepitheliomatous hyperplasia is present
- Flea is 1–2 mm in size with exoskeleton encircling internal organs and characteristic developing eggs
- Flea communicate with outside to breath and lay eggs

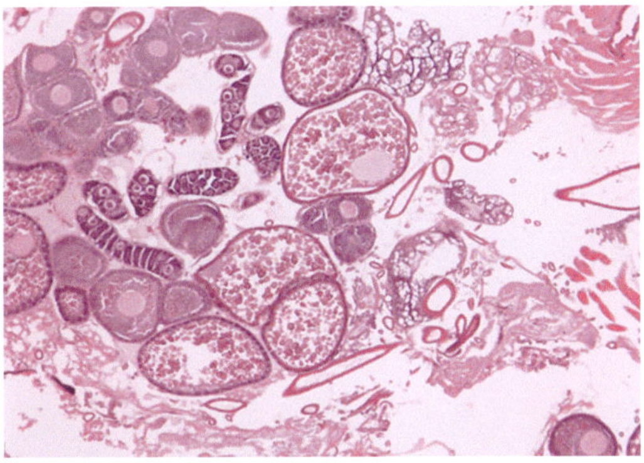

Fig. 19.154 Flea's internal organs

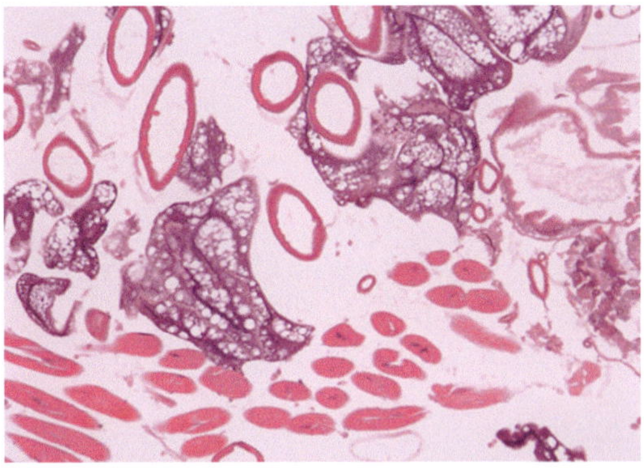

Fig. 19.155 Parts of trachea, intestine and skeletal muscle

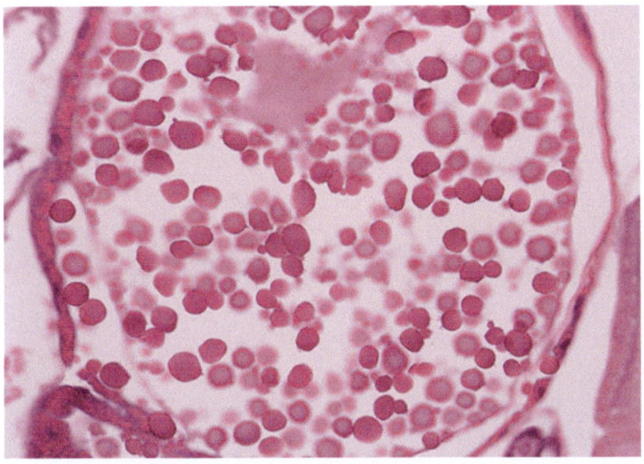

Fig. 19.156 Numerous developing eggs are present within ova

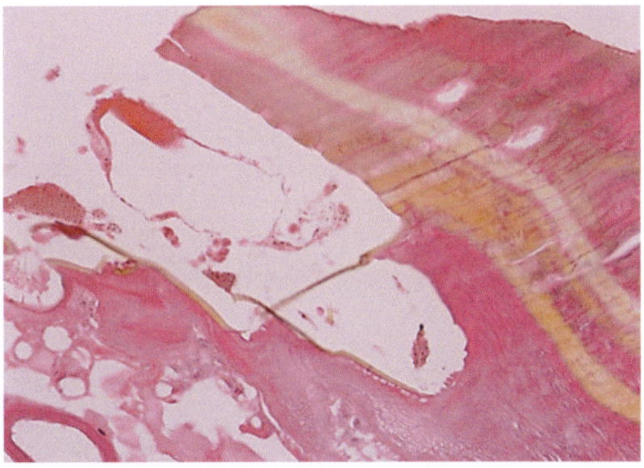

Fig. 19.157 Portion of the head and proboscis (stylet)

20 Dermatopathology U

V. Vincek, *Dermatopathology A–Z*, https://doi.org/10.1007/978-3-319-89486-7_20

Urachal Cyst

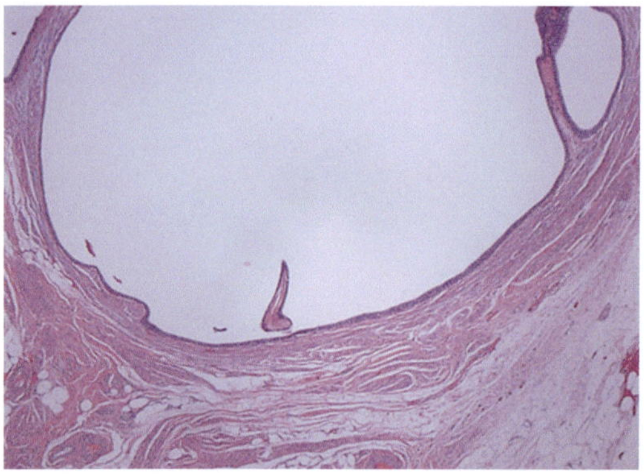

Fig. 20.1 Cyst with thin lining and no content

Synonym: Urachal Remnant

Histopathology (Figs. 20.1, 20.2, and 20.3)
- Periumbilical cyst that might have epidermal opening
- Cyst lining is made of transitional epithelium with submucosal connective tissue and smooth muscle
- Cyst lumen is clear of any material

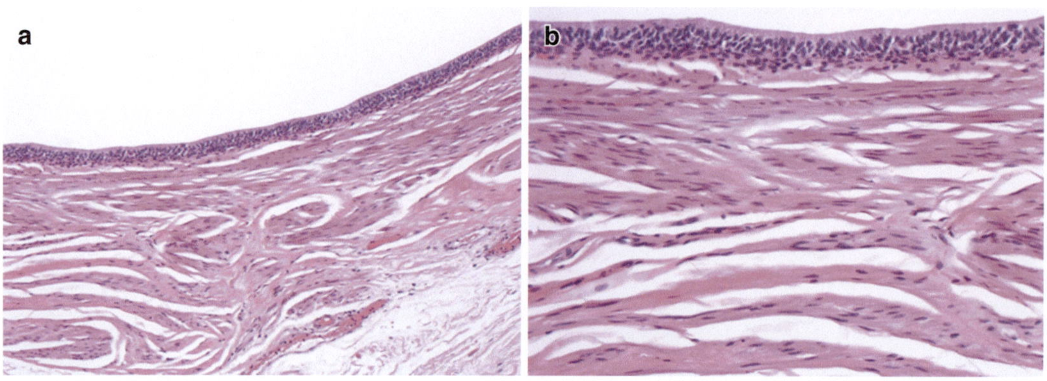

Fig. 20.2 (a, b) Cyst walled made of three layers: transitional epithelium, submucosal connective tissue, and smooth muscle

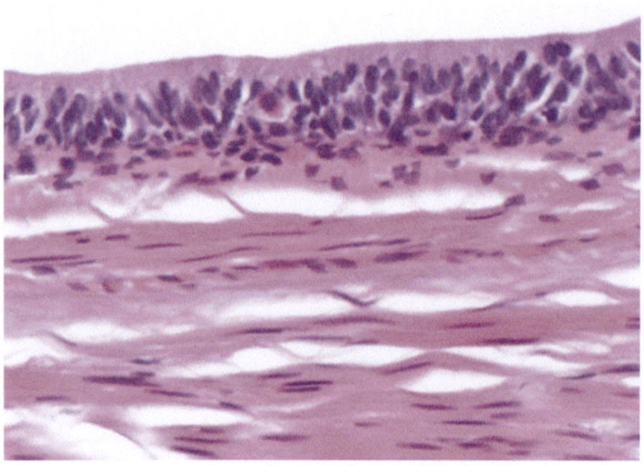

Fig. 20.3 Transitional epithelial lining

Urticaria

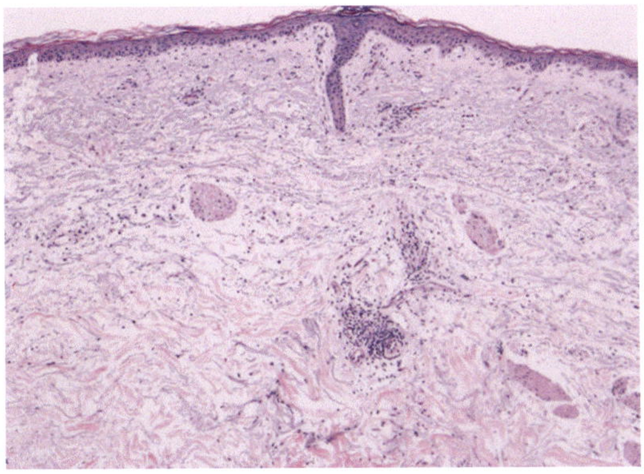

Fig. 20.4 Pale dermis with scattered inflammatory cells

Histopathology (Figs. 20.4, 20.5, and 20.6)

- Unremarkable epidermis
- Dermal edema with separation of collagen bundles
- Sparse perivascular and interstitial inflammation made of lymphocytes and scattered eosinophils
- Scattered neutrophils can be present in cold, pressure, solar, and cholinergic urticaria

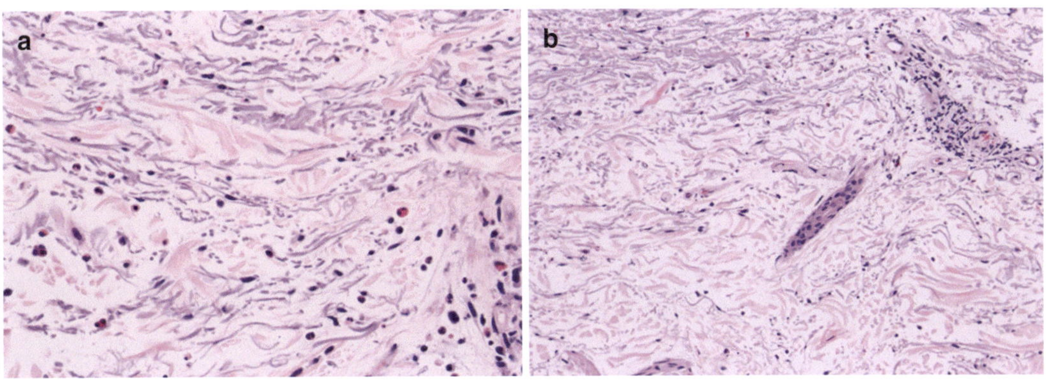

Fig. 20.5 (**a**, **b**) Dermal edema with scattered lymphocytes and eosinophils

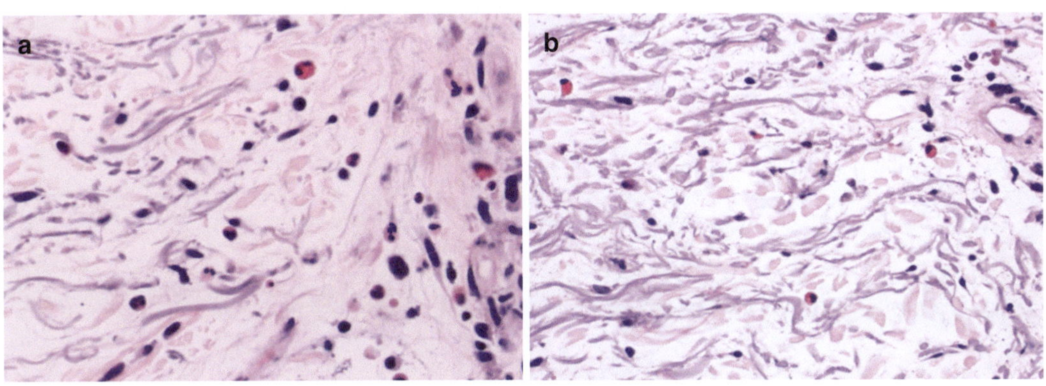

Fig. 20.6 (**a**, **b**) Scattered neutrophils can be seen in some form of urticaria

Urticarial Vasculitis

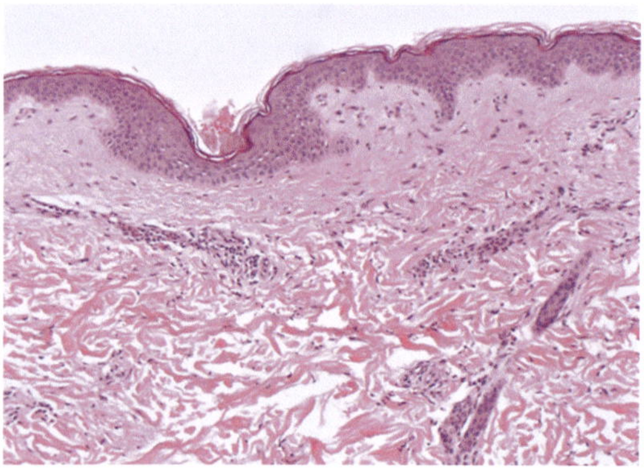

Fig. 20.7 Dermal edema and perivascular inflammation

Histopathology (Figs. 20.7, 20.8, 20.9, 20.10, and 20.11)

- Dermal edema but milder than in urticaria
- Vascular damage with swollen endothelial cells but no microthrombi
- Perivascular lymphocytic, neutrophilic, and eosinophilic infiltrate with variable ratio
- No obvious neutrophilic leukocytoclasia
- Neutrophils present within capillaries
- Scattered interstitial eosinophils

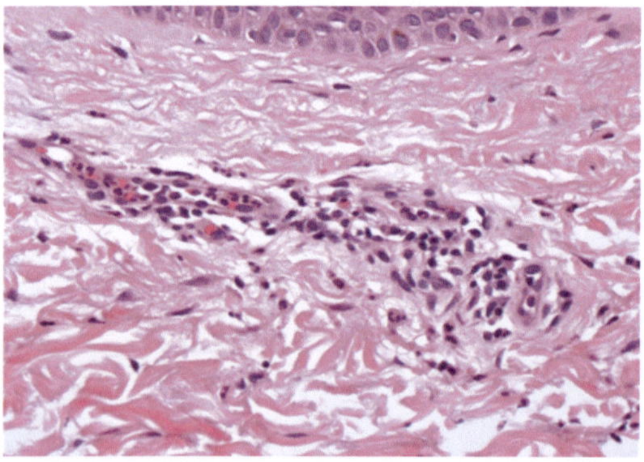

Fig. 20.8 Perivascular neutrophils, lymphocytes, and eosinophils

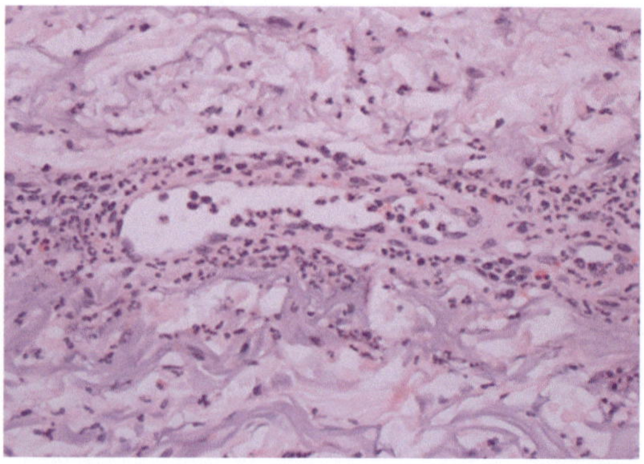

Fig. 20.9 An example with more neutrophils some of which are within the capillary

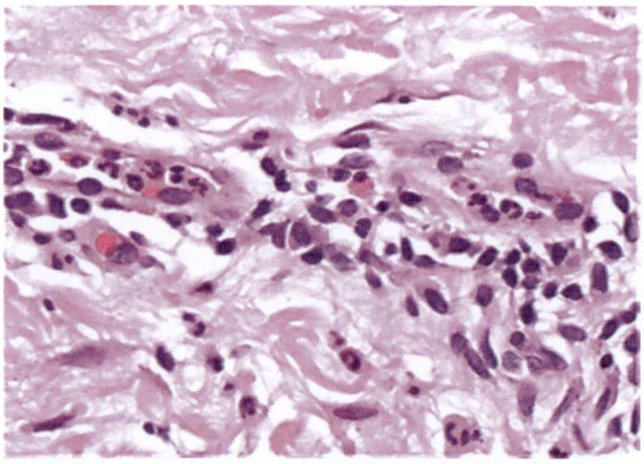

Fig. 20.10 Endothelial cells are swollen

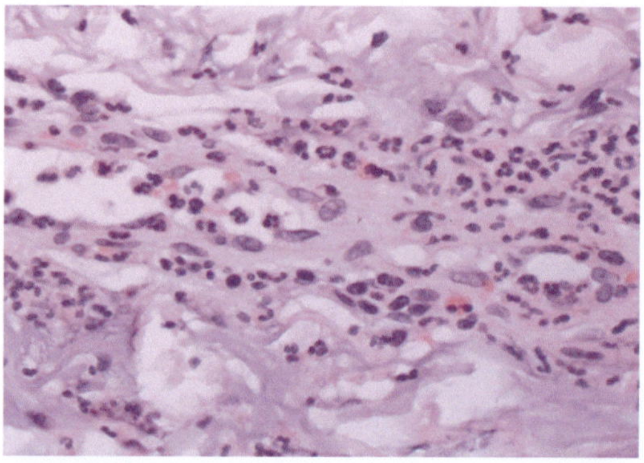

Fig. 20.11 Scattered eosinophils and no significant leukocytoclasia

Urticaria Pigmentosa

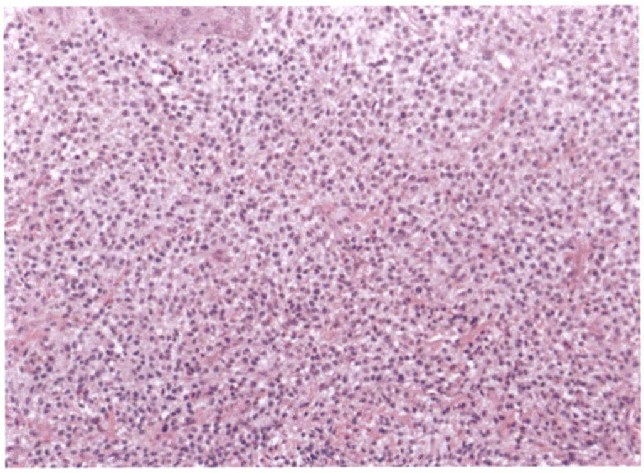

Fig. 20.12 Dermal infiltrate of uniform appearing cells

Solitary Mastocytoma shows identical **histopathology** (Figs. 20.12, 20.13, and 20.14)

- Infant/child with diffuse dermal mast cells
- Mast cells are uniform with "fried egg" appearance (dark central nucleus and purple finely granulated cytoplasm)
- Mast cells stain with Giemsa stain and toluidine blue stain special stains and mast cell tryptase and CD117 immunostains

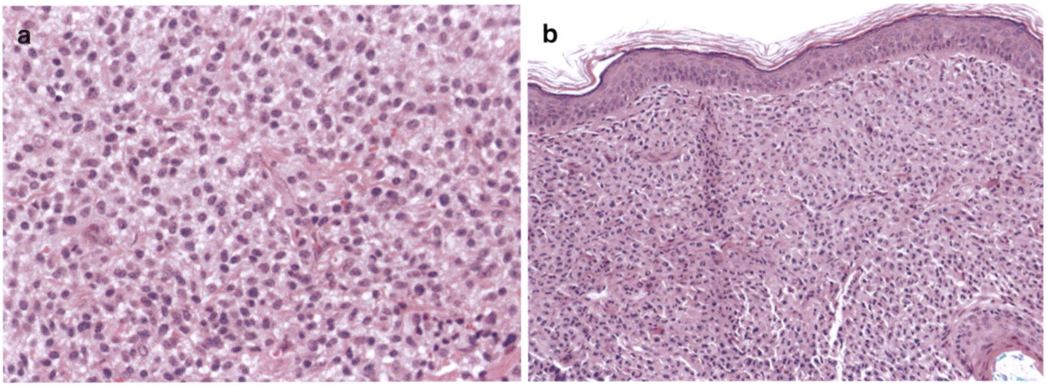

Fig. 20.13 (**a**, **b**) "Fried egg" appearing cells with dark nuclei and purple finely granular cytoplasm

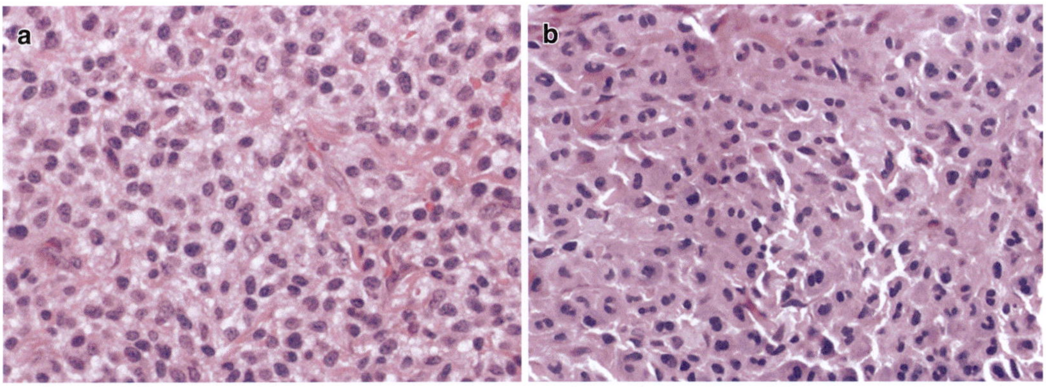

Fig. 20.14 (**a**, **b**) To better appreciate cytoplasmic granularity microscope's condenser should be moved up and down

21 Dermatopathology V

V. Vincek, *Dermatopathology A–Z*, https://doi.org/10.1007/978-3-319-89486-7_21

Vasculopathy

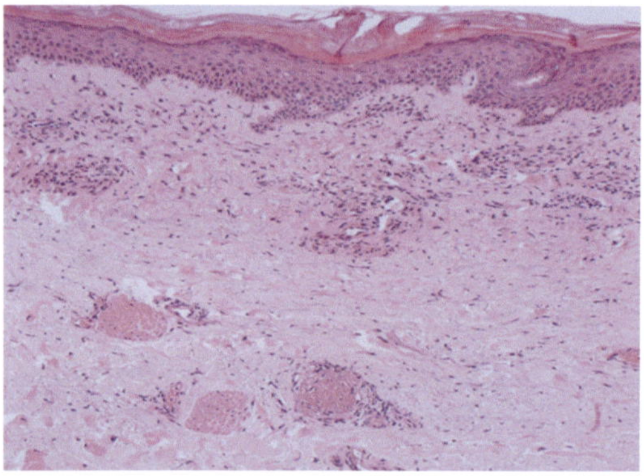

Fig. 21.1 Dermal microthrombi

Disseminated intravascular coagulopathy, sickle cell disease, idiopathic thrombocytopenic purpura, and thrombotic thrombocytopenic purpura show similar **histopathological** findings (Figs. 21.1, 21.2, and 21.3)

- RBC congestion of dermal capillaries
- Numerous small thrombi within capillaries
- Mild perivascular lymphocytic inflammation
- Variable dermal red blood cell extravasation

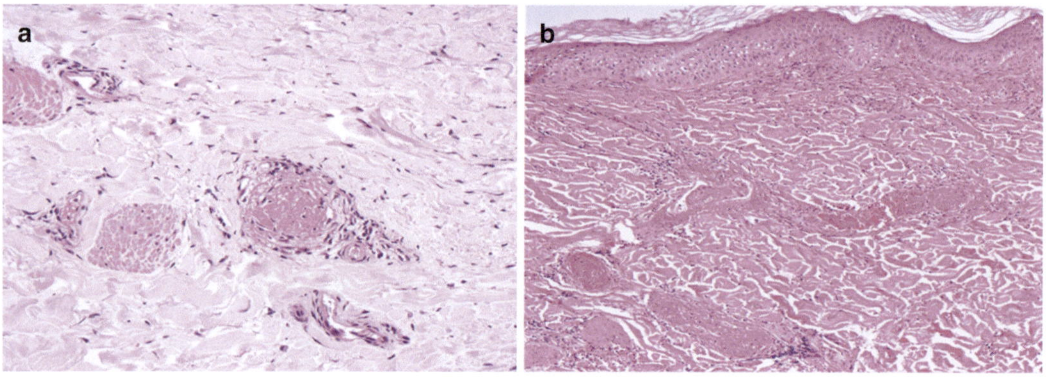

Fig. 21.2 (**a**, **b**) Multiple thrombi within dermal capillaries

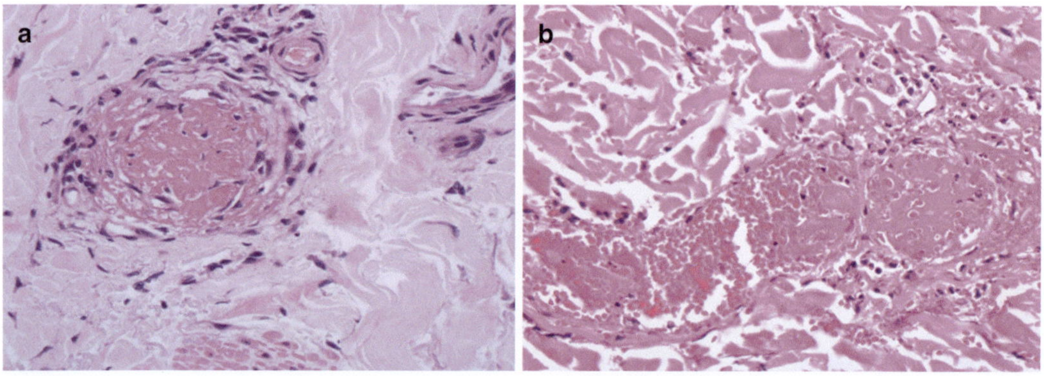

Fig. 21.3 (**a**, **b**) Microthrombi with perivascular lymphocytic inflammation and red blood cell extravasation

Vellus Hair Cyst

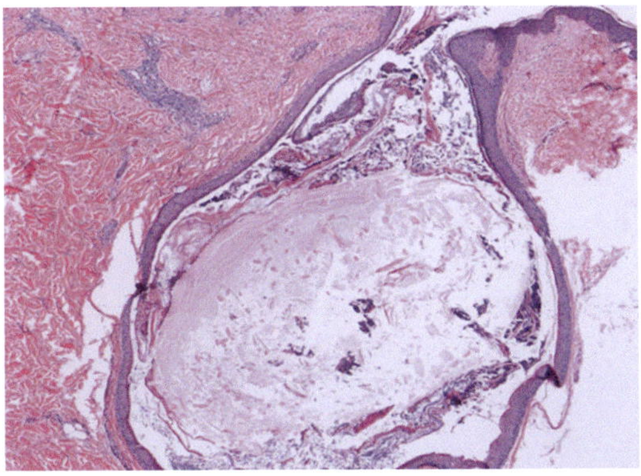

Fig. 21.4 Cyst can demonstrate a connection to vellus hair or to the skin surface

Histopathology (Figs. 21.4, 21.5, 21.6, and 21.7)

- Small cyst located in the upper dermis
- Connection to vellus hair or outer surface can be found
- Cyst lining consists of flattened squamous epithelium without adnexal appendages
- Cyst lumen contains flaky loose keratin and multiple vellus hairs

P.S. rarely associated with Lowe syndrome

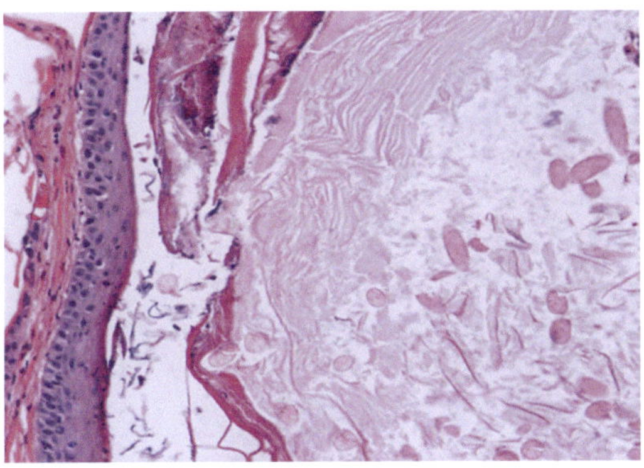

Fig. 21.5 Cyst wall is thin with no appendages

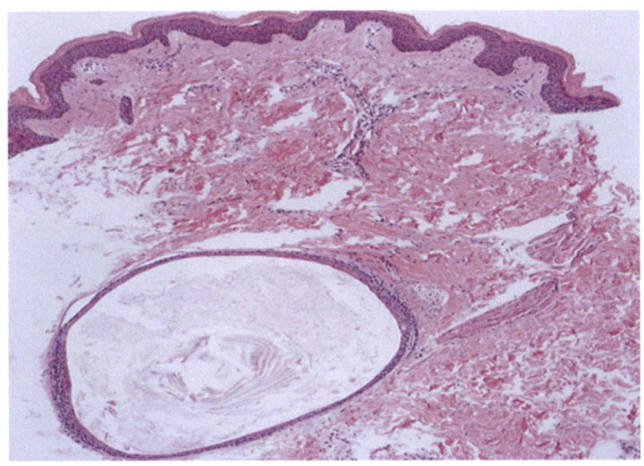

Fig. 21.6 Small dermal cyst with flattened epithelial lining

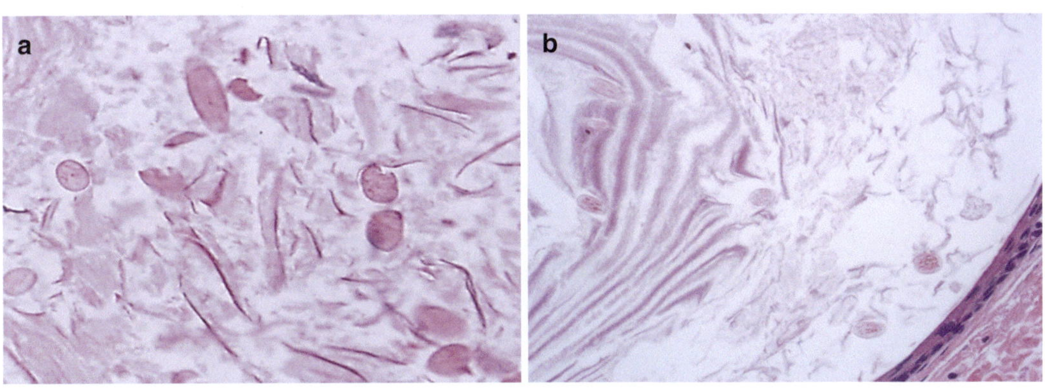

Fig. 21.7 (**a**, **b**) Cyst lumen filled with keratin and multiple vellus hairs

Venous Lake

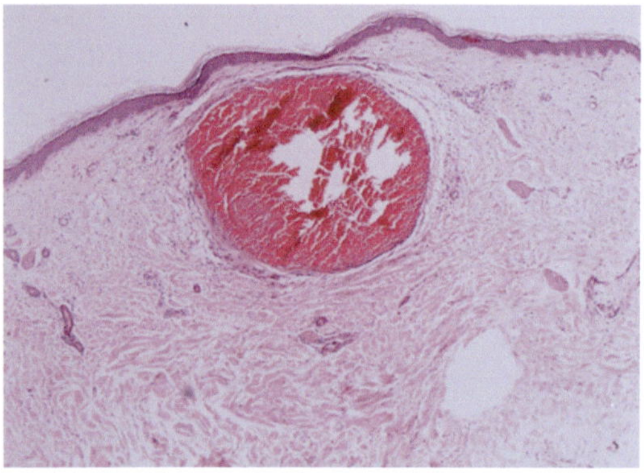

Fig. 21.8 Round dilated vascular channel

Histopathology (Figs. 21.8, 21.9, and 21.10)

- Dilated vascular channel in the dermis
- The lake is filled with red blood cells
- Thin endothelial vascular lining
- Surrounding dermal solar elastosis and edema

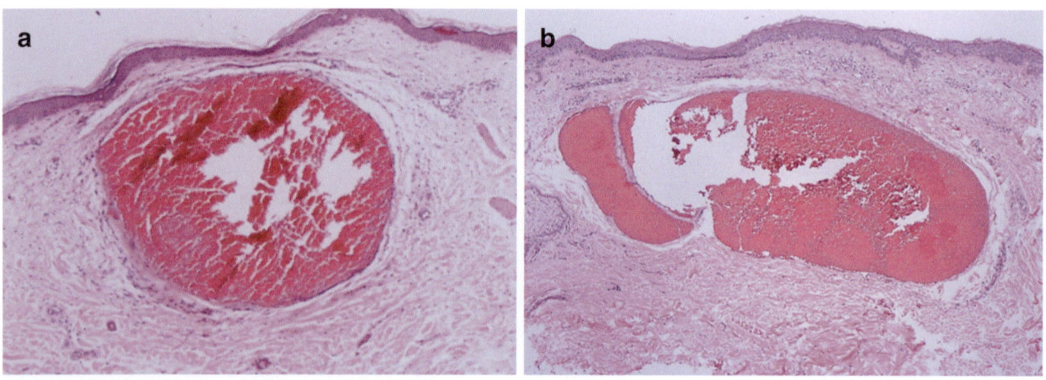

Fig. 21.9 (**a**, **b**) Thin wall made of single layer of endothelial cells encircle a lake of RBCs

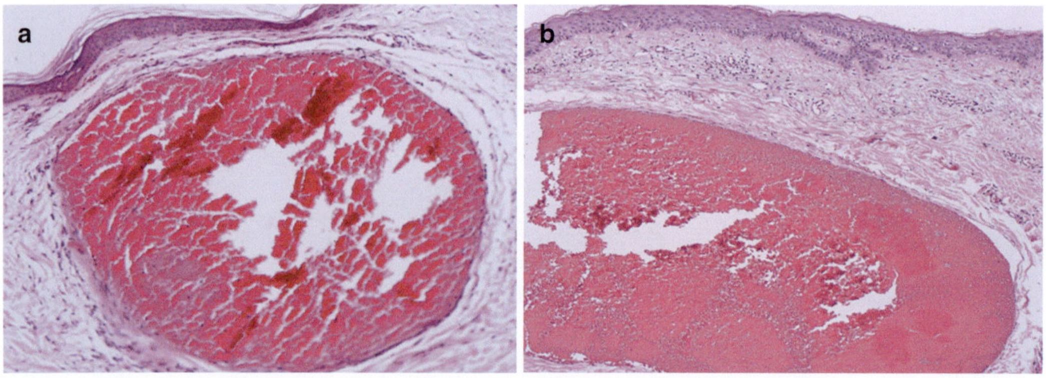

Fig. 21.10 (**a**, **b**) Surrounding dermal solar elastosis and edema

Verruca Plana

Synonym: Flat Wart

Histopathology (Figs. 21.11, 21.12, and 21.13)

- Wavy hyperkeratotic epidermis
- Epidermal hyperkeratosis and hypergranulosis
- Mild to moderate papillomatosis
- Usually absent parakeratosis
- Vacuolated keratinocytes with viral koilocytic changes

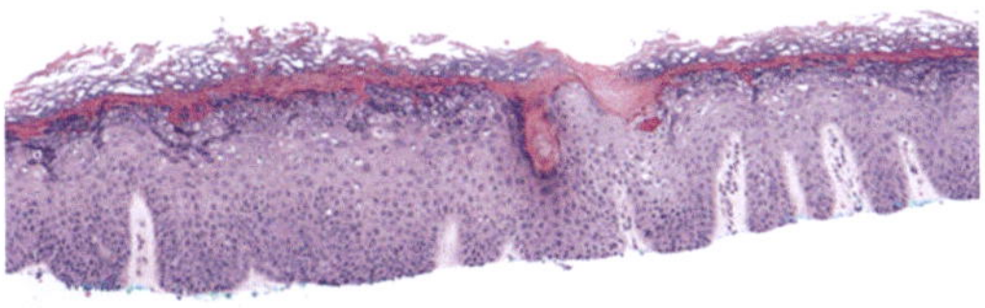

Fig. 21.11 "Basketwoven" acanthotic epidermis

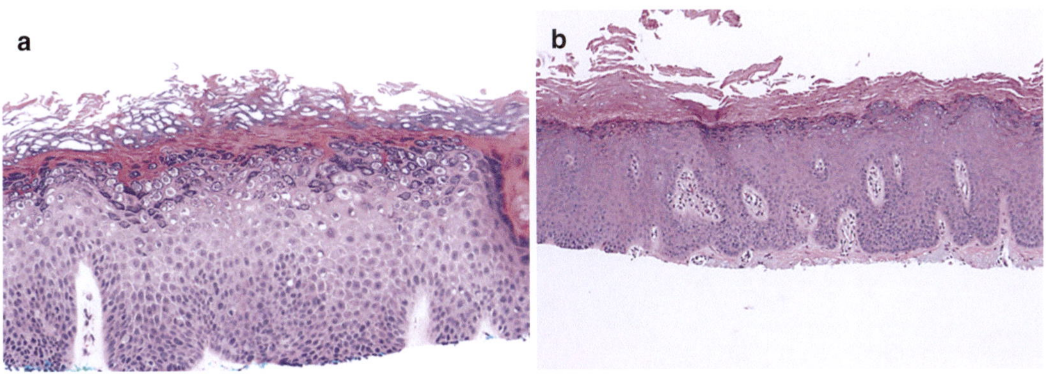

Fig. 21.12 (**a**, **b**) Epidermal hyperkeratosis and hypergranulosis with mild papillomatosis

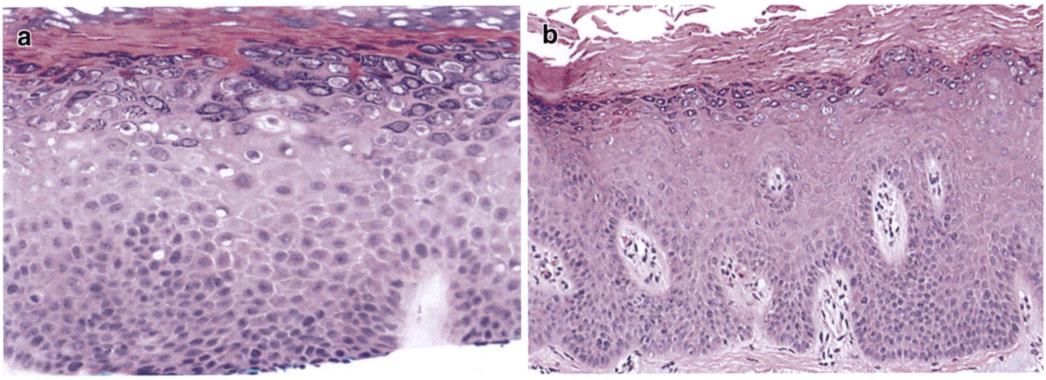

Fig. 21.13 (**a**, **b**) Vacuolated keratinocytes and koilocytes with minimal parakeratosis

Verruca Vulgaris

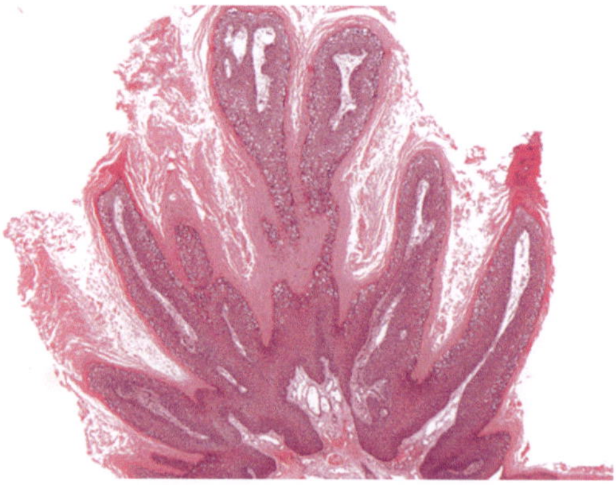

Fig. 21.14 "Church spire-like" epidermal proliferation

Synonyms: Common Wart, Wart

Histopathology (Figs. 21.14, 21.15, 21.16, and 21.17)

- "Church spire-like" epidermal proliferation
- Epidermal hyperkeratosis and hypergranulosis with mounds of parakeratosis extending up from the top of exophytic projections
- Vacuolization of upper layer keratinocytes with prominent keratinohyalin granules
- Viral koilocytes with dark nuclei and perinuclear white halo present in the upper portion of the epidermis

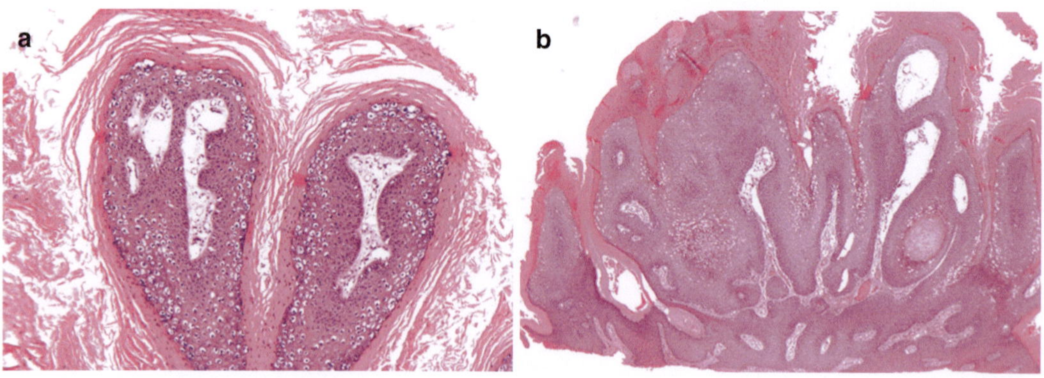

Fig. 21.15 (**a**, **b**) Epidermal hyperkeratosis and hypergranulosis

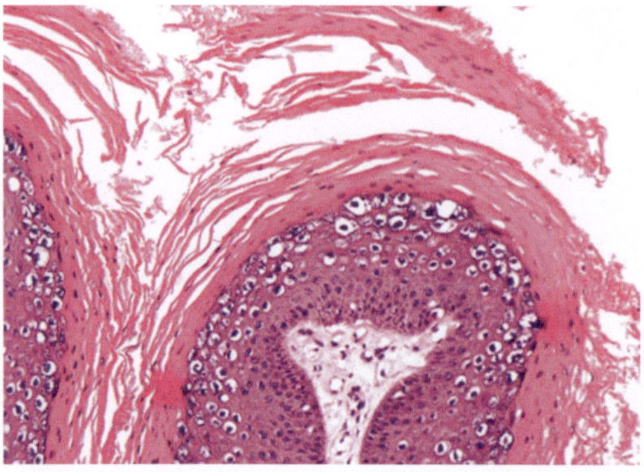

Fig. 21.16 Prominent keratohyalin granules and koilocytes

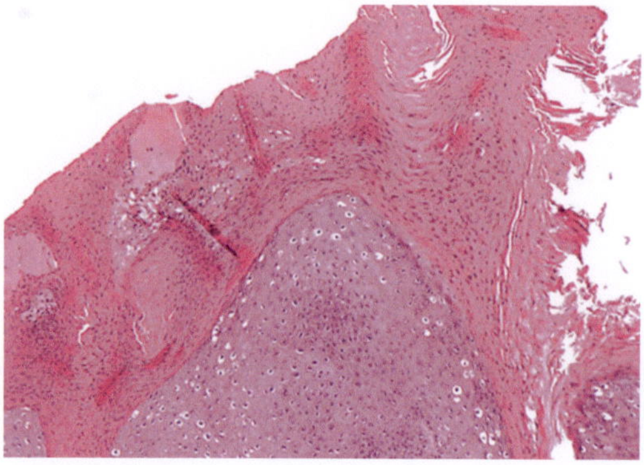

Fig. 21.17 Mounds of parakeratosis

Verrucous Carcinoma

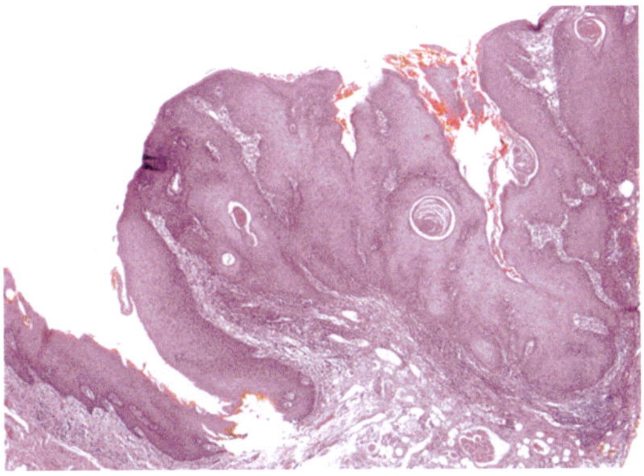

Fig. 21.18 Exophytic and endophytic verrucous epidermal proliferation

Histopathology (Figs. 21.18, 21.19, 21.20, 21.21, and 21.22)
- Verruciform epidermal hyperkeratosis and papillomatosis with exophytic and endophytic epidermal proliferation
- Minimal cytological atypia with few mitoses limited to the basal layer
- Endophytic portion has pushing non infiltrating borders with broad retes
- Keratinous cysts and microabscesses can be present but koilocytes are absent

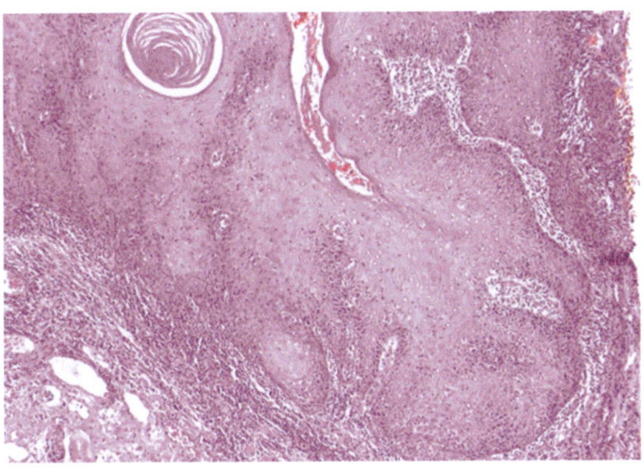

Fig. 21.19 Endophytic portion with keratinous cyst

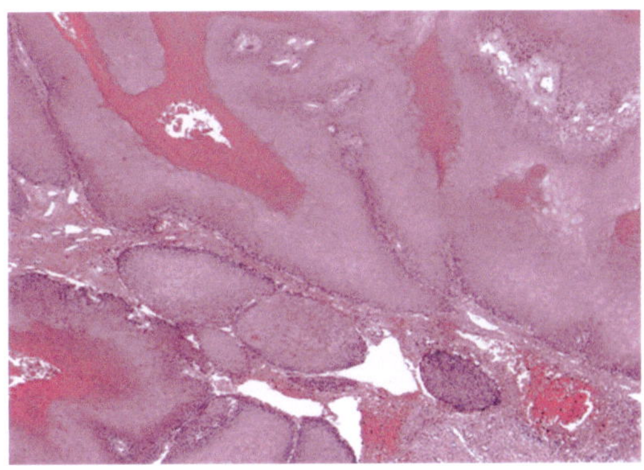

Fig. 21.20 Endophytic portion has pushing borders

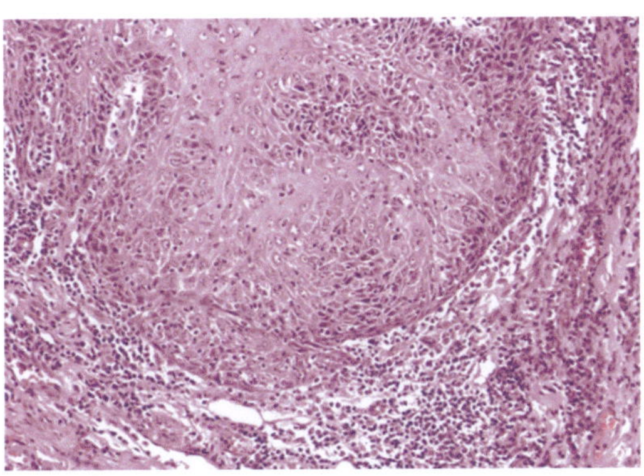

Fig. 21.21 Mitoses are few and limited to the basal layer. Dermal lymphocytic inflammation is present

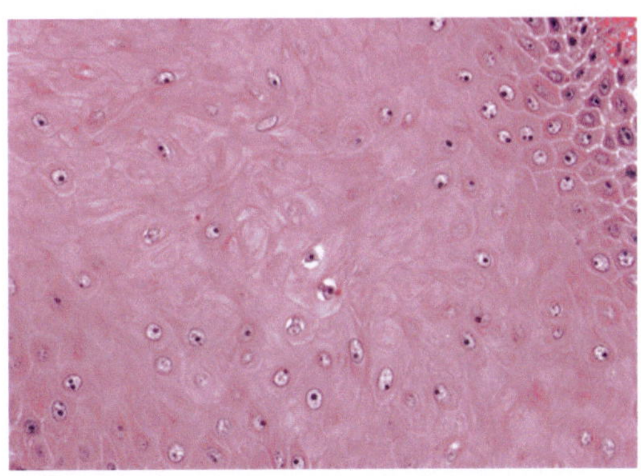

Fig. 21.22 Glassy keratinocytes with minimal atypia

Viral Exanthema

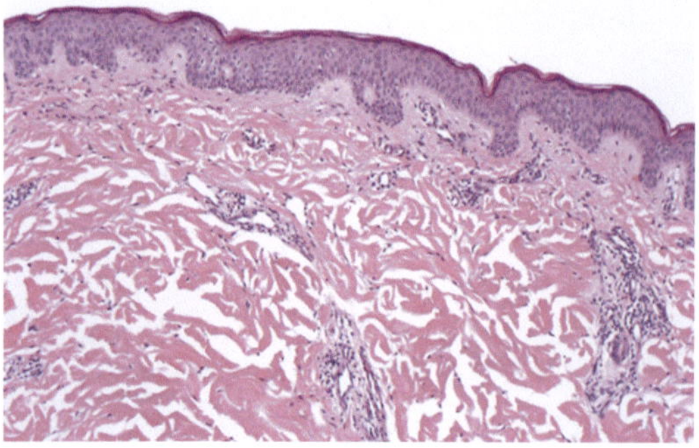

Fig. 21.23 Mild perivascular inflammation

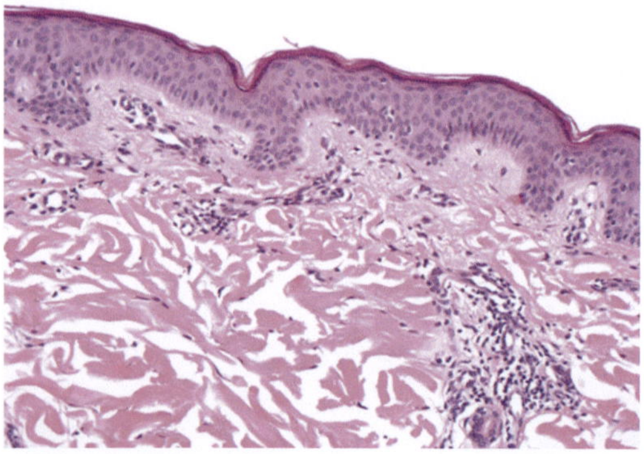

Fig. 21.24 Mild perivascular lymphocytes infiltrate

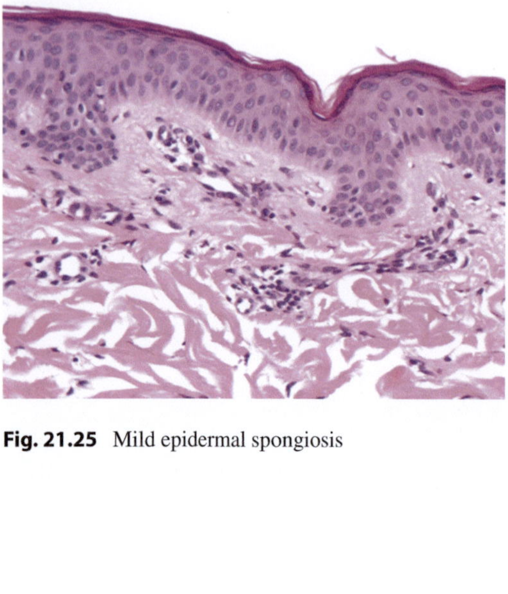

Fig. 21.25 Mild epidermal spongiosis

Measles, Rubella, Fifth disease (Erythema Infectiosum), Roseola (Exanthema Subitum), Dengue fever, HIV exanthem, and Zika exanthem show similar **histopathology:**

- Mild epidermal spongiosis and superficial perivascular lymphocytic inflammation. (Figs. 21.23, 21.24, and 21.25)

In addition, the following can be seen:

- In *Measles*—giant Warthin-Finkeldey keratinocytes with 3–20 nuclei
- In *Rubella*—Turk cells (atypical lymphocytes) in the dermis
- In *Dengue fever*—numerous extravasated red blood cells in the hemorrhagic form
- In *HIV exanthem*—scattered necrotic keratinocytes
- In *Zika exanthem*—few dermal neutrophils in addition to dermal perivascular lymphocytes

Vitiligo

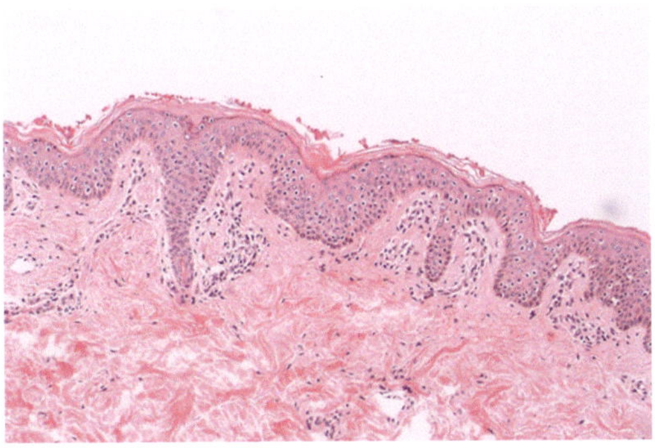

Fig. 21.26 At low power on H&E slide the skin appears normal

Histopathology of Vitiligo and Piebaldism is identical: (Figs. 21.26, 21.27, 21.28, and 21.29)

- Absence of melanocytes and melanin in well-established lesion
- Decreased number of melanocytes and melanin at the periphery of the lesion and in the trichrome vitiligo

P.S. in **Vogt-Koyanagi-Harada syndrome** the skin changes are identical in addition to hypomelanosis of the leptomeninges, uvea, and stria vascularis

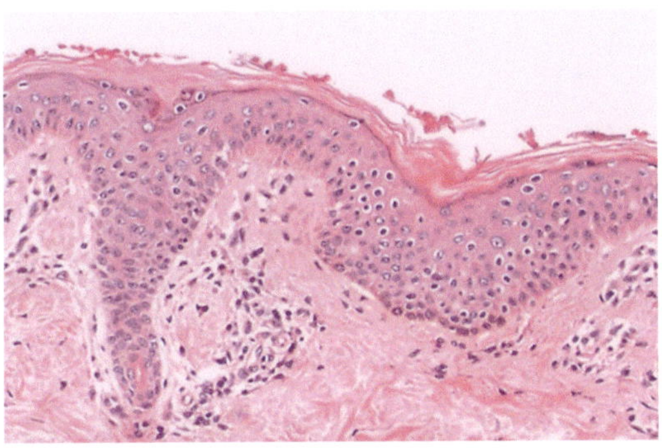

Fig. 21.27 Knowing that the biopsy is from African-American person the left side of the epidermis is missing melanin and the right side is hypopigmented (the biopsy was taken from the edge of the lesion)

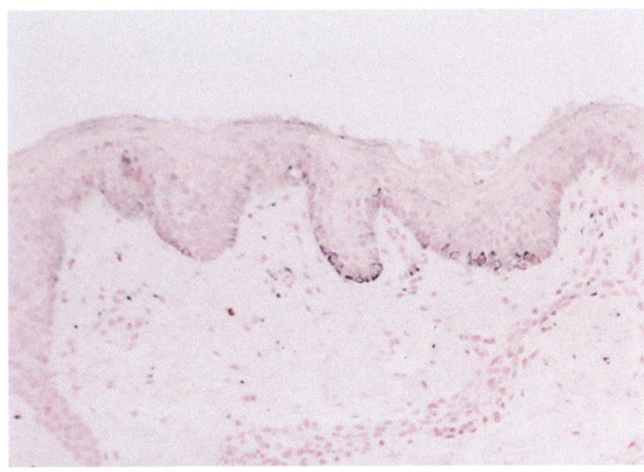

Fig. 21.28 Fontana Masson confirms the absence of epidermal melanin on the left and melanin presence on the right

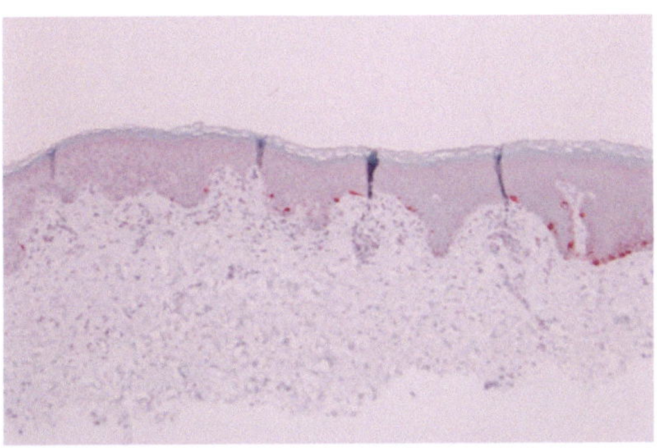

Fig. 21.29 MART1 stain confirms the absence of melanocytes on the left and presence on the right side

22 Dermatopathology W

V. Vincek, *Dermatopathology A–Z*, https://doi.org/10.1007/978-3-319-89486-7_22

Warty Dyskeratoma

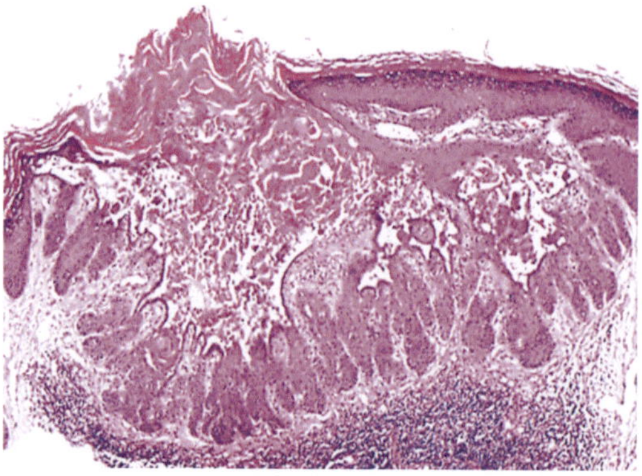

Fig. 22.1 Cup shaped warty lesion

Histopathology (Figs. 22.1, 22.2, and 22.3)

- Often associated with hair follicle
- Cup shaped lesion filled with parakeratotic keratin debris
- Suprabasal acantholysis with formation of villi
- Corp ronds and grains are present
- Mild dermal lymphocytic inflammation

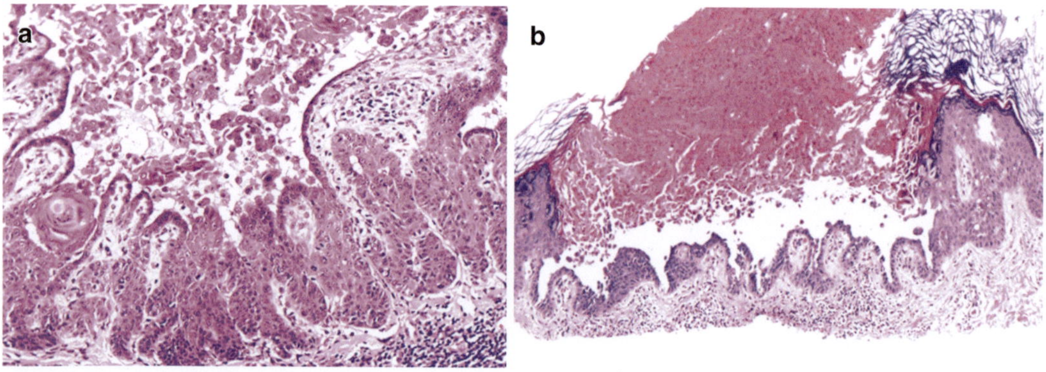

Fig. 22.2 (**a**, **b**) Lesion is filled with keratin debris and parakeratosis

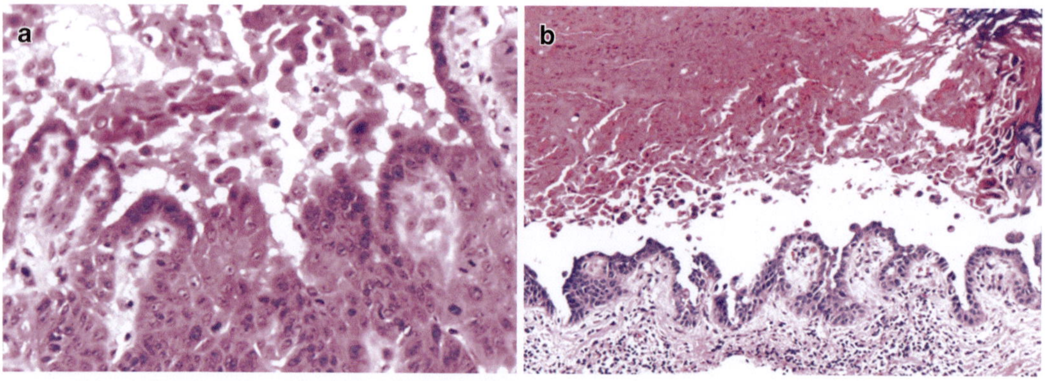

Fig. 22.3 (**a**, **b**) Suprabasal acantholysis with formation of villi and corp ronds and grains

Weber-Christian Disease

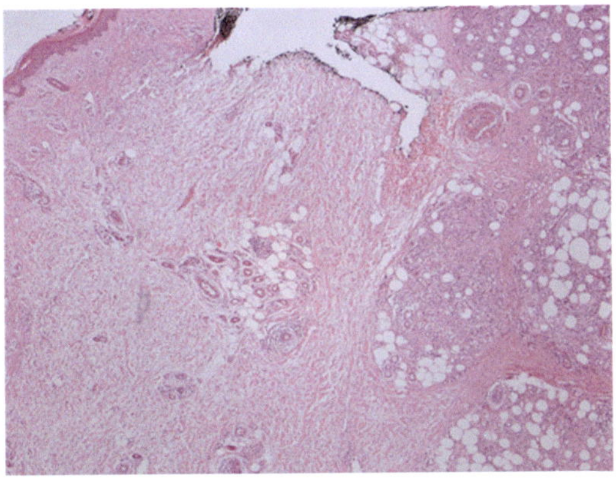

Fig. 22.4 Lobular panniculitis

Synonym: Relapsing Febrile Nodular Nonspecific Panniculitis
Many believe that this is non-specific reaction pattern and not a distinct entity. Therefore, it was suggested instead to use term *lobular panniculitis of unknown etiology*.

Histopathology (Figs. 22.4, 22.5, and 22.6)
- Lobular panniculitis with neutrophils in the early stages
- Lymphocytes, foamy histiocytes, and giant cells in the later stages

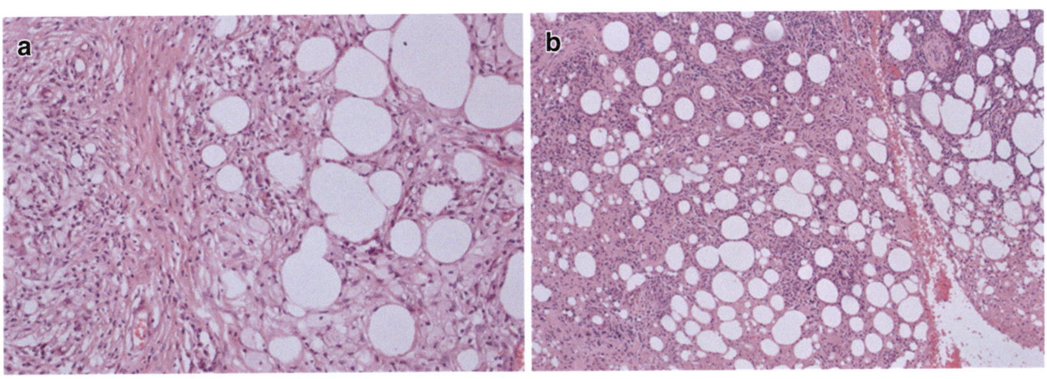

Fig. 22.5 (**a**, **b**) Inflamed lobules with spillover of inflammation into septae

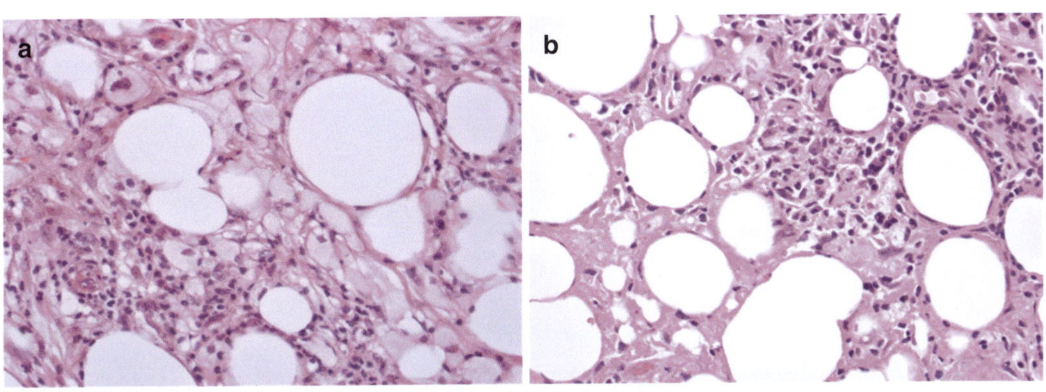

Fig. 22.6 (**a**, **b**) Adipocytes are admixed with neutrophils and foamy histiocytes; focal fat necrosis is present

Wegener's Granulomatosis

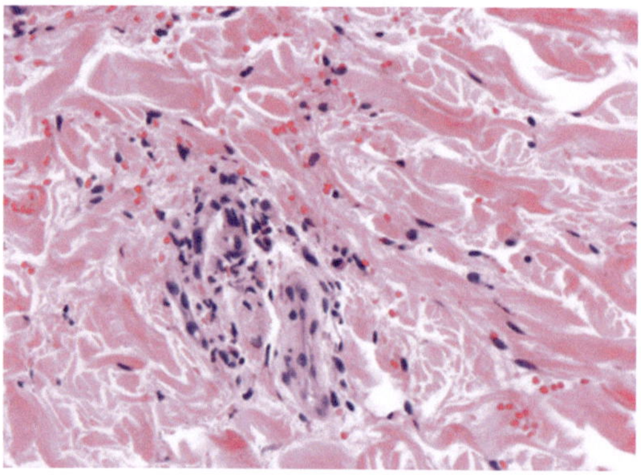

Fig. 22.7 Skin lesion with leukocytoclastic vasculitis

Synonym: Granulomatosis with Polyangiitis

Histopathology (Figs. 22.7, 22.8, 22.9, and 22.10)

- Skin lesions demonstrate non-specific leukocytoclastic vasculitis
- Nasal lesions show ill-defined extravascular granulomas in mixed inflammatory background with numerous eosinophils
- Polyangiitis of medium size vessels with granulomas are seen mostly in lungs and kidneys

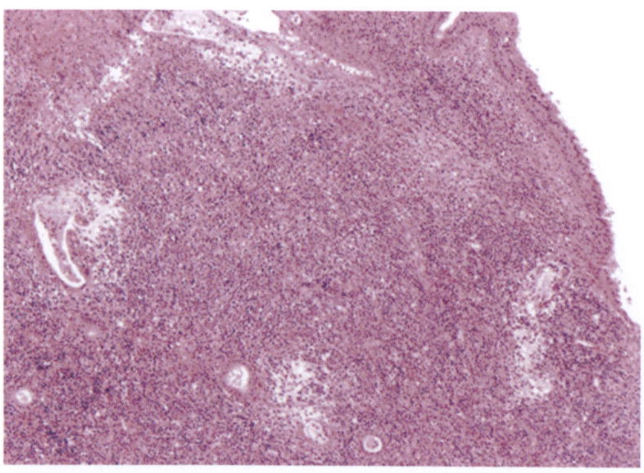

Fig. 22.8 Nasal respiratory mucosa with dense inflammation

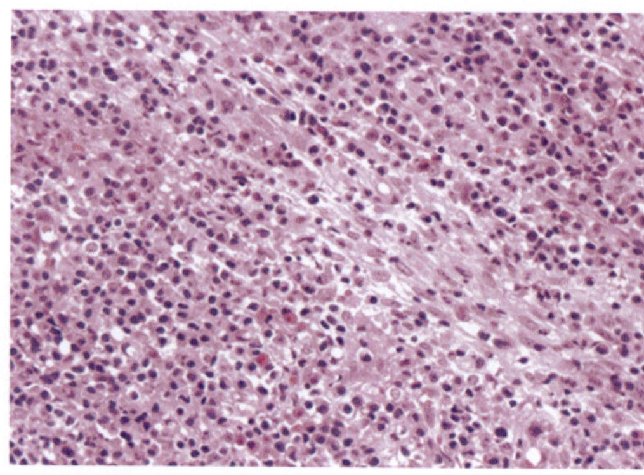

Fig. 22.9 Ill-defined granuloma is present

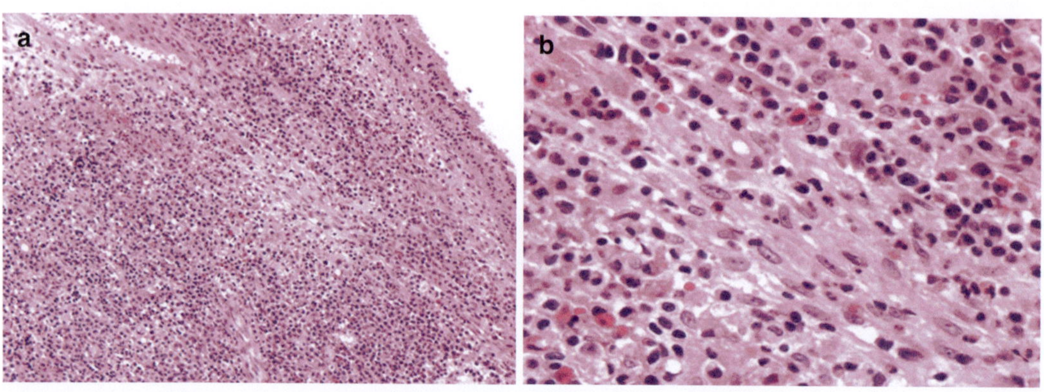

Fig. 22.10 (**a**, **b**) Histiocytes with lymphocytes, neutrophils and numerous eosinophils

Wells Syndrome

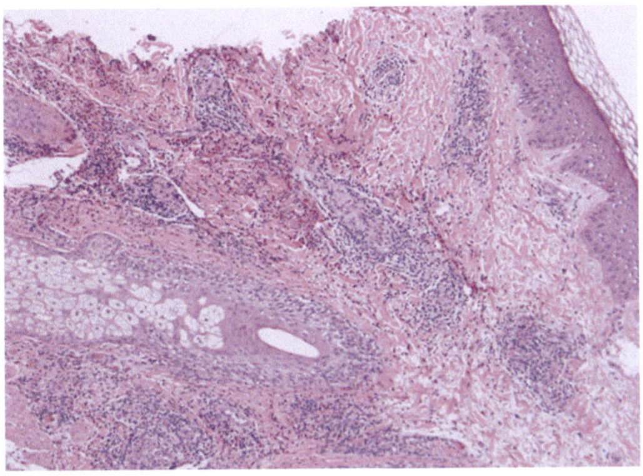

Fig. 22.11 Superficial and deep inflammation

Synonym: Eosinophilic Cellulitis

Histopathology (Figs. 22.11, 22.12, and 22.13)

- Superficial and deep perivascular and interstitial mixed inflammation with numerous eosinophils
- Edema can be present in early lesions
- Characteristic "flame figures" made of degranulated eosinophils deposited on the top of collagen bundles

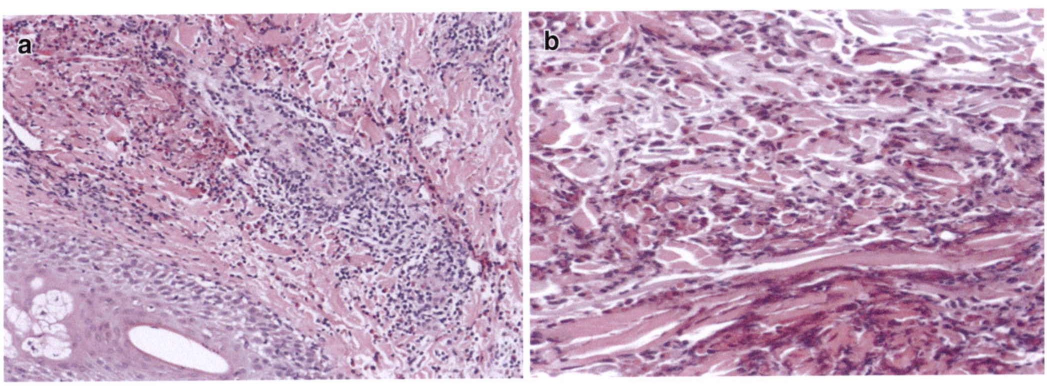

Fig. 22.12 (**a**, **b**) Mostly perivascular mixed inflammation with numerous eosinophils

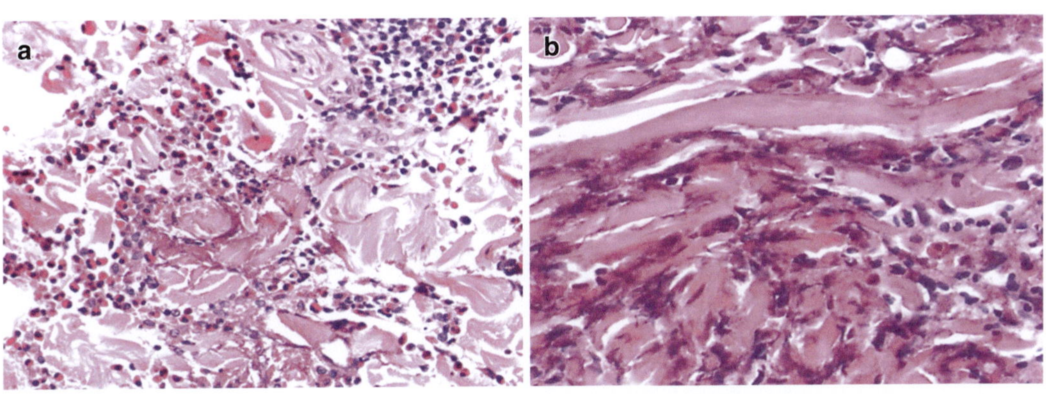

Fig. 22.13 (**a**, **b**) Many eosinophils have degranulated on the top of collagen bundles forming "flame figures"

White Sponge Nevus

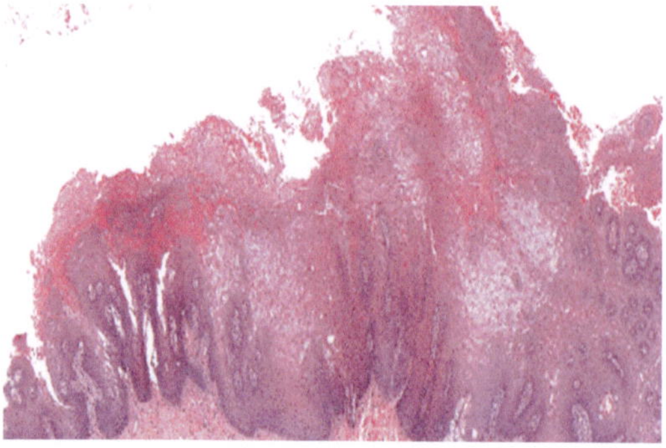

Fig. 22.14 Verruciform pale mucosal epithelium

Synonym: Nevus of Cannon

Histopathology (Figs. 22.14, 22.15, 22.16, and 22.17)

- Hyperplasia of oral mucosa with focal parakeratosis, mild spongiosis, and no inflammation
- Vacuolization of the keratinocyte with perinuclear eosinophilic condensation

P.S. autosomal dominant condition caused by mutations of keratin 4 and 13

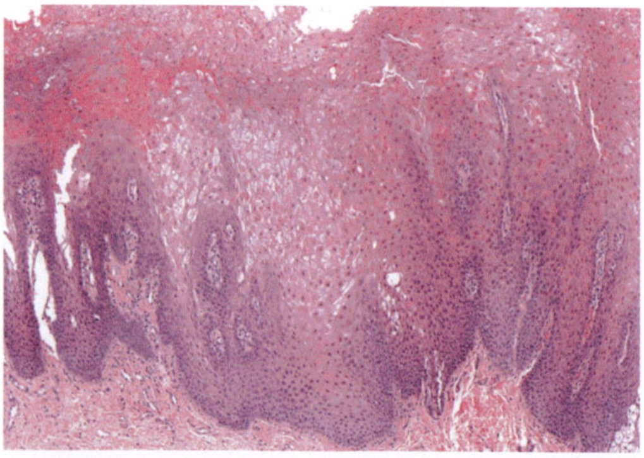

Fig. 22.15 Focal parakeratosis and no submucosal inflammation

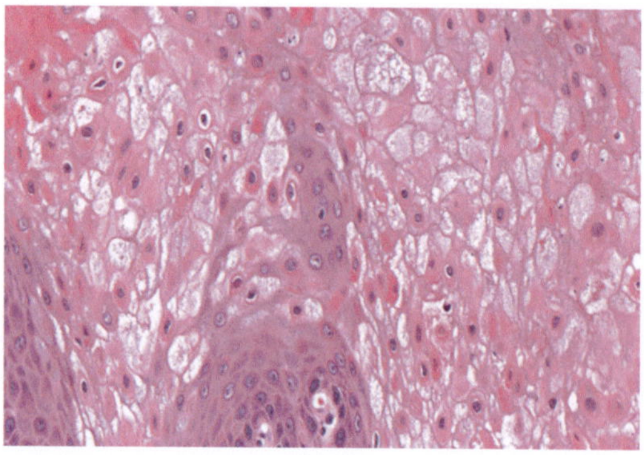

Fig. 22.16 Cytoplasmic vacuolization of keratinocytes

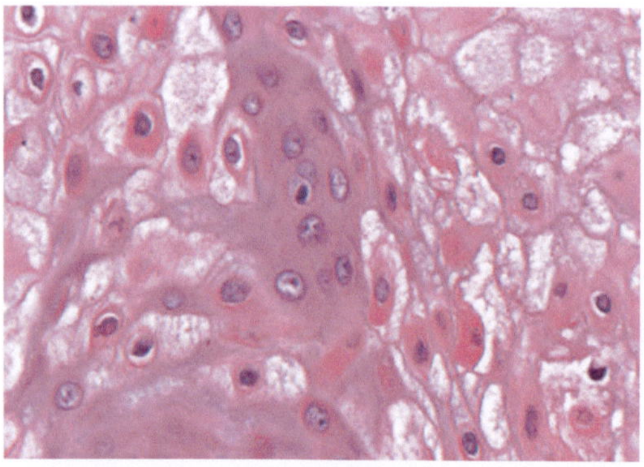

Fig. 22.17 Perinuclear eosinophilic condensation

23 Dermatopathology X

V. Vincek, *Dermatopathology A–Z*, https://doi.org/10.1007/978-3-319-89486-7_23

Xanthogranuloma

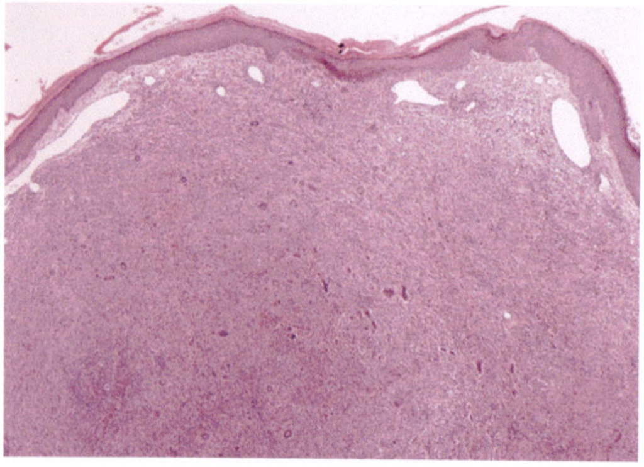

Fig. 23.1 Dermal and subcutaneous nodule

Adult Xanthogranuloma, Juvenile Xanthogranuloma, Benign Cephalic Histiocytosis, and Xanthoma Disseminatum demonstrate identical **histopathology** (Figs. 23.1, 23.2, 23.3, and 23.4) and clinical correlation is required for diagnosis:

- Diffuse histiocytic proliferation (CD68+) filling dermis and abutting but not involving epidermis
- Histiocytes have foamy xanthomatous cytoplasm and there are scattered Touton giant cells
- Admixed lymphocytes and some eosinophils

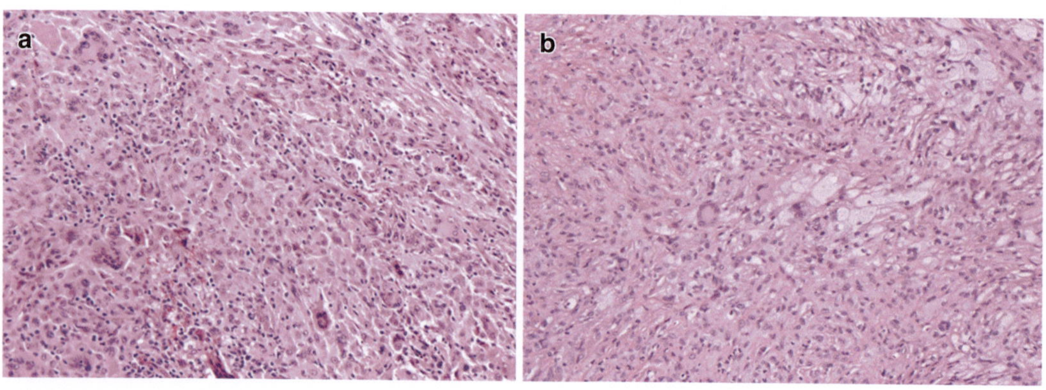

Fig. 23.2 (**a**, **b**) Diffuse proliferation of pale foamy histiocytes many of which are xanthomatized

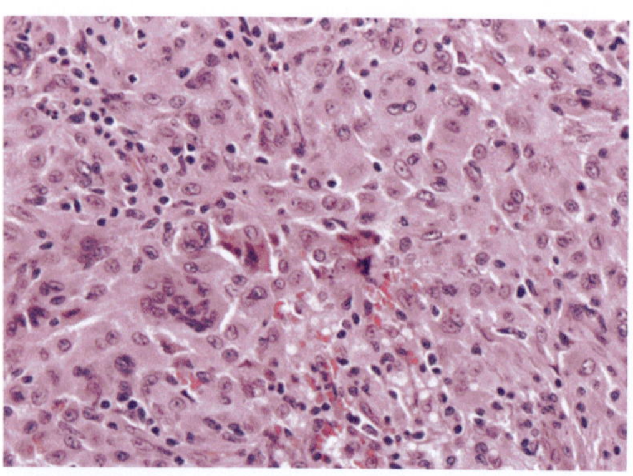

Fig. 23.3 Giant cell with histiocytes and lymphocytes

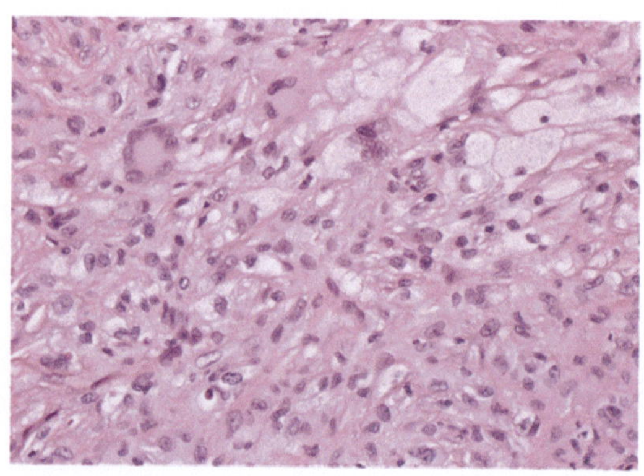

Fig. 23.4 Touton giant cells and xanthoma cells with foamy pale cytoplasm

Xanthoma/Xanthelasma

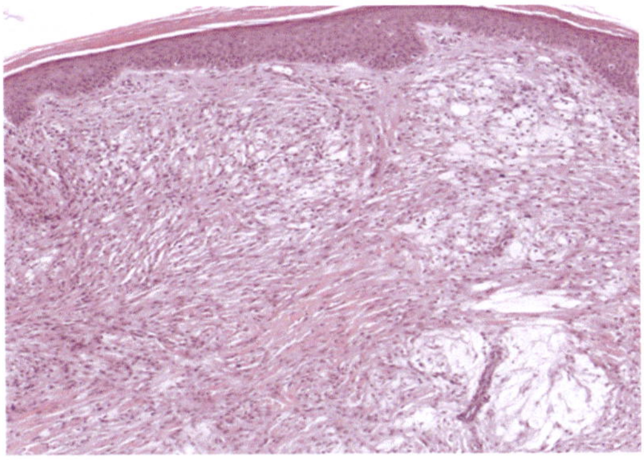

Fig. 23.5 **Eruptive xanthoma** with foamy cells and vague granulomatous appearance

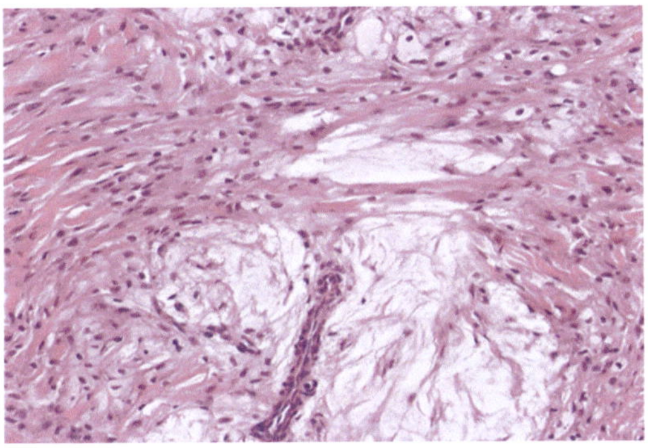

Fig. 23.6 Eruptive xanthoma with fewer xanthoma cells and more histiocytes, lymphocytes and fibrosis

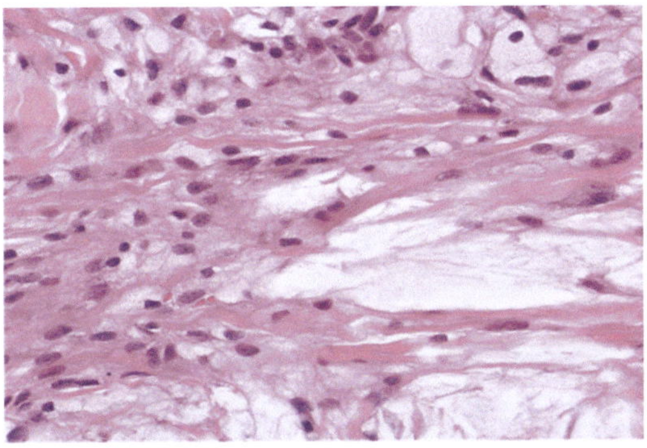

Fig. 23.7 Intracellular and extracellular lipid is present in fibrotic background

The name xanthoma generically applies to the lesions containing foamy histiocytes (xanthoma cells) filled with lipids. The nuclei of xanthoma cells are uniform and usually dark and cytoplasm is smooth, foamy, and pink.

Histopathology

Eruptive xanthoma (Figs 23.5, 23.6, and 23.7)
- Foamy and non-foamy histiocytes with admixed lymphocytes.
- Extracellular lipid is present.
- Can appear vaguely granulomatous.

Tendinous xanthoma (Figs. 23.8 and 23.9)
- Sheets of uniform xanthoma cells with collagen bundles in between
- Few or no lymphocytes

Tuberous xanthoma: (Figs. 23.10, 23.11, and 23.12)
- Several dermal and subcutaneous nodules in skin over pressure areas
- Nodules are made of xanthoma cells with marked scarring in older lesions

Verruciform xanthoma: (Figs. 23.13, 23.14, and 23.15)
- Verruciform epidermis with xanthoma cells in dermal papillae

Xanthelasma **(present on eyelid, otherwise called** *xanthoma plana*)**:** (Figs. 23.16, 23.17, and 23.18)
- Xanthoma cells that vary in size but have very uniform nuclei and cytoplasm
- Few lymphocytes and dermal telangiectasias

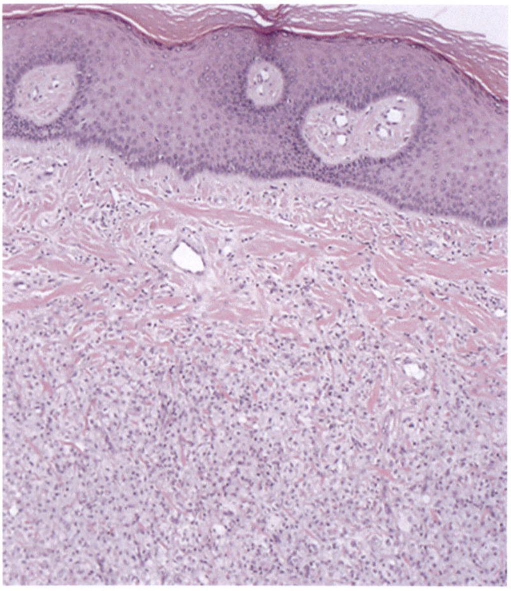

Fig. 23.8 **Tendinous xanthoma**

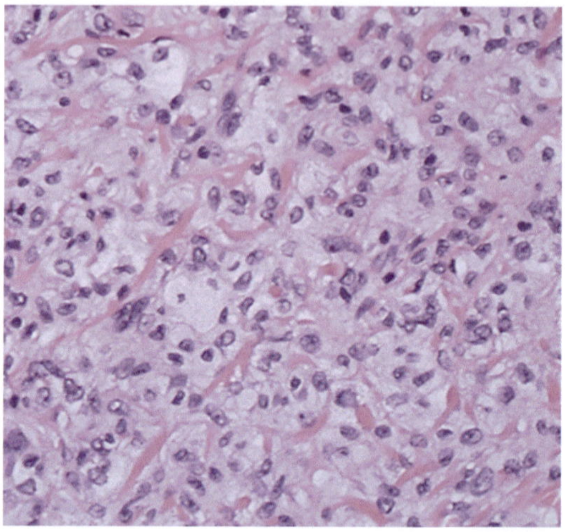

Fig. 23.9 Sheets of foamy macrophages with collagen in between

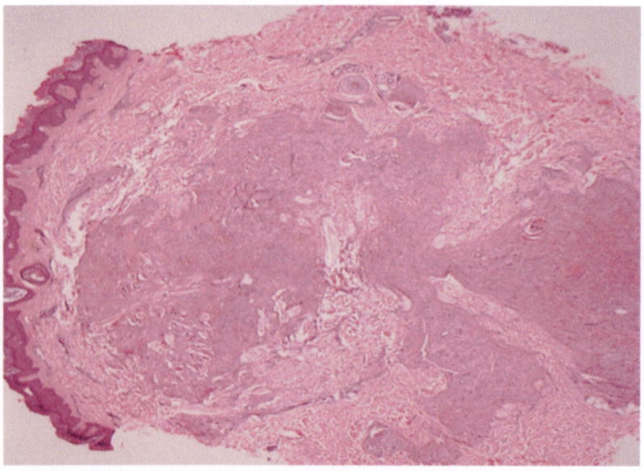

Fig. 23.10 **Tuberous xanthoma** consisting of several dermal and subcutaneous nodules

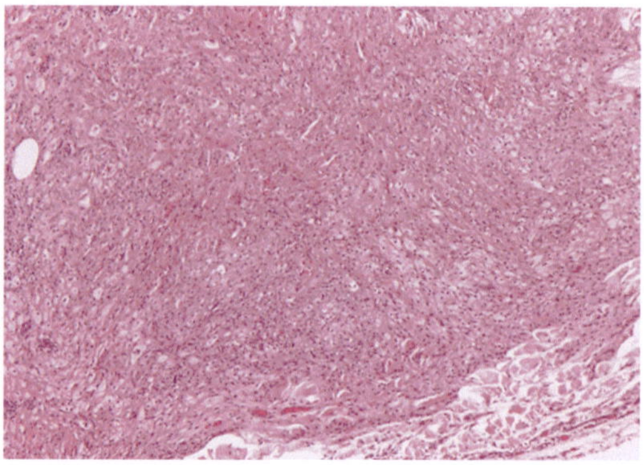

Fig. 23.11 Nodules are made of xanthoma cells with marked scarring in the older lesions

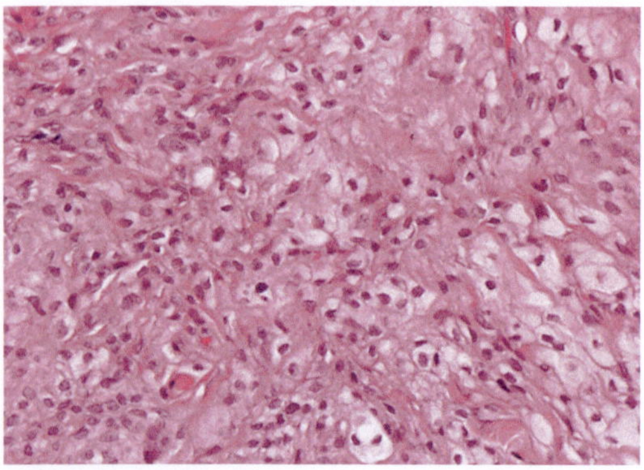

Fig. 23.12 Xanthoma cells are uniformed with pale, foamy cytoplasm and dark central nuclei

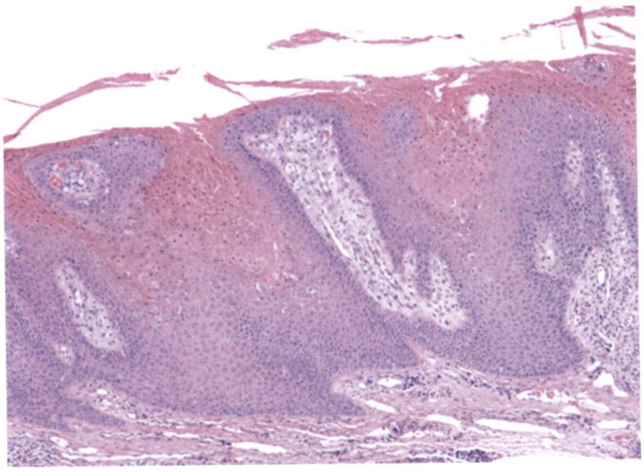

Fig. 23.13 **Verruciform xanthoma** with epidermal acanthosis, papillomatosis, and common superficial excoriation

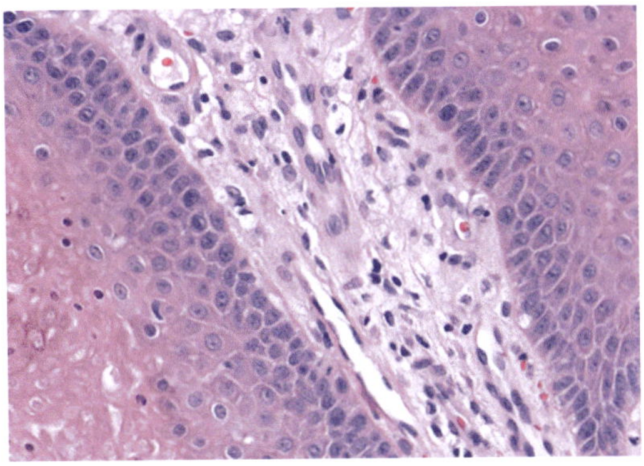

Fig. 23.14 Dermal papillae contain foamy and non-foamy histiocytes

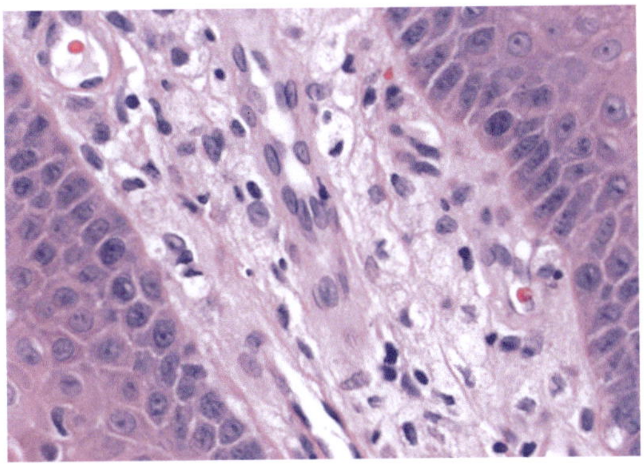

Fig. 23.15 Xanthoma cells are admixed with scatted lymphocytes

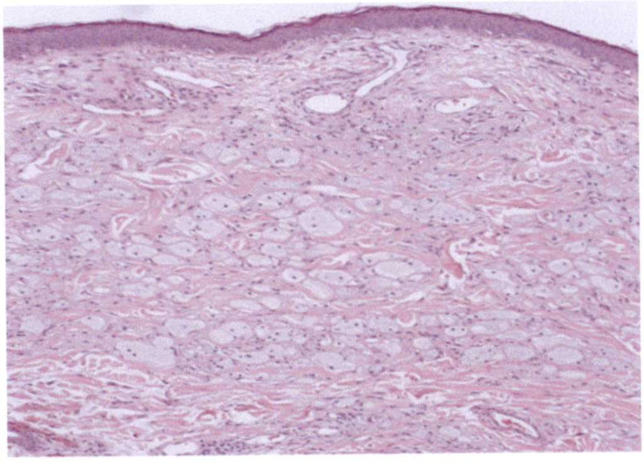

Fig. 23.16 **Xanthelasma** shows pale, monotonous histology

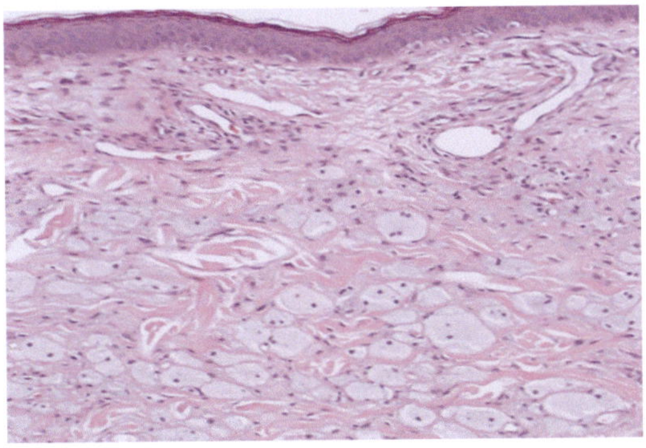

Fig. 23.17 Xanthoma cells with few lymphocytes and dermal telangiectasias

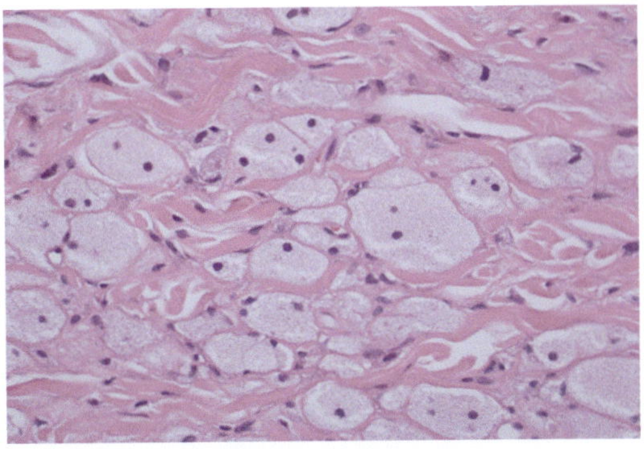

Fig. 23.18 Xanthoma cells are intact and vary in size; they have dark regular nuclei and smooth pink cytoplasm

Dermatopathology Z

24

V. Vincek, *Dermatopathology A–Z*, https://doi.org/10.1007/978-3-319-89486-7_24

Zoon's Balanitis/Vulvitis

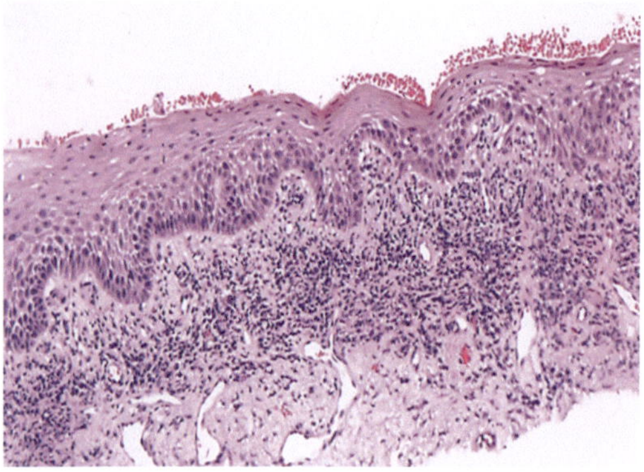

Fig. 24.1 Band-like lichenoid dermal infiltrate

Histopathology (Figs. 24.1, 24.2, and 24.3)
- Atrophic mildly spongiotic epidermis with scattered neutrophils
- Dermal lichenoid infiltrate made of plasma cells and lymphocytes
- Vascular ectasia is common

P.S. epidermis is commonly excoriated

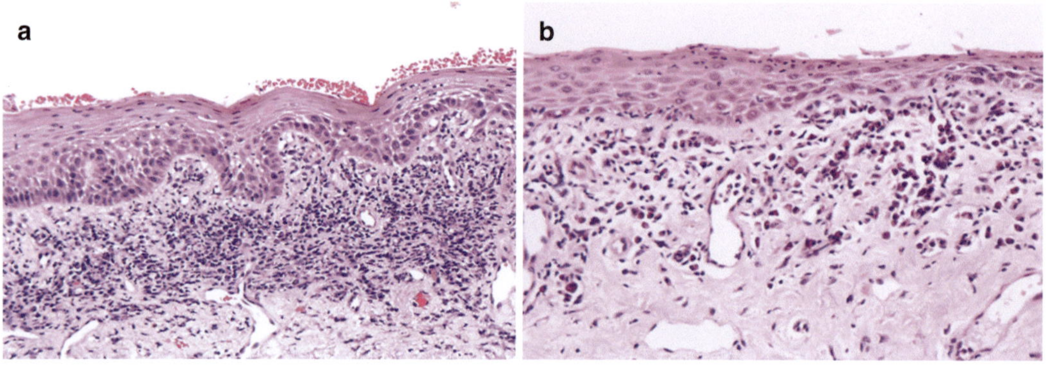

Fig. 24.2 (**a**, **b**) Epidermal spongiosis, focal atrophy, and intraepidermal neutrophils

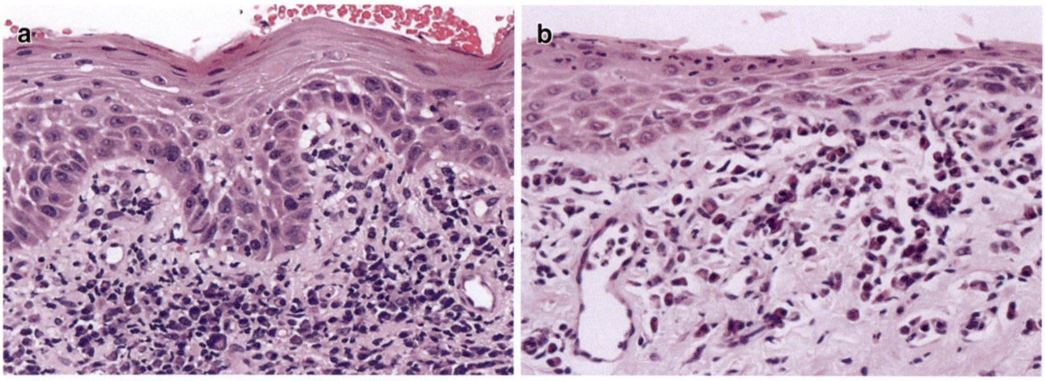

Fig. 24.3 (**a**, **b**) Mostly plasmocytic inflammation with scattered lymphocytes and dilated dermal vessels

Index

V. Vincek, *Dermatopathology A–Z*, https://doi.org/10.1007/978-3-319-89486-7

M

MIX
Papier aus verantwortungsvollen Quellen
Paper from responsible sources
FSC® C105338

If you have any concerns about our products,
you can contact us on
ProductSafety@springernature.com

In case Publisher is established outside the EU,
the EU authorized representative is:
Springer Nature Customer Service Center GmbH
Europaplatz 3, 69115 Heidelberg, Germany

Printed by Libri Plureos GmbH
in Hamburg, Germany